SAUNDERS
Q&A REVIEW

for the
NCLEX-RN®
EXAMINATION

SAUNDERS
Q&A REVIEW

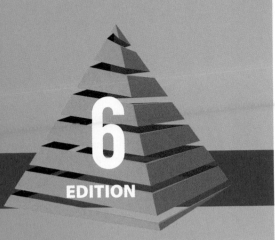

6 EDITION

for the NCLEX-RN®
the EXAMINATION

Linda Anne Silvestri, PhD, RN

Instructor of Nursing
Salve Regina University
Newport, Rhode Island

President
Nursing Reviews, Inc.
Las Vegas, Nevada
Nursing Reviews, Inc.
Charlestown, Rhode Island
Professional Nursing Seminars, Inc.
Charlestown, Rhode Island

Elsevier Consultant
HESI NCLEX-RN® and NCLEX-PN® Live Review Courses

ELSEVIER

SAUNDERS

3251 Riverport Lane
St. Louis, Missouri 63043

SAUNDERS Q&A REVIEW FOR THE NCLEX-RN®
EXAMINATION, SIXTH EDITION

ISBN: 978-1-4557-5373-4

Library of Congress Cataloging-in-Publication Data
Silvestri, Linda Anne, author.
  Saunders Q & A review for the NCLEX-RN examination / Linda Anne Silvestri. – Edition 6.
    p. ; cm.
  Q & A review for the NCLEX-RN examination
  Saunders Q and A review for the NCLEX-RN examination
  Includes bibliographical references and index.
  ISBN 978-1-4557-5373-4 (paperback : alk. paper)
  I. Title. II. Title: Q & A review for the NCLEX-RN examination. III. Title: Saunders Q and A review for the NCLEX-RN examination.
  [DNLM: 1. Nursing Care–Examination Questions. 2. Nursing Process–Examination Questions. 3. Test Taking Skills–Examination Questions. WY 18.2]
  RT55
  610.73076–dc23
                                                                    2014023364

Content Strategist: Yvonne Alexopoulos
Content Developmental Manager: Laurie Gower
Content Development Specialist: Laura Goodrich
Marketing Manager: Danielle LeCompte
Marketing Coordinator: Julie Mark
Publishing Services Manager: Jeff Patterson
Project Manager: Bill Drone
Senior Designer: Christian Bilbow

Printed in USA

Last digit is the print number: 9 8 7 6 5 4 3 2

To my father,

ARNOLD LAWRENCE

*My memories of his love, support, and words of encouragement
will remain in my heart forever!*

and

*To my many nursing students, past, present, and future: their inspiration has brought
many personal and professional rewards to my life!*

To All Future Registered Nurses,

Congratulations to you!

You should be very proud and pleased with yourself on your nursing school accomplishments and well-deserved success of completing your nursing program to become a registered nurse. I know that you have worked very hard to become successful and that you have proven to yourself that indeed you can achieve your goals.

In my opinion, you are about to enter the most wonderful and rewarding profession that exists. Your willingness, desire, and ability to assist those who need nursing care will bring great satisfaction to your life. In the profession of nursing, learning is a lifelong process, which makes the profession stimulating and dynamic and ensures that your learning will continue to expand and grow as the profession continues to evolve. Your next very important endeavor will be the learning process needed to achieve success in your examination to become a registered nurse.

I am excited and pleased to be able to provide you with the *Saunders Pyramid to Success* products, which will help you prepare for your next important professional goal: becoming a registered nurse. I want to thank all of my former nursing students whom I have assisted in their studies for the NCLEX-RN exam for their willingness to offer ideas regarding their needs in preparing for licensure. Student ideas have certainly added a special uniqueness to all of the products available in the *Saunders Pyramid to Success.*

Saunders Pyramid to Success products provide you with everything that you need to ready yourself for the NCLEX-RN exam. These products include material that is required for the NCLEX-RN exam for all nursing students regardless of educational background, specific strengths, areas in need of improvement, or clinical experience during the nursing program.

So let's get started and begin our journey through the *Saunders Pyramid to Success,* and welcome to the wonderful profession of nursing!

Sincerely,

Linda Anne Silvestri

Linda Anne Silvestri, PhD, RN

About the Author

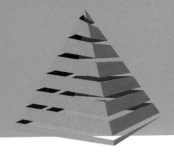

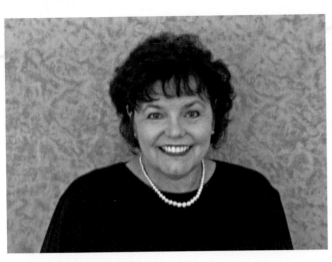

Linda Anne Silvestri

(Photo by Laurent W. Valliere)

As a child, I always dreamed of becoming either a nurse or a teacher. Initially I chose to become a nurse because I really wanted to help others, especially those who were ill. Then I realized that both of my dreams could come true; I could be both a nurse and a teacher. So I pursued my dreams.

I received my diploma in nursing at Cooley Dickinson Hospital School of Nursing in Northampton, Massachusetts. Afterward, I worked at Baystate Medical Center in Springfield, Massachusetts, where I cared for clients in acute medical-surgical units, the intensive care unit, the emergency department, pediatric units, and other acute care units. Later, I received an associate degree from Holyoke Community College in Holyoke, Massachusetts, my BSN from American International College in Springfield, Massachusetts, and my MSN from Anna Maria College in Paxton, Massachusetts, with a dual major in Nursing Management and Patient Education. I received my PhD in Nursing from the University of Nevada, Las Vegas (UNLV), and conducted research on self-efficacy and the predictors of NCLEX success. In 2012, I received the UNLV School of Nursing, Alumna of the Year Award. I am also a member of the Honor Society of Nursing, Sigma Theta Tau International, Phi Kappa Phi, the Western Institute of

Nursing, the Eastern Nursing Research Society, the Golden Key International Honour Society, the National League for Nursing, and the America Nurses Association.

As a native of Springfield, Massachusetts, I began my teaching career as an instructor of medical-surgical nursing and leadership-management nursing in 1981 at Baystate Medical Center School of Nursing. In 1989, I relocated to Rhode Island and began teaching advanced medical-surgical nursing and psychiatric nursing to RN and LPN students at the Community College of Rhode Island. While teaching there, a group of students approached me for assistance in preparing for the NCLEX examination. I have always had a very special interest in test success for nursing students because of my own personal experiences with testing. Taking tests was never easy for me, and as a student I needed to find methods and strategies that would bring success. My own difficult experiences, desire, and dedication to assist nursing students to overcome the obstacles associated with testing inspired me to develop and write the many products that would foster success with testing. My experiences as a student, nursing educator, and item writer for the NCLEX exams aided me as I developed a comprehensive review course to prepare nursing graduates for the NCLEX examination.

Later, in 1994, I began teaching medical-surgical nursing at Salve Regina University in Newport, Rhode Island, and remain there as an adjunct faculty member. I also prepare nursing students at Salve Regina University for the NCLEX-RN examination.

I established Professional Nursing Seminars, Inc., in 1991 and Nursing Reviews, Inc., in 2000. These companies are located in Charlestown, Rhode Island. In 2012, I established an additional company, Nursing Reviews, Inc. in Las Vegas, Nevada. Both companies are dedicated to helping nursing graduates achieve their goals of becoming registered nurses, licensed practical/vocational nurses, or both.

Today, I am the successful author of numerous review products. Also, I serve as an Elsevier Consultant for HESI live reviews, the review courses for the NCLEX examination conducted throughout the country. I am so pleased that you have decided to join me on your journey to success in testing for nursing examinations and for the NCLEX-RN examination!

Contributors

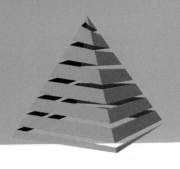

Barbara Callahan, BSN, MEd
ADN Program
Lenoir Community College
Kinston, North Carolina

Miranda Cox, RN, BSN
Graduate
Chamberlain College of Nursing
Jacksonville, Florida

Mattie Davis, DNP, MSN, RN
Nursing Instructor
JF Drake
Huntsville, Alabama

Marilyn Johnessee Greer, MS, RN
Associate Professor of Nursing
Rockford College
Rockford, Illinois

Linda Turchin, RN, BSN, MSN
Assistant Professor of Nursing
Fairmont State University
Fairmont, West Virginia

Laurent W. Valliere, BS, DD
Vice President
Professional Nursing Seminars, Inc.
Charlestown, Rhode Island

Michael Walls, MSN, PhD, RN

Donna E. Wilsker, MSN, BSN
Assistant Professor
Lamar University
Beaumont, Texas

SPECIAL CONTRIBUTOR

Eileen H. Gray, DNP, RN, CPNP
Chair, Department of Nursing
Salve Regina University
Newport, Rhode Island

CONSULTANTS

Allison Bowser
Researcher and Proofreader
Leesburg, Georgia

Dianne E. Fiorentino
Research Coordinator
Nursing Reviews, Inc.
Las Vegas, Rhode Island

James Guibault Jr., BS, PharmD
Clinical Pharmacist
Wilbraham, Massachusetts

Nicholas L. Silvestri, BA
Editorial and Communications Analyst
Nursing Reviews, Inc.
Las Vegas, Rhode Island

Angela Silvestri-Elmore, MSN, RN, BAS
Doctoral Student
University of Nevada, Las Vegas
Las Vegas, Nevada

ITEM WRITERS

Amber Ballard, MSN, RN
Sparrow Health System
Lansing, Michigan

Kim Clevenger, EdD, MSN, RN, BC
Baccalaureate & RN-BSN Program Coordinator
Associate Professor of Nursing
Morehead State University
Morehead, Kentucky

Mary L. Dowell, PhD, RN, BC
Assistant Professor
San Antonio College
San Antonio, Texas

Mary Ann Kennedy, RNC, BSN, MSN
Nursing Instructor
Bullard Havens Technical School
Bridgeport, Connecticut

Erin Roberts, MSN, RN, ONC, CDE
Nurse Clinician and Diabetes Educator
Sparrow Hospital
Lansing, Michigan

Valerie Talenda, MSN, RN-BC
Instructor
Lamar University
Beaumont, Texas

Olga Van Dyke, MSN, CAGS, RN
Assistant Professor
MCPHS University
Boston, Massachusetts

The author and publisher would also like to acknowledge the following individuals for contributions to the previous editions of this book:

Marianne P. Barba, MS, RN
Coventry, Rhode Island

Nancy Blasdell, PhD, RN
Kingston, Rhode Island

Rebecca S. Blaszczak, RN
Newport, Rhode Island

Barbara Bono-Snell, MS, RN, CS
Liverpool, New York

Netta Moncur Bowen, MSN, RN
Sanford, Florida

Carolyn Pierce Buckelew, RNCS, NC, CHyp
Perth Amboy, New Jersey

Janis M. Byers, MSN, RNC
Sewickley, Pennsylvania

Penny S. Cass, PhD, RN
Kokomo, Indiana

Deborah H. Chatham, RN, MS, CS
Gulfport, Mississippi

Tom Christenbery, MSN, RN
Nashville, Tennessee

Anita M. Creamer, RN, MS, CS
Warwick, Rhode Island

Barbara A. Dagastine, EdMSN, RN
Troy, New York

Jean DeCoffe, MSN, RN
Milton, Massachusetts

Katherine Dimmock, JD, EdD, MSN, RN
Milwaukee, Wisconsin

DeAnna Jan Emory, MS, RN
Muskogee, Oklahoma

Mary E. Farrell, MS, RN, CCRN
Salem, Massachusetts

Patsy H. Fasnacht, MSN, RN, CCRN
Lancaster, Pennsylvania

Dona Ferguson, MSN, RN, C
Mays Landing, New Jersey

Thomas E. Folcarelli, MSN, RN
Newport, Rhode Island

Florence Hayes Gibson, MSN, CNS
Monroe, Louisiana

Alma V. Harkey, RNC, MSN, ACCE
Cape Girardeau, Missouri

Joyce Ellen Heil, BSN, CCRN
Pittsburgh, Pennsylvania

Barbara Hicks, DSN, RN
Sylacauga, Alabama

Mary Ann Hogan, RN, MSN
Amherst, Massachusetts

Noreen M. Houck, MS, RN
Syracuse, New York

Amy Lawyer Hudson, RN, MSN
Helene, Arkansas

Frances E. Johnson, MS, RNC
Berrien Springs, Michigan

Deborah Klaas, RN, PhD
Flagstaff, Arizona

June Peterson Larson, RN, MS
Vermillion, South Dakota

Suzanne K. Marnocha, RN, MSN, CCRN
Oshkosh, Wisconsin

Ellen Frances McCarty, PhD, RN, CS
Newport, Rhode Island

Connie M. Metzler, MSN, RN
Lancaster, Pennsylvania

Patricia A. Miller, MSN, RN
Springfield, Massachusetts

Jo Ann Barnes Mullaney, PhD, RN, CS
Newport, Rhode Island

Giuliana Nava, RN, BSN
Graduate, Salve Regina University, Newport, Rhode Island

Kathleen Ann Ohman, RN, MS, EdD
St. Joseph, Minnesota

Lynda C. Opdyke, RN, MSN
Charlotte, North Carolina

MaeDella Perry, RN, MSN
Augusta, Georgia

Donna Russo, RN, MSN, CCRN
Philadelphia, Pennsylvania

Lisa A. Ruth-Sahd, MSN, RN, CEN, CCRN
York, Pennsylvania

Jeanine T. Seguin, MS, RN, CS
Keuka Park, New York

Alberta Elaine Severs, MSN, MA, RN
Lincoln, Rhode Island

Kimberly Sharpe, MS, RN
Syracuse, New York

Susan Sienkiewicz, MA, RN, CS
Lincoln, Rhode Island

Angela E. Silvestri-Elmore, RN, MSN, BAS
Las Vegas, Nevada

Yvonne Marie Smith, MSN, RN, CCRN
Canton, Ohio

Sharon Souter, RN, PhD
Abilene, Texas

Judith Stamp, MS, RN
Troy, New York

Yvonne Nazareth Stringfield, EdD, RN
Nashville, Tennessee

Mattie Tolley, RN, MS
Weatherford, Oklahoma

Johanna M. Tracy, MSN, RN, CS
Trenton, New Jersey

Joyce I. Turnbull, RN, MN
San Jose, California

Paula A. Viau, PhD, RN
Kingston, Rhode Island

Carol Warner, RN, CPN, MSN
Bethlehem, Pennsylvania

Cheryle I. Whitney, RN, MSN, BC
The Woodlands, Texas

Deborah Williams, EdD, RN
Bowling Green, Kentucky

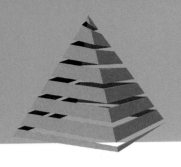

Reviewers

Mary C. Carrico, MS, RN
Associate Professor of Nursing
West Kentucky Community and Technical College
Paducah, Kentucky

Nancee Croatt Wozney, PhD, RN
Dean of Nursing
Minnesota State College – Southeast Technical
Winona, Minnesota

Mattie Davis, DNP, FNP-C
Nursing Instructor
J. F. Drake State Community and Technical College
Huntsville, Alabama

Sherry Donovan, MSN, RN-C
Nursing Faculty
Yakima Valley Community College
Yakima, Washington

Alise Farrell, RN, MSN, CPN, CNL
Instructor
University of Tennessee Health Science Center
Memphis, Tennessee

Mary Ford, MSN, RN
Instructor
Lamar University
Beaumont, Texas

Sarah Gabua, DNP, RN
Adjunct Professor of Nursing
Rasmussen College
Rockford, Illinois

Crystal Gazda, RN, MSN, MPH
Nursing Faculty
Brookhaven College
Dallas, Texas

Sheila Grossman, Ph.D. APRN, FNP-BC, FAAN
Professor & Coordinator FNP Track
Fairfield University School of Nursing, Fairfield
Connecticut

Rose Harding, MSN, RN
Instructor, Coordinator of Standardized Test
Evaluation Committee
Lamar University
Beaumont, Texas

Thuy Lam, Ph.D., RN
Nursing Faculty
J. F. Drake State Community and Technical College
Huntsville, Alabama

Dawn Le Porte, MSN, RN
Nursing Supervisor
Northeast Rehabilitation Hospital
Salem, New Hampshire

Sara A. Melendez, MSN, RN, CCNS-BC
Clinical Nurse Specialist
Doctors Hospital of Laredo
Laredo, Texas

Laure J Miller, MSN, RN
Associate Professor Nursing
Iowa Lakes Community College
Emmetsburg, Iowa

Rebecca Personett, PhD, RN, NEA-BC
Dallas County Community College
North Central Texas College
Gainesville, Texas

Colleen Reid, MSN, Ed, CCNS, CCRN
Senior Clinical Educator, Critical Care Emergency Course
Blanchfield Army Medical Center
Fort Sam, Houston, Texas

Johnnie Robbins, MSN, RN, CCRN, CCNS
Clinical Nurse Specialist
US Army Institute of Surgical Research
Fort Sam, Houston, TX

Katherine Roberts, MSN, RN
Assistant Professor of Nursing
Lamar University
Beaumont, Texas

Joyce Swegle, RN, PhD
Nursing Professor
El Centro College
Dallas, Texas

Theresa Villarreal, MSN, RN
Clinical Professor
University of Texas Health Science Center at San Antonio
San Antonio, Texas

Daryle Wane, PhD, ARNP, FNP-BC
Professor of Nursing
RN to BSN Coordinator, Pasco-Hernando State College
New Port Richey, Florida

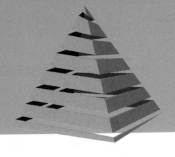

Preface

"Success is climbing a mountain, facing the challenge of obstacles, and reaching the top of the mountain."

Linda Anne Silvestri, PhD, RN

Welcome to *Saunders Pyramid to Success!*

AN ESSENTIAL RESOURCE FOR TEST SUCCESS

Saunders Q&A Review for the NCLEX-RN® Examination is one in a series of products designed to assist you in achieving your goal of becoming a registered nurse. This text and Evolve site package provide you with more than 6000 practice NCLEX-RN test questions based on the current NCLEX-RN test plan.

The current test plan for the NCLEX-RN identifies a framework based on *Client Needs*. The Client Needs categories include Physiological Integrity, Safe and Effective Care Environment, Health Promotion and Maintenance, and Psychosocial Integrity. *Integrated Processes* are also identified as a component of the test plan. These include Caring, Communication and Documentation, Nursing Process, and Teaching and Learning. This book has been uniquely designed and includes chapters that describe each specific component of the NCLEX-RN test plan framework and six practice tests that contain NCLEX-style questions specific to each component.

NCLEX-RN® TEST PREPARATION

This book begins with information regarding NCLEX-RN preparation. **Chapter 1** addresses all of the information related to the NCLEX-RN test plan and the testing procedures related to the examination. This chapter answers all of the questions that you may have regarding the testing procedures.

Chapter 2 provides information to the foreign-educated nurse about the process of obtaining a license to practice as a registered nurse in the United States.

Chapter 3 discusses the NCLEX-RN from a nonacademic viewpoint and emphasizes a holistic approach for your individual test preparation. This chapter identifies the components of a structured study plan, anxiety-reducing techniques, and personal focus issues. Nursing students also want to hear what other students have to say about their experiences with the NCLEX-RN and what it is really like to take this examination. **Chapter 4** is a story of success written by a nursing graduate who recently took the NCLEX-RN and addresses the issue of what the examination is all about.

Chapter 5 includes all of the important strategies that will assist in teaching you how to read a question, how not to read into a question, and how to use the process of elimination and various other strategies to select the correct response from the options presented.

CLIENT NEEDS

Chapter 6 and Tests 1 through 4 address the NCLEX-RN test plan component, *Client Needs*. **Chapter 6** describes each category of Client Needs as identified by the test plan and lists any subcategories, the percentage of test questions for each category, and some of the content included on the NCLEX-RN. **Tests 1 through 4** contain practice test questions related specifically to each category of Client Needs. Test 1 comprises questions related to Physiological Integrity; Test 2 contains questions dealing with Safe and Effective Care Environment; Test 3 is made up of questions concerned with Health Promotion and Maintenance; and Test 4 contains Psychosocial Integrity questions.

INTEGRATED PROCESSES

Chapter 7 and Test 5 address the *Integrated Processes* as identified in the NCLEX-RN test plan. **Chapter 7** describes each Integrated Process. **Test 5** contains practice test questions related specifically to each Integrated Process, including Caring, Communication and Documentation, Nursing Process, and Teaching and Learning.

COMPREHENSIVE TEST

A comprehensive test, **Test 6,** is included at the end of this book. It consists of 300 practice questions representative of the components of the test plan framework for the NCLEX-RN.

SPECIAL FEATURES OF THE BOOK

Book Design

The book is designed with a unique two-column format. The left column presents the practice questions, answer options, and coding areas while the right column provides the corresponding answers, rationales, priority nursing tips, test-taking strategies, and references. The two-column format makes the review easier because you do not have to flip through pages in search of answers and rationales.

SPECIAL FEATURES FOUND ON EVOLVE

Pretest and Study Calendar

The accompanying Evolve site contains a 75-question pretest that provides you with feedback on your strengths and weaknesses. The results of your pretest will generate an individualized study calendar to guide you in your preparation for the NCLEX examination.

Heart, Lung, and Bowel Sound Questions

The accompanying Evolve site contains *Audio Questions* representative of content addressed in the current test plan for the NCLEX-RN exam. These questions are in NCLEX-style format, and each question presents an audio sound as a component of the question.

Video Questions

The accompanying Evolve site also contains new *Video Questions* representative of content addressed in the current test plan for the NCLEX-RN exam. These questions are in NCLEX-style format, and each question presents a video clip as a component of the question.

Testlet Questions

The accompanying Evolve site contains testlet questions. These question types include a client scenario and several accompanying practice questions that relate to the content of the scenario.

Audio Review Summaries

The companion Evolve site includes three *Audio Review Summaries* that cover challenging subject areas under the current NCLEX-RN test plan, including *Pharmacology*, *Acid-Base Balance*, and *Fluids and Electrolytes*.

PRACTICE QUESTIONS

Multiple Choice and Alternate Item Format Questions

While preparing for the NCLEX-RN, students have a strong need to review practice test questions. This book contains practice questions that are in the multiple-choice format or in alternate item test question formats used in the NCLEX-RN examination. In the book, alternate item format questions are marked by a special symbol: ❖. Each practice test contains several multiple-choice questions and an alternate item format question.

The accompanying Evolve site contains more than 6000 questions: all of the questions from the book, plus new questions, including all types of alternate item formats. The alternate item format questions in the book and on the accompanying Evolve site may be presented as one of the following:

- Fill-in-the-blank question
- Multiple response question
- Prioritizing (ordered response) question, also known as a drag-and-drop question
- Figure/illustration question, also known as a hot spot question
- Graphic options question, in which each option contains a figure or illustration
- Chart/exhibit question
- Audio question that includes a heart, lung, or bowel sound
- Video question
- Testlet question

These questions provide you with practice in prioritizing, decision-making, and critical thinking skills. In addition, questions that require knowledge of common laboratory values have a review button for your reference while studying on the Evolve site.

Answer Sections for Practice Questions

Each practice question is accompanied by the correct answer, rationale, priority nursing tip, test-taking strategy, question categories, and reference source. The structure of the answer section is unique and provides the following information for every question:

- **Rationale:** The rationale provides you significant information regarding both correct and incorrect options.
- **Priority Nursing Tip:** The priority nursing tip provides you with an important piece of information that will be helpful to you when answering practice questions and questions on the NCLEX.
- **Test-Taking Strategy:** The test-taking strategy provides a logical path for selecting the correct option and helps you select an answer to a question on which you might have to guess. In each practice question, the specific strategy that will assist in answering the question correctly is highlighted in bold blue type. Specific suggestions for review are identified in the test-taking strategy and are highlighted in bold magenta type to provide you direction for locating the specific content for review. The highlighting of the specific test-taking strategies and specific content areas in the practice questions will provide you with guidance on what topics to review for further remediation in *Saunders Strategies for Test Success: Passing Nursing School and the NCLEX® Exam* and *Saunders Comprehensive Review for the NCLEX-RN® Exam.*
- **Question Categories:** Each question in the book and on the accompanying Evolve site is identified based on the categories used by the NCLEX-RN test plan. Additional content area categories are provided with each question to assist you in identifying areas in need of review. The categories identified with each question include Level of Cognitive Ability, Client Needs, Integrated Process, and the specific nursing Content Area. New to this edition is a Priority Concepts code, which provides you with the specific concept related to nursing practice. All categories are identified by their full names so that you do not need to memorize codes or abbreviations.
- **Reference:** The reference source and page number are listed for you so that you can easily find the information you need to review in your undergraduate nursing textbooks.

HOW TO USE THIS BOOK

Saunders Q&A Review for the NCLEX-RN® Examination is specially designed to help you with your successful journey to the peak of the Pyramid to Success: becoming a registered nurse. As you begin your journey through this book, you will be introduced to all of the important points regarding the NCLEX-RN examination, the process of testing, and the unique and special tips regarding how to prepare yourself both academically and nonacademically for this important examination. Read the chapter from the nursing graduate who recently passed the NCLEX-RN and consider what the graduate had to say about the examination. The test-taking strategy chapter will provide you with important strategies that will guide you in selecting the correct option or assist you in guessing the answer. Read this chapter and practice these strategies as you proceed through your journey with this book.

Once you have read the introductory components of this book, it is time to begin the practice questions. As you read through each question and select an answer, be sure to read the rationale, the priority nursing tip, and the test-taking strategy. The rationale provides you with significant information regarding both the correct and incorrect options. The priority nursing tip provides you with a piece of important information to remember that will help answer questions on the NCLEX, and the test-taking strategy provides you with the logic for selecting the correct option. The strategy also identifies the content area that you need to review if you had difficulty with the question. Use the reference source provided so that you can easily find the information you need to review.

CLIMBING THE PYRAMID TO SUCCESS

This step on the *Pyramid to Success* is to get additional practice with a **Q&A review** product. *Saunders Q&A Review for the NCLEX-RN® Examination* offers more than 6000 unique practice questions in the book and on the companion Evolve site. The questions are focused on the Client Needs and Integrated Processes of the NCLEX test plan, making it easy to access your study area of choice. For on-the-go Q&A review, you can pick up *Saunders Q&A Review Cards for the NCLEX-RN® Examination*, or, if you own an iPhone or iPod Touch, you can search for "Saunders Q&A Review" in Apple's App Store.

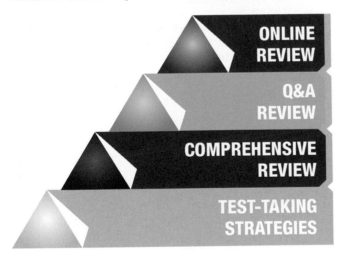

As you work your way through *Saunders Q&A Review for the NCLEX-RN® Examination* and identify your areas of strength and weakness, you can return to the companion book, *Saunders Comprehensive Review for the NCLEX-RN® Examination*, to focus your study on these areas. The purpose of the *Saunders Comprehensive Review for the NCLEX-RN® Examination* is to provide a **comprehensive review** of the nursing content you will be tested on during the NCLEX-RN examination. However, *Saunders Comprehensive Review for the NCLEX-RN® Examination* is intended to do more than simply prepare you for the rigors of the NCLEX; this book is also meant to serve as a valuable study tool that you can refer to throughout your nursing program, with customizable Evolve site selections to help identify and reinforce key content areas. Your final step on the Pyramid to Success is to master the **online review**. *HESI/Saunders Online Review for the NCLEX-RN® Examination* provides an interactive and individualized platform to get you ready for your final licensure exam. This online course provides 10 high-level content modules, supplemented with instructional videos, animations, audio, illustrations, testlets, and several subject matter exams. End of module practice tests are provided along with several Crossing the Finish Line: Practice Tests. In addition, you can assess your progress with a pre-test and comprehensive exam in a computerized environment that prepares you for the actual NCLEX-RN exam.

At the base of the Pyramid to Success are my **test-taking strategies**, which provide a foundation for understanding and unpacking the complexities of NCLEX exam questions, including alternate item formats. *Saunders Strategies for Test Success: Passing Nursing School and the NCLEX® Exam* takes a detailed look at all the test-taking strategies you will need to know in order to pass any nursing examination, including the NCLEX. Special tips are integrated for beginning nursing students, and there are 1000 practice questions included so you can apply the testing strategies.

To obtain any of these resources that will prepare you for your nursing exams and the NCLEX-RN exam, visit the Elsevier Health Sciences Web site at elsevierhealth.com.

Good Luck with your journey through the *Saunders Pyramid to Success*. I wish you continued success throughout your new career as a Registered Nurse!

Linda Anne Silvestri, PhD, RN

Acknowledgments

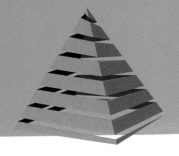

There are many individuals who in their own ways have contributed to my success in making my professional dreams become a reality. My sincere appreciation and warmest thanks are extended to all of them.

First, I want to acknowledge my parents, who opened my door of opportunity in education. I thank my mother, Frances Mary, for all of her love, support, and assistance as I continuously worked to achieve my professional goals. I thank my father, Arnold Lawrence, who always provided insightful words of encouragement. My memories of his love and support will always remain in my heart. I also thank my best friend and love of my life, my husband, Larry; my sister, Dianne Elodia and her husband Lawrence; my brother, Lawrence Peter; and my nieces and nephews: Gina, Karen, Angela, Katie, Gabrielle, Brianna, Nicholas, Anthony, and Nathan, who were continuously supportive, giving, and helpful during my research and preparation of this publication. They were always there and by my side whenever I needed them.

I want to thank my nursing students at the Community College of Rhode Island who approached me in 1991 and persuaded me to assist them in preparing to take the NCLEX-RN examination. Their enthusiasm and inspiration led to the commencement of my professional endeavors in conducting review courses for the NCLEX-RN exam for nursing students. I also thank the numerous nursing students who have attended my review courses for their willingness to share their needs and ideas. Their input has certainly added a special uniqueness to this publication.

I wish to acknowledge all of the nursing faculty who taught in my review courses for the NCLEX-RN exam. Their commitment, dedication, and expertise have certainly assisted nursing students in achieving success with the NCLEX-RN exam. Additionally, I want to especially acknowledge my husband, Laurent W. Valliere, for his contribution to this publication, for teaching in my review courses for the NCLEX-RN exam, and for his commitment and dedication in assisting my nursing students to prepare for the exam from a nonacademic point of view. I also want to extend a very special thank you to my niece, Angela E. Silvestri-Elmore, for her assistance in writing many of the priority nursing tips. I also sincerely thank Miranda Cox, RN, BSN, for writing a chapter for this book about her experiences with preparing for and taking the NCLEX-RN examination.

A special thank you and acknowledgment also goes to all of the contributors and item writers who updated and provided many of the practice questions and all of the previous contributors who provided contributions to this book. A very special thank you to all of you!

I also want to thank my husband Larry for all of his continuous support as I moved through my personal challenges and professional endeavors; he has been my rock of support! I thank Dianne E. Fiorentino for her continuous support and dedication to my work in both the NCLEX exam review courses and in reference support and other secretarial responsibilities for the sixth edition of this book. I thank Allison Bowser for her dedication to my work as she researched and proofread manuscript, Jimmy Guibault for providing medication research support, and Nick Silvestri for his communication and proofreading skills as he reviewed manuscript.

I also want to extend a special acknowledgment and thank you to Dr. Eileen Gray for her special contributing and super-editing skills as she reviewed the manuscript for this book and Evolve site. Thank you, Dr. Gray!

I sincerely acknowledge and thank three very important individuals from Elsevier. I thank Kristin Geen, Director of Traditional Education, and Yvonne Alexopoulos, Content Strategist, for their continuous support, enthusiasm, and expert professional guidance throughout the preparation of this edition. Thank you also to Laura Goodrich, Content Developmental Specialist, who provided me with a tremendous amount of support throughout this publication. Laura generated creative ideas for the book and did outstanding work in strategizing and maintaining order for all of the work that I submitted for manuscript production and all of the work submitted by contributors. Thank you, Kristin, Yvonne, and Laura; I could not have completed this publication without you! In addition, I also extend a special thank you to Hannah Corrier, Content Coordinator, who assisted Laura Goodrich with many of the tasks associated with preparing the manuscript for production.

I want to acknowledge all of the staff at Elsevier for their tremendous help throughout the preparation and production of this publication. A special thanks to all of them. I thank all of the special people in the production and marketing department: Danielle LeCompte, Marketing Manager; Bill Drone, Project Manager; Jeff Patterson, Publishing Services Manager; David Rushing and Jason Gonulsen, Multimedia Producers; and Christian Bilbow, Designer, all of whom played such significant roles in finalizing this publication. I would also like to acknowledge Patricia Mieg, former Educational Sales Representative, who encouraged me to submit my ideas and initial work for the first edition of this book to the W.B. Saunders Company.

I also need to thank Salve Regina University for the opportunity to educate nursing students in the baccalaureate nursing program and for its encouragement and support as I researched and wrote this publication.

I wish to acknowledge the Community College of Rhode Island, which provided me the opportunity to educate nursing students in the Associate Degree of Nursing Program, and a special thank you to Patricia Miller, MSN, RN, and Michelina McClellan, MS, RN, from Baystate Medical Center School of Nursing in Springfield, Massachusetts, who were my first mentors in nursing education.

Lastly, a very special thank you to all my nursing students: past, present, and future. All of you light up my life! Your love and dedication to the profession of nursing and your commitment to provide health care will bring never-ending rewards!

Linda Anne Silvestri, PhD, RN

Contents

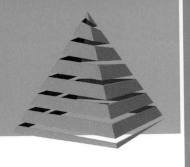
NCLEX-RN® Preparation

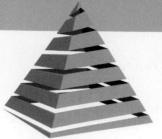

CHAPTER 1

The NCLEX-RN® Examination

Pyramid to Success

Welcome to *Saunders Q&A Review for the NCLEX-RN® Examination,* the second component of the Pyramid to Success! At this time, you have completed your first path toward the peak of the pyramid with *Saunders Comprehensive Review for the NCLEX-RN® Examination.* Now it is time to continue that journey to become a registered nurse with *Saunders Q&A Review for the NCLEX-RN® Examination.*

As you begin your journey through this book, you will be introduced to all of the important points regarding the NCLEX-RN examination, the types of questions on the NCLEX, the process of testing, and unique and special tips regarding how to prepare yourself both academically and nonacademically for this very important examination. You will read what a nursing graduate who passed the NCLEX-RN examination has to say about the examination. Important test-taking strategies are detailed that will guide you in selecting the correct option or in selecting an answer when you need to guess.

About This Resource

Saunders Q&A Review for the NCLEX-RN® Examination contains more than 6000 NCLEX-RN–style practice questions. Question types include multiple choice; multiple response; fill-in-the-blank; prioritizing (ordered-response), also known as drag and drop; image ("hot spot") questions; chart/exhibit questions; graphic options; testlets (case studies); and audio and video questions. The Evolve site also includes audios on test-taking strategies, pharmacology strategies, and fluids and electrolytes and acid-base balance. The chapters in the book have been developed to provide a description of the components of the NCLEX-RN test plan, including Client Needs and the Integrated Processes. In addition, chapters have been prepared to contain practice questions specific to each category of Client Needs and the Integrated Processes.

A rationale, priority nursing tip, test-taking strategy, and reference source containing a page number are provided with each question. Each question is coded on the basis of the Level of Cognitive Ability, Client Needs category, Integrated Process, and the Content Area being tested. In addition, two Priority Concepts that relate to the content of the question are identified. This code is helpful specifically for students whose curriculum is concept-based. The rationale contains significant information regarding both the correct and incorrect options. The priority nursing tip provides you with key information about a nursing point to remember. The test-taking strategy maps out a logical path for selecting the correct option and identifies the content area to review, if necessary. The reference source and page number provide easy access to the information that you need to review.

Other Parts of the Pyramid to Success
Saunders Comprehensive Review for the NCLEX-RN® Examination

Saunders Comprehensive Review for the NCLEX-RN® Examination is a "must-have" book and is specially designed to help you begin your successful journey to the peak of the pyramid, becoming a registered nurse. Each of the units in this book begins with the Pyramid to Success. The Pyramid to Success addresses specific points related to the NCLEX-RN examination, including the Pyramid Terms and the Client Needs as identified in the test plan framework for the examination. *Pyramid Terms* are key words that are defined and set in bold-face throughout each chapter to direct your attention to those significant points for the examination. The Client Needs specific to the content of the chapter are identified.

Throughout each chapter, you will find Pyramid Point bullets that identify areas most likely to be tested on the NCLEX-RN examination. You can test your strengths and abilities by taking all the practice tests provided in this book and on the accompanying Evolve site. Be sure to read all the rationales and test-taking strategies. The rationale provides you with significant information regarding the correct and incorrect options. The test-taking strategy provides you with the logical path to selecting the correct option. The test-taking strategy also identifies the content area to review, if required. The reference source and page number are provided so that you can easily find the information that you need to review. Each question is coded based on the Level of Cognitive Ability, the Client Needs category, the Integrated Process, and the nursing content area. In addition to all question types, this book also contains "Critical Thinking: What Should You Do?" boxes, "Priority Nursing Action" boxes that provide clinical situations and the actions that the nurse should take in order of priority, and Pyramid Alerts that provide you with important information about nursing care information.

HESI/Saunders Online Review for the NCLEX-RN® Examination

HESI/Saunders Online Review for the NCLEX-RN® Examination addresses all areas of the test plan identified by the National Council of State Boards of Nursing (NCSBN). The course contains a pretest that provides feedback regarding your strengths and weaknesses. After taking the pretest, an individualized study schedule in a calendar format is generated to provide guidance in preparing for the NCLEX. Content review is in an outline format and includes self-check practice questions and testlets, figures and illustrations, a glossary, and animations and videos. Additional practice exams include 100–question end-of-module exams, five

"Crossing the Finish Line" 100-question exams, and a comprehensive exam. Types of practice questions in this course include multiple choice; multiple response; fill-in-the-blank; ordered-response (prioritizing), also known as drag and drop; image ("hot spot") questions; chart/exhibit questions; graphic options; testlets; heart and lung sound questions; and video questions. There are 2500 practice test questions in *HESI/Saunders Online Review for the NCLEX-RN® Examination.*

Saunders Strategies for Test Success: Passing Nursing School and the NCLEX® Exam

Saunders Strategies for Test Success: Passing Nursing School and the NCLEX® Exam focuses on the test-taking strategies that will help you pass your nursing examinations while in nursing school and will prepare you for the NCLEX-RN examination. The chapters describe all the test-taking strategies and include several sample questions that illustrate how to use each test-taking strategy. There are a total of 1000 NCLEX style questions, including multiple choice and alternate item format questions. NCLEX tips and tips for the beginning nursing student are offered, as well as information on cultural characteristics and practices, pharmacology strategies, medication and intravenous calculations, laboratory values, positioning guidelines, and therapeutic diets.

Saunders Q&A Review Cards for the NCLEX-RN® Exam

The *Saunders Q&A Review Cards for the NCLEX-RN® Exam* is organized specifically by nursing content areas and the test plan framework of the current NCLEX-RN test plan. This product provides you with 1200 practice test questions on portable and easy to use cards. The question is on the front of the card and the answer, rationale, and test-taking strategy are on the back of the card. This product includes both multiple choice questions and alternate item format questions including fill-in-the-blank, multiple response, prioritizing (ordered response), figure, and chart/exhibit questions. All the products in Saunders Pyramid to Success can be obtained online by visiting http://www.elsevierhealth.com or by calling 800-426-4545.

Let's begin our journey through the Pyramid to Success.

The Examination Process

An important step in the Pyramid to Success is to become as familiar as possible with the examination process. Candidates facing the challenge of this examination may experience a significant amount of anxiety. Knowing what the examination is all about and knowing what you will encounter during the process of testing will assist in alleviating fear and anxiety. The information contained in this chapter addresses the procedures related to the development of the NCLEX-RN examination test plan, the components of the test plan, and the answers to the questions most commonly asked by nursing students and graduates preparing to take the NCLEX-RN examination. The information contained in this chapter related to the test plan was obtained from the NCSBN Web site (http://www.ncsbn.org) and the National Council of State Boards of Nursing Test Plan for the NCLEX-RN Examination (effective date, April 2013). You can obtain additional information regarding the test and its development by accessing the NCSBN Web site at www.ncsbn.org or by writing to the National Council of State Boards of Nursing, 111 East Wacker Drive, Suite 2900, Chicago, IL 60601. You are encouraged to access the NCSBN Web site because the site provides you with valuable information about the NCLEX and other resources available to an NCLEX candidate.

Computer Adaptive Testing

The acronym *CAT* stands for computer adaptive test, which means that the examination is created as the test-taker answers each question. All the test questions are categorized based on the test plan structure and the level of difficulty of the question. As you answer a question, the computer determines your competency based on the answer you selected. If you selected a correct answer to a question, the computer scans the question bank and selects a more difficult question. If you selected an incorrect answer, the computer scans the question bank and selects an easier question. This process continues until the test plan requirements are met and a reliable pass-or-fail decision is made. Additional information about computer adaptive testing can be located at the NCSBN Web site.

When a test question is presented on the computer screen, you must answer it or the test will not move on. This means that you will not be able to skip questions, go back and review questions, or go back and change answers. Remember that in a CAT examination, once an answer is recorded, all subsequent questions administered depend, to an extent, on the answer selected for that question. Skipping and returning to earlier questions are not compatible with the logical methodology of a computer adaptive test. The inability to skip questions or go back to change previous answers will not be a disadvantage to you because you will not fall into the "trap" of changing a correct answer to an incorrect one with the CAT system.

If you are faced with a question that contains unfamiliar content, you may need to guess at the answer. There is no penalty for guessing on this examination. Remember, with most of the questions, the answer will be obvious. If you need to guess, use your nursing knowledge and clinical experiences to their fullest extent, as well as all the test-taking strategies that you have practiced in this review program.

You do not need any computer experience to take this examination. A keyboard tutorial is provided and administered to all test-takers at the start of the examination. The tutorial will instruct you on the use of the on-screen optional calculator, the use of the mouse, and how to record an answer. In addition to the traditional four-option multiple choice question, the tutorial also provides instructions on how to respond to alternate item format questions. This tutorial is provided on the NCSBN Web site, and you are encouraged to view the tutorial when you are preparing for the NCLEX. Additionally, at the testing site, a test administrator is present to assist in explaining the use of the computer to ensure your full understanding of how to proceed.

Development of the Test Plan

The test plan for the NCLEX-RN examination is developed by the NCSBN. The NCLEX examination is a national examination; therefore, the NCSBN considers the legal scope of nursing practice as governed by state laws and regulations, including the Nurse Practice Act, and uses these laws to define the areas on the examination that will assess the competence of the test taker for licensure.

The NCSBN also conducts a very important study every 3 years, known as a practice analysis study, to determine the framework for the test plan for the examination. The participants in this study include newly licensed registered nurses from all types of basic nursing education programs. From a list of nursing activities provided, the participants are asked about the frequency and importance of performing them in relation to client safety and the setting in which they are performed. A panel of content experts at the NCSBN analyzes the results of the study and makes decisions regarding the test plan framework. The results of this recently conducted study provided the structure for the test plan implemented in April 2013.

Item Writers

The NCSBN selects question (item) writers after an extensive application process. The writers are registered nurses who hold a master's or higher degree and many of the writers are nursing educators. Question writers voluntarily submit an application to become a writer and must meet specific criteria established by the council to be accepted as participants in the process.

The Test Plan

The content of the NCLEX-RN examination reflects the activities identified in the practice analysis study conducted by the NCSBN. The questions are written to address the Levels of Cognitive Ability, Client Needs, and Integrated Processes as identified in the test plan developed by the NCSBN.

Levels of Cognitive Ability

The practice of nursing requires critical thinking in decision making. Therefore, most questions on the NCLEX examination are written at the application level or higher levels of cognitive ability, such as the analyzing, synthesizing, evaluating, and creating levels. Box 1-1 presents an example of a question that requires you to apply data.

Client Needs

In the test plan implemented in April 2013, the NCSBN applied a test plan framework based on Client Needs. The NCSBN identifies four major categories of Client Needs including Safe and Effective Care Environment, Health Promotion and Maintenance, Psychosocial Integrity, and Physiological Integrity. Some of these categories are further divided into subcategories. Refer to Chapter 6 for a detailed description of the categories of Client Needs and the NCLEX-RN examination, and refer to Table 1-1 for the percentages of questions from each Client Needs category.

Integrated Processes

The NCSBN identifies four processes that are fundamental to the practice of nursing. These processes are a component of the test plan and are incorporated throughout the major categories of Client Needs. The subcategories of the Integrated Processes include Caring, Communication and

---

BOX 1-1	Level of Cognitive Ability Question

A woman at 32 weeks' gestation is brought into the emergency department after an automobile accident. The client is bleeding vaginally and fetal assessment indicates moderate fetal distress. Which action should the nurse take **first** in an attempt to reduce the stress on the fetus?

1. Start intravenous (IV) fluids at a keep open rate.
2. Set up for an immediate cesarean section delivery.
3. Elevate the head of the bed to a semi-Fowler's position.
4. Administer oxygen via a face mask at 7 to 10 liters per minute.

Answer: 4

Note the strategic word, *first*. This question requires you to identify the *first* nursing action that you will take. Also use the ABCs—airway, breathing, and circulation—to answer correctly. Administering oxygen will increase the amount of oxygen for transport to the fetus, partially compensating for the loss of circulating blood volume. This action is essential regardless of the cause or amount of bleeding. IV fluids will also be initiated. Although a cesarean delivery may be needed, there are no data that indicate it is necessary at this time. The client will be positioned per health care provider's prescription. Review: nursing care if **fetal distress** occurs.

Level of Cognitive Ability: Applying

TABLE 1-1 Client Needs Categories and Percentage of Questions on the NCLEX-RN® Examination

Client Needs Category	Percentage of Questions
Safe and Effective Care Environment	
Management of Care	17%-23%
Safety and Infection Control	9%-15%
Health Promotion and Maintenance	6%-12%
Psychosocial Integrity	6%-12%
Physiological Integrity	
Basic Care and Comfort	6%-12%
Pharmacological and Parenteral Therapies	12%-18%
Reduction of Risk Potential	9%-15%
Physiological Adaptation	11%-17%

From National Council of State Boards of Nursing: *2013 NCLEX-RN® detailed test plan*, Chicago, 2013, National Council of State Boards of Nursing.

Documentation, Nursing Process (Assessment, Analysis, Planning, Implementation, Evaluation), and Teaching and Learning. Refer to Chapter 7 for a detailed description of the Integrated Processes and the NCLEX-RN examination.

Types of Questions on the Examination

The types of questions that may be administered on the examination include multiple choice; fill-in-the-blank; multiple response; prioritizing (ordered response), also known as drag and drop; and questions that contain a figure, chart/exhibit, graphic option items, and audio or video item formats. Some questions may require you to use the mouse and cursor on the computer. For example, you may be presented with a visual that displays the heart of an adult client. In this visual, you may be asked to "point and click" (using the mouse) on the area where you would place the stethoscope to count the apical heart rate. In all types of questions, the answer is scored as either right or wrong. In other words, credit is not given for a partially correct answer. Additionally, all question types may include pictures, graphics, tables, charts, sound, or video. The NCSBN provides specific directions for you to follow with all question types to guide you in your process of testing. Be sure to read these directions as they appear on the computer screen. Examples of some of these types of questions are noted in this chapter. Most question types are placed in this book, and all types including testlets, are on the accompanying Evolve site.

Multiple Choice Questions

Most of the questions that you will be asked to answer are in the multiple choice format. These questions provide you with data about a client situation and four answers or options. There is only one correct answer.

Fill-in-the-Blank Questions

Fill-in-the-blank questions may ask you to perform a medication calculation, determine an intravenous flow rate, or calculate an intake or output record on a client. You will need to type only a number (your answer) in the answer box. The unit of measure for your answer will already be noted for you outside of the answer box. If the question requires rounding the answer, this needs to be performed at the end of the calculation. The rules for rounding an answer are provided in the tutorial provided by the NCSBN and are also provided in the specific question. Additionally, you must type in a decimal point if necessary; however, it is not necessary to type a "0" before the decimal point. See Box 1-2 for an example.

Multiple Response Questions (Select All That Apply)

For a multiple response question, you will be asked to select or check all the options, such as nursing interventions, that relate to the information in the question. No partial credit is given for correct selections. You need to do exactly as the question asks, which is to select all the options that apply. See Box 1-3 for an example.

BOX 1-2   Fill-in-the-Blank Question

The health care provider prescribes 12 mEq of liquid potassium chloride. The medication label reads 20 mEq/15 mL. The nurse needs to administer how many milliliters (mL) to the client?

Answer: $\boxed{9}$ *mL*

Focus on the subject, the amount of mL to be administered. For this fill-in-the-blank question, use the formula for calculating medication doses. Once the dose is determined, you will need to type your numeric answer in the answer box. Always follow the specific directions noted on the computer screen when answering a question. Also, remember that there will be an on-screen calculator on the computer for your use to confirm your answer. Review: **medication calculations.**

Formula:

$$\frac{Desired}{Available} \times mL = mL \text{ per dose}$$

$$\frac{12\ mEq}{20\ mEq} \times 15\ mL = 9\ mL$$

Prioritizing (Ordered Response) Questions

In this type of question, you are asked to use the computer mouse to drag and drop your nursing actions in order of priority. Information is presented in a question, and based on the data, you need to determine what you will do first, second, third, and so forth. The unordered options are located in boxes on the left side of the screen and you need to move all options in order of priority to ordered response boxes on the right side of the screen. Specific directions for moving the options are provided with the question. See Box 1-4 for an example. More examples of this question type are located on the Evolve site.

Figure Questions

A question with a picture or graphic asks you to answer the question based on the picture or graphic. The question could contain a chart, table, or a figure or illustration. You also may be asked to use the computer mouse to point and click on a specific area in the visual. A figure or illustration may appear in any type of question, including a multiple choice question. See Box 1-5 for an example.

BOX 1-3   Multiple Response Question

The nurse is caring for a client with a terminal condition who is dying. Which respiratory assessment findings would indicate to the nurse that death is imminent? **Select all that apply.**

- ☑ 1. Dyspnea
- ☑ 2. Cyanosis
- ☐ 3. Kussmaul's respiration
- ☐ 4. Tachypnea without apnea
- ☑ 5. Irregular respiratory pattern
- ☑ 6. Adventitious bubbling lung sounds

Focus on the subject, assessment findings in a client who is dying. In a multiple response question, you will be asked to select or check all the options, such as interventions, that relate

to the information in the question. Be sure to follow the specific directions given on the computer screen. To answer this question think about the respiratory assessment findings that indicate death is imminent. These include altered patterns of respiration, such as slow, labored, irregular, or Cheyne-Stokes pattern (alternating periods of apnea and deep, rapid breathing); increased respiratory secretions and adventitious bubbling lung sounds (death rattle); irritation of the tracheobronchial airway as evidenced by hiccups, chest pain, fatigue, or exhaustion; and poor gas exchange as evidenced by hypoxia, dyspnea, or cyanosis. Kussmaul's respirations are abnormally deep, very rapid sighing respirations characteristic of diabetic ketoacidosis. Review: assessment findings in a **dying client.**

BOX 1-4   **Prioritizing (Ordered Response) Question**

The nurse is preparing to insert a nasogastric (NG) tube in a client. Arrange in order of priority the actions that the nurse should take to perform this procedure. **All options must be used.**

Unordered Options

- Verify tube placement.
- Anchor the tube to the nose.
- Position the client in high-Fowler's position.
- Document the tube length in the client's record.
- Measure the distance to insert the tube and mark the length of the tube with tape; lubricate the end of the tube with water-soluble lubricating jelly.
- Insert the tube through the naris and instruct the client to take a sip of water and swallow, continuing to advance the tube until the tape mark is reached.

Ordered Response

- Position the client in high-Fowler's position.
- Measure the distance to insert the tube and mark the distance of the tube with tape; lubricate the end of the tube with water-soluble lubricating jelly.
- Insert the tube through the naris and instruct the client to take a sip of water and swallow, continuing to advance the tube until the tape mark is reached.
- Verify tube placement.
- Anchor the tube to the nose.
- Document the tube length in the client's record.

Focus on the **subject**, the procedure for inserting an NG tube. This question requires you to arrange in order of priority the nursing actions that should be taken to insert an NG tube. To insert an NG tube, the nurse first performs hand hygiene and explains the procedure to the client. The nurse applies gloves and positions the client in high-Fowler's position, then places a bath towel over the client's chest. The nurse next measures the distance to insert the tube (the distance from the tip of the nose to the earlobe to the xiphoid process), marks the distance of the tube, and lubricates the end of the tube with water-soluble lubricating jelly. The nurse inserts the tube through the naris and, with the tube just above the oropharynx, instructs the client to flex the head forward and take a sip of water and swallow. The nurse continues to advance the tube until the tape mark is reached. The nurse then verifies tube placement and anchors the tube to the nose. Once the procedure is complete, the nurse documents the tube distance inserted and other appropriate data in the client's record. Also, remember that on the NCLEX examination, you will use the computer mouse to place the unordered options in an ordered response. Review: procedure for **inserting an NG tube.**

BOX 1-5   **Figure Question**

The nurse performs client rounds and notes that a client with a respiratory disorder is wearing this oxygen device (refer to figure). The nurse should document that the client is receiving oxygen by which type of low-flow oxygen delivery system? **Refer to figure.**

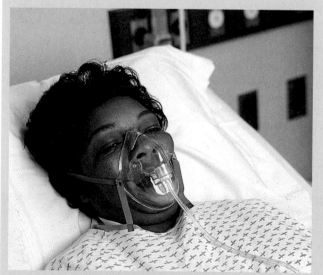

From Potter P, Perry A, Stockert P, Hall A: *Fundamentals of nursing*, ed 8, St. Louis, 2013, Mosby.

1. Venturi mask
2. Nasal cannula
3. Simple face mask
4. Partial rebreather mask

Answer: 3

Focus on the **subject**, the type of face mask that the client is wearing. For some of these question types you need to use the computer mouse and point and click at a designated area to answer the question. For this question, use of the computer mouse is not necessary. A simple face mask is used to deliver oxygen concentrations of 40% to 60% for short-term oxygen therapy. It also may be used in an emergency. A minimum flow rate of 5 L/min is needed to prevent the rebreathing of exhaled air. The simple face mask fits over the nose and mouth, has exhalation ports, and has a tube that connects to the oxygen source. A Venturi mask is a high-flow oxygen delivery system that delivers an accurate oxygen concentration. An adaptor is located between the bottom of the mask and the oxygen source. The adaptor contains holes of different sizes that allow specific amounts of air to mix with the oxygen. The nasal cannula contains nasal prongs that are used to deliver oxygen flow rates at 1 to 6 L/min. A partial rebreather mask is a mask with a reservoir bag without flaps. It provides oxygen concentrations of 60% to 75% with flow rates of 6 to 11 L/min. Review: **oxygen delivery systems.**

Chart/Exhibit Questions

In this type of question, you are presented with a question and a chart or exhibit. You are provided with three tabs or buttons that you need to click to obtain the information needed to answer the question. A prompt or message will appear that will indicate the need to click on a tab or button. See Box 1-6 for an example.

Graphic Options Questions

In this type of question, the option selections are pictures rather than text. Each option is preceded by a circle, and you will need to use the computer mouse to click in the circle that represents your answer choice. See Box 1-7 for an example.

BOX 1-6 Chart/Exhibit Question

Oral prednisone is prescribed for a hospitalized client. The nurse reviews the client's medical record and is **most** concerned about this prescription because of which documented item? **Refer to chart.**

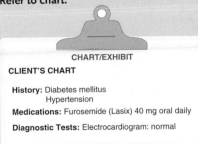

CHART/EXHIBIT

CLIENT'S CHART

History: Diabetes mellitus
Hypertension

Medications: Furosemide (Lasix) 40 mg oral daily

Diagnostic Tests: Electrocardiogram: normal

1. Hypertension
2. Diabetes mellitus
3. Furosemide (Lasix)
4. Normal electrocardiogram

Answer: **2**

Note the strategic word, *most*. This chart/exhibit question provides you with data from a client's medical chart, identifies a prescribed medication, and asks about a concern related to this medication. Read all the data in the question and the client's chart. Use nursing knowledge about the interactions and effects of prednisone and recall that this medication may increase the blood glucose level. This will assist in directing you to option 2, diabetes mellitus. For these question types, be certain to read all of the data in the client's chart before selecting the answer. Review: concerns related to administering **prednisone.**

Audio Questions

Audio questions require listening to a sound in order to answer the question. These questions prompt you to use the headset provided and to click on the sound icon. You are able to click on the volume button to adjust the volume to your comfort level and you may listen to the sound as many times as necessary. Content examples include but are not limited to various lung, heart, or bowel sounds. These question types are located on the accompanying Evolve site. See Figure 1-1 for an example.

Video Questions

Video questions require viewing an animation or video clip in order to answer the question. These questions prompt you to click on the video icon. There may be sound associated with the animation and video, in which case you will be prompted to use the headset. Content examples include but are not limited to assessment techniques, nursing procedures, or communication skills. These question types are located on the accompanying Evolve site. See Figure 1-2 for an example.

Registering to Take the Examination

It is important to obtain an NCLEX examination candidate bulletin from the NCSBN Web site at http://www.ncsbn.org because this bulletin provides all the information that you need to register for and schedule your examination. It also provides you with Web site and telephone information for NCLEX examination contacts. The initial step in the registration process is to submit an application to the state board of nursing in the state in which you intend to obtain licensure. You need to obtain information from the board of nursing

BOX 1-7 Graphic Options Question

The health care provider prescribes a tuberculin skin test to be done on a client. Which syringe should the nurse select to perform the test? **Refer to Figures 1 to 4.**

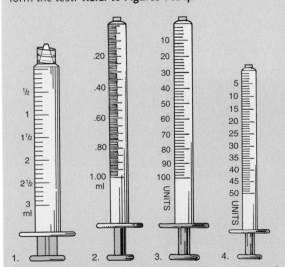

Figure from Potter P, Perry A, Stockert P, Hall A: *Fundamentals of nursing,* ed 8, St. Louis, 2013, Mosby.

Answer: **2**

Focus on the subject, the procedure for administering a tuberculin skin test. This question requires you to select the picture that represents your answer choice. To perform a tuberculin skin test, the nurse would use a tuberculin syringe that is marked in 0.01 (hundredths) because the dose for administration is less than 1 mL. Option 1 is a 3-mL syringe and is marked in 0.1 (tenths) and is used for most subcutaneous or intramuscular injections. Insulin syringes are available in 50 and 100 units and are used to administer insulin. Review: procedure for administering a **tuberculin skin test.**

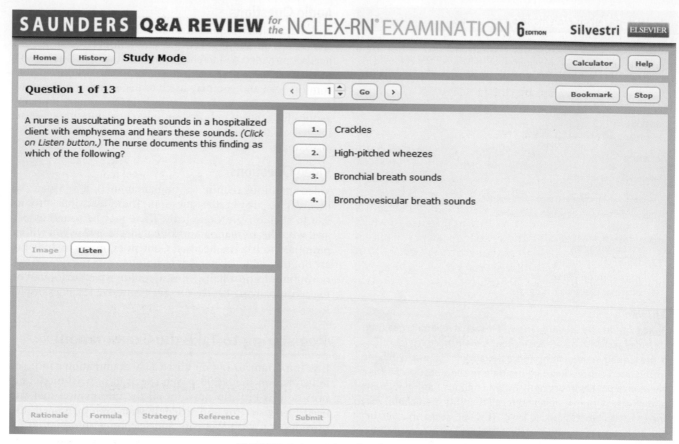

FIGURE 1-1 Screenshot of an audio question.

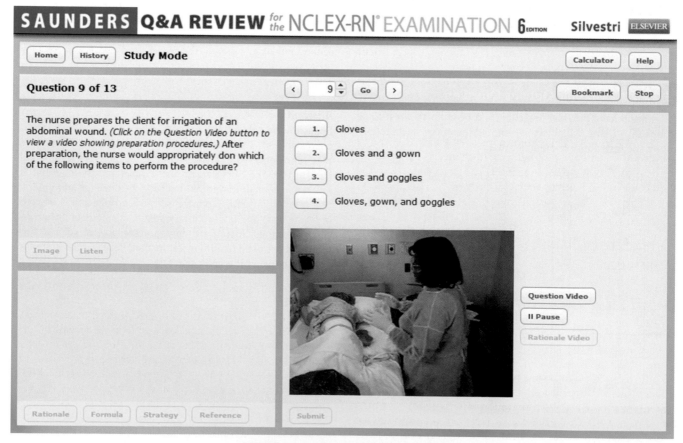

FIGURE 1-2 Screenshot of a video question.

regarding the specific registration process because the process may vary from state to state. Once you receive confirmation from the board of nursing that you have met all of the state requirements, you can register to take the NCLEX examination with Pearson Vue. You may register for the examination through the Internet, by United States (U.S.) mail, or by telephone. The NCLEX candidate Web site is http://www.pearsonvue.com/nclex.

Following the registration instructions and completing the registration forms precisely and accurately are important. Registration forms not properly completed or not accompanied by the proper fees in the required method of payment will be returned to you and will delay testing. You must pay a fee for taking the examination, and you also may have to pay additional fees to the board of nursing in the state in which you are applying. You will then be made eligible by the licensure board and will receive an Authorization to Test (ATT). If you do not receive an ATT within 2 weeks of registration, you should contact the candidate services at 1-866-496-2539 (U.S. candidates).

Authorization to Test Form and Scheduling an Appointment

You cannot make an appointment until the board of nursing declares eligibility and you receive an Authorization to Test (ATT) form. You will not receive an ATT form until you have been deemed eligible and have completed all necessary forms and have paid all required fees. Note the validity dates on the ATT form and schedule a date and time when you receive the ATT. The examination will take place at a Pearson Professional Center, and U.S. candidates can make an appointment through the Internet (http://www.pearsonvue.com/nclex) or by telephone (1-866-496-2539). You can schedule an appointment at any Pearson Professional Center. You do not have to take the examination in the same state in which you are seeking licensure. A confirmation of your appointment with the appointment date and time and the directions to the testing center will be sent to you.

The ATT form contains important information, including your test authorization number, candidate identification number, and validity date. You need to take your ATT form to the test center on the day of your examination. You will not be admitted to the examination if you do not have it.

Canceling or Rescheduling the Appointment

If for any reason you need to cancel or reschedule your appointment to test, you can make the change on the candidate Web site (http://www.pearsonvue.com/nclex) or by calling candidate services. The change needs to be made 1 full business day (24 hours) before your scheduled appointment. If you fail to arrive for the examination or fail to cancel your appointment to test without providing appropriate notice, you will forfeit your examination fee and your ATT will be invalidated. This information will be reported to the board of nursing in the state in which you have applied for licensure, and you will be required to register and pay the testing fees again.

The Day of the Examination

It is important that you arrive at the testing center at least 30 minutes before the test is scheduled. If you arrive late for the scheduled testing appointment, you may be required to forfeit your examination appointment. If it is necessary to forfeit your appointment, you will need to reregister for the examination and pay an additional fee. The board of nursing will be notified that you did not take the test. A few days before your scheduled date of testing, take the time to drive to the testing center to determine its exact location, the length of time required to arrive to that destination, and any potential obstacles that might delay you, such as road construction, traffic, or parking sites. You must have the ATT and proper identification (ID) to be admitted to take the examination. The ATT form will clearly list the types of acceptable identification. Acceptable identification includes U.S. driver's license, passport, U.S. state ID, or U.S. military ID. All acceptable identification must be valid and not expired and contain a photograph and signature (in English). Additionally, the first and last names on the ID must match the ATT. According to the NCSBN guidelines, any name discrepancies require legal documentation, such as a marriage license, divorce decree, or court action legal name change.

Special Testing Circumstances

If you require special testing accommodations, you should contact the board of nursing before submitting a registration form. The board of nursing will provide the procedures for the request. The board of nursing must authorize special testing accommodations. Following board of nursing approval, the NCSBN reviews the requested accommodations and also must approve the request. If the request is approved, the candidate will be notified and provided the procedure for registering for and scheduling the examination.

The Testing Center

The testing center is designed to ensure complete security of the testing process. Strict candidate identification requirements have been established. You must bring the ATT and required forms of identification. You will be asked to read the rules related to testing. A digital fingerprint and palm vein print will be taken, and this procedure is usually done twice. A digital signature and photograph will also be taken at the test center. These identity confirmations will accompany the NCLEX exam results. Additionally, if you leave the testing room for any reason, you may be required to perform these identity confirmation procedures again to be readmitted to the room.

Personal belongings are not allowed in the testing room. Secure storage, such as a locker and locker key, will be provided for you; however, storage space is limited, so you must plan accordingly. In addition, the testing center will not assume responsibility for your personal belongings. All electronic devices, such as cell phones, must be placed in a sealable bag provided by the test administrator and kept in the locker. Any evidence of tampering of the bag could result in an incident and a result cancellation. The testing waiting areas are generally small; therefore, friends or family members who accompany you are not permitted to wait in the testing center while you are taking the examination.

Once you have completed the admission process, the test administrator will escort you to the assigned computer. You will be seated at an individual work space area that includes computer equipment, appropriate lighting, and an erasable note board or white board and a marker. No items, including unauthorized scratch paper, are allowed into the testing room. Eating, drinking, or the use of tobacco is not allowed in the testing room. You will be observed at all times by the test administrator while taking the examination. Additionally, video and audio recordings of all test sessions are made. Pearson Professional Centers have no control over the sounds made by others typing on the computer. If these sounds are distracting, raise your hand to summon the test administrator. Earplugs are available on request.

You must follow the directions given by the testing center staff and must remain seated during the test, except when authorized to leave. If you think that you have a problem with the computer, need an additional erasable or white board, need to take a break, or need the test administrator for any reason, you must raise your hand. You are also encouraged to access the candidate Web site (http://www.pearsonvue.com/nclex) to obtain additional information about the physical environment of the testing center. A virtual tour is available at this site.

Testing Time

The maximum testing time is 6 hours; this period includes the tutorial, the sample items, all breaks, and the examination. All breaks are optional. The first optional break will be offered after 2 hours of testing. The second optional break is offered after 3½ hours of testing. Remember that all breaks count against testing time. If you take a break, you must leave the testing room and, when you return, you may be required to perform identity confirmation procedures to be readmitted.

Length of the Examination

The minimum number of questions that you will need to answer is 75. Of these 75 questions, 60 will be operational (scored) questions and 15 will be pretest (unscored) questions. The maximum number of questions in the test is 265. Fifteen of the total number of questions that you need to answer will be pretest (unscored) questions.

The pretest questions are questions that may be presented as scored questions on future examinations. These pretest questions are not identified as such. In other words, you do not know which questions are the pretest (unscored) questions.

Pass-or-Fail Decisions

All the examination questions are categorized by test plan area and level of difficulty. This is an important point to keep in mind when you consider how the computer makes a pass-or-fail decision because a pass-or-fail decision is not based on a percentage of correctly answered questions.

The NCSBN indicates that a pass-or-fail decision is governed by three different scenarios. The first scenario is the 95% Confidence Interval Rule, in which the computer stops administering test questions when it is 95% certain that the test-taker's ability is clearly above the passing standard or clearly below the passing standard. The second scenario is known as the Maximum-Length Exam, in which the final ability estimate of the test-taker is considered. If the final ability estimate is above the passing standard, the test-taker passes; if it is below the passing standard, the test-taker fails.

The third scenario is the Run-Out-Of-Time rule (R.O.O.T). If the examination ends because the test-taker ran out of time, the computer may not have enough information with 95% certainty to make a clear pass-or-fail decision. If this is the case, the computer will review the test-taker's performance during testing. If the test-taker has not answered the minimum number of required questions, the test-taker fails. If the test-taker's ability estimate was consistently above the passing standard on the last 60 questions, the test-taker passes. If the test-taker's ability estimate falls to or below the passing standard, even once, the test-taker fails. Additional information about pass-or-fail decisions can be found in the 2013 NCLEX examination candidate bulletin located at www.ncsbn.org.

Completing the Examination

Once the examination has ended, you will complete a brief computer-delivered questionnaire about your testing experience. After you complete this questionnaire, you need to raise your hand to summon the test administrator. The test administrator will collect and inventory all erasable or white boards and then permit you to leave.

Processing Results

Every computerized examination is scored twice, once by the computer at the testing center and then again after the examination is transmitted to Pearson Professional Centers. No results are released at the test center; test center staff do not have access to examination results. The board of nursing receives your result and your result will be mailed to you approximately 1 month after you take the examination. In some states, an unofficial result can be obtained via the Quick Results Service 2 business days after taking the examination. This can be done through the Internet or telephone, and there is a fee for this service. Information about obtaining your NCLEX result by this method can be obtained on the NCSBN Web site under candidate services.

Candidate Performance Report

A candidate performance report is provided to a test-taker who failed the examination. This report provides the test-taker with information about her or his strengths and weaknesses in relation to the test plan framework and provides a guide for studying and retaking the examination. If a retake is necessary, the candidate must wait 45 to 90 days between examination administration, depending on state policy. This waiting period provides the test-taker time to remediate. Test-takers should refer to the state board of nursing in the state in which licensure is sought for procedures regarding when the examination can be taken again.

Interstate Endorsement

Because the NCLEX-RN examination is a national examination, you can apply to take the examination in any state. Once licensure is received, you can apply for interstate endorsement, which is obtaining another license in another state to practice nursing in that state. The procedures and requirements for interstate endorsement may vary from state to state, and these procedures can be obtained from the state board of nursing in the state in which endorsement is sought. You may also be allowed to practice nursing in another state if the state has enacted a Nurse Licensure Compact. The state boards of nursing can be accessed via the NCSBN Web site at http://www.ncsbn.org. Additionally those states that participate in the Nurse Licensure Compact can be located on this Web site.

Nurse Licensure Compact

It may be possible to hold one license from the state of residency and practice nursing in another state under the mutual recognition model of nursing licensure if the state has enacted a Nurse Licensure Compact. To obtain information about the Nurse Licensure Compact and the states that are part of this interstate compact, access the National Council of State Boards of Nursing Web site at http://www.ncsbn.org.

Additional Information about the Examination

Additional information regarding the NCLEX-RN examination can be obtained through the NCLEX examination candidate bulletin located on the NCSBN Web site and from the National Council of State Boards of Nursing, 111 East Wacker Drive, Suite 2900, Chicago, IL 60601. The telephone number for the NCLEX examinations department is (866) 293-9600. The Web site is http://www.ncsbn.org.

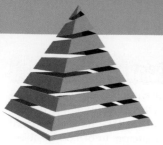

CHAPTER 2

NCLEX-RN® Preparation for Foreign-Educated Nurses: Transitional Issues for Foreign-Educated Nurses

You have taken an important first step—seeking the information that you need to know to become a registered nurse (RN) in the United States (U.S.). The challenge that is presented to you is one that requires great patience and endurance. The positive result of your endeavor will reward you professionally, however, and give you the personal satisfaction of knowing that you have become part of a family of highly skilled professionals, registered nurses.

National Council of State Boards of Nursing

The National Council of State Boards of Nursing (NCSBN) is the agency that develops and administers the NCLEX-RN examination, the examination that you need to pass to become licensed as a registered nurse in the United States. Guidelines and procedures must be followed and documents must be sought and submitted to become eligible to take this examination. This chapter provides general information regarding the process you need to pursue to become a registered nurse in the United States. An important first step in the process of obtaining information about becoming a registered nurse in the United States is to access the NCSBN Web site at http://www.ncsbn.org and obtain information provided for international nurses in the NCLEX Web site link. The NCSBN provides information about some of the documents you need to obtain as an international nurse seeking licensure in the United States and about credentialing agencies. The NCSBN also provides a resource manual for international nurses that contains all of the necessary licensure information regarding the requirements for education, English proficiency, and immigration requirements, such as visas and VisaScreens. You are encouraged to access the NCSBN Web site to obtain the most current information about seeking licensure as a registered nurse in the United States.

⚠ A first step is to access the NCSBN Web site at http://www.ncsbn.org and obtain information provided for international nurses in the NCLEX Web site link. This information can be located at https://www.ncsbn.org/171.htm

State Requirements for Licensure

An important factor to consider as you pursue this process is that some requirements may vary from state to state. You need to contact the board of nursing in the state in which you are planning to obtain licensure to determine the specific requirements and documents that you need to submit. Boards of nursing can decide either to use a credentialing agency to evaluate your documents or to review your documents at the specific state board, known as in-house evaluation. When you contact the board of nursing in the state in which you intend to work as a nurse, inform them that you were educated outside of the United States and ask that they send you an application to apply for licensure by examination. Be sure to specify that you are applying for registered nurse (RN) licensure. You should also ask about the specific documents needed to become eligible to take the NCLEX exam. You can obtain contact information for each state board of nursing through the NCSBN Web site at http://www.ncsbn.org. When you have accessed the NCSBN Web site, select the link titled "Boards of Nursing." Additionally, you can write to the NCSBN regarding the NCLEX exam. The address is 111 East Wacker Drive, Suite 2900, Chicago, IL 60601. The telephone number for the NCSBN is (866) 293-9600; the fax number is (312) 279-1036.

⚠ Contact the board of nursing in the state in which you are planning to obtain licensure to determine the specific requirements and documents that you need to submit. Documents that you need to submit vary state by state.

Credentialing Agencies

The state board of nursing in the state in which you are seeking licensure may choose to use a credentialing agency to review your documents. If so, it is necessary that you use the credentialing agency that the state requires. The state board of nursing will provide you with the name and contact information of the credentialing agency. Seeking this information is important because you need to know where to send your required documents. Additionally, the NCSBN Web site (http://www.ncsbn.org) can provide information about credentialing agencies.

General Licensure Requirements

Required documents may vary depending on the state requirements. These documents must be sent to either the state board of nursing or the credentialing agency specified by the state. Neither the credentialing agency nor the state board of nursing

---

BOX 2-1   Some Documents Needed to Obtain Licensure

1. Proof of citizenship or lawful alien status
2. Work visa
3. VisaScreen certificate
4. Commission on Graduates of Foreign Nursing Schools (CGFNS) certificate
5. Criminal background check documents
6. Official transcripts of educational credentials sent directly to credentialing agency or board of nursing from home country school of nursing
7. Validation of a comparable nursing education as that provided in U.S. nursing programs; this may include theoretical instruction and clinical practice in a variety of nursing areas including but not limited to medical nursing, surgical nursing, pediatric nursing, maternity and newborn nursing, community and public health nursing, and mental health nursing
8. Validation of safe professional nursing practice in home country
9. Copy of nursing license or diploma or both
10. Proof of proficiency in the English language
11. Photograph(s)
12. Social security number
13. Application and fees

BOX 2-2   General Steps in the Licensure Process

1. Access the NCSBN Web site at http://www.ncsbn.org and read the literature provided for international nurses.
2. Contact the board of nursing in the state in which you are planning to obtain licensure to determine the specific requirements and documents that you need to submit.
3. Have the required documents sent from the appropriate agency in your home country.
4. When you are notified about eligibility to take the NCLEX exam, obtain the application form from the state in which you intend to obtain licensure, complete the form, and submit it with required fees.
5. Schedule an appointment to take the NCLEX exam when you receive your Authorization to Test (ATT) form.
6. Take the NCLEX exam.
7. Become a registered nurse in the United States.

---

will accept these documents if they are sent directly from you. These documents must be official documents sent directly from the licensing authority or other agency in your home country to verify validity. Some of the general documents required are listed in Box 2-1; however, remember that the documents you need to submit vary state by state. Use the list provided in Box 2-1 as a checklist for yourself after you have found out about the documents you are required to submit.

When all of your documents have been submitted, they will be reviewed. If you have met the eligibility requirements to take the NCLEX examination, you will be notified that you are eligible. Then you need to obtain an application to take the NCLEX exam from the state in which you intend to seek licensure and submit the required fees. Your application will be reviewed and processed, and you will be notified that you can make an appointment to take the NCLEX exam. Additional information about the application process for the NCLEX exam can be obtained at the NCSBN Web site at www.ncsbn.org. Box 2-2 provides a brief guide of the general steps to take in the licensure process.

⚠ Official documents must be sent directly from the licensing authority or other agency in your home country.

Work Visa

A foreign-educated nurse who wants to work in the United States needs to obtain the proper work visa or visas. Obtaining the work visa is a U.S. federal government requirement. To obtain information about the work visa and the application process, contact the Department of Homeland Security (DHS), Office of U.S. Citizenship and Immigration Services (USCIS). The Web site is http://www.immigrationdirect.com.

VisaScreen

U.S. immigration law requires certain health care professionals to complete a screening program successfully before receiving an occupational (work) visa (Section §343 of the Illegal Immigration Reform and Immigration Responsibility Act of 1996). To become a registered nurse in the United States, you are required to obtain a VisaScreen certificate. You can ask about the VisaScreen certificate when you make your initial contact with the state board of nursing in which you are seeking licensure. The VisaScreen is a federal screening program, and the certificate needs to be obtained through an organization that offers this program.

⚠ Obtaining the work visa and the VisaScreen is a U.S. federal government requirement.

The Commission on Graduates of Foreign Nursing Schools (CGFNS) is an organization that offers federal screening programs. The VisaScreen components of this program include an educational analysis, license verification, assessment of proficiency in the English language, and an examination that tests nursing knowledge. When the applicant successfully achieves each component, the applicant is presented with a VisaScreen certificate. You can obtain information related to the VisaScreen through the CGFNS Web site at http://www.cgfns.org. The CGFNS Web site also provides you with specific information about the components of this program.

The CGFNS is also a credentialing agency and awards a CGFNS certificate to the applicant when all eligibility requirements are met. Some state boards of nursing use the CGFNS as a credentialing agency and require a CGFNS certificate, whereas others do not. Check with the state board of nursing regarding this certificate. The CGFNS certification program contains three parts, and you must complete all parts successfully to be awarded a CGFNS certificate. The three parts include a credentials review, a qualifying examination that tests nursing knowledge, and an English language proficiency examination. These components are similar to those needed to obtain the VisaScreen certificate.

You can obtain information related to the CGFNS certificate through the CGFNS Web site at http://www.cgfns.org.

⚠ The NCLEX examination is administered in English only.

Registering to Take the NCLEX Exam

When you have completed all state and federal requirements and received documentation that you are eligible to take the NCLEX examination, you can register for the exam. You need to obtain information from the state board of nursing in the state in which you are seeking licensure regarding the specific registration process because the process may vary from state to state. The NCLEX candidate Web site is http://www.pearsonvue.com/nclex, and you are encouraged to access this site for additional information. Following the registration instructions and completing the registration forms precisely and accurately are important. You must pay a fee for taking the examination, and you may have to pay additional fees to the board of nursing in the state in which you are applying. When your eligibility is determined by the state licensure board, you will receive an Authorization to Test (ATT) form. You cannot make an appointment to test until the board of nursing declares eligibility and you receive an ATT form.

⚠ Registration forms for taking the NCLEX exam that are not properly completed or not accompanied by the proper fees in the required method of payment will be returned to you and will delay testing.

The examination takes place at a Pearson Professional Center, and you can make an appointment through the Internet or by telephone. You can schedule an appointment at any Pearson Professional Center. You do not have to take the exam in the state in which you are seeking licensure. NCLEX exam testing abroad is also available in some countries, and it is recommended that you visit the NCLEX Web site for current information about international testing sites. Chapter 1 contains additional information regarding the NCLEX exam and testing procedures. You can also obtain information about the registration process and testing procedures from the NCSBN Web site at http://www.ncsbn.org.

Preparing to Take the NCLEX Exam

When you have successfully completed the requirements to become eligible to take the NCLEX exam, you have one more important goal to achieve: to pass the NCLEX exam.

⚠ Begin preparing for the NCLEX exam as soon as possible; start preparing even before you begin the licensure process.

I highly recommend adequate preparation for the NCLEX exam because the examination is difficult. An important step that you have taken in preparing is that you are using this book, *Saunders Q&A Review for the NCLEX-RN®*

Examination; this book provides you with more than 6000 practice questions based on the NCLEX-RN examination test plan framework, with a specific focus on Client Needs and Integrated Processes. The *Saunders Comprehensive Review for the NCLEX-RN® Examination* is also a "MUST HAVE" book for you to use in preparation for the NCLEX examination. This book contains both content review in an outline format and over 5100 practice NCLEX-style questions. Then you will be ready for *HESI/Saunders Online Review for the NCLEX-RN® Examination*. Additional products in Saunders Pyramid to Success include *Saunders Strategies for Test Success: Passing Nursing School and the NCLEX® Exam* and *Saunders Q&A Review Cards for the NCLEX-RN® Exam*. These additional products are described next.

HESI/Saunders Online Review for the NCLEX-RN® Examination addresses all areas of the test plan identified by the NCSBN. The course contains a pretest that provides feedback regarding your strengths and weaknesses and that generates an individualized study schedule in a calendar format. Content review is in an outline format and includes self-check practice questions and case studies, figures and illustrations, a glossary, animations, videos, and testlets (case studies). Numerous practice exams are included. There are more than 2500 practice questions, and the types of questions in this course include multiple choice and alternate item formats.

Saunders Strategies for Test Success: Passing Nursing School and the NCLEX® Exam focuses on the test-taking strategies that will prepare you for the NCLEX-RN exam. The chapters describe all the test-taking strategies and include several sample questions that illustrate how to use the test-taking strategy. This book has over 1000 practice questions. All the practice questions reflect the framework and the content identified in the NCLEX-RN test plan and include multiple choice and alternate item format questions. Also included in this book is information on cultural characteristics and practices, pharmacology strategies, medication and intravenous calculations, laboratory values, positioning guidelines, and therapeutic diets.

Saunders Q&A Review Cards for the NCLEX-RN® Exam is organized by content areas and the test plan framework of the NCLEX-RN test plan. This product provides you with 1200 practice test questions on portable and easy to use cards. The question is on the front of the card and the answer, rationale, and test-taking strategy is on the back of the card. This product includes both multiple choice questions and alternate item format questions including fill-in-the-blank, multiple response, prioritizing (ordered response), figure, and chart/exhibit questions.

All the products in Saunders Pyramid to Success can be obtained online by visiting http://elsevierhealth.com or by calling 800-545-2522.

⚠ Stay positive and confident, and believe that you can achieve your goal.

Finally, never lose sight of your goal. Patience and dedication contribute significantly to your achieving the status of registered nurse. Remember, success is climbing a mountain, facing the challenge of obstacles, and reaching the top of the mountain. I wish you the best success in your journey and beginning your career as a registered nurse in the United States.

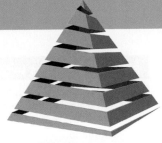
CHAPTER 3

Profiles to Success

Laurent W. Valliere, BS, DD

The Pyramid to Success

Preparing to take the National Council Licensure Examination (NCLEX-RN®) can produce a great deal of anxiety in the nursing graduate. You may be thinking that the NCLEX-RN is the most important examination that you will ever have to take and that it reflects the culmination of everything for which you have worked so hard. The NCLEX-RN is an important examination because achieving that nursing license defines the beginning of your career as a registered nurse. A vital ingredient to your success on the NCLEX is examining your profile to success and avoiding negative thoughts that allow this examination to seem overwhelming and intimidating. Such thoughts will take full control over your destiny (Fig. 3-1).

Your Profile to Success (Box 3-1)

Developing Your Preparation Plan

Nursing graduates preparing for the NCLEX must develop a comprehensive plan to prepare for this examination. The most important component in developing a plan is identifying the study patterns that guided you to your nursing degree. It is important to begin your planning by reflecting on all of the personal and academic challenges you experienced during your nursing education. Take time to focus on the thoughts, feelings, and emotions that you experienced before taking an examination while in your nursing program. Examine the methods that you used in preparing for that examination both academically and from the standpoint of how you dealt with the anxiety that parallels the experience of facing an examination. These factors are very important considerations in preparing for the NCLEX because they identify the patterns that worked for you. Think about this for a moment. Your own methods of study must have worked, or you would not be at the point of preparing for the NCLEX-RN.

Each individual requires his or her own methods of preparing for an examination. Graduate nurses who have taken the NCLEX-RN will probably share their experiences and methods of preparing for this challenge with you. It is very helpful to listen to what they tell you. These graduates can provide you with important strategies that they have used. Listen closely to what they have to say, but remember that this examination is all about you. Your identity and what you require in terms of preparation are most important.

Reflect on the methods and strategies that worked for you throughout your nursing program. Do not think that you need to develop new methods and strategies to prepare for

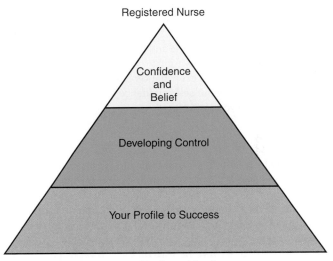

Registered Nurse

Confidence and Belief

Developing Control

Your Profile to Success

FIGURE 3-1 The Pyramid to Success.

the NCLEX. Use what has worked for you. Take some time to reflect on these strategies, write them down on a large blank card, sign your name, and write RN after your name. Post this card in a place where you will see it every morning. Commit to your own special strategies. These strategies reflect your profile and identity, and will lead you to a successful outcome—Registered Nurse!

A frequent concern of graduates preparing for the NCLEX relates to deciding whether they should study alone or become a part of a study group. Examining your profile will easily direct you in making this decision. Again, reflect on what has worked for you throughout your nursing program as you prepared for examinations. Remember, your needs are most important. Address your own needs and do not become pressured by peers who are encouraging you to join a study group if this is not your normal pattern for study. Additional pressure is not what you need at this important time of your life.

You may ask, "What is the best method of preparing?" First, remember that you are prepared. In fact, you began preparing for this examination on the first day that you entered your nursing program. The task you are faced with is to review, in a comprehensive manner, all of the nursing content that you learned in your nursing program. It can become totally overwhelming to look at your bookshelf, which is overflowing with the nursing books you used during nursing school, and your challenge becomes monumental when you look at the boxes of nursing lecture notes that you have accumulated. It is unrealistic to even think that you could read all of those nursing books and lecture notes in preparation for the NCLEX.

BOX 3-1   Profiles to Success

- Avoid negative thoughts that allow the examination to seem overwhelming and intimidating.
- Develop a comprehensive plan to prepare for the examination.
- Examine the study methods and strategies that you used in preparing for examinations during nursing school.
- Develop realistic time goals.
- Select a study time period and study place that will be most conducive to your success.
- Commit to your own special study methods and strategies.
- Incorporate a balance of exercise with adequate rest and relaxation time in your preparation schedule.
- Maintain healthy eating habits.
- Learn to control anxiety.
- Remember that discipline and perseverance will automatically bring control.
- Remember that this examination is all about you.
- Remember that your self-confidence and the belief in yourself will lead you to success!

These books and lecture notes should be used as reference sources, if needed, during your preparation for the NCLEX.

Saunders Comprehensive Review for the NCLEX-RN® Examination has identified for you all of the important nursing content areas relevant to the examination. During the comprehensive review, you should have noted the areas that are unfamiliar or unclear to you. Be sure that you have taken the time to become familiar with these areas. Now, you are progressing through the Pyramid to Success and testing your knowledge in this book, *Saunders Q&A Review for the NCLEX-RN® Examination*. Answer all of the practice questions provided in this book and on the Evolve site: practice question, after question, after question! You may identify nursing content areas that require further review. Take the time to review these nursing content areas, as you are guided to do in this book.

Identifying Your Goals for Success

Your profile to success requires that you develop realistic time goals to prepare for the NCLEX. It is necessary to take the time to examine your life and all of the commitments you may have. These commitments may include family, work, and friends. As you develop your goals, remember to plan time for fun and exercise. To achieve success, you require a balance of time for both work and enjoyment. If you do not plan for some leisure time, you will become frustrated and perhaps even angry. These sorts of feelings will block your ability to focus and concentrate. Remember that you need time for yourself.

Goal development may be a relatively easy process because you have probably been juggling your life commitments ever since you entered nursing school. Remember that your goal is to identify a daily time frame and time period for you to use in reviewing and preparing for the NCLEX. Open your calendar and identify days on which life commitments will not allow you to spend this time preparing. Block those days off and do not consider them as a part of your review time. Identify the time that is best for you in terms of your ability to concentrate and focus, so that you can accomplish the most in your identified time frame. Be sure you consider a time that is quiet and free of distractions. Many individuals find the morning hours most productive, whereas others may find the afternoon and evening hours most productive. Remember that this examination is all about you, so select the time period that will be most conducive to your success.

Selecting Your Study Place

The place of study is very important. Select a place that is quiet and comfortable for study—where you normally do your studying and preparing. If studying at home in your own environment is your normal pattern, be sure to free yourself of distractions during your scheduled preparation time. If you are not able to free yourself of distractions, you may consider spending your preparation time in a library. When selecting your place of study, reflect on what worked best for you during your nursing program.

Deciding on Your Amount of Daily Study Time

Selecting the amount of daily preparation time can be a dilemma for many graduates preparing for the NCLEX. It is very important to set a realistic time period that can be adhered to on a daily basis. Set a time frame that will provide you with quality time and a time frame that can be achieved. If you set a time frame that is not realistic and cannot be achieved every day, you will become frustrated. This frustration will block your journey toward the peak of the Pyramid to Success.

The best suggestion is to spend at least 2 hours daily for NCLEX preparation. Two hours is a realistic time period, both in terms of spending quality time and adhering to a time frame. You may find that after 2 hours your ability to focus and concentrate is diminished. You may, however, find that on some days you are able to spend more than the scheduled 2 hours. If you can and feel as though your ability to concentrate and focus is still present, then do so.

Developing Control

Discipline and perseverance will automatically bring control. Control will provide you with the momentum that will sweep you to the peak in the Pyramid to Success.

Discipline yourself to spend time preparing for the NCLEX every day. Daily preparation is very important because it maintains a consistent pattern and keeps you in synchrony with the mind flow needed on the day you are scheduled to take the NCLEX examination. Some days you may think about skipping your scheduled preparation time because you are not in the mood for study or because you just do not feel like studying. On these days, practice discipline and persevere. Stand yourself up, shake off those thoughts of skipping a day of preparation, take a deep breath, and get the oxygen flowing throughout your body. Look in the mirror, smile, and say to yourself, "This time is for me and I can do this!" Look at your card that displays your name with "RN" after it, and get yourself to that special study place. Remember that discipline and perseverance will bring control!

Dealing with Anxiety

In the profile to success, academic preparation directs the path to the peak of the Pyramid to Success. There are, however, additional factors that will influence successful achievement to the peak. These factors include your ability to control anxiety, physical stamina, the amount of rest and relaxation you get, your self-confidence, and the belief in yourself that you will achieve success on the NCLEX. You need to take time to think about these important factors and incorporate these factors into your daily preparation schedule.

Anxiety is a common concern among students preparing to take the NCLEX. Feeling some anxiety is normal and will keep your senses sharp and alert. A great deal of anxiety, however, can block your process of thinking and hamper your ability to focus and concentrate. You have already practiced the task of controlling anxiety when you took examinations in nursing school. Now you need to continue with this practice and incorporate this control on a daily basis. Each day, before beginning your scheduled preparation time, sit in your quiet special study place, close your eyes, and take a slow deep breath. Fill your body with oxygen, hold your breath to a count of four, and then exhale slowly through your mouth. Continue with this exercise and repeat it four to six times. This exercise helps relieve your mind of any unnecessary chatter and delivers oxygen to all of your body tissues and your brain. On your scheduled day for taking the NCLEX, after the necessary pretesting procedures, you will be escorted to your test computer. Practice this breathing exercise before beginning the examination. Use this exercise during the examination if you feel yourself becoming anxious and distracted and if you are having difficulty focusing or concentrating. Remember that breathing will move that oxygen to your brain!

Ensuring Physical Readiness

Physical stamina is a necessary component of readiness for the NCLEX. Plan to incorporate a balance of exercise with adequate rest and relaxation time in your preparation schedule. It is also important that you maintain healthy eating habits. Begin to practice these healthy habits now, if you have not already done so. There are a few points to keep in mind each day as you plan your daily meals. Three balanced meals are important, with snacks, such as fruits, included between meals. Remember that food items that contain fat will slow you down, and food items that contain caffeine could cause increased nervousness. These items need to be avoided. Healthy foods that are high in complex carbohydrates work best to supply your energy needs. Remember that your brain works like a muscle. It requires those carbohydrates (Box 3-2).

If you are the type of individual who is not a breakfast eater, work on changing that habit. Practice the habit of eating breakfast now as you are preparing for the NCLEX. Attempt to provide your brain with energy in the morning with some form of complex carbohydrate food. It will make a difference. On your scheduled day for the NCLEX, feed your brain and eat a healthy breakfast. In addition, on this very important day, bring some form of healthy snack and feed your brain

again so that you will have the energy to concentrate, focus, and complete your examination.

Adequate rest, relaxation, and exercise are important in your preparation process. Many graduates preparing for the NCLEX have difficulty sleeping, particularly the night before the examination. Begin now to develop methods that will assist in relaxing your body and mind and allow you to obtain a restful sleep. You may have already developed a particular method to help you sleep. If not, it may be helpful to try the breathing exercise while you lie in bed to assist in eliminating any "mind chatter" that is present. It is also helpful to visualize your favorite and most peaceful place while you do these breathing exercises. Graduates have also stated that listening to quiet music and relaxation tapes has assisted in helping them relax and sleep. Begin to practice some of these helpful methods now while you are preparing for the NCLEX. Identify those that work best for you. The night before your scheduled examination is an important one. Spend time having some fun, get to bed early, and incorporate the relaxation method that you have been using to help you sleep.

Confidence and Belief in Yourself

Confidence and belief that you have the ability to achieve success will bring your goals to fruition. Reflect on your profile maintained during your nursing education. Your confidence and belief in yourself, along with your academic achievements, have brought you to the status of graduate nurse. Now you are facing one more important challenge (Box 3-3).

Can you meet this challenge successfully? Yes, you can! There is no reason to think otherwise, if you have taken all of the necessary steps to ensure that profile to success. Each morning, place your feet on the floor, stand tall, take a deep breath, and smile. Take both hands and imagine yourself brushing off any negative feelings. Look at your card that bears your name with the letters "RN" after it, and tell yourself, **"Yes, I can!!!!"**

Believe in yourself, and you will reach the peak of the Pyramid to Success!

Congratulations, and I wish you continued success in your career as a registered nurse!

BOX 3-2 Healthy Eating Habits

Eat three balanced meals each day.
Include snacks, such as fruits and vegetables, between meals.
Avoid food items that contain fat.
Avoid food items that contain caffeine.
Consume healthy foods that are high in complex carbohydrates.

BOX 3-3 Meeting the Challenge

Believe
In your success every day.

Plan
The study strategies that work for you.

Control
Always maintain command of your emotions, and breathe.

Practice
Review, review, review: Practice questions, practice questions, and more practice questions!

Succeed
Believe, plan, control, and practice: "Yes, I can!"

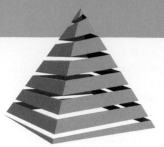

CHAPTER 4

The NCLEX-RN® Examination: A Graduate's Perspective

Miranda Cox, RN, BSN

The NCLEX-RN examination can be very intimidating to most new graduates. It most definitely was to me! By far, it is one of the hardest, most important, and life-changing exams that I have had to take in my lifetime. The exam required me to compile and piece together everything that I had learned from day one of nursing school until graduation. Although this was a scary concept, I knew that all of my hard work, determination, and sacrifice up until this point would pay off once I passed the NCLEX-RN. Studying seemed like such a tedious task at this point, but I knew it was so important! Some of my former classmates chose to take some time off to go on vacation and do things that they could not do while in nursing school. I was tempted to do the same thing, but instead I chose to get right back to it, and I continued to study for my test. I knew that the NCLEX-RN examination was the only thing that stood between me and my lifelong dream of becoming a registered nurse.

Preparing Myself for the NCLEX-RN Examination

The NCLEX-RN examination was different from any other exam that I had taken in nursing school. In contrast to some, I found that some of the things that had worked for me as a study routine during school did not work out well for me as I studied for the NCLEX-RN examination. If this happens to you, try to keep in mind that it's okay if you have to change things up a bit. I tried different strategies based on how I learn best. For example, I learn best when I do things hands on. If I am unsure of something, I will remember and retain it better if I am the one who looks it up and finds the answer versus someone telling me. You have to find what works for you. If you learn best by bouncing ideas off of someone or having questions answered by a person rather than doing the research yourself, find a reliable resource like a professor or a family member to help you. I like to compare studying for the NCLEX-RN to going on a trip. If I'm unsure of where I'm going or how to get there, I ask for directions to my destination or use a GPS to find my way. The same concept proved true for me when planning a study routine for the NCLEX-RN. In order to reach my goal of passing, I needed to develop a study plan to get me there.

Planning a Study Routine That Works

I planned my study routine in two phases. Phase one for me consisted of organization and self-assessment. Phase two consisted of planning, preparation, and practice.

Phase One

In phase one, I set up a series of action steps that had certain dates and a timeline attached to them. I developed a binder organizational system that I used to collect and secure all NCLEX-RN–related materials and information. Next, I established a dedicated exam study space or location that was quiet and free from distraction. I then conducted a thorough self-assessment to identify my areas of strengths and weaknesses. I reflected on past nursing courses, and I figured out the subject matter I understood and which subjects I did not understand as well. I also used my past exams to remediate any deficiencies they revealed. Doing this helped me target some of my recurring areas of weakness. After doing all of this, I printed out the NCLEX-RN detailed test plan that can be located at the National Council of State Boards of Nursing (NCSBN) Web site at www.ncsbn.org. I found that using this test plan helped me keep my studying focused. Finally, I identified and obtained NCLEX-RN exam resources, such as the *Saunders Comprehensive Review for the NCLEX-RN® Exam*; the *Saunders Q&A Review for NCLEX-RN® Exam*; the *HESI/Saunders Online Review for the NCLEX-RN® Exam*, resources available at www.YourBestGrade.com/hesi/ and the *Saunders Q&A Review NCLEX* app for my phone, which helped facilitate on-the-go studying. Once phase one preparation was complete, it was time to move on to phase two.

Phase Two

This phase consisted of planning, preparation, and practice. During this time I used *HESI/Saunders Online Review for the NCLEX-RN Exam* review course. I completed the pretest at the beginning to see what I really knew and to see the areas I needed to review. I then read the NCLEX-RN Detailed Test Plan. From there I began to prioritize and list subject matter of specific content areas of weakness, starting with my weakest areas first. Next, I planned out a study schedule to review and study my subject matter of specific areas of weakness. Part of the preparation to take the NCLEX-RN exam, aside from just studying, was to maintain a healthy lifestyle that included healthy eating, exercise, adequate rest, stress management, and my favorite part—relaxation and fun! A healthy balance among these things ensured my success, as it will yours.

Answering Question After Question

The number of questions on the NCLEX-RN examination ranges from 75 to 265 questions. In order for me to successfully complete and pass this exam, I had to build up my testing endurance by practicing an incrementally higher number of NCLEX-type questions every day. I committed myself to 2 hours of uninterrupted study time each day. I used the previously mentioned resources for access to questions to help facilitate my study time. Once the 2 hours were over, I would jot down my incorrect answers and look up and review the content area connected to those questions.

It's also really important to read and study the rationale and test-taking strategy for each question that you answer. Even if you chose the correct response, still go back and read why your choice was the correct answer. I found that by doing this, I learned and reinforced my understanding of content, and the questions became easier and easier to answer. Although all questions are not the same, some address the same general topic. If you have read the rationales to previously answered questions, it may help you work through the question you're currently on, even if you are unsure of the correct answer. My goal was to have answered 3500 questions before my NCLEX-RN exam. My recommendation would be to study subject matter you are weak in **first** and practice answering questions in a content-specific way. I focused on one area at a time. My school offered a 3-day intensive review course for the NCLEX-RN, which also provided me with valuable information on how to answer NCLEX questions.

The NCLEX-RN Application Process

The NCLEX-RN application process was stressful for me to even think about. It all sounded so overwhelming, and I was tempted to wait and start the process after I had taken a short break. I am so glad that I didn't! My school's Center for Academic Success (CAS) manager gave me the best advice. She told me to keep studying and take the NCLEX-RN while the content was fresh in my mind.

Applying for NCLEX-RN is a step-by-step process. You have to be finger-printed and have a background check done. I chose to do this first. I then applied for licensure with my state's board of nursing. Each state's fees and requirements are different. Make sure that you use your state's board of nursing Web site to check on the appropriate fees and documentation needed. I also registered and paid the applicable fees through Pearson Vue online. The turn-around time between registering to take NCLEX-RN and the Board of Nursing making me eligible in the Pearson Vue system was fairly quick. I chose to receive my Authorization to Test (ATT) via email. When you receive your ATT, they provide you with a range of validity dates during which you can take the test. Mine was valid for 90 days. The night Pearson Vue emailed my ATT letter, I scheduled my exam appointment. My exam date was 9 days away. After I hit submit, I started thinking to myself that it was too soon and

that I should probably reschedule. Instead of rescheduling, I kept that date and kept reassuring myself that I had been studying diligently and that I knew the content. I even took several blank pieces of paper and in permanent marker I wrote, "I will be successful!" I made several and posted them throughout my house. This helped to build my self-confidence.

The Final Steps

Before my testing date, I sat down and began to gather everything that I would need for exam day. When scheduling to take the NCLEX-RN, I made my exam time in the morning. I'm not necessarily a morning person, but I feel more refreshed after a good night's sleep, so I felt that would be better for me. I picked a testing center close to my house and decided to do a test drive the day before my exam. It is recommended to take a test drive to the testing center a day to a week before your test date at the same time your exam will be. Pearson Vue allows you to come in and look around to get a feel for the exam environment and orient yourself to the testing center. I chose not to do this because I felt that it would further increase my testing anxiety. Everyone is different so if you think going inside the testing center will put your mind at ease, I encourage you to do so.

I reserved the night before the exam for rest and relaxation! I went to a nice, relaxing dinner with my family, rented a movie to watch at home, popped some popcorn, and relaxed! I tried to avoid any last minute cramming. If you do this, it can increase your stress level by causing you to second guess things you already know. I also got all necessary documentation and identification (ID) together in a plastic bag. In addition to your ATT letter, acceptable identification such as a valid driver's license is also needed as a form of ID. You must have everything that they require you to bring at the time of your appointment; if not, they will require you to reschedule and pay the testing fees again. I also took the online NCLEX-RN examination tutorial beforehand. You can locate this tutorial on the NCSBN and Pearson Vue Web sites. You will still have to take the tutorial the day of your exam, but the NCLEX-RN is a timed exam. If you do the tutorial and familiarize yourself beforehand, you aren't wasting your time the day of the exam.

I went to bed early and made sure to get a good night's rest so that I would feel refreshed. The morning of the exam, I made sure to eat a light and nutritious breakfast. I dressed comfortably and left with my husband to make the drive. During the entire ride he was boosting my confidence by telling me how smart I am. The last thing he said to me, as he was grinning from ear to ear was, "You got this, girl!" His sense of humor and support eased some of my worries.

I arrived at the testing center 30 minutes early so I could start the paperwork and orient myself to my surroundings. When you arrive, they provide you with registration paperwork and a locker for your things. They also require you to turn your cell phone completely off and place it in a sealed, tamper-proof bag that they check at the end of your exam. If the bag has been opened or tampered with, you automatically fail the exam. They don't even allow you to chew gum! I sat in the waiting room and when they called my name, I started sweating bullets! I thought to myself, "This is it, the moment of truth!" Before you enter the testing room they check your ID and scan your palm. You are allowed breaks during the exam, but your testing time keeps running, so keep track of your time if you take a break. You can't bring anything into the exam room. They provide you with everything you need, including a marker and dry erase board on which to do medication calculations. You are in your own cubicle and when you enter the exam room, the proctor sits you down, logs you in, and instructs you to raise your hand if you need anything and to stay seated until they come to you. Then, they start your exam.

During the NCLEX-RN Examination

At the start of the exam, you receive the tutorial. Because I had previously reviewed it at home, I was able to breeze right through it. When the tutorial ended and the exam started, I stopped, closed my eyes, and took deep breaths in and out. I tried to clear my mind of anything that would cause me to become distracted. After that I was ready to begin. Question after question began to pop up on the screen, and anytime I started feeling myself lose focus, I would close my eyes and take some deep breaths again. I was anxious as I approached the 75-question mark. I had spoken with numerous people who had reached question number 75, the exam shut off, and they received a passing score. Question number 75 came and went for me. I could feel the anxiety building, so I raised my hand to take a break. I walked out of the room and attempted to clear my head and did some deep breathing to refocus myself. After a short break I was ready to begin again. I re-entered the testing room, the proctor logged me back in, and I began to answer questions. The computer shut off after

110 questions. I sat there for a minute to gather my thoughts and then left the room. The testing center attendant gave me instructions for obtaining my results, which unfortunately would not be available for a few days. I could have obtained them sooner, but I would have had to pay an additional fee. I was a nervous wreck! I felt somewhat indifferent because all of my former classmates that I had spoken with told me that their exams shut off at 75 questions and my exam went up to 110 questions. I continued to check Pearson Vue and the National Council of State Boards of Nursing's (NCSBN) Web sites for my exam results. True to their word, a few days later I saw the word, "PASS" on Pearson Vue's Web site! I was so excited that it took my breath away. Even with all of the odds and obstacles stacked against me during the past several years, I had done it! I was finally able to complete my journey and become a registered nurse.

Passing the NCLEX-RN Examination

The feelings that I had after I passed the NCLEX-RN were fulfillment, excitement, and accomplishment all mixed up into one. Once you pass, and of course you *WILL* pass, I'm sure you will feel the same. This is the part of your story when all of your sacrifice, hard work, and determination pay off. I hope that some of my experiences and suggestions will help guide you as you prepare for this exam. They worked wonders for me and can help keep you on the right track to success! Congratulations for all that you have and will accomplish. Good luck as you practice and find your way in your exciting, new career!

CHAPTER 5

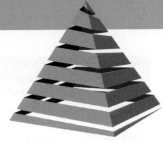

Test-Taking Strategies

If you would like to read more about test-taking strategies after completing this chapter, *Saunders Strategies for Test Success: Passing Nursing School and the NCLEX® Exam* focuses on the test-taking strategies that will help you pass your nursing examinations while in nursing school and will prepare you for the NCLEX-RN examination.

I. Key Test-Taking Strategies (Box 5-1)

II. How to Avoid Reading into the Question (Box 5-2)

A. Pyramid Points

1. Avoid asking yourself the forbidden words, "Well, what if …?" because this will lead you right into the "forbidden" area of reading into the question.
2. Focus only on the information in the question, read every word, and make a decision about what the question is asking.
3. Look for the strategic words in the question, such as *immediate, initial, first, priority*. Strategic words clarify what the question is asking.
4. Focus on the subject of the question, such as *a nursing action, assessment findings, complications, side effects, adverse effects,* or *toxic effects of a medication*.
5. In multiple choice questions, multiple response questions, or questions that require you to arrange nursing interventions or other data in order of priority, read every choice or option presented before answering.
6. Always use the process of elimination when choices or options are presented; after you have eliminated

options, reread the question before selecting your final choice or choices.

7. With questions that require you to fill in the blank, focus on the information in the question and determine what the question is asking; if the question requires you to calculate a medication dose, an intravenous flow rate, or intake and output amounts, recheck your work in calculating and always use the on-screen calculator to verify the answer.

B. Ingredients of a question (Box 5-3)

1. The *ingredients of a question* include the event; the event query; and the options or answers.
2. The *event* provides you with the content about the client or clinical situation that you need to think about when answering the question.

BOX 5-1 Key Test-Taking Strategies

- Avoid asking yourself, "Well, what if …?" because this will lead you right into reading into the question.
- Focus only on the information in the question, read every word, and make a decision regarding what the question is asking.
- Look for the strategic words in the question; strategic words clarify what the question is asking.
- Determine whether the question is a positive or negative event query.
- Always use the process of elimination when choices or options are presented; when you have eliminated options, reread the question before selecting your final choice or choices.
- Use all your nursing knowledge, your clinical experiences, and your test-taking skills and strategies to answer the question.

BOX 5-2 Practice Question: Avoiding the "What if …" Syndrome and Reading into the Question

The nurse is changing the tapes on a tracheostomy tube. The client coughs and the tube is dislodged. What is the **initial** nursing action?

1. Call the health care provider to reinsert the tube.
2. Ventilate the client using a manual resuscitation bag and face mask.
3. Cover the tracheostomy site with a sterile dressing to prevent infection.
4. Call the respiratory therapy department to reinsert the tracheostomy tube.

Answer: 2

Test-Taking Strategy: Now you may immediately think, "The tube is dislodged and I need the health care provider!" Read the question carefully and note the strategic word *initial*. Focus on the subject, the tube is dislodged. The question is asking you for a nursing action so that is what you need to look for as you eliminate the incorrect options. Eliminate options 1 and 4 because they are comparable or alike and delay the *initial* intervention needed. Eliminate option 3 because this action will block the airway. If the tube is dislodged, the *initial* nursing action is to ventilate the client using a manual resuscitation bag and face mask. Additionally, use of the ABCs—airway, breathing, and circulation—will direct you to the correct option. Remember: Avoid the "What if…?" syndrome and reading into the question! Review: care of the client with a **tracheostomy tube**.

BOX 5-3   Ingredients of a Question: Event, Event Query, and Options

Event: The clinic nurse instructs an adolescent with iron deficiency anemia about the administration of oral iron preparations.

Event Query: The nurse should tell the adolescent that it is **best** to take the iron with which item?

Options:
1. Cola
2. Soda
3. Water
4. Tomato juice

Answer: 4

Test-Taking Strategy: Note the strategic word, *best*. Remember that vitamin C enhances the absorption of the iron preparation. Tomato juice has a high ascorbic acid (vitamin C) content, whereas cola, soda, and water do not contain vitamin C. Note that options 1 and 2 are comparable or alike, so eliminate these options. Next, recalling that vitamin C increases the absorption of iron will direct you to option 4, tomato juice. As you read a question, remember to note its ingredients: the event, event query, and options! Review: procedures for administering **oral iron preparations.**

---

3. The *event query* asks something specific about the content of the event.
4. The *options* are all the answers provided with the question.
5. In a multiple choice question, there are four options and you must select one; read every option carefully and think about the event and the event query as you use the process of elimination.
6. In a multiple response question, there are several correct options and you must select all options that apply to the event in the question; visualize the event and use your nursing knowledge and clinical experiences to answer the question.
7. In a prioritizing (ordered response)/drag-and-drop question, you are required to arrange in order of priority nursing interventions or other data; visualize the event and use your nursing knowledge and clinical experiences to answer the question.
8. A fill-in-the-blank question will not contain options, and some figure/illustration questions and audio or video item formats may or may not contain options. A graphic option item will contain options in the form of a picture or graphic.
9. A chart/exhibit question will most likely contain options; read the question carefully and all of the information in the chart or exhibit before selecting an answer.
10. Testlet (case study) questions are accompanied by several questions that relate to the information in the question; these questions can be in a multiple choice format or an alternate item format.

III. Strategic Words (Boxes 5-4 and 5-5)

A. *Strategic words* focus your attention on a critical point to consider when answering the question and will assist you in eliminating the incorrect options.

BOX 5-4   Common Strategic Words and Assessment Words

Words That Indicate the Need to Prioritize
Best
Early or late
Essential
First
Highest priority
Immediate
Initial
Next
Most
Most appropriate or least appropriate
Most important
Most likely or least likely
Priority
Primary
Vital

Words That Reflect Assessment
Ascertain
Assess
Check
Collect
Determine
Find out
Gather
Identify
Monitor
Observe
Obtain information
Recognize

BOX 5-5   Practice Question: Strategic Words

The home care nurse visits a client with chronic obstructive pulmonary disease (COPD) who is on home oxygen at 2 L per minute. The client's respiratory rate is 22 breaths per minute, and the client is complaining of increased dyspnea. The nurse should take which **initial** action?
1. Determine the need to increase the oxygen.
2. Call emergency services to come to the home.
3. Reassure the client that there is no need to worry.
4. Collect more information about the client's respiratory status.

Answer: 4

Test-Taking Strategy: Note the strategic word, *initial*. Completing the assessment and collecting additional information regarding the client's respiratory status is the *initial* nursing action. The oxygen is not increased without validation of the need for further oxygen and the approval of the health care provider, especially because clients with COPD can retain carbon dioxide. Calling emergency services is a premature action. Reassuring the client is appropriate, but it is inappropriate to tell the client not to worry. Use the steps of the nursing process to answer correctly and remember that assessment is the first step. Also, use the ABCs—airway, breathing, and circulation—to direct you to option 4. Remember to look for strategic words! Review: care of the client with **chronic obstructive pulmonary disease.**

B. Some strategic words may indicate that all options are correct and that it will be necessary to prioritize to select the correct option; words that reflect the process of assessment are also important to note (see Box 5-4).

C. As you read the question, look for the strategic words, which clarify the focus of the question. Throughout this book, *strategic words* presented in the question, such as those that indicate the need to prioritize, are **bolded**. If the test-taking strategy is to focus on *strategic words*, then *strategic words* is highlighted in blue where it appears in the test-taking strategy.

IV. Subject of the Question (Box 5-6)

A. The *subject of the question* is the specific topic that the question is asking about.

B. Identifying the subject of the question will assist in eliminating the incorrect options and direct you in selecting the correct option. Throughout this book, if the *subject* of the question is a specific strategy to use in answering the question correctly, it is highlighted in blue in the test-taking strategy. Also, the specific content area to review, such as *heart failure,* is highlighted in **magenta** where it appears in the test-taking strategy.

C. The highlighting of the strategy and specific content areas provides you with guidance on what topics to review for further remediation in *Saunders Strategies for Test Success: Passing Nursing School and the NCLEX® Exam* and *Saunders Comprehensive Review for the NCLEX-RN® Examination.*

V. Positive and Negative Event Queries (Boxes 5-7 and 5-8)

A. A *positive event query* uses strategic words that ask you to select an option that is correct; for example, the event query may read, "Which statement by a client *indicates an understanding* of the side effects of the prescribed medication?"

B. A *negative event query* uses strategic words that ask you to select an option that is an incorrect item or statement; for example, the event query may read, "Which statement by a client *indicates a need for further teaching* about the side effects of the prescribed medication?"

VI. Questions That Require Prioritizing

A. Many questions in the examination will require you to use the skill of prioritizing nursing actions.

B. Look for the strategic words in the question that indicate the need to prioritize (see Box 5-4).

C. Remember that when a question requires prioritization, all options may be correct and you need to determine the correct order of action.

BOX 5-6 Practice Question: Subject of the Question

The nurse should implement which measures to prevent infection in a hospitalized immunocompromised client? **Select all that apply.**
- ☐ 1. Use strict aseptic technique for all invasive procedures.
- ☐ 2. Insert a Foley catheter to eliminate the need to use a bedpan.
- ☐ 3. Use good hand-washing technique before touching the client.
- ☐ 4. Keep fresh flowers and potted plants out of the client's room.
- ☐ 5. Place the client in a semiprivate room with another client who is immunocompromised.
- ☐ 6. Keep frequently used equipment such as a blood pressure cuff in the client's room for use by the client.

Answer: 1, 3, 4, 6
Test-Taking Strategy: Focus on the subject, measures to prevent infection. An immunocompromised client is at high risk for infection, and specific measures are taken to prevent infection. Strict aseptic technique is necessary for all invasive procedures; however, invasive procedures are avoided as much as possible. Foley catheters are avoided because of the risk of infection associated with their use. Good hand-washing technique is used before touching the client. Fresh fruits, fresh flowers, and potted plants are kept out of the client's room because they harbor organisms, placing the client at risk for infection. The client is placed in a private room. Frequently used equipment such as a blood pressure cuff, stethoscope, or thermometer is kept in the client's room for use by the client only. The client is also monitored daily for any signs of infection. Remember to focus on the subject of the question! Review: care of the **immunocompromised client.**

BOX 5-7 Practice Question: Positive Event Query

The nurse is teaching a postpartum woman how to bathe her newborn. The nurse should provide which instructions to the mother? **Select all that apply.**
- ☐ 1. Support the newborn's body during the bath.
- ☐ 2. Clean any eye discharge using a wet cotton ball.
- ☐ 3. Fill the bathtub with no more than 10 inches of water.
- ☐ 4. Clean the eyes, moving from the outer canthus to the inner canthus.
- ☐ 5. Cover the newborn's body except for the part being washed or rinsed.
- ☐ 6. Begin the bath with the face, and clean the newborn's diaper area next.

Answer: 1, 2, 5
Test-Taking Strategy: Focus on the subject, instructions for bathing the newborn. Note that the question identifies a positive event query, and you need to select the correct instructions for bathing a newborn. Visualize each option carefully, keeping the principles of safety and infection control in mind. During bathing, the newborn's body is supported at all times by placing a hand under the newborn's head and neck. If the newborn is bathed in a bathtub, the tub should be lined with a towel to provide comfort and traction to prevent slipping, and it is filled with no more than 3 inches of water. The newborn's body is covered except for the part being washed or rinsed. Any eye discharge is cleaned using a wet cotton ball moving from the inner canthus to the outer canthus. The bath is started with the face, then other body areas are washed, and the diaper area is cleaned last. Remember to read the event query and note if it is a positive event type. Review: procedure for **bathing a newborn.**

BOX 5-8   Practice Question: Negative Event Query

The nurse provides home care instructions to a client who is taking lithium carbonate (Lithobid). Which statement by the client indicates a **need for further instructions?**
1. "I need to take the lithium with meals."
2. "My blood levels must be monitored very closely."
3. "I need to decrease my salt and fluid intake while taking the lithium."
4. "I need to withhold the medication if I have excessive diarrhea, vomiting, or sweating."

Answer: 3

Test-Taking Strategy: This question identifies an example of a negative event query question. Note the strategic words, *need for further instructions*. These strategic words indicate that you need to select an option that identifies an incorrect client statement. Lithium is irritating to the gastric mucosa; therefore, lithium should be taken with meals. Because therapeutic and toxic dosage ranges are so close, lithium blood levels must be monitored very closely, more frequently at first, then once every several months after that. The client should be instructed to withhold the medication if excessive diarrhea, vomiting, or diaphoresis occurs, and to inform the health care provider if any of these problems occur. A normal diet and normal salt and fluid intake (1500 to 3000 mL per day) should be maintained because lithium decreases sodium reabsorption by the renal tubules, which could cause sodium depletion. A low-sodium intake causes a relative increase in lithium retention and could lead to toxicity. Watch for negative event queries! Remember that negative event queries ask you to select an option that is an *incorrect* item or statement! Review: **lithium carbonate.**

D. Strategies to use to prioritize include the ABCs (airway, breathing, and circulation), Maslow's Hierarchy of Needs theory, and the steps of the nursing process.
E. The ABCs (Box 5-9)
 1. Use the ABCs—airway, breathing, and circulation—when selecting an answer or determining the order of priority.
 2. Remember the order of priority—airway, breathing, and circulation.
 3. Airway is always the first priority. Note that an exception is the performance of cardiopulmonary resuscitation; in this situation the nurse follows the CAB (circulation, airway, breathing) guidelines.
F. Maslow's Hierarchy of Needs theory (Box 5-10; Fig. 5-1)
 1. According to Maslow's Hierarchy of Needs theory, physiological needs are the priority, followed by safety and security needs, love and belonging needs, self-esteem needs, and, finally, self-actualization needs; select the option or determine the order of priority by addressing physiological needs first.
 2. When a physiological need is not addressed in the question or noted in one of the options, continue to use Maslow's Hierarchy of Needs theory as a guide and look for the option that addresses safety.
G. Steps of the nursing process
 1. Use the steps of the nursing process to prioritize.
 2. The steps include assessment, analysis, planning, implementation, and evaluation and are followed in this order.

---

3. Assessment
 a. Assessment questions address the process of gathering subjective and objective data relative to the client, confirming the data, and communicating and documenting the data.

BOX 5-9   Practice Question: Use of the ABCs

A client is admitted to the emergency department with complaints of severe chest pain. The client is extremely restless, frightened, and dyspneic. Immediate admission prescriptions include oxygen by nasal cannula at 4 L per minute, troponin, creatinine phosphokinase and isoenzymes blood levels, a chest x-ray, and a 12-lead electrocardiogram (ECG). Which action should the nurse take **first?**
1. Obtain the 12-lead ECG.
2. Draw the blood specimens.
3. Apply the oxygen to the client.
4. Call radiology to obtain the chest x-ray study.

Answer: 3

Test-Taking Strategy: Note the strategic word *first* and use the ABCs—airway, breathing, and circulation. The *first* action would be to apply the oxygen because the client can be experiencing myocardial ischemia. The ECG can provide evidence of cardiac damage and the location of myocardial ischemia. However, oxygen is the priority to prevent further cardiac damage. Drawing the blood specimens would be done after oxygen administration and just before or after the ECG, depending on the situation. Although the chest x-ray can show cardiac enlargement, having the chest x-ray would not influence immediate treatment. Remember to use the ABCs—airway, breathing, and circulation—to prioritize! Review: nursing care for a client experiencing **chest pain.**

BOX 5-10   Practice Question: Maslow's Hierarchy of Needs Theory

A female client arrives at the emergency department and states she was just raped. In preparing a plan of care, which is the **priority** intervention?
1. Providing instructions for medical follow-up
2. Obtaining appropriate counseling for the victim
3. Providing anticipatory guidance for police investigations, medical questions, and court proceedings
4. Exploring safety concerns by obtaining permission to notify significant others who can provide shelter

Answer: 4

Test-Taking Strategy: Note the strategic word, *priority*. Use Maslow's Hierarchy of Needs theory. After the provision of medical treatment, the nurse's next *priority* would be obtaining support and planning for safety. Option 1 is concerned with ensuring that the victim understands the importance of and commits to the need for medical follow-up. Options 2 and 3 seek to meet the emotional needs related to the rape and emotional readiness for the process of discovery and legal action. From the options provided, these are not *priority* interventions. Remember that physiological needs are the *priority*, followed by safety needs. Therefore, select option 4 because it addresses the client's safety needs. Remember to use Maslow's Hierarchy of Needs theory to prioritize! Review: care of the **rape victim.**

Nursing Priorities from Maslow's Hierarchy

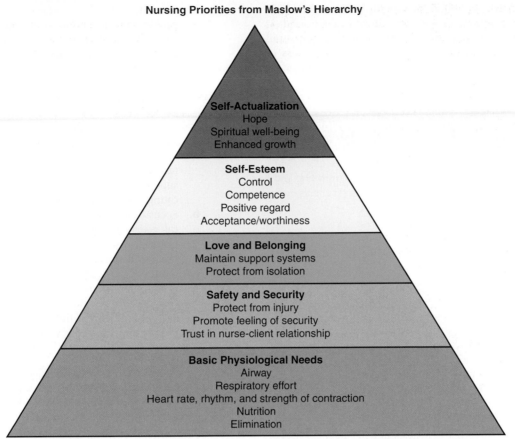

FIGURE 5-1 Use Maslow's Hierarchy of Needs to establish priorities. (From Harkreader H, Hogan MA, Thobaben M: *Fundamentals of nursing: caring and clinical judgment*, ed 3, St. Louis, 2007, Saunders.)

b. Remember that assessment is the first step in the nursing process.

c. When you are asked to select your first, immediate, or initial nursing action, follow the steps of the nursing process to prioritize when selecting the correct option.

d. Look for strategic words in the options that reflect assessment (see Box 5-4).

e. If an option contains the concept of assessment or the collection of client data, the best choice is to select that option (Box 5-11).

f. If an assessment action is not one of the options, follow the steps of the nursing process as your guide to select your first, immediate, or initial action.

g. Possible exception to the guideline—if the question presents an emergency situation, read carefully; in an emergency situation, an intervention may be the priority.

4. Analysis (Box 5-12)

a. Analysis questions are the most difficult questions because they require understanding of the principles of physiological responses and require interpretation of the data based on assessment.

b. Analysis questions require critical thinking and determining the rationale for therapeutic prescriptions or interventions that may be addressed in the question.

BOX 5-11 Practice Question: The Nursing Process—Assessment

The clinic nurse prepares to develop a diabetic teaching program. To meet the clients' needs, the nurse should take which action **first**?

1. Assess the clients' functional abilities.
2. Ensure that insurance will pay for participation in the program.
3. Discuss the focus of the program with the interprofessional team.
4. Include everyone who comes into the clinic in the teaching sessions.

Answer: 1

Test-Taking Strategy: Note the strategic word, *first*, which indicates the need to prioritize. Use the steps of the nursing process to answer the question, remembering that assessment is the first step. The only option that addresses assessment is option 1. The nurse should focus on individualized disease prevention and health promotion and maintenance. Therefore, the nurse must *first* assess the clients and their needs so as to effectively plan the program. Options 2, 3, and 4 do not address the clients' needs. Remember that assessment is the first step in the nursing process! Review: **teaching and learning** principles.

c. Analysis questions may address the formulation of a statement that identifies a client need or problem and include the communication and documentation of the results of the process of analysis.

5. Planning (Box 5-13)

BOX 5-12 Practice Question: The Nursing Process—Analysis

The nurse reviews the arterial blood gas results of a client and notes the following: pH of 7.30, Pco_2 of 50 mm Hg, and HCO_3^- of 22 mEq/L. The nurse analyzes these results as indicating which condition?

1. Metabolic acidosis, compensated
2. Respiratory alkalosis, compensated
3. Metabolic alkalosis, uncompensated
4. Respiratory acidosis, uncompensated

Answer: *4*

Test-Taking Strategy: Focus on the subject, interpreting arterial blood gas results. The normal pH is 7.35 to 7.45. In a respiratory condition, an opposite effect will be seen between the pH and the Pco_2. In this situation, the pH is lower than the normal value, and the Pco_2 is elevated. In an acidotic condition, the pH is low. Therefore, the values identified in the question indicate respiratory acidosis. Compensation occurs when the pH returns to a normal value. Because the pH is not normal, compensation has not occurred. Remember that in a respiratory imbalance you will find an opposite response between the pH and the Pco_2 as indicated in the question. Therefore, you can eliminate options 1 and 3. Also, remember that the pH decreases in an acidotic condition and compensation occurs, as evidenced by a normal pH. Remember that analysis is the second step in the nursing process! Review: steps for interpreting **arterial blood gas** results.

BOX 5-13 Practice Question: The Nursing Process—Planning

A client with active tuberculosis (TB) is to be admitted to a medical-surgical unit. Which action should the nurse take when planning a bed assignment?

1. Tell the admitting office to send the client to the intensive care unit.
2. Place the client in a private, airborne infection isolation room (AIIR).
3. Assign the client to a room with another client because intravenous antibiotics will be administered.
4. Assign the client to a room with another client and place a "strict hand washing" sign outside the door.

Answer: *2*

Test-Taking Strategy: Focus on the subject, planning nursing care and identifying the safe bed assignment. Note that the question states "active tuberculosis." Tuberculosis is spread via the airborne route. Preventing the spread of infection requires the use of special air handling and ventilation in an AIIR. Therefore, option 2 is the only correct option when planning a bed assignment for this client. Remember that planning is the third step in the nursing process. Review: care of the client with **tuberculosis.**

---

a. Planning questions require prioritizing client problems, determining goals and outcome criteria for goals of care, developing the plan of care, and communicating and documenting the plan of care.

b. Remember that actual client problems rather than potential client problems will most likely be the priority.

6. Implementation (Box 5-14)

a. Implementation questions address the process of organizing and managing care, counseling and teaching, providing care to achieve established goals, supervising and coordinating care, and communicating and documenting nursing interventions.

b. Focus on a nursing action rather than on a medical action when you are answering a question, unless the question is asking you what prescribed medical action is anticipated.

c. On the NCLEX-RN exam, the only client that you need to be concerned about is the client in the current question; avoid the "What if …?" syndrome and remember that the client in the question on the computer screen is your only assigned client.

BOX 5-14 Practice Question: The Nursing Process—Implementation

The nurse is performing range-of-motion (ROM) exercises on a client when the client unexpectedly develops spastic muscle contractions. The nurse should implement which interventions? **Select all that apply.**

❑ 1. Stop movement of affected part.
❑ 2. Massage the affected part vigorously.
❑ 3. Notify the health care provider immediately.
❑ 4. Force movement of the joint supporting the muscle.
❑ 5. Ask the client to stand and walk rapidly around the room.
❑ 6. Place continuous gentle pressure on the muscle group until it relaxes.

Answer: *1, 6*

Test-Taking Strategy: Implementation questions address the process of organizing and managing care. Focus on the subject, interventions to relieve spastic muscle contractions. ROM exercises should put each joint through as full a range of motion as possible without causing discomfort. An unexpected outcome is the development of spastic muscle contraction during ROM exercises. If this occurs, the nurse should stop movement of the affected part and place continuous gentle pressure on the muscle group until it relaxes. Once the contraction subsides, the exercises are resumed using slower, steady movement. Massaging the affected part vigorously may worsen the contraction. There is no need to notify the health care provider unless intervention is ineffective. The nurse should never force movement of a joint. Asking the client to stand and walk rapidly around the room is an inappropriate measure. Additionally, if the client is able to walk, ROM exercises are probably unnecessary. Remember that implementation is the fourth step in the nursing process. Review: procedure for performing **range-of-motion exercises.**

d. Answer the question from a textbook and ideal point of view; remember that the nurse has all the time and all of the equipment needed to care for the client readily available at the bedside; remember that you do not need to run to the treatment room to obtain, for example, sterile gloves or wound dressing materials because these items will be at the client's bedside.

7. Evaluation (Box 5-15)

a. Evaluation questions focus on comparing the actual outcomes of care with the expected outcomes and on communicating and documenting findings.

b. These questions focus on assisting in determining the client's response to care and identifying factors that may interfere with achieving expected outcomes.

c. In an evaluation question, watch for negative event queries because they are frequently used in evaluation-type questions.

BOX 5-15	Practice Question: The Nursing Process—Evaluation

The nurse instructs a client receiving external radiation therapy about skin care. Which statements by the client indicate an understanding of the instructions? **Select all that apply.**

☐ **1.** "I can lie in the sun as long as I limit the time to 2 hours daily."

☐ **2.** "I should wear snug clothing to support the irradiated skin area."

☐ **3.** "I should wash the irradiated area gently each day with a mild soap and water."

☐ **4.** "After bathing I should dry the area with a patting motion using a clean soft towel."

☐ **5.** "I should avoid the use of powders, lotions, or creams on the skin area being irradiated."

☐ **6.** "I should avoid removing the markings on the skin when bathing until the entire course of radiation is complete."

Answer: 3, 4, 5, 6

Test-Taking Strategy: Focus on the subject, client understanding of the instructions. The subject specifies that this is an evaluation-type question. Recall that external radiation therapy can cause altered skin integrity and special measures need to be taken to protect the skin. These measures include washing the irradiated area gently (using the hand rather than a wash cloth) each day with either water alone or water and a mild soap (rinse soap thoroughly); drying the area with a patting motion (not a rubbing motion) with a clean soft towel; avoiding removing the markings on the skin when bathing until the entire course of radiation is complete because these markings indicate exactly where the beam of radiation is to be focused; avoiding the use of powders, lotions, or creams on the skin area being irradiated unless prescribed by the health care provider; avoiding wearing clothing or items that bind or rub the irradiated skin area; and avoiding heat exposure or sun exposure to the irradiated area. Remember that evaluation is the fifth step in the nursing process. Review: **external radiation therapy.**

VII. Client Needs

A. Safe and Effective Care Environment

1. According to the National Council of State Boards of Nursing (NCSBN), these questions test the concepts that the nurse provides nursing care; collaborates with interprofessional team members to facilitate effective client care; and protects clients, significant others, and health care personnel from environmental hazards.

2. Focus on safety with these types of questions, and remember the importance of hand washing, call bells, bed positioning, appropriate use of side rails, asepsis, use of standard and other precautions; prioritizing, triage principles, and emergency response planning are also areas of focus.

B. Physiological Integrity

1. The NCSBN indicates that these questions test the concepts that the nurse provides comfort and assistance in the performance of activities of daily living and provides care related to the administration of medications and parenteral therapies.

2. These questions also address the nurse's ability to reduce the client's potential for developing complications or health problems related to treatments, procedures, or existing conditions and to provide care to clients with acute, chronic, or life-threatening physical health conditions.

3. Focus on Maslow's Hierarchy of Needs theory in these types of questions and remember that physiological needs are a priority and are addressed first.

4. Use the ABCs—airway, breathing, and circulation—and the steps of the nursing process when selecting an option addressing Physiological Integrity.

C. Psychosocial Integrity

1. The NCSBN notes that these questions test the concepts that the nurse provides nursing care that promotes and supports the emotional, mental, and social well-being of the client and significant others.

2. Content addressed in these questions relates to supporting and promoting the client's or significant others' ability to cope, adapt, or problem solve in situations such as illnesses; disabilities; or stressful events including abuse, neglect, or violence.

3. In this Client Needs category, you may be asked communication-type questions that relate to how you would respond to a client, a client's family member or significant other, or other health care team members.

4. Use therapeutic communication techniques to answer communication questions because of their effectiveness in the communication process.

5. Remember to select the option that focuses on the thoughts, feelings, concerns, anxieties, or fears of the client, client's family member, or significant other (Box 5-16).

D. Health Promotion and Maintenance

1. According to the NCSBN, these questions test the concepts that the nurse provides and assists in directing nursing care to promote and maintain health.

2. Content addressed in these questions relates to assisting the client and significant others during the normal expected stages of growth and development, and providing client care related to the prevention and early detection of health problems.

BOX 5-16   Practice Question: Communication

A client with a diagnosis of major depression says to the nurse, "I should have died. I've always been a failure." The nurse should make which therapeutic response to the client?

1. "I see a lot of positive things in you."
2. "You still have a great deal to live for."
3. "Feeling like a failure is part of your illness."
4. "You've been feeling like a failure for some time now?"

Answer: 4

Test-Taking Strategy: Use therapeutic communication techniques to answer this question. Remember to address the client's feelings and concerns. Option 4 is the only option that is stated in the form of a question and is open-ended, thus encouraging the verbalization of feelings. Remember to use therapeutic communication techniques and focus on the client. Review: **therapeutic communication techniques.**

---

3. Use the Teaching and Learning theory if the question addresses client teaching, remembering that the client's willingness, desire, and readiness to learn are the first priorities.
4. Watch for negative event queries because they are frequently used in questions that address Health Promotion and Maintenance and client education.

VIII. Eliminating Comparable or Alike Options (Box 5-17)

A. When reading the options in multiple choice questions, look for options that are comparable or alike.
B. Comparable or alike options can be eliminated as possible answers because it is impossible for both options to be correct.

BOX 5-17   Practice Question: Eliminate Comparable or Alike Options

The nurse is assessing the leg pain of a client who has just undergone right femoral-popliteal artery bypass grafting. Which question would be **most** useful in determining whether the client is experiencing graft occlusion?

1. "Can you describe what the pain feels like?"
2. "Can you rate the pain on a scale of 1 to 10?"
3. "Did you get any relief from the last dose of pain medication?"
4. "Can you compare this pain to the pain you felt before surgery?"

Answer: 4

Test-Taking Strategy: Note the strategic word, *most*, and focus on the subject, differentiating expected postoperative pain from pain that indicates graft occlusion. The most frequent indication that a graft is occluding is the return of pain that is similar to that experienced preoperatively. Eliminate options 1, 2, and 3 because they are comparable or alike and are standard pain assessment questions. Remember to eliminate comparable or alike options! Review: manifestations of **graft occlusion.**

BOX 5-18   Practice Question: Eliminate Options That Contain Closed-Ended Words

A client is to undergo a barium swallow and the nurse provides preprocedure instructions. The nurse should instruct the client to take which action in the preprocedure period?

1. Avoid eating or drinking after midnight before the test.
2. Limit self to only two cigarettes on the morning of the test.
3. Have a clear liquid breakfast only on the morning of the test.
4. Take all routine medications with a glass of water on the morning of the test.

Answer: 1

Test-Taking Strategy: Note the closed-ended words *only* in options 2 and 3 and *all* in option 4. Eliminate options that contain closed-ended words because these options are usually incorrect. Also, note that options 2, 3, and 4 are comparable or alike options in that they all involve taking in something on the morning of the test. Remember to eliminate options that contain closed-ended words. Review: preprocedure care for a client undergoing **barium swallow.**

IX. Eliminate Options Containing Closed-Ended Words (Box 5-18)

A. Some closed-ended words include *all, always, every, must, none, never,* and *only.*
B. Eliminate options that contain closed-ended words because these words infer a fixed or extreme meaning; these types of options are usually incorrect.
C. Options that contain open-ended words, such as *may, usually, normally, commonly,* or *generally,* should be considered as possible correct options.

X. Look for the Umbrella Option (Box 5-19)

A. When answering a question, look for the umbrella option.
B. The umbrella option is one that is a broad or universal statement and that usually contains the concepts of the other options within it.
C. The umbrella option will be the correct answer.

XI. Use the Guidelines for Delegating and Making Assignments (Box 5-20)

A. You may be asked a question that will require you to decide how you will delegate a task or assign clients to other health care providers.
B. Focus on the information in the question and what task or assignment is to be delegated.
C. When you have determined what task or assignment is to be delegated, consider the client's needs and match the client's needs with the scope of practice of the health care providers identified in the question.
D. The Nurse Practice Act and any practice limitations define which aspects of care can be delegated and which must be performed by a registered nurse. Use nursing scope of practice as a guide to assist in answering questions.
E. In general, noninvasive interventions, such as skin care, range-of-motion exercises, ambulation, grooming, and hygiene measures, can be assigned to unlicensed assistive personnel (UAP).

BOX 5-19   Practice Question: Look for the Umbrella Option

The home care nurse is caring for a client who has just been discharged from the hospital after implantation of a permanent pacemaker. The nurse should assess the client's home for the presence of which **priority** item?

1. Hair dryer
2. Electric blanket
3. Electric toothbrush with holder
4. Electrical items with strong magnetic fields

Answer: 4

Test-Taking Strategy: Note the strategic word, *priority*, and the umbrella option. A pacemaker is shielded from interference from most electrical devices. Radios, televisions, electric blankets, toasters, microwave ovens, heating pads, and hair dryers are considered to be safe. Devices to be forewarned about include those with a strong electric current or magnetic field, such as antitheft devices in stores, metal detectors used in airports, and radiation therapy (if applicable and which might require relocation of the pacemaker). Note that option 4 uses the word "strong" and is the umbrella option addressing items with strong electric currents or magnetic fields. Remember that the umbrella option is a broad or universal option that includes the concepts of the other options in it! Review: home care instructions for a client with a **pacemaker**.

BOX 5-20   Practice Question: Use Guidelines for Delegating and Assignment-Making

The nurse is planning the client assignments for the day and has a licensed practical nurse (LPN) and an unlicensed assistive personnel (UAP) on the nursing team. Which client should the nurse **most appropriately** assign to the LPN?

1. A client with stable heart failure who has early-stage Alzheimer's disease
2. A client who is scheduled for an electrocardiogram and a chest radiograph
3. A client who was treated for dehydration and is weak and needs assistance with bathing
4. A client with emphysema who is receiving oxygen at 2 L by nasal cannula and becomes dyspneic on exertion

Answer: 4

Test-Taking Strategy: Note the strategic words, *most appropriately*, and focus on the subject, the assignment to be delegated to the LPN. When asked questions related to delegation, think about the role description of the employee and the needs of the client. The nurse would most appropriately assign the client with emphysema to the LPN. This client has an airway problem and has the highest priority needs of the clients presented in the options. The clients described in options 1, 2, and 3 can be cared for appropriately by the UAP. Remember to match the client's needs with the scope of practice of the health care provider! Review: **delegating principles.**

F. A licensed practical nurse can perform the tasks that UAP can perform and can usually perform certain invasive tasks, such as dressings, suctioning, urinary catheterization, and administering medications orally or by the subcutaneous or intramuscular route; some selected piggyback intravenous medications may also be administered.

G. A registered nurse can perform the tasks that a licensed practical nurse can perform and is responsible for assessment and planning care, analyzing client data, implementing and evaluating client care, supervising care, initiating teaching, and administering medications intravenously.

XII. Answering Pharmacology Questions (Box 5-21)

A. If you are familiar with the medication, use nursing knowledge to answer the question.

B. Remember that the question will identify the generic name and the trade name of the medication.

C. If the question identifies a medical diagnosis, try to form a relationship between the medication and the diagnosis; for example, you can determine that cyclophosphamide is an antineoplastic medication if the question refers to a client with breast cancer who is taking this medication.

D. Try to determine the classification of the medication being addressed to assist in answering the question. Identifying the classification will assist in determining a medication's action or side/adverse effects or both; for example, diltiazem (*Cardizem*) is a cardiac medication.

E. Recognize the common side/adverse effects associated with each medication classification and relate the appropriate nursing interventions to each effect; for example, if a side effect is hypertension, the associated nursing intervention would be to monitor the blood pressure.

F. Focus on what the question is asking: intended effect, side effect, adverse effect, or toxic effect.

G. Learn medications that belong to a classification by commonalities in their medication names; for example, medications that act as beta blockers end with "*-lol*" (e.g., ateno*lol*).

H. Look at the medication name and use medical terminology to assist in determining the medication action; for example, *Lopressor* lowers *(lo)* the blood pressure *(pressor)*.

I. If the question requires a medication calculation, remember that a calculator is available on the computer; talk yourself through each step to be sure the answer makes sense, and recheck the calculation before answering the question, particularly if the answer seems like an unusual dosage.

BOX 5-21   Practice Question: Answering Pharmacology Questions

The nurse is preparing to administer atenolol (Tenormin) to a client. The nurse should check which **priority** item before administering the medication?

1. Temperature
2. Blood pressure
3. Potassium level
4. Blood glucose level

Answer: 2

Test-Taking Strategy: Note the strategic word, *priority*. Focus on the name of the medication. Recall that most beta-blocker medication names end with the letters *-lol* and that these medications are used to treat hypertension. This will direct you to option 2. Remember to use pharmacology guidelines to assist you in answering questions about medications! Review: **atenolol (Tenormin).**

J. Pharmacology: Pyramid Points to Remember

1. In general, the client should not take an antacid with medication because the antacid will affect the absorption of the medication.
2. Enteric-coated and sustained-release tablets should not be crushed; also, capsules should not be opened.
3. The client should never adjust or change a medication dose or abruptly stop taking a medication.
4. The nurse never adjusts or changes the client's medication dosage and never discontinues a medication.
5. The client needs to avoid taking any over-the-counter medications or any other medications, such as herbal preparations, unless they are approved for use by the health care provider.
6. The client needs to avoid consuming alcohol.
7. Medications are never administered if the prescription is difficult to read, is unclear, or identifies a medication dose that is not a normal one.
8. Additional strategies for answering pharmacology are presented in *Saunders Strategies for Test Success: Passing Nursing School and the NCLEX® Exam.*

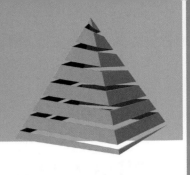

UNIT II

Client Needs

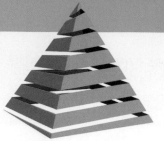

CHAPTER 6

Client Needs and the NCLEX-RN® Test Plan

In the new test plan, which was implemented in April 2013, the National Council of State Boards of Nursing (NCSBN) identified a test plan framework that was based on Client Needs. This framework was selected on the basis of the findings in a practice analysis study of newly licensed registered nurses in the United States. This study identified the nursing activities performed by entry-level nurses. Also, according to the NCSBN, the Client Needs categories provide a structure for defining nursing actions and competencies across all settings for all clients. The NCSBN identifies four major categories of Client Needs. Some of these categories are further divided into subcategories, and the percentage of test questions in each subcategory is identified in Table 6-1.

The information in this chapter related to the test plan was obtained from the NCSBN Web site at www.ncsbn.org and from the NCSBN *2013 NCLEX-RN® Detailed Test Plan*. Additional information regarding the test and its development can be obtained by accessing the NCSBN Web site at www.ncsbn.org or by writing to the National Council of State Boards of Nursing, 111 E. Wacker Drive, Suite 2900, Chicago, IL 60601.

TABLE 6-1 Client Needs Categories and Percentage of Questions on the NCLEX-RN® Examination

Client Needs Category	Percentage of Questions
Safe and Effective Care Environment	
Management of Care	17%-23%
Safety and Infection Control	9%-15%
Health Promotion and Maintenance	6%-12%
Psychosocial Integrity	6%-12%
Physiological Integrity	
Basic Care and Comfort	6%-12%
Pharmacological and Parenteral Therapies	12%-18%
Reduction of Risk Potential	9%-15%
Physiological Adaptation	11%-17%

From National Council of State Boards of Nursing: *2013 NCLEX-RN detailed test plan*, Chicago, 2013, National Council of State Boards of Nursing.

Physiological Integrity

The Physiological Integrity category includes four subcategories: Basic Care and Comfort, Pharmacological and Parenteral Therapies, Reduction of Risk Potential, and Physiological Adaptation. The NCSBN describes the content tested in each subcategory. Basic Care and Comfort (6% to 12%) addresses content that tests the knowledge, skills, and ability required to provide basic care and comfort measures and assistance to the client in performing activities of daily living. Pharmacological and Parenteral Therapies (12% to 18%) addresses content that tests the knowledge, skills, and ability required to administer medications and parenteral therapies. Reduction of Risk Potential (9% to 15%) addresses content that tests the knowledge, skills, and ability required to prevent complications or health problems related to the client's condition, or any prescribed treatments or procedures. Physiological Adaptation (11% to 17%) addresses content that tests the knowledge, skills, and ability required to provide care to clients with acute, chronic, or life-threatening conditions.

The NCSBN identifies related content and specific nursing activities for the subcategories of the Physiological Integrity category. For specific content and nursing activities, refer to the NCSBN test plan that can be located at the NCSBN Web site at

www.ncsbn.org. See Box 6-1 for examples of questions in this Client Needs category, and refer to Test 1 for practice questions reflective of this Client Needs category.

Safe and Effective Care Environment

The Safe and Effective Care Environment category includes two subcategories: (1) Management of Care and (2) Safety and Infection Control. The NCSBN describes the content tested in each subcategory. Management of Care (17% to 23%) addresses content that tests the knowledge, skills, and ability required to provide and direct nursing care that will enhance the care delivery setting to protect clients, health care personnel, and others. Safety and Infection Control (9% to 15%) addresses content that tests the knowledge, skills, and ability required to protect clients, health care personnel, and others from health and environmental hazards.

The NCSBN identifies related content and nursing activities for the subcategories of the Safe and Effective Care Environment category. For specific content and nursing activities, refer to the NCSBN test plan. See Box 6-2 for examples of questions in this Client Needs category, and refer to Test 2 for practice questions reflective of this Client Needs category.

BOX 6-1 Physiological Integrity Questions

Basic Care and Comfort

A client with right-sided weakness needs to learn how to use a cane for home maintenance of mobility. The nurse should teach the client to position the cane by holding it in which way?

1. Left hand and 6 inches lateral to the left foot
2. Right hand and 6 inches lateral to the right foot
3. Left hand and placing the cane in front of the left foot
4. Right hand and placing the cane in front of the right foot

Answer: 1

This question addresses content related to the use of an assistive device. Focus on the subject, use of a cane for a client with right-sided weakness. The client is taught to hold the cane on the opposite side of the weakness, because with normal walking the opposite arm and leg move together (called *reciprocal motion*). The cane is placed 6 inches lateral to the fifth toe. Review: procedures for the safe use of a **cane.**

Pharmacological and Parenteral Therapies

A client with hypertension is receiving torsemide (Demadex) 5 mg orally daily. Which finding would indicate to the nurse that the client is experiencing an adverse effect related to the medication?

1. A chloride level of 98 mEq/L
2. A sodium level of 135 mEq/L
3. A potassium level of 3.1 mEq/L
4. A blood urea nitrogen (BUN) of 15 mg/dL

Answer: 3

This question addresses content related to a medication. Focus on the subject, an adverse effect. Torsemide is a loop diuretic. The medication can produce acute, profound water loss; volume and electrolyte depletion; dehydration; decreased blood volume; and circulatory collapse. Option 3 is the only option that indicates an electrolyte depletion because the normal potassium level is 3.5 to 5.0 mEq/L. The normal chloride level is 98 to 107 mEq/L. The normal sodium level is 135 to 145 mEq/L. The normal BUN is 5 to 20 mg/dL. Review: adverse effects of **torsemide.**

Reduction of Risk Potential

A client is scheduled to undergo a renal biopsy. To minimize the risk of postprocedure complications, the nurse should report which laboratory result to the health care provider before the procedure?

1. Potassium: 3.8 mEq/L
2. Serum creatinine: 1.2 mg/dL
3. Prothrombin time: 15 seconds
4. Blood urea nitrogen (BUN): 18 mg/dL

Answer: 3

This question addresses a potential postprocedure complication of a diagnostic test (renal biopsy). Focus on the subject, an abnormal laboratory result. Postprocedure hemorrhage is a complication after renal biopsy. Because of this, prothrombin time is assessed before the procedure. The normal prothrombin time range is 9.5 to 11.8 seconds. The nurse ensures that these results are available and reports abnormalities promptly. The normal potassium is 3.5 to 5.0 mEq/L, the normal serum creatinine is 0.6 to 1.3 mg/dL, and the normal BUN is 5 to 20 mg/dL. Review: preprocedure care for **renal biopsy.**

Physiological Adaptation

A pregnant client tells the nurse that she felt wetness on her peri-pad and that she found some clear fluid. The nurse immediately inspects the perineum and notes the presence of the umbilical cord. The nurse should take which **immediate** action?

1. Monitor the fetal heart rate.
2. Notify the health care provider.
3. Transfer the client to the delivery room.
4. Place the client in Trendelenburg position.

Answer: 4

This question addresses an acute and life-threatening physical health condition. Note the strategic word, *immediate*. On inspection of the perineum, if the umbilical cord is noted, the nurse immediately places the client in Trendelenburg position while holding the presenting part upward to relieve the cord compression. This position is maintained, the health care provider is notified, and the nurse monitors the fetal heart rate. The client is transferred to the delivery room when prescribed by the health care provider. Review: immediate care for **prolapsed cord.**

Health Promotion and Maintenance

The Health Promotion and Maintenance category (6% to 12%) addresses the principles related to growth and development. According to the NCSBN, this Client Needs category also addresses content that tests the knowledge, skills, and ability required to assist the client, family members, and/or significant others to prevent health problems, recognize alterations in health to detect health problems early, and develop health practices and strategies that promote and support wellness and achieve optimal health.

The NCSBN identifies related content and specific nursing activities for the Health and Promotion and Maintenance category. For specific content and nursing activities, refer to the NCSBN test plan. See Box 6-3 for examples of questions in this Client Needs category, and refer to Test 3 for practice questions reflective of this Client Needs category.

Psychosocial Integrity

The Psychosocial Integrity category (6% to 12%) addresses content that tests the knowledge, skills, and ability required to promote and support the client, family, and/or significant other's ability to cope, adapt, and/or solve problems during stressful events. According to the NCSBN, this Client Needs category also addresses the emotional, mental, and social well-being of the client, family, or significant other,

BOX 6-2   Safe and Effective Care Environment Questions

Management of Care

The registered nurse is planning the client assignments for the day. Which is the appropriate assignment for the unlicensed assistive personnel (UAP)?

1. A client requiring colostomy irrigation
2. A client receiving continuous tube feedings
3. A client who requires stool specimen collections
4. A client who has difficulty swallowing food and fluids

Answer: 3

This question addresses content related to delegation. Focus on the subject, the appropriate assignment for the UAP. Work that is delegated to others must be done consistent with the individual's level of expertise and licensure or lack of licensure. In this situation, the most appropriate assignment for the UAP is to care for the client who requires stool specimen collections. Colostomy irrigations and tube feedings are not performed by unlicensed personnel. The client with difficulty swallowing food and fluids is at risk for aspiration. Remember, the health care provider needs to be competent and skilled to perform the assigned task or activity. Review: **delegation guidelines.**

Safety and Infection Control

A client diagnosed with tuberculosis (TB) is scheduled to go to the radiology department for a chest radiograph. The nurse should take which action when preparing to transport the client?

1. Apply a mask to the client.
2. Apply a mask and gown to the client.
3. Apply a mask, gown, and gloves to the client.
4. Notify the radiology department so that the personnel can be sure to wear masks when the client arrives.

Answer: 1

This question addresses content related to airborne precautions. Focus on the subject, transporting a client with TB. Clients known or suspected of having TB should wear a mask when out of the hospital room to prevent the spread of the infection to others. Gown and gloves are not necessary. Others are not protected unless the infected client wears the mask. Review: infection control measures for a client with **tuberculosis.**

BOX 6-3   Health Promotion and Maintenance Questions

The postpartum nurse has instructed a new mother on how to bathe her newborn. The nurse demonstrates the procedure to the mother and on the following day asks the mother to perform the procedure. Which observation by the nurse indicates that the mother is performing the procedure correctly?

1. The mother washes the ears and then moves to the eyes and the face.
2. The mother washes the newborn by starting with the eyes and face.
3. The mother washes the arms, chest, and back followed by the neck, arms, and face.
4. The mother washes the entire newborn's body and then washes the eyes, face, and scalp.

Answer: 2

This question addresses the postpartum period. Focus on the subject, that the mother can perform the bathing procedure for her newborn. Bathing should start at the eyes and face and with the cleanest area first. Next, the external ears and behind the ears are cleaned. The newborn's neck should be washed because formula, lint, or breast milk often accumulates in the folds of the neck. Hands and arms are then washed. The newborn's legs are washed next, with the diaper area washed last. Remember to always start with the cleanest area of the body first and proceed to the dirtiest area. Review: bathing procedure for a newborn and **newborn care.**

A client with atherosclerosis asks the nurse about dietary modifications to lower the risk of heart disease. The nurse should encourage the client to eat which food that will lower this risk?

1. Fresh cantaloupe
2. Broiled cheeseburger
3. Mashed potato with gravy
4. Fried chicken without skin

Answer: 1

This question addresses health and wellness. Focus on the subject, the food item lowest in fat. To lower the risk of heart disease, the diet should be low in saturated fat, with the appropriate number of total calories. The diet should include fewer red meats and more white meat, with the skin removed. Fried foods are high in fat. Dairy products used should be low in fat, and foods with large amounts of empty calories should be avoided. Fresh fruits and vegetables are naturally low in fat. Review: **high and low-fat foods.**

and the knowledge, skills, and ability required to care for the client with an acute or chronic mental illness.

The NCSBN identifies related content and specific nursing activities for the Psychosocial Integrity category. For specific content and nursing activities, refer to the NCSBN test plan. See Box 6-4 for examples of questions in this Client Needs category, and refer to Test 4 for practice questions reflective of this Client Needs category.

BOX 6-4 Psychosocial Integrity Questions

The nurse is planning care for a client who is experiencing anxiety following a myocardial infarction. Which nursing intervention should be included in the plan of care?

1. Answer questions with factual information.
2. Provide detailed explanations of all procedures.
3. Limit family involvement during the acute phase.
4. Administer an antianxiety medication to promote relaxation.

Answer: 1

This question addresses content related to fear and anxiety. Focus on the subject, an intervention that will alleviate anxiety. Accurate and factual information reduces fear, strengthens the nurse–client relationship, and assists the client in dealing realistically with the situation. Providing detailed information may increase the client's anxiety. Information should be provided simply and clearly. The client's family may be a source of support for the client. Limiting family involvement may or may not be helpful. Medication should not be used unless necessary. Review: interventions to alleviate **anxiety.**

The nurse in the mental health clinic is performing an initial assessment of a family with a diagnosis of domestic violence. Which factor should the nurse **initially** include in the assessment?

1. The coping style of each family member
2. The family's ability to use community resources
3. The family's anger toward the intrusiveness of the nurse
4. The family's denial of the violent nature of their behavior

Answer: 1

This question addresses domestic violence. Note the strategic word, *initially*. The initial family assessment includes a careful history of each family member. Options 2, 3, and 4 address the family. Option 1 addresses each family member. Review: nursing care procedures for **domestic violence.**

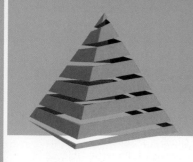

Physiological Integrity

❖ **1.** The nurse is caring for a client who is receiving blood transfusion therapy. Which clinical manifestations should alert the nurse to a hemolytic transfusion reaction? **Select all that apply.**
  ❑ 1. Headache
  ❑ 2. Tachycardia
  ❑ 3. Hypertension
  ❑ 4. Apprehension
  ❑ 5. Distended neck veins
  ❑ 6. A sense of impending doom

Level of Cognitive Ability: Analyzing
Client Needs: Physiological Integrity
Integrated Process: Nursing Process/Assessment
Content Area: Critical Care: Blood Administration
Priority Concepts: Clinical Judgment; Immunity

Answer: 1, 2, 4, 6
Rationale: Hemolytic transfusion reactions are caused by blood type or Rh incompatibility. When blood containing antigens different from the client's own antigens are infused, antigen-antibody complexes are formed in the client's blood. These complexes destroy the transfused cells and start inflammatory responses in the client's blood vessel walls and organs. The reaction may include fever and chills or may be life threatening with disseminated intravascular coagulation and circulatory collapse. Other manifestations include headache, tachycardia, apprehension, a sense of impending doom, chest pain, low back pain, tachypnea, hypotension, and hemoglobinuria. The onset may be immediate or may not occur until subsequent units have been transfused. Distended neck veins are characteristics of circulatory overload.
Priority Nursing Tip: The nurse should suspect a transfusion reaction if the client develops any symptom or complains of anything unusual while receiving the blood transfusion.
Test-Taking Strategy: Focus on the subject, a hemolytic transfusion reaction. Recall the pathophysiology of this type of reaction to select the correct options. Also think about other types of transfusion reactions that can occur, and recall that distended neck veins are characteristic of circulatory overload. Review: the clinical manifestations of a hemolytic transfusion reaction.
Reference(s): Ignatavicius, Workman (2013), p. 901.

2. A client has an arteriovenous (AV) fistula in place in the right upper extremity for hemodialysis treatments. When planning care for this client, which measure should the nurse implement to promote client safety?
1. Take blood pressures only on the right arm to ensure accuracy.
2. Use the fistula for all venipunctures and intravenous infusions.
3. Ensure that small clamps are attached to the AV fistula dressing.
4. Assess the fistula for the presence of a bruit and thrill every 4 hours.

Level of Cognitive Ability: Applying
Client Needs: Physiological Integrity
Integrated Process: Nursing Process/Planning
Content Area: Adult Health: Renal and Urinary
Priority Concepts: Perfusion; Safety

Answer: 4
Rationale: Arteriovenous fistulas are created by anastomosis of an artery and a vein within the subcutaneous tissues to create access for hemodialysis. Fistulas should be evaluated for presence of thrills (palpate over the area) and bruits (auscultate with a stethoscope) as an assessment of patency. Blood pressures or venipunctures are not done on the extremity with the fistula because of the risk for clotting, infection, or damage to the fistula. The fistula is not used for venipunctures or intravenous infusions for the same reason. Clamps may be needed for an external device such as an AV shunt, but the AV fistula is internal.
Priority Nursing Tip: For the client receiving hemodialysis, the AV fistula is the client's lifeline. The client's hemodynamic status should be closely monitored. Clients need teaching on which medications to avoid before dialysis.
Test-Taking Strategy: Focus on the subject, an AV fistula and safety. Eliminate option 3 first because this refers to care of an AV shunt, in which there is an external cannula that can become disconnected. If accidental disconnection occurs, the small clamps can be used to occlude the ends of the cannula. Blood pressure measurement, insertion of intravenous access, and venipuncture should never be performed on the affected extremity because of the potential for infection and clotting of the fistula; therefore, eliminate options 1 and 2. The only option that relates to the subject of this question is option 4. Review: care of the client with an **arteriovenous (AV) fistula**.
Reference(s): Ignatavicius, Workman (2013), p. 1561.

3. A client with a wound infection and osteomyelitis is to receive hyperbaric oxygen therapy. During the therapy, which **priority** intervention should the nurse implement?
1. Maintain an intravenous access.
2. Ensure that oxygen is being delivered.
3. Administer sedation to prevent claustrophobia.
4. Provide emotional support to the client's family.

Level of Cognitive Ability: Applying
Client Needs: Physiological Integrity
Integrated Process: Nursing Process/Implementation
Content Area: Adult Health: Immune
Priority Concepts: Clinical Judgment; Gas Exchange

Answer: 2
Rationale: Hyperbaric oxygen therapy is a process by which oxygen is administered at greater than atmospheric pressure. When oxygen is inhaled under pressure, the level of tissue oxygen is greatly increased. The high levels of oxygen promote the action of phagocytes and promote healing of the wound. Because the client is placed in a closed chamber, the administration of oxygen is of primary importance. Although options 1, 3, and 4 may be appropriate interventions, option 2 is the priority.
Priority Nursing Tip: Hyperbaric oxygen therapy may be a treatment measure for chronic osteomyelitis to increase tissue perfusion and promote healing.
Test-Taking Strategy: Note the strategic word, *priority.* Use the ABCs—airway, breathing, and circulation—to direct you to option 2, which addresses oxygen. Also note the relationship of the words *hyperbaric oxygen* in the question and *oxygen* in the correct option. Review: care of the client receiving **hyperbaric oxygen therapy**.
Reference(s): Bryant, Nix (2012), pp. 348-350; Ignatavicius, Workman (2013), pp. 1132-1133.

4. A client is scheduled for hydrotherapy for a burn dressing change. Which action should the nurse take to ensure that the procedure is **most** tolerable for the client?

1. Ensure that the client has a robe and slippers.
2. Administer an analgesic 20 minutes before therapy.
3. Send dressing supplies with the client to hydrotherapy.
4. Administer the intravenous antibiotic 30 minutes before therapy.

Level of Cognitive Ability: Applying
Client Needs: Physiological Integrity
Integrated Process: Nursing Process/Implementation
Content Area: Adult Health: Integumentary
Priority Concepts: Pain; Tissue Integrity

Answer: 2
Rationale: The client should receive pain medication approximately 20 minutes before a burn dressing change. This will help the client tolerate an otherwise painful procedure. A robe and slippers are beneficial for the client's comfort if traveling by wheelchair, but pain medication is more essential. Dressing supplies are generally available in the hydrotherapy area and do not need to be sent with the client. Antibiotics are timed evenly around the clock and not necessarily in relation to timing of burn dressing changes. Additionally, antibiotics do not affect pain level.
Priority Nursing Tip: A burn injury is extremely painful, and the client is adequately medicated before a burn dressing change to reduce pain and prevent fear of future dressing changes. Strict aseptic technique is used for dressing changes because of the risk of infection.
Test-Taking Strategy: Use Maslow's Hierarchy of Needs theory (physiological needs are the priority) and focus on the strategic word, *most*. This will direct you to option 2, which addresses pain management. Review: care of the **burn** client.
Reference(s): Bryant, Nix (2012), pp. 452-453; Ignatavicius, Workman (2013), p. 531.

5. The nurse is caring for a client with heart failure who has a magnesium level of 0.75 mg/dL. Which action should the nurse take?

1. Monitor the client for irregular heart rhythms.
2. Encourage the intake of antacids with phosphate.
3. Teach the client to avoid foods high in magnesium.
4. Provide a diet of ground beef, eggs, and chicken breast.

Level of Cognitive Ability: Applying
Client Needs: Physiological Integrity
Integrated Process: Nursing Process/Implementation
Content Area: Fundamental Skills: Laboratory Values
Priority Concepts: Clinical Judgment; Fluid and Electrolyte Balance

Answer: 1
Rationale: The normal magnesium level ranges from 1.2 to 2.6 mg/dL; therefore, this client is experiencing hypomagnesemia. The client should be monitored for dysrhythmias because magnesium plays an important role in myocardial nerve cell impulse conduction; thus, hypomagnesemia increases the client's risk of ventricular dysrhythmias. The nurse avoids administering phosphate in the presence of hypomagnesemia because it aggravates the condition. The nurse instructs the client to consume foods high in magnesium; ground beef, eggs, and chicken breast are low in magnesium.
Priority Nursing Tip: The client with hypomagnesemia is at risk for seizures. Therefore the nurse needs to initiate seizure precautions if the magnesium level is low.
Test-Taking Strategy: Focus on the subject, a client with heart failure who has a magnesium level of 1.4 mg/dL. Recalling the normal magnesium level and noting that the client is experiencing hypomagnesemia will direct you to option 1. Also, use of the ABCs—airway, breathing, and circulation—will direct you to the correct option. Review: the normal **magnesium** level and the treatment for high and low levels.
Reference(s): Ignatavicius, Workman (2013), p. 193; Pagana, Pagana (2013), pp. 626-627.

❖ **6.** The nurse is assessing a pregnant client with a diagnosis of abruptio placentae. Which manifestations of this condition should the nurse expect to note? **Select all that apply.**
- ❏ 1. Uterine irritability
- ❏ 2. Uterine tenderness
- ❏ 3. Bright red vaginal bleeding
- ❏ 4. Abdominal and low back pain
- ❏ 5. Strong and frequent contractions
- ❏ 6. Nonreassuring fetal heart rate patterns

Level of Cognitive Ability: Analyzing
Client Needs: Physiological Integrity
Integrated Process: Nursing Process/Assessment
Content Area: Critical Care: Emergency Situations
Priority Concepts: Perfusion; Reproduction

Answer: 1, 2, 4, 6
Rationale: Placental abruption, also referred to as abruptio placentae, is the separation of a normally implanted placenta before the fetus is born. It occurs when there is bleeding and formation of a hematoma on the maternal side of the placenta. Manifestations include uterine irritability with frequent low-intensity contractions, uterine tenderness that may be localized to the site of the abruption, aching and dull abdominal and low back pain, painful vaginal bleeding, and a high uterine resting tone identified by the use of an intrauterine pressure catheter. Additional signs include nonreassuring fetal heart rate patterns, signs of hypovolemic shock, and fetal death. Painless and bright red vaginal bleeding is a sign of placenta previa.
Priority Nursing Tip: It is important to know the differences between the manifestations of abruptio placentae and placenta previa. In abruptio placentae, dark red vaginal bleeding, uterine pain and/or tenderness, and uterine rigidity are characteristic. In placenta previa, there is painless, bright red vaginal bleeding, and the uterus is soft, relaxed, and nontender.
Test-Taking Strategy: Focus on the subject, manifestations of abruptio placentae. Think about the word, *abrupt*. Recalling the pathophysiology associated with this hemorrhagic condition will assist in selecting the correct options. Remember that placental abruption occurs when there is separation of the placenta and bleeding and formation of a hematoma on the maternal side of the placenta. Review: the manifestations of abruptio placentae.
Reference(s): McKinney et al (2013), pp. 585-586.

7. The nurse is caring for a client with a herniated lumbar intervertebral disk who is experiencing low back pain. Which position should the nurse place the client in to minimize the pain?
1. Flat with the knees raised
2. High Fowler's position with the foot of the bed flat
3. Semi-Fowler's position with the foot of the bed flat
4. Semi-Fowler's position with the knees slightly raised

Level of Cognitive Ability: Applying
Client Needs: Physiological Integrity
Integrated Process: Nursing Process/Implementation
Content Area: Adult Health: Neurological
Priority Concepts: Caregiving; Pain

Answer: 4
Rationale: Clients with low back pain are often more comfortable in the semi-Fowler's position with the knees raised sufficiently to flex the knees (William's position). This relaxes the muscles of the lower back and relieves pressure on the spinal nerve root. Keeping the bed flat with the knees raised would excessively stretch the lower back. Keeping the foot of the bed flat will enhance extension of the spine.
Priority Nursing Tip: A physical therapist will work with a client with a herniated lumbar intervertebral disk to develop an individualized exercise program, and the type of exercises prescribed depends on the location and nature of the injury and the type of pain. The client does not begin exercise until acute pain is reduced.
Test-Taking Strategy: Focus on the subject, a client with a herniated lumbar intervertebral disk who is experiencing low back pain. Visualize each of the positions, noting that option 4 places the least amount of pressure on the spine. Review: care of the client with a herniated lumbar intervertebral disk.
Reference(s): Ignatavicius, Workman (2013), p. 962.

8. A client with myasthenia gravis is admitted to the hospital, and the nursing history reveals that the client is taking pyridostigmine (Mestinon). When assessing the client for side effects of the medication, the nurse should ask the client about the presence of which occurrence?

1. Mouth ulcers
2. Muscle cramps
3. Feelings of depression
4. Unexplained weight gain

Level of Cognitive Ability: Applying
Client Needs: Physiological Integrity
Integrated Process: Nursing Process/Assessment
Content Area: Pharmacology: Neurological Medications
Priority Concepts: Clinical Judgment; Safety

Answer: 2
Rationale: Pyridostigmine is an acetylcholinesterase inhibitor used to treat myasthenia gravis, a neuromuscular disorder. Muscle cramps and small muscle contractions are side effects and occur as a result of overstimulation of neuromuscular receptors. Mouth ulcers, depression, and weight gain are not associated with this medication.
Priority Nursing Tip: Indicators of a therapeutic response to pyridostigmine (Mestinon) include increased muscle strength, decreased fatigue, and improved chewing and swallowing functions.
Test-Taking Strategy: Focus on the subject, the side effects of pyridostigmine (Mestinon). Recall that myasthenia gravis is a neuromuscular disorder. Select the option that is most closely associated with this disorder. This will direct you to the correct option. Review: the side effects associated with **pyridostigmine (Mestinon)**.
Reference(s): Hodgson, Kizior (2014), pp. 1004-1006.

9. A client with a fractured right ankle has a short leg cast applied in the emergency department. During discharge teaching, which information should the nurse provide to the client to prevent complications?

1. Trim the rough edges of the cast after it is dry.
2. Weight bearing on the right leg is allowed once the cast feels dry.
3. Expect burning and tingling sensations under the cast for 3 to 4 days.
4. Keep the right ankle elevated above the heart level with pillows for 24 hours.

Level of Cognitive Ability: Applying
Client Needs: Physiological Integrity
Integrated Process: Teaching and Learning
Content Area: Adult Health: Musculoskeletal
Priority Concepts: Client Education; Perfusion

Answer: 4
Rationale: Leg elevation is important to increase venous return and decrease edema. Edema can cause compartment syndrome, a major complication of fractures and casting. The client and/or family may be taught how to "petal" the cast to prevent skin irritation and breakdown, but rough edges, if trimmed, can fall into the cast and cause a break in skin integrity. Weight bearing on a fractured extremity is prescribed by the health care provider during follow-up examination, after radiographs are obtained. Additionally, a walking heel or cast shoe may be added to the cast if the client is allowed to bear weight and walk on the affected leg. Although the client may feel heat after the cast is applied, burning and/or tingling sensations indicate nerve damage or ischemia and are not expected. These complaints should be reported immediately.
Priority Nursing Tip: Circulation impairment and peripheral nerve damage can result from tightness of the cast applied to an extremity. The client needs to be taught to assess for adequate circulation, including the ability to move the area distal to the casted extremity.
Test-Taking Strategy: Focus on the subject, measures to prevent complications with a short leg cast. Recall the ABCs—airway, breathing, and circulation. Option 4 is associated with maintenance of circulation. Review: client teaching points related to **cast care**.
Reference(s): Ignatavicius, Workman (2013), pp. 1152-1153; Lewis et al (2011), p. 1601.

10. An adult client with a fractured left tibia has a long leg cast and is using crutches to ambulate. In caring for the client, the nurse assesses for which sign/symptom that indicates a complication associated with crutch walking?
1. Left leg discomfort
2. Weak biceps brachii
3. Triceps muscle spasms
4. Forearm muscle weakness

Level of Cognitive Ability: Analyzing
Client Needs: Physiological Integrity
Integrated Process: Nursing Process/Assessment
Content Area: Adult Health: Musculoskeletal
Priority Concepts: Clinical Judgment; Mobility

Answer: 4
Rationale: Forearm muscle weakness is a sign of radial nerve injury caused by crutch pressure on the axillae. When a client lacks upper body strength, especially in the flexor and extensor muscles of the arms, he or she frequently allows weight to rest on the axillae and on the crutch pads instead of using the arms for support while ambulating with crutches. Leg discomfort is expected as a result of the injury. Weak biceps brachii is not a complication of crutch walking. Triceps muscle spasms may occur as a result of increased muscle use but is not a complication of crutch walking.
Priority Nursing Tip: To prevent pressure on the axillary nerve from the use of crutches, there should be two to three finger breadths between the axilla and the top of the crutch when the crutch tip is at least 6 inches diagonally in the front of the foot. The crutch is adjusted so that the elbow is flexed no more than 30 degrees when the palm is on the handle.
Test-Taking Strategy: Focus on the subject, a complication of crutch walking. When asked about a complication of the use of crutches, think about nerve injury caused by crutch pressure on the axillae. This will direct you to option 4. Review: the complications associated with the use of **crutches**.
Reference(s): Ignatavicius, Workman (2013), pp. 1157-1158; Potter et al (2013), p. 761.

11. A client with myasthenia gravis is experiencing prolonged periods of weakness, and the health care provider prescribes an edrophonium (Enlon) test, also known as a Tensilon test. A test dose is administered and the client becomes weaker. How should the nurse interpret these results?
1. This result is a normal finding.
2. This result is a positive finding.
3. Myasthenic crisis is present.
4. Cholinergic crisis is present.

Level of Cognitive Ability: Analyzing
Client Needs: Physiological Integrity
Integrated Process: Nursing Process/Analysis
Content Area: Adult Health: Neurological
Priority Concepts: Clinical Judgment; Functional Ability

Answer: 4
Rationale: An edrophonium test may be performed to determine whether increasing weakness in a previously diagnosed myasthenic client is a result of cholinergic crisis (overmedication with anticholinesterase medications or myasthenic crisis (undermedication). Worsening of the symptoms after the test dose of medication is administered indicates a cholinergic crisis.
Priority Nursing Tip: Although rare, the edrophonium test, also known as the Tensilon test, can cause ventricular fibrillation and cardiac arrest. Atropine sulfate is the antidote for edrophonium and should be available when the test is performed in case these complications occur.
Test-Taking Strategy: Focus on the subject, a client who becomes weaker after edrophonium is administered. Recalling that edrophonium is a short-acting anticholinesterase and that the treatment for myasthenia gravis includes administration of an anticholinesterase will assist in answering the question. If the client's symptoms worsen after administration of edrophonium, then the client is likely experiencing overmedication. Review: **myasthenia gravis and the edrophonium test**.
Reference(s): Ignatavicius, Workman (2013), pp. 992-993.

❖ **12.** Tranylcypromine (Parnate) is prescribed for a client with depression. Which food items should the nurse instruct the client to avoid? **Select all that apply.**
- ❑ 1. Figs
- ❑ 2. Apples
- ❑ 3. Bananas
- ❑ 4. Broccoli
- ❑ 5. Sauerkraut
- ❑ 6. Baked chicken

Level of Cognitive Ability: Applying
Client Needs: Physiological Integrity
Integrated Process: Teaching and Learning
Content Area: Pharmacology: Psychiatric Medications
Priority Concepts: Client Education; Safety

Answer: 1, 3, 5
Rationale: Tranylcypromine is a monoamine oxidase inhibitor (MAOI). Foods that contain tyramine need to be avoided because of the risk of hypertensive crisis associated with use of this medication. Foods to avoid include figs; bananas; sauerkraut; avocados; soybeans; meats or fish that are fermented, smoked, or otherwise aged; some cheeses; yeast extract; and some beers and wine.
Priority Nursing Tip: Hypertensive crisis is characterized by an extreme increase in blood pressure resulting in an increased risk for stroke, headache, anxiety, and shortness of breath.
Test-Taking Strategy: Focus on the subject, foods to avoid with an MAOI. Focus on the name of the medication and recall that tranylcypromine is an MAOI. Next, recall the foods that contain tyramine to answer the question. Remember that figs, bananas, and sauerkraut are high in tyramine. Review: the effects of **tranylcypromine (Parnate)** and the foods high in **tyramine**.
Reference(s): Hodgson, Kizior (2014), p. 1201; Lehne (2013), p. 370.

13. The nurse notes an isolated premature ventricular contraction (PVC) on the cardiac monitor. Which action should the nurse take?
1. Prepare for defibrillation.
2. Continue to monitor the rhythm.
3. Notify the health care provider immediately.
4. Prepare to administer lidocaine hydrochloride (Xylocaine).

Level of Cognitive Ability: Applying
Client Needs: Physiological Integrity
Integrated Process: Nursing Process/Implementation
Content Area: Adult Health: Cardiovascular
Priority Concepts: Clinical Judgment; Perfusion

Answer: 2
Rationale: As an isolated occurrence, the PVC is not life threatening. In this situation, the nurse should continue to monitor the client. Frequent PVCs, however, may be precursors of more life-threatening rhythms, such as ventricular tachycardia and ventricular fibrillation. If this occurs, the health care provider needs to be notified. Defibrillation is done to treat ventricular fibrillation. Lidocaine hydrochloride is not needed to treat isolated PVCs; it may be used to treat frequent PVCs in a client who is symptomatic and is experiencing decreased cardiac output.
Priority Nursing Tip: Ventricular tachycardia can progress to ventricular fibrillation, a life-threatening condition.
Test-Taking Strategy: Focus on the subject, the action to take for an isolated PVC. This should direct you to the option that addresses continued monitoring. Also, use of the ABCs—airway, breathing, and circulation—will direct you to the correct option. Review: the implications of **premature ventricular contraction (PVC)**.
Reference(s): Ignatavicius, Workman (2013), p. 728.

14. The clinic nurse prepares to assess the fundal height on a client who is in the second trimester of pregnancy. When measuring the fundal height, what should the nurse expect to note with this measurement?
1. It is less than gestational age.
2. It correlates with gestational age.
3. It is greater than gestational age.
4. It has no correlation with gestational age.

Level of Cognitive Ability: Applying
Client Needs: Physiological Integrity
Integrated Process: Nursing Process/Assessment
Content Area: Maternity: Antepartum
Priority Concepts: Clinical Judgment; Reproduction

Answer: 2
Rationale: Until the third trimester, the measurement of fundal height will, on average, correlate with the gestational age. Therefore, options 1, 3, and 4 are incorrect.
Priority Nursing Tip: Usually a paper tape is used to measure fundal height. Consistency in performing the measurement technique is important to ensure reliability in the findings. If possible, the same person should examine the pregnant woman at each of her prenatal visits.
Test-Taking Strategy: Focus on the subject, fundal height in the second trimester. Recall the correlation of fundal height and gestational age to direct you to correct option. Review: **fundal height**.
Reference(s): McKinney et al (2013), pp. 250-251.

15. A pregnant client tells the nurse that she felt wetness on her peri-pad and found some clear fluid. The nurse inspects the perineum and notes the presence of the umbilical cord. What is the **immediate** nursing action?

1. Monitor the fetal heart rate.
2. Notify the health care provider.
3. Transfer the client to the delivery room.
4. Place the client in the Trendelenburg position.

Level of Cognitive Ability: Applying
Client Needs: Physiological Integrity
Integrated Process: Nursing Process/Implementation
Content Area: Critical Care: Emergency Situations
Priority Concepts: Clinical Judgment; Reproduction

Answer: 4
Rationale: On inspection of the perineum, if the umbilical cord is noted, the nurse immediately places the client in the Trendelenburg position while gently holding the presenting part upward to relieve the cord compression. This position is maintained and the health care provider is notified. The fetal heart rate also needs to be monitored to assess for fetal distress. The client is transferred to the delivery room when prescribed by the health care provider.
Priority Nursing Tip: Relieving cord compression is the priority goal if the umbilical cord is protruding from the vagina. The nurse never attempts to push the cord back into the vagina.
Test-Taking Strategy: Note the strategic word, *immediate*, which indicates the immediate action on the nurse's part to prevent or relieve cord compression. The only action that will achieve this is option 4. Review: **prolapsed umbilical cord.**
Reference(s): McKinney et al (2013), pp. 659-660.

16. The nurse admits a newborn to the nursery. On assessment of the newborn, the nurse palpates the anterior fontanel and notes that it feels soft. The nurse determines that this finding indicates which condition?

1. Dehydration
2. A normal finding
3. Increased intracranial pressure
4. Decreased intracranial pressure

Level of Cognitive Ability: Applying
Client Needs: Physiological Integrity
Integrated Process: Nursing Process/Assessment
Content Area: Maternity: Newborn
Priority Concepts: Clinical Judgment; Development

Answer: 2
Rationale: The anterior fontanel is normally 2 to 3 cm in width, 3 to 4 cm in length, and diamond-like in shape. It can be described as soft, which is normal, or full and bulging, which could indicate increased intracranial pressure. Conversely a depressed fontanel could mean that the infant is dehydrated.
Priority Nursing Tip: The anterior fontanel is a diamond-shaped area where the frontal and parietal bones meet. It closes between 12 and 18 months of age. Vigorous crying may cause the fontanel to bulge, which is a normal finding.
Test-Taking Strategy: Focus on the subject, an anterior fontanel that is soft. Recalling the normal physiological finding in the newborn will direct you to the correct option. Review: **normal newborn findings.**
Reference(s): Hockenberry, Wilson (2013), pp. 195-196; Potter et al (2013), p. 141.

17. A client with acquired immunodeficiency syndrome (AIDS) is admitted to the hospital for chills, fever, nonproductive cough, and pleuritic chest pain. A diagnosis of *Pneumocystis jiroveci* pneumonia is made, and the client is started on intravenous (IV) pentamidine (Pentam 300). What should the nurse plan to do to safely administer the medication?

1. Infuse over 1 hour and allow the client to ambulate.
2. Infuse over 1 hour with the client in a supine position.
3. Administer over 30 minutes with the client in a reclining position.
4. Administer by IV push over 15 minutes with the client in a supine position.

Level of Cognitive Ability: Applying
Client Needs: Physiological Integrity
Integrated Process: Nursing Process/Planning
Content Area: Adult Health: Immune
Priority Concepts: Clinical Judgment; Safety

Answer: 2
Rationale: Intravenous pentamidine is infused over 1 hour with the client supine to minimize severe hypotension and dysrhythmias. Options 1, 3, and 4 are inaccurate in either the length of time that pentamidine is administered or the client's position.
Priority Nursing Tip: During the administration of intravenous (IV) pentamidine (Pentam 300) the client should remain supine and the nurse should monitor the blood pressure for hypotension and the cardiac pattern for dysrhythmias.
Test-Taking Strategy: Focus on the subject, the procedure for administering pentamidine (Pentam 300). Eliminate options 3 and 4 first because these time frames are short for an IV medication. From the remaining options, recalling that the medication causes hypotension will direct you to option 2, which addresses both the supine position and the longest time of administration. Review: the procedure for administering intravenous (IV) **pentamidine (Pentam 300).**
Reference(s): Gahart, Nazareno (2012), p. 1083; Hodgson, Kizior (2014), pp. 930-931.

18. The nurse is caring for a client who has been transferred to the surgical unit after a pelvic exenteration. During the postoperative period, the client complains of pain in the calf area. What action should the nurse take?
1. Ask the client to walk and observe the gait.
2. Lightly massage the calf area to relieve the pain.
3. Check the calf area for temperature, color, and size.
4. Administer PRN morphine sulfate as prescribed for postoperative pain.

Level of Cognitive Ability: Applying
Client Needs: Physiological Integrity
Integrated Process: Nursing Process/Implementation
Content Area: Fundamental Skills: Perioperative Care
Priority Concepts: Clinical Judgment; Clotting

Answer: 3
Rationale: The nurse monitors the postoperative client for complications such as deep vein thrombosis, pulmonary emboli, and wound infection. Pain in the calf area could indicate a deep vein thrombosis. Change in color, temperature, or size of the client's calf could also indicate this complication. Options 1 and 2 could result in an embolus if in fact the client had a deep vein thrombosis. Administering pain medication for this client complaint is not the appropriate nursing action. Further assessment needs to take place.
Priority Nursing Tip: The primary signs of deep vein thrombosis are calf or groin tenderness and pain and sudden onset of unilateral swelling of the leg.
Test-Taking Strategy: Focus on the information in the question and use the steps of the nursing process. Assessment is the first step. Option 3 is the only option that addresses assessment. Review: pelvic exenteration and deep vein thrombosis.
Reference(s): Ignatavicius, Workman (2013), pp. 799-800; Lewis et al (2011), p. 1370.

19. A health care provider prescribes acetaminophen (Tylenol) liquid, 450 mg orally every 4 hours PRN for pain. The medication label reads: 160 mg/5 mL. The nurse prepares how many milliliters (mL) to administer one dose? **Fill in the blank.**
Answer: _____ mL

Level of Cognitive Ability: Applying
Client Needs: Physiological Integrity
Integrated Process: Nursing Process/Implementation
Content Area: Fundamental Skills: Medication/IV Calculations
Priority Concepts: Clinical Judgment; Safety

Answer: 14 mL
Rationale: Use the formula for calculating medication dosages.
Formula:
$$\frac{\text{Desired} \times \text{Volume}}{\text{Available}} = \text{mL per dose}$$
$$\frac{450\,\text{mg} \times 5\,\text{mL}}{160\,\text{mg}} = 14\,\text{mL}$$

Priority Nursing Tip: After performing a medication calculation, make sure that the amount calculated is a reasonable amount.
Test-Taking Strategy: Focus on the subject, a medication calculation. Identify the components of the question and what the question is asking. In this case, the question asks for milliliters per dose. Set up the formula knowing that the desired dose is 450 mg and that what is available is 160 mg per 5 mL. Verify the answer using a calculator and be sure that the answer makes sense. Review: medication calculations.
Reference(s): Potter et al (2013), pp. 574-577.

20. The nurse is performing an assessment on a client with a diagnosis of chronic angina pectoris who is receiving sotalol (Betapace) 80 mg orally twice daily. Which assessment finding indicates that the client is experiencing an adverse effect of the medication?
1. Dry mouth
2. Palpitations
3. Diaphoresis
4. Difficulty swallowing

Level of Cognitive Ability: Analyzing
Client Needs: Physiological Integrity
Integrated Process: Nursing Process/Assessment
Content Area: Pharmacology: Cardiovascular Medications
Priority Concepts: Clinical Judgment; Safety

Answer: 2
Rationale: Sotalol is a beta-adrenergic blocking agent. Adverse effects include palpitations, bradycardia, an irregular heartbeat, difficulty breathing, signs of heart failure, and cold hands and feet. Gastrointestinal disturbances, anxiety and nervousness, and unusual tiredness and weakness can also occur. Options 1, 3, and 4 are not adverse effects of this medication.
Priority Nursing Tip: For the client taking a beta-adrenergic blocking agent, monitor the blood pressure for hypotension and the apical pulse rate for bradycardia. If the client's blood pressure is lower that the client's baseline or the heart rate is below 60 beats per minute, notify the health care provider before administration.
Test-Taking Strategy: Focus on the subject, adverse effects of sotalol. Note that the question presents a client with chronic angina pectoris, a cardiac disorder. Remember that medication names ending with the letters -lol (sotalol) are beta blockers, which are commonly used for cardiac disorders. Note that option 2 is the only option that is directly cardiac related. Review: the adverse effects of sotalol (Betapace).
Reference(s): Hodgson, Kizior (2014), pp. 1100-1102.

21. Which action should the nurse take before performing a venipuncture to initiate continuous intravenous (IV) therapy?
1. Apply a cool compress to the affected area.
2. Inspect the IV solution and expiration date.
3. Secure a padded armboard above the IV site.
4. Apply a tourniquet below the venipuncture site.

Level of Cognitive Ability: Applying
Client Needs: Physiological Integrity
Integrated Process: Nursing Process/Implementation
Content Area: Fundamental Skills: Safety
Priority Concepts: Clinical Judgment; Safety

Answer: 2
Rationale: IV solutions should be free of particles or precipitates to prevent trauma to veins or a thromboembolic event; in addition, the nurse avoids administering IV solutions whose expiration date has passed to prevent infection. Cool compresses cause vasoconstriction, making the vein less visible, smaller, and more difficult to puncture. Arm boards are applied after the IV is started and are used only if necessary. A tourniquet is applied above the chosen vein site to halt venous return and engorge the vein; this makes the vein easier to puncture.
Priority Nursing Tip: Administration of an IV solution provides immediate access to the vascular system. Check the health care provider's prescription and ensure that the correct solution and flow rate are administered as prescribed.
Test-Taking Strategy: Note the word "before" and use the steps of the nursing process. Option 2 is the only option that reflects assessment, the first step of the nursing process. Review: nursing interventions related to **initiating an IV.**
Reference(s): Potter et al (2013), pp. 918-919.

22. The nurse is caring for a client who had an allogenic liver transplant and is receiving tacrolimus (Prograf) daily. Which finding indicates to the nurse that the client is experiencing an adverse effect of the medication?
1. Hypotension
2. Photophobia
3. Profuse sweating
4. Decrease in urine output

Level of Cognitive Ability: Analyzing
Client Needs: Physiological Integrity
Integrated Process: Nursing Process/Assessment
Content Area: Pharmacology: Cardiovascular
Priority Concepts: Clinical Judgment; Safety

Answer: 4
Rationale: Tacrolimus is an immunosuppressant medication used in the prophylaxis of organ rejection in clients receiving allogenic liver transplants. Adverse reactions and toxic effects include nephrotoxicity and pleural effusion. Nephrotoxicity is characterized by an increasing serum creatinine level and a decrease in urine output. Frequent side effects include headache, tremor, insomnia, paresthesia, diarrhea, nausea, constipation, vomiting, abdominal pain, and hypertension.
Priority Nursing Tip: Assess the renal status of the client before administering tacrolimus (Prograf) because the medication is nephrotoxic.
Test-Taking Strategy: Focus on the subject, an adverse effect of tacrolimus (Prograf). First, determine the medication classification. Note the client's diagnosis and look at the medication name, Prograf (*pro-* meaning "for" and *-graf* meaning "graft") to identify the action of the medication, which is to prevent transplant rejection. This will assist in identifying the medication classification as immunosuppressant. Next, recalling that nephrotoxicity is an adverse effect of the medication will direct you to the correct option. Review: **tacrolimus (Prograf).**
Reference(s): Hodgson, Kizior (2014), p. 1120.

23. A client was admitted to the hospital 24 hours ago after sustaining blunt chest trauma. Which **earliest** clinical manifestation of acute respiratory distress syndrome (ARDS) should the nurse monitor for?
1. Cyanosis and pallor
2. Diffuse crackles and rhonchi on chest auscultation
3. Increase in respiratory rate from 18 to 30 breaths per minute
4. Haziness or "white-out" appearance of lungs on chest radiograph

Level of Cognitive Ability: Analyzing
Client Needs: Physiological Integrity
Integrated Process: Nursing Process/Assessment
Content Area: Adult Health: Respiratory
Priority Concepts: Clinical Judgment; Gas Exchange

Answer: 3
Rationale: ARDS usually develops within 24 to 48 hours after an initiating event, such as chest trauma. In most cases, tachypnea and dyspnea are the earliest clinical manifestations as the body compensates for mild hypoxemia through hyperventilation. Cyanosis and pallor are late findings and are the result of severe hypoxemia. Breath sounds in the early stages of ARDS are usually clear but then progress to diffuse crackles and rhonchi as pulmonary edema occurs. Chest radiographic findings may be normal during the early stages but will show diffuse haziness or "white-out" appearance in the later stages.
Priority Nursing Tip: If the client sustains a chest injury, assess the respiratory status of the client. This assessment is followed by the treatment of life-threatening conditions.
Test-Taking Strategy: Note the strategic word, *earliest*. Remember that with ARDS initial presenting symptoms are tachypnea, dyspnea, and restlessness as hypoxia develops. Knowing the definition of tachypnea and possible etiologies will direct you to the correct option. Review: the early clinical manifestations of **acute respiratory distress syndrome (ARDS).**
Reference(s): Ignatavicius, Workman (2013), pp. 671-672; Lewis et al (2011), pp. 1758-1759.

24. The nurse is caring for a client with Buck's traction and is monitoring the client for complications of the traction. Which assessment finding indicates a complication?
1. Weak pedal pulses
2. Drainage at the pin sites
3. Complaints of discomfort
4. Warm toes with brisk capillary refill

Level of Cognitive Ability: Analyzing
Client Needs: Physiological Integrity
Integrated Process: Nursing Process/Assessment
Content Area: Adult Health: Musculoskeletal
Priority Concepts: Mobility; Perfusion

Answer: 1
Rationale: Buck's traction is skin traction. Weak pedal pulses are a sign of vascular compromise, which can be caused by pressure on the tissues of the leg by the elastic bandage or prefabricated boot used to secure this type of traction. Skeletal (not skin) traction uses pins. Discomfort is expected. Warm toes with brisk capillary refill is a normal finding.
Priority Nursing Tip: If the client in traction exhibits signs of neurovascular compromise such as changes in temperature, sensation, or the ability to move digits of the affected extremity, the health care provider is notified immediately.
Test-Taking Strategy: Use the ABCs—airway, breathing, and circulation—to direct you to option 1, indicative of vascular compromise. Also eliminate option 2 because Buck's traction does not use pins. Options 3 and 4 can be eliminated because they are comparable and alike and are both normal findings. Review: care of the client with **Buck's traction.**
Reference(s): Ignatavicius, Workman (2013), pp. 1153-1154.

25. A prenatal client has been diagnosed with a vaginal infection from the organism *Candida albicans*. What should the nurse expect to note on assessment of the client?
1. Costovertebral angle pain
2. Pain, itching, and vaginal discharge
3. Absence of any signs and symptoms
4. Proteinuria, hematuria, and hypertension

Level of Cognitive Ability: Analyzing
Client Needs: Physiological Integrity
Integrated Process: Nursing Process/Assessment
Content Area: Maternity: Antepartum
Priority Concepts: Infection; Sexuality

Answer: 2
Rationale: Clinical manifestations of a *Candida* infection include pain; itching; and a thick, white vaginal discharge. Proteinuria and hypertension are signs of preeclampsia. Costovertebral angle pain, proteinuria, and hematuria are clinical manifestations associated with upper urinary tract infections.
Priority Nursing Tip: *Candida albicans* is a fungal infection of the skin and mucous membranes. Common areas of occurrence include the mucous membranes of the mouth, perineum, vagina, axilla, and under the breasts.
Test-Taking Strategy: Focus on the subject, vaginal infection. Note the relationship between the subject and option 2. Review: the signs of a **vaginal *Candida albicans* infection.**
Reference(s): Lowdermilk, Perry, Cashion, Alden (2012), p. 161; McKinney et al (2013), pp. 235-236.

26. A prenatal client is suspected of having iron deficiency anemia. On assessment, which finding should the nurse expect to note regarding the client's status?
1. Dehydration
2. Overhydration
3. A high hematocrit level
4. A low hemoglobin level

Level of Cognitive Ability: Applying
Client Needs: Physiological Integrity
Integrated Process: Nursing Process/Assessment
Content Area: Adult Health: Hematological
Priority Concepts: Cellular Regulation; Reproduction

Answer: 4
Rationale: Pathological anemia of pregnancy is primarily caused by iron deficiency. When the hemoglobin level is below 11 mg/dL, iron deficiency is suspected. An indirect index of the oxygen-carrying capacity is determined via a packed red blood cell volume or hematocrit level. Dehydration and overhydration are not specifically associated with iron deficiency anemia.
Priority Nursing Tip: The ferritin level is a laboratory test that is used to diagnose iron deficiency anemia. A ferritin level of less than 10 to 15 mcg/L confirms the diagnosis.
Test-Taking Strategy: Focus on the subject, manifestations of iron deficiency anemia. Note the relationship between the words "deficiency" in the diagnosis and "low" in the correct option. Review: the manifestations of iron deficiency anemia.
Reference(s): Lowdermilk, Perry, Cashion, Alden (2012), pp. 314-315; McKinney et al (2013), pp. 621-622.

27. The nurse is caring for a postpartum client. Which finding should make the nurse suspect endometritis in this client?
1. Breast engorgement
2. Elevated white blood cell count
3. Lochia rubra on the second day postpartum
4. Fever over 38° C, beginning 2 days postpartum

Level of Cognitive Ability: Analyzing
Client Needs: Physiological Integrity
Integrated Process: Nursing Process/Assessment
Content Area: Maternity: Postpartum
Priority Concepts: Infection; Reproduction

Answer: 4
Rationale: Endometritis is a common cause of postpartum infection. The presence of fever of 38° C or more on 2 successive days of the first 10 postpartum days (not counting the first 24 hours after birth) is indicative of a postpartum infection. Breast engorgement is a normal response in the postpartum period and is not associated with endometritis. The white blood cell count of a postpartum woman is normally elevated; thus, this method of detecting infection is not of great value in the puerperium. Lochia rubra on the second day postpartum is a normal finding.
Priority Nursing Tip: A postpartum infection may also be termed a puerperal infection and is described as an infection of the genital canal that occurs within 28 days after a miscarriage, induced abortion, or childbirth.
Test-Taking Strategy: Focus on the subject, endometritis. Recalling the normal findings in the postpartum period will assist in eliminating options 1, 2, and 3. Review: the signs of endometritis.
Reference(s): McKinney et al (2013), pp. 678-679.

28. The nurse is performing an assessment on a postterm infant. Which physical characteristic should the nurse expect to observe in this infant?
1. Peeling of the skin
2. Smooth soles without creases
3. Lanugo covering the entire body
4. Vernix that covers the body in a thick layer

Level of Cognitive Ability: Analyzing
Client Needs: Physiological Integrity
Integrated Process: Nursing Process/Assessment
Content Area: Maternity: Newborn
Priority Concepts: Development; Health Promotion

Answer: 1
Rationale: The postterm infant (born after the 42nd week of gestation) exhibits dry, peeling, cracked, almost leatherlike skin over the body, which is called desquamation. The preterm infant (born between 24 and 37 weeks of gestation) exhibits smooth soles without creases, lanugo covering the entire body, and thick vernix covering the body.
Priority Nursing Tip: The postterm infant may exhibit meconium staining on the fingernails, long nails and hair, and the absence of vernix.
Test-Taking Strategy: Focus on the subject, the postterm infant. Think about the physiology associated with the postterm infant. Recalling that the postterm infant is born after the 42nd week of gestation will assist in directing you to the correct option. Review: the characteristics of preterm and postterm infants.
Reference(s): McKinney et al (2013), pp. 710-711.

29. A postterm infant, delivered vaginally, is exhibiting tachypnea, grunting, retractions, and nasal flaring. The nurse interprets that these assessment findings are indicative of which condition?
1. Hypoglycemia
2. Respiratory distress syndrome
3. Meconium aspiration syndrome
4. Transient tachypnea of the newborn

Level of Cognitive Ability: Analyzing
Client Needs: Physiological Integrity
Integrated Process: Nursing Process/Analysis
Content Area: Maternity: Newborn
Priority Concepts: Development; Gas Exchange

Answer: 3
Rationale: Tachypnea, grunting, retractions, and nasal flaring are symptoms of respiratory distress related to meconium aspiration syndrome (MAS). MAS occurs often in postterm infants and develops when meconium in the amniotic fluid enters the lungs during fetal life or at birth. The symptoms noted in the question are unrelated to hypoglycemia. Respiratory distress syndrome is a complication of preterm infants. Transient tachypnea of the newborn is primarily found in infants delivered via cesarean section.
Priority Nursing Tip: The health care provider is notified if meconium is noted in the amniotic fluid during labor. Although meconium is sterile, aspiration can lead to lung damage, which promotes the growth of bacteria; thus, the newborn needs to be closely monitored for infection.
Test-Taking Strategy: Focus on the subject, a postterm infant and note the symptoms identified in the question. Option 1 is eliminated first because hypoglycemia is not a respiratory condition. From the remaining options, recalling the complications that can occur in a postterm infant will direct you to the correct option. Review: the complications that can occur in the **postterm infant**.
Reference(s): McKinney et al (2013), pp. 719-720.

30. The nurse is caring for a client who had an orthopedic injury of the leg requiring surgery and application of a cast. Postoperatively, which nursing assessment is of **highest priority**?
1. Monitoring for heel breakdown
2. Monitoring for bladder distention
3. Monitoring for extremity shortening
4. Monitoring for loss of blanching ability of toe nail beds

Level of Cognitive Ability: Analyzing
Client Needs: Physiological Integrity
Integrated Process: Nursing Process/Assessment
Content Area: Adult Health: Musculoskeletal
Priority Concepts: Mobility; Perfusion

Answer: 4
Rationale: With cast application, concern for compartment syndrome development is of the highest priority. If postsurgical edema compromises circulation, the client will demonstrate numbness, tingling, loss of blanching of toenail beds, and pain that will not be relieved by opioids. Although heel breakdown, bladder distention, or extremity lengthening or shortening can occur, these complications are not potentially life-threatening complications.
Priority Nursing Tip: Monitor the client with a cast for early signs of compartment syndrome. Assess the client for the "six Ps," which include pain, pressure, paralysis, paresthesia, pallor, and pulselessness.
Test-Taking Strategy: Note the strategic words, *highest priority.* Use the ABCs—airway, breathing, and circulation—to answer the question. Assessment for circulation to the foot, including observations for numbness and tingling and the ability of the nail beds to blanch, will direct you to the correct option. Review: **compartment syndrome**.
Reference(s): Ignatavicius, Workman (2013), pp. 1145-1146.

❖ **31.** The nurse is sending an arterial blood gas (ABG) specimen to the laboratory for analysis. Which pieces of information should the nurse write on the laboratory requisition? **Select all that apply.**
- ❑ 1. Ventilator settings
- ❑ 2. A list of client allergies
- ❑ 3. The client's temperature
- ❑ 4. The date and time the specimen was drawn
- ❑ 5. Any supplemental oxygen the client is receiving
- ❑ 6. Extremity from which the specimen was obtained

Level of Cognitive Ability: Applying
Client Needs: Physiological Integrity
Integrated Process: Communication and Documentation
Content Area: Fundamental Skills: Diagnostic Tests
Priority Concepts: Clinical Judgment; Communication

Answer: 1, 3, 4, 5
Rationale: An ABG requisition usually contains information about the date and time the specimen was drawn, the client's temperature, whether the specimen was drawn on room air or using supplemental oxygen, and the ventilator settings if the client is on a mechanical ventilator. The client's allergies and the extremity from which the specimen was drawn do not have a direct bearing on the laboratory results.
Priority Nursing Tip: An arterial blood gas (ABG) specimen must be transported to the laboratory for processing within 15 minutes from the time that it was obtained.
Test-Taking Strategy: Focus on the subject, procedures for preparing an arterial blood gas draw. Review the pieces of information from the viewpoint of the relevance of the item to the client's airway status or oxygen use. The only pieces of information that do not relate to airway status or oxygen use are the client's allergies and the extremity from which the specimen was drawn. Review: the procedure related to drawing an **arterial blood gas (ABG)**.
Reference(s): Chernecky, Berger (2013), pp. 212-213; Pagana, Pagana (2013), pp. 117-118.

32. The nurse is caring for a client with hypertension receiving torsemide (Demadex) 5 mg orally daily. What value should indicate to the nurse that the client might be experiencing an adverse effect of the medication?
1. A chloride level of 98 mEq/L
2. A sodium level of 135 mEq/L
3. A potassium level of 3.1 mEq/L
4. A blood urea nitrogen (BUN) level of 15 mg/dL

Level of Cognitive Ability: Analyzing
Client Needs: Physiological Integrity
Integrated Process: Nursing Process/Analysis
Content Area: Pharmacology; Cardiovascular Medications
Priority Concepts: Clinical Judgment; Fluid and Electrolyte Balance

Answer: 3
Rationale: Torsemide (Demadex) is a loop diuretic. The medication can produce acute, profound water loss; volume and electrolyte depletion; dehydration; decreased blood volume; and circulatory collapse. Option 3 is the only option that indicates electrolyte depletion because the normal potassium level is 3.5 to 5.0 mEq/L. The normal chloride level is 98 to 107 mEq/L. The normal sodium level is 135 to 145 mEq/L. The normal BUN level ranges from 8 to 25 mg/dL.
Priority Nursing Tip: Nursing interventions for a client taking a loop diuretic include monitoring the blood pressure, weight, intake and output, and serum electrolytes (especially potassium), and assessing the client for any hearing abnormality.
Test-Taking Strategy: Focus on the subject, adverse effects of torsemide (Demadex). Recall knowledge of normal laboratory values to assist in selecting option 3, which is the only abnormal laboratory value presented. Review: **normal laboratory values** and the side effects and adverse effects of **torsemide (Demadex)**.
Reference(s): Hodgson, Kizior (2014), p. 1194; Potter et al (2013), p. 883.

33. During history taking of a client admitted with newly diagnosed Hodgkin's disease, which symptom should the nurse expect the client to report?
1. Weight gain
2. Night sweats
3. Severe lymph node pain
4. Headache with minor visual changes

Level of Cognitive Ability: Analyzing
Client Needs: Physiological Integrity
Integrated Process: Nursing Process/Assessment
Content Area: Adult Health: Oncology
Priority Concepts: Cellular Regulation; Clinical Judgment

Answer: 2
Rationale: Assessment of a client with Hodgkin's disease most often reveals night sweats, enlarged, painless lymph nodes, fever, and malaise. Weight loss may be present if metastatic disease occurs. Headache and visual changes may occur if brain metastasis is present.
Priority Nursing Tip: The most common assessment finding in Hodgkin's disease is the presence of a large and painless lymph node(s), often located in the neck. Biopsy of the node reveals the presence of Reed-Sternberg cells.
Test-Taking Strategy: Focus on the subject, symptoms associated with Hodgkin's disease. Eliminate options 3 and 4 first because they are comparable or alike in that they relate to discomfort. Weight gain is rarely the symptom of a cancer diagnosis, so eliminate option 1. Review: content related to **Hodgkin's disease**.
Reference(s): Ignatavicius, Workman (2013), pp. 892-893.

34. The nurse is assessing a 3-day-old preterm neonate with a diagnosis of respiratory distress syndrome (RDS). Which assessment finding indicates that the neonate's respiratory status is improving?
1. Edema of the hands and feet
2. Urine output of 3 mL/kg/hour
3. Presence of a systolic murmur
4. Respiratory rate between 60 and 70 breaths per minute

Level of Cognitive Ability: Evaluating
Client Needs: Physiological Integrity
Integrated Process: Nursing Process/Evaluation
Content Area: Maternity: Newborn
Priority Concepts: Clinical Judgment; Gas Exchange

Answer: 2
Rationale: RDS is a serious lung disorder caused by immaturity and the inability to produce surfactant, resulting in hypoxia and acidosis. Lung fluid, which occurs in RDS, moves from the lungs into the bloodstream as the condition improves and the alveoli open. This extra fluid circulates to the kidneys, which results in increased voiding. Therefore, normal urination is an early sign that the neonate's respiratory condition is improving (normal urinary output is 2 to 5 mL/kg/hour). Edema of the hands and feet occurs within the first 24 hours after the development of RDS as a result of low protein concentrations, a decrease in colloidal osmotic pressure, and transudation of fluid from the vascular system to the tissues. Systolic murmurs usually indicate the presence of a patent ductus arteriosus, which is a common complication of RDS. Respiratory rates above 60 are indicative of tachypnea, which is a sign of respiratory distress.
Priority Nursing Tip: Surfactant replacement therapy is used to treat respiratory distress syndrome. The surfactant is instilled into the endotracheal tube.
Test-Taking Strategy: Note the subject, preterm neonate with a diagnosis of RDS. Option 2 is the only normal finding and indicates a normal urine output, which would indicate resolution of excess lung fluid. Review: the pathophysiology related to **respiratory distress syndrome (RDS)**.
Reference(s): McKinney et al (2013), p. 695.

35. The nurse is caring for a term newborn. Which assessment finding would predispose the newborn to the occurrence of jaundice?
1. Presence of a cephalhematoma
2. Infant blood type of O negative
3. Birth weight of 8 pounds 6 ounces
4. A negative direct Coombs' test result

Level of Cognitive Ability: Analyzing
Client Needs: Physiological Integrity
Integrated Process: Nursing Process/Assessment
Content Area: Maternity: Newborn
Priority Concepts: Clinical Judgment; Development

Answer: 1
Rationale: A cephalhematoma is swelling caused by bleeding into an area between the bone and its periosteum (does not cross over the suture line). Enclosed hemorrhage, such as with cephalhematoma, predisposes the newborn to jaundice by producing an increased bilirubin load as the cephalhematoma resolves (usually within 6 weeks) and is absorbed into the circulatory system. The classic Rh incompatibility situation involves an Rh-negative mother with an Rh-positive fetus/newborn. The birth weight in option 3 is within the acceptable range for a term newborn and therefore does not contribute to an increased bilirubin level. A negative direct Coombs' test result indicates that there are no maternal antibodies on fetal erythrocytes.
Priority Nursing Tip: Normal or physiological jaundice appears after the first 24 hours in a full-term newborn. Jaundice occurring before this time is known as pathological jaundice and warrants health care provider notification.
Test-Taking Strategy: Focus on the subject, a term newborn's predisposition to jaundice. Recalling the risk factors associated with jaundice and the association between hemorrhage and jaundice will direct you to the correct option. Review: the risk factors associated with **newborn jaundice.**
Reference(s): Hockenberry, Wilson (2013), pp. 229-230, 256; McKinney et al (2013), p. 487.

36. Which assessment is **most important** for the nurse to make before advancing a client from liquid to solid food?
1. Bowel sounds
2. Chewing ability
3. Current appetite
4. Food preferences

Level of Cognitive Ability: Applying
Client Needs: Physiological Integrity
Integrated Process: Nursing Process/Assessment
Content Area: Fundamental Skills: Nutrition
Priority Concepts: Nutrition; Safety

Answer: 2
Rationale: The nurse needs to assess the client's chewing ability before advancing a client from liquid to solid food. It may be necessary to modify a client's diet to a soft or mechanical chopped diet if the client has difficulty chewing because of the risk of aspiration. Bowel sounds should be present before introducing any diet, including liquids. Appetite will affect the amount of food eaten, but not the type of diet prescribed. Food preferences should be ascertained on admission assessment.
Priority Nursing Tip: The consistency of food should be altered based on the client's ability to chew or swallow. Liquid can be added to food to alter its consistency, but the liquid used should complement the food and its original flavor.
Test-Taking Strategy: Focus on the strategic words, *most important.* Also, focusing on the subject, advancing a diet from liquid to solid, will direct you to the correct option because the primary difference between a liquid and a solid diet is that the food needs mechanical processing (chewing) before it can be safely swallowed. Review: nursing considerations related to a **liquid diet** and a **solid diet.**
Reference(s): Perry, Potter, Ostendorf (2014), pp. 765, 767; Potter et al (2013), pp. 1026-1027.

37. The nurse is caring for a client who is in the active stage of labor. The nurse is monitoring the fetal status and notes that the monitor strip shows a late deceleration. Based on this observation, which action should the nurse plan to take **immediately**?
1. Document the findings.
2. Prepare for immediate birth.
3. Administer oxygen via face mask.
4. Increase the rate of an oxytocin (Pitocin) infusion.

Level of Cognitive Ability: Analyzing
Client Needs: Physiological Integrity
Integrated Process: Nursing Process/Implementation
Content Area: Maternity: Intrapartum
Priority Concepts: Perfusion; Reproduction

Answer: 3
Rationale: Late decelerations are caused by uteroplacental insufficiency as the result of decreased blood flow and oxygen transfer to the fetus through the intervillous space during the uterine contractions. This causes hypoxemia; therefore, oxygen is necessary. Although the finding needs to be documented, documentation is not the priority action in this situation. Late decelerations are considered an ominous sign but do not necessarily require immediate birth of the baby. The oxytocin infusion should be discontinued when a late deceleration is noted. The oxytocin would cause further hypoxemia because the medication stimulates contractions and leads to increased uteroplacental insufficiency.
Priority Nursing Tip: Late decelerations are nonreassuring patterns that reflect impaired placental exchange or uteroplacental insufficiency. The patterns look similar to early decelerations, but they begin well after the contraction begins and return to baseline after the contraction ends.
Test-Taking Strategy: Note the strategic word, *immediately.* Use the ABCs—airway, breathing, and circulation—to direct you to option 3. Review: **late decelerations.**
Reference(s): McKinney et al (2013), pp. 376-377.

38. The nurse is caring for an obese client on a weight loss program. Which method should the nurse use to **most** accurately assess the program's **effectiveness**?
1. Weigh the client.
2. Monitor intake and output.
3. Check serum protein levels.
4. Calculate daily caloric intake.

Level of Cognitive Ability: Evaluating
Client Needs: Physiological Integrity
Integrated Process: Nursing Process/Evaluation
Content Area: Fundamental Skills: Nutrition
Priority Concepts: Clinical Judgment; Nutrition

Answer: 1
Rationale: The most accurate measurement of weight loss is weighing of the client. This should be done at the same time of the day, in the same clothes, and using the same scale. Options 2, 3, and 4 measure nutrition and hydration status.
Priority Nursing Tip: Clothing and shoes affect the obtained weight measurement. It is important to make a notation about any clothing, shoes, accessories (heavy jewelry), or other items such as casts or braces worn by the client while obtaining the weight.
Test-Taking Strategy: Focus on the subject, weight loss, and note the strategic words, *most* and *effectiveness*. Assessing weight will most accurately identify weight changes. Also note that options 2, 3, and 4 are comparable or alike and measure nutrition and hydration status. Review: care of the client on a **weight loss** program.
Reference(s): Perry, Potter, Ostendorf (2014), pp. 761-762.

39. A client has fallen and sustained a leg injury. Which question should the nurse ask the client to help determine if the client sustained a fracture from the fall?
1. "Is the pain a dull ache?"
2. "Is the pain sharp and continuous?"
3. "Does the discomfort feel like a cramp?"
4. "Does the pain feel like the muscle was stretched?"

Level of Cognitive Ability: Applying
Client Needs: Physiological Integrity
Integrated Process: Nursing Process/Assessment
Content Area: Fundamental Skills: Pain
Priority Concepts: Mobility; Pain

Answer: 2
Rationale: Fracture pain is generally described as sharp, continuous, and increasing in frequency. Bone pain is often described as a dull, deep ache. Muscle injury is often described as an aching or cramping pain, or soreness. Strains result from trauma to a muscle body or the attachment of a tendon from overstretching or overextension.
Priority Nursing Tip: Some fractures can be identified on inspection and exhibit manifestations such as an obvious deformity, edema, and bruising; others are detected only on x-ray examination.
Test-Taking Strategy: Focus on the subject, manifestations of a fracture. Recalling that pain from a new injury such as a fracture is more likely to be described as sharp will direct you to the correct option. Review: the clinical manifestations of a **fracture**.
Reference(s): Ignatavicius, Workman (2013), p. 1149; Perry, Potter, Ostendorf (2014), p. 256.

40. Which arterial blood gases (ABGs) values should the nurse anticipate in the client with a nasogastric tube attached to continuous suction?
1. pH 7.25, Pco_2 55, HCO_3 24
2. pH 7.30, Pco_2 38, HCO_3 20
3. pH 7.48, Pco_2 30, HCO_3 23
4. pH 7.49, Pco_2 38, HCO_3 30

Level of Cognitive Ability: Analyzing
Client Needs: Physiological Integrity
Integrated Process: Nursing Process/Analysis
Content Area: Fundamental Skills: Acid-Base
Priority Concepts: Acid-Base Balance; Clinical Judgment

Answer: 4
Rationale: The anticipated ABG finding in the client with a nasogastric tube to continuous suction is metabolic alkalosis resulting from loss of acid. In uncompensated metabolic alkalosis, the pH will be elevated (greater than 7.45), bicarbonate will be elevated (greater than 27 mEq/mL), and the Pco_2 will most likely be within normal limits (35 to 45 mm Hg). Therefore, options 1, 2, and 3 are incorrect.
Priority Nursing Tip: The normal pH is 7.35 to 7.45. A pH level below 7.35 indicates an acidotic condition. A pH greater than 7.45 indicates an alkalotic condition.
Test-Taking Strategy: Focus on the subject, the acid-base imbalance that occurs in a client with continuous nasogastric suctioning. Note that the question addresses a gastrointestinal situation. Eliminate options 1 and 3 because they both identify a respiratory imbalance (opposite effects between the pH and the Pco_2). From the remaining options, remember that acid will be removed with nasogastric suctioning, so an alkalotic condition will result. This will direct you to the correct option. Review: **arterial blood gas (ABG)** and **nasogastric suctioning**.
Reference(s): Ignatavicius, Workman (2013), p. 207; Potter et al (2013), p. 894.

41. The nurse obtains a finger-stick glucose reading of 425 mg/dL on a client who was recently started on total parenteral nutrition (TPN). Which action should the nurse take at this time?
1. Stop the TPN.
2. Administer insulin.
3. Notify the health care provider.
4. Decrease the flow rate of the TPN.

Level of Cognitive Ability: Applying
Client Needs: Physiological Integrity
Integrated Process: Nursing Process/Implementation
Content Area: Fundamental Skills: Nutrition
Priority Concepts: Collaboration; Glucose Regulation

Answer: 3
Rationale: Hyperglycemia is a complication of TPN, and the nurse should report abnormalities to the health care provider. Options 1, 2, and 4 are not done without a health care provider's prescription.
Priority Nursing Tip: When a client is receiving total parenteral nutrition (TPN), the risk of hyperglycemia exists because of the high concentration of dextrose (glucose) in the solution.
Test-Taking Strategy: Focus on the subject, a finger-stick glucose reading of 425 mg/dL. Note that options 1, 2, and 4 are comparable or alike and are not within the scope of nursing practice and require a health care provider's prescription. A blood glucose of 425 mg/dL requires notification of the health care provider. Review: the complications associated with **total parenteral nutrition (TPN).**
Reference(s): Ignatavicius, Workman (2013), p. 1421; Potter et al (2013), pp. 1023-1024.

42. The nurse provides information to a preoperative client who will be receiving relaxation therapy. The nurse should tell the client that which effects occur from this type of therapy? **Select all that apply.**
☐ 1. Increased heart rate
☐ 2. Improved well-being
☐ 3. Lowered blood pressure
☐ 4. Increased respiratory rate
☐ 5. Decreased muscle tension
☐ 6. Increased neural impulses to the brain

Level of Cognitive Ability: Applying
Client Needs: Physiological Integrity
Integrated Process: Teaching and Learning
Content Area: Fundamental Skills: Perioperative Care
Priority Concepts: Health Promotion; Stress

Answer: 2, 3, 5
Rationale: Relaxation is the state of generalized decreased cognitive, physiological, and/or behavioral arousal. Relaxation elongates the muscle fibers, reduces the neural impulses to the brain, and thus decreases the activity of the brain and other systems. The effects of relaxation therapy include improved well-being; lowered blood pressure, heart rate, and respiratory rate; decreased muscle tension; and reduced symptoms of distress in persons who need to undergo treatments, those experiencing complications from medical treatment or disease, or those grieving the loss of a significant other. This therapy does not cause an increased heart rate, increased respiratory rate, or increased neural impulses to the brain.
Priority Nursing Tip: A simple relaxation exercise should be incorporated into the daily routine of an individual's life to decrease stress levels; stress can be a significant factor in the development of disease.
Test-Taking Strategy: Focus on the subject, the effects of relaxation therapy. Thinking about the definition of relaxation and recalling that it is the state of generalized decreased cognitive, physiological, and/or behavioral arousal will assist in directing you to the correct options. Review: the effects of **relaxation therapy.**
Reference(s): Potter et al (2013), pp. 644, 646-647.

43. A client has developed atrial fibrillation and has a ventricular rate of 150 beats per minute. The nurse should assess the client for which effects of this cardiac occurrence?
1. Flat neck veins
2. Nausea and vomiting
3. Hypotension and dizziness
4. Hypertension and headache

Level of Cognitive Ability: Analyzing
Client Needs: Physiological Integrity
Integrated Process: Nursing Process/Assessment
Content Area: Adult Health: Cardiovascular
Priority Concepts: Clinical Judgment; Perfusion

Answer: 3
Rationale: The client with uncontrolled atrial fibrillation with a ventricular rate over 100 beats per minute is at risk for low cardiac output caused by loss of atrial kick. The nurse should assess the client for palpitations, chest pain or discomfort, hypotension, pulse deficit, fatigue, weakness, dizziness, syncope, shortness of breath, and distended neck veins.
Priority Nursing Tip: Clients with atrial fibrillation are at risk for thromboembolism. Monitor the client closely for signs of this life-threatening situation.
Test-Taking Strategy: Focus on the subject, the effects of uncontrolled atrial fibrillation. Recalling that flat neck veins are normal or indicate hypovolemia will assist in eliminating option 1. Remembering that nausea and vomiting are associated with vagus nerve activity, not a tachycardic state, will assist you in eliminating option 2. From the remaining options, thinking of the effects of a falling cardiac output will direct you to the correct option. Review: the symptoms related to **atrial fibrillation.**
Reference(s): Ignatavicius, Workman (2013), p. 722.

44. A preschooler with a history of cleft palate repair comes to the clinic for a routine well-child checkup. To determine whether this child is experiencing a long-term effect of cleft palate, which question should the nurse ask the parent?
1. "Does the child play with an imaginary friend?"
2. "Was the child recently treated for pneumonia?"
3. "Is the child unresponsive when given directions?"
4. "Has the child had any difficulty swallowing food?"

Level of Cognitive Ability: Analyzing
Client Needs: Physiological Integrity
Integrated Process: Nursing Process/Assessment
Content Area: Child Health: Gastrointestinal
Priority Concepts: Development; Sensory Perception

Answer: 3
Rationale: A child with cleft palate is at risk for developing frequent otitis media, which can result in hearing loss. Unresponsiveness may be an indication that the child is experiencing hearing loss. Option 1 is normal behavior for a preschool child. Many preschoolers with vivid imaginations have imaginary friends. Options 2 and 4 are unrelated to cleft palate after repair.
Priority Nursing Tip: After a cleft palate repair, avoid the use of oral suction or placing objects in the child's mouth such as a tongue depressor, thermometer, straws, spoons, forks, or pacifiers.
Test-Taking Strategy: Focus on the subject, a long-term effect of cleft palate. Think about the anatomy of this disorder and the pathophysiology associated with it. Recalling that hearing loss can occur in a child with cleft palate will direct you to the correct option. Review: the long-term effects of cleft palate.
Reference(s): McKinney et al (2013), p. 1073.

45. The nurse is performing a respiratory assessment on a client being treated for an asthma attack. The nurse determines that the client's respiratory status is worsening if which occurs?
1. Loud wheezing
2. Wheezing on expiration
3. Noticeably diminished breath sounds
4. Wheezing during inspiration and expiration

Level of Cognitive Ability: Evaluating
Client Needs: Physiological Integrity
Integrated Process: Nursing Process/Evaluation
Content Area: Adult Health: Respiratory
Priority Concepts: Clinical Judgment; Gas Exchange

Answer: 3
Rationale: Noticeably diminished breath sounds are an indication of severe obstruction and impending respiratory failure. Wheezing is not a reliable manifestation to determine the severity of an asthma attack. Clients with minor attacks may experience loud wheezes, whereas others with severe attacks may not wheeze. The client with severe asthma attacks may have no audible wheezing because of the decrease of airflow. For wheezing to occur, the client must be able to move sufficient air to produce breath sounds.
Priority Nursing Tip: During an acute asthma attack, position the client in a high-Fowler's or sitting position to aid in breathing.
Test-Taking Strategy: Use the ABCs—airway, breathing, and circulation. Note the subject, evidence of worsening respiratory status in a client being treated for an asthma attack. Remember that diminished breath sounds indicate obstruction and impending respiratory failure; this will direct you to the correct option. Also note that options 1, 2, and 4 are comparable or alike and address wheezing. Review: care of the client experiencing an asthma attack.
Reference(s): Perry, Potter, Ostendorf (2014), p. 89.

46. The nurse is assessing the casted extremity of a client for signs of infection. Which finding is indicative of infection?
1. Dependent edema
2. Diminished distal pulse
3. Coolness and pallor of the skin
4. Presence of warm areas on the cast

Level of Cognitive Ability: Analyzing
Client Needs: Physiological Integrity
Integrated Process: Nursing Process/Assessment
Content Area: Adult Health: Musculoskeletal
Priority Concepts: Infection; Mobility

Answer: 4
Rationale: Manifestations of infection under a casted area include a musty odor or purulent drainage from the cast or the presence of areas on the cast that are warmer than others. The health care provider should be notified if any of these occur. Dependent edema, diminished arterial pulse, and coolness and pallor of the skin all signify impaired circulation in the distal extremity.
Priority Nursing Tip: Teach the client and family to monitor for signs of infection under a casted area. Teach them to monitor for warm areas on the cast and to smell the area for a musty or unpleasant odor, which would indicate the presence of infected material.
Test-Taking Strategy: Focus on the subject, manifestations of infection under the cast. Eliminate options 1, 2, and 3 because edema, diminished distal pulse, and coolness and pallor of the skin are comparable or alike and all signify impaired circulation in the distal extremity. Also thinking about the signs of infection (i.e., redness, swelling, heat, and drainage) will direct you to option 4. Review: the signs and symptoms of **infection** under a **cast**.
Reference(s): Ignatavicius, Workman (2013), p. 1153.

47. The home care nurse assesses a client with chronic obstructive pulmonary disease (COPD) who is complaining of increased dyspnea. The client is on home oxygen via a concentrator at 2 L per minute, and the client's respiratory rate is 22 breaths per minute. Which action should the nurse take?
1. Determine the need to increase the oxygen.
2. Reassure the client that there is no need to worry.
3. Conduct further assessment of the client's respiratory status.
4. Call emergency services to take the client to the emergency department.

Level of Cognitive Ability: Applying
Client Needs: Physiological Integrity
Integrated Process: Nursing Process/Implementation
Content Area: Adult Health: Respiratory
Priority Concepts: Clinical Judgment; Gas Exchange

Answer: 3
Rationale: With the client's respiratory rate at 22 breaths per minute, the nurse should obtain further assessment. Oxygen is not increased without the approval of the health care provider, especially because the client with COPD can retain carbon dioxide. Reassuring the client that there is "no need to worry" is inappropriate. Calling emergency services is a premature action.
Priority Nursing Tip: For the client with chronic obstructive pulmonary disease (COPD), a low concentration of oxygen is prescribed (1 to 2 L/min) because the stimulus to breathe is a low arterial Po_2 instead of an increased Pco_2.
Test-Taking Strategy: Focus on the subject, the action to take for a client with COPD experiencing increased dyspnea. Eliminate option 2 first because it is an inappropriate communication technique and dismisses the client's complaint of dyspnea. Option 4 can be eliminated because calling emergency services is a premature action and there is no data to support the notion that an emergency exists. Remember that oxygen is not increased without health care provider approval, and there is no evidence to support that the client is exhibiting tissue hypoxia. Also, use of the steps of the nursing process will direct you to the correct option. Review: care of the client with **chronic obstructive pulmonary disease (COPD)**.
Reference(s): Ignatavicius, Workman (2013), p. 616; Perry, Potter, Ostendorf (2014), p. 589.

❖ **48.** The nurse reviews the client's vital signs in the client's chart. Based on this data, what is the client's pulse pressure? **Refer to chart. Fill in the blank.**

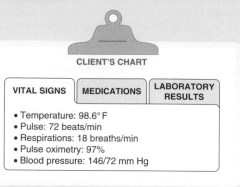

CLIENT'S CHART

| VITAL SIGNS | MEDICATIONS | LABORATORY RESULTS |

- Temperature: 98.6° F
- Pulse: 72 beats/min
- Respirations: 18 breaths/min
- Pulse oximetry: 97%
- Blood pressure: 146/72 mm Hg

Answer: _____

Level of Cognitive Ability: Applying
Client Needs: Physiological Integrity
Integrated Process: Nursing Process/Assessment
Content Area: Adult Health: Cardiovascular
Priority Concepts: Clinical Judgment; Perfusion

Answer: **74**
Rationale: The difference between the systolic and diastolic blood pressure is the pulse pressure. Therefore, if the client has a blood pressure of 146/72 mm Hg, then the pulse pressure is 74.
Priority Nursing Tip: The pulse pressure value is an indirect measure of cardiac output. A narrow pulse pressure is seen in clients with heart failure, hypovolemia, or shock. An increased pulse pressure is noted in clients with hypertension, increased intracranial pressure, slow heart rate, aortic regurgitation, atherosclerosis, and aging.
Test-Taking Strategy: Focus on the subject, determining the pulse pressure. Recall that the pulse pressure is the difference between the systolic and diastolic blood pressure, and then use simple mathematics to subtract 72 from 146 to yield 74. Review: the procedure for determining the **pulse pressure**.
Reference(s): Ignatavicius, Workman (2013), p. 698; Lewis et al (2011), p. 719; Potter et al (2013), pp. 458-459.

49. The home care nurse is making follow-up visits to a client after renal transplant. The nurse should assess the client for which manifestations of acute graft rejection?
1. Hypotension, graft tenderness, and anemia
2. Hypertension, oliguria, thirst, and hypothermia
3. Fever, hypertension, graft tenderness, and malaise
4. Fever, vomiting, hypotension, and copious amounts of dilute urine output

Level of Cognitive Ability: Analyzing
Client Needs: Physiological Integrity
Integrated Process: Nursing Process/Assessment
Content Area: Adult Health: Renal and Urinary
Priority Concepts: Cellular Regulation, Immunity

Answer: **3**
Rationale: Acute rejection usually occurs within the first 3 months after transplant, although it can occur for up to 2 years after transplant. The client exhibits fever, hypertension, malaise, and graft tenderness. Treatment is immediately begun with corticosteroids and possibly also with monoclonal antibodies and antilymphocytic agents.
Priority Nursing Tip: The priority focus of care for the renal transplant recipient is the prevention and early recognition of graft rejection. Goals of care include preventing infection and rejection, maintaining hydration, promoting diuresis, and avoiding fluid overload.
Test-Taking Strategy: Focus on the subject, the manifestations of acute graft rejection. Think about the pathophysiology that occurs with acute graft rejection. Eliminate options 1 and 4 first because hypotension is not part of the clinical picture with graft rejection. Additionally, option 4 can be eliminated because the client rejecting a transplanted kidney would experience oliguria versus copious amounts of urine output. From the remaining options, recalling that fever rather than hypothermia accompanies this complication will direct you to the correct option. Review: the signs of **acute graft rejection**.
Reference(s): Ignatavicius, Workman (2013), p. 1570; Lewis et al (2011), p. 1193.

50. The nurse is caring for a client diagnosed with a skin infection who is receiving tobramycin sulfate (Nebcin) intravenously every 8 hours. Which result should indicate to the nurse that the client is experiencing an adverse effect of the medication?
1. A total bilirubin of 0.5 mg/dL.
2. A sedimentation rate of 15 mm/hour
3. A blood urea nitrogen (BUN) of 30 mg/dL.
4. A white blood cell count (WBC) of 6000 cells/mm³

Level of Cognitive Ability: Analyzing
Client Needs: Physiological Integrity
Integrated Process: Nursing Process/Analysis
Content Area: Pharmacology: Immune Medications
Priority Concepts: Clinical Judgment; Safety

Answer: 3
Rationale: Tobramycin sulfate (Nebcin) is an aminoglycoside antibiotic. Adverse effects or toxic effects of tobramycin sulfate include nephrotoxicity as evidenced by an increased BUN and serum creatinine; irreversible ototoxicity as evidenced by tinnitus, dizziness, ringing or roaring in the ears, and reduced hearing; and neurotoxicity as evidenced by headaches, dizziness, lethargy, tremors, and visual disturbances. The normal BUN ranges from 8 to 25 mg/dL, depending on the laboratory. The normal total bilirubin level is less than 1.5 mg/dL. The normal sedimentation rate is 0 to 30 mm/hour. A normal WBC is 4500 to 11,000 cells/mm³.
Priority Nursing Tip: Aminoglycoside antibiotics are potentially nephrotoxic substances.
Test-Taking Strategy: Focus on the subject, an adverse effect of tobramycin sulfate (Nebcin). Think about these adverse effects and recall knowledge of normal laboratory values to assist in directing you to the correct option, which is the only abnormal laboratory value presented in the options. Review: the adverse effects of **tobramycin sulfate (Nebcin)** and the normal laboratory values.
Reference(s): Hodgson, Kizior (2014), p. 1179; Pagana, Pagana (2013), p. 944.

51. The nurse hears the alarm sound on the telemetry monitor, looks at the monitor, and notes that the client is in ventricular tachycardia. The nurse rushes to the client's room. Upon reaching the client's bedside, which action should the nurse take **first**?
1. Call a code.
2. Prepare for cardioversion.
3. Prepare to defibrillate the client.
4. Check the client's level of consciousness.

Level of Cognitive Ability: Applying
Client Needs: Physiological Integrity
Integrated Process: Nursing Process/Implementation
Content Area: Critical Care: Emergency Situations
Priority Concepts: Clinical Judgment; Perfusion

Answer: 4
Rationale: Determining unresponsiveness is the first assessment action to take. When a client is in ventricular tachycardia, there is a significant decrease in cardiac output. However, assessing for unresponsiveness helps determine whether the client is affected by the decreased cardiac output. If the client is unconscious, then cardiopulmonary resuscitation is initiated.
Priority Nursing Tip: For the client with stable ventricular tachycardia (with a pulse and no signs or symptoms of decreased cardiac output), oxygen and antidysrhythmics may be prescribed.
Test-Taking Strategy: Note the strategic word, *first*. Use the steps of the nursing process, remembering that assessment is the first action. Review: the nursing actions that you should take if a client experiences **ventricular tachycardia**.
Reference(s): Ignatavicius, Workman (2013), pp. 728-729.

52. The nurse assesses a preoperative client. Which question should the nurse ask the client, to help determine the client's risk for developing malignant hyperthermia in the perioperative period?
1. "Have you ever had heat exhaustion or heat stroke?"
2. "What is the normal range for your body temperature?"
3. "Do you or any of your family members have frequent infections?"
4. "Do you or any of your family members have problems with general anesthesia?"

Level of Cognitive Ability: Applying
Client Needs: Physiological Integrity
Integrated Process: Nursing Process/Assessment
Content Area: Fundamental Skills: Perioperative Care
Priority Concepts: Clinical Judgment; Thermoregulation

Answer: 4
Rationale: Malignant hyperthermia is a genetic disorder in which a combination of anesthetic agents (the muscle relaxant succinylcholine and inhalation agents such as halothanes) triggers uncontrolled skeletal muscle contractions that can quickly lead to a potentially fatal hyperthermia. Questioning the client about the family history of general anesthesia problems may reveal this as a risk for the client. Options 1, 2, and 3 are unrelated to this surgical complication.
Priority Nursing Tip: Early indicators of malignant hyperthermia include masseter muscle contractions and tachycardia. An elevated temperature is a late sign.
Test-Taking Strategy: Focus on the subject, malignant hyperthermia. Think about the pathophysiology associated with this disorder. Recalling that this disorder is genetic will direct you to the correct option. Review: the characteristics of **malignant hyperthermia**.
Reference(s): Ignatavicius, Workman (2013), p. 273.

53. A client has developed oral mucositis as a result of radiation to the head and neck. Which measure should the nurse teach the client to incorporate in a daily home care routine?
1. Oral hygiene should be performed in the morning and evening.
2. A glass of wine per day will not pose any further harm to the oral cavity.
3. High-protein foods such as peanut butter should be incorporated in the diet.
4. A combination of frequent teeth cleaning and rinsing with a weak saline and water solution before and after each meal.

Level of Cognitive Ability: Applying
Client Needs: Physiological Integrity
Integrated Process: Teaching and Learning
Content Area: Adult Health: Oncology
Priority Concepts: Client Education; Inflammation

Answer: 4
Rationale: Oral mucositis (irritation, inflammation, and/or ulceration of the mucosa) also known as stomatitis, commonly occurs in clients receiving radiation to the head and neck. Measures need to be taken to soothe the mucosa and provide effective cleansing of the oral cavity. A combination of a weak saline and water solution is an effective cleansing agent. Oral hygiene should be performed more frequently than in the morning and evening. Alcohol would dry and irritate the mucosa. Peanut butter has a thick consistency and will stick to the irritated mucosa.
Priority Nursing Tip: Special "swish and spit" mixtures are available to treat mucositis (stomatitis) and many contain a local anesthetic combined with anti-inflammatory agents. The client should be taught not to swallow these mixtures.
Test-Taking Strategy: Focus on the subject, oral mucositis. Knowing the definition of mucositis will help you eliminate the incorrect options. First, eliminate option 2, knowing that alcohol will have a further drying and irritating effect on the mucosa. Next, eliminate option 3, knowing that although high-protein foods are necessary, peanut butter would not be a good choice because of its consistency. From the remaining options, choose option 4 over option 1 because of the frequency noted in option 1. Review: the care of the client experiencing oral **mucositis**.
Reference(s): Ignatavicius, Workman (2013), p. 422.

54. A client who is being treated for acute heart failure has the following vital signs: blood pressure (BP), 85/50 mm Hg; pulse, 96 beats per minute; respirations, 26 breaths per minute. The health care provider prescribes digoxin (Lanoxin). To evaluate a therapeutic response to this medication, which changes in the client's vital signs should the nurse expect?

1. BP 85/50 mm Hg, pulse 60 beats per minute, respirations 26 breaths per minute
2. BP 98/60 mm Hg, pulse 80 beats per minute, respirations 24 breaths per minute
3. BP 130/70 mm Hg, pulse 104 beats per minute, respirations 20 breaths per minute
4. BP 110/40 mm Hg, pulse 110 beats per minute, respirations 20 breaths per minute

Level of Cognitive Ability: Evaluating
Client Needs: Physiological Integrity
Integrated Process: Nursing Process/Evaluation
Content Area: Pharmacology: Cardiovascular Medications
Priority Concepts: Perfusion; Safety

Answer: 2
Rationale: The main function of digoxin is inotropic. It produces increased myocardial contractility that is associated with an increased cardiac output. This causes a rise in the BP in a client with heart failure. Digoxin also has a negative chronotropic effect (decreases heart rate) and will therefore cause a slowing of the heart rate. As cardiac output improves, there should be an improvement in respirations as well. The remaining choices do not reflect the physiological changes attributed to this medication.
Priority Nursing Tip: The nurse should monitor the client taking digoxin for digoxin toxicity. A normal serum digoxin level is 0.5 to 2 ng/mL.
Test-Taking Strategy: Focus on the subject, the physiologic changes that occur with digoxin administration. Recalling that digoxin slows the heart rate will assist in eliminating options 3 and 4 that show an increase in the heart rate. Next recalling that digoxin improves cardiac output will assist in eliminating option 1, which does not show improvement in blood pressure. Review: the therapeutic effects of digoxin (Lanoxin).
Reference(s): Ignatavicius, Workman (2013), pp. 753, 757; Lehne (2013), pp. 566-567; Perry, Potter, Elkin (2012), pp. 457, 459.

55. A client has been taking an antihypertensive medication for approximately 2 months. The home care nurse monitoring the effects of therapy should determine that drug tolerance has developed if which is noted in the client?

1. Decrease in weight
2. Output greater than intake
3. Decrease in blood pressure
4. Gradual rise in blood pressure

Level of Cognitive Ability: Analyzing
Client Needs: Physiological Integrity
Integrated Process: Nursing Process/Assessment
Content Area: Pharmacology: Cardiovascular Medications
Priority Concepts: Clinical Judgment; Safety

Answer: 4
Rationale: Drug tolerance can develop in a client taking an antihypertensive, which is evident by rising blood pressure levels. The health care provider should be notified, who may then increase the medication dosage, change medication, or add a diuretic to the medication regimen. The client is also at risk of developing fluid retention, which would be manifested as dependent edema, intake greater than output, and an increase in weight. This would also warrant adding a diuretic to the course of therapy.
Priority Nursing Tip: Hypertension is a major risk factor for coronary, cerebral, renal, and peripheral vascular disease.
Test-Taking Strategy: Focus on the subject, drug tolerance with antihypertensives. Recall the definition of drug tolerance; that is, as one adjusts to a medication, the therapeutic effect diminishes. These concepts will direct you to the correct option. Review: the definition of drug tolerance.
Reference(s): Hammond, Zimmermann (2013), p. 135; Potter et al (2013), pp. 988-989.

56. A client with a known history of panic disorder comes to the emergency department and states to the nurse, "Please help me. I think I'm having a heart attack." What is the **priority** nursing action?
1. Check the client's vital signs.
2. Encourage the client to use relaxation techniques.
3. Identify the manifestations related to the panic disorder.
4. Determine what the client's activity involved when the pain started.

Level of Cognitive Ability: Applying
Client Needs: Physiological Integrity
Integrated Process: Nursing Process/Implementation
Content Area: Mental Health
Priority Concepts: Anxiety; Clinical Judgment

Answer: 1
Rationale: Clients with a panic disorder can experience acute physical symptoms, such as chest pain and palpitations. The priority is to assess the client's physical condition to rule out a physiological disorder. Although options 2, 3, and 4 may be appropriate at some point in the care of the client, they are not the priority.
Priority Nursing Tip: A client complaint of chest pain is always a priority. Immediate assessment and treatment is needed.
Test-Taking Strategy: Note the strategic word, *priority*. Focus on Maslow's Hierarchy of Needs theory, recalling that physiological needs are the priority. Also, use of the ABCs—airway, breathing, and circulation—will direct you to the correct option. Review: care of the client with a **panic disorder** who develops physiological manifestations.
Reference(s): Hammond, Zimmermann (2013), p. 508; Varcarolis (2013), pp. 176-177.

57. A client with trigeminal neuralgia (tic douloureux) asks the nurse for a snack and something to drink. Which is the **best** selection the nurse should provide for the client?
1. Hot cocoa with honey and toast
2. Vanilla pudding and lukewarm milk
3. Hot herbal tea with graham crackers
4. Iced coffee and peanut butter and crackers

Level of Cognitive Ability: Applying
Client Needs: Physiological Integrity
Integrated Process: Nursing Process/Implementation
Content Area: Adult Health: Neurological
Priority Concepts: Clinical Judgment; Pain

Answer: 2
Rationale: Because mild tactile stimulation of the face of clients with trigeminal neuralgia can trigger pain, the client needs to eat or drink lukewarm, nutritious foods that are soft and easy to chew. Extremes of temperature will cause trigeminal pain.
Priority Nursing Tip: Monitor the nutritional status of the client with trigeminal neuralgia closely. Because of the facial pain associated with the disorder, the client may not eat enough to meet his or her daily nutritional needs.
Test-Taking Strategy: Focus on the strategic word, *best*. Note that options 1, 3, and 4 are comparable or alike because these options contain hot or iced items and foods that are mechanically difficult to chew and swallow. Review: care of the client with **trigeminal neuralgia**.
Reference(s): Ignatavicius, Workman (2013), p. 1001; Nix (2013), p. 462.

58. An adolescent is admitted to the orthopedic nursing unit after spinal rod insertion for the treatment of scoliosis. Which assessment is **most important** in the immediate postoperative period?
1. Pain level
2. Ability to flex and extend the feet
3. Ability to turn using the logroll technique
4. Capillary refill, sensation, and motion in all extremities

Level of Cognitive Ability: Analyzing
Client Needs: Physiological Integrity
Integrated Process: Nursing Process/Assessment
Content Area: Child Health: Neurological/Musculoskeletal
Priority Concepts: Mobility; Perfusion

Answer: 4
Rationale: When the spinal column is manipulated during surgery, altered neurovascular status is a possible complication; therefore, neurovascular checks including circulation, sensation, and motion should be done at least every 2 hours. Level of pain is an important postoperative assessment, but circulatory status is more important. Assessment of flexion and extension of the lower extremities is a component of option 4, which includes checking motion. Logrolling is performed by nurses.
Priority Nursing Tip: Contact the health care provider immediately if signs of neurovascular impairment are noted in a postoperative client or a client with a cast, traction, or brace.
Test-Taking Strategy: Note the strategic words, *most important.* Use the ABCs—airway, breathing, and circulation—to lead you to option 4 because it addresses circulatory status. Review: priority nursing assessments after spinal rod insertion.
Reference(s): McKinney et al (2013), p. 1358.

59. The nurse has just finished assisting the health care provider in placing a central intravenous (IV) line. Which is a **priority** intervention after central line insertion?
1. Prepare the client for a chest radiograph.
2. Assess the client's temperature to monitor for infection.
3. Label the dressing with the date and time of catheter insertion.
4. Monitor the blood pressure (BP) to assess for fluid volume overload.

Level of Cognitive Ability: Applying
Client Needs: Physiological Integrity
Integrated Process: Nursing Process/Implementation
Content Area: Critical Care: Medications and Intravenous Therapy
Priority Concepts: Clinical Judgment; Safety

Answer: 1
Rationale: A major risk associated with central line placement is the possibility of a pneumothorax developing from an accidental puncture of the lung. Assessing the results of a chest radiograph is one of the best methods to determine if this complication has occurred and verify catheter tip placement before initiating intravenous (IV) therapy. A temperature elevation related to central line insertion would not likely occur immediately after placement. Labeling the dressing site is important but is not the priority. Although BP assessment is always important in assessing a client's status after an invasive procedure, fluid volume overload is not a concern until IV fluids are started.
Priority Nursing Tip: A chest x-ray is needed to ensure that the tip of a newly inserted central IV catheter resides in the superior vena cava. IV solutions should not be infused into the catheter until this is verified.
Test-Taking Strategy: Note the strategic word, *priority.* Recall that assessment of accurate placement is essential before initiating IV therapy. Review: care of the client after central line placement.
Reference(s): Ignatavicius, Workman (2013), p. 216.

❖ **60.** A child sustains a greenstick fracture of the humerus from a fall out of a tree house. The nurse describes this type of fracture to the parents and should provide them with which picture? **Refer to figures 1-4.**

1.

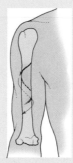

2.

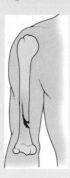

3.

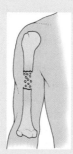

4.

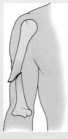

Figures from Ignatavicius D, Workman M: *Medical-surgical nursing: patient-centered collaborative care*, ed 7, St. Louis, 2013, Saunders.

Level of Cognitive Ability: Applying
Client Needs: Physiological Integrity
Integrated Process: Nursing Process/Implementation
Content Area: Child Health: Musculoskeletal
Priority Concepts: Client Education; Mobility

Answer: 1
Rationale: A greenstick fracture is a break that occurs through the periosteum on one side of the bone with only bowing or buckling on the other side. A spiral fracture (option 2) is characterized by a twisted or circular break that affects the length rather than the width. In a comminuted fracture (option 3), the bone is splintered into pieces. In an open (compound) fracture (option 4), the skin surface over the fracture is disrupted causing an external wound.
Priority Nursing Tip: The nurse should closely monitor the client's affected extremity. Of particular importance are color, sensation, and motion of the affected limb. Compartment syndrome, which occurs when pressure builds within the muscle causing decreased blood flow and oxygen delivery, is a common complication associated with breaks and fractures.
Test-Taking Strategy: Focus on the subject, greenstick fracture. Recalling that the definition of a greenstick fracture is a break that occurs through the periosteum on one side of the bone with only bowing or buckling on the other side will assist in directing you to the correct option. Review: the characteristics of a **greenstick fracture**.
Reference(s): McKinney et al (2013), p. 1348.

61. A child has just returned from surgery and has a hip spica cast. What is the **priority** nursing action at this time?
1. Elevate the head of the bed.
2. Abduct the hips, using pillows.
3. Turn the child on the right side.
4. Assess the child's circulatory status.

Level of Cognitive Ability: Applying
Client Needs: Physiological Integrity
Integrated Process: Nursing Process/Implementation
Content Area: Child Health: Musculoskeletal
Priority Concepts: Mobility; Perfusion

Answer: 4
Rationale: During the first few hours after a cast is applied, the chief concern is swelling that may cause the cast to act as a tourniquet and obstruct circulation, resulting in compartment syndrome; therefore, circulatory assessment is the priority. Elevating the head of the bed of a child in a hip spica cast would cause discomfort. Using pillows to abduct the hips is not necessary because a hip spica cast immobilizes the hip and knee. Turning the child side to side at least every 2 hours is important because it allows the body cast to dry evenly and prevents complications related to immobility; however, it is not a higher priority than checking circulation.
Priority Nursing Tip: If a hip spica cast is placed, the cast edges around the perineum and buttocks may need to be taped with waterproof tape to prevent the cast from becoming wet or soiled during elimination.
Test-Taking Strategy: Note the strategic word, *priority*. Recall the ABCs—airway, breathing, and circulation—to answer this question. Also, use the steps of the nursing process to answer this question. Because assessment is the first step in the nursing process, it is likely that the priority is to assess. Review: nursing care after application of a hip spica cast.
Reference(s): Hockenberry, Wilson (2013), pp. 1059-1061; McKinney et al (2013), p. 1343.

62. The nurse is assessing a client with a brainstem injury. What else should the nurse do in addition to performing the Glasgow Coma Scale?
1. Perform arterial blood gases.
2. Assist with a lumbar puncture.
3. Perform a pulmonary wedge pressure.
4. Assess cranial nerve functioning and respiratory rate and rhythm.

Level of Cognitive Ability: Applying
Client Needs: Physiological Integrity
Integrated Process: Nursing Process/Implementation
Content Area: Adult Health: Neurological
Priority Concepts: Clinical Judgment; Intracranial Regulation

Answer: 4
Rationale: Assessment should be specific to the area of the brain involved. Assessing the respiratory status and cranial nerve function is a critical component of the assessment process in a client with a brainstem injury because the respiratory center is located in the brainstem. Options 1, 2, and 3 are not necessary based on the data in the question.
Priority Nursing Tip: For a client with a head injury, priority is given to maintaining a patent airway, breathing, and circulation.
Test-Taking Strategy: Focus on the ABCs—airway, breathing, and circulation. Recall the anatomical location of the respiratory center to direct you to option 4. Remember that the respiratory center is located in the brainstem. Review: content and nursing care related to brainstem injuries.
Reference(s): Ignatavicius, Workman (2013), pp. 1020, 1025-1026.

63. A client has had a Miller-Abbott tube in place for 24 hours. Which assessment finding indicates that the tube is properly located in the intestine?
1. The client is nauseous.
2. Bowel sounds are absent.
3. Aspirate from the tube has a pH of 7.
4. The abdominal radiograph report indicates that the end of the tube is above the pylorus.

Level of Cognitive Ability: Analyzing
Client Needs: Physiological Integrity
Integrated Process: Nursing Process/Assessment
Content Area: Adult Health: Gastrointestinal
Priority Concepts: Clinical Judgment; Safety

Answer: 3
Rationale: The Miller-Abbott tube is a nasoenteric tube that is used to decompress the intestine and correct a bowel obstruction. The pH of the gastric fluid is acidic, and the pH of the intestinal fluid is alkaline (7 or higher). Nausea should subside as decompression is accomplished. Although bowel sounds will be abnormal in the presence of obstruction, the presence or absence of bowel sounds is not associated with the location of the tube. The end of the tube should be located in the intestine (below the pylorus). Location of the tube can also be determined by radiographs.
Priority Nursing Tip: The client who has had an intestinal tube inserted should be positioned on his or her right side to facilitate passage of the weighted bag in the tube through the pylorus of the stomach and into the small intestine.
Test-Taking Strategy: Focus on the subject, a Miller-Abbott tube and its intestinal location. Recalling that intestinal fluid is alkaline will direct you to the correct option. Review: the purpose and nursing care of a client with a Miller-Abbott tube.
Reference(s): Potter et al (2013), pp. 1029, 1031.

64. While a client with myxedema is being admitted to the hospital, the client reports having experienced a lack of energy, cold intolerance, and puffiness around the eyes and face. The nurse plans care knowing that these clinical manifestations are caused by a lack of production of which hormones?
  1. Luteinizing hormone (LH)
  2. Adrenocorticotropic hormone (ACTH)
  3. Triiodothyronine (T₃) and thyroxine (T₄)
  4. Prolactin (PRL) and growth hormone (GH)

Level of Cognitive Ability: Applying
Client Needs: Physiological Integrity
Integrated Process: Nursing Process/Planning
Content Area: Adult Health: Endocrine
Priority Concepts: Clinical Judgment; Thermoregulation

Answer: 3
Rationale: Although all of these hormones originate from the anterior pituitary, only T₃ and T₄ are associated with the client's symptoms. Myxedema results from inadequate thyroid hormone levels (T₃ and T₄). Low levels of thyroid hormone result in an overall decrease in the basal metabolic rate, affecting virtually every body system and leading to weakness, fatigue, and a decrease in heat production. A decrease in LH results in the loss of secondary sex characteristics. A decrease in ACTH is seen in Addison's disease. PRL stimulates breast milk production by the mammary glands, and GH affects bone and soft tissue by promoting growth through protein anabolism and lipolysis.
Priority Nursing Tip: Myxedema is a rare but serious disorder that results from severe or prolonged thyroid deficiency.
Test-Taking Strategy: Focus on the subject, myxedema. Recalling that myxedema is associated with the thyroid gland (hypothyroidism) will assist in connecting the subject of the question, the client's symptoms, and option 3. Review: **myxedema.**
Reference(s): Ignatavicius, Workman (2013), p. 1402.

65. A client is admitted to the hospital with a suspected diagnosis of Graves' disease. On assessment, which manifestation related to the client's menstrual cycle should the nurse expect the client to **most likely** report?
  1. Amenorrhea
  2. Menorrhagia
  3. Metrorrhagia
  4. Dysmenorrhea

Level of Cognitive Ability: Applying
Client Needs: Physiological Integrity
Integrated Process: Nursing Process/Assessment
Content Area: Adult Health: Endocrine
Priority Concepts: Clinical Judgment; Thermoregulation

Answer: 1
Rationale: Amenorrhea or a decreased menstrual flow is common in the client with Graves' disease. Menorrhagia, metrorrhagia, and dysmenorrhea are also disorders related to the female reproductive system; however, they do not manifest in the presence of Graves' disease.
Priority Nursing Tip: Graves' disease is also known as toxic diffuse goiter and results in a hyperthyroid state from the hypersecretion of thyroid hormones.
Test-Taking Strategy: Note the strategic words, *most likely*, and focus on the subject of Graves' disease. Thinking about the pathophysiology associated with Graves' disease will direct you to the correct option. Review: the clinical manifestations of **Graves' disease.**
Reference(s): Ignatavicius, Workman (2013), p. 1394.

66. A client with gestational hypertension is in active labor. Which assessment finding should the nurse **most likely** expect to note?
  1. Increased urine output
  2. Increased blood pressure
  3. Increased fetal heart rate
  4. Decreased brachial reflexes

Level of Cognitive Ability: Analyzing
Client Needs: Physiological Integrity
Integrated Process: Nursing Process/Assessment
Content Area: Maternity: Intrapartum
Priority Concepts: Perfusion; Reproduction

Answer: 2
Rationale: The major manifestation of gestational hypertension is increased blood pressure. As the disease progresses, it is possible that increased brachial reflexes, decreased fetal heart rate and variability, and decreased urine output will occur, particularly during labor.
Priority Nursing Tip: Gestational hypertension can lead to preeclampsia. Manifestations of preeclampsia are hypertension and proteinuria.
Test-Taking Strategy: Note the strategic words, *most likely*, and focus on the subject of gestational hypertension. Noting the name of the disorder will easily direct you to the correct option. Review: **gestational hypertension.**
Reference(s): McKinney et al (2013), pp. 590-591.

67. The nurse has just administered a purified protein derivative (PPD) tuberculin skin test (Mantoux test) to a client who is at low risk for developing tuberculosis. The nurse determines that the test is positive if which occurs?
1. An induration of 15 mm
2. The presence of a wheal
3. A large area of erythema
4. Complaints of itching at the injection site

Level of Cognitive Ability: Analyzing
Client Needs: Physiological Integrity
Integrated Process: Nursing Process/Assessment
Content Area: Adult Health: Respiratory
Priority Concepts: Clinical Judgment; Infection

Answer: 1
Rationale: An induration of 10 mm or more is considered positive for clients in low-risk groups. The presence of a wheal would indicate that the skin test was administered appropriately. Erythema or itching at the site is not indicative of a positive reaction.
Priority Nursing Tip: A positive Mantoux test does not mean that active tuberculosis is present, but rather indicates previous exposure to tuberculosis or the presence of inactive (dormant) disease.
Test-Taking Strategy: Focus on the subject, a positive Mantoux test, and note that the client is at low risk for developing tuberculosis. This will direct you to the correct option. Review: **Mantoux tuberculin skin test.**
Reference(s): Potter et al (2013), pp. 630, 835.

68. The nurse is performing an otoscopic examination on a client with a suspected diagnosis of mastoiditis. Which finding should the nurse expect to note if this disorder was present?
1. A mobile tympanic membrane
2. A transparent tympanic membrane
3. A pearly colored tympanic membrane
4. A thick and immobile tympanic membrane

Level of Cognitive Ability: Applying
Client Needs: Physiological Integrity
Integrated Process: Nursing Process/Assessment
Content Area: Adult Health: Ear
Priority Concepts: Clinical Judgment; Sensory Perception

Answer: 4
Rationale: Otoscopic examination of a client with mastoiditis reveals a red, dull, thick, and immobile tympanic membrane with or without perforation. Options 1, 2, and 3 indicate normal findings in an otoscopic examination.
Priority Nursing Tip: Mastoiditis may be acute or chronic and results from untreated or inadequately treated chronic or acute otitis media. Interventions focus on stopping the infection before it spreads to other structures.
Test-Taking Strategy: Focus on the subject, manifestations of mastoiditis. Recall knowledge of normal assessment findings on an ear examination to direct you to the correct option, the only abnormal finding. Review: **mastoiditis.**
Reference(s): Ignatavicius, Workman (2013), p. 1094.

69. The nurse is reviewing the record of a client with a disorder involving the inner ear. Which finding should the nurse **most likely** note as an assessment finding in this client?
1. Complaints of tinnitus
2. Complaints of burning in the ear
3. Complaints of itching in the affected ear
4. Complaints of severe pain in the affected ear

Level of Cognitive Ability: Applying
Client Needs: Physiological Integrity
Integrated Process: Nursing Process/Assessment
Content Area: Adult Health: Ear
Priority Concepts: Clinical Judgment; Sensory Perception

Answer: 1
Rationale: Tinnitus is the most common complaint of clients with ear disorders, especially disorders involving the inner ear. Manifestations of tinnitus can range from mild ringing in the ear that can go unnoticed during the day to a loud roaring in the ear that can interfere with the client's thinking process and attention span. The assessment findings noted in options 2, 3, and 4 are not specifically noted in the client with an inner ear disorder.
Priority Nursing Tip: The inner ear contains the semicircular canals, cochlea, and the distal end of the eight cranial nerves, and maintains a sense of balance or equilibrium.
Test-Taking Strategy: Note the strategic words, *most likely.* Focus on the subject, inner ear disorder. Recalling the function of the inner ear will direct you to the correct option. Review: **inner ear disorders.**
Reference(s): Ignatavicius, Workman (2013), p. 1095.

70. The nurse has a prescription to administer hydroxyzine (Vistaril) to a client by the intramuscular route. Before administering the medication, what should the nurse tell the client?
1. Excessive salivation is a side effect.
2. There will be some pain at the injection site.
3. There will be relief from nausea within 5 minutes.
4. The client will have increased alertness for about 2 hours.

Level of Cognitive Ability: Applying
Client Needs: Physiological Integrity
Integrated Process: Nursing Process/Implementation
Content Area: Pharmacology: Gastrointestinal Medications
Priority Concepts: Clinical Judgment; Safety

Answer: 2
Rationale: Hydroxyzine is an antiemetic and sedative/hypnotic that may be used in conjunction with opioid analgesics for added effect. The injection can be painful. Hydroxyzine causes dry mouth and drowsiness as side effects. Medications administered by the intramuscular route generally take 20 to 30 minutes to become effective.
Priority Nursing Tip: In an adult, a maximum of 3 mL of solution should be administered by the intramuscular route. Larger volumes are difficult for the injection site to absorb and, if prescribed, need to be verified.
Test-Taking Strategy: Focus on the subject, intramuscular injection of hydroxyzine (Vistaril). Read each option carefully. Recalling that the medication is an antiemetic and sedative/hypnotic, eliminate options 1 and 4 first because they are the least likely effects. From the remaining options, noting that the medication is administered by the intramuscular route will direct you to the correct option. Review: **hydroxyzine (Vistaril).**
Reference(s): Hodgson, Kizior (2014), p. 578.

71. A client with diabetes mellitus has a blood glucose level of 644 mg/dL. The nurse interprets that this client is **most** at risk of developing which type of acid-base imbalance?
1. Metabolic acidosis
2. Metabolic alkalosis
3. Respiratory acidosis
4. Respiratory alkalosis

Level of Cognitive Ability: Analyzing
Client Needs: Physiological Integrity
Integrated Process: Nursing Process/Analysis
Content Area: Adult Health: Endocrine
Priority Concepts: Acid-Base Balance; Glucose Regulation

Answer: 1
Rationale: Diabetes mellitus can lead to metabolic acidosis. When the body does not have sufficient circulating insulin, the blood glucose level rises. At the same time, the cells of the body use all available glucose. The body then breaks down glycogen and fat for fuel. The by-products of fat metabolism are acidotic and can lead to the condition known as diabetic ketoacidosis. Options 2, 3, and 4 are incorrect.
Priority Nursing Tip: In metabolic acidosis, to compensate for the acidosis, hyperpnea with Kussmaul's respiration occurs as the lungs attempt to exhale excess carbon dioxide (CO_2), an acidotic by-product of respiration.
Test-Taking Strategy: Note the strategic word, *most.* Focus on the subject, diabetes mellitus. Noting the client's diagnosis will assist in eliminating options 3 and 4. From the remaining options, remember that the client with diabetes mellitus is at risk for developing acidosis. Review: **metabolic acidosis** and **diabetes mellitus.**
Reference(s): Ignatavicius, Workman (2013), pp. 202-203, 1456.

72. The nurse reviews the client's most recent blood gas results that include a pH of 7.43, Pco_2 of 31 mm Hg, and HCO_3 of 21 mEq/L. Based on these results, the nurse determines that which acid-base imbalance is present?
1. Compensated metabolic acidosis
2. Compensated respiratory alkalosis
3. Uncompensated respiratory acidosis
4. Uncompensated metabolic alkalosis

Level of Cognitive Ability: Analyzing
Client Needs: Physiological Integrity
Integrated Process: Nursing Process/Analysis
Content Area: Fundamental Skills: Acid-Base
Priority Concepts: Acid-Base Balance; Clinical Judgment

Answer: 2
Rationale: The normal pH is 7.35 to 7.45, the normal Pco_2 is 35 to 45 mm Hg, and the normal HCO_3 is 22 to 27 mEq/L. The pH is elevated in alkalosis and low in acidosis. In a respiratory condition, the pH and the Pco_2 move in opposite directions; that is, the pH rises and the Pco_2 drops (alkalosis) or vice versa (acidosis). In a metabolic condition, the pH and the bicarbonate move in the same direction; if the pH is low, the bicarbonate level will be low also. In this client, the pH is at the high end of normal, indicating compensation and alkalosis. The Pco_2 is low, indicating a respiratory condition (opposite direction of the pH).
Priority Nursing Tip: If the client has a condition that causes over-stimulation of the respiratory system, monitor the client for respiratory alkalosis.
Test-Taking Strategy: Focus on the subject, an acid-base imbalance. Remember that in a respiratory imbalance you will find that the pH and Pco_2 move in opposite directions. Therefore, options 1 and 4 are eliminated first. Next, remember that the pH is elevated with alkalosis, but compensation has occurred if the pH is within normal range. Option 2 reflects a respiratory alkalotic condition and compensation because the Pco_2 is below normal, but the pH is at the high end of normal. Review: **compensated respiratory alkalosis.**
Reference(s): Ignatavicius, Workman (2013), pp. 205, 207-208; Potter et al (2013), p. 892.

73. The nurse is caring for a client with a nasogastric tube that is attached to low suction. Which acid-base disorder is **most likely** to occur in this client?
1. Metabolic acidosis
2. Metabolic alkalosis
3. Respiratory acidosis
4. Respiratory alkalosis

Level of Cognitive Ability: Analyzing
Client Needs: Physiological Integrity
Integrated Process: Nursing Process/Analysis
Content Area: Fundamental Skills: Acid-Base
Priority Concepts: Acid-Base Balance; Clinical Judgment

Answer: 2
Rationale: Loss of gastric fluid via nasogastric suction or vomiting causes metabolic alkalosis because of the loss of hydrochloric acid (HCl), an acid secreted in the stomach. Thus, the loss of hydrogen ions in the HCl results in alkalosis. Because the respiratory system is not involved, the alkalosis must be metabolic.
Priority Nursing Tip: Monitor the client experiencing excessive vomiting or the client with gastrointestinal suctioning for manifestations of metabolic alkalosis.
Test-Taking Strategy: Note the strategic words, *most likely.* Focus on the subject, complications of gastrointestinal suctioning and acid-base disorders. Eliminate options 1 and 3 first because the loss of HCl would cause an alkalotic condition. Because the question addresses a situation other than a respiratory one, the acid-base disorder would be metabolic alkalosis. Review: the causes of **metabolic alkalosis.**
Reference(s): Ignatavicius, Workman (2013), pp. 207, 1254; Potter et al (2013), pp. 892-893.

74. The nurse reviews the results of a blood chemistry profile for a client who has late-stage salicylate poisoning and metabolic acidosis. Which serum study should the nurse review for data about the client's acid-base balance?
1. Sodium
2. Potassium
3. Magnesium
4. Phosphorus

Level of Cognitive Ability: Applying
Client Needs: Physiological Integrity
Integrated Process: Nursing Process/Assessment
Content Area: Fundamental Skills: Acid-Base
Priority Concepts: Acid-Base Balance; Clinical Judgment

Answer: 2
Rationale: A client with late-stage salicylate poisoning is at risk for metabolic acidosis because acetylsalicylic acid increases the client's hydrogen ion (H^+) concentration, decreases the pH, and creates a bicarbonate deficit. Hyperkalemia develops as the body attempts to compensate for the influx of H^+ by moving H^+ into the cell and potassium out of the cell; thus, potassium accumulates in the extracellular space. Clinical manifestations of metabolic acidosis include the clinical indicators of hyperkalemia, including hyperpnea, central nervous system depression, twitching, and seizures. Options 1, 3, and 4 are not primary concerns.
Priority Nursing Tip: In acidosis, the potassium moves out of the cell to make room for the hydrogen ions; thus, the potassium level increases. In alkalosis, the potassium moves into the cell and the potassium level decreases.
Test-Taking Strategy: Focus on the subject, an acid-base imbalance and salicylate poisoning. Specific knowledge about the effect of an influx of H^+ in an acid-base disorder and the potassium shifts that occur will direct you to the correct option. Review: **salicylate poisoning and metabolic acidosis.**
Reference(s): Ignatavicius, Workman (2013), pp. 202-203, 205.

75. An emergency department nurse prepares to treat a child with acetaminophen (Tylenol) overdose. The nurse reviews the health care provider's prescriptions and prepares to administer which medication?
1. Acetylcysteine
2. Protamine sulfate
3. Succimer (Chemet)
4. Vitamin K (phytonadione, Mephyton, Aquamephyton)

Level of Cognitive Ability: Applying
Client Needs: Physiological Integrity
Integrated Process: Nursing Process/Planning
Content Area: Critical Care: Emergency Situations
Priority Concepts: Clinical Judgment; Safety

Answer: 1
Rationale: Acetylcysteine is the antidote for acetaminophen overdose. It is administered orally or via nasogastric tube in a diluted form with water, juice, or soda. It can also be administered intravenously (undiluted). Protamine sulfate is the antidote for heparin. Succimer (Chemet) is used in the treatment of lead poisoning. Vitamin K is the antidote for warfarin (Coumadin).
Priority Nursing Tip: When used as an antidote via oral administration, dilute acetylcysteine (Mucomyst) in juice or soda because of its offensive odor.
Test-Taking Strategy: Focus on the subject, acetaminophen overdose management. Specific knowledge regarding the antidote for acetaminophen overdose is required to answer this question. Remember that acetylcysteine is the antidote for acetaminophen overdose. Review: **acetaminophen (Tylenol) overdose.**
Reference(s): Hodgson, Kizior (2014), p. 11; McKinney et al (2013), p. 862.

❖ **76.** What should the nurse consider when determining whether a client with respiratory disease could tolerate and benefit from active progressive relaxation? **Select all that apply.**
   ❑ 1. Social status
   ❑ 2. Financial status
   ❑ 3. Functional status
   ❑ 4. Medical diagnosis
   ❑ 5. Ability to expend energy
   ❑ 6. Motivation of the individual

Level of Cognitive Ability: Applying
Client Needs: Physiological Integrity
Integrated Process: Nursing Process/Planning
Content Area: Adult Health: Respiratory
Priority Concepts: Clinical Judgment; Gas Exchange

Answer: 3, 4, 5, 6
Rationale: Active progressive relaxation training teaches the client how to effectively rest and reduce tension in the body. Some important considerations when choosing the type of relaxation technique is the client's physiological and psychological status. Because active progressive relaxation training requires a moderate expenditure of energy, the nurse needs to consider the client's functional status, medical diagnosis, and ability to expend energy. For example, a client with advanced respiratory disease may not have sufficient energy reserves to participate in active progressive relaxation techniques. The client needs to be motivated to participate in this form of alternative therapy to obtain beneficial results. The client's social or financial status has no relationship with his or her ability to tolerate and benefit from active progressive relaxation (options 1 and 2).
Priority Nursing Tip: Relaxation techniques are important to learn and integrate into daily activities to aid in the prevention of potential stress-related disease processes.
Test-Taking Strategy: Focus on the subject, determining whether a client could tolerate and benefit from active progressive relaxation. Use teaching and learning principles to determine that client motivation is a key factor in the learning process (option 6). From the remaining options, noting the word "active" will assist in determining that options 3, 4, and 5 should be considered. Review: the characteristics of **active progressive relaxation**.
Reference(s): Potter et al (2013), pp. 647-648.

77. An adult client has undergone a lumbar puncture to obtain cerebrospinal fluid (CSF) for analysis. The nurse reviews the results of the analysis and should anticipate which values to be negative if the CSF is normal?
   1. Protein
   2. Glucose
   3. Red blood cells
   4. White blood cells

Level of Cognitive Ability: Applying
Client Needs: Physiological Integrity
Integrated Process: Nursing Process/Assessment
Content Area: Fundamental Skills: Laboratory Values
Priority Concepts: Clinical Judgment; Intracranial Regulation

Answer: 3
Rationale: The adult with a normal CSF has no red blood cells in the CSF. Protein (15 to 45 mg/dL) and glucose (45 to 74 mg/dL) are normally present in CSF. The client may have small levels of white blood cells (0 to 8 cells/mm^3).
Priority Nursing Tip: Cerebrospinal fluid is normally clear. A pink or red-colored specimen may be caused by the presence of red blood cells.
Test-Taking Strategy: Focus on the subject, normal CSF analysis. Recalling that the presence of red blood cells is abnormal and would indicate blood vessel rupture or meningeal irritation will direct you to the correct option. Review: **cerebrospinal fluid (CSF)**.
Reference(s): Chernecky, Berger (2013), pp. 319-321; Ignatavicius, Workman (2013), p. 924.

78. A client with a burn injury receives a prescription for a regular diet. Which is the **best** meal for the nurse to provide to the client to promote wound healing?
1. Peanut butter and jelly sandwich, apple, tea
2. Chicken breast, broccoli, strawberries, milk
3. Veal chop, boiled potatoes, Jell-O, orange juice
4. Pasta with tomato sauce, garlic bread, ginger ale

Level of Cognitive Ability: Applying
Client Needs: Physiological Integrity
Integrated Process: Nursing Process/Implementation
Content Area: Fundamental Skills: Nutrition
Priority Concepts: Health Promotion; Nutrition

Answer: 2
Rationale: The meal with the best potential to promote wound healing includes nutrient-rich food choices including protein, such as chicken and milk, and vitamin C, such as broccoli and strawberries. The remaining options include one or more items with a low nutritional value, especially the tea, jelly, Jell-O, and ginger ale.
Priority Nursing Tip: Depending on the extent of the injury, the basal metabolic rate is 40 to 100 times higher than normal in a client with a burn.
Test-Taking Strategy: Focus on the subject, nutrition for a client with a burn injury. Knowledge that protein and vitamin C are necessary for wound healing assists in selecting the option that contains those nutrients, and the option with the most nutrients is the best choice. Eliminate options 1 and 3 first because jelly, tea, and Jell-O have no nutritional value related to healing. From the remaining options, select option 2 over option 4 because option 2 contains foods with greater nutritional value. Review: **foods high in protein** and **vitamin C**.
Reference(s): Ignatavicius, Workman (2013), p. 536; Nix (2013), pp. 467-468.

---

79. The nurse is developing a care plan for a client with urge urinary incontinence. Which interventions would be **most** helpful for this type of incontinence? **Select all that apply.**
☐ 1. Surgery
☐ 2. Bladder retraining
☐ 3. Scheduled toileting
☐ 4. Dietary modifications
☐ 5. Pelvic muscle exercises
☐ 6. Intermittent catheterization

Level of Cognitive Ability: Applying
Client Needs: Physiological Integrity
Integrated Process: Nursing Process/Planning
Content Area: Adult Health: Renal and Urinary
Priority Concepts: Clinical Judgment; Elimination

Answer: 2, 3, 4, 5
Rationale: Urge incontinence is the involuntary passage of urine after a strong sense of the urgency to void. It is characterized by urinary urgency, often with frequency (more often than every 2 hours); bladder spasm or contraction; and voiding in either small amounts (less than 100 mL) or large amounts (greater than 500 mL). It can be caused by decreased bladder capacity, irritation of the bladder stretch receptors, infection, and alcohol or caffeine ingestion. Interventions to assist the client with urge incontinence include bladder retraining, scheduled toileting, dietary modifications such as eliminating alcohol and caffeine intake, and pelvic muscle exercises to strengthen the muscles. Surgery and urinary catheterization are invasive measures and will not assist in the treatment of urge incontinence.
Priority Nursing Tip: During bladder retraining, to aid in ensuring complete bladder emptying, teach the client to urinate as much as possible, relax for a few moments, then attempt to urinate again. This is known as "double-voiding."
Test-Taking Strategy: Note the strategic word, *most*. Focus on the subject, urge urinary incontinence and recall the definition of this type of incontinence. Also note that options 1 and 6 are invasive measures, and these types of measures are avoided. Review: the interventions for **urge urinary incontinence**.
Reference(s): Ignatavicius, Workman (2013), p. 1504; Potter et al (2013), p. 1060.

80. The nurse caring for a client with a neurological disorder is planning care to maintain nutritional status. The nurse is concerned about the client's swallowing ability. Which food item should the nurse eliminate from this client's diet?
1. Spinach
2. Custard
3. Scrambled eggs
4. Mashed potatoes

Level of Cognitive Ability: Applying
Client Needs: Physiological Integrity
Integrated Process: Nursing Process/Planning
Content Area: Adult Health: Neurological
Priority Concepts: Nutrition; Safety

Answer: 1
Rationale: Raw vegetables; chunky vegetables such as diced beets; and stringy vegetables such as spinach, corn, and peas are foods commonly excluded from the diet of a client with a poor swallowing reflex. In general, flavorful, warm, or well-chilled foods with texture stimulate the swallowing reflex. Soft and semisoft foods such as custards or puddings, egg dishes, and potatoes are usually effective.
Priority Nursing Tip: Pureed foods may be necessary as a means of providing nutritional intake to a client with an altered swallowing ability. Molding the pureed food into the shape of the original food can enhance the appeal of the food item and thus enhance the client's appetite.
Test-Taking Strategy: Focus on the subject, altered swallowing ability. Select option 1 as the food that is stringy and with the least amount of substance or consistency. Review: feeding measures for a client with **altered swallowing ability.**
Reference(s): Ignatavicius, Workman (2013), p. 1028; Nix (2013), p. 355.

81. An adult client arrives in the emergency department with burns to both entire legs and the perineal area. Using the rule of nines, the nurse should determine that approximately what percentage of the client's body surface has been burned? **Fill in the blank.**
Answer: ____%

Level of Cognitive Ability: Understanding
Client Needs: Physiological Integrity
Integrated Process: Nursing Process/Assessment
Content Area: Adult Health: Integumentary
Priority Concepts: Clinical Judgment; Tissue Integrity

Answer: 37%
Rationale: The most rapid method used to calculate the size of a burn injury in adult clients whose weights are in normal proportion to their heights is the rule of nines. This method divides the body into areas that are multiples of 9%, except for the perineum. Each entire leg is 18%, each arm is 9%, and the head is 9%. The trunk is 36%, and the perineal area is 1%. Both legs and perineal area equal 37%.
Priority Nursing Tip: The rule of nines gives an inaccurate estimate of the extent of the burn injury in a child because of the difference in body proportion between children and adults. Instead, the extent of the burn is expressed as a percent of the total body surface area using age-related charts.
Test-Taking Strategy: Focus on the subject, rule of nines. Knowledge regarding the percentages associated with this method of calculating burn injuries is required to answer this question. Remember that each leg is 18%, each arm is 9%, the head is 9%, the trunk is 36%, and the perineal area is 1%. Review: **rule of nines.**
Reference(s): Ignatavicius, Workman (2013), p. 523.

82. A client is resuming a diet after a Billroth II procedure. To minimize complications from eating, which actions should the nurse teach the client to do? **Select all that apply.**
☐ 1. Lay down after eating
☐ 2. Eat a diet high in protein
☐ 3. Drink liquids with meals
☐ 4. Eat six small meals per day
☐ 5. Eat concentrated sweets between meals only

Level of Cognitive Ability: Applying
Client Needs: Physiological Integrity
Integrated Process: Nursing Process/Implementation
Content Area: Adult Health: Gastrointestinal
Priority Concepts: Client Education; Elimination

Answer: 1, 2, 4
Rationale: The client who has had a Billroth II procedure is at risk for dumping syndrome. The client should lie down after eating and avoid drinking liquids with meals to prevent this syndrome. The client should be placed on a dry diet that is high in protein, moderate in fat, and low in carbohydrates. Frequent small meals are encouraged, and the client should avoid concentrated sweets.
Priority Nursing Tip: Dumping syndrome is a complication of gastric resection and results from the rapid emptying of the gastric contents into the small intestine after eating.
Test-Taking Strategy: Focusing on the subject, Billroth II procedure, and recalling that dumping syndrome is a complication of this surgical procedure will direct you to the correct options. Eliminate option 5 because of the closed-ended word only. Also thinking about the pathophysiology associated with dumping syndrome will assist in answering correctly. Review: **Billroth II procedure.**
Reference(s): Ignatavicius, Workman (2013), pp. 1236-1237.

❖ **83.** The nurse is getting a client out of bed for the first time after having abdominal surgery. What clinical manifestations should indicate to the nurse that the client may be experiencing orthostatic hypotension? **Select all that apply.**
- ❑ 1. Nausea
- ❑ 2. Dizziness
- ❑ 3. Bradycardia
- ❑ 4. Lightheadedness
- ❑ 5. Flushing of the face
- ❑ 6. Reports of seeing spots

Level of Cognitive Ability: Analyzing
Client Needs: Physiological Integrity
Integrated Process: Nursing Process/Assessment
Content Area: Adult Health: Cardiovascular
Priority Concepts: Clinical Judgment; Perfusion

Answer: 1, 2, 4, 6
Rationale: Orthostatic hypotension occurs when a normotensive person develops symptoms of low blood pressure when rising to an upright position. Whenever the nurse gets a client up and out of a bed or chair, there is a risk for orthostatic hypotension. Symptoms of nausea, dizziness, lightheadedness, tachycardia, pallor, and reports of seeing spots are characteristic of orthostatic hypotension. A drop of approximately 15 mm Hg in the systolic blood pressure and 10 mm Hg in the diastolic blood pressure also occurs. Fainting can result without intervention, which includes immediately assisting the client to a lying position.
Priority Nursing Tip: Baroreceptors (located in the walls of the aortic arch and carotid sinuses) are specialized nerve endings affected by changes in the blood pressure. Increases in the arterial pressure stimulate baroreceptors to decrease the pressure. Conversely, decreases in arterial pressure reduce stimulation and the blood pressure increases.
Test-Taking Strategy: Focus on the subject, the manifestations of orthostatic hypotension. As you read each option, think about the physiological changes that occur when the blood pressure drops. This will assist in answering the question. Review: the manifestations of orthostatic hypotension.
Reference(s): Ignatavicius, Workman (2013), p. 698; Perry, Potter, Ostendorf (2014), pp. 236-238.

84. The nurse is closely monitoring a child with increased intracranial pressure who has been exhibiting decorticate (flexor) posturing. The nurse notes that the child suddenly exhibits decerebrate (extensor) posturing and interprets that this change in the child's condition indicates which finding?
1. An insignificant finding
2. An improvement in condition
3. Decreasing intracranial pressure
4. Deteriorating neurological function

Level of Cognitive Ability: Analyzing
Client Needs: Physiological Integrity
Integrated Process: Nursing Process/Analysis
Content Area: Child Health: Neurological
Priority Concepts: Clinical Judgment; Intracranial Regulation

Answer: 4
Rationale: The progression from decorticate to decerebrate posturing usually indicates deteriorating neurological function and warrants health care provider notification. Options 1, 2, and 3 are inaccurate interpretations.
Priority Nursing Tip: Posturing indicates deterioration in the client's neurological status.
Test-Taking Strategy: Focus on the subject, decorticate and decerebrate posturing. Eliminate options 2 and 3 first because they are comparable or alike. From the remaining options, recalling the significance of decerebrate posturing will assist in eliminating option 1. Review: the significance of decorticate and decerebrate posturing.
Reference(s): McKinney et al (2013), pp. 1419-1420.

85. The nurse caring for a hospitalized infant is monitoring for increased intracranial pressure (ICP) and notes that the anterior fontanel bulges when the infant cries. Based on this assessment finding, which action should the nurse take?
1. Document the findings.
2. Lower the head of the bed.
3. Place the infant on NPO status.
4. Notify the health care provider immediately.

Level of Cognitive Ability: Applying
Client Needs: Physiological Integrity
Integrated Process: Nursing Process/Implementation
Content Area: Fundamental Skills: Safety
Priority Concepts: Clinical Judgment; Development

Answer: 1
Rationale: The anterior fontanel is diamond shaped and located on the top of the head. It should be soft and flat in a normal infant, and it normally closes by 12 to 18 months of age. The posterior fontanel closes by 2 to 3 months of age. A bulging or tense fontanel may result from crying or increased ICP. Noting a bulging fontanel when the infant cries is a normal finding that should be documented and monitored. It is not necessary to notify the health care provider. Options 2 and 3 are inappropriate actions.
Priority Nursing Tip: A full or bulging anterior fontanel in a quiet infant may indicate increased intracranial pressure (ICP).
Test-Taking Strategy: Focus on the subject, bulging anterior fontanel. Note that the question states the anterior fontanel bulges when the infant cries. Remember that a bulging or tense fontanel may result from crying; therefore, it is a normal finding. Review: **anterior fontanel** and **infant assessment.**
Reference(s): Hockenberry, Wilson (2013), pp. 195-196, 928-929.

86. The nurse is assessing the vital signs of a 3-year-old child hospitalized with a diagnosis of croup and notes that the respiratory rate is 28 breaths per minute. Based on this finding, which nursing action is appropriate?
1. Administer oxygen.
2. Document the findings.
3. Notify the health care provider.
4. Reassess the respiratory rate in 15 minutes.

Level of Cognitive Ability: Applying
Client Needs: Physiological Integrity
Integrated Process: Nursing Process/Implementation
Content Area: Child Health: Throat/Respiratory
Priority Concepts: Development; Gas Exchange

Answer: 2
Rationale: The normal respiratory rate for a 3-year-old child is approximately 20 to 30 breaths per minute. Because the respiratory rate is normal, options 1, 3, and 4 are unnecessary actions. The nurse would document the findings.
Priority Nursing Tip: Nasal flaring, sternal retractions, and inspiratory stridor are signs of a compromised airway and respiratory distress.
Test-Taking Strategy: Focus on the subject, pediatric vital signs. Recalling that the normal respiratory rate for a 3-year-old child is approximately 20 to 30 breaths per minute will direct you to the correct option. Review: the **normal vital signs** in a 3-year-old child.
Reference(s): McKinney et al (2013), p. 808.

87. The nurse is performing an assessment on a female client who is suspected of having mittelschmerz. On assessment of the client, which finding does the nurse expect to note?
1. Experiences pain during intercourse
2. Has pain at the onset of menstruation
3. Experiences profuse vaginal bleeding
4. Has sharp pelvic pain during ovulation

Level of Cognitive Ability: Understanding
Client Needs: Physiological Integrity
Integrated Process: Nursing Process/Assessment
Content Area: Adult Health: Health Assessment/Physical Exam
Priority Concepts: Pain; Reproduction

Answer: 4
Rationale: Mittelschmerz (middle pain) refers to pelvic pain that occurs midway between menstrual periods or at the time of ovulation. The pain is caused by a growth follicle within the ovary, or rupture of the follicle and subsequent spillage of follicular fluid and blood into the peritoneal space. The pain is fairly sharp and is felt on the right or left side of the pelvis. It generally lasts 1 to 3 days, and slight vaginal bleeding may accompany the discomfort.
Priority Nursing Tip: The discomfort that occurs with mittelschmerz is usually relieved with a mild analgesic.
Test-Taking Strategy: Focus on the subject, mittelschmerz. Recalling that mittelschmerz is "middle pain" will direct you to the correct option. Review: **mittelschmerz.**
Reference(s): Dolan, Holt (2013), p. 452.

88. During a health assessment, the client tells the nurse that she was diagnosed with endometriosis and asks the nurse to describe this condition. How should the nurse explain endometriosis to the client?
1. Endometriosis is extrauterine endometrial tissue.
2. Endometriosis is known as primary dysmenorrhea.
3. Endometriosis is a process that halts menstruation.
4. Endometriosis is pain that occurs during ovulation.

Level of Cognitive Ability: Understanding
Client Needs: Physiological Integrity
Integrated Process: Nursing Process/Implementation
Content Area: Adult Health: Health Assessment/Physical Exam
Priority Concepts: Client Education; Reproduction

Answer: 1
Rationale: Endometriosis is defined as the presence of tissue outside the uterus that resembles the endometrium in structure, function, and response to estrogen and progesterone during the menstrual cycle. *Primary dysmenorrhea* refers to menstrual pain without identified pathology. *Amenorrhea*, the cessation of menstruation for a period of at least three cycles or 6 months in a woman who has established a pattern of menstruation, can result from a variety of causes. *Mittelschmerz* refers to pelvic pain that occurs midway between menstrual periods coinciding with ovulation.
Priority Nursing Tip: Nonpharmacologic measures such as rest and the application of heat to the lower abdomen will assist in relieving the discomfort associated with menstrual discomfort.
Test-Taking Strategy: Focus on the subject, endometriosis. Note the relationship between "endometriosis" in the question and "endometrium" in the correct option. Review: the endometriosis.
Reference(s): Hammond, Zimmermann (2013), p. 499.

❖ **89.** The health care provider prescribes 250 mg of amikacin sulfate (Amikin) every 12 hours to treat a skin infection and the nurse determines that the dosage prescribed is safe. How many milliliters (mL) should the nurse prepare to administer one dose? **Refer to the figure. Fill in the blank.**

Answer: _____ mL

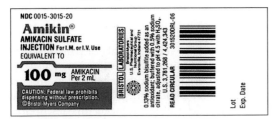

From Kee J, Marshall S: *Clinical calculations*, ed 7, St. Louis, 2012, Saunders.

Level of Cognitive Ability: Applying
Client Needs: Physiological Integrity
Integrated Process: Nursing Process/Implementation
Content Area: Fundamental Skills: Medication/IV Calculations
Priority Concepts: Clinical Judgment; Safety

Answer: 5
Rationale: Use the medication calculation formula.
Formula:

$$\frac{Desired \times mL}{Available} = mL\,per\,dose$$

$$\frac{250\,mg \times 2\,mL}{100\,mg} = 5\,mL\,per\,dose$$

Priority Nursing Tip: Amikacin sulfate (Amikin) is an aminoglycoside that can cause ototoxicity and renal toxicity as adverse effects.
Test-Taking Strategy: Focus on the subject, amikacin sulfate (Amikin) and note the data on the medication label. Follow the formula for calculating the correct dose. Once you have performed the calculation, recheck your work with a calculator and make sure that the answer makes sense. Review: **medication calculation** problems.
Reference(s): Potter et al (2013), pp. 573-574.

90. A hepatitis B screen is performed on a post-partum client and the results indicate the presence of antigens in the maternal blood. Which intervention should the nurse anticipate to be prescribed to protect the neonate?
1. Obtain serum liver enzymes.
2. Repeat hepatitis B screen in 1 week.
3. Administer antibiotics during pregnancy.
4. Administer hepatitis vaccine and hepatitis B immune globulin to the neonate.

Level of Cognitive Ability: Analyzing
Client Needs: Physiological Integrity
Integrated Process: Nursing Process/Analysis
Content Area: Maternity: Newborn
Priority Concepts: Infection; Safety

Answer: 4
Rationale: A hepatitis B screen is performed to detect the presence of antigens in maternal blood. If antigens are present, the neonate should receive the hepatitis vaccine and hepatitis B immune globulin within 12 hours after birth. Obtaining serum liver enzymes, retesting the maternal blood in a week, and administering antibiotics are inappropriate actions and would not decrease the chance of the neonate contracting the hepatitis B virus.
Priority Nursing Tip: The risks of prematurity, low birth weight, and neonatal death increase if the mother has hepatitis B infection.
Test-Taking Strategy: Focus on the subject, hepatitis B in pregnancy and the data in the question. Eliminate options 1, 2, and 3 because they are actions that would not decrease a chance of the neonate contracting the hepatitis B virus. Recall that the concern is the effect on the fetus and neonate, which will lead you to the correct option. Review: the purpose and the significance of the hepatitis B screen during pregnancy.
Reference(s): Lowdermilk, Perry, Cashion, Alden (2012), p. 850; McKinney et al (2013), p. 249.

❖ **91.** The nurse is counseling the family of a client who has terminal cancer about palliative care. The nurse explains that which are goals of palliative care? **Select all that apply.**
❏ 1. Delays death
❏ 2. Offers a support system
❏ 3. Provides relief from pain
❏ 4. Enhances the quality of life
❏ 5. Focuses only on the client, not the family
❏ 6. Manages symptoms of disease and therapies

Level of Cognitive Ability: Applying
Client Needs: Physiological Integrity
Integrated Process: Caring
Content Area: Developmental Stages: End-of-Life Care
Priority Concepts: Caregiving; Palliation

Answer: 2, 3, 4, 6
Rationale: Palliative care is a philosophy of total care. Palliative care goals include the following: offering a support system to help the client live as actively as possible until death; providing relief from pain and other distressing symptoms; enhancing the quality of life; offering a support system to help families cope during the client's illness and their own bereavement; affirming life and regarding dying as a normal process, neither hastening nor postponing death; and integrating psychological and spiritual aspects of client care.
Priority Nursing Tip: Palliative care is designed to assist the client and family in achieving the best quality of life during the entire course of an illness.
Test-Taking Strategy: Focus on the subject, goals of palliative care. Recall that palliative care interventions are designed to relieve or reduce the intensity of uncomfortable symptoms but not to produce a cure, and that palliative care is a philosophy of total care. With this in mind, read each option and determine if it meets this description. Review: the goals of palliative care.
Reference(s): Ignatavicius, Workman (2013), p. 110; Potter et al (2013), pp. 989-990.

92. The nurse is performing an assessment on a client seen in the health care clinic for a first prenatal visit. The nurse asks the client when the first day of the last menstrual period (LMP) was and the client reports February 9, 2015. Using Näegele's rule, what should the nurse determine is the estimated date of birth?

1. October 7, 2015
2. October 16, 2015
3. November 7, 2015
4. November 16, 2015

Level of Cognitive Ability: Understanding
Client Needs: Physiological Integrity
Integrated Process: Nursing Process/Assessment
Content Area: Maternity: Antepartum
Priority Concepts: Clinical Judgment; Reproduction

Answer: 4
Rationale: Accurate use of Näegele's rule requires that the woman have a regular 28-day menstrual cycle. To calculate the estimated date of birth, the nurse would subtract 3 months from the first day of the LMP, add 7 days, and then adjust the year as appropriate. First day of last menstrual period: February 9, 2015; subtract 3 months: November 9, 2014; add 7 days: November 16, 2014; and add 1 year, November 16, 2015.
Priority Nursing Tip: There are several formulas that can be used by the health care provider to determine the estimated date of birth. Näegele's rule is reasonably accurate and is the method that is usually used.
Test-Taking Strategy: Focus on the subject, Näegele's rule to answer this question. Be careful when following the steps to determine the estimated date of birth using this rule. Read all of the options carefully, noting the dates and years before selecting an option. Review: Näegele's rule.
Reference(s): McKinney et al (2013), p. 247.

93. The nurse prepares to access an implanted vascular access port. Which should the nurse implement **first**?

1. Palpate the vascular port.
2. Anchor the vascular port.
3. Cleanse the site with alcohol.
4. Apply a cool compress to the site.

Level of Cognitive Ability: Applying
Client Needs: Physiological Integrity
Integrated Process: Nursing Process/Implementation
Content Area: Critical Care: Medications and Intravenous Therapy
Priority Concepts: Clinical Judgment; Safety

Answer: 1
Rationale: Before accessing an implanted vascular access port, the nurse must palpate the port to locate the center of the septum because the nurse needs to know where to insert the needle to avoid more than one needle stick for the client. The nurse then applies the cool compress to the insertion site to ease any discomfort that occurs from the needle stick, cleanses the site with alcohol, anchors the port with the nondominant hand avoiding contamination of the septum, and accesses the site.
Priority Nursing Tip: An implanted vascular access port is surgically implanted under the skin and is used for long-term administration of repeated intravenous therapy.
Test-Taking Strategy: Note the strategic word, *first*. Use the steps of the nursing process, remembering that assessment is the first step. Palpation is an assessment technique. Review: the concepts related to accessing **implanted vascular access ports**.
Reference(s): Ignatavicius, Workman (2013), pp. 218-219.

94. The nurse is preparing to measure the fundal height of a client whose fetus is 28 weeks' gestation. In what position should the nurse place the client to perform the procedure?

1. In a standing position
2. In the Trendelenburg position
3. Supine with the head of the bed elevated to 45 degrees
4. Supine with her head on a pillow and knees slightly flexed

Level of Cognitive Ability: Applying
Client Needs: Physiological Integrity
Integrated Process: Nursing Process/Assessment
Content Area: Maternity: Antepartum
Priority Concepts: Clinical Judgment; Reproduction

Answer: 4
Rationale: When measuring fundal height, the client lies in a supine (back) position with her head on a pillow and knees slightly flexed. The standing position, Trendelenburg (head lowered), or supine with the head of the bed elevated to 45 degrees would not give an accurate measurement.
Priority Nursing Tip: During the second and third trimesters of pregnancy (weeks 18 to 30), fundal height in centimeters (cm) approximately equals fetal age in weeks plus 2 cm.
Test-Taking Strategy: Focus on the subject, measuring fundal height. Visualize this assessment technique to direct you to the correct option. Options 1, 2, or 3 would not give an accurate measurement. Review: the procedure for measuring **fundal height**.
Reference(s): McKinney et al (2013), pp. 250-251.

95. The nurse is measuring the fundal height on a client who is 36 weeks' gestation when the client complains of feeling lightheaded. The nurse should determine that the client's complaint is **most likely** caused by which condition?

1. Fear
2. Anemia
3. A full bladder
4. Compression of the vena cava

Level of Cognitive Ability: Analyzing
Client Needs: Physiological Integrity
Integrated Process: Nursing Process/Analysis
Content Area: Maternity: Antepartum
Priority Concepts: Perfusion; Reproduction

Answer: 4
Rationale: Compression of the inferior vena cava and aorta by the uterus may cause supine hypotension syndrome (vena cava syndrome) late in pregnancy. Having the client turn onto her left side or elevating the left buttock during fundal height measurement will prevent the problem. Options 1, 2, and 3 are unrelated to this syndrome.
Priority Nursing Tip: Signs of supine hypotension (vena cava syndrome) in a pregnant client include pallor, lightheadedness, breathlessness, tachycardia, hypotension, sweating, cool and damp skin, and fetal distress.
Test-Taking Strategy: Note the strategic words, *most likely.* Focus on the subject, vena cava syndrome. Recalling that compression of the inferior vena cava and aorta by the uterus may cause supine hypotension syndrome will direct you to the correct option. Review: **vena cava syndrome.**
Reference(s): McKinney et al (2013), p. 237.

96. The nurse in the prenatal clinic is monitoring a client who is pregnant with twins. The nurse monitors the client closely for which **priority** complication that is associated with a twin pregnancy?

1. Hemorrhoids
2. Postterm labor
3. Maternal anemia
4. Costovertebral angle tenderness

Level of Cognitive Ability: Applying
Client Needs: Physiological Integrity
Integrated Process: Nursing Process/Assessment
Content Area: Maternity: Antepartum
Priority Concepts: Clinical Judgment; Reproduction

Answer: 3
Rationale: Maternal anemia often occurs in twin pregnancies because of a greater demand for iron by the fetuses. Options 1 and 4 occur in a twin pregnancy but would not be as high a priority as anemia. Option 2 is incorrect because twin pregnancies often end in prematurity.
Priority Nursing Tip: The woman with a multifetal pregnancy needs to be monitored closely for signs of anemia. Adequate nutrition is critical, and supplemental vitamins are prescribed to meet the needs of each fetus without depleting maternal stores.
Test-Taking Strategy: Focus on the subject, twin pregnancy, and note the strategic word, *priority.* Thinking about the physiological occurrences of a twin pregnancy will direct you to the correct option. Review: the risks associated with a **twin pregnancy.**
Reference(s): Lowdermilk, Perry, Cashion, Alden (2012), pp. 362-363; McKinney et al (2013), pp. 251-252.

97. A clinic nurse is assessing a prenatal client with heart disease. The nurse carefully assesses the client's vital signs, weight, and fluid and nutritional status to detect for complications caused by which pregnancy-related concern?

1. Rh incompatibility
2. Fetal cardiomegaly
3. The increase in circulating blood volume
4. Hypertrophy and increased contractility of the heart

Level of Cognitive Ability: Applying
Client Needs: Physiological Integrity
Integrated Process: Nursing Process/Assessment
Content Area: Maternity: Antepartum
Priority Concepts: Perfusion; Reproduction

Answer: 3
Rationale: Pregnancy taxes the circulating system of every woman because the blood volume increases, which causes the cardiac output to increase. Stroke volume × heart rate = cardiac output (SV × HR = CO). Options 1, 2, and 4 are not directly associated with pregnancy in a client with a cardiac condition.
Priority Nursing Tip: A pregnant client with cardiac disease may be unable to physiologically cope with the added blood volume that occurs during pregnancy.
Test-Taking Strategy: Focus on the subject, a prenatal client with heart disease. Eliminate options 1 and 2 first because they address the fetus, not the prenatal client. From the remaining options, recalling the changes that take place in the woman during pregnancy will direct you to the correct option. Also, remember that hypertrophy of the heart may occur in cardiac disease, but the outcome would be a decrease in contractility, not an increase. Review: the pathophysiology in relation to **cardiac disease in the pregnant client.**
Reference(s): Lowdermilk, Perry, Cashion, Alden (2012), pp. 715, 717; McKinney et al (2013), p. 619.

98. The nurse assists the health care provider with a liver biopsy performed at the bedside. Which position should the nurse place the client in after the biopsy?

1. Supine with the head elevated on one pillow
2. Semi-Fowler's with two pillows under the legs
3. Left side-lying with a small pillow under the puncture site
4. Right side-lying with a folded towel under the puncture site

Level of Cognitive Ability: Applying
Client Needs: Physiological Integrity
Integrated Process: Nursing Process/Implementation
Content Area: Adult Health: Gastrointestinal
Priority Concepts: Clinical Judgment; Clotting

Answer: 4
Rationale: The liver is located on the right side of the body. After a liver biopsy, the nurse positions the client on the right side with a small pillow or folded towel under the puncture site for 2 hours. This position compresses the liver against the abdominal wall at the biopsy site to tamponade bleeding from the puncture site.
Priority Nursing Tip: Because of the concern for bleeding after a liver biopsy, coagulation blood studies (prothrombin time, partial thromboplastin time, platelet count) are performed before the procedure is done.
Test-Taking Strategy: Focus on the subject, liver biopsy. Use knowledge regarding the anatomy of the body and principles of hemostasis to answer this question. Remember that the liver is on the right side of the body, and by applying pressure at the puncture site, the nurse helps prevent the escape of blood or bile. Review: care of the client after a liver biopsy.
Reference(s): Pagana, Pagana (2013), p. 604.

❖ **99.** A client has a prescription to receive an enema before bowel surgery. The nurse assists the client into which position to administer the enema? **Refer to figures 1-4.**

1.

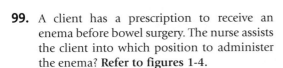

2.

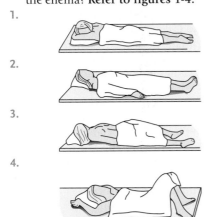

3.

4.

Figures from Potter P, Perry A, Stockert P, Hall A: *Fundamentals of nursing*, 8e, St. Louis, 2013, Mosby.

Level of Cognitive Ability: Applying
Client Needs: Physiological Integrity
Integrated Process: Nursing Process/Implementation
Content Area: Adult Health: Gastrointestinal
Priority Concepts: Clinical Judgment; Elimination

Answer: 3
Rationale: When administering an enema, the nurse places the client in a left-lateral Sims' position (option 3) exposing the rectal area and allowing the enema solution to flow by gravity in the natural direction of the colon. In the prone position (option 1), the client is lying on the stomach. In the supine position (option 2), the client is lying on the back. The dorsal recumbent position (option 4) is used for abdominal assessment because it promotes relaxation of abdominal muscles.
Priority Nursing Tip: Administering an enema with the client sitting on the toilet can cause injury to the rectal mucosa because the rectal tubing is curved and could scratch the tissue.
Test-Taking Strategy: Focus on the subject, enema administration. Use knowledge regarding the anatomy of the bowel to answer the question. This will assist in eliminating options 2 and 4. From the remaining options, visualize the procedure for administering an enema and eliminate option 1 because in the prone position, the client is lying on the stomach. Review: the procedure for administering an enema.
Reference(s): Potter et al (2013), pp. 490, 1112-1114.

100. The nurse is caring for a client who is receiving cyclosporine (Sandimmune). Which indicates to the nurse that the client is experiencing an adverse effect of the medication?
1. Acne
2. Sweating
3. Joint pain
4. Hyperkalemia

Level of Cognitive Ability: Analyzing
Client Needs: Physiological Integrity
Integrated Process: Nursing Process/Analysis
Content Area: Pharmacology: Immune Medications
Priority Concepts: Clinical Judgment; Safety

Answer: 4
Rationale: Cyclosporine is an immunosuppressant medication used in the prophylaxis of organ rejection. Adverse effects include nephrotoxicity, infection, hepatotoxicity, hypomagnesemia, coma, hypertension, tremor, and hirsutism. Additionally, neurotoxicity, gastrointestinal effects, hyperkalemia, and hyperglycemia can occur. Options 1, 2, and 3 are not associated with this medication.
Priority Nursing Tip: Monitor the urine output and the potassium level if a client is receiving a medication that is nephrotoxic.
Test-Taking Strategy: Focus on the subject, cyclosporine (Sandimmune). Recall that this medication is an immunosuppressant used to prevent organ rejection. Next, remember that this medication is nephrotoxic and causes hyperkalemia. This will direct you to the correct option. Review: the adverse effects of cyclosporine (Sandimmune).
Reference(s): Hodgson, Kizior (2014), p. 293.

101. A childbirth educator tells a class of expectant parents that it is standard routine to instill a medication into the eyes of a newborn infant as a preventive measure against ophthalmia neonatorum. The educator should tell the class that which medication is currently used for the prophylaxis of ophthalmia neonatorum?
1. Penicillin ophthalmic eye ointment
2. Neomycin ophthalmic eye ointment
3. Vitamin K injection (Aquamephyton)
4. Erythromycin ophthalmic eye ointment

Level of Cognitive Ability: Applying
Client Needs: Physiological Integrity
Integrated Process: Teaching and Learning
Content Area: Maternity: Newborn
Priority Concepts: Infection; Safety

Answer: 4
Rationale: Ophthalmic erythromycin 0.5% ointment is a broad-spectrum antibiotic and is used prophylactically to prevent ophthalmia neonatorum, an eye infection acquired from the newborn infant's passage through the birth canal. Infection from these organisms can cause blindness or serious eye damage. Erythromycin is effective against *Neisseria gonorrhoeae* and *Chlamydia trachomatis*. Vitamin K is administered to the newborn infant to prevent abnormal bleeding, and it promotes liver formation of the clotting factors II, VII, IX, and X. Options 1 and 2 are incorrect and are not medications routinely used in the newborn.
Priority Nursing Tip: Administer prophylactic eye medication to a newborn within 1 hour after birth.
Test-Taking Strategy: Focus on the subject, eye medication used for the prophylaxis of ophthalmia neonatorum. This will assist in eliminating option 3, an injection. From the remaining options, recalling that erythromycin is a broad-spectrum antibiotic will direct you to the correct option. Review: ophthalmia neonatorum.
Reference(s): McKinney et al (2013), pp. 509-510.

102. The nurse is reviewing the records of recently admitted clients to the postpartum unit. The nurse determines that which new client would be at least risk for developing a puerperal infection?
1. A client with a history of previous infections
2. A client who had an excessive number of vaginal exams
3. A client who underwent a vaginal delivery of the newborn
4. A client who experienced prolonged rupture of the membranes

Level of Cognitive Ability: Analyzing
Client Needs: Physiological Integrity
Integrated Process: Nursing Process/Assessment
Content Area: Maternity: Antepartum
Priority Concepts: Infection; Reproduction

Answer: 3
Rationale: A vaginal delivery would put the client at least risk for developing a puerperal infection. Risk factors associated with puerperal infection include a history of previous infections, excessive number of vaginal examinations, cesarean births, prolonged rupture of the membranes, prolonged labor, trauma, and retained placental fragments.
Priority Nursing Tip: The temperature may be elevated during the first 24 hours postpartum because of the dehydrating effects of labor. However, a temperature higher than 100.4° F needs to be reported to the health care provider because it is an indication of infection.
Test-Taking Strategy: Note the words "least risk" and focus on the subject, developing a puerperal infection. Eliminate option 1 first because of its relationship to infection. Next, eliminate option 4 because of the word "prolonged" and option 2 because of the word "excessive." Review: the risk factors associated with puerperal infection.
Reference(s): McKinney et al (2013), p. 678.

103. The nurse in the delivery room assists with the delivery of a newborn. After delivery, what should the nurse do to prevent heat loss via conduction in the newborn?
1. Wrap the newborn in a blanket
2. Close the doors to the delivery room
3. Dry the newborn with a warm blanket
4. Place a warm pad on the crib before placing the newborn in the crib

Level of Cognitive Ability: Applying
Client Needs: Physiological Integrity
Integrated Process: Nursing Process/Implementation
Content Area: Maternity: Newborn
Priority Concepts: Development; Thermoregulation

Answer: 4
Rationale: Hypothermia caused by conduction occurs when the newborn is on a cold surface, such as a cold pad or mattress. Warming the crib pad will assist in preventing hypothermia by conduction. Radiation occurs when heat from the newborn radiates to a colder surface. Convection occurs as air moves across the newborn's skin from an open door and heat is transferred to the air. Evaporation of moisture from a wet body dissipates heat along with the moisture. Keeping the newborn dry by drying the wet newborn at birth will prevent hypothermia via evaporation.
Priority Nursing Tip: Newborns do not shiver to produce heat. Instead, they have brown fat deposits, which produce heat.
Test-Taking Strategy: Focus on the subject, preventing heat loss in the newborn. Note the word "conduction" in the question to assist in selecting the correct option. Recalling that conduction occurs when a baby is on a cold surface will assist in directing you to the correct option. Review: **conduction.**
Reference(s): McKinney et al (2013), pp. 470-471.

104. After assessment and diagnostic evaluation, it has been determined that the client has Lyme disease, stage II. The nurse assesses the client for which manifestation that is **most** indicative of this stage?
1. Lethargy
2. Headache
3. Erythematous rash
4. Neurological deficits

Level of Cognitive Ability: Analyzing
Client Needs: Physiological Integrity
Integrated Process: Nursing Process/Assessment
Content Area: Adult Health: Immune
Priority Concepts: Clinical Judgment; Immunity

Answer: 4
Rationale: Stage II of Lyme disease develops within 1 to 3 months in most untreated individuals. The most serious problems in this stage include cardiac dysrhythmias, dyspnea, dizziness, and neurological disorders such as Bell's palsy and paralysis. These problems are not usually permanent. Flulike symptoms (headache and lethargy), muscle pain and stiffness, and a rash appear in stage I.
Priority Nursing Tip: The typical ring-shaped rash of Lyme disease does not occur in all clients. Additionally if a rash does occur, it can occur anywhere on the body, not only at the site of the tick bite.
Test-Taking Strategy: Note the strategic word, *most.* Focus on the subject, Lyme disease. Recalling that a rash and flulike symptoms occur in stage I will assist you in eliminating options 1, 2, and 3 and direct you to the correct option. Review: **Lyme disease.**
Reference(s): Hammond, Zimmermann (2013), p. 347; Ignatavicius, Workman (2013), pp. 352-353.

105. The nurse is caring for a client with a diagnosis of pemphigus vulgaris. On assessment of the client, the nurse should look for which sign characteristic of this condition?
1. Turner's sign
2. Chvostek's sign
3. Nikolsky's sign
4. Trousseau's sign

Level of Cognitive Ability: Analyzing
Client Needs: Physiological Integrity
Integrated Process: Nursing Process/Assessment
Content Area: Adult Health: Integumentary
Priority Concepts: Clinical Judgment; Tissue Integrity

Answer: 3
Rationale: A hallmark sign of pemphigus vulgaris is Nikolsky's sign, which occurs when the epidermis can be rubbed off by slight friction or injury. Other characteristics include flaccid bullae that rupture easily and emit a foul-smelling drainage, leaving crusted, denuded skin. The lesions are common on the face, back, chest, and umbilicus. Even slight pressure on an intact blister may cause spread to adjacent skin. *Turner's sign* refers to a grayish discoloration of the flanks and is seen in clients with acute pancreatitis. *Chvostek's sign,* seen in tetany, is a spasm of the facial muscles elicited by tapping the facial nerve in the region of the parotid gland. *Trousseau's sign* is a sign for tetany, in which carpal spasm can be elicited by compressing the upper arm with a blood pressure cuff inflated above the systolic pressure and causing ischemia to the nerves distally.
Priority Nursing Tip: Pemphigus vulgaris is a rare autoimmune disease that causes blister (bullae) formation. The nurse needs to provide gentle care to prevent disruption of the skin lesions.
Test-Taking Strategy: Focus on the subject, pemphigus vulgaris. Eliminate options 2 and 4 first because they are comparable or alike and both relate to tetany. From the remaining options, recalling that Turner's sign is related to pancreatitis will direct you to the correct option. Review: the characteristics of **pemphigus vulgaris.**
Reference(s): Ignatavicius, Workman (2013), p. 508; Medline Plus: Nikolsky's Sign (2013), available at http://www.nlm.nih.gov/medlineplus/ency/article/003285.htm.

106. After tonsillectomy, which fluid or food item is **most appropriate** to offer to the child?
1. Green Jell-O
2. Cold soda pop
3. Butterscotch pudding
4. Cool raspberry Kool-Aid

Level of Cognitive Ability: Applying
Client Needs: Physiological Integrity
Integrated Process: Nursing Process/Implementation
Content Area: Child Health: Throat/Respiratory
Priority Concepts: Nutrition; Safety

Answer: 1
Rationale: After tonsillectomy, clear, cool liquids should be administered. Citrus, carbonated, and extremely hot or cold liquids need to be avoided because they may irritate the throat. Milk and milk products (pudding) are avoided because they coat the throat and cause the child to clear the throat, thus increasing the risk of bleeding. Red liquids need to be avoided because they give the appearance of blood if the child vomits.
Priority Nursing Tip: After tonsillectomy, position the client prone or side-lying to facilitate mouth drainage.
Test-Taking Strategy: Note the strategic words, *most appropriate.* Avoiding foods and fluids that may irritate or cause bleeding is the concern. This will assist in eliminating options 2 and 3. The word "raspberry" in option 4 should be the clue that this is not an appropriate food item. Review: **tonsillectomy.**
Reference(s): McKinney et al (2013), p. 1158.

107. The nurse provides a class to new mothers on newborn care. When teaching cord care, the nurse should instruct mothers to take which action?
1. If antibiotic ointment has been applied to the cord, it is not necessary to do anything else to it.
2. All that is necessary is to wash the cord with antibacterial soap and allow it to air dry once a day.
3. Apply alcohol thoroughly to the cord, being careful not to move the cord because it will cause the newborn infant pain.
4. Apply the prescribed cleansing agent to the cord, ensuring that all areas around the cord are cleaned two to three times a day.

Level of Cognitive Ability: Applying
Client Needs: Physiological Integrity
Integrated Process: Teaching and Learning
Content Area: Maternity: Newborn
Priority Concepts: Client Education; Infection

Answer: 4
Rationale: The cord and base should be cleansed with alcohol (or another substance as prescribed) thoroughly, two to three times per day. The steps are (1) lift the cord; (2) wipe around the cord, starting at the top; (3) clean the base of the cord; and (4) fold the diaper below the umbilical cord to allow the cord to air dry and prevent contamination from urine. Antibiotic ointment is not normally prescribed. Continuation of cord care is necessary until the cord falls off within 7 to 14 days. Water and soap are not necessary; in fact, the cord should be kept from getting wet. The infant does not feel pain in this area.
Priority Nursing Tip: The nurse needs to teach the parents of a newborn about the importance of providing cord care because the umbilical cord stump provides a medium for bacterial growth and can easily become infected.
Test-Taking Strategy: Focus on the subject, umbilical cord care. Simply recalling that the cord should be cleansed two to three times a day will direct you to the correct option. Also, note the words "prescribed cleansing agent" in the correct option. Review: **cord care.**
Reference(s): Lowdermilk, Perry, Cashion, Alden (2012), p. 596; McKinney et al (2013), pp. 515, 522.

108. The nurse is monitoring a preterm newborn infant for manifestations of respiratory distress syndrome (RDS). The nurse should monitor the infant for which manifestations?
1. Acrocyanosis, emphysema, and interstitial edema
2. Acrocyanosis, apnea, pneumothorax, and grunting
3. Barrel-shaped chest, acrocyanosis, and bradycardia
4. Cyanosis, tachypnea, retractions, grunting respirations, and nasal flaring

Level of Cognitive Ability: Applying
Client Needs: Physiological Integrity
Integrated Process: Nursing Process/Assessment
Content Area: Maternity: Newborn
Priority Concepts: Clinical Judgment; Gas Exchange

Answer: 4
Rationale: The newborn infant with RDS may present with clinical manifestation of cyanosis, tachypnea or apnea, chest wall retractions, audible grunts, or nasal flaring. Acrocyanosis, the bluish discoloration of the hands and feet, is associated with immature peripheral circulation and is not uncommon in the first few hours of life. Options 1, 2, and 3 do not indicate clinical signs of RDS.
Priority Nursing Tip: The presence of retractions indicates respiratory distress and possible hypoxemia.
Test-Taking Strategy: Focus on the subject, respiratory distress syndrome. Recalling that acrocyanosis may be a normal sign in a newborn infant will assist in eliminating options 1, 2, and 3. Also, note the relationship between the diagnosis and the signs noted in option 4. Review: the signs of **respiratory distress syndrome (RDS).**
Reference(s): Hockenberry, Wilson (2013), p. 269; McKinney et al (2013), pp. 708-709.

109. The nurse is preparing to assess the apical heart rate of a newborn infant. The nurse performs the procedure and notes that the heart rate is normal if which value is noted?
1. A heart rate of 90 beats per minute
2. A heart rate of 140 beats per minute
3. A heart rate of 180 beats per minute
4. A heart rate of 190 beats per minute

Level of Cognitive Ability: Understanding
Client Needs: Physiological Integrity
Integrated Process: Nursing Process/Assessment
Content Area: Maternity: Newborn
Priority Concepts: Development; Perfusion

Answer: 2
Rationale: The normal heart rate in a newborn infant is approximately 100 to 160 beats per minute. Options 1, 3, and 4 are incorrect. Option 1 indicates bradycardia, and options 3 and 4 indicate tachycardia (greater than 100 beats per minute).
Priority Nursing Tip: To measure the apical heart rate of a newborn infant, the nurse should place the stethcope at the fourth intercostal space and auscultate for 1 full minute.
Test-Taking Strategy: Focus on the subject, a newborn infant heart rate. Recalling the normal heart rate for a newborn infant will direct you to the correct option. Review: **newborn vital signs.**
Reference(s): McKinney et al (2013), p. 808.

110. The nurse reviews the electrolyte values of a client with heart failure, notes that the potassium level is low, and notifies the health care provider. The health care provider prescribes a dose of intravenous (IV) potassium chloride. When administering the IV potassium chloride, which action should the nurse take?
1. Inject it as a bolus.
2. Use a filter in the IV line.
3. Dilute it per medication instructions.
4. Apply cool compresses to the IV site during administration.

Level of Cognitive Ability: Applying
Client Needs: Physiological Integrity
Integrated Process: Nursing Process/Planning
Content Area: Pharmacology: Cardiovascular Medications
Priority Concepts: Clinical Judgment; Safety

Answer: 3
Rationale: Potassium chloride is very irritating to the vein and must be diluted to prevent phlebitis and is administered using an IV pump. Potassium chloride is never administered as a bolus injection because it can cause cardiac arrest. A filter is not necessary for potassium solutions. Cool compresses would constrict the blood vessel, which could possibly be more irritating to the vein.
Priority Nursing Tip: After adding potassium to an intravenous (IV) solution, rotate and invert the solution bag to ensure that the potassium is distributed evenly throughout the IV solution.
Test-Taking Strategy: Focus on the subject, potassium administration. Recalling that potassium chloride is always diluted before administration will eliminate option 1. From the remaining options, noting the words "per medication instructions" in option 3 will direct you to the correct option. Review: the procedure for administering IV **potassium chloride.**
Reference(s): Gahart, Nazareno (2012), p. 1132; Hodgson, Kizior (2014), pp. 963-965.

111. The nurse is caring for a client after a supratentorial craniotomy. The nurse places a sign above the client's bed stating that the client should be maintained in which position?
1. Prone
2. Supine
3. Semi-Fowler's
4. Dorsal recumbent

Level of Cognitive Ability: Applying
Client Needs: Physiological Integrity
Integrated Process: Nursing Process/Implementation
Content Area: Adult Health: Neurological
Priority Concepts: Clinical Judgment; Safety

Answer: 3
Rationale: After supratentorial surgery (surgery above the brain's tentorium), the client's head is usually elevated 30 degrees to promote venous outflow through the jugular veins and modulate intracranial pressure (ICP). Options 1, 2, and 4 are incorrect positions after this surgery because they are likely to increase ICP.
Priority Nursing Tip: To prevent increased intracranial pressure (ICP), position the client to avoid extreme hip or neck flexion and maintain the head in a midline, neutral position.
Test-Taking Strategy: Focus on the subject, supratentorial craniotomy. A helpful strategy is to remember: supra, above the brain's tentorium, head up. Also note that options 1 and 2 are comparable or alike in that they are flat positions; option 4 is eliminated because the increased intraabdominal pressure from this position is more likely to inhibit venous return from the brain. Review: **supratentorial craniotomy.**
Reference(s): Ignatavicius, Workman (2013), p. 1034.

112. An infant has been found to be human immunodeficiency virus (HIV) positive. When teaching the infant's mother, which action should the nurse instruct the mother to take?
1. Check the anterior fontanel for bulging and the sutures for widening each day.
2. Feed the infant in an upright position with the head and chest tilted slightly back to avoid aspiration.
3. Provide meticulous skin care to the infant and change the infant's diaper after each voiding or stool.
4. Feed the infant with a special nipple and burp the infant frequently to decrease the tendency to swallow air.

Level of Cognitive Ability: Applying
Client Needs: Physiological Integrity
Integrated Process: Teaching and Learning
Content Area: Child Health: Immune
Priority Concepts: Client Education; Immunity

Answer: 3
Rationale: Meticulous skin care helps protect the HIV-infected infant from secondary infections. Bulging fontanels, feeding the infant in an upright position, and using a special nipple are unrelated to the pathology associated with HIV.
Priority Nursing Tip: Newborns born to human immunodeficiency virus (HIV)-positive clients may test positive because the mother's antibodies may persist in the newborn for 18 months after birth.
Test-Taking Strategy: Focus on the subject, a newborn with HIV. Read the question carefully. The question specifically asks for instructions to be given to the mother regarding HIV. Although options 1, 2, and 4 may be correct or partially correct, the content does not specifically relate to care of the infant infected with HIV. Review: care of an infant infected with **human immunodeficiency virus (HIV)**.
Reference(s): McKinney et al (2013), pp. 725, 727.

113. The nurse is checking postoperative prescriptions and planning care for a 110-pound child after spinal fusion. Morphine sulfate, 8 mg subcutaneously every 4 hours PRN for pain, is prescribed. The pediatric medication reference states that the safe dose is 0.1 to 0.2 mg/kg/dose every 3 to 4 hours. From this information, the nurse determines what about the prescription?
1. The dose is too low.
2. The dose is too high.
3. The dose is within the safe dosage range.
4. There is not enough information to determine the safe dose.

Level of Cognitive Ability: Analyzing
Client Needs: Physiological Integrity
Integrated Process: Nursing Process/Planning
Content Area: Fundamental Skills: Medication/IV Calculations
Priority Concepts: Clinical Judgment; Safety

Answer: 3
Rationale: Use the formula to determine the dosage parameters. Convert pounds to kilograms by dividing weight by 2.2. Therefore, $110 \text{ lb} \div 2.2 = 50 \text{ kg}$.

Dosage parameters:
$$0.1 \text{ mg} / \text{kg} / \text{dose} \times 50 \text{ kg} = 5 \text{ mg}$$
$$0.2 \text{ mg} / \text{kg} / \text{dose} \times 50 \text{ kg} = 10 \text{ mg}$$

Dosage is within the safe dosage range.
Priority Nursing Tip: Conversion is the first step in the calculation of medication doses.
Test-Taking Strategy: Focus on the subject, a medication calculation. Identify the important components of the question and what the question is asking. In this case, the question asks for the safe dosage range for medication. Change pounds to kilograms. Calculate the dosage parameters using the safe dose range identified in the question and the child's weight in kilograms. Use a calculator to verify the answer. Review: **medication calculations**.
Reference(s): McKinney et al (2013), p. 952; Potter et al (2013), pp. 574-577.

114. The nurse is performing a physical assessment on a client and is testing the client's reflexes. What action should the nurse take to assess the pharyngeal reflex?
1. Ask the client to swallow.
2. Pull down on the lower eyelid.
3. Shine a light toward the bridge of the nose.
4. Stimulate the back of the throat with a tongue depressor.

Level of Cognitive Ability: Applying
Client Needs: Physiological Integrity
Integrated Process: Nursing Process/Assessment
Content Area: Adult Health: Health Assessment/Physical Exam
Priority Concepts: Clinical Judgment; Health Promotion

Answer: 4
Rationale: The pharyngeal (gag) reflex is tested by touching the back of the throat with an object, such as a tongue depressor. A positive response to this reflex is considered normal. Asking the client to swallow assesses the swallowing reflex. To assess the palpebral conjunctiva, the nurse would pull down and evert the lower eyelid. The corneal light reflex is tested by shining a penlight toward the bridge of the nose at a distance of 12 to 15 inches (light reflection should be symmetrical in both corneas).
Priority Nursing Tip: If a client receives a local throat anesthetic for a diagnostic or other procedure, the client must remain NPO until the gag reflex returns.
Test-Taking Strategy: Focus on the subject, pharyngeal reflex. Recalling that "pharyngeal" refers to the pharynx, or back of the throat, will assist in determining how this reflex is tested and direct you to the correct option. Review: assessment of the pharyngeal reflex.
Reference(s): Jarvis (2012), p. 367.

115. The pediatric nurse specialist provides an educational session to the nursing students about childhood communicable diseases, mumps. The pediatric nurse informs the students that which clinical manifestation is indicative of the **most** common complication of this communicable disease?
1. Pain
2. Deafness
3. Nuchal rigidity
4. A red swollen testicle

Level of Cognitive Ability: Analyzing
Client Needs: Physiological Integrity
Integrated Process: Teaching and Learning
Content Area: Child Health: Communicable and Infectious Diseases
Priority Concepts: Clinical Judgment; Infection

Answer: 3
Rationale: The most common complication of mumps is aseptic meningitis, with the virus being identified in the cerebrospinal fluid. Common signs include nuchal rigidity, lethargy, and vomiting. Muscular pain, parotid pain, or testicular pain may occur, but pain does not indicate a sign of a common complication. Although mumps is one of the leading causes of unilateral nerve deafness, it does not occur frequently. A red swollen testicle may be indicative of orchitis. Although this complication appears to cause most concern among parents, it is not the most common complication. Swollen and tender salivary glands under the ears on one or both sides of the head (parotitis) is the most common sign of the most common complication.
Priority Nursing Tip: Transmission of mumps is via direct contact or droplet spread from an infected person.
Test-Taking Strategy: Focus on the subject, mumps and the strategic word, *most*. Recalling that aseptic meningitis is the most common complication of mumps will direct you to the correct option. Review: mumps.
Reference(s): McKinney et al (2013), p. 1021.

116. A 5-year-old child is hospitalized with Rocky Mountain spotted fever (RMSF). The nursing assessment reveals that the child was bitten by a tick 2 weeks ago. The child presents with complaints of headache, fever, and anorexia, and the nurse notes a rash on the palms of the hands and soles of the feet. The nurse reviews the health care provider's prescriptions and anticipates that which medication will be prescribed?
1. Ganciclovir
2. Amantadine (Symmetrel)
3. Doxycycline (Vibramycin)
4. Amphotericin B (Fungizone)

Level of Cognitive Ability: Analyzing
Client Needs: Physiological Integrity
Integrated Process: Nursing Process/Analysis
Content Area: Child Health: Infectious and Communicable Diseases
Priority Concepts: Clinical Judgment; Immunity

Answer: 3
Rationale: The nursing care of a child with RMSF includes the administration of doxycycline. An alternative medication is chloramphenicol. Ganciclovir is used to treat cytomegalovirus. Amantadine is used to treat Parkinson's disease. Amphotericin B is used for fungal infections.
Priority Nursing Tip: The agent that causes Rocky Mountain spotted fever is *Rickettsia rickettsii;* transmission is via the bite of an infected tick.
Test-Taking Strategy: Focus on the subject, Rocky Mountain Spotted Fever (RMSF). Knowledge regarding the treatment plan associated with RMSF is required to answer this question. Remember that RMSF is treated with doxycycline. Review: **Rocky Mountain spotted fever.**
Reference(s): McKinney et al (2013), pp. 1028-1029.

117. A nursing instructor assigns a student nurse to present a clinical conference to the student group about brain tumors in children younger than 3 years of age. The student nurse prepares for the conference and should include which information in the presentation?
1. Radiation is the treatment of choice.
2. The most significant symptoms are headache and vomiting.
3. Head shaving is not required before removal of the brain tumor.
4. Surgery is not normally performed because of the risk of functional deficits occurring as a result of the surgery.

Level of Cognitive Ability: Applying
Client Needs: Physiological Integrity
Integrated Process: Teaching and Learning
Content Area: Child Health: Oncological
Priority Concepts: Cellular Regulation; Development

Answer: 2
Rationale: The classic symptoms of children with brain tumors are headaches and vomiting. The treatment of choice is total surgical removal of the tumor. Before surgery, the child's head will be shaved, although every effort is made to shave only as much hair as is necessary. Radiation therapy is avoided in children younger than 3 years of age because of the toxic side effects on the developing brain, particularly in very young children.
Priority Nursing Tip: The headache associated with a brain tumor in a child is worse on awakening and improves during the day.
Test-Taking Strategy: Focus on the subject, brain tumors in children. Eliminate options 3 and 4 first because of the closed-ended word "not." From the remaining options, recalling that radiation therapy is avoided in children younger than 3 years of age because of the toxic side effects on the developing brain will lead you to the correct option. Review: **brain tumors in children.**
Reference(s): McKinney et al (2013), p. 1280.

118. The nurse is caring for a child admitted to the hospital with a diagnosis of viral pneumonia. The nurse describes the treatment plan to the parents and determines the **need for further teaching** if the parents indicate that which is part of the treatment?

1. Oxygen
2. Antibiotics
3. Intravenous fluids
4. Chest physiotherapy

Level of Cognitive Ability: Evaluating
Client Needs: Physiological Integrity
Integrated Process: Teaching and Learning
Content Area: Child Health: Throat/Respiratory
Priority Concepts: Client Education; Gas Exchange

Answer: 2
Rationale: The therapeutic management for viral pneumonia is supportive. Antibiotics are not given unless the pneumonia is bacterial. More severely ill children may be hospitalized and given oxygen, chest physiotherapy, and intravenous fluids.
Priority Nursing Tip: If a specimen culture is prescribed, the culture is obtained before prescribed antibiotics are initiated.
Test-Taking Strategy: Note the strategic words, *need for further teaching*. These words indicate a negative event query and ask you to select an option that is an incorrect statement. Also note the word "viral" in the question. Recalling that viral infections are not treated with antibiotics will direct you to option 2. Oxygen, intravenous fluids, and chest physiotherapy are all appropriate interventions for this child. Review: the treatment measures for **viral pneumonia**.
Reference(s): Hockenberry, Wilson (2013), p. 726.

119. Tretinoin (Retin-A) gel is prescribed for a client with acne. The client calls the clinic nurse and tells the nurse that her skin has become very red and is beginning to peel. The nurse should make which statement to the client?

1. "Discontinue the medication."
2. "Come to the clinic immediately."
3. "Notify the health care provider."
4. "This is a normal occurrence with the use of this medication."

Level of Cognitive Ability: Applying
Client Needs: Physiological Integrity
Integrated Process: Nursing Process/Implementation
Content Area: Pharmacology: Integumentary
Priority Concepts: Client Education; Safety

Answer: 4
Rationale: Tretinoin decreases cohesiveness of the epithelial cells, increasing cell mitosis and turnover. It is potentially irritating, particularly when used correctly. Within 48 hours of use, the skin generally becomes red and begins to peel. Options 1, 2, and 3 are incorrect statements to the client.
Priority Nursing Tip: Tretinoin (Retin-A) is a derivative of vitamin A; therefore, vitamin A supplements need to be discontinued during therapy with tretinoin.
Test-Taking Strategy: Focus on the subject, tretinoin (Retin-A). Options 2 and 3 can be eliminated first because they are comparable or alike. Eliminate option 1 next because it is not within the scope of nursing practice to advise a client to discontinue a medication. Review: tretinoin (Retin-A).
Reference(s): Hodgson, Kizior (2014), p. 1207.

120. A child is hospitalized with a diagnosis of lead poisoning, and chelation therapy is prescribed. The nurse caring for the child should prepare to administer which medication?

1. Ipecac syrup
2. Activated charcoal
3. Sodium bicarbonate
4. Calcium disodium edetate (EDTA)

Level of Cognitive Ability: Applying
Client Needs: Physiological Integrity
Integrated Process: Nursing Process/Planning
Content Area: Critical Care: Emergency Situations
Priority Concepts: Clinical Judgment; Safety

Answer: 4
Rationale: EDTA is a chelating agent that is used to treat lead poisoning. Ipecac syrup may be prescribed by the health care provider for use in the hospital setting but would not be used to treat lead poisoning. Activated charcoal is used to decrease absorption in certain poisoning situations. Sodium bicarbonate may be used in salicylate poisoning.
Priority Nursing Tip: During chelation therapy, provide adequate hydration and monitor kidney function for nephrotoxicity because the medication is excreted via the kidneys.
Test-Taking Strategy: Focus on the subject, treatment related to lead poisoning. Think about the classifications of the medications in the options. Recalling that EDTA is a chelating agent will direct you to the correct option. Review: the treatment for **lead poisoning**.
Reference(s): McKinney et al (2013), p. 863.

121. The nurse is performing pin site care on a client in skeletal traction. Which normal finding should the nurse expect to note when assessing the pin sites?
1. Loose pin sites
2. Clear drainage from the pin sites
3. Purulent drainage from the pin sites
4. Redness and swelling around the pin sites

Level of Cognitive Ability: Analyzing
Client Needs: Physiological Integrity
Integrated Process: Nursing Process/Assessment
Content Area: Adult Health: Musculoskeletal
Priority Concepts: Clinical Judgment; Mobility

Answer: 2
Rationale: A small amount of clear drainage ("weeping") may be expected after cleaning and removing crusting around the pin sites of skeletal traction. Pins should not be loose; if this is noted the health care provider should be notified. Purulent drainage and redness and swelling around the pin sites may be indicative of an infection.
Priority Nursing Tip: Skeletal traction is applied mechanically to the bone with pins, wires, or tongs. Because skin integrity is disrupted, the client is at risk for infection.
Test-Taking Strategy: Focus on the subject, pin site care. Option 1 is not an expected finding and can be eliminated first because loose pins would not provide a secure hold with the traction. Eliminate options 3 and 4 next because they are comparable or alike and indicate signs of infection. Review: assessment of pin sites in the client with skeletal traction.
Reference(s): Ignatavicius, Workman (2013), pp. 1153-1154; Perry, Potter, Ostendorf (2014), p. 266.

122. The nurse is caring for a client who has been placed in Buck's extension traction while awaiting surgical repair of a fractured femur. What should the nurse check to perform a complete neurovascular assessment of the affected extremity?
1. Vital signs and bilateral lung sounds
2. Warmth of the skin and the temperature in the affected extremity
3. Pain level and for the presence of edema in the affected extremity
4. Color, sensation, movement, capillary refill, and pulse of the affected extremity

Level of Cognitive Ability: Applying
Client Needs: Physiological Integrity
Integrated Process: Nursing Process/Assessment
Content Area: Adult Health: Musculoskeletal
Priority Concepts: Mobility; Perfusion

Answer: 4
Rationale: A complete neurovascular assessment of an extremity includes color, sensation, movement, capillary refill, and pulse of the affected extremity. Option 1 is not related to neurovascular assessment. Options 2 and 3 identify components of neurovascular assessment but not of a complete assessment.
Priority Nursing Tip: Buck's extension traction is a type of skin traction used to alleviate muscle spasms and immobilize a lower limb. It is applied by using elastic bandages or adhesive, a foam boot, or a sling, and counter weights, and the foot of the bed is elevated to provide the traction.
Test-Taking Strategy: Focus on the subject, complete neurovascular assessment. Options 2 and 3 identify only some of the components of a neurovascular assessment while option 1 does not identify any. Also, use the ABCs—airway, breathing, and circulation—to direct you to the correct option. Review: the components of a neurovascular assessment.
Reference(s): Ignatavicius, Workman (2013), p. 1154.

123. A client in the emergency department has a cast applied. The client arrives at the nursing unit, and the nurse prepares to transfer the client into the bed using which method?
1. Placing ice on top of the cast
2. Supporting the cast with the fingertips only
3. Asking the client to support the cast during transfer
4. Using the palms of the hands and soft pillows to support the cast

Level of Cognitive Ability: Applying
Client Needs: Physiological Integrity
Integrated Process: Nursing Process/Planning
Content Area: Adult Health: Musculoskeletal
Priority Concepts: Mobility; Tissue Integrity

Answer: 4
Rationale: The palms or the flat surface of the extended fingers should be used when moving a wet cast to prevent indentations. Pillows are used to support the curves of the cast to prevent cracking or flattening of the cast from the weight of the body. Half-full bags of ice may be placed next to the cast to prevent swelling, but this would be done after the client is placed in bed. Asking the client to support the cast during transfer is inappropriate.
Priority Nursing Tip: Instruct the client with a cast not to stick objects inside the cast because the object can disrupt skin integrity and result in infection. If the skin under the cast is itchy, instruct the client to direct cool air from a hair dryer inside the cast.
Test-Taking Strategy: Focus on the subject, cast care. Eliminate option 1 because ice can be used for swelling after the client is placed in bed. Eliminate option 2 because of the closed-ended word "only" in this option. Eliminate option 3 because it is inappropriate to ask the client to support the cast. Review: care of the client in a newly applied plaster cast.
Reference(s): Ignatavicius, Workman (2013), p. 1151.

124. A magnetic resonance imaging (MRI) scan is prescribed for a client with a suspected brain tumor. Which prescription should the nurse prepare to administer to the client before the procedure?
1. An opioid
2. A sedative
3. A corticosteroid
4. An antihistamine

Level of Cognitive Ability: Analyzing
Client Needs: Physiological Integrity
Integrated Process: Nursing Process/Planning
Content Area: Fundamental Skills: Diagnostic Tests
Priority Concepts: Clinical Judgment; Safety

Answer: 2
Rationale: An MRI scan is a noninvasive diagnostic test that visualizes the body's tissues, structure, and blood flow. For an MRI, the client is positioned on a padded table and moved into a cylinder-shaped scanner. Relaxation techniques, an eye mask, and sedation are used before the procedure to reduce claustrophobic effects; however, because the client must remain very still during the scan, the nurse avoids oversedating the client to ensure client cooperation. There is no useful purpose for administering an opioid, corticosteroid, or antihistamine. Open MRI systems are available in some diagnostic facilities and this method of testing can be used for clients with claustrophobia.
Priority Nursing Tip: In a magnetic resonance scan, magnetic fields are used to produce an image. Therefore, all metallic objects such as a watch, other jewelry, clothing with metal fasteners, and metal hair fasteners must be removed.
Test-Taking Strategy: Focus on the subject, magnetic resonance imaging (MRI) scan. Recalling that claustrophobia is a concern will direct you to the correct option. Review: **magnetic resonance imaging (MRI) scans.**
Reference(s): Pagana, Pagana (2013), pp. 631-633.

125. A low dose of ondansetron (Zofran) is prescribed for relief of nausea in a client receiving chemotherapy. The nurse anticipates that the health care provider will **most likely** prescribe the medication by which route?
1. Oral
2. Intranasal
3. Intravenous
4. Subcutaneous

Level of Cognitive Ability: Analyzing
Client Needs: Physiological Integrity
Integrated Process: Nursing Process/Analysis
Content Area: Pharmacology: Gastrointestinal Medications
Priority Concepts: Cellular Regulation; Safety

Answer: 3
Rationale: Ondansetron (Zofran) is an antiemetic used to control nausea, vomiting, and motion sickness. It is available for administration by the oral, intramuscular (IM), or intravenous (IV) routes. The IV route is the route used when relief of nausea is needed in the client receiving chemotherapy. The IM route may be used when the medication is used as an adjunct to anesthesia. Option 1 should not be used in clients who are nauseated. Options 2 and 4 are not routes of administration of this medication.
Priority Nursing Tip: Antiemetics can cause drowsiness and hypotension; therefore, a priority intervention is to protect the client from injury.
Test-Taking Strategy: Note the strategic words, *most likely.* Focus on the subject, ondansetron (Zofran) administration to a client receiving chemotherapy. Noting that the client is receiving chemotherapy will direct you to the correct option. Review: the methods of administration of **ondansetron (Zofran).**
Reference(s): Hodgson, Kizior (2014), pp. 875-876.

126. The nurse is teaching the parents of a child with celiac disease about dietary measures. In the teaching plan, the nurse should instruct the parents to take which appropriate measure?
1. Restrict corn and rice in the diet.
2. Restrict fresh vegetables in the diet.
3. Substitute grain cereals with pasta products.
4. Read all label ingredients carefully to avoid hidden sources of gluten.

Level of Cognitive Ability: Applying
Client Needs: Physiological Integrity
Integrated Process: Teaching and Learning
Content Area: Child Health: Gastrointestinal
Priority Concepts: Client Education; Nutrition

Answer: 4
Rationale: Gluten is found primarily in the grains of wheat, rye, barley, and oats. Gluten is added to many foods as hydrolyzed vegetable protein that is derived from cereal grains; therefore, labels need to be read. Corn and rice, as well as vegetables, are acceptable in a gluten-free diet, and corn and rice become substitute foods. Many pasta products contain gluten. Grains are frequently added to processed foods for thickness or fillers.
Priority Nursing Tip: Celiac crisis is precipitated by fasting, infection, or the ingestion of gluten. It causes profuse watery diarrhea and vomiting, leading to rapid dehydration, electrolyte imbalance, and severe acidosis.
Test-Taking Strategy: Focus on the subject, celiac diet. Recall that a gluten-free diet is required in celiac disease. Select option 4 because it is the umbrella option. Review: the dietary measures in celiac disease.
Reference(s): McKinney et al (2013), p. 1105.

127. A 45-year-old client is admitted to the hospital for evaluation of recurrent runs of ventricular tachycardia noted on Holter monitoring. The client is scheduled for electrophysiology studies (EPS) the following morning. Which statement should the nurse include in a teaching plan for this client?

1. "You will continue to take your medications until the morning of the test."
2. "You will be sedated during the procedure and will not remember what has happened."
3. "This test is a noninvasive method of determining the effectiveness of your medication regimen."
4. "During the procedure, a special wire is used to increase the heart rate and produce the irregular beats that caused your signs and symptoms."

Level of Cognitive Ability: Applying
Client Needs: Physiological Integrity
Integrated Process: Nursing Process/Implementation
Content Area: Adult Health: Cardiovascular
Priority Concepts: Client Education; Perfusion

Answer: 4
Rationale: The purpose of EPS is to study the heart's electrical system. During this invasive procedure, a special wire is introduced into the heart to produce dysrhythmias. To prepare for this procedure, the client should be NPO for 6 to 8 hours before the test, and all antidysrhythmics are held for at least 24 hours before the test to study the dysrhythmias without the influence of medications. Because the client's verbal responses to the rhythm changes are extremely important, sedation is avoided if possible.
Priority Nursing Tip: Inducing a dysrhythmia during electrophysiology studies assists the health care provider in making a diagnosis and determining the appropriate treatment.
Test-Taking Strategy: Focus on the subject, electrophysiology studies (EPS). Note the relationship between the words "recurrent runs of ventricular tachycardia" in the question and "produce the irregular beats" in option 4. Review: the procedure for performing electrophysiology studies (EPS).
Reference(s): Ignatavicius, Workman (2013), p. 706; Pagana, Pagana (2013), pp. 382-385.

128. The nurse is providing diet teaching to a client with heart failure. The nurse tells the client to avoid which food item?

1. Sherbet
2. Steak sauce
3. Apple juice
4. Leafy green vegetables

Level of Cognitive Ability: Applying
Client Needs: Physiological Integrity
Integrated Process: Teaching and Learning
Content Area: Adult Health: Cardiovascular
Priority Concepts: Client Education; Nutrition

Answer: 2
Rationale: Steak sauce is high in sodium. Leafy green vegetables, any juice (except tomato or V8 brand vegetable), and sherbet are all low in sodium. Clients with heart failure should monitor sodium intake.
Priority Nursing Tip: Clients with heart failure need to monitor sodium intake because sodium causes the retention of fluid.
Test-Taking Strategy: Focus on the subject, a client with heart failure. Note the word "avoid." This word asks you to select an inappropriate food choice. Note that options 1, 3, and 4 are comparable or alike in that they are low-sodium foods. Recalling that the client with heart failure should limit sodium intake will direct you to the correct option. Review: dietary measures for the client with heart failure.
Reference(s): Ignatavicius, Workman (2013), pp. 751-752; Nix (2013), p. 389.

129. The home care nurse is developing a plan of care for an older client with type 1 diabetes mellitus who has gastroenteritis. To maintain food and fluid intake to prevent dehydration, which action should the nurse plan to take?

1. Offer water only until the client is able to tolerate solid foods.
2. Withhold all fluids until vomiting has ceased for at least 4 hours.
3. Encourage the client to take 8 to 12 ounces of fluid every hour while awake.
4. Maintain a clear liquid diet for at least 5 days before advancing to solids to allow inflammation of the bowel to dissipate.

Level of Cognitive Ability: Applying
Client Needs: Physiological Integrity
Integrated Process: Nursing Process/Planning
Content Area: Adult Health: Endocrine
Priority Concepts: Glucose Regulation; Fluid and Electrolyte Balance

Answer: 3
Rationale: Dehydration needs to be prevented in the client with type 1 diabetes mellitus because of the risk of diabetic ketoacidosis (DKA). Small amounts of fluid may be tolerated, even when vomiting is present. The client should be offered liquids containing both glucose and electrolytes. The diet should be advanced as tolerated and include a minimum of 100 to 150 g of carbohydrates daily. Offering water only and maintaining liquids for 5 days will not prevent dehydration but may promote it in this client.
Priority Nursing Tip: Diabetic ketoacidosis is a life-threatening complication of type 1 diabetes mellitus that develops when a severe insulin deficiency occurs.
Test-Taking Strategy: Focus on the subject, type 1 diabetes mellitus. Eliminate options 1 and 2 because of the words "only" and "all" in these options, respectively. From the remaining options, note the words "for at least 5 days" in option 4. Thinking about the subject, a client with diabetes mellitus and preventing dehydration, will assist in eliminating this option. Review: sick day rules for a client with diabetes mellitus.
Reference(s): Ignatavicius, Workman (2013), pp. 173, 1412-1413.

❖ **130.** The nurse in the postpartum unit is assessing a newborn for signs of breast-feeding problems. Which findings indicate a problem? **Select all that apply.**
- ❑ 1. The infant exhibits dimpling of the cheeks.
- ❑ 2. The infant makes smacking or clicking sounds.
- ❑ 3. The mother's breast gets softer during a feeding.
- ❑ 4. Milk drips from the mother's breast occasionally.
- ❑ 5. The infant falls asleep after feeding less than 5 minutes.
- ❑ 6. The infant can be heard swallowing frequently during a feeding.

Level of Cognitive Ability: Analyzing
Client Needs: Physiological Integrity
Integrated Process: Nursing Process/Assessment
Content Area: Maternity: Postpartum
Priority Concepts: Nutrition; Reproduction

Answer: 1, 2, 5
Rationale: It is important for the nurse to identify breast-feeding problems while the mother is hospitalized so that the nurse can teach the mother how to prevent and treat any problems. Infant signs of breast-feeding problems include dimpling of the cheeks; making smacking or clicking sounds; falling asleep after feeding less than 5 minutes; refusing to breast-feed; tongue thrusting; failing to open the mouth at latch-on; turning the lower lip in; making short, choppy motions of the jaw; and not swallowing audibly. Softening of the breast during feeding, noting milk in the infant's mouth or dripping from the mother's breast occasionally, and hearing the infant swallow are signs that the infant is receiving adequate nutrition.
Priority Nursing Tip: If the mother is breast-feeding, calorie needs increase by 200 to 500 calories per day; increased fluids and the continuance of prenatal vitamins and minerals are important.
Test-Taking Strategy: Focus on the subject, signs of breast-feeding problems. Think about the process of feeding and visualize the effect of each observation identified in the options. This will direct you to the correct options. Review: the signs of **breast-feeding** problems.
Reference(s): McKinney et al (2013), p. 539.

131. The nurse has completed tracheostomy care for a client whose tracheostomy tube has a nondisposable inner cannula. Immediately before reinserting the inner cannula, which is the **best** nursing action for the nurse to take?
1. Rinsing it in sterile water
2. Suctioning the client's airway
3. Drying it with loosely woven gauze
4. Tapping it against a sterile basin and using pipe cleaners to dry it

Level of Cognitive Ability: Applying
Client Needs: Physiological Integrity
Integrated Process: Nursing Process/Implementation
Content Area: Adult Health: Respiratory
Priority Concepts: Clinical Judgment; Safety

Answer: 4
Rationale: After washing and rinsing the inner cannula, the nurse taps it dry to remove large water droplets and uses pipe cleaners specifically for use with a tracheostomy to dry it; then the nurse inserts the cannula into the tracheostomy and turns it clockwise to lock it into place. The nurse should avoid shaking the inner cannula to prevent contamination. A wet cannula should not be inserted into a tracheostomy because water is a lung irritant. Suctioning is not performed without an inner cannula in place. Fine-mesh sterile gauze may be used to dry the inner cannula because it is less likely than loosely woven gauze to deposit debris on the cannula.
Priority Nursing Tip: Keep a tracheostomy obturator and a tracheostomy tube of the same size for emergency replacement if the tracheostomy is dislodged.
Test-Taking Strategy: Note the strategic word, *best*. Also note the word "nondisposable" and visualize the procedure. Eliminate option 1 because a wet cannula should not be inserted and option 2 because you would not suction a client without the inner cannula in place. Eliminate option 3 because loosely woven gauze would deposit debris. Review: the procedure for **tracheostomy** care.
Reference(s): Ignatavicius, Workman (2013), p. 576; Potter et al (2013), p. 865.

132. The nurse suspects that an air embolism has occurred when the client's central venous catheter disconnects from the intravenous (IV) tubing. The nurse **immediately** places the client in which position?
1. Trendelenburg's on the left side
2. Trendelenburg's on the right side
3. Reverse Trendelenburg's on the left side
4. Reverse Trendelenburg's on the right side

Level of Cognitive Ability: Applying
Client Needs: Physiological Integrity
Integrated Process: Nursing Process/Implementation
Content Area: Critical Care: Emergency Situations
Priority Concepts: Clinical Judgment; Gas Exchange

Answer: 1
Rationale: If the client develops an air embolism, the immediate action is to place the client in Trendelenburg's position on the left side. This position raises the client's feet higher than the head and traps any air in the right atrium. If necessary, the air can then be directly removed by intracardiac aspiration. Options 2, 3, and 4 are incorrect positions because reverse Trendelenburg's position elevates the head, puts the air in a dependent position, and increases the risk of a cerebral embolism; lying on the right side places the air in a dependent position, rendering it more likely to migrate.
Priority Nursing Tip: If an air embolism is suspected, the intravenous tubing is clamped off immediately.
Test-Taking Strategy: Focus on the subject, air embolism. Note the strategic word, *immediately*. Visualize each position in the options and recall cardiac anatomy. Recalling that the goal of action is to trap air in the right atrium will direct you to the correct option. Review: immediate care of a client with an **air embolism**.
Reference(s): Ignatavicius, Workman (2013), p. 231.

133. An anxious client enters the emergency department seeking treatment for a laceration of the finger. The client's vital signs are pulse 106 beats per minute, blood pressure (BP) 158/88 mm Hg, and respirations 28 breaths per minute. After cleansing the injury and reassuring the client, the nurse rechecks the vital signs and notes a pulse of 82 beats per minute, BP 130/80 mm Hg, and respirations 20 breaths per minute. Which accounts for the change in vital signs?
1. Cooling effects of the cleansing agent
2. Client's adaptation to the air conditioning
3. Early clinical indicators of cardiogenic shock
4. Fall in sympathetic nervous system discharge

Level of Cognitive Ability: Understanding
Client Needs: Physiological Integrity
Integrated Process: Nursing Process/Planning
Content Area: Adult Health: Cardiovascular
Priority Concepts: Perfusion; Stress

Answer: 4
Rationale: Physical or emotional stress triggers sympathetic nervous system stimulation. Increased epinephrine and norepinephrine cause tachycardia, high blood pressure, and tachypnea. Stress reduction then returns these parameters to baseline as the sympathetic discharge falls. Options 1 and 2 are unrelated to the changes in vital signs. Because the client's vital signs remain within normal limits, the client exhibits no indication of cardiogenic shock.
Priority Nursing Tip: Anxiety can cause an increase in the pulse rate, respiratory rate, and blood pressure.
Test-Taking Strategy: Focus on the subject, stress effects on vital signs. Eliminate options 1 and 2 first because they are comparable or alike. Next, note that the client is anxious and has an injury. These two pieces of information guide you to think about the body's response to stress. Recalling the relationship of stress to the sympathetic nervous system will direct you to the correct option. Review: the effects of physical stress on the **vital signs**.
Reference(s): Hammond, Zimmermann (2013), p. 214; Potter et al (2013), p. 459.

134. The nurse schedules multiple diagnostic procedures for the client with heart failure who has activity intolerance. The procedures prescribed include an echocardiogram, a chest radiograph (CXR), and a computed axial tomography (CAT) scan. Which is the **best** schedule for the nurse to plan to meet the needs of this client safely and **effectively**?

1. CAT scan and CXR in the morning, and echocardiogram on the following morning
2. CXR and echocardiogram together in the morning, and CAT scan in the afternoon of the same day
3. Echocardiogram in the morning, and CXR and CAT scans together in the afternoon of the same day
4. CXR in the morning, echocardiogram in the afternoon, and CAT scan in the morning of the following day

Level of Cognitive Ability: Analyzing
Client Needs: Physiological Integrity
Integrated Process: Nursing Process/Planning
Content Area: Adult Health: Cardiovascular
Priority Concepts: Functional Ability; Perfusion

Answer: 4
Rationale: CAT scans are always performed in radiology, and CXR and echocardiograms can be done at the bedside; however, the best results usually occur when the test is performed in the related department. As long as the client is stable and transportation is provided, the nurse can schedule each procedure in its department with two procedures on 1 day separated by a rest period, and the remaining procedure the next day. The nurse should plan the CXR and echocardiogram on the same day because if the client's condition deteriorates after the first procedure, the nurse can obtain a portable CXR or echocardiogram.
Priority Nursing Tip: The nurse should instruct the client with heart failure to balance periods of rest and activity and avoid performing isometric activities because they increase pressure in the heart.
Test-Taking Strategy: Focus on the subject, scheduling multiple diagnostic procedures for the client with heart failure who has activity intolerance. Note the strategic words, *best* and *effectively*. Recalling that the client will do best if activities are spaced will direct you to the correct option. Review: interventions for the client with **activity intolerance**.
Reference(s): Ignatavicius, Workman (2013), pp. 840-841; Potter et al (2013), pp. 755-756.

135. The nurse is preparing to initiate an intravenous nitroglycerin drip on a client with acute myocardial infarction. In the absence of an invasive (arterial) monitoring line, the nurse prepares to have which piece of equipment for use at the bedside?

1. Defibrillator
2. Pulse oximeter
3. Central venous pressure (CVP) tray
4. Noninvasive blood pressure monitor

Level of Cognitive Ability: Applying
Client Needs: Physiological Integrity
Integrated Process: Nursing Process/Planning
Content Area: Critical Care: Emergency Situations
Priority Concepts: Perfusion; Safety

Answer: 4
Rationale: Nitroglycerin dilates arteries and veins (vasodilator), causing peripheral blood pooling, thus reducing preload, afterload, and myocardial workload. This action accounts for the primary side effect of nitroglycerin, which is hypotension. In the absence of an arterial monitoring line, the nurse should have a noninvasive blood pressure monitor for use at the bedside.
Priority Nursing Tip: An intravenous infusion device such as a pump or controller must be used when administering nitroglycerin via the intravenous route.
Test-Taking Strategy: Focus on the subject, initiating an intravenous nitroglycerin drip on a client with acute myocardial infarction. Note the words "absence of an invasive (arterial) monitoring line." Recalling the purpose of this type of monitoring device and the action of nitroglycerin will direct you to the correct option. Review: nursing responsibilities when administering a **nitroglycerin** drip.
Reference(s): Ignatavicius, Workman (2013), p. 837; Hodgson, Kizior (2014), p. 847.

136. A client in labor has a concurrent diagnosis of sickle cell anemia. Which action has **priority** to assist in preventing a sickling crisis from occurring during labor?
1. Reassuring the client
2. Administering oxygen
3. Preventing bearing down
4. Maintaining strict asepsis

Level of Cognitive Ability: Applying
Client Needs: Physiological Integrity
Integrated Process: Nursing Process/Implementation
Content Area: Maternity: Intrapartum
Priority Concepts: Clinical Judgment; Gas Exchange

Answer: 2
Rationale: During the labor process, the client with sickle cell anemia is at high risk for being unable to meet the oxygen demands of labor. Administering oxygen will prevent sickle cell crisis during labor. Intravenous (IV) fluid therapy will also reduce the risk of a sickle cell crisis. Options 1 and 4 are appropriate actions but are unrelated to sickle cell crisis. Option 3 is inappropriate.
Priority Nursing Tip: During labor, the client with sickle cell anemia needs to receive oxygen and fluids to prevent hypoxemia and dehydration because these conditions stimulate the sickling process.
Test-Taking Strategy: Note the strategic word, *priority*. Focus on the client's diagnosis and use the ABCs—airway, breathing, and circulation—to direct you to the correct option. Review: care of the client with sickle cell anemia.
Reference(s): McKinney et al (2013), pp. 622-623.

137. A client is scheduled for computed tomography (CT) of the kidneys to rule out renal disease. Which history component should the nurse ask the client about before the procedure?
1. Allergies
2. Familial renal disease
3. Frequent antibiotic use
4. Long-term diuretic therapy

Level of Cognitive Ability: Applying
Client Needs: Physiological Integrity
Integrated Process: Nursing Process/Assessment
Content Area: Fundamental Skills: Diagnostic Tests
Priority Concepts: Clinical Judgment; Safety

Answer: 1
Rationale: The client undergoing any type of diagnostic testing involving possible dye administration should be questioned about allergies, specifically an allergy to shellfish or iodine. This is essential to identify the risk for potential allergic reaction to contrast dye, which may be used. The other items are also useful as part of the assessment but are not as critical as the allergy determination in the preprocedure period.
Priority Nursing Tip: The nurse should ask the client if he or she ever had an allergic reaction to contrast media used for diagnostic testing. If so, the client is at high risk for experiencing another reaction if contrast media is administered.
Test-Taking Strategy: Focus on the subject, preprocedural CT scan. Because the question indicates that CT of the kidneys is planned, the items in the options are evaluated against their potential connection to this aspect of care. Recalling that contrast dye may be used during CT to enhance visualization of the kidneys will direct you to the correct option. Review: **computed tomography (CT).**
Reference(s): Ignatavicius, Workman (2013), p. 1543; Pagana, Pagana (2013), p. 282.

138. The nurse assists a client with a renal disorder in collecting a 24-hour urine specimen. Which does the nurse implement to ensure proper collection of the 24-hour urine specimen?
1. Have the client void at the start time and discard the specimen.
2. Strain the specimen before pouring the urine into the container.
3. Save all urine, beginning with the urine voided at the start time.
4. Once completed, refrigerate the urine collection until picked up by the laboratory.

Level of Cognitive Ability: Applying
Client Needs: Physiological Integrity
Integrated Process: Nursing Process/Implementation
Content Area: Fundamental Skills: Diagnostic Tests
Priority Concepts: Clinical Judgment; Elimination

Answer: 1
Rationale: The nurse asks the client to void at the beginning of the collection period and discards this urine sample because this urine has been stored in the bladder for an undetermined length of time. All urine thereafter is saved in an iced or refrigerated container. The client is asked to void at the finish time, and this sample is the last specimen added to the collection. Straining the urine is contraindicated for timed urine collections. The container is labeled, placed on fresh ice, and sent to the laboratory immediately after the 24-hour urine collection has ended.
Priority Nursing Tip: If the client is collecting a 24-hour urine specimen, check with the laboratory about the need to restrict certain foods or avoid taking certain medications before and during the collection. Some foods and medications affect test results.
Test-Taking Strategy: Focusing on the subject, a 24-hour urine collection, will assist in eliminating options 2 and 4. Straining the urine is contraindicated, and the urine must be sent to the laboratory immediately after the collection time has ended. For the remaining options, think about the procedure. Remember that it is best to discard the first specimen. Review: the procedure for collecting a 24-**hour urine specimen.**
Reference(s): Ignatavicius, Workman (2013), p. 1479.

139. The nurse is caring for a client in active labor. Which **priority** action should the nurse perform to prevent fetal heart rate decelerations?
1. Prepare the client for a cesarean delivery.
2. Monitor the fetal heart rate every 30 minutes.
3. Increase the rate of the oxytocin (Pitocin) infusion.
4. Encourage upright or side-lying maternal positions.

Level of Cognitive Ability: Applying
Client Needs: Physiological Integrity
Integrated Process: Nursing Process/Implementation
Content Area: Maternity: Intrapartum
Priority Concepts: Perfusion; Reproduction

Answer: 4
Rationale: Side-lying and upright positions such as walking, standing, and squatting can improve venous return and encourage effective uterine activity. There are many nursing actions to prevent fetal heart rate decelerations without necessitating surgical intervention. Monitoring the fetal heart rate every 30 minutes will not prevent fetal heart rate decelerations. The nurse should discontinue an oxytocin infusion in the presence of fetal heart rate decelerations, thereby reducing uterine activity and increasing uteroplacental perfusion.
Priority Nursing Tip: Early fetal heart rate decelerations are not associated with fetal compromise and require no intervention. Late decelerations indicate impaired placental exchange or uteroplacental insufficiency.
Test-Taking Strategy: Note the strategic word, *priority*, and the subject, to prevent fetal heart rate decelerations. Options 1, 2, and 3 will not prevent fetal heart rate decelerations. Side-lying and upright positions will improve venous return and encourage effective uterine activity. Review: nursing interventions for the client in **labor**.
Reference(s): McKinney et al (2013), p. 377.

140. A client with diabetes mellitus is at 36 weeks' gestation. The client has had weekly nonstress tests for the last 3 weeks, and the results have been reactive. This week, the nonstress test was nonreactive after 40 minutes. Based on these results, the nurse should prepare the client for which intervention?
1. A contraction stress test
2. Immediate induction of labor
3. Hospitalization with continuous fetal monitoring
4. A return appointment in 2 to 7 days to repeat the nonstress test

Level of Cognitive Ability: Analyzing
Client Needs: Physiological Integrity
Integrated Process: Nursing Process/Planning
Content Area: Maternity: Antepartum
Priority Concepts: Clinical Judgment; Reproduction

Answer: 1
Rationale: A nonreactive nonstress test needs further assessment. A contraction stress test is the next test needed to further assess the fetal status. There are not enough data in the question to indicate that the procedures in options 2 and 3 are necessary at this time. To send the client home for 2 to 7 days may place the fetus in jeopardy.
Priority Nursing Tip: A nonstress test is performed to assess placental function and oxygenation and evaluate the fetal heart rate response to fetal movement.
Test-Taking Strategy: Focus on the subject, a change in nonstress test results from reactive to nonreactive. Options 2 and 3 can be eliminated first because they are unnecessary at this time. Option 4 can be eliminated next because repeating the test at a later time is not a safe intervention, especially considering the fact that previous test results were reactive. Review: **nonstress test**.
Reference(s): McKinney et al (2013), pp. 309-311.

141. The nurse is administering magnesium sulfate to a client for severe preeclampsia. What intervention should the nurse take during the administration of magnesium sulfate for this client?
1. Schedule a daily ultrasound to assess fetal movement.
2. Schedule a nonstress test every 4 hours to assess fetal well-being.
3. Assess the client's temperature every 2 hours because the client is at high risk for infection.
4. Assess for signs and symptoms of labor because the client's level of consciousness may be altered.

Level of Cognitive Ability: Applying
Client Needs: Physiological Integrity
Integrated Process: Nursing Process/Implementation
Content Area: Pharmacology: Reproductive/Maternity/Newborn Medications
Priority Concepts: Reproduction; Safety

Answer: 4
Rationale: Magnesium sulfate is a central nervous system depressant and anticonvulsant. Because of the sedative effect of the magnesium sulfate, the client may not perceive labor. Daily ultrasounds are not necessary for this client. A nonstress test may be done, but not every 4 hours. This client is not at high risk for infection.
Priority Nursing Tip: Calcium gluconate is the antidote to magnesium sulfate.
Test-Taking Strategy: Focus on the subject, magnesium sulfate administration. Use the steps of the nursing process to answer the question. Assessment is the first step; therefore, eliminate options 1 and 2. From the remaining options, knowledge that the client is not at high risk for infection will assist in directing you to the correct option. Review: nursing responsibilities when administering magnesium sulfate.
Reference(s): McKinney et al (2013), pp. 594-595.

142. A client's nasogastric (NG) tube stops draining. Which should the nurse implement **first** to maintain client safety?
1. Verify the tube placement.
2. Instill 30 to 60 mL of fluid.
3. Clamp the tube for 2 hours.
4. Retract the tube by 2 inches.

Level of Cognitive Ability: Applying
Client Needs: Physiological Integrity
Integrated Process: Nursing Process/Implementation
Content Area: Fundamental Skills: Safety
Priority Concepts: Clinical Judgment; Safety

Answer: 1
Rationale: If a client's nasogastric tube stops draining, the nurse verifies placement first to ensure that the tube remains in the stomach. After checking placement and verifying a prescription for tube irrigation, the nurse irrigates the tube with 30 to 60 mL of the fluid per agency procedure. Clamping the tube increases the risk of aspiration and is contraindicated; besides, this intervention cannot unclog a tube. Retracting the tube may displace the tube and place the client at risk for aspiration. Replacement of the tube is the last step if other actions are unsuccessful.
Priority Nursing Tip: Accurate placement of a gastrointestinal tube is always checked before instilling feeding solutions, medications, or any other solution.
Test-Taking Strategy: Focus on the subject, the NG tube stopped draining, and note the strategic word, *first*. Eliminate options 2, 3, and 4 because these interventions increase client risk of aspiration. Also use the steps of the nursing process; option 1 is the only assessment action. Review: care of the client with a nasogastric (NG) tube.
Reference(s): Ignatavicius, Workman (2013), p. 290.

143. The nurse is planning to give a tepid tub bath to a child who has hyperthermia. Which action should the nurse plan to perform?
1. Obtain isopropyl alcohol to add to the bath water.
2. Allow 5 minutes for the child to soak in the bath water.
3. Have cool water available to add to the warm bath water.
4. Warm the water to the same body temperature as the child's.

Level of Cognitive Ability: Applying
Client Needs: Physiological Integrity
Integrated Process: Nursing Process/Planning
Content Area: Child Health: Metabolic/Endocrine
Priority Concepts: Clinical Judgment; Thermoregulation

Answer: 3
Rationale: Adding cool water to an already warm bath allows the water temperature to slowly drop. The child is able to gradually adjust to the changing water temperature and will not experience chilling. Alcohol is toxic, can cause peripheral vasoconstriction, and is contraindicated for tepid sponge or tub baths. The child should be in a tepid tub bath for 20 to 30 minutes to achieve maximum results. To achieve the best cooling results, the water temperature should be at least 2 degrees lower than the child's body temperature.
Priority Nursing Tip: Perform a complete assessment on a child with a fever. Assessment findings associated with the fever provide important indications of the seriousness of the fever.
Test-Taking Strategy: Focus on the subject, tepid water bath. Eliminate option 1, recalling that alcohol is toxic, as well as irritating, to the skin. Eliminate option 4 because water that is the same as body temperature will not reduce hyperthermia. Eliminate option 2 because of the 5-minute time frame. Review: measures for hyperthermia and the procedure for giving a tepid bath to a child.
Reference(s): Hockenberry, Wilson (2013), p. 651.

144. The nurse is assigned to care for an infant on the first postoperative day after a surgical repair of a cleft lip. Which nursing intervention is appropriate when caring for this child's surgical incision?

1. Rinse the incision with sterile water after feeding.
2. Clean the incision only when serous exudate forms.
3. Rub the incision gently with a sterile cotton-tipped swab.
4. Replace the Logan bar carefully after cleaning the incision.

Level of Cognitive Ability: Applying
Client Needs: Physiological Integrity
Integrated Process: Nursing Process/Implementation
Content Area: Child Health: Gastrointestinal
Priority Concepts: Clinical Judgment; Development

Answer: 1
Rationale: The incision should be rinsed with sterile water after every feeding. Rubbing alters the integrity of the suture line. Rather, the incision should be patted or dabbed. The purpose of the Logan bar is to maintain the integrity of the suture line. Removing the Logan bar on the first postoperative day would increase tension on the surgical incision.
Priority Nursing Tip: After cleft lip repair, avoid positioning the infant on the side of the repair or in the prone position because these positions can cause rubbing of the surgical site on the mattress.
Test-Taking Strategy: Focus on the subject, cleft lip repair. Eliminate options 2 and 3 first because of the word "only" in option 2 and "rub" in option 3. Focus on the words "first postoperative day." This should assist in eliminating option 4. Review: **cleft lip.**
Reference(s): McKinney et al (2013), p. 1073.

145. A client is in ventricular tachycardia and the health care provider prescribes intravenous (IV) lidocaine (Xylocaine). The nurse should dilute the concentrated solution of lidocaine with which solution?

1. Lactated Ringer's
2. Normal saline 0.9%
3. 5% Dextrose in water
4. Normal saline 0.45%

Level of Cognitive Ability: Applying
Client Needs: Physiological Integrity
Integrated Process: Nursing Process/Implementation
Content Area: Critical Care: Medications and Intravenous Therapy
Priority Concepts: Clinical Judgment; Safety

Answer: 3
Rationale: Lidocaine (Xylocaine) for IV administration is dispensed in concentrated and dilute formulations. The concentrated formulation must be diluted with 5% dextrose in water. Therefore options 1, 2, and 4 are incorrect.
Priority Nursing Tip: When administering lidocaine (Xylocaine), be sure that resuscitative equipment is readily available.
Test-Taking Strategy: Focus on the subject, (IV) lidocaine (Xylocaine). Eliminate options 2 and 4 first because they are similar solutions. From the remaining options, it is necessary to know that the concentrated formulation must be diluted with 5% dextrose in water. Review: **(IV) lidocaine (Xylocaine).**
Reference(s): Hodgson, Kizior (2014), pp. 687-689; Ignatavicius, Workman (2013), p. 723.

146. A client receiving total parenteral nutrition (TPN) via a central venous catheter (CVC) is scheduled to receive an intravenous (IV) antibiotic. Which should the nurse implement before administering the antibiotic?

1. Turn off the TPN for 30 minutes.
2. Ensure a separate IV access route.
3. Flush the CVC with normal saline.
4. Check for compatibility with TPN.

Level of Cognitive Ability: Applying
Client Needs: Physiological Integrity
Integrated Process: Nursing Process/Implementation
Content Area: Critical Care: Medications and Intravenous Therapy
Priority Concepts: Clinical Judgment; Safety

Answer: 2
Rationale: The TPN line is used only for the administration of the TPN solution to prevent crystallization in the CVC tubing and disruption of the TPN infusion. Any other IV medication must be administered through a separate IV access site, including a separate infusion port of the CVC catheter. Therefore, options 1, 3, and 4 are incorrect actions.
Priority Nursing Tip: Parenteral nutrition solutions that are cloudy or darkened should not be used for administration and should be returned to the pharmacy.
Test-Taking Strategy: Focus on the subject, total parenteral nutrition. Eliminate options 1, 3, and 4 because they are comparable or alike in that they involve using the TPN line for the administration of the antibiotic. Review: **parenteral nutrition.**
Reference(s): Potter et al (2013), p. 632.

❖ **147.** The nurse is monitoring a postoperative client for behavioral indicators of the effects of pain. Which are indicators that the client is in pain? **Select all that apply.**
   ❑ 1. Gasping
   ❑ 2. Lip biting
   ❑ 3. Muscle tension
   ❑ 4. Pacing activities
   ❑ 5. Conversing with the roommate
   ❑ 6. Enjoying social interaction with visitors

Level of Cognitive Ability: Analyzing
Client Needs: Physiological Integrity
Integrated Process: Nursing Process/Assessment
Content Area: Fundamental Skills: Pain
Priority Concepts: Clinical Judgment; Pain

Answer: 1, 2, 3, 4
Rationale: The nurse should assess verbalization, vocal response, facial and body movements, and social interaction as indicators of pain. Behavioral indicators of pain include gasping, lip biting (facial expressions), muscle tension, pacing activities, moaning, crying, grunting (vocalizations), grimacing, clenching teeth, wrinkling the forehead, tightly closing or widely opening the eyes or mouth, restlessness, immobilization, increased hand and finger movements, rhythmic or rubbing motions, protective movements of body parts (body movement), avoidance of conversation, focusing only on activities for pain relief, avoiding social contacts and interactions, and reduced attention span.
Priority Nursing Tip: It is important for the nurse to monitor for behavioral indicators of pain, particularly if the client is unable to verbalize the presence of pain.
Test-Taking Strategy: Focus on the subject, behavioral indicators of pain. Think about the physiological and psychosocial responses that occur during the pain experience as you read each option. This will assist in answering correctly. Review: the behavioral indicators of **pain**.
Reference(s): Potter et al (2013), p. 974.

❖ **148.** The nurse is developing a care plan for a client receiving enteral nutrition and identifies the situations that place the client at risk for aspiration. Which conditions place the client at increased risk for aspiration? **Select all that apply.**
   ❑ 1. Sedation
   ❑ 2. Coughing
   ❑ 3. An artificial airway
   ❑ 4. Head elevated position
   ❑ 5. Nasotracheal suctioning
   ❑ 6. Decreased level of consciousness

Level of Cognitive Ability: Analyzing
Client Needs: Physiological Integrity
Integrated Process: Nursing Process/Planning
Content Area: Fundamental Skills: Safety
Priority Concepts: Gas Exchange; Safety

Answer: 1, 2, 3, 5, 6
Rationale: A serious complication associated with enteral feedings is aspiration of formula into the tracheobronchial tree. Some common conditions that increase the risk for aspiration include sedation, coughing, an artificial airway, nasotracheal suctioning, decreased level of consciousness, and lying flat. A head-elevated position does not increase the risk of aspiration.
Priority Nursing Tip: The nurse must assess the client for conditions that place him or her at risk for aspiration. Aspiration can result in airway obstruction.
Test-Taking Strategy: Focus on the subject, the risks associated with aspiration. Recall that aspiration is the inhalation of foreign material into the tracheobronchial tree. Next read each option and think about the effect it produces with regard to aspiration. This will direct you to the correct options. Review: the risks associated with **aspiration** and **enteral nutrition.**
Reference(s): Perry, Potter, Ostendorf (2014), pp. 504, 792; Potter et al (2013), pp. 1026-1027; Swearingen (2012), pp. 525-526.

149. A client, without history of respiratory disease, has experienced sudden onset of chest pain and dyspnea and is diagnosed with a pulmonary embolus. The nurse **immediately** implements which expected prescription for this client?

1. Semi-Fowler's position, oxygen, and morphine sulfate intravenously (IV)
2. Supine position, oxygen, and meperidine hydrochloride (Demerol) intramuscularly (IM)
3. High Fowler's position, oxygen, and two tablets of acetaminophen with codeine (Tylenol #3)
4. High Fowler's position, oxygen, and meperidine hydrochloride (Demerol) intravenously (IV)

Level of Cognitive Ability: Applying
Client Needs: Physiological Integrity
Integrated Process: Nursing Process/Implementation
Content Area: Critical Care: Emergency Situations
Priority Concepts: Gas Exchange; Perfusion

Answer: 1
Rationale: Standard therapeutic intervention for the client with pulmonary embolus includes proper positioning, oxygen, and intravenous analgesics. The head of the bed is placed in semi-Fowler's position. The supine position will increase the dyspnea that occurs with pulmonary embolism. High Fowler's is avoided because extreme hip flexure slows venous return from the legs and increases the risk of new thrombi. The usual analgesic of choice is morphine sulfate administered IV. This medication reduces pain, alleviates anxiety, and can diminish congestion of blood in the pulmonary vessels because it causes peripheral venous dilation.
Priority Nursing Tip: Clients prone to pulmonary embolism are those at risk for deep vein thrombosis.
Test-Taking Strategy: Note the strategic word, *immediately*. Eliminate option 2 first because a supine position will exacerbate the dyspnea. From the remaining options, recall that a high Fowler's position is avoided because extreme hip flexure slows venous return from the legs and increases the risk of new thrombi. This will assist in eliminating options 3 and 4. Review: **pulmonary embolus.**
Reference(s): Dolan, Holt (2013), pp. 411-412; Ignatavicius, Workman (2013), p. 665.

150. A client who recently experienced a myocardial infarction is scheduled to have a percutaneous transluminal coronary angioplasty (PTCA). The nurse should plan to teach the client about which aspect of a balloon-tipped catheter?

1. A meshlike device will be inflated that will spring open.
2. The catheter will be used to compress the plaque against the coronary blood vessel wall.
3. The catheter will cut away the plaque from the coronary vessel wall using a cutting blade.
4. The catheter will be positioned in a coronary artery to take pressure measurements in the vessel.

Level of Cognitive Ability: Applying
Client Needs: Physiological Integrity
Integrated Process: Teaching and Learning
Content Area: Adult Health: Cardiovascular
Priority Concepts: Client Education; Perfusion

Answer: 2
Rationale: In PTCA, a balloon-tipped catheter is used to compress the plaque against the coronary blood vessel wall. Option 1 describes placement of a coronary stent, option 3 describes coronary atherectomy, and option 4 describes part of the process used in cardiac catheterization.
Priority Nursing Tip: Complications of percutaneous transluminal coronary angioplasty (PTCA) include arterial dissection or rupture, embolization of plaque fragments, spasm, and acute myocardial infarction.
Test-Taking Strategy: Focus on the subject, percutaneous transluminal coronary angioplasty (PTCA). Look at the name of the procedure. "Angioplasty" refers to repair of a blood vessel; this will assist in eliminating options 1 and 4. From the remaining options, recalling that a procedure that cuts something away would have the suffix *-ectomy* will assist in eliminating option 3. Review: **percutaneous transluminal coronary angioplasty (PTCA).**
Reference(s): Ignatavicius, Workman (2013), pp. 844-845; Pagana, Pagana (2013), p. 216.

151. The nurse is caring for a client who has been placed in Buck's extension traction. Which action by the nurse provides for countertraction to reduce shear and friction?
1. Using a footboard
2. Providing an overhead trapeze
3. Slightly elevating the foot of the bed
4. Slightly elevating the head of the bed

Level of Cognitive Ability: Applying
Client Needs: Physiological Integrity
Integrated Process: Nursing Process/Implementation
Content Area: Adult Health: Musculoskeletal
Priority Concepts: Clinical Judgment; Mobility

Answer: 3
Rationale: The part of the bed under an area in traction is usually elevated to aid in countertraction. For the client in Buck's extension traction (which is applied to a leg), the foot of the bed is elevated. Option 3 provides a force that opposes the traction force effectively without harming the client. A footboard, an overhead trapeze, or elevating the head of the bed are not used to provide countertraction.
Priority Nursing Tip: The health care provider's prescription is always followed regarding the amount of weight applied to the traction device. For Buck's extension traction usually not more than 8 to 10 pounds is prescribed.
Test-Taking Strategy: Focus on the subject, countertraction for Buck's traction. Eliminate option 4, recalling that Buck's extension traction is applied to the leg. From the remaining options, focus on the subject to eliminate options 1 and 2. Review: **Buck's extension traction**.
Reference(s): Ignatavicius, Workman (2013), p. 1154; Perry, Potter, Ostendorf (2014), pp. 258-259.

152. The nurse is preparing to initiate bolus enteral feedings via nasogastric (NG) tube to a client. Which action represents safe practice by the nurse?
1. Checks the volume of the residual after administering the bolus feeding
2. Aspirates gastric contents before initiating the feeding and ensures that pH is greater than 9
3. Elevates the head of the bed to 25 degrees and maintains for 30 minutes after instillation of feeding
4. Verifies correct nasogastric tube position with aspiration and administration of air bolus with auscultation

Level of Cognitive Ability: Applying
Client Needs: Physiological Integrity
Integrated Process: Nursing Process/Implementation
Content Area: Fundamental Skills: Safety
Priority Concepts: Nutrition; Safety

Answer: 4
Rationale: After initial radiographic confirmation of NG tube placement, methods used to verify nasogastric tube placement include measuring the length of the tube from the point it protrudes from the nose to the end, injecting 10 to 30 mL of air into the tube and auscultating over the left upper quadrant of the abdomen, and aspirating the secretions and checking to see if the pH is less than 3.5 (safest method). Residual should be assessed before administration of the next feeding. Fowler's position is recommended for bolus feedings, if permitted, and should be maintained for 1 hour after instillation.
Priority Nursing Tip: Residual volumes are checked every 4 hours, before each feeding or the instillation of any solution, and before giving medications.
Test-Taking Strategy: Focus on the subject, bolus enteral feedings via nasogastric (NG) tube. Note the words "safe practice." Knowing that the pH of gastric contents should be between 1 and 5 will assist you in eliminating option 2. Option 3 can be eliminated because the head of the bed elevation should be at a minimum of 30 degrees for all types of enteral feedings to prevent aspiration. From the remaining two options, use knowledge of when to check residuals to assist you in eliminating option 1. Review: procedures related to administration of **enteral feedings via nasogastric tube**.
Reference(s): Ignatavicius, Workman (2013), p. 1344; Potter et al (2013), pp. 1028-1029.

153. The nurse has inserted a nasogastric (NG) tube to the level of the oropharynx and has repositioned the client's head in a flexed-forward position. The client has been asked to begin swallowing, and as the nurse starts to slowly advance the NG tube with each swallow, the client begins to gag. Which nursing action would **least likely** result in proper tube insertion and promote client relaxation?

1. Pulling the tube back slightly
2. Instructing the client to breathe slowly
3. Continuing to advance the tube to the desired distance
4. Checking the back of the pharynx using a tongue blade and flashlight

Level of Cognitive Ability: Applying
Client Needs: Physiological Integrity
Integrated Process: Nursing Process/Implementation
Content Area: Fundamental Skills: Safety
Priority Concepts: Clinical Judgment; Safety

Answer: 3
Rationale: As the NG tube is passed through the oropharynx, the gag reflex is stimulated, which may cause gagging. Instead of passing through to the esophagus, the NG tube may coil around itself in the oropharynx, or it may enter the larynx and obstruct the airway. Because the tube may enter the larynx, advancing the tube may position it in the trachea. The nurse should check the back of the pharynx using a tongue blade and flashlight to check for coiling and then pull the tube back slightly to prevent entrance into the larynx. Slow breathing helps the client relax to reduce the gag response. The tube may be advanced after the client relaxes.
Priority Nursing Tip: To determine the insertion length of a nasogastric tube, measure the length of the tube from the bridge of the nose to the earlobe to the xiphoid process and indicate this length with a piece of tape.
Test-Taking Strategy: Note the strategic words, *least likely*. These words indicate a negative event query and the need to select the incorrect nursing action. Focusing on these words and noting that the client is gagging will direct you to the correct option. Review: the procedure for inserting a **nasogastric (NG) tube.**
Reference(s): Potter et al (2013), pp. 1116-1117.

❖ **154.** The nurse is caring for a client with a terminal condition who is dying. Which respiratory assessment findings should indicate to the nurse that death is imminent? **Select all that apply.**

❑ 1. Dyspnea
❑ 2. Cyanosis
❑ 3. Tachypnea
❑ 4. Kussmaul's respiration
❑ 5. Irregular respiratory pattern
❑ 6. Adventitious bubbling lung sounds

Level of Cognitive Ability: Analyzing
Client Needs: Physiological Integrity
Integrated Process: Nursing Process/Assessment
Content Area: Developmental Stages: End-of-Life Care
Priority Concepts: Clinical Judgment; Gas Exchange

Answer: 1, 2, 5, 6
Rationale: Respiratory assessment findings that indicate death is imminent include poor gas exchange as evidenced by hypoxia, dyspnea, or cyanosis; altered patterns of respiration, such as slow, labored, irregular, or Cheyne-Stokes pattern (alternating periods of apnea and deep, rapid breathing); increased respiratory secretions and adventitious bubbling lung sounds (death rattle); and irritation of the tracheobronchial airway as evidenced by hiccups, chest pain, fatigue, or exhaustion. Kussmaul's respirations are abnormally deep, very rapid sighing respirations characteristic of diabetic ketoacidosis. Tachypnea is defined as rapid breathing. In an adult, it would indicate a respiratory rate of over 20 breaths per minute.
Priority Nursing Tip: As death approaches, metabolism is reduced, and the body gradually slows down until all function ends.
Test-Taking Strategy: Focus on the subject, respiratory assessment findings near death. Think about the physiological processes that occur in the dying person as you read each option. This will assist in answering the question correctly. Review: these **respiratory assessment** findings.
Reference(s): Potter et al (2013), pp. 721, 723.

155. The nurse is caring for an infant with spina bifida cystica (meningomyelocele type) who had the sac surgically removed. The nurse plans which intervention in the postoperative period to maintain the infant's safety?
1. Covering the back dressing with a binder
2. Placing the infant in a head-down position
3. Strapping the infant in a baby seat sitting up
4. Elevating the head with the infant in the prone position

Level of Cognitive Ability: Applying
Client Needs: Physiological Integrity
Integrated Process: Nursing Process/Planning
Content Area: Child Health: Neurological/Musculoskeletal
Priority Concepts: Intracranial Regulation; Safety

Answer: 4
Rationale: Spina bifida is a central nervous system defect that results from failure of the neural tube to close during embryonic development. Care of the operative site is carried out under the direction of the surgeon and includes close observation for signs of leakage of cerebrospinal fluid. The prone position is maintained after surgical closure to decrease the pressure on the surgical site on the back; however, many neurosurgeons allow side-lying or partial side-lying positions unless it aggravates a coexisting hip dysplasia or permits undesirable hip flexion. This offers an opportunity for position changes, which reduces the risk of pressure sores and facilitates feeding. Elevating the head will decrease the chance of cerebrospinal fluid collecting in the cranial cavity. If permitted, the infant can be held upright against the body with care taken to avoid pressure on the operative site. Binders and a baby seat should not be used because of the pressure they would exert on the surgical site.
Priority Nursing Tip: In the preoperative period, the myelomeningocele sac is protected by covering with a sterile, moist (normal saline), nonadherent dressing to maintain the moisture of the sac and contents.
Test-Taking Strategy: Focus on the subject, postoperative care for an infant with spina bifida who had the sac removed. Recall that preventing pressure on the surgical site and preventing intracranial cerebrospinal fluid collection are goals for the postoperative period. Options 1 and 3 would increase pressure on the surgical site, and option 2 would not promote drainage of cerebrospinal fluid from the cranial cavity. Review: **spina bifida.**
Reference(s): Hockenberry, Wilson (2013), p. 1103.

156. The nurse is assessing a client who is being treated with a beta-adrenergic blocker. Which assessment findings would indicate that the client may be experiencing dose-related side effects of the medication? **Select all that apply.**
☐ 1. Dizziness
☐ 2. Bradycardia
☐ 3. Reflex tachycardia
☐ 4. Sexual dysfunction
☐ 5. Cardiac dysrhythmias

Level of Cognitive Ability: Analyzing
Client Needs: Physiological Integrity
Integrated Process: Nursing Process/Assessment
Content Area: Pharmacology: Cardiovascular Medications
Priority Concepts: Clinical Judgment; Safety

Answer: 1, 2, 4
Rationale: Beta-adrenergic blockers, commonly called beta blockers, are useful in treating cardiac dysrhythmias, mild hypertension, mild tachycardia, and angina pectoris. Side effects commonly associated with beta blockers are usually dose related and include dizziness (hypotensive effect), bradycardia, hypotension, and sexual dysfunction (impotence). Options 3 and 5 are reasons for prescribing a beta blocker; however, these are general side effects of alpha-adrenergic blockers.
Priority Nursing Tip: Advise the client with diabetes mellitus who is taking beta-adrenergic blockers that the medication can mask the early signs of hypoglycemia such as nervousness and tachycardia.
Test-Taking Strategy: Focus on the subject, beta blockers. Specific knowledge regarding the side effects of beta blockers is needed to select the correct options. However, if you can remember that beta blockers are useful in treating cardiac dysrhythmias, mild hypertension, mild tachycardia, and angina pectoris, you will be able to eliminate the incorrect options. Review: the side effects of a beta-adrenergic blocker.
Reference(s): Ignatavicius, Workman (2013), p. 757; Lehne (2013), pp. 175-176.

157. A client at risk for respiratory failure is receiving oxygen via nasal cannula at 6 L per minute. Arterial blood gas (ABG) results indicate: pH 7.29, P_{CO_2} 49 mm Hg, P_{O_2} 58 mm Hg, HCO_3 18 mEq/L. What should the nurse anticipate that the health care provider will prescribe for respiratory support?

1. Intubation and mechanical ventilation
2. Keeping the oxygen at 6 L per minute via nasal cannula
3. Lowering the oxygen to 4 L per minute via nasal cannula
4. Adding a partial rebreather mask to the current prescription

Level of Cognitive Ability: Analyzing
Client Needs: Physiological Integrity
Integrated Process: Nursing Process/Planning
Content Area: Critical Care: Emergency Situations
Priority Concepts: Clinical Judgment; Gas Exchange

Answer: 1
Rationale: If respiratory failure occurs and supplemental oxygen cannot maintain acceptable Pa_{O_2} and Pa_{CO_2} levels, endotracheal intubation and mechanical ventilation are necessary. The client is exhibiting respiratory acidosis, metabolic acidosis, and hypoxemia. Lowering or keeping the oxygen at the same liter flow will not improve the client's condition. A partial rebreather mask will raise CO_2 levels even further.
Priority Nursing Tip: The manifestations of respiratory failure are related to the extent and rapidity of change in the Pa_{O_2} and Pa_{CO_2}.
Test-Taking Strategy: Focus on the **subject,** ABG analysis in a client at risk for respiratory failure. Note the ABG values. Noting that the oxygen level is low will eliminate options 2 and 3. Knowing that the P_{CO_2} is high will eliminate option 4 because a partial rebreather mask will raise CO_2 levels even further. Review: **arterial blood gas (ABG)** and the treatment for **respiratory failure.**
Reference(s): Ignatavicius, Workman (2013), pp. 672, 674-675.

158. The nurse is preparing to assess the respirations of a newborn just admitted to the nursery. The nurse performs the procedure and determines that the respiratory rate is normal if which finding is noted?

1. A respiratory rate of 20 breaths per minute
2. A respiratory rate of 40 breaths per minute
3. A respiratory rate of 90 breaths per minute
4. A respiratory rate of 100 breaths per minute

Level of Cognitive Ability: Understanding
Client Needs: Physiological Integrity
Integrated Process: Nursing Process/Assessment
Content Area: Maternity: Newborn
Priority Concepts: Development; Gas Exchange

Answer: 2
Rationale: Normal respiratory rate varies from 30 to 50 breaths per minute when the infant is not crying. Respirations should be counted for 1 full minute to ensure an accurate measurement because the newborn infant may be a periodic breather. Observing and palpating respirations while the infant is quiet promotes accurate assessment. Palpation aids observation in determining the respiratory rate. Option 1 indicates bradypnea, and options 3 and 4 indicate tachypnea.
Priority Nursing Tip: The newborn infant's respiratory rate and apical heart rate are counted for 1 full minute to detect irregularities in rate or rhythm.
Test-Taking Strategy: Focus on the **subject,** newborn respiratory rate. Recall knowledge regarding the normal respiratory rate for a newborn infant to answer this question. Remember that the normal respiratory rate varies from 30 to 50 breaths per minute. Review: **newborn respiratory rate.**
Reference(s): Potter et al (2013), p. 457.

159. During a routine prenatal visit, a client in her second trimester of pregnancy reports having frequent calf pain when she walks. The nurse suspects superficial thrombophlebitis and checks for which sign associated with this condition?

1. Severe chills
2. Kernig's sign
3. Brudzinski's sign
4. Palpable thrombus that feels hard

Level of Cognitive Ability: Analyzing
Client Needs: Physiological Integrity
Integrated Process: Nursing Process/Assessment
Content Area: Maternity: Antepartum
Priority Concepts: Clinical Judgment; Clotting

Answer: 4
Rationale: Pain in the calf during walking could indicate venous thrombosis or peripheral arterial disease. The manifestations of superficial thrombophlebitis include a palpable thrombus that feels bumpy and hard, tenderness and pain in the affected lower extremity, and a warm and pinkish red color over the thrombus area. Severe chills can occur in a variety of inflammatory or infectious conditions and are also a manifestation of pelvic thrombophlebitis. Brudzinski's sign and Kernig's sign test for meningeal irritability.
Priority Nursing Tip: If a thrombus is suspected, never massage the site because of the risk of dislodging it and causing it to travel to the pulmonary system.
Test-Taking Strategy: Focus on the **subject,** thrombophlebitis. Eliminate options 2 and 3 first because they both test for meningeal irritation. From the remaining options, focus on the words "frequent calf pain when she walks" and "thrombophlebitis" to assist in directing you to the correct option. Review: the signs of superficial **thrombophlebitis.**
Reference(s): McKinney et al (2013), p. 253.

160. The nurse evaluates the patency of a peripheral intravenous (IV) site and suspects an infiltration. Which action should the nurse take to determine if the IV has infiltrated?
1. Strip the tubing and assess for a blood return.
2. Check the regional tissue for redness and warmth.
3. Increase the infusion rate and observe for swelling.
4. Gently palpate regional tissue for edema and coolness.

Level of Cognitive Ability: Applying
Client Needs: Physiological Integrity
Integrated Process: Nursing Process/Implementation
Content Area: Fundamental Skills: Safety
Priority Concepts: Clinical Judgment; Safety

Answer: 4
Rationale: When assessing an IV for clinical indicators of infiltration, it is important to assess the site for edema and coolness, signifying leakage of the IV fluid into the surrounding tissues. Stripping the tubing will not cause a blood return but will force IV fluid into the surrounding tissues, which can increase the risk of tissue damage. Redness and warmth are more likely to indicate infection or phlebitis. Increasing the IV flow rate can further damage the tissues if the IV has infiltrated. Additionally, a health care provider's prescription is needed to increase an IV flow rate.
Priority Nursing Tip: If an intravenous (IV) infiltration occurs, the IV device is removed from the client's vein; if IV therapy is still needed, a new IV device is inserted into a vein in a different extremity.
Test-Taking Strategy: Focus on the subject, IV infiltration. Recalling that the site will feel cool will direct you to the correct option. Also note the word "gently" in the correct option. Review: the signs of infiltration.
Reference(s): Ignatavicius, Workman (2013), p. 228; Potter et al (2013), p. 910.

161. A client who is unresponsive and pulseless and who has a possible neck injury is brought into the emergency department after a motor vehicle crash. What should the nurse do to open the client's airway?
1. Insert oropharyngeal airway.
2. Tilt the head and lift the chin.
3. Place in the recovery position.
4. Stabilize the skull and push up the jaw.

Level of Cognitive Ability: Applying
Client Needs: Physiological Integrity
Integrated Process: Nursing Process/Implementation
Content Area: Critical Care: Emergency Situations
Priority Concepts: Gas Exchange; Safety

Answer: 4
Rationale: The health care team uses the jaw-thrust maneuver to open the airway until a radiograph confirms that the client's cervical spine is stable to avoid potential aggravation of a cervical spine injury. Options 1 and 2 require manipulation of the spine to open the airway, and option 3 can be ineffective for opening the airway.
Priority Nursing Tip: If a neck injury is suspected in a victim who sustained an injury, the jaw-thrust maneuver (rather than the head-tilt chin-lift) is used to open the airway to prevent further spine damage.
Test-Taking Strategy: Focus on the ABCs—airway, breathing, and circulation. Recalling the principles related to airway management will assist in eliminating options 1 and 2. From the remaining options, visualize each and eliminate option 3 because this action can be ineffective if the client is unable to maintain the airway. Review: open airway in a client with a neck injury.
Reference(s): Dolan, Holt (2013), pp. 114-115, 126.

162. The nurse is caring for a child with Reye's syndrome. The nurse monitors for manifestations of which **primary** problem associated with this syndrome?
1. Protein in the urine
2. Symptoms of hyperglycemia
3. Increased intracranial pressure
4. A history of a staphylococcus infection

Level of Cognitive Ability: Analyzing
Client Needs: Physiological Integrity
Integrated Process: Nursing Process/Assessment
Content Area: Child Health: Neurological
Priority Concepts: Clinical Judgment; Intracranial Regulation

Answer: 3
Rationale: Reye's syndrome is an acute encephalopathy that follows a viral illness and is characterized pathologically by cerebral edema and fatty changes in the liver. Intracranial pressure and encephalopathy are major problems associated with Reye's syndrome. Protein is not present in the urine. Reye's syndrome is related to a history of viral infections, and hypoglycemia is a symptom of this disease.
Priority Nursing Tip: The administration of aspirin and non–aspirin-containing salicylates is not recommended for a child with a febrile illness or a child with varicella or influenza because of its association with Reye's syndrome.
Test-Taking Strategy: Focus on the subject, Reye's syndrome. Note the strategic word, primary. Recalling that Reye's syndrome is an acute encephalopathy will assist in directing you to the correct option. Review: Reye's syndrome.
Reference(s): Hockenberry, Wilson (2013), p. 956.

163. The nurse analyzed an electrocardiogram (ECG) strip **(refer to figure)** for a client with left-sided heart failure and interprets the ECG strip as which rhythm?

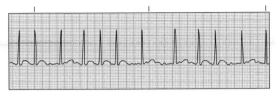

Figure from Ignatavicius D, Workman M: *Medical-surgical nursing: patient-centered collaborative care*, ed 7, Philadelphia, 2013, Saunders.

1. Atrial fibrillation
2. Sinus dysrhythmia
3. Ventricular fibrillation
4. Third-degree heart block

Level of Cognitive Ability: Analyzing
Client Needs: Physiological Integrity
Integrated Process: Nursing Process/Analysis
Content Area: Adult Health: Cardiovascular
Priority Concepts: Clinical Judgment; Perfusion

Answer: 1
Rationale: Atrial fibrillation is characterized by rapid, chaotic atrial depolarization. Ventricular rates may be less than 100 beats per minute (controlled) or greater than 100 beats per minute (uncontrolled). The ECG reveals chaotic or no identifiable P waves and an irregular ventricular rhythm. A sinus dysrhythmia has a normal P wave and PR interval and QRS complex. In ventricular fibrillation, there are no identifiable P waves, QRS complexes, or T waves. In third-degree heart block, the atria and ventricles beat independently, and the PR interval varies in length.
Priority Nursing Tip: The client with atrial fibrillation is at risk for pulmonary embolism because thrombi can form in the right atrium as a result of atrial quivering and travel to the right atrium to the lungs.
Test-Taking Strategy: Focus on the subject, ECG interpretation. Look at the rhythm and compare it to what a normal rhythm would look like. Recall that in atrial fibrillation the P wave is usually absent or chaotic and the ventricular rhythm is irregular. This will direct you to the correct option. Review: **cardiac dysrhythmias.**
Reference(s): Ignatavicius, Workman (2013), pp. 722, 727-728.

164. The nurse admits a client to the hospital with a suspected diagnosis of bulimia nervosa. While performing the admission assessment, the nurse asks questions and expects to elicit which data about bulimia?

1. Binge eats, then purges
2. Is accepting of body size
3. Overeats for the enjoyment of eating food
4. Overeats in response to losing control of diet

Level of Cognitive Ability: Applying
Client Needs: Physiological Integrity
Integrated Process: Nursing Process/Assessment
Content Area: Mental Health
Priority Concepts: Clinical Judgment; Nutrition

Answer: 1
Rationale: Individuals with bulimia nervosa develop cycles of binge eating, followed by purging. They seldom attempt to diet and have no sense of loss of control. Options 2, 3, and 4 are true of the obese person who may binge eat (not purge).
Priority Nursing Tip: The client with an eating disorder experiences an altered body image.
Test-Taking Strategy: Focus on the subject, bulimia nervosa. Eliminate options 3 and 4 because they are comparable or alike. From the remaining options, recalling the definition of bulimia will direct you to the correct option. Review: **bulimia nervosa.**
Reference(s): Fortinash, Holoday-Worret (2012), pp. 422-423; Varcarolis (2013), p. 239.

165. The nurse is caring for a client who develops compartment syndrome from a severely fractured arm. The client asks the nurse how this can happen. Which response by the nurse is **most appropriate**?
1. A bone fragment has injured the nerve supply in the area.
2. An injured artery causes impaired arterial perfusion through the compartment.
3. Bleeding and swelling cause increased pressure in an area that cannot expand.
4. The fascia expands with injury, causing pressure on underlying nerves and muscles.

Level of Cognitive Ability: Applying
Client Needs: Physiological Integrity
Integrated Process: Nursing Process/Implementation
Content Area: Adult Health: Musculoskeletal
Priority Concepts: Mobility; Perfusion

Answer: 3
Rationale: Compartment syndrome is caused by bleeding and swelling within a compartment, which is lined by fascia that does not expand. The bleeding and swelling place pressure on the nerves, muscles, and blood vessels in the compartment, triggering the symptoms. Therefore options 1, 2, and 4 are incorrect statements.
Priority Nursing Tip: Within 4 to 6 hours after the onset of compartment syndrome, neurovascular damage is irreversible if not treated.
Test-Taking Strategy: Focus on the subject, compartment syndrome. Also, note the strategic words, most appropriate. Option 2 is eliminated first because this syndrome is not caused by an arterial injury. Knowing that the fascia cannot expand eliminates option 4. From the remaining options, it is necessary to know that bleeding and swelling (not a nerve injury) cause the symptoms. Review: **compartment syndrome.**
Reference(s): Ignatavicius, Workman (2013), pp. 1145-1146.

166. A client with an extremity burn injury has undergone fasciotomy to treat compartment syndrome of the leg. The nurse prepares to provide which type of wound care to the fasciotomy site?
1. Dry sterile dressings
2. Hydrocolloid dressings
3. Wet, sterile saline dressings
4. One-half strength Betadine dressings

Level of Cognitive Ability: Applying
Client Needs: Physiological Integrity
Integrated Process: Nursing Process/Planning
Content Area: Adult Health: Integumentary
Priority Concepts: Clinical Judgment; Tissue Integrity

Answer: 3
Rationale: A fasciotomy is an incision made extending through the subcutaneous tissue and fascia. The fasciotomy site is not sutured but is left open to relieve pressure and edema. The site is covered with wet sterile saline dressings. After 3 to 5 days, when perfusion is adequate and edema subsides, the wound is debrided and closed. A hydrocolloid dressing is not indicated for use with clean, open incisions. The incision is clean, not dirty, so there should be no reason to require Betadine. Additionally, Betadine can be irritating to normal tissues.
Priority Nursing Tip: After fasciotomy, assess pulses, color, movement, and sensation of the affected extremity, and control any bleeding with pressure.
Test-Taking Strategy: Focus on the subject, fasciotomy. Recall knowledge of what a fasciotomy involves and the basics of wound care. Recall that the skin is not sutured closed but left open for pressure relief. Remembering that moist tissue needs to remain moist will direct you to the correct option. Review: **fasciotomy.**
Reference(s): Bryant, Nix (2012), p. 452; Ignatavicius, Workman (2013), pp. 1156-1157; Potter et al (2013), pp. 1219-1220.

167. The nurse is caring for a female client who was recently admitted to the hospital with a diagnosis of anorexia nervosa. When the nurse enters the room, the client is engaged in rigorous push-ups. Which nursing action would be therapeutic?

1. Allow the client to complete the exercise program.
2. Interrupt the client and weigh the client immediately.
3. Interrupt the client and offer to take the client for a walk.
4. Tell the client that she is not allowed to exercise rigorously.

Level of Cognitive Ability: Applying
Client Needs: Physiological Integrity
Integrated Process: Nursing Process/Implementation
Content Area: Mental Health
Priority Concepts: Anxiety; Nutrition

Answer: 3
Rationale: Clients with anorexia nervosa are frequently preoccupied with rigorous exercise and push themselves beyond normal limits to work off caloric intake. The nurse must provide for appropriate exercise, as well as place limits on rigorous activities. Allowing the client to complete the exercise program could be harmful. Weighing the client reinforces the altered self-concept that the client experiences and the client's need to control weight. Telling the client that she is not allowed to exercise rigorously will increase her anxiety.
Priority Nursing Tip: The client with an eating disorder experiences an altered body image.
Test-Taking Strategy: Focus on the subject, a client with anorexia nervosa. Note the word "therapeutic." Focus on the need for the nurse to set limits with clients who have this disorder. Also, recalling that the nurse needs to provide and guide the client to perform appropriate exercise will direct you to the correct option. Review: **anorexia nervosa.**
Reference(s): Fortinash, Holoday-Worret (2012), pp. 426-428; Stuart (2013), p. 490.

168. The nurse assesses a peripheral intravenous (IV) dressing and notes that it is damp and the tape is loose. Which is the **best** action for the nurse to take?

1. Stop the infusion immediately.
2. Apply a sterile, occlusive dressing.
3. Ensure tight IV tubing connections.
4. Remove the IV and insert a new IV.

Level of Cognitive Ability: Applying
Client Needs: Physiological Integrity
Integrated Process: Nursing Process/Implementation
Content Area: Fundamental Skills: Safety
Priority Concepts: Clinical Judgment; Safety

Answer: 3
Rationale: To determine subsequent nursing interventions, the nurse checks all connections to ensure tight seals while the IV infuses to help locate the source of the leak. If the leak is at the insertion site, the nurse stops the infusion, removes the IV, and inserts a new IV catheter. The nurse applies a new sterile occlusive dressing after resolving the source of the leak.
Priority Nursing Tip: Administration of an IV solution provides immediate access to the vascular system. Always ensure that the correct solution is administered as prescribed.
Test-Taking Strategy: Note the strategic word, best, and recall that the nurse needs to determine the cause of the leaking. Use the steps of the nursing process and remember that assessment is the first step. Read each option carefully to determine which option indicates assessment to direct you to the correct option. Review: care of the client with a **peripheral intravenous (IV).**
Reference(s): Potter et al (2013), pp. 934-936.

169. The nurse assists the health care provider with the removal of a chest tube. During removal of the chest tube, the nurse instructs the client to perform which action?

1. Breathe in deeply.
2. Breathe normally.
3. Breathe out forcefully.
4. Exhale and bear down.

Level of Cognitive Ability: Applying
Client Needs: Physiological Integrity
Integrated Process: Nursing Process/Implementation
Content Area: Adult Health: Respiratory
Priority Concepts: Clinical Judgment; Gas Exchange

Answer: 4
Rationale: The client is instructed to perform the Valsalva maneuver (take a deep breath, exhale, and bear down) for chest tube removal. This maneuver will increase intrathoracic pressure, thereby lessening the potential for air to enter the pleural space. Therefore, options 1, 2, and 3 are incorrect.
Priority Nursing Tip: Never clamp a chest tube without a written prescription from the health care provider. Additionally, agency policy regarding clamping a chest tube needs to be followed.
Test-Taking Strategy: Focus on the subject, chest tube removal. Eliminate options 1 and 2 because they are comparable or alike in that breathing will cause air to enter the pleural space. From the remaining options, eliminate option 3 because of the word "forcefully." Review: the procedure for the removal of a **chest tube.**
Reference(s): Perry, Potter, Ostendorf (2014), p. 670.

170. The nurse assesses the water seal chamber of a closed chest drainage system and notes fluctuations in the chamber. What does this finding indicate?
1. The tubing is kinked.
2. An air leak is present.
3. The lung has reexpanded.
4. The system is functioning as expected.

Level of Cognitive Ability: Analyzing
Client Needs: Physiological Integrity
Integrated Process: Nursing Process/Analysis
Content Area: Adult Health: Respiratory
Priority Concepts: Clinical Judgment; Gas Exchange

Answer: 4
Rationale: Fluctuations (tidaling) in the water seal chamber are normal during inhalation and exhalation until the lung reexpands and the client no longer requires chest drainage. If fluctuations are absent, it could indicate occlusion of the tubing or that the lung has reexpanded. Excessive bubbling in the water seal chamber indicates that an air leak is present.
Priority Nursing Tip: In the water seal chamber, the tip of the tube is underwater, allowing fluid and air to drain from the pleural space and preventing air from entering the pleural space.
Test-Taking Strategy: Focus on the subject, chest tube system. Recalling the normal expectations related to the functioning of chest tube drainage systems will direct you to the correct option. Review: care of the client with a **chest tube**.
Reference(s): Perry, Potter, Ostendorf (2014), p. 666.

❖ **171.** The nurse is developing a care plan for an older client being admitted to a long-term care facility. Which information should the nurse use to plan interventions for this client? **Select all that apply.**
1. Most older clients are incontinent.
2. Older clients are at risk for dehydration.
3. Depression is a normal part of the aging process.
4. Age-related skin changes require special monitoring.
5. Older clients are at risk for complications of immobility.
6. Confusion and cognitive changes are common findings in the older population.

Level of Cognitive Ability: Applying
Client Needs: Physiological Integrity
Integrated Process: Nursing Process/Planning
Content Area: Developmental Stages: Early Adulthood to Later Adulthood
Priority Concepts: Development; Health Promotion

Answer: 2, 4, 5
Rationale: Older clients are at risk for dehydration and complications related to immobility. Another normal physiological change that occurs during the aging process is loss of skin integrity. Incontinence, depression, confusion, and cognitive changes are not normal parts of the aging process.
Priority Nursing Tip: During the aging process, normal physiological body changes occur.
Test-Taking Strategy: Focus on the subject, an older client being admitted to a long-term care facility. Read each option carefully and recall normal manifestations of the aging process to lead you to the correct options. Review: the **aging process**.
Reference(s): Potter et al (2013), pp. 176, 186-187.

Test 1

172. The nurse plans care for a client requiring intravenous (IV) fluids and electrolytes understanding that which are findings that correlate with the need for this type of therapy? **Select all that apply.**
☐ 1. Bounding pulse rate
☐ 2. Chronic kidney disease
☐ 3. Isolated syncope episodes
☐ 4. Rapid, weak, and thready pulse
☐ 5. Serum electrolyte abnormalities
☐ 6. Abnormal serum and urine osmolality levels

Level of Cognitive Ability: Applying
Client Needs: Physiological Integrity
Integrated Process: Nursing Process/Planning
Content Area: Fundamental Skills: Fluids & Electrolytes
Priority Concepts: Clinical Judgment; Fluid and Electrolyte Balance

Answer: 4, 5, 6
Rationale: Abnormal assessment findings of major body systems offer clues to fluid and electrolyte imbalances. Rapid, weak, and thready pulse is an assessment abnormality found with fluid and electrolyte imbalances, such as hyponatremia. Abnormal serum and urine osmolality are laboratory tests that are helpful in identifying the presence of or risk of fluid imbalances. Isolated episodes of syncope are not indicators for intravenous therapy unless fluid and electrolyte imbalances are identified. A bounding pulse rate is a manifestation of fluid volume excess; therefore, IV fluids are not indicated. Clients with chronic kidney disease experience the inability of the kidneys to regulate the body's water balance; fluid restrictions may be used.
Priority Nursing Tip: Clinical data noted from the assessment process are necessary to consider before intravenous therapy is initiated.
Test-Taking Strategy: Focus on the subject, clinical indicators of intravenous fluid and electrolyte therapy. Think about the purpose of IV therapy and circumstances in which it is prescribed to lead you to the correct options. Review: the principles of intravenous therapy.
Reference(s): Potter et al (2013), pp. 896-897.

173. A child is admitted to the hospital with a diagnosis of rheumatic fever. The nurse reviews the blood laboratory findings, knowing that which finding will confirm the likelihood of this disorder?
1. Increased leukocyte count
2. Decreased hemoglobin count
3. Increased antistreptolysin-O (ASO titer)
4. Decreased erythrocyte sedimentation rate

Level of Cognitive Ability: Analyzing
Client Needs: Physiological Integrity
Integrated Process: Nursing Process/Assessment
Content Area: Child Health: Cardiovascular
Priority Concepts: Clinical Judgment; Inflammation

Answer: 3
Rationale: Children suspected of having rheumatic fever are tested for streptococcal antibodies. The most reliable and best standardized test to confirm the diagnosis is the ASO titer. An elevated level indicates the presence of rheumatic fever. The remaining options are unrelated to diagnosing rheumatic fever. Additionally, an increased leukocyte count indicates the presence of infection but is not specific in confirming a particular diagnosis.
Priority Nursing Tip: Rheumatic fever manifests 2 to 6 weeks after a group A beta-hemolytic streptococcal infection of the upper respiratory tract.
Test-Taking Strategy: Note the word "confirm." Focusing on the subject of rheumatic fever will assist in eliminating options 2 and 4. From the remaining options, recall that an increased leukocyte count indicates the presence of infection but is not specific in confirming a particular diagnosis. Review: the diagnostic tests for rheumatic fever.
Reference(s): McKinney et al (2013), pp. 1229-1230.

174. A 5-year-old child is admitted to the hospital for heart surgery to repair the tetralogy of Fallot. The nurse reviews the child's record and notes that the child has clubbed fingers. This finding is indicative of which condition?
1. Tissue hypoxia
2. Chronic hypertension
3. Delayed physical growth
4. Destruction of bone marrow

Level of Cognitive Ability: Analyzing
Client Needs: Physiological Integrity
Integrated Process: Nursing Process/Analysis
Content Area: Child Health: Cardiovascular
Priority Concepts: Gas Exchange; Perfusion

Answer: 1
Rationale: Clubbing, a thickening and flattening of the tips of the fingers and toes, is thought to occur because of chronic tissue hypoxia and polycythemia. Options 2, 3, and 4 do not cause clubbing.
Priority Nursing Tip: Hypercyanotic spells (acute episodes of cyanosis and hypoxia) are also called *blue spells* or *tet spells* and occur when the child's oxygen requirements exceed the blood supply, such as during feeding, crying, or defecating.
Test-Taking Strategy: Focus on the child's diagnosis. Use the ABCs—airway, breathing, and circulation. Hypoxia relates to oxygenation, which is a concern with this disorder. Review: tetralogy of Fallot.
Reference(s): Hockenberry, Wilson (2013), p. 830.

❖ **175.** The nurse plans care for a client diagnosed with end-stage renal disease (ESRD). Which findings does the nurse expect to find documented in the client's medical record? **Select all that apply.**
- ❑ 1. Edema
- ❑ 2. Anemia
- ❑ 3. Polyuria
- ❑ 4. Bradycardia
- ❑ 5. Hypotension
- ❑ 6. Osteoporosis

Level of Cognitive Ability: Analyzing
Client Needs: Physiological Integrity
Integrated Process: Nursing Process/Assessment
Content Area: Adult Health: Renal and Urinary
Priority Concepts: Elimination; Fluid and Electrolyte Balance

Answer: 1, 2
Rationale: The manifestations of ESRD are the result of impaired kidney function. Two functions of the kidney are maintenance of water balance in the body and the secretion of erythropoietin, which stimulates red blood cell formation in bone marrow. Impairment of these functions results in edema and anemia. Kidney failure results in decreased urine production and increased blood pressure. Tachycardia is a result of increased fluid load on the heart. Osteoporosis is not a common finding with ESRD.
Priority Nursing Tip: The manifestations of kidney failure are primarily caused by the retention of nitrogenous wastes, the retention of fluids, and the inability of the kidneys to regulate electrolytes.
Test-Taking Strategy: Focus on the subject, ESRD. Recalling the anatomy and physiology of the renal system and focusing on how the kidney functions and pathophysiology of ESRD will lead you to the correct options. Review: the clinical manifestations of end-stage renal disease.
Reference(s): Ignatavicius, Workman (2013), p. 1549.

❖ **176.** The nurse is performing range-of-motion (ROM) exercises on a client when the client unexpectedly develops spastic muscle contractions. Which interventions should the nurse implement? **Select all that apply.**
- ❑ 1. Stop movement of the affected part.
- ❑ 2. Massage the affected part vigorously.
- ❑ 3. Notify the health care provider immediately.
- ❑ 4. Force movement of the joint supporting the muscle.
- ❑ 5. Ask the client to stand and walk rapidly around the room.
- ❑ 6. Place continuous gentle pressure on the muscle group until it relaxes.

Level of Cognitive Ability: Applying
Client Needs: Physiological Integrity
Integrated Process: Nursing Process/Implementation
Content Area: Adult Health: Musculoskeletal
Priority Concepts: Mobility; Pain

Answer: 1, 6
Rationale: ROM exercises should put each joint through as full a range of motion as possible without causing discomfort. An unexpected outcome is the development of spastic muscle contraction during ROM exercises. If this occurs, the nurse should stop movement of the affected part and place continuous gentle pressure on the muscle group until it relaxes. Once the contraction subsides, the exercises are resumed using slower, steady movement. Massaging the affected part vigorously may worsen the contraction. There is no need to notify the health care provider unless intervention is ineffective. The nurse should never force movement of a joint. Asking the client to stand and walk rapidly around the room is an inappropriate measure. Additionally, if the client is able to walk, ROM exercises are probably unnecessary.
Priority Nursing Tip: Range-of-motion (ROM) exercises provide adequate muscle use and maintain strength and flexibility of the muscles and joints.
Test-Taking Strategy: Focus on the subject, interventions to relieve spastic muscle contractions. Eliminate option 2 because of the word *vigorously,* option 3 because of the word *immediately,* and option 4 because of the word *force.* Next eliminate option 5 because if the client is able to walk, ROM exercises are probably unnecessary. Review: the unexpected outcomes related to range-of-motion (ROM) exercises and their treatment.
Reference(s): Perry, Potter, Ostendorf (2014), pp. 158-159, 230.

177. A client has been admitted to the hospital with a diagnosis of acute glomerulonephritis. During history taking, the nurse should ask the client about a recent history of which event?
1. Bleeding ulcer
2. Myocardial infarction
3. Deep vein thrombosis
4. Streptococcal infection

Level of Cognitive Ability: Applying
Client Needs: Physiological Integrity
Integrated Process: Nursing Process/Assessment
Content Area: Adult Health: Renal and Urinary
Priority Concepts: Fluid and Electrolyte Balance; Infection

Answer: 4
Rationale: The predominant cause of acute glomerulonephritis is infection with beta-hemolytic *Streptococcus* 3 weeks before the onset of symptoms. In addition to bacteria, other infectious agents that could trigger the disorder include viruses, fungi, and parasites. Bleeding ulcer, myocardial infarction, and deep vein thrombosis are not precipitating causes.
Priority Nursing Tip: Edema, hematuria, and proteinuria are manifestations of glomerulonephritis.
Test-Taking Strategy: Focus on the subject, glomerulonephritis. Recalling that infection is a common trigger for glomerulonephritis assists in eliminating options 1, 2, and 3. It is also necessary to know that streptococcal infections are a common cause of this problem. Review: the causes of acute **glomerulonephritis**.
Reference(s): Ignatavicius, Workman (2013), p. 1527.

178. A client has just been admitted to the emergency department with chest pain. Serum cardiac enzyme levels are drawn, and the results indicate an elevated serum creatine kinase (CK)-MB isoenzyme, troponin T, and troponin I. The nurse concludes that these results are compatible with what diagnosis?
1. Stable angina
2. Unstable angina
3. Prinzmetal's angina
4. New-onset myocardial infarction (MI)

Level of Cognitive Ability: Analyzing
Client Needs: Physiological Integrity
Integrated Process: Nursing Process/Analysis
Content Area: Adult Health: Cardiovascular
Priority Concepts: Clinical Judgment; Perfusion

Answer: 4
Rationale: Creatine kinase (CK)-MB isoenzyme is a sensitive indicator of myocardial damage. Levels begin to rise 3 to 6 hours after the onset of chest pain, peak at approximately 24 hours, and return to normal in about 3 days. Troponin is a regulatory protein found in striated muscle (skeletal and myocardial). Increased amounts of troponins are released into the bloodstream when an infarction causes damage to the myocardium. Troponin I is particularly sensitive to myocardial muscle injury; therefore, the client's results are compatible with new-onset MI. Options 1, 2, and 3 all refer to angina. These levels would not be elevated in angina.
Priority Nursing Tip: Troponin I has a high affinity for myocardial injury. The level rises within 3 hours after injury and persists up to 7 to 10 days.
Test-Taking Strategy: Focus on the subject, cardiac enzymes. Eliminate options 1, 2, and 3 because they are comparable or alike and all refer to angina. Review: **cardiac enzymes** and **myocardial infarction (MI)**.
Reference(s): Dolan, Holt (2013), pp. 396-397; Ignatavicius, Workman (2013), p. 835.

179. As part of cardiac assessment, the nurse palpates the apical pulse. To perform this assessment, the nurse places the fingertips at which location?
1. At the left midclavicular line at the fifth intercostal space
2. At the left midclavicular line at the third intercostal space
3. To the right of the left midclavicular line at the fifth intercostal space
4. To the right of the left midclavicular line at the third intercostal space

Level of Cognitive Ability: Applying
Client Needs: Physiological Integrity
Integrated Process: Nursing Process/Assessment
Content Area: Developmental Stages: Health Assessment/Physical Exam
Priority Concepts: Clinical Judgment; Perfusion

Answer: 1
Rationale: The point of maximal impulse (PMI), where the apical pulse is palpated, is normally located in the fourth or fifth intercostal space, at the left midclavicular line. Options 2, 3, and 4 are not descriptions of the location for palpation of the apical pulse.
Priority Nursing Tip: The apical impulse may not be palpable in obese clients or clients with thick chest walls.
Test-Taking Strategy: Focus on the subject, point of maximal impulse (PMI). Recalling that the PMI corresponds to the left ventricular apex and visualizing each position in the options will direct you to the correct option. Review: **point of maximal impulse (PMI)**.
Reference(s): Jarvis (2012), p. 474.

180. The nurse is caring for a client receiving bolus feedings via a nasogastric (NG) tube. Which position should the nurse use to administer the feeding?
1. Supine
2. Semi-Fowler's
3. Trendelenburg's
4. Lateral recumbent

Level of Cognitive Ability: Applying
Client Needs: Physiological Integrity
Integrated Process: Nursing Process/Implementation
Content Area: Fundamental Skills: Safety
Priority Concepts: Nutrition; Safety

Answer: 2
Rationale: Clients are at high risk for aspiration during an NG tube feeding because the tube bypasses a protective mechanism, the gag reflex. The head of the bed is elevated 35 to 40 degrees to prevent this complication by facilitating gastric emptying. The remaining options increase the risk of aspiration by blunting the effect of gravity on gastric emptying.
Priority Nursing Tip: Check the expiration date on the formula before administering the nasogastric tube feeding.
Test-Taking Strategy: Focus on the subject, nasogastric (NG) tube feeding. Eliminate options 1, 3, and 4 because they are comparable or alike and increase the risk of aspiration. Review: care of the client receiving nasogastric (NG) tube feeding.
Reference(s): Ignatavicius, Workman (2013), p. 1345.

181. The nurse is caring for a client with acute pancreatitis who has a history of alcoholism. The nurse closely monitors the client for paralytic ileus, knowing that which assessment data indicate this complication of pancreatitis?
1. Inability to pass flatus
2. Loss of anal sphincter control
3. Severe, constant pain with rapid onset
4. Firm, nontender mass palpable at the lower right costal margin

Level of Cognitive Ability: Applying
Client Needs: Physiological Integrity
Integrated Process: Nursing Process/Assessment
Content Area: Adult Health: Gastrointestinal
Priority Concepts: Clinical Judgment; Elimination

Answer: 1
Rationale: An inflammatory reaction such as acute pancreatitis can cause paralytic ileus, the common form of nonmechanical obstruction. Inability to pass flatus is a clinical manifestation of paralytic ileus. Loss of sphincter control is not a sign of paralytic ileus. Pain is associated with paralytic ileus, but the pain usually presents as a more constant generalized discomfort. Pain that is severe, constant, and rapid in onset is more likely caused by strangulation of the bowel. Option 4 is the description of the physical finding of liver enlargement. The liver is usually enlarged in the client with cirrhosis or hepatitis. Although this client may have an enlarged liver, an enlarged liver is not a sign of paralytic ileus.
Priority Nursing Tip: Cullen's sign (discoloration of the abdomen and periumbilical area) and Turner's sign (bluish discoloration of the flanks) are indicative of pancreatitis.
Test-Taking Strategy: Focus on the subject, a sign of paralytic ileus. Recalling the definition of this complication and noting the word, "paralytic," will direct you to the correct option. Review: the signs of paralytic ileus.
Reference(s): Dolan, Holt (2013), p. 433; Ignatavicius, Workman (2013), p. 1245.

182. After performing an initial abdominal assessment on a client with a diagnosis of cholelithiasis, the nurse documents that the bowel sounds are normal. Which description describes this assessment finding?
1. Waves of loud gurgles auscultated in all four quadrants
2. Soft gurgling or clicking sounds auscultated in all four quadrants
3. Low-pitched swishing sounds auscultated in one or two quadrants
4. Very high-pitched loud rushes auscultated, especially in one or two quadrants

Level of Cognitive Ability: Understanding
Client Needs: Physiological Integrity
Integrated Process: Nursing Process/Assessment
Content Area: Adult Health: Gastrointestinal
Priority Concepts: Clinical Judgment; Health Promotion

Answer: 2
Rationale: Although frequency and intensity of bowel sounds will vary depending on the phase of digestion, normal bowel sounds are relatively soft gurgling or clicking sounds that occur irregularly 5 to 35 times per minute. Loud gurgles (borborygmi) indicate hyperperistalsis. A swishing or buzzing sound represents turbulent blood flow associated with a bruit. No aortic bruits should be heard. Bowel sounds will be higher pitched and loud (hyperresonance) when the intestines are under tension, such as in intestinal obstruction.
Priority Nursing Tip: Murphy's sign (the client cannot take a deep breath when the examiner's fingers are passed below the hepatic margin because of pain) is a characteristic of cholecystitis.
Test-Taking Strategy: Focus on the subject, normal bowel sounds. Normally bowel sounds should be audible in all four quadrants; therefore, options 3 and 4 can be eliminated. From the remaining options, select option 2 because of the word "soft" in this option. Review: bowel sounds.
Reference(s): Ignatavicius, Workman (2013), pp. 1184, 1317-1318; Jarvis (2012), p. 539.

183. The nurse is assigned to care for a client with nephrotic syndrome. Which important parameter should the nurse assess on a daily basis?
1. Weight
2. Albumin levels
3. Activity tolerance
4. Blood urea nitrogen (BUN) level

Level of Cognitive Ability: Applying
Client Needs: Physiological Integrity
Integrated Process: Nursing Process/Assessment
Content Area: Adult Health: Renal and Urinary
Priority Concepts: Clinical Judgment; Fluid and Electrolyte Balance

Answer: 1
Rationale: The client with nephrotic syndrome typically presents with edema, hypoalbuminemia, and proteinuria. The nurse carefully assesses the fluid balance of the client, which includes daily monitoring of weight, intake and output, edema, and girth measurements. Albumin levels are monitored as they are prescribed, as are the BUN and creatinine levels. The client's activity level is adjusted according to the amount of edema and water retention. As edema increases, the client's activity level should be restricted.
Priority Nursing Tip: In nephrotic syndrome, the blood pressure may be normal or slightly decreased from normal.
Test-Taking Strategy: Focus on the subject, a client with nephrotic syndrome. Note the words "daily basis." Recalling that the typical signs of nephrotic syndrome are edema, hypoalbuminemia, and proteinuria will direct you to the correct option. Review: the characteristics of nephrotic syndrome.
Reference(s): Ignatavicius, Workman (2013), pp. 1529-1530.

184. A client is being admitted to the hospital with a diagnosis of urolithiasis and ureteral colic. The nurse expects to note which finding on pain assessment?
1. Dull and aching pain in the costovertebral area
2. Aching and cramplike pain throughout the abdomen
3. Pain that is sharp and radiating posteriorly to the spinal column
4. Pain that is excruciating, wavelike, and radiating toward the genitalia

Level of Cognitive Ability: Analyzing
Client Needs: Physiological Integrity
Integrated Process: Nursing Process/Assessment
Content Area: Fundamental Skills: Pain
Priority Concepts: Clinical Judgment; Pain

Answer: 4
Rationale: The pain of ureteral colic is caused by movement of a stone through the ureter and is sharp, excruciating, and wavelike, radiating to the genitalia and thigh. The stone causes reduced flow of urine, and the urine also contains blood because of the stone's abrasive action on urinary tract mucosa. Stones in the renal pelvis cause pain that is a dull ache in the costovertebral area. Renal colic is characterized by pain that is acute, with tenderness over the costovertebral area. Options 1, 2, and 3 are not characteristics of urolithiasis and ureteral colic.
Priority Nursing Tip: For the client with renal calculi, strain all urine for the presence of stones and send the stones to the laboratory for analysis.
Test-Taking Strategy: Focus on the subject, urolithiasis and ureteral colic. Recall the anatomical location of the kidneys and the ureters. Because the kidneys are located in the posterior abdomen near the ribcage, pain in the costovertebral area is more likely to be associated with stones in the renal pelvis. On the other hand, sharp wavelike pain that radiates toward the genitalia is more consistent with the location of the ureters in the abdomen. Review: **urolithiasis and ureteral colic.**
Reference(s): Ignatavicius, Workman (2013), pp. 1508-1509.

185. The nurse is assessing the client with left-sided heart failure. The client states that he needs to use three pillows under the head and upper torso at night to be able to breathe comfortably while sleeping. The nurse documents that the client is experiencing which clinical finding?

1. Orthopnea
2. Dyspnea at rest
3. Dyspnea on exertion
4. Paroxysmal nocturnal dyspnea

Level of Cognitive Ability: Understanding
Client Needs: Physiological Integrity
Integrated Process: Communication and Documentation
Content Area: Adult Health: Cardiovascular
Priority Concepts: Functional Ability; Gas Exchange

Answer: 1
Rationale: Dyspnea is a subjective complaint that can range from an awareness of breathing to physical distress and does not necessarily correlate with the degree of heart failure. Dyspnea can be exertional or at rest. Orthopnea is a more severe form of dyspnea, requiring the client to assume a "three-point" position while upright and use pillows to support the head and upper torso at night. Paroxysmal nocturnal dyspnea is a severe form of dyspnea occurring suddenly at night because of rapid fluid reentry into the vasculature from the interstitium during sleep.
Priority Nursing Tip: Signs of left-sided heart failure are evident in the pulmonary system. Signs of right-sided heart failure are evident in the systemic circulation.
Test-Taking Strategy: Focus on the subject, a client with left-sided heart failure who has trouble breathing while sleeping. Recall knowledge of the different degrees of dyspnea. Eliminate options 3 and 4 because the question mentions nothing about exertion or a sudden (paroxysmal) event. From the remaining options, select option 1 because the client is breathing "comfortably" with the use of pillows. Review: **dyspnea** and **orthopnea.**
Reference(s): Ignatavicius, Workman (2013), pp. 551, 614.

186. The nurse admits a client who is in sickle cell crisis to the hospital. Which should the nurse prepare for as the **priority** in the management of the client?

1. Pain management
2. Iron administration
3. Oxygen administration
4. Red blood cell transfusion

Level of Cognitive Ability: Applying
Client Needs: Physiological Integrity
Integrated Process: Nursing Process/Planning
Content Area: Adult Health: Hematological
Priority Concepts: Caregiving; Gas Exchange

Answer: 3
Rationale: The priority nursing intervention for a client in sickle cell crisis is to administer supplemental oxygen because the client is hypoxemic, and as a result, the red blood cells change to the sickle shape. In addition, oxygen is the priority because airway and breathing are more important than circulatory needs. The nurse also plans for fluid therapy to promote hydration and reverse the agglutination of sickled cells, opioid analgesics for relief from severe pain, and, blood transfusions (rather than iron administration) to increase the blood's oxygen-carrying capacity.
Priority Nursing Tip: In sickle cell anemia, situations that precipitate sickling include fever, dehydration, and emotional and physical stress.
Test-Taking Strategy: Focus on the subject, sickle cell crisis and focus on the strategic word, *priority.* Recalling the ABCs—airway, breathing, and circulation—will assist in answering correctly. Recalling that clumping of sickled cells occurs when the sickle cell client is hypoxemic will direct you to the correct option. Review: the treatment for sickle cell crisis.
Reference(s): Ignatavicius, Workman (2013), pp. 871, 874.

187. The nurse suspects that a client who had a myocardial infarction is developing cardiogenic shock. The nurse should assess for which peripheral vascular manifestation of this complication?

1. Flushed, dry skin with bounding pedal pulses
2. Warm, moist skin with irregular pedal pulses
3. Cool, clammy skin with weak or thready pedal pulses
4. Cool, dry skin with alternating weak and strong pedal pulses

Level of Cognitive Ability: Analyzing
Client Needs: Physiological Integrity
Integrated Process: Nursing Process/Assessment
Content Area: Critical Care: Emergency Situations
Priority Concepts: Gas Exchange; Perfusion

Answer: 3
Rationale: Some of the manifestations of cardiogenic shock include increased pulse (weak and thready); decreased blood pressure; decreasing urinary output; signs of cerebral ischemia (confusion, agitation); and cool, clammy skin.
Priority Nursing Tip: The goals of treatment for cardiogenic shock are to maintain tissue oxygenation and perfusion and improve the pumping ability of the heart.
Test-Taking Strategy: Focus on the subject, cardiogenic shock. Recall the signs and symptoms of shock. The word "clammy" in option 3 should direct you to the correct option. Review: the signs of **cardiogenic shock.**
Reference(s): Ignatavicius, Workman (2013), p. 842.

188. The nurse is teaching a client about general hygienic measures for foot and nail care. Which instructions should the nurse provide to the client? **Select all that apply.**
  ❑ 1. Wear knee-high hose to prevent edema.
  ❑ 2. Soak and wash the feet daily using cool water.
  ❑ 3. Use commercial removers for corns or calluses.
  ❑ 4. Use over-the-counter preparations to treat ingrown nails.
  ❑ 5. Apply lanolin or baby oil if dryness is noted along the feet.
  ❑ 6. Pat the feet dry thoroughly after washing and dry well between toes.

Level of Cognitive Ability: Applying
Client Needs: Physiological Integrity
Integrated Process: Teaching and Learning
Content Area: Adult Health: Integumentary
Priority Concepts: Client Education; Health Promotion

Answer: 5, 6
Rationale: The nurse should offer the following guidelines in a general hygienic foot and nail care program: Inspect the feet daily, including the tops and soles of the feet, the heels, and the areas between the toes; wash the feet daily using lukewarm water, and avoid soaks to the feet, thoroughly patting the feet dry and drying well between toes; and avoid cutting corns or calluses or using commercial removers. Additional general hygienic measures include gently rubbing lanolin, baby oil, or corn oil into the skin if dryness is noted along the feet or between the toes; filing the toe nails straight across and square (do not use scissors or clippers); avoiding the use of over-the-counter preparations to treat ingrown toenails and consulting a health care provider or for these problems; and avoiding wearing elastic stockings, knee-high hose, or constricting garters.
Priority Nursing Tip: A complication of diabetes mellitus is peripheral neuropathy, which results in decreased sensation, particularly in the feet. A client with diabetes mellitus needs to be cautious about temperature exposure and injuries to the feet because they may not be felt because of the decreased sensation.
Test-Taking Strategy: Focus on the subject, general hygienic measures for foot and nail care. Eliminate option 1, recalling that constricting items need to be avoided. Eliminate option 2 because of the words "soak" and "cool." Eliminate options 3 and 4 because of the words "commercial removers" and "over-the-counter," respectively. Review: general hygienic measures for foot and nail care.
Reference(s): Perry, Potter, Ostendorf (2014), pp. 420-425.

189. A client with renal cancer is being treated preoperatively with radiation therapy. The nurse evaluates that the client has an understanding of proper care of the skin over the treatment field when the client states to perform which action?
  1. Wash the ink marks off the skin.
  2. Avoid skin exposure to direct sunlight.
  3. Apply perfumed lotion to the affected skin.
  4. Wear tight clothing over the skin site to provide support.

Level of Cognitive Ability: Evaluating
Client Needs: Physiological Integrity
Integrated Process: Nursing Process/Evaluation
Content Area: Adult Health: Oncology
Priority Concepts: Cellular Regulation; Tissue Integrity

Answer: 2
Rationale: The client undergoing radiation therapy must keep the affected skin protected from temperature extremes, direct sunlight, and chlorinated water (as from swimming pools). The client should wash the site using mild soap and warm or cool water and pat the area dry. Lines or ink marks that are placed on the skin to guide the radiation therapy should be left in place. No lotions, creams, alcohol, perfumes, or deodorants should be placed on the skin over the treatment site. The client should wear cotton clothing over the skin site and guard against irritation from tight or rough clothing such as belts or bras.
Priority Nursing Tip: Radiation therapy is effective on tissues directly within the path of the radiation beam.
Test-Taking Strategy: Focus on the subject, care of the skin over the treatment field after radiation therapy. Note the words "understanding of proper care." Recalling that the goal of care is to prevent skin irritation will direct you to the correct option. Review: client teaching related to radiation therapy.
Reference(s): Ignatavicius, Workman (2013), p. 413.

190. A client with chronic kidney disease is receiving epoetin alfa (Epogen, Procrit) to support erythropoiesis. The nurse should question the client about compliance with taking which medication that supports red blood cell (RBC) production?
1. Iron supplement
2. Zinc supplement
3. Calcium supplement
4. Magnesium supplement

Level of Cognitive Ability: Applying
Client Needs: Physiological Integrity
Integrated Process: Nursing Process/Assessment
Content Area: Pharmacology: Hematological Medications
Priority Concepts: Adherence; Safety

Answer: 1
Rationale: Iron is needed for RBC production; otherwise, the body cannot produce sufficient erythrocytes. In either case the client is not receiving the full benefit of epoetin alfa therapy if iron is not taken. Options 2, 3, or 4 are not needed for RBC production.
Priority Nursing Tip: A side effect of epoetin alfa (Epogen) is hypertension.
Test-Taking Strategy: Focus on the subject, red blood cell (RBC) production. Note the relationship of RBC production in the question and iron in the correct option. Review: **epoetin alfa (Epogen, Procrit).**
Reference(s): Hodgson, Kizior (2014), p. 424.

191. The home health nurse is performing an initial assessment on a client who has arrived home after insertion of a permanent pacemaker. Which client statement indicates that an understanding of self-care is evident?
1. "I will never be able to operate a microwave oven again."
2. "I should expect occasional feelings of dizziness and fatigue."
3. "I will take my pulse in the wrist or neck daily and record it in a log."
4. "Moving my arms and shoulders vigorously helps check pacemaker functioning."

Level of Cognitive Ability: Evaluating
Client Needs: Physiological Integrity
Integrated Process: Nursing Process/Evaluation
Content Area: Adult Health: Cardiovascular
Priority Concepts: Client Education; Perfusion

Answer: 3
Rationale: Clients with permanent pacemakers must be able to take their pulse in the wrist and/or neck accurately so as to note any variation in the pulse rate or rhythm that may need to be reported to the health care provider. Clients can safely operate most appliances and tools, such as microwave ovens, video recorders, AM-FM radios, electric blankets, lawn mowers, and leaf blowers, as long as the devices are grounded and in good repair. If the client experiences any feelings of dizziness, fatigue, or an irregular heartbeat, the health care provider is notified. The arms and shoulders should not be moved vigorously for 6 weeks after insertion.
Priority Nursing Tip: A responsibility of the nurse is to teach a client with a pacemaker how to measure the pulse rate.
Test-Taking Strategy: Focus on the subject, client understanding about care to a pacemaker. Recalling that a pacemaker assists in controlling cardiac rate and rhythm will direct you to the correct option. Review: client teaching points related to a **pacemaker.**
Reference(s): Ignatavicius, Workman (2013), p. 741.

192. A client with a severe major depressive episode is unable to address activities of daily living (ADL). Which is the appropriate nursing intervention?
  1. Have the client's peers confront the client about how noncompliance in addressing ADL affects the milieu.
  2. Structure the client's day so that adequate time can be devoted to the client's assuming responsibility for ADL.
  3. Offer the client choices and describe the consequences for the failure to comply with the expectation of maintaining his/her own ADL.
  4. Feed, bathe, and dress the client as needed until the client's condition improves so that he/she can perform these activities independently.

Level of Cognitive Ability: Applying
Client Needs: Physiological Integrity
Integrated Process: Nursing Process/Implementation
Content Area: Mental Health
Priority Concepts: Caregiving; Functional Ability

Answer: 4
Rationale: The symptoms of major depression include depressed mood, loss of interest or pleasure, changes in appetite and sleep patterns, psychomotor agitation or retardation, fatigue, feelings of worthlessness or guilt, diminished ability to think or concentrate, and recurrent thoughts of death. Often, the client does not have the energy or interest to complete activities of daily living. Option 1 will increase the client's feelings of poor self-esteem and of unworthiness. Option 2 is incorrect because the client still lacks the energy and motivation to do these independently. Option 3 may lead to increased feelings of worthlessness as the client fails to meet expectations.
Priority Nursing Tip: For the client with depression, the nurse needs to avoid pushing the client to make decisions that the client is not ready to make.
Test-Taking Strategy: Focus on the subject, major depression. Use Maslow's Hierarchy of Needs theory and remember that physiological needs are the priority. This will direct you to the correct option. Review: care of the client with depression.
Reference(s): Varcarolis (2013), pp. 233-234, 261.

193. A pregnant client of 32 weeks' gestation is admitted to the obstetrical unit for observation after a motor vehicle crash. The client is experiencing slight vaginal bleeding and mild cramps. Which action should the nurse take to determine the viability of the fetus?
  1. Insert an intravenous line and begin an infusion at 125 mL per hour.
  2. Administer oxygen to the woman via a face mask at 7 to 10 liters per minute.
  3. Position and connect the ultrasound transducer to the external fetal monitor.
  4. Position and connect a spiral electrode to the fetal monitor for internal fetal monitoring.

Level of Cognitive Ability: Applying
Client Needs: Physiological Integrity
Integrated Process: Nursing Process/Implementation
Content Area: Maternity: Antepartum
Priority Concepts: Perfusion; Reproduction

Answer: 3
Rationale: External fetal monitoring will allow the nurse to determine any change in the fetal heart rate and rhythm that would indicate that the fetus is in jeopardy. The amount of bleeding described is insufficient to require intravenous fluid replacement. Because fetal distress has not been determined at this time, oxygen administration is premature. Internal monitoring is contraindicated when there is vaginal bleeding, especially in preterm labor.
Priority Nursing Tip: Internal fetal monitoring is invasive and requires rupturing of the membranes and attaching an electrode to the presenting part of the fetus.
Test-Taking Strategy: Focus on the subject, to determine viability of the fetus. Next use the steps of the nursing process, and note that option 3 is an assessment and a noninvasive measure. Review: fetal assessment techniques.
Reference(s): McKinney et al (2013), pp. 662-663.

194. The nurse is reviewing the results of a sweat test performed on a child with cystic fibrosis (CF). Which finding should the nurse expect to note?
  1. A sweat sodium concentration less than 40 mEq/L
  2. A sweat potassium concentration less than 40 mEq/L
  3. A sweat chloride concentration greater than 60 mEq/L
  4. A sweat potassium concentration greater than 40 mEq/L

Level of Cognitive Ability: Understanding
Client Needs: Physiological Integrity
Integrated Process: Nursing Process/Assessment
Content Area: Fundamental Skills: Diagnostic Tests
Priority Concepts: Clinical Judgment; Development

Answer: 3
Rationale: Cystic fibrosis is a chronic multisystem disorder characterized by exocrine gland dysfunction. A consistent finding of abnormally high chloride concentrations in the sweat is a unique characteristic of CF. Normally the sweat chloride concentration is less than 40 mEq/L. A sweat chloride concentration greater than 60 mEq/L is diagnostic of CF. Potassium concentration is unrelated to the sweat test.
Priority Nursing Tip: Usually more than 75 mg of sweat is needed to perform the sweat test. This amount is difficult to obtain from an infant; therefore an immunoreactive trypsinogen analysis and direct deoxyribonucleic acid (DNA) analysis for mutant genes may be done to test for cystic fibrosis.
Test-Taking Strategy: Focus on the subject, sweat test. Eliminate options 2 and 4 first because they are comparable and alike and the potassium level is unrelated to the sweat test. From the remaining options, note that option 3 indicates a greater value. Review: the sweat test.
Reference(s): Hockenberry, Wilson (2013), pp. 748-749.

195. The emergency department nurse is assessing a client who abruptly discontinued benzodiazepine therapy and is experiencing withdrawal. Which manifestations of withdrawal should the nurse expect to note? **Select all that apply.**
  ❑ 1. Tremors
  ❑ 2. Sweating
  ❑ 3. Lethargy
  ❑ 4. Agitation
  ❑ 5. Nervousness
  ❑ 6. Muscle weakness

Level of Cognitive Ability: Analyzing
Client Needs: Physiological Integrity
Integrated Process: Nursing Process/Assessment
Content Area: Pharmacology: Psychiatric Medications
Priority Concepts: Clinical Judgment; Safety

Answer: 1, 2, 4, 5
Rationale: Benzodiazepines should not be abruptly discontinued because withdrawal symptoms are likely to occur. Withdrawal symptoms include tremor, sweating, agitation, nervousness, insomnia, anorexia, and muscular cramps. Withdrawal symptoms from long-term, high-dose benzodiazepine therapy include paranoia, delirium, panic, hypertension, and status epilepticus.
Priority Nursing Tip: Abrupt withdrawal of benzodiazepines can be potentially life threatening, and withdrawal should occur only under medical supervision.
Test-Taking Strategy: Focus on the subject, benzodiazepines. Specific knowledge regarding the withdrawal symptoms of benzodiazepines is needed to select the correct options. However, if you can remember that the therapeutic effect of benzodiazepines is anxiolytic, you will be able to eliminate the incorrect options because abrupt withdrawal will produce the opposite effect of an anxiolytic. Review: the withdrawal symptoms of benzodiazepines.
Reference(s): Kee, Hayes, McCuistion (2012), p. 394.

196. The nurse performs a neurovascular assessment on a client with a newly applied cast. The nurse should determine that there is a need for close observation and a **need for follow-up** if which is noted?

1. Palpable pulses distal to the cast
2. Capillary refill greater than 6 seconds
3. Blanching of the nail bed when it is depressed
4. Sensation when the area distal to the cast is pinched

Level of Cognitive Ability: Analyzing
Client Needs: Physiological Integrity
Integrated Process: Nursing Process/Assessment
Content Area: Adult Health: Musculoskeletal
Priority Concepts: Clinical Judgment; Perfusion

Answer: 2
Rationale: To assess for adequate circulation, the nail bed of each finger or toe is depressed until it blanches, and then the pressure is released. This is known as capillary refill time. Optimally, the color will change from white to pink rapidly (less than 3 seconds). If this does not occur, the toes or fingers will require close observation and follow-up. Palpable pulses and sensations distal to the cast are expected. However, if pulses could not be palpated or if the client complained of numbness or tingling, the health care provider should be notified.
Priority Nursing Tip: For the client with a cast applied to an extremity, if pulses could not be palpated or the client complains of numbness or tingling, the health care provider should be notified.
Test-Taking Strategy: Focus on the subject, client assessment after cast application. Note the strategic words, *need for follow-up*. This creates a negative event query and requires you to select a finding that is not normal. Eliminate options 1, 3, and 4 because these options identify normal expected findings. Option 2 identifies an abnormal or unexpected finding. Review: assessment of **capillary refill**.
Reference(s): Ignatavicius, Workman (2013), p. 1149.

197. The nurse is caring for a client with a head injury and is monitoring the client for decerebrate posturing. Which is characteristic of this type of posturing?

1. Abnormal involuntary flexion of the extremities
2. Abnormal involuntary extension of the extremities
3. Upper extremity extension with lower extremity flexion
4. Upper extremity flexion with lower extremity extension

Level of Cognitive Ability: Analyzing
Client Needs: Physiological Integrity
Integrated Process: Nursing Process/Assessment
Content Area: Adult Health: Neurological
Priority Concepts: Clinical Judgment; Intracranial Regulation

Answer: 2
Rationale: Decerebrate posturing, which can occur with upper brainstem injury, is characterized by abnormal involuntary extension of the extremities. Options 1, 3, and 4 are incorrect descriptions of this type of posturing.
Priority Nursing Tip: Decerebrate or decorticate posturing is an indication of neurological deterioration warranting immediate notification of the health care provider.
Test-Taking Strategy: Focus on the subject, decerebrate posturing. Remember that decerebrate may also be known as extension. Recalling this concept will direct you to the correct option. Review: decerebrate posturing.
Reference(s): Ignatavicius, Workman (2013), pp. 918, 1026.

198. The nurse is caring for a client admitted to the surgical nursing unit following right radical mastectomy to treat breast cancer. The nurse includes which intervention in the nursing plan of care for this client?
1. Take blood pressures in the right arm only.
2. Draw serum laboratory samples from the right arm only.
3. Position the client supine and flat with the right arm elevated on a pillow.
4. Check the right posterior axilla area when assessing the surgical dressing.

Level of Cognitive Ability: Applying
Client Needs: Physiological Integrity
Integrated Process: Nursing Process/Planning
Content Area: Adult Health: Oncology
Priority Concepts: Cellular Regulation; Safety

Answer: 4
Rationale: If there is drainage or bleeding from the surgical site after mastectomy, gravity will cause the drainage to seep down and soak the posterior axillary portion of the dressing first. The nurse checks this area to detect early bleeding. Blood pressure measurement, venipuncture, and intravenous sites should not involve use of the operative arm. The client should be positioned with the head in semi-Fowler's position and the arm on the operative side elevated on pillows to decrease edema. Edema is likely to occur because lymph drainage channels have been resected during the surgical procedure.
Priority Nursing Tip: Breast self-examination should be done monthly, 7 to 10 days after menses. Postmenopausal clients should select a specific day of the month and perform BSE monthly on that day.
Test-Taking Strategy: Focus on the subject, postmastectomy care. Eliminate options 1 and 2 first because of the words "right arm only." From the remaining options, use knowledge of the effects of gravity to direct you to the correct option. Review: care of the client after mastectomy.
Reference(s): Ignatavicius, Workman (2013), p. 1602.

199. The nurse is assisting the client with hepatic encephalopathy to fill out the dietary menu. The nurse advises the client to avoid which entree items that could aggravate the client's condition?
1. Tomato soup
2. Fresh fruit plate
3. Vegetable lasagna
4. Ground beef patty

Level of Cognitive Ability: Applying
Client Needs: Physiological Integrity
Integrated Process: Nursing Process/Implementation
Content Area: Adult Health: Gastrointestinal
Priority Concepts: Nutrition; Safety

Answer: 4
Rationale: Clients with hepatic encephalopathy have impaired ability to convert ammonia to urea and must limit intake of protein and ammonia-containing foods in the diet. The client should avoid foods such as chicken, beef, ham, cheese, milk, peanut butter, and gelatin. The food items in options 1, 2, and 3 are acceptable to eat.
Priority Nursing Tip: Some food sources of protein include bread and cereal products, dairy products, beans, eggs, meats, fish, and poultry.
Test-Taking Strategy: Focus on the subject, hepatic encephalopathy and note the word "avoid." Note that options 1, 2, and 3 are comparable or alike in that they address food items of a fruit and vegetable nature. Review: dietary measures for the client with hepatic encephalopathy.
Reference(s): Ignatavicius, Workman (2013), p. 1295; Nix (2013), pp. 372-373.

❖ **200.** A client with a colostomy is complaining of gas building up in the colostomy bag. The nurse instructs the client that which food items should be consumed to best prevent this problem? **Select all that apply.**
❑ 1. Yogurt
❑ 2. Broccoli
❑ 3. Cabbage
❑ 4. Crackers
❑ 5. Cauliflower
❑ 6. Toasted bread

Level of Cognitive Ability: Applying
Client Needs: Physiological Integrity
Integrated Process: Teaching and Learning
Content Area: Adult Health: Gastrointestinal
Priority Concepts: Elimination; Nutrition

Answer: 1, 4, 6
Rationale: Consumption of yogurt, crackers, and toast or crackers can help prevent gas. Gas-forming foods include broccoli, mushrooms, cauliflower, onions, peas, and cabbage. These should be avoided by the client with a colostomy until tolerance to them is determined.
Priority Nursing Tip: The best way for a client with a colostomy to control flatus is through diet. Every client is different, and the client must learn which foods will be problematic.
Test-Taking Strategy: Focus on the subject, prevention of gas build-up in the colostomy bag. Note the similarity between options 2, 3, and 5 in terms of their food substance to assist you in eliminating these options. Review: gas-forming foods and colostomy.
Reference(s): Ignatavicius, Workman (2013), pp. 1252-1253.

201. A client receiving total parenteral nutrition (TPN) complains of nausea, excessive thirst, and increased frequency of voiding. The nurse should **initially** assess which client data?
1. Rectal temperature
2. Last serum potassium
3. Capillary blood glucose
4. Serum blood urea nitrogen and creatinine

Level of Cognitive Ability: Analyzing
Client Needs: Physiological Integrity
Integrated Process: Nursing Process/Assessment
Content Area: Critical Care: Parenteral Nutrition
Priority Concepts: Glucose Regulation; Nutrition

Answer: **3**
Rationale: Clients receiving TPN are at risk for hyperglycemia related to the increased glucose load of the solution. The symptoms exhibited by the client are consistent with hyperglycemia. The nurse would need to assess the client's blood glucose level to verify these data. The other options would not provide any information that would correlate with the client's symptoms.
Priority Nursing Tip: Hyperglycemia occurs in the client receiving total parenteral nutrition because of the high concentration of dextrose (glucose) in the solution.
Test-Taking Strategy: Note the strategic word, *initially*. Focus on the subject, total parenteral nutrition (TPN) therapy. Review the client's symptoms and think about the complications of TPN. Recalling that hyperglycemia is a complication will direct you to the correct option. Review: **total parenteral nutrition (TPN)** and **hyperglycemia**.
Reference(s): Perry, Potter, Ostendorf (2014), p. 798.

202. A client admitted to the hospital with a diagnosis of cirrhosis has massive ascites and difficulty breathing. The nurse performs which intervention as a **priority** measure to assist the client with breathing?
1. Repositions side to side every 2 hours
2. Elevates the head of the bed 60 degrees
3. Auscultates the lung fields every 4 hours
4. Encourages deep breathing exercises every 2 hours

Level of Cognitive Ability: Applying
Client Needs: Physiological Integrity
Integrated Process: Nursing Process/Implementation
Content Area: Adult Health: Gastrointestinal
Priority Concepts: Caregiving; Gas Exchange

Answer: **2**
Rationale: The client is having difficulty breathing because of upward pressure on the diaphragm from the ascitic fluid in the abdomen. Elevating the head of the bed enlists the aid of gravity in relieving pressure on the diaphragm. The other options are general measures in the care of a client with ascites, but the priority measure is the one that relieves diaphragmatic pressure.
Priority Nursing Tip: A paracentesis may be performed to remove abdominal fluid in a client with cirrhosis and ascites.
Test-Taking Strategy: Note the strategic word, *priority*, and the subject, to assist with breathing in a client with massive ascites. Recalling that elevating the head will provide immediate relief of symptoms associated with difficulty breathing will direct you to the correct option. Review: care of the client with **ascites** who is having **difficulty breathing**.
Reference(s): Ignatavicius, Workman (2013), p. 1300.

❖ **203.** The nurse who practices culturally sensitive nursing care incorporates which characteristics? **Select all that apply.**
❑ 1. The expression of pain is affected by learned behaviors.
❑ 2. Physiologically, all individuals experience pain in a similar manner.
❑ 3. Ethnic culture has an effect on the physiological response to pain medications.
❑ 4. Clients should be assessed for pain regardless of a lack of overt symptomatology.
❑ 5. The use of a standardized pain assessment tool ensures unbiased pain assessment.

Level of Cognitive Ability: Analyzing
Client Needs: Physiological Integrity
Integrated Process: Nursing Process/Planning
Content Area: Fundamental Skills: Cultural Awareness
Priority Concepts: Culture; Pain

Answer: **1, 3, 4**
Rationale: Pain and its expression are often affected by an individual's ethnic culture in ways that include learned means of pain expression, the physiological response to pain medications, and attitudes regarding acceptable ways of dealing with pain. Physiologically not all individuals, even those of the same ethnic culture, will respond to pain in a similar manner, and so a standardized pain assessment tool is not effective in measuring pain in all clients.
Priority Nursing Tip: Pain and the expression of pain are individual specific responses that are greatly influenced by an individual's ethnic culture.
Test-Taking Strategy: Focus on the subject, pain and cultural awareness. Considering the effects of culture on pain will direct you to the correct options. Also note the closed-ended word "all" in option 2 and the words "ensures unbiased" in option 5. Review: the concepts related to **pain** and **culture**.
Reference(s): Potter et al (2013), p. 107.

204. The nurse is gathering data from a client about the client's medication history and notes that the client is taking tolterodine tartrate (Detrol LA). The nurse should determine that the client is taking the medication to treat which disorder?
1. Glaucoma
2. Pyloric stenosis
3. Renal insufficiency
4. Urinary frequency and urgency

Level of Cognitive Ability: Analyzing
Client Needs: Physiological Integrity
Integrated Process: Nursing Process/Analysis
Content Area: Pharmacology: Renal and Urinary Medications
Priority Concepts: Clinical Judgment; Safety

Answer: 4
Rationale: Tolterodine tartrate (Detrol LA) is an antispasmodic used to treat overactive bladder and symptoms of urinary frequency, urgency, or urge incontinence. It is contraindicated in urinary retention and uncontrolled narrow-angle glaucoma. It is used with caution in renal function impairment, bladder outflow obstruction, and gastrointestinal obstructive disease such as pyloric stenosis.
Priority Nursing Tip: Extended-release capsules of tolterodine tartrate (Detrol LA) should not be split, chewed, or crushed.
Test-Taking Strategy: Focus on the subject, the action and use of tolterodine tartrate (Detrol LA). Recalling that tolterodine tartrate is an antispasmodic will direct you to the correct option. Review: tolterodine tartrate (Detrol LA).
Reference(s): Hodgson, Kizior (2014), p. 1185.

❖ **205.** The nurse provides discharge instructions for a client beginning oral hypoglycemic therapy. Which statements if made by the client indicate a **need for further teaching**? **Select all that apply.**
☐ 1. "If I am ill, I should skip my daily dose."
☐ 2. "If I overeat, I will double my dosage of medication."
☐ 3. "Oral agents are effective in managing type 2 diabetes."
☐ 4. "If I become pregnant, I will discontinue my medication."
☐ 5. "Oral hypoglycemic medications will cause my urine to turn orange."
☐ 6. "My medications are used to manage my diabetes along with diet and exercise."

Level of Cognitive Ability: Evaluating
Client Needs: Physiological Integrity
Integrated Process: Teaching and Learning
Content: Adult Health: Endocrine
Priority Concepts: Client Education; Glucose Regulation

Answer: 1, 2, 4, 5
Rationale: Clients are instructed that oral agents are used in addition to diet and exercise as therapy for diabetes mellitus. During illness or periods of intense stress, the client should be instructed to monitor his or her blood glucose level frequently and should contact the health care provider if the blood glucose is elevated because insulin may be needed to prevent symptoms of acute hyperglycemia. The medication should not be skipped or the dosage should not be doubled. Taking extra medication should be avoided unless specifically prescribed by the health care provider. Medication should never be discontinued unless instructed to do so by the health care provider. However, the diabetic who becomes pregnant will need to contact her health care provider because the oral diabetic medication may have to be changed to insulin therapy because some oral hypoglycemics can be harmful to the fetus. These medications do not change the color of the urine.
Priority Nursing Tip: Any changes to prescribed medication usage or amounts should not be made by clients without prior health care provider approval.
Test-Taking Strategy: Focus on the subject, oral hypoglycemic therapy. Note the strategic words, *need for further teaching*. These words indicate a negative event query and the need to select the incorrect options. Think about the pathophysiology of diabetes mellitus and its treatment, and use general medication guidelines to select the correct options. Review: the characteristics of **oral hypoglycemics**.
Reference(s): Lehne (2013), pp. 718-719; Lilley, Rainforth Collins, Harrington, Snyder (2014), pp. 505-506.

206. The nurse evaluates a client following treatment for carbon monoxide poisoning. The nurse should document that the treatment was **effective** if which finding was present?
1. The client is sleeping soundly.
2. The client is awake and talking.
3. The heart monitor shows sinus tachycardia.
4. Carboxyhemoglobin levels are less than 5%.

Level of Cognitive Ability: Evaluating
Client Needs: Physiological Integrity
Integrated Process: Nursing Process/Evaluation
Content Area: Adult Health: Respiratory
Priority Concepts: Gas Exchange; Perfusion

Answer: 4
Rationale: Normal carboxyhemoglobin levels are less than 5% for an adult (0.05% to 2.5% for a nonsmoker and 5% to 10% for a heavy smoker). Clients can be awake and talking with abnormally high levels. The symptoms of carbon monoxide poisoning are tachycardia, tachypnea, and central nervous system depression.
Priority Nursing Tip: A carbon monoxide level of 61% or above is fatal poisoning.
Test-Taking Strategy: Focus on the subject, carbon monoxide poisoning. Note the strategic word, *effective*. Note the relationship between the words "carbon monoxide poisoning" in the question and option 4. Option 4 is the only option that specifically addresses this subject. Review: **carbon monoxide poisoning**.
Reference(s): Hammond, Zimmermann (2013), pp. 195-196; Ignatavicius, Workman (2013), p. 522.

207. The nurse instructs a preoperative client in the proper use of an incentive spirometer. What should the nurse use to determine that the client is using the incentive spirometer **effectively**?
1. Cloudy sputum
2. Shallow breathing
3. Unilateral wheezing
4. Productive coughing

Level of Cognitive Ability: Evaluating
Client Needs: Physiological Integrity
Integrated Process: Nursing Process/Evaluation
Content Area: Fundamental Skills: Perioperative Care
Priority Concepts: Client Education; Gas Exchange

Answer: 4
Rationale: Incentive spirometry helps reduce atelectasis, open airways, stimulate coughing, and help mobilize secretions for expectoration, via vital client participation in recovery. Cloudy sputum, shallow breathing, and wheezing indicate that the incentive spirometry is not effective because they point to infection, counterproductive depth of breathing, and bronchoconstriction, respectively.
Priority Nursing Tip: The client should assume a sitting or upright position when using an incentive spirometer.
Test-Taking Strategy: Focus on the subject, incentive spirometer. Note the strategic word, *effectively*. Think about the purpose of an incentive spirometer. Eliminate options 1, 2, and 3, which indicate abnormal findings. Review: the purpose of an **incentive spirometer**.
Reference(s): Potter et al (2013), pp. 848, 1288-1289.

208. A client is to be started on prazosin hydrochloride (Minipress). The client asks the nurse why the first dose must be taken at bedtime. Which response by the nurse is based on the understanding of the early use of prazosin?
1. Treatment with prazosin hydrochloride (Minipress) results in extreme drowsiness.
2. Treatment with prazosin hydrochloride (Minipress) can cause significant dependent edema.
3. Prazosin hydrochloride (Minipress) should be taken when the stomach is empty.
4. Treatment with prazosin hydrochloride (Minipress) can cause dizziness, lightheadedness, or possible syncope.

Level of Cognitive Ability: Applying
Client Needs: Physiological Integrity
Integrated Process: Teaching and Learning
Content Area: Pharmacology: Cardiovascular Medications
Priority Concepts: Client Education; Safety

Answer: 4
Rationale: Prazosin is an alpha-adrenergic blocking agent. "First-dose hypotensive reaction" may occur during early therapy, which is characterized by dizziness, lightheadedness, and possible loss of consciousness. The occurrence of these effects is better tolerated if the client is in bed. This also can occur when the dosage is increased. This effect usually disappears with continued use or the dosage is decreased. Options 1, 2, and 3 are not characteristics of the medication.
Priority Nursing Tip: When prescribed, the first dose of prazosin hydrochloride (Minipress) should be given at bedtime. If the first dose needs to be given during the daytime, the client must remain supine for 3 to 4 hours.
Test-Taking Strategy: Focus on the subject, prazosin hydrochloride (Minipress). Note the name of the medication. This will assist in determining that the medication is an antihypertensive agent. Recalling that orthostatic hypotension occurs with the use of antihypertensives will direct you to the correct option. Review: **prazosin hydrochloride (Minipress)**.
Reference(s): Hodgson, Kizior (2014), pp. 973-974.

209. The nurse has applied the prescribed dressing to the leg of a client with an ischemic arterial leg ulcer. Which method should the nurse use to cover the dressing?

1. Apply a Kerlix roll and tape it to the skin.
2. Apply a large, soft pad and tape it to the skin.
3. Apply small Montgomery straps and tie the edges together.
4. Apply a Kling roll and tape the edge of the roll onto the bandage.

Level of Cognitive Ability: Applying
Client Needs: Physiological Integrity
Integrated Process: Nursing Process/Implementation
Content Area: Adult Health: Cardiovascular
Priority Concepts: Perfusion; Tissue Integrity

Answer: 4
Rationale: Standard dressing technique includes the use of Kling rolls on circumferential dressings. With an arterial leg ulcer, the nurse applies tape only to the bandage. Tape is never used directly on the skin because it could cause further tissue damage. For the same reason, Montgomery straps should not be applied to the skin (although these are generally intended for use on abdominal wounds, anyway).
Priority Nursing Tip: Because swelling in the extremities prevents arterial blood flow, the client with peripheral arterial disease is instructed to elevate the feet at rest but to avoid elevating them above the level of the heart because extreme elevation slows arterial blood flow to the feet.
Test-Taking Strategy: Focus on the subject, care of ischemic arterial leg ulcers. Note that options 1, 2, and 3 are comparable or alike. In options 1 and 2, tape is applied to the skin. For the same reason, eliminate option 3, because the Montgomery straps would need to be adhered to the skin as well. Review: care of the client with an arterial leg ulcer.
Reference(s): Bryant, Nix (2012), pp. 190-191; Ignatavicius, Workman (2013), p. 486; Perry, Potter, Ostendorf (2014), p. 448.

210. A child is admitted to the pediatric unit with a diagnosis of celiac disease. Based on this diagnosis, the nurse expects that the child's stools will have which characteristic?

1. Malodorous
2. Dark in color
3. Unusually hard
4. Abnormally small in amount

Level of Cognitive Ability: Analyzing
Client Needs: Physiological Integrity
Integrated Process: Nursing Process/Assessment
Content Area: Child Health: Gastrointestinal
Priority Concepts: Elimination; Nutrition

Answer: 1
Rationale: Celiac disease is a disorder in which the child has intolerance to gluten, the protein component of wheat, barley, rye, and oats. The stools of a child with celiac disease are characteristically malodorous, pale, large (bulky), and soft (loose). Excessive flatus is common, and bouts of diarrhea may occur.
Priority Nursing Tip: Teach the parents of a child with celiac disease to read all food labels for the presence of gluten; if the food contains gluten, it needs to be avoided.
Test-Taking Strategy: Focus on the subject, celiac disease. Thinking about the pathophysiology that occurs in celiac disease and the manifestations will direct you to the correct option. Review: celiac disease.
Reference(s): Hockenberry, Wilson (2013), pp. 1325-1327; Jarvis (2012), pp. 716-717.

211. A clinic nurse is caring for a client with a suspected diagnosis of gestational hypertension. The nurse assesses the client, expecting to note which set of findings if gestational hypertension is present?

1. Hypertension and proteinuria
2. Edema, ketonuria, and obesity
3. Edema, tachycardia, and ketonuria
4. Glycosuria, hypertension, and obesity

Level of Cognitive Ability: Analyzing
Client Needs: Physiological Integrity
Integrated Process: Nursing Process/Assessment
Content Area: Maternity: Antepartum
Priority Concepts: Perfusion; Reproduction

Answer: 1
Rationale: Gestational hypertension is the most common hypertensive disorder in pregnancy. It is characterized by the development of hypertension and proteinuria. Glycosuria and ketonuria occur in diabetes mellitus. Tachycardia and obesity are not specifically related to diagnosing gestational hypertension. Edema is not specific to gestational hypertension and can occur in many disorders.
Priority Nursing Tip: Gestational hypertension can be mild or severe and can lead to preeclampsia and then eclampsia (seizures).
Test-Taking Strategy: Focus on the subject, gestational hypertension. Eliminate options 2 and 3 because they do not address hypertension. From the remaining options, recalling that glycosuria is an indication of diabetes mellitus will assist in directing you to the correct option. Review: gestational hypertension.
Reference(s): McKinney et al (2013), pp. 590-593; Swearingen (2012), pp. 647-648.

212. A client who undergoes a gastric resection is at risk for developing dumping syndrome. Which manifestation should the nurse monitor the client for?
1. Dizziness
2. Bradycardia
3. Constipation
4. Extreme thirst

Level of Cognitive Ability: Applying
Client Needs: Physiological Integrity
Integrated Process: Nursing Process/Assessment
Content Area: Adult Health: Gastrointestinal
Priority Concepts: Clinical Judgment; Elimination

Answer: 1
Rationale: Dumping syndrome is the rapid emptying of the gastric contents into the small intestine that occurs after gastric resection. Early manifestations of dumping syndrome occur 5 to 30 minutes after eating. Manifestations also include vasomotor disturbances such as dizziness, tachycardia, syncope, sweating, pallor, palpitations, and the desire to lie down.
Priority Nursing Tip: The client with dumping syndrome should eat small meals and avoid consuming fluids with meals.
Test-Taking Strategy: Focus on the subject, dumping syndrome. Recalling that the symptoms of this disorder are vasomotor in nature will direct you to the correct option. Review: **dumping syndrome.**
Reference(s): Ignatavicius, Workman (2013), pp. 1236-1237.

❖ **213.** The nurse is monitoring a client in the telemetry unit who has recently been admitted with the diagnosis of chest pain and notes this heart rate pattern on the monitoring strip (**refer to figure**). What is the **initial** action to be taken by the nurse?

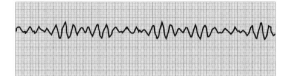

Figure from Ignatavicius D, Workman M: *Medical-surgical nursing: patient-centered collaborative care,* ed 7, Philadelphia, 2013, Saunders.

1. Notify the health care provider.
2. Initiate cardiopulmonary resuscitation (CPR).
3. Continue to monitor the client and the heart rate patterns.
4. Administer oxygen with a face mask at 8 to 10 L per minute.

Level of Cognitive Ability: Applying
Client Needs: Physiological Integrity
Integrated Process: Nursing Process/Implementation
Content Area: Critical Care: Emergency Situations
Priority Concepts: Gas Exchange; Perfusion

Answer: 2
Rationale: The monitor is showing ventricular fibrillation, a life-threatening dysrhythmia that requires cardiopulmonary resuscitation and defibrillation to maintain life. Although the health care provider must be notified, CPR is the initial action. Oxygen is necessary, but again the initiation of CPR is the priority because it will provide more than just oxygen to the client. Monitoring the client is necessary, but not as an initial action; emergency resuscitative treatment must be provided to the client immediately.
Priority Nursing Tip: There is no cardiac output with ventricular fibrillation, and it must be treated immediately to save the client's life.
Test-Taking Strategy: Knowledge regarding emergency care is essential. Note the strategic word, *initial*. Recalling that ventricular fibrillation is a life-threatening dysrhythmia that requires cardiopulmonary resuscitation and defibrillation to maintain life will direct you to the correct option. Review: **cardiopulmonary resuscitation** and **ventricular fibrillation.**
Reference(s): Ignatavicius, Workman (2013), pp. 729-730.

214. A clinic nurse is performing an assessment on a child. Which finding indicates the presence of an inguinal hernia?
1. Complaints of difficulty defecating
2. Complaints of a dribbling urinary stream
3. Absence of the testes within the scrotum
4. Painless inguinal swelling that appears when the child cries or strains

Level of Cognitive Ability: Analyzing
Client Needs: Physiological Integrity
Integrated Process: Nursing Process/Assessment
Content Area: Developmental Stages: Health Assessment/Physical Exam
Priority Concepts: Clinical Judgment; Elimination

Answer: 4
Rationale: Inguinal hernia is a common defect that appears as a painless inguinal swelling when the child cries or strains. Option 1 is a symptom indicating a partial obstruction of the herniated loop of intestine. Option 2 describes a sign of phimosis, a narrowing or stenosis of the preputial opening of the foreskin. Option 3 describes cryptorchidism.
Priority Nursing Tip: An inguinal hernia is characterized by painless inguinal swelling that is reducible. Swelling may disappear during periods of rest and is most noticeable when the infant cries or coughs.
Test-Taking Strategy: Focus on the subject, assessment of an inguinal hernia. Note the relationship between the child's diagnosis, inguinal hernia, and the words "inguinal swelling" in option 4. Review: the characteristics related to **inguinal hernia.**
Reference(s): Hockenberry, Wilson (2013), p. 912.

215. A client with heart failure was experiencing difficulty breathing and increased pulmonary congestion. The health care provider prescribed furosemide (Lasix) 40 mg to be given intravenously, and it was given an hour ago by the nurse. Which indicates the therapy has been **effective**?
1. The lungs are now clear to auscultation.
2. The urine output has increased by 400 mL.
3. The serum potassium has decreased from 4.7 mEq to 4.1 mEq.
4. The blood pressure has decreased from 118/64 mm Hg to 106/62 mm Hg.

Level of Cognitive Ability: Evaluating
Client Needs: Physiological Integrity
Integrated Process: Nursing Process/Evaluation
Content Area: Pharmacology: Cardiovascular Medications
Priority Concepts: Perfusion; Safety

Answer: 1
Rationale: Furosemide (Lasix) is a diuretic. In this situation, it was given to decrease preload and reduce the pulmonary congestion and associated difficulty in breathing. Although all options may occur, option 1 is the reason the furosemide was administered.
Priority Nursing Tip: When administering a medication, knowing its purpose will assist in evaluating its effectiveness.
Test-Taking Strategy: Focus on the subject, furosemide (Lasix) administration in a client with heart failure who was experiencing difficulty breathing and increased pulmonary congestion. Note the strategic word, *effective.* Specific knowledge of the use of furosemide in heart failure and its side effects is essential. Note the relationship between the words "pulmonary congestion" in the question and option 1. Review: **heart failure** and **furosemide (Lasix).**
Reference(s): Gahart, Nazareno (2012), p. 662; Ignatavicius, Workman (2013), p. 752.

216. Skin closure with heterograft will be performed on a client with a burn injury, and the client asks the nurse about the meaning of a heterograft. The nurse should tell the client that a heterograft is from which source?
1. A cadaver
2. Another species
3. The burned client
4. A synthetic source

Level of Cognitive Ability: Applying
Client Needs: Physiological Integrity
Integrated Process: Nursing Process/Implementation
Content Area: Adult Health: Integumentary
Priority Concepts: Client Education; Tissue Integrity

Answer: 2
Rationale: Biologic dressings are usually heterograft or homograft material. Heterograft is skin from another species. The most commonly used type of heterograft is pig skin because of its availability and its relative compatibility with human skin. Homograft is skin from another human, which is usually obtained from a cadaver and is provided through a skin bank. Autograft is skin from the client. Synthetic dressings are also available for covering burn wounds.
Priority Nursing Tip: Autografting provides permanent wound coverage.
Test-Taking Strategy: Focus on the subject, a heterograft. Also, note that options 1 and 3 are comparable or alike and relate to grafts from human skin. Next it is necessary to know that heterograft is skin from another species. Review: the various types of **skin closure grafts.**
Reference(s): Ignatavicius, Workman (2013), p. 532.

217. The nurse is caring for a client admitted to the hospital after sustaining a head injury. In which position should the nurse place the client to prevent increased intracranial pressure (ICP)?
1. In left Sims' position
2. In reverse Trendelenburg
3. With the head elevated on a pillow
4. With the head of the bed elevated at least 30 degrees

Level of Cognitive Ability: Applying
Client Needs: Physiological Integrity
Integrated Process: Nursing Process/Implementation
Content Area: Adult Health: Neurological
Priority Concepts: Clinical Judgment; Intracranial Regulation

Answer: 4
Rationale: The client with a head injury is positioned to avoid extreme flexion or extension of the neck and to maintain the head in the midline, neutral position. The head of the bed is elevated to at least 30 degrees or as recommended by the health care provider. The client is log rolled when turned to avoid extreme hip flexion. Therefore, options 1, 2, and 3 are incorrect.
Priority Nursing Tip: Altered level of consciousness is the most sensitive and earliest indication of increased intracranial pressure.
Test-Taking Strategy: Focus on the subject, head injury. Recall that the client with a head injury is at risk for increased ICP. Bearing this in mind and considering the principles of gravity will direct you to the correct option. Review: care of the client following a **head injury**.
Reference(s): Ignatavicius, Workman (2013), p. 1027.

218. A newborn infant is diagnosed with esophageal atresia. Which assessment finding should the nurse typically find in this client?
1. Slowed reflexes
2. Continuous drooling
3. Diaphragmatic breathing
4. Passage of large amounts of frothy stool

Level of Cognitive Ability: Analyzing
Client Needs: Physiological Integrity
Integrated Process: Nursing Process/Assessment
Content Area: Child Health: Gastrointestinal
Priority Concepts: Development; Elimination

Answer: 2
Rationale: In esophageal atresia, the esophagus terminates before it reaches the stomach, ending in a blind pouch. This condition prevents the passage of swallowed mucus and saliva into the stomach. After fluid has accumulated in the pouch, it flows from the mouth and the infant then drools continuously. Responsiveness of the infant to stimulus would depend on the overall condition of the infant and is not considered a classic sign of esophageal atresia. Diaphragmatic breathing is not associated with this disorder. The inability to swallow amniotic fluid in utero prevents the accumulation of normal meconium, and lack of stools results.
Priority Nursing Tip: Tracheoesophageal fistula should be suspected if the child exhibits the "3 Cs"—coughing, choking with feedings, and cyanosis.
Test-Taking Strategy: Focus on the subject, esophageal atresia. Review the anatomical location of the disorder to eliminate options 1 and 4 first. From the remaining options, recalling the pathophysiology associated with esophageal atresia and recalling that the word "atresia" indicates narrowing will direct you to the correct option. Review: **esophageal atresia**.
Reference(s): McKinney et al (2013), p. 1071.

219. The nurse is determining the need for suctioning in a client with an endotracheal (ET) tube attached to a mechanical ventilator. Which observation by the nurse indicates this need?
1. Clear breath sounds
2. Visible mucus bubbling in the ET tube
3. Apical pulse rate of 72 beats per minute
4. Low peak inspiratory pressure on the ventilator

Level of Cognitive Ability: Analyzing
Client Needs: Physiological Integrity
Integrated Process: Nursing Process/Assessment
Content Area: Adult Health: Respiratory
Priority Concepts: Clinical Judgment; Gas Exchange

Answer: 2
Rationale: Indications for suctioning include visible mucus bubbling in the ET tube, wet respirations, restlessness, rhonchi or crackles on auscultation of the lungs, increased pulse and respiratory rates, and increased peak inspiratory pressures on the ventilator and high pressure alarms on the ventilator. A low peak inspiratory pressure indicates a leak in the mechanical ventilation system.
Priority Nursing Tip: The nurse needs to hyperoxygenate the client before and after performing respiratory suctioning.
Test-Taking Strategy: Focus on the subject, the need for suctioning in a client with an endotracheal (ET) tube attached to a mechanical ventilator. Eliminate options 1 and 3 first because they are normal findings. From the remaining options, focus on the subject and note the word "mucus" in option 2. Review: **mechanical ventilation** and the indications for the need for **suctioning**.
Reference(s): Hammond, Zimmermann (2013), pp. 85-87; Potter et al (2013), pp. 860-861, 872.

220. A client is intubated and receiving mechanical ventilation. The health care provider has added 7 cm of positive end-expiratory pressure (PEEP) to the ventilator settings of the client. The nurse should assess for which expected but adverse effect of PEEP?

1. Decreased peak pressure on the ventilator
2. Increased rectal temperature from 98° F to 100° F
3. Decreased heart rate from 78 to 64 beats per minute
4. Systolic blood pressure decrease from 122 to 98 mm Hg

Level of Cognitive Ability: Analyzing
Client Needs: Physiological Integrity
Integrated Process: Nursing Process/Assessment
Content Area: Critical Care: Emergency Situations
Priority Concepts: Gas Exchange; Perfusion

Answer: 4
Rationale: PEEP improves oxygenation by enhancing gas exchange and preventing atelectasis. PEEP leads to increased intrathoracic pressure, which in turn leads to decreased cardiac output. This is manifested in the client by decreased systolic blood pressure and increased pulse (compensatory). Peak pressures on the ventilator should not be affected, although the pressure at the end of expiration remains positive at the level set for the PEEP. Fever indicates respiratory infection or infection from another source.
Priority Nursing Tip: The need for positive end-expiratory pressure (PEEP) indicates a severe gas exchange disturbance.
Test-Taking Strategy: Focus on the subject, expected but adverse effect of positive end-expiratory pressure (PEEP). Knowing that PEEP increases intrathoracic pressure leads you to look for the option that reflects a consequence of this event. Fever is irrelevant, and option 2 is eliminated first. From the remaining options, think about the effects of PEEP to direct you to the correct option. Review: the effects of positive end-expiratory pressure (PEEP).
Reference(s): Hammond, Zimmermann (2013), pp. 86, 197; Ignatavicius, Workman (2013), p. 677.

221. The nurse is assessing the respiratory status of the client after thoracentesis. The nurse would become **most** concerned with which assessment finding?

1. Equal bilateral chest expansion
2. Respiratory rate of 22 breaths per minute
3. Diminished breath sounds on the affected side
4. Few scattered wheezes, unchanged from baseline

Level of Cognitive Ability: Analyzing
Client Needs: Physiological Integrity
Integrated Process: Nursing Process/Analysis
Content Area: Adult Health: Respiratory
Priority Concepts: Clinical Judgment; Gas Exchange

Answer: 3
Rationale: After thoracentesis, the nurse assesses vital signs and breath sounds. The nurse especially notes increased respiratory rates, dyspnea, retractions, diminished breath sounds, or cyanosis, which could indicate pneumothorax. Any of these manifestations should be reported to the health care provider. Options 1 and 2 are normal findings. Option 4 indicates a finding that is unchanged from the baseline.
Priority Nursing Tip: For a thoracentesis, the client is positioned sitting upright, with the arms and shoulders supported by a bedside table. If the client cannot sit up, the client is placed lying in bed on the unaffected side, with the head of the bed elevated.
Test-Taking Strategy: Note the strategic word, *most*. Eliminate options 1 and 2 first because they are normal findings. Option 4 is an abnormality, but note that the wheezes are unchanged from the client's baseline. Option 3 is the abnormal finding. Review: the signs of complications after a **thoracentesis**.
Reference(s): Pagana, Pagana (2013), p. 890.

222. The nurse is preparing to administer a Mantoux tuberculin skin test to a client. The nurse determines that which area is **most appropriate** for injection of the medication?

1. Dorsal aspect of the upper arm near a mole
2. Inner aspect of the forearm that is close to a burn scar
3. Inner aspect of the forearm that is not heavily pigmented
4. Dorsal aspect of the upper arm that has a small amount of hair

Level of Cognitive Ability: Applying
Client Needs: Physiological Integrity
Integrated Process: Nursing Process/Implementation
Content Area: Fundamental Skills: Diagnostic Tests
Priority Concepts: Clinical Judgment; Safety

Answer: 3
Rationale: Intradermal injections are most commonly given in the inner surface of the forearm. Other sites include the dorsal area of the upper arm or the upper back beneath the scapulae. The nurse finds an area that is not heavily pigmented and is clear of hairy areas or lesions that could interfere with reading the results.
Priority Nursing Tip: After administering a skin test, document the date and time of administration and the test site. Interpret the reaction at the injection site 48 to 72 hours after administration of the test antigen.
Test-Taking Strategy: Focus on the subject, Mantoux tuberculin skin test. Note the strategic words, *most appropriate*. Note that options 1, 2, and 4 are comparable or alike in that they indicate areas that are not clear of lesions or hair. Review: **Mantoux tuberculin skin test**.
Reference(s): Chernecky, Berger (2013), p. 765; Potter et al (2013), pp. 608, 629-630.

❖ **223.** Which questions should the nurse ask when assessing a client for possibly manifestations of Ménière's disease? **Select all that apply.**
- ❏ 1. "Do you experience ringing in your ears?"
- ❏ 2. "Are you prone to vertigo that can last for days?"
- ❏ 3. "Can you hear better out of one ear than the other?"
- ❏ 4. "Is there a history of Ménière's disease in your family?"
- ❏ 5. "Have you ever experienced a head injury in the area of your ears?"

Level of Cognitive Ability: Analyzing
Client Needs: Physiological Integrity
Integrated Process: Nursing Process/Assessment
Content Area: Adult Health: Ear
Priority Concepts: Clinical Judgment; Sensory Perception

Answer: 1, 2, 3
Rationale: Ménière's disease is characterized by dilation of the endolymphatic system by overproduction or decreased reabsorption of endolymphatic fluid. Manifestations include tinnitus, vertigo that can last for days, and one-sided sensorineural hearing loss. Although the exact cause of the disease is unknown, there does not seem to be a connection with either genetics or head trauma.
Priority Nursing Tip: Ménière's disease has characteristic manifestations that include tinnitus, unilateral hearing impairment, and severe episodes of vertigo.
Test-Taking Strategy: Focus on the subject, Ménière's disease. Specific knowledge regarding the manifestations of Ménière's disease will direct you to the correct options 1, 2, and 3. Remember that tinnitus, hearing loss, and vertigo are characteristic of this disease. Review: the symptoms of Ménière's disease.
Reference(s): Ignatavicius, Workman (2013), p. 1096.

224. A hospitalized client is dyspneic and has been diagnosed with left tension pneumothorax by chest x-ray after insertion of a central venous catheter. Which finding observed by the nurse indicates that the pneumothorax is rapidly worsening?
1. Hypertension
2. Flat neck veins
3. Pain with respiration
4. Tracheal deviation to the right

Level of Cognitive Ability: Analyzing
Client Needs: Physiological Integrity
Integrated Process: Nursing Process/Assessment
Content Area: Critical Care: Emergency Situations
Priority Concepts: Gas Exchange; Perfusion

Answer: 4
Rationale: A tension pneumothorax is characterized by distended neck veins, displaced point of maximal impulse (PMI), tracheal deviation to the unaffected side, asymmetry of the thorax, decreased to absent breath sounds on the affected side, worsening cyanosis, and worsening dyspnea. The increased intrathoracic pressure causes the blood pressure to fall, not rise. The client could have pain with respiration.
Priority Nursing Tip: After insertion of a central venous catheter, catheter placement must be confirmed by radiography before infusing fluids into it.
Test-Taking Strategy: Focus on the subject, tension pneumothorax, and note the words "rapidly worsening." Pain and hypertension are the least specific indicators and are eliminated first. From the remaining options, remember that a tension pneumothorax causes the trachea to be pushed in the opposite direction, to the unaffected side. Review: the complications of tension pneumothorax.
Reference(s): Ignatavicius, Workman (2013), pp. 683-684.

225. A client is admitted to the hospital with a diagnosis of right lower lobe pneumonia. The nurse auscultates the right lower lobe, expecting to note which type of breath sounds?
1. Absent
2. Vesicular
3. Bronchial
4. Bronchovesicular

Level of Cognitive Ability: Analyzing
Client Needs: Physiological Integrity
Integrated Process: Nursing Process/Assessment
Content Area: Adult Health: Respiratory
Priority Concepts: Clinical Judgment; Gas Exchange

Answer: 3
Rationale: Bronchial sounds are normally heard over the trachea. The client with pneumonia will have bronchial breath sounds over area(s) of consolidation because the consolidated tissue carries bronchial sounds to the peripheral lung fields. The client may also have crackles in the affected area resulting from fluid in the interstitium and alveoli. Absent breath sounds are not likely to occur unless a serious complication of the pneumonia occurs. Vesicular sounds are normally heard over the lesser bronchi, bronchioles, and lobes. Bronchovesicular sounds are normally heard over the main bronchi.
Priority Nursing Tip: Pneumonia can be community acquired or hospital acquired. The sputum culture identifies organisms that may be present and assists in determining appropriate treatment.
Test-Taking Strategy: Focus on the subject, breath sounds in a client with lower lobe pneumonia. Recalling that vesicular breath sounds are normal in the lung periphery and bronchovesicular sounds are normally heard over the main bronchi helps eliminate options 2 and 4. From the remaining options, recall that the pneumonia transmits bronchial breath sounds, so they are heard over the area of consolidation. Review: assessment findings in pneumonia.
Reference(s): Ignatavicius, Workman (2013), p. 650.

226. The nurse assesses the client with acquired immunodeficiency syndrome (AIDS) for early signs of Kaposi's sarcoma. The nurse anticipates the lesions to have which appearance?
1. Unilateral, raised, and bluish-purple in color
2. Unilateral, red, raised, and resembling a blister
3. Bilateral, flat, and brownish and scaly in appearance
4. Bilateral, flat, and pink, turning to dark violet or black in color

Level of Cognitive Ability: Analyzing
Client Needs: Physiological Integrity
Integrated Process: Nursing Process/Assessment
Content Area: Adult Health: Immune
Priority Concepts: Clinical Judgment; Tissue Integrity

Answer: 4
Rationale: Kaposi's sarcoma generally starts with an area that is flat and pink that changes to a dark violet or black color. The lesions are usually present bilaterally. They may appear in many areas of the body and are treated with radiation, chemotherapy, and cryotherapy.
Priority Nursing Tip: Kaposi's sarcoma is characterized by skin lesions that occur in individuals with a compromised immune system.
Test-Taking Strategy: Focus on the subject, Kaposi's sarcoma. Recalling that Kaposi's sarcoma occurs in a bilateral pattern eliminates options 1 and 2. From the remaining options, recalling the character of the lesions will direct you to the correct option. Review: the characteristics of **Kaposi's sarcoma**.
Reference(s): Ignatavicius, Workman (2013), pp. 367, 1196.

227. A client is suspected of having a pleural effusion. The nurse should assess the client for which typical manifestations of this respiratory problem?
1. Dyspnea at rest and moist, productive cough
2. Dyspnea at rest and dry, nonproductive cough
3. Dyspnea on exertion and moist, productive cough
4. Dyspnea on exertion and dry, nonproductive cough

Level of Cognitive Ability: Analyzing
Client Needs: Physiological Integrity
Integrated Process: Nursing Process/Assessment
Content Area: Adult Health: Respiratory
Priority Concepts: Clinical Judgment; Gas Exchange

Answer: 4
Rationale: A pleural effusion is the collection of fluid in the pleural space. Typical assessment findings in the client with a pleural effusion include dyspnea, which usually occurs with exertion, and a dry, nonproductive cough. The cough is caused by bronchial irritation and possible mediastinal shift.
Priority Nursing Tip: Any condition that interferes with the secretion or drainage of pleural fluid will lead to pleural effusion.
Test-Taking Strategy: Focus on the subject, pleural effusion. Specific knowledge that pleural effusion is in the pleural space and not the airway helps eliminate options 1 and 3 (moist productive cough does not occur). Remembering that dyspnea occurs on exertion before it occurs at rest will direct you to the correct option from the remaining options. Review: the manifestations of **pleural effusion**.
Reference(s): Hammond, Zimmermann (2013), pp. 190-191.

228. A client with pleural effusion had a thoracentesis, and a sample of fluid was sent to the laboratory. Analysis of the fluid reveals a high red blood cell count. Which condition is this test result most consistent with?
1. Trauma
2. Infection
3. Liver failure
4. Heart failure

Level of Cognitive Ability: Analyzing
Client Needs: Physiological Integrity
Integrated Process: Nursing Process/Analysis
Content Area: Adult Health: Respiratory
Priority Concepts: Clinical Judgment; Gas Exchange

Answer: 1
Rationale: Pleural fluid from an effusion that has a high red blood cell count may result from trauma and may be treated with placement of a chest tube for drainage. Other causes of pleural effusion include infection, heart failure, liver or renal failure, malignancy, or inflammatory processes. Infection would be accompanied by white blood cells. The fluid portion of the serum would accumulate with liver failure and heart failure.
Priority Nursing Tip: With a pleural effusion, the client experiences pleuritic pain that is sharp and increases with inspiration.
Test-Taking Strategy: Focus on the subject, pleural effusion with a high red blood cell count. Recall that infection would be accompanied by white blood cells, not red, to eliminate option 2. Remember that in liver and heart failure, the fluid portion of the serum would accumulate to direct you to eliminate options 3 and 4. Review: the causes of **pleural effusion**.
Reference(s): Hammond, Zimmermann (2013), p. 191; Ignatavicius, Workman (2013), pp. 553, 638.

229. The nurse is scheduling a client for diagnostic studies of the gastrointestinal (GI) system. Which studies, if prescribed, should the nurse schedule last?
1. Ultrasound
2. Colonoscopy
3. Barium enema
4. Computed tomography

Level of Cognitive Ability: Applying
Client Needs: Physiological Integrity
Integrated Process: Nursing Process/Planning
Content Area: Leadership: Management: Prioritizing
Priority Concepts: Care Coordination; Elimination

Answer: 3
Rationale: When barium is instilled into the lower GI tract, it may take up to 72 hours to clear the GI tract. The presence of barium could cause interference with obtaining clear visualization and accurate results of the other tests listed if performed before the client has fully excreted the barium. For this reason, diagnostic studies that involve barium contrast are scheduled at the conclusion of other medical imaging studies.
Priority Nursing Tip: After a barium enema, the client is instructed to increase oral fluid intake to help pass the barium.
Test-Taking Strategy: Focus on the subject, diagnostic studies of the gastrointestinal (GI) system. Note the word "last." Recall that barium shows up on x-ray as opaque and that this substance would impair visualization during other tests. Review: **barium enema.**
Reference(s): Ignatavicius, Workman (2013), pp. 1186-1187.

230. The nurse is caring for a client who is scheduled to have a liver biopsy. Before the procedure, it is **most important** for the nurse to assess which parameter of the client?
1. Tolerance for pain
2. Allergy to iodine or shellfish
3. History of nausea and vomiting
4. Ability to lie still and hold the breath

Level of Cognitive Ability: Applying
Client Needs: Physiological Integrity
Integrated Process: Nursing Process/Assessment
Content Area: Fundamental Skills: Diagnostic Tests
Priority Concepts: Clinical Judgment; Safety

Answer: 4
Rationale: It is most important for the nurse to assess the client's ability to lie still and hold the breath for the procedure. This helps the health care provider avoid complications, such as puncturing the lung or other organs. The client's tolerance for pain is a useful item to know. However, the area will receive a local anesthetic. Assessment of allergy to iodine or shellfish is unnecessary for this procedure because no contrast dye is used. Knowledge of the history related to nausea and vomiting is generally a part of assessment of the gastrointestinal system but has no relationship to the procedure.
Priority Nursing Tip: Bleeding is a concern after a liver biopsy. Assess the results of coagulation tests (prothrombin time, partial thromboplastin time, platelet count) before a liver biopsy is performed and report abnormal results to the health care provider.
Test-Taking Strategy: Focus on the subject, a liver biopsy. Note the strategic words, *most important.* Visualizing this procedure and thinking about its complications will direct you to the correct option. Review: care to the client during a **liver biopsy.**
Reference(s): Pagana, Pagana (2013), pp. 602-603.

231. The nurse is caring for a client diagnosed with pneumonia. The nurse plans which as the **best** time to take the client for a short walk?
1. After the client eats lunch
2. After the client has a brief nap
3. After the client uses the metered-dose inhaler
4. After recording oxygen saturation on the bedside flow sheet

Level of Cognitive Ability: Applying
Client Needs: Physiological Integrity
Integrated Process: Nursing Process/Planning
Content Area: Adult Health: Respiratory
Priority Concepts: Gas Exchange; Mobility

Answer: 3
Rationale: The nurse should schedule activities for the client with pneumonia after the client has received respiratory treatments or medications. After the administration of bronchodilators (often administered by metered-dose inhaler), the client has the best oxygen exchange possible and would tolerate the activity best. Still, the nurse implements activity cautiously, so as not to increase the client's dyspnea. The client would become fatigued after eating; therefore, this is not a good time to ambulate the client. Although the client may be rested somewhat after a nap, from the options provided, this is not the best time to ambulate. Option 4 is unrelated to the client's ability to tolerate ambulation.
Priority Nursing Tip: Clients with a respiratory disorder should be positioned with the head of the bed elevated.
Test-Taking Strategy: Note the strategic word, *best.* Use the ABCs—airway, breathing, and circulation. The use of bronchodilator medication would widen the air passages, allowing for more air to enter the client's lungs. Review: care of the client with **pneumonia.**
Reference(s): Ignatavicius, Workman (2013), p. 652.

232. The nurse inserts an indwelling Foley catheter into the bladder of a postoperative client who has not voided for 8 hours and has a distended bladder. After the tubing is secured and the collection bag is hung on the bed frame, the nurse notices that 900 mL of urine has drained into the collection bag. What is the appropriate nursing action for the safety of this client?

1. Check the specific gravity of the urine.
2. Clamp the tubing for 30 minutes and then release.
3. Provide suprapubic pressure to maintain a steady flow of urine.
4. Raise the collection bag high enough to slow the rate of drainage.

Level of Cognitive Ability: Applying
Client Needs: Physiological Integrity
Integrated Process: Nursing Process/Implementation
Content Area: Adult Health: Renal and Urinary
Priority Concepts: Elimination; Safety

Answer: 2
Rationale: Rapid emptying of a large volume of urine may cause engorgement of pelvic blood vessels and hypovolemic shock, prolapse of the bladder, or bladder spasms. Clamping the tubing for 30 minutes allows for equilibration to prevent complications. Option 1 is an assessment and would not affect the flow of urine or prevent possible hypovolemic shock. Option 3 would increase the flow of urine, which could lead to hypovolemic shock. Option 4 could cause backflow of urine. Infection is likely to develop if urine is allowed to flow back into the bladder.
Priority Nursing Tip: The total bladder capacity is approximately 1 L and normal adult urine output is 1500 mL/day.
Test-Taking Strategy: Focus on the subject, slowing the urine drainage in a postoperative client with an indwelling Foley catheter. Note the amount "900 mL." Recall the physiology of the hemodynamic changes after the rapid collapse of an overdistended bladder. Eliminate options 3 and 4; these actions will increase flow rate. Note that option 1 is an assessment action rather than an action that affects the amount of urine drainage. Review: **distended bladder.**
Reference(s): Potter et al (2013), pp. 1062, 1083-1084.

233. The nurse has a prescription to administer amphotericin B intravenously to the client with histoplasmosis. Which action should the nurse plan to do during administration of the medication?

1. Monitor for hypothermia.
2. Monitor for an excessive urine output.
3. Administer a concurrent fluid challenge.
4. Assess the intravenous (IV) infusion site.

Level of Cognitive Ability: Applying
Client Needs: Physiological Integrity
Integrated Process: Nursing Process/Planning
Content Area: Pharmacology: Immune Medications
Priority Concepts: Clinical Judgment; Safety

Answer: 4
Rationale: Amphotericin B is an antifungal medication and is a toxic medication, which can produce symptoms during administration such as chills, fever (hyperthermia), headache, vomiting, and impaired renal function (decreased urine output). The medication is also very irritating to the IV site, commonly causing thrombophlebitis. The nurse administering this medication monitors for these complications. Administering a concurrent fluid challenge is not necessary.
Priority Nursing Tip: If a medication is nephrotoxic, assess kidney function before, during, and after administration. The health care provider may prescribe blood urea nitrogen (BUN) and creatinine studies. Urine output is also monitored closely.
Test-Taking Strategy: Focus on the subject, amphotericin B administration. Recall the toxic effects of this medication. Knowing that fever and chills can occur eliminates option 1. Recalling that the medication can be toxic to the kidneys eliminates option 2. From the remaining options, knowing that there is no rationale for giving concurrent fluids will direct you to the correct option. Review: **amphotericin B.**
Reference(s): Gahart, Nazareno (2012), pp. 108, 111; Hodgson, Kizior (2014), pp. 59-60.

234. A client who experiences repeated pleural effusions from inoperable lung cancer is to undergo pleurodesis. What should the nurse plan to assist with after the health care provider injects the sclerosing agent through the chest tube?
1. Ambulate the client.
2. Clamp the chest tube.
3. Ask the client to cough and deep breathe.
4. Ask the client to remain in one position only.

Level of Cognitive Ability: Applying
Client Needs: Physiological Integrity
Integrated Process: Nursing Process/Planning
Content Area: Adult Health: Respiratory
Priority Concepts: Collaboration; Gas Exchange

Answer: 2
Rationale: After injection of the sclerosing agent, the chest tube is clamped to prevent the agent from draining back out of the pleural space. Depending on health care provider preference, a repositioning schedule is used to disperse the substance. Ambulation, coughing, and deep breathing have no specific purpose in the immediate period after injection.
Priority Nursing Tip: The agent injected during pleurodesis creates an inflammatory response that scleroses pleural tissue together.
Test-Taking Strategy: Focus on the subject, pleurodesis. This will assist in eliminating option 1. Eliminate option 4 because of the closed-ended word "only." From the remaining options, recall the purpose of the procedure. It is most reasonable to clamp the chest tube so that the sclerosing agent cannot flow back out of the tube. Coughing and deep breathing have no specific purpose in this situation. Review: the procedure for **pleurodesis**.
Reference(s): Ignatavicius, Workman (2013), pp. 553, 638.

235. A client with a posterior wall bladder injury has had surgical repair and placement of a suprapubic catheter. What should the nurse plan to do to prevent complications with the use of this catheter?
1. Monitor urine output every shift.
2. Measure specific gravity once a shift.
3. Encourage a high intake of oral fluids.
4. Prevent kinking of the catheter tubing.

Level of Cognitive Ability: Applying
Client Needs: Physiological Integrity
Integrated Process: Nursing Process/Planning
Content Area: Adult Health: Renal and Urinary
Priority Concepts: Clinical Judgment; Elimination

Answer: 4
Rationale: A complication after surgical repair of the bladder is disruption of sutures caused by tension on them from urine buildup. The nurse prevents this from happening by ensuring that the catheter is able to drain freely. This involves basic catheter care, including keeping the tubing free from kinks, keeping the tubing below the level of the bladder, and monitoring the flow of urine frequently. Monitoring urine output every shift is insufficient to detect decreased flow from catheter kinking. Measurement of urine specific gravity and a high oral fluid intake do not prevent complications of bladder surgery.
Priority Nursing Tip: A blunt or penetrating injury to the lower abdomen can cause bladder trauma. Monitor the client for hematuria and pain below the level of the umbilicus, which can radiate to the shoulders.
Test-Taking Strategy: Focus on the subject, suprapubic catheter. Eliminate option 1 first, because once-a-shift measurement is not a preventive action and is also insufficient in frequency. Eliminate option 2 next because specific gravity measurement is not a preventive action. From the remaining options, knowing that a high oral fluid intake will not prevent complications with the catheter directs you to the correct option. Review: care of the client with a **suprapubic catheter**.
Reference(s): Potter et al (2013), p. 1063.

242. The nurse is assisting a client with a chest tube to get out of bed, and the chest tubing accidentally gets caught in the bed rail and disconnects. While trying to reestablish the connection, the Pleur-Evac drainage system falls over and cracks. The nurse should take which **immediate** action?

1. Clamp the chest tube.
2. Call the health care provider.
3. Apply a petroleum gauze over the end of the chest tube.
4. Immerse the chest tube in a bottle of sterile water or normal saline.

Level of Cognitive Ability: Applying
Client Needs: Physiological Integrity
Integrated Process: Nursing Process/Implementation
Content Area: Critical Care: Emergency Situations
Priority Concepts: Clinical Judgment; Gas Exchange

Answer: 4
Rationale: If a chest tube accidentally disconnects from the tubing of the drainage apparatus, the nurse should first reestablish an underwater seal to prevent tension pneumothorax and mediastinal shift. This can be accomplished by reconnecting the chest tube, or in this case, immersing the end of the chest tube 1 to 2 inches below the surface of a 250-mL bottle of sterile water or normal saline until a new chest tube can be set up. The health care provider should be notified after taking corrective action. If the health care provider is called first, tension pneumothorax has time to develop. Clamping the chest tube could also cause tension pneumothorax. A petroleum gauze would be applied to the skin over the chest tube insertion site if the entire chest tube was accidentally removed from the chest.
Priority Nursing Tip: If a closed chest tube drainage system cracks or breaks, insert the chest tube into a bottle of sterile water, remove the cracked or broken system, and replace it with a new system.
Test-Taking Strategy: Note the strategic word, *immediate*. Option 1 would create a tension pneumothorax because this action does not reestablish an underwater seal. Eliminate option 2 because it is too time consuming to be the immediate action. From the remaining options, noting that an underwater seal must be established will direct you to the correct option. Review: care of the client with a **chest tube**.
Reference(s): Ignatavicius, Workman (2013), p. 637; Perry, Potter, Ostendorf (2014), p. 665.

243. The nurse is caring for a client with a diagnosis of Cushing's syndrome. The nurse should plan which of these measures to prevent complications from this medical condition?

1. Monitoring glucose levels
2. Encouraging daily jogging
3. Monitoring epinephrine levels
4. Encouraging visits from friends

Level of Cognitive Ability: Analyzing
Client Needs: Physiological Integrity
Integrated Process: Nursing Process/Planning
Content Area: Adult Health: Endocrine
Priority Concepts: Clinical Judgment; Glucose Regulation

Answer: 1
Rationale: Cushing's syndrome is a metabolic disorder resulting from the chronic and excessive production of cortisol by the adrenal cortex or the administration of glucocorticoids in large doses for several weeks or longer. In the client with Cushing's syndrome, increased levels of glucocorticoids can result in hyperglycemia and signs and symptoms of diabetes mellitus. Clients experience activity intolerance related to muscle weakness and fatigue; therefore, option 2 is incorrect. Epinephrine levels are not affected. Visitors should be limited because of the client's impaired immune response.
Priority Nursing Tip: Hyperglycemia, hypernatremia, hypokalemia, and hypocalcemia occur in Cushing's syndrome. The opposite effects occur in Addison's disease.
Test-Taking Strategy: Focus on the subject, complications of Cushing's syndrome. Recalling that increased levels of glucocorticoids can result in hyperglycemia will direct you to the correct option. Review: the clinical manifestations associated with **Cushing's syndrome**.
Reference(s): Hammond, Zimmermann (2013), pp. 310-311; Ignatavicius, Workman (2013), pp. 1385-1386.

244. A client with a central venous catheter who is receiving total parenteral nutrition (TPN) suddenly becomes short of breath; complains of chest pain; and is tachycardic, pale, and anxious. The nurse, suspecting an air embolism, clamps the catheter and places the client in Trendelenburg position on the left side and then takes which step **next**?

1. Monitors vital signs
2. Checks the lines for air
3. Notifies the health care provider
4. Boluses the client with 500 mL normal saline

Level of Cognitive Ability: Applying
Client Needs: Physiological Integrity
Integrated Process: Nursing Process/Implementation
Content Area: Critical Care: Emergency Situations
Priority Concepts: Gas Exchange; Perfusion

Answer: 3
Rationale: If the client experiences air embolus, the client is placed in the lateral Trendelenburg position on the left side to trap the air in the right atrium. The nurse should also clamp the catheter and notify the health care provider. Vital signs are monitored continuously. A fluid bolus would cause the air embolus to travel.
Priority Nursing Tip: Air embolism can be caused by an inadequately primed intravenous (IV) line or a loose connection. Air embolism may occur during tubing change or during removal of the IV.
Test-Taking Strategy: Focus on the subject, suspected air embolism. Note the strategic word, *next*. Recall that air embolism is a life-threatening condition and that the health care provider needs to be notified. This will direct you to the correct option. Review: the interventions for an **air embolism**.
Reference(s): Ignatavicius, Workman (2013), p. 231; Perry, Potter, Ostendorf (2014), p. 798.

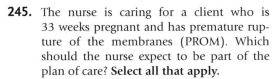

245. The nurse is caring for a client who is 33 weeks pregnant and has premature rupture of the membranes (PROM). Which should the nurse expect to be part of the plan of care? **Select all that apply.**
- [ ] 1. Perform frequent biophysical profiles.
- [ ] 2. Monitor for elevated serum creatinine.
- [ ] 3. Monitor for manifestations of infection.
- [ ] 4. Teach the client how to count fetal movements.
- [ ] 5. Use strict sterile technique for vaginal examinations.
- [ ] 6. Inform the client about the need for tocolytic therapy.

Level of Cognitive Ability: Analyzing
Client Needs: Physiological Integrity
Integrated Process: Nursing Process/Planning
Content Area: Maternity: Antepartum
Priority Concepts: Caregiving; Reproduction

Answer: 1, 3, 4, 5
Rationale: PROM is membrane rupture before 37 weeks of gestation. Frequent biophysical profiles are performed to determine fetal health status and estimate amniotic fluid volume. Monitoring for signs of infection is a major part of the nursing care. The woman should also be taught how to count fetal movements daily, because slowing of fetal movement has been shown to be a precursor to severe fetal compromise. Whenever PROM is suspected, strict sterile technique should be used in any vaginal examination to prevent infection. Elevated serum creatinine does not occur in PROM but may be noted in severe preeclampsia. Tocolytic therapy is used for women in preterm labor (not for PROM).
Priority Nursing Tip: An assessment finding in premature rupture of the membranes (PROM) is the evidence of fluid pooling in the vaginal vault. The fluid tests positive with the Nitrazine test.
Test-Taking Strategy: Focus on the subject, premature rupture of the membranes (PROM). Think about the pathophysiology of this condition. Select options 3 and 5 because they relate to preventing infection. Next select options 1 and 4 because they relate to determining fetal health status. Recalling the causes of an elevated serum creatinine and the purpose of tocolytic therapy will assist in eliminating these options. Review: the care plan for a client with **premature rupture of the membranes (PROM)**.
Reference(s): Lowdermilk, Perry, Cashion, Alden (2012), p. 791; McKinney et al (2013), pp. 645-646.

246. The nurse is monitoring the laboratory results for the client who has been diagnosed with carbon monoxide poisoning and is asking for the oxygen mask to be removed. The nurse determines that the oxygen may be safely removed once the carboxyhemoglobin level decreases to less than which level?

1. 5%
2. 10%
3. 15%
4. 25%

Level of Cognitive Ability: Understanding
Client Needs: Physiological Integrity
Integrated Process: Nursing Process/Planning
Content Area: Adult Health: Respiratory
Priority Concepts: Clinical Judgment; Gas Exchange

Answer: 1
Rationale: Oxygen may be removed safely from the client with carbon monoxide poisoning once carboxyhemoglobin levels are less than 5%. Options 2, 3, and 4 are elevated levels.
Priority Nursing Tip: Carbon monoxide is a colorless, odorless, and tasteless gas.
Test-Taking Strategy: Focus on the subject, safely removing the oxygen in CO poisoning. If you are unsure, it would be best to select the lowest level as identified in the correct option. Review: the normal **carboxyhemoglobin levels** and **carbon monoxide poisoning.**
Reference(s): Hammond, Zimmermann (2013), p. 196; Ignatavicius, Workman (2013), p. 524.

247. The nurse is teaching a pregnant client about nutrition. The nurse should include which information in the client's teaching plan?

1. All mothers are at high risk for nutritional deficiencies.
2. Calcium intake is not necessary until the third trimester.
3. Iron supplements are not necessary unless the mother has iron deficiency anemia.
4. The nutritional status of the mother significantly influences fetal growth and development.

Level of Cognitive Ability: Applying
Client Needs: Physiological Integrity
Integrated Process: Nursing Process/Implementation
Content Area: Fundamental Skills: Nutrition
Priority Concepts: Client Education; Nutrition

Answer: 4
Rationale: Poor nutrition during pregnancy can negatively influence fetal growth and development. Although pregnancy poses some nutritional risk for the mother, not all clients are at high risk. Calcium intake is critical during the third trimester but must be increased from the onset of pregnancy. Intake of dietary iron is insufficient for the majority of pregnant women, and iron supplements are routinely prescribed.
Priority Nursing Tip: An increase of about 300 calories/day is needed during the last 6 months of pregnancy.
Test-Taking Strategy: Focus on the subject, nutrition during pregnancy. Option 1 uses the closed-ended word "all"; therefore, eliminate this option. Options 2 and 3 offer specific time frames or conditions for interventions; therefore, eliminate these options. Option 4 is also a general statement that is true for any stage of pregnancy. Review: the importance of **nutrition during pregnancy.**
Reference(s): Lowdermilk, Perry, Cashion, Alden (2012), pp. 312, 321-323; McKinney et al (2013), pp. 296-297.

❖ **248.** A client is admitted to the hospital with a diagnosis of acute bacterial pericarditis, and the nurse prepares to perform an assessment on the client. Which findings are associated with this inflammatory heart disease? **Select all that apply.**
  ❑ 1. Fever
  ❑ 2. Leukopenia
  ❑ 3. Bradycardia
  ❑ 4. Pericardial friction rub
  ❑ 5. Decreased erythrocyte sedimentation rate
  ❑ 6. Severe precordial chest pain that intensifies when in the supine position

Level of Cognitive Ability: Analyzing
Client Needs: Physiological Integrity
Integrated Process: Nursing Process/Assessment
Content Area: Adult Health: Cardiovascular
Priority Concepts: Infection; Inflammation

Answer: 1, 4, 6
Rationale: In acute bacterial pericarditis, the membranes surrounding the heart become inflamed and rub against each other, producing the classic pericardial friction rub. Fever typically occurs and is accompanied by leukocytosis and an elevated erythrocyte sedimentation rate. The client complains of severe precordial chest pain that intensifies when lying supine and decreases in a sitting position. The pain also intensifies when the client breathes deeply. Malaise, myalgia, and tachycardia are common.
Priority Nursing Tip: Monitor the client with pericarditis for signs of heart failure or cardiac tamponade as complications.
Test-Taking Strategy: Focus on the subject, bacterial pericarditis. The diagnosis will assist in determining that the client has a fever (option 1); the compensatory response to fever is an increased metabolic rate and tachycardia. Also remember that when the client has an inflammatory disease, the erythrocyte sedimentation rate will increase, as will the white blood cell count (leukocytosis, not leukopenia). Lastly, focusing on the diagnosis will assist in determining that a pericardial friction rub and severe precordial chest pain are present (options 4 and 6). Review: **acute bacterial pericarditis.**
Reference(s): Dolan, Holt (2013), pp. 401-402; Ignatavicius, Workman (2013), p. 765.

249. A client is admitted to the hospital with a diagnosis of Cushing's syndrome. The nurse monitors the client for which problem that is likely to occur with this diagnosis?
  1. Hypovolemia
  2. Hypoglycemia
  3. Mood disturbances
  4. Deficient fluid volume

Level of Cognitive Ability: Applying
Client Needs: Physiological Integrity
Integrated Process: Nursing Process/Assessment
Content Area: Adult Health: Endocrine
Priority Concepts: Clinical Judgment; Mood and Affect

Answer: 3
Rationale: Cushing's syndrome is a metabolic disorder resulting from the chronic and excessive production of cortisol. When Cushing's syndrome develops, the normal function of the glucocorticoids becomes exaggerated and the classic picture of the syndrome emerges. This exaggerated physiological action can cause mood disturbances, including memory loss, poor concentration and cognition, euphoria, and depression. It can also cause persistent hyperglycemia along with sodium and water retention (hypernatremia), producing edema (hypervolemia; fluid volume excess) and hypertension.
Priority Nursing Tip: Cushing's disease is characterized by the hypersecretion of glucocorticoids, whereas Addison's disease is characterized by a hyposecretion of adrenal cortex hormones (glucocorticoids and mineralocorticoids).
Test-Taking Strategy: Focus on the subject, Cushing's syndrome. Eliminate options 1 and 4 first because they are comparable or alike. Recalling that hyperglycemia rather than hypoglycemia occurs in this condition will direct you to the correct option. Review: the manifestations of **Cushing's syndrome.**
Reference(s): Ignatavicius, Workman (2013), p. 1386.

250. A health care provider is performing indirect visualization of the larynx on a client to assess the function of the vocal cords. Which action should the nurse instruct the client to do during the procedure?

1. Try to swallow.
2. Hold the breath.
3. Breathe normally.
4. Roll the tongue to the back of the mouth.

Level of Cognitive Ability: Applying
Client Needs: Physiological Integrity
Integrated Process: Nursing Process/Implementation
Content Area: Adult Health: Respiratory
Priority Concepts: Clinical Judgment; Gas Exchange

Answer: 3

Rationale: Indirect laryngoscopy is done to assess the function of the vocal cords or obtain tissue for biopsy. Observations are made during rest and phonation by using a laryngeal mirror, head mirror, and light source. The client is placed in an upright position to facilitate passage of the laryngeal mirror into the mouth and is instructed to breathe normally. Swallowing cannot be done with the mirror in place. The procedure takes longer than the time the client would be able to hold the breath, and this action is ineffective, anyway. The tongue cannot be moved back because it would occlude the airway.

Priority Nursing Tip: After laryngoscopy, maintain an NPO status until the gag reflex returns.

Test-Taking Strategy: Focus on the subject, indirect laryngoscopy. Option 4 is eliminated first because it is not possible to move the tongue back with the mirror in place. It would also cause the airway to become occluded. Given the length of time needed to do the procedure, the client could not realistically hold the breath, so option 2 is eliminated next. Trying to swallow would actually cause the larynx to move against the mirror and could cause gagging; therefore, eliminate option 1. Review: care of the client during **indirect laryngoscopy.**

Reference(s): Ignatavicius, Workman (2013), p. 590; Pagana, Pagana (2013), pp. 193-194.

251. The nurse is caring for a client scheduled for a bilateral adrenalectomy for treatment of an adrenal tumor that is producing excessive aldosterone (primary hyperaldosteronism). What should the nurse tell the client about the surgery?

1. "You will need to wear an abdominal binder after surgery."
2. "You will **most** likely need to undergo chemotherapy after surgery."
3. "You will not require any special long-term treatment after surgery."
4. "You will need to take hormone replacements for the rest of your life."

Level of Cognitive Ability: Applying
Client Needs: Physiological Integrity
Integrated Process: Nursing Process/Implementation
Content Area: Adult Health: Endocrine
Priority Concepts: Client Education; Cellular Regulation

Answer: 4

Rationale: The major cause of primary hyperaldosteronism is an aldosterone-secreting tumor called an aldosteronoma. Surgery is the treatment of choice. Clients undergoing a bilateral adrenalectomy require permanent replacement of adrenal hormones. Options 1, 2, and 3 are inaccurate.

Priority Nursing Tip: Following adrenalectomy, monitor for signs of acute adrenal insufficiency, which is also known as Addisonian crisis.

Test-Taking Strategy: Focus on the subject, bilateral adrenalectomy. Recalling the function of the adrenal glands and that glucocorticoids and mineralocorticoids are essential to sustain life will direct you to the correct option. Review: care after **bilateral adrenalectomy.**

Reference(s): Ignatavicius, Workman (2013), pp. 1387-1388.

252. The nurse is caring for a client who is scheduled for an adrenalectomy. The nurse plans to administer which medication in the preoperative period to prevent Addisonian crisis?
1. Prednisone orally
2. Fludrocortisone (Florinef) orally
3. Spironolactone (Aldactone) intramuscularly
4. Methylprednisolone sodium succinate (Solu-Medrol) intravenously

Level of Cognitive Ability: Analyzing
Client Needs: Physiological Integrity
Integrated Process: Nursing Process/Planning
Content Area: Adult Health: Endocrine
Priority Concepts: Clinical Judgment; Fluid and Electrolyte Balance

Answer: 4
Rationale: A glucocorticoid preparation will be administered intravenously or intramuscularly in the immediate preoperative period to a client scheduled for an adrenalectomy. Methylprednisolone sodium succinate protects the client from developing acute adrenal insufficiency (Addisonian crisis) that can occur as a result of the adrenalectomy. Prednisone is an oral corticosteroid. Fludrocortisone is a mineralocorticoid. Aldactone is a potassium-sparing diuretic.
Priority Nursing Tip: Emergency care of the client with Addisonian crisis includes hormone replacement and hyperkalemia and hypoglycemia management.
Test-Taking Strategy: Focus on the subject, preventing Addisonian crisis in a client scheduled for adrenalectomy. Recalling the function of the adrenals will assist in eliminating options 2 and 3. From the remaining options, select option 4 because the client is preoperative and should receive medications via routes other than orally. Review: preoperative care for the client scheduled for **adrenalectomy**.
Reference(s): Ignatavicius, Workman (2013), p. 1387; Lehne (2013), p. 916.

253. The nurse is preparing a client with Graves' disease to receive radioactive iodine therapy. What should the nurse tell the client about the therapy?
1. After the initial dose, subsequent treatments must continue lifelong.
2. The radioactive iodine is designed to destroy the entire thyroid gland with just one dose.
3. It takes 6 to 8 weeks after treatment to experience relief from the symptoms of the disease.
4. The high levels of radioactivity prohibit contact with family for 4 weeks after initial treatment.

Level of Cognitive Ability: Applying
Client Needs: Physiological Integrity
Integrated Process: Nursing Process/Implementation
Content Area: Adult Health: Endocrine
Priority Concepts: Cellular Regulation; Client Education

Answer: 3
Rationale: Graves' disease is also known as toxic diffuse goiter and is characterized by a hyperthyroid state resulting from hypersecretion of thyroid hormones. After treatment with radioactive iodine therapy, a decrease in the thyroid hormone level should be noted, which helps alleviate symptoms. Relief of symptoms does not occur until 6 to 8 weeks after initial treatment. Occasionally, a client may require a second or third dose, but treatments are not lifelong. This form of therapy is not designed to destroy the entire gland; rather, some of the cells that synthesize thyroid hormone will be destroyed by the local radiation. The nurse must reassure the client and family that unless the dosage is extremely high, clients are not required to observe radiation precautions. The rationale for this is that the radioactivity quickly dissipates.
Priority Nursing Tip: The consumption or administration of any substance that contains a stimulant needs to be avoided in the client with hyperthyroidism.
Test-Taking Strategy: Focus on the subject, Graves' disease. Recall knowledge regarding this treatment. Note the closed-ended words "must," "entire," and "prohibit" in the incorrect options. Review: treatment with radioactive iodine therapy for **Graves' disease**.
Reference(s): Ignatavicius, Workman (2013), pp. 1397-1398.

254. A client arrives at the emergency department with upper gastrointestinal (GI) bleeding and is in moderate distress. What is the **priority** action?
1. Obtain vital signs.
2. Ask the client about the precipitating events.
3. Complete an abdominal physical assessment.
4. Insert a nasogastric (NG) tube and test the emesis for the presence of blood.

Level of Cognitive Ability: Applying
Client Needs: Physiological Integrity
Integrated Process: Nursing Process/Implementation
Content Area: Critical Care: Emergency Situations
Priority Concepts: Clotting; Perfusion

Answer: 1
Rationale: The priority action for the client with GI bleeding is to obtain vital signs to determine whether the client is in shock from blood loss and obtain a baseline by which to monitor the progress of treatment. The client may not be able to provide subjective data until the immediate physical needs are met. A complete abdominal physical assessment must be performed but is not the priority. Insertion of an NG tube may be prescribed but is not the priority action.
Priority Nursing Tip: For the client experiencing active gastrointestinal bleeding, assess for signs of dehydration and hypovolemic shock.
Test-Taking Strategy: Note the strategic word, priority. Recall that the client with a GI bleed is at risk for shock. Also, the correct option addresses the ABCs—airway, breathing, and circulation. Review: care of the client with an **upper gastrointestinal (GI) bleeding**.
Reference(s): Hammond, Zimmermann (2013), p. 295; Ignatavicius, Workman (2013), p. 1228.

255. A client with acute kidney injury is prescribed to be on a fluid restriction of 1500 mL per day. Which step is **best** for the nurse to take in assisting the client in maintaining this restriction?
1. Removing the water pitcher from the bedside
2. Using mouthwash with alcohol for mouth care
3. Prohibiting beverages with sugar to minimize thirst
4. Asking the client to calculate the IV fluids into the total daily allotment

Level of Cognitive Ability: Applying
Client Needs: Physiological Integrity
Integrated Process: Nursing Process/Implementation
Content Area: Fundamental Skills: Fluids and Electrolytes
Priority Concepts: Clinical Judgment; Fluid and Electrolyte Balance

Answer: 1
Rationale: The nurse can help the client maintain fluid restriction through a variety of means. The water pitcher should be removed from the bedside to aid in compliance. Frequent mouth care is important; however, alcohol-based products should be avoided because they are drying to mucous membranes. Beverages that the client enjoys are provided and are not restricted based on sugar content. The client is not asked to keep track of IV fluid intake; this is the nurse's responsibility. The use of ice chips and lip ointments is another intervention that may be helpful to the client on fluid restriction.
Priority Nursing Tip: As long as the beverage is not contraindicated, allow the client on fluid restriction to select preferred beverages.
Test-Taking Strategy: Focus on the subject, a client with acute kidney injury who is on fluid restriction. Eliminate option 4 because this is a nursing responsibility. Eliminate option 2 next, because alcohol-based products are drying to oral mucous membranes and could exacerbate thirst. From the remaining options, focus on the strategic word, *best*, to direct you to the correct option. Review: measures to promote compliance with **fluid restrictions.**
Reference(s): Ignatavicius, Workman (2013), p. 1553; Perry, Potter, Ostendorf (2014), p. 765.

256. The nurse has administered approximately half of a high cleansing enema when the client complains of pain and cramping. Which nursing action is appropriate?
1. Reassuring the client and continuing the flow
2. Discontinuing the enema and notifying the health care provider
3. Raising the enema bag so the solution can be completed quickly
4. Clamping the tubing for 30 seconds and restarting the flow at a slower rate

Level of Cognitive Ability: Applying
Client Needs: Physiological Integrity
Integrated Process: Nursing Process/Implementation
Content Area: Fundamental Skills: Elimination
Priority Concepts: Clinical Judgment; Elimination

Answer: 4
Rationale: The enema fluid should be administered slowly. If the client complains of pain or cramping, the flow is stopped for 30 seconds and restarted at a slower rate. Slow enema administration and stopping the flow temporarily, if necessary, will decrease the likelihood of intestinal spasm and premature ejection of the solution. The higher the solution container is held above the rectum, the faster the flow and the greater the force in the rectum. There is no need to discontinue the enema and notify the health care provider at this time.
Priority Nursing Tip: During enema administration, ask the client to breathe slowly in through the nose and out through the mouth. This will assist the client in tolerating the instillation of the solution.
Test-Taking Strategy: Focus on the subject, alleviating pain and cramping with enema instillation. Eliminate options 1 and 3 first because they are comparable or alike. From the remaining options, noting that there is no need to notify the health care provider will direct you to the correct option. Review: the procedure for **enema administration.**
Reference(s): Perry, Potter, Ostendorf (2014), p. 856; Potter et al (2013), p. 1115.

257. The client with chronic kidney disease who is scheduled for hemodialysis this morning is due to receive a daily dose of enalapril (Vasotec). When should the nurse plan to administer this medication?
1. During dialysis
2. Just before dialysis
3. The day after dialysis
4. Upon return from dialysis

Level of Cognitive Ability: Applying
Client Needs: Physiological Integrity
Integrated Process: Nursing Process/Planning
Content Area: Pharmacology: Cardiovascular Medications
Priority Concepts: Clinical Judgment; Fluid and Electrolyte Balance

Answer: 4
Rationale: Antihypertensive medications, such as enalapril (Vasotec), are administered to the client after hemodialysis. This prevents the client from becoming hypotensive during dialysis and also from having the medication removed from the bloodstream by dialysis. There is no rationale for waiting a full day to resume the medication. This would lead to ineffective control of the blood pressure.
Priority Nursing Tip: In addition to antihypertensive medications, water-soluble vitamins, certain antibiotics, and digoxin (Lanoxin) are withheld before a hemodialysis treatment because they can be removed by dialysis.
Test-Taking Strategy: Focus on the subject, medication administration with hemodialysis. Think about the effects of an antihypertensive medication on the blood pressure when fluid is being removed from the body. Because hypotension is much more likely to occur in this circumstance, eliminate options 1 and 2. Most clients are hemodialyzed three times a week, so if the medication were held for dialysis until the following day, the client would miss three of the seven doses that would usually be given in a week. This would lead to ineffective blood pressure control; therefore, eliminate option 3. Review: the procedure for preparing a client for **dialysis.**
Reference(s): Ignatavicius, Workman (2013), p. 1562.

258. The nurse is assessing a client's cigarette smoking habit, and the client states that he has smoked three-fourths of a pack per day over the last 10 years. The nurse calculates that the client has a smoking history of how many pack-years? **Fill in the blank and record your answer using one decimal place.**
Answer: _____ pack-years

Level of Cognitive Ability: Applying
Client Needs: Physiological Integrity
Integrated Process: Nursing Process/Assessment
Content Area: Developmental Stages: Health Assessment/Physical Exam
Priority Concepts: Clinical Judgment; Health Promotion

Answer: 7.5 pack-years
Rationale: The standard method for quantifying smoking history is to multiply the number of packs smoked per day by the number of years of smoking. The number is recorded as the number of pack-years. The calculation for the number of pack-years for the client who has smoked three-fourths of a pack per day for 10 years is 0.75 pack × 10 years = 7.5 pack-years.
Priority Nursing Tip: When obtaining a smoking history, ask the client about possible exposure to passive smoke.
Test-Taking Strategy: Focus on the subject, number of pack-years. Review the information in the question and multiply the number of packs of cigarettes smoked per day by the number of years of smoking. Review: **pack-years.**
Reference(s): Ignatavicius, Workman (2013), pp. 549-550, 693.

259. The nurse is preparing to care for a client returning from the operating room after a subtotal thyroidectomy. The nurse anticipates the need for which item to be placed at the bedside?
1. Hypothermia blanket
2. Emergency tracheostomy kit
3. Magnesium sulfate in a ready-to-inject vial
4. Ampule of saturated solution of potassium iodide (SSKI) (ThyroShield)

Level of Cognitive Ability: Applying
Client Needs: Physiological Integrity
Integrated Process: Nursing Process/Planning
Content Area: Adult Health: Endocrine
Priority Concepts: Caregiving; Safety

Answer: 2
Rationale: Respiratory distress can occur after thyroidectomy as a result of swelling in the tracheal area. The nurse would ensure that an emergency tracheostomy kit is available. Surgery on the thyroid does not alter the heat control mechanism of the body. Magnesium sulfate would not be indicated because the incidence of hypomagnesemia is not a common problem after thyroidectomy. SSKI is typically administered preoperatively to block thyroid hormone synthesis and release and to place the client in a euthyroid state.
Priority Nursing Tip: After thyroidectomy, maintain the client is a semi-Fowler's position to assist in preventing edema at the operative site.
Test-Taking Strategy: Focus on the subject, postoperative thyroidectomy. Recall the anatomical location of the thyroid gland to direct you to the correct option. Also, use the ABCs—airway, breathing, and circulation. Maintaining a patent airway is critical. Review: care of the client after **thyroidectomy.**
Reference(s): Ignatavicius, Workman (2013), p. 1399.

260. In caring for a client with myasthenia gravis, the nurse should be alert for which manifestations of myasthenic crisis? **Select all that apply.**
- ❑ 1. Bradycardia
- ❑ 2. Increased diaphoresis
- ❑ 3. Decreased lacrimation
- ❑ 4. Bowel and bladder incontinence
- ❑ 5. Absent cough and swallow reflex
- ❑ 6. Sudden marked rise in blood pressure

Level of Cognitive Ability: Analyzing
Client Needs: Physiological Integrity
Integrated Process: Nursing Process/Assessment
Content Area: Adult Health: Neurological
Priority Concepts: Clinical Judgment; Safety

Answer: 2, 4, 5, 6
Rationale: Myasthenic crisis is caused by undermedication or can be precipitated by an infection or sudden withdrawal of anticholinesterase medications. It may also occur spontaneously. Clinical manifestations include increased diaphoresis, bowel and bladder incontinence, absent cough and swallow reflex, sudden marked rise in blood pressure because of hypoxia, increased heart rate, severe respiratory distress and cyanosis, increased secretions, increased lacrimation, restlessness, and dysarthria.
Priority Nursing Tip: Myasthenic crisis is an acute exacerbation of myasthenia gravis; one cause is undermedication. Cholinergic crisis is caused by overmedication with an anticholinesterase. It is imperative that the nurse documents the time of medication administration, as well as the time of any change in client condition.
Test-Taking Strategy: Focus on the subject, myasthenia gravis. Specific knowledge regarding the manifestations of myasthenic crisis is needed to answer this question. Recall that myasthenic crisis is caused by undermedication. With this in mind, think about the manifestations of myasthenia gravis to assist in selecting the correct options. Review: the manifestations of **myasthenic crisis.**
Reference(s): Hammond, Zimmermann (2013), pp. 272-273; Ignatavicius, Workman (2013), p. 991.

261. The nurse is encouraging the client to cough and deep breathe after cardiac surgery. The nurse ensures that which item is available to maximize the **effectiveness** of this procedure?
1. Nebulizer
2. Ambu bag
3. Suction equipment
4. Incisional splinting pillow

Level of Cognitive Ability: Applying
Client Needs: Physiological Integrity
Integrated Process: Nursing Process/Implementation
Content Area: Fundamental Skills: Perioperative Care
Priority Concepts: Gas Exchange; Health Promotion

Answer: 4
Rationale: The use of an incisional splint such as a "cough pillow" can ease discomfort during coughing and deep breathing. The client who is comfortable will do more effective deep breathing and coughing exercises. Use of an incentive spirometer is also indicated. Options 1, 2, and 3 will not encourage the client to cough and deep breathe.
Priority Nursing Tip: If a surgical incision is located in the abdominal or thoracic area, instruct the client to place a folded towel or pillow, or one hand with the other on top, over the incisional area to splint it during coughing and deep breathing.
Test-Taking Strategy: Focus on the subject, coughing and deep breathing after cardiac surgery. Note the strategic word, *effectiveness.* The cough pillow is an item that will maximize effectiveness. Eliminate options 2 and 3, which are items used by the nurse. A nebulizer (option 1) is used to deliver medication. Review: assisting the **postoperative client** with **coughing and deep breathing.**
Reference(s): Ignatavicius, Workman (2013), p. 256.

262. The nurse is preparing to administer an intermittent tube feeding through a nasogastric (NG) tube and assesses for residual volume. What is the purpose of the nurse assessing the residual volume before administering tube feeding?
  1. Confirm proper NG tube placement.
  2. Determine the client's nutritional status.
  3. Evaluate the adequacy of gastric emptying.
  4. Assess the client's fluid and electrolyte status.

Level of Cognitive Ability: Applying
Client Needs: Physiological Integrity
Integrated Process: Nursing Process/Implementation
Content Area: Fundamental Skills: Safety
Priority Concepts: Clinical Judgment; Nutrition

Answer: 3
Rationale: All stomach contents are aspirated and measured before administering a tube feeding to determine the gastric residual volume. If the stomach fails to empty and propel its contents forward, the tube feeding accumulates in the stomach and increases the client's risk of aspiration. If the aspirated gastric contents exceed the predetermined limit, the nurse withholds the tube feeding and collaborates with the health care provider on a plan of care. Assessing gastric residual volume does not confirm placement or assess fluid and electrolyte status. The nurse uses clinical indicators including serum albumin levels to determine the client's nutritional status.
Priority Nursing Tip: When administering a nasogastric tube feeding, warm the feeding to room temperature to prevent stomach cramps and diarrhea.
Test-Taking Strategy: Focus on the subject, the purpose for assessing the gastric residual volume. Eliminate options 1 and 4 because assessing gastric residual volume does not confirm proper tube placement or assess fluid and electrolyte status. Other clinical indicators will determine client nutritional status, so therefore eliminate option 2. Note the relationship between the subject and option 3 to direct you to this option. Review: the purpose of assessing gastric residual volume.
Reference(s): Perry, Potter, Ostendorf (2014), pp. 776, 790.

263. The nurse is caring for a client scheduled to undergo a renal biopsy. To minimize the risk of postprocedure complications, the nurse reports which laboratory results to the health care provider before the procedure?
  1. Potassium: 3.8 mEq/L
  2. Serum creatinine: 1.2 mg/dL
  3. Prothrombin time: 15 seconds
  4. Blood urea nitrogen (BUN): 18 mg/dL

Level of Cognitive Ability: Applying
Client Needs: Physiological Integrity
Integrated Process: Nursing Process/Implementation
Content Area: Fundamental Skills: Diagnostic Tests
Priority Concepts: Collaboration; Safety

Answer: 3
Rationale: Postprocedure hemorrhage is a complication after renal biopsy. Because of this, prothrombin time is assessed before the procedure. The normal prothrombin time range is 9.5 to 11.8 seconds. The nurse ensures that these results are available and reports abnormalities promptly. Options 1, 2, and 4 identify normal values. The normal potassium is 3.5 to 5.0 mEq/L; the normal serum creatinine is 0.6 to 1.3 mg/dL; and the normal BUN is 8 to 25 mg/dL.
Priority Nursing Tip: After renal biopsy, monitor for bleeding. Provide pressure to the site and check the biopsy site and under the client for bleeding.
Test-Taking Strategy: Focus on the subject, renal biopsy. When a client is to have a biopsy, remember that bleeding is a concern. This will direct you to the correct option. Also note that options 1, 2, and 4 identify normal values. Review: the complications of renal biopsy and normal laboratory values.
Reference(s): Ignatavicius, Workman (2013), pp. 1486-1487; Pagana, Pagana (2013), p. 795.

264. A client involved in a house fire is experiencing respiratory distress, and an inhalation injury is suspected. What should the nurse monitor to check for the presence of carbon monoxide poisoning?
1. Pulse oximetry
2. Urine myoglobin
3. Sputum carbon levels
4. Serum carboxyhemoglobin levels

Level of Cognitive Ability: Applying
Client Needs: Physiological Integrity
Integrated Process: Nursing Process/Assessment
Content Area: Critical Care: Emergency Situations
Priority Concepts: Gas Exchange: Perfusion

Answer: 4
Rationale: Serum carboxyhemoglobin levels are the most direct measure of carbon monoxide poisoning, provide the level of poisoning, and thus determine the appropriate treatment measures. The carbon monoxide molecule has a 200 times greater affinity for binding with hemoglobin than an oxygen molecule, causing decreased availability of oxygen to the cells. Clients are treated with 100% oxygen under pressure (hyperbaric oxygen therapy). Options 1, 2, and 3 would not identify carbon monoxide poisoning.
Priority Nursing Tip: The normal range for the carboxyhemoglobin level is 0% to 10%. It elevates as a result of inhalation of smoke and carbon monoxide.
Test-Taking Strategy: Focus on the subject, carbon monoxide poisoning. Note the relationship between "carbon monoxide" and the correct option. Review: **carbon monoxide poisoning.**
Reference(s): Hammond, Zimmermann (2013), p. 196; Ignatavicius, Workman (2013), p. 522.

265. The nurse is assigned to care for a client with hypertonic labor contractions. The nurse plans to conserve the client's energy and promote rest by performing which intervention?
1. Keeping the TV or radio on to provide distraction
2. Assisting the client with breathing and relaxation techniques
3. Keeping the room brightly lit so the client can watch her monitor
4. Avoiding uncomfortable procedures such as intravenous infusions or epidural anesthesia

Level of Cognitive Ability: Applying
Client Needs: Physiological Integrity
Integrated Process: Nursing Process/Planning
Content Area: Maternity: Antepartum
Priority Concepts: Health Promotion; Reproduction

Answer: 2
Rationale: Breathing and relaxation techniques aid the client in coping with the discomfort of labor and conserving energy. Noise from a TV or radio and light stimulation does not promote rest. A quiet, dim environment would be more advantageous. Intravenous or epidural pain relief can be useful. Intravenous hydration can increase perfusion and oxygenation of maternal and fetal tissues and provide glucose for energy needs.
Priority Nursing Tip: In hypertonic labor contractions, the uterine resting tone between contractions is high, reducing uterine blood flow and decreasing fetal oxygen supply.
Test-Taking Strategy: Focus on the subject, hypertonic labor contractions. Review conserving energy and promoting rest for the client. Noting the word "assisting" in option 2 will direct you to the correct option. Review: care of the client with **hypertonic labor contractions.**
Reference(s): Lowdermilk, Perry, Cashion, Alden (2012), p. 792; McKinney et al (2013), pp. 637-638.

266. A client with acute pyelonephritis has nausea and is vomiting and is scheduled for an intravenous pyelogram. The nurse places **priority** on which action?
1. Ask the client to sign the informed consent.
2. Explain the procedure thoroughly to the client.
3. Place the client on hourly intake and output measurements.
4. Request a prescription for an intravenous infusion from the health care provider.

Level of Cognitive Ability: Applying
Client Needs: Physiological Integrity
Integrated Process: Nursing Process/Implementation
Content Area: Fundamental Skills: Diagnostic Tests
Priority Concepts: Fluid and Electrolyte Balance; Safety

Answer: 4
Rationale: The highest priority of the nurse would be to request a prescription for an intravenous infusion. This is needed to replace fluid lost with vomiting, will be necessary for dye injection for the procedure, and will assist with the elimination of the dye after the procedure. Explanation of the procedure and obtaining the signed informed consent are done once the client's physiological needs are met. The intake and output should be measured, but this will not assist in preventing dehydration.
Priority Nursing Tip: Inform the client who will undergo an intravenous pyelogram (IVP) about the possibility of experiencing throat irritation, flushing of the face, warmth, or a salty or metallic taste during the test.
Test-Taking Strategy: Focus on strategic word, *priority.* Using Maslow's Hierarchy of Needs theory will assist in eliminating options 1 and 2. From the remaining options, noting that the client is vomiting will direct you to the correct option. Review: care of the client who is **vomiting** and **intravenous pyelogram.**
Reference(s): Ignatavicius, Workman (2013), pp. 1482-1484; Pagana, Pagana (2013), p. 783; Potter et al (2013), p. 1055.

267. The nurse is planning care for a client with a T3 spinal cord injury. The nurse should include which intervention in the plan to prevent autonomic dysreflexia (hyperreflexia)?

1. Assist the client to develop a daily bowel routine to prevent constipation.
2. Teach the client that this condition is relatively minor with few symptoms.
3. Assess vital signs and observe for hypotension, tachycardia, and tachypnea.
4. Administer dexamethasone (Decadron) per the health care provider's prescription.

Level of Cognitive Ability: Applying
Client Needs: Physiological Integrity
Integrated Process: Nursing Process/Planning
Content Area: Adult Health: Neurological
Priority Concepts: Caregiving; Intracranial Regulation

Answer: 1
Rationale: Autonomic dysreflexia is a potentially life-threatening condition and may be triggered by bladder distention, bowel distention, visceral distention, or stimulation of pain receptors in the skin. A daily bowel program eliminates this trigger. Option 4 is unrelated to this specific condition. A client with autonomic hyperreflexia would be severely hypertensive and bradycardic. Removal of the stimuli results in prompt resolution of the signs and symptoms.
Priority Nursing Tip: Autonomic dysreflexia is a neurological emergency and must be treated immediately to prevent a hypertensive stroke.
Test-Taking Strategy: Focus on the subject, autonomic dysreflexia. Focus on the word "prevent" to eliminate options 2 and 3. From the remaining options, remembering that this condition may be triggered by bowel distention will direct you to the correct option. Review: the causes of **autonomic dysreflexia**.
Reference(s): Ignatavicius, Workman (2013), p. 974.

268. A client taking diuretics is at risk for hypokalemia. The nurse monitors for which clinical manifestations of hypokalemia? **Select all that apply.**
1. Muscle twitches
2. Tall T waves on electrocardiogram (ECG)
3. Deep tendon hyporeflexia
4. Prominent U wave on ECG
5. General skeletal muscle weakness
6. Hypoactive to absent bowel sounds

Level of Cognitive Ability: Analyzing
Client Needs: Physiological Integrity
Integrated Process: Nursing Process/Assessment
Content Area: Fundamental Skills: Fluids & Electrolytes
Priority Concepts: Clinical Judgment; Fluid and Electrolyte Balance

Answer: 3, 4, 5, 6
Rationale: Hypokalemia is a serum potassium level less than 3.5 mEq/L. Clinical manifestations include ECG abnormalities such as ST depression, inverted T wave, prominent U wave, and heart block. Other manifestations include deep tendon hyporeflexia, general skeletal muscle weakness, decreased bowel motility and hypoactive to absent bowel sounds, shallow ineffective respirations and diminished breath sounds, polyuria, decreased ability to concentrate urine, and decreased urine specific gravity. Tall T waves and muscle twitches are manifestations of hyperkalemia.
Priority Nursing Tip: A potassium deficit is potentially life threatening because every body system is affected.
Test-Taking Strategy: Focus on the subject, the manifestations of hypokalemia. Note that options 3, 5, and 6 are comparable or alike in that they identify a decreased, or hypo-, response; these are manifestations of hypokalemia. Next remember that a prominent U wave on ECG is a manifestation of hypokalemia. Review: the manifestations of **hypokalemia**.
Reference(s): Ignatavicius, Workman (2013), pp. 184-185.

269. A client has a left pleural effusion that has not yet been treated. The nurse should plan to have which item available for **immediate** use?
1. Intubation tray
2. Paracentesis tray
3. Thoracentesis tray
4. Central venous line insertion tray

Level of Cognitive Ability: Applying
Client Needs: Physiological Integrity
Integrated Process: Nursing Process/Planning
Content Area: Adult Health: Respiratory
Priority Concepts: Clinical Judgment; Gas Exchange

Answer: 3
Rationale: The client with a significant pleural effusion is usually treated by thoracentesis. This procedure allows drainage of the fluid from the pleural space, which may then be analyzed to determine the precise cause of the effusion. The nurse ensures that a thoracentesis tray is readily available in case the client's symptoms should rapidly become more severe. A paracentesis tray is needed for the removal of abdominal effusion. Options 1 and 4 are not specifically indicated for this procedure.
Priority Nursing Tip: Instruct the client undergoing thoracentesis not to cough, breathe deeply, or move during the procedure.
Test-Taking Strategy: Focus on the subject, pleural effusion and thoracentesis. Note the strategic word, *immediate*. Recall knowledge regarding the usual treatment for pleural effusion. Note the relationship between the word "pleural" in the question and "thoracentesis" in the correct option. Review: the treatment for **pleural effusion**.
Reference(s): Hammond, Zimmermann (2013), pp. 190-191.

270. A client has been taking procainamide. The nurse understands that the **priority** intervention before administering the medication is which step?
1. Obtain a chest x-ray.
2. Check the blood pressure and pulse.
3. Obtain a complete blood cell count and liver function studies.
4. Schedule the client for a drug level to be drawn 1 hour after the dose.

Level of Cognitive Ability: Applying
Client Needs: Physiological Integrity
Integrated Process: Nursing Process/Implementation
Content Area: Pharmacology: Cardiovascular Medications
Priority Concepts: Clinical Judgment; Safety

Answer: 2
Rationale: Procainamide is an antidysrhythmic medication. Before the medication is administered, the client's blood pressure and pulse are checked. This medication can cause toxic effects, and serum blood levels would be checked before administering the medication (therapeutic serum level is 3 to 10 mcg/mL). A chest x-ray and obtaining a complete blood cell count and liver function studies are unnecessary.
Priority Nursing Tip: Antidysrhythmic medications suppress dysrhythmias by inhibiting abnormal pathways of electrical conduction through the heart.
Test-Taking Strategy: Note the strategic word, *priority*. Use the steps of the nursing process. This will direct you to option 2 because it is the only assessment action. Also recalling that this medication is an antidysrhythmic will direct you to the correct option. Review: **procainamide**.
Reference(s): Hodgson, Kizior (2014), p. 984.

271. A client with urolithiasis is being evaluated to determine the type of urinary calculi that might be excreted. The nurse should plan to keep which item available in the client's room to assist in this process?
1. A strainer
2. A calorie count sheet
3. A vital signs graphic sheet
4. An intake and output record

Level of Cognitive Ability: Applying
Client Needs: Physiological Integrity
Integrated Process: Nursing Process/Planning
Content Area: Adult Health: Renal and Urinary
Priority Concepts: Caregiving; Elimination

Answer: 1
Rationale: The urine is strained until the stone is passed, obtained, and analyzed. Straining the urine will catch small stones that should be sent to the laboratory for analysis. Once the type of stone is determined, an individualized plan of care for prevention and treatment is developed. Options 2, 3, and 4 are unrelated to the question.
Priority Nursing Tip: Urolithiasis refers to the formation of urinary calculi and these calculi form in the ureters.
Test-Taking Strategy: Focus on the subject, urolithiasis. You will need an item that will help determine the type of stone. Eliminate options 2, 3, and 4 because these items give information about food intake, vital signs, and fluid balance, but they will not provide data that will help determine the type of stone. Review: care of the client with **urolithiasis**.
Reference(s): Ignatavicius, Workman (2013), p. 1510.

272. The nurse provides dietary instructions to a client who needs to limit intake of sodium. The nurse instructs the client that which food items must be avoided because of their high-sodium content? **Select all that apply.**
❑ 1. Ham
❑ 2. Apples
❑ 3. Broccoli
❑ 4. Soy sauce
❑ 5. Asparagus
❑ 6. Cantaloupe

Level of Cognitive Ability: Applying
Client Needs: Physiological Integrity
Integrated Process: Teaching and Learning
Content Area: Fundamental Skills: Nutrition
Priority Concepts: Client Education; Nutrition

Answer: 1, 4
Rationale: Foods highest in sodium include table salt, some cheeses, soy sauce, cured pork, canned foods because of the preservatives, and foods such as cold cuts. Fruits and vegetables contain minimal amounts of sodium.
Priority Nursing Tip: Sodium causes the retention of fluid, and the health care provider may prescribe limited sodium intake for clients with hypertension, heart disease, respiratory disease, and certain gastrointestinal and neurological disorders.
Test-Taking Strategy: Focus on the subject, foods high in sodium. Eliminate options 2, 3, 5, and 6 because they are comparable or alike in that they are fruits and vegetables and are low in sodium. Review: **high-sodium foods**.
Reference(s): Ignatavicius, Workman (2013), p. 181; Nix (2013), pp. 136-137.

273. The nurse is preparing to care for a client after ureterolithotomy who has a ureteral catheter in place. The nurse should plan to implement which action in the management of this catheter when the client arrives from the recovery room?
1. Clamp the catheter
2. Place tension on the catheter
3. Check the drainage from the catheter
4. Irrigate the catheter using 10 mL sterile normal saline

Level of Cognitive Ability: Applying
Client Needs: Physiological Integrity
Integrated Process: Nursing Process/Implementation
Content Area: Adult Health: Renal and Urinary
Priority Concepts: Caregiving; Elimination

Answer: 3
Rationale: Drainage from the ureteral catheter should be checked when the client returns from the recovery room and at least every 1 to 2 hours thereafter. The catheter drains urine from the renal pelvis, which has a capacity of 3 to 5 mL. If the volume of urine or fluid in the renal pelvis increases, tissue damage to the pelvis will result from pressure. Therefore, the ureteral tube is never clamped. Additionally, irrigation is not performed unless there is a specific health care provider's prescription to do so.
Priority Nursing Tip: If the client has a ureteral catheter, monitor urine output closely. If the urine output is less than 30 mL per hour or there is a lack of urine output for more than 15 minutes, the health care provider should be notified immediately.
Test-Taking Strategy: Focus on the subject, a ureteral catheter, and think about the anatomy of the kidney. Recalling both that the ureteral catheter is placed in the renal pelvis and the anatomy of this anatomical location will assist in eliminating options 1, 2, and 4. Review: care of the client with a **ureteral catheter**.
Reference(s): Perry, Potter, Ostendorf (2014), pp. 813, 826.

274. Before administering an intermittent tube feeding, the nurse aspirates 40 mL of undigested formula from the client's nasogastric tube. Which should the nurse implement as a result of this finding?
1. Discard the aspirate and record as client output.
2. Mix with new formula to administer the feeding.
3. Dilute with water and inject into the nasogastric tube.
4. Reinstill the aspirate through the nasogastric tube via gravity using a syringe.

Level of Cognitive Ability: Applying
Client Needs: Physiological Integrity
Integrated Process: Nursing Process/Implementation
Content Area: Fundamental Skills: Fluids & Electrolytes
Priority Concepts: Clinical Judgment; Fluid and Electrolyte Balance

Answer: 4
Rationale: After checking residual feeding contents, the nurse reinstills the gastric contents into the stomach by removing the syringe bulb or plunger and pouring the gastric contents via the syringe into the nasogastric tube. Gastric contents should be reinstilled (unless they exceed an amount of 100 mL or as defined by agency policy) to maintain the client's fluid and electrolyte balance. The nurse avoids mixing gastric aspirate with fresh formula to prevent contamination. Because the gastric aspirate is a small volume, it should be reinstilled; however, mixing the formula with water can also disrupt the client's fluid and electrolyte balance unless the client is dehydrated.
Priority Nursing Tip: If the client is receiving nasogastric tube feedings, check the gastric residual volume before each feeding if the client is receiving intermittent feedings, and every 4 to 6 hours if the client is receiving continuous feedings.
Test-Taking Strategy: Focus on the subject, residual tube feeding. Eliminate option 1 because it increases the risk of dehydration and disrupts the client's fluid and electrolyte balance. Also, recalling that aspirated gastric contents are not mixed with formula will assist in directing you to the correct option. Review: **tube feeding**.
Reference(s): Ignatavicius, Workman (2013), p. 1345; Potter et al (2013), p. 1020; Perry, Potter, Ostendorf (2014), p. 860.

275. To increase medication **effectiveness**, the nurse should instruct the client taking oral bisacodyl (Dulcolax) to take the medication via which procedure?
1. At bedtime
2. With a large meal
3. With a glass of milk
4. On an empty stomach

Level of Cognitive Ability: Applying
Client Needs: Physiological Integrity
Integrated Process: Nursing Process/Implementation
Content Area: Pharmacology: Gastrointestinal Medications
Priority Concept: Clinical Judgment; Elimination

Answer: 4
Rationale: Bisacodyl (Dulcolax) is a laxative. The most rapid effect from bisacodyl occurs when it is taken on an empty stomach. If it is taken at bedtime, the client will have a bowel movement in the morning. It will not have a rapid effect if taken with a large meal. Taking the medication with a glass of milk will not speed up its effect.
Priority Nursing Tip: The client taking a laxative needs to increase fluid intake to prevent dehydration.
Test-Taking Strategy: Focus on the subject, bisacodyl (Dulcolax). Note the strategic word, *effectiveness*. Recalling that medications generally are more effective if taken on an empty stomach will direct you to the correct option. Review: **bisacodyl (Dulcolax)**.
Reference(s): Hodgson, Kizior (2014), p. 134.

276. A client with acute respiratory distress syndrome has a prescription to be placed on a continuous positive airway pressure (CPAP) face mask. What should the nurse implement for this procedure to be **most effective**?

1. Obtain baseline arterial blood gases
2. Obtain baseline pulse oximetry levels
3. Apply the mask to the face with a snug fit
4. Encourage the client to remove the mask frequently for coughing and deep breathing exercises

Level of Cognitive Ability: Applying
Client Needs: Physiological Integrity
Integrated Process: Nursing Process/Implementation
Content Area: Adult Health: Respiratory
Priority Concepts: Caregiving; Gas Exchange

Answer: 3
Rationale: The CPAP face mask must be applied over the nose and mouth with a snug fit, which is necessary to maintain positive pressure in the client's airways. The nurse obtains baseline respiratory assessments and arterial blood gases to evaluate the effectiveness of therapy, but these are not done to increase the effectiveness of the procedure. A disadvantage of the CPAP face mask is that the client must remove it for coughing, eating, or drinking. This removes the benefit of positive pressure in the airway each time it is removed.
Priority Nursing Tip: In acute respiratory distress syndrome, the major site of injury is the alveolar capillary membrane.
Test-Taking Strategy: Focus on the subject, continuous positive airway pressure (CPAP). Note the strategic words, *most effective*. Options 1 and 2 do not make the therapy more effective and are eliminated. From the remaining options, knowing that positive pressure must be maintained to be effective will direct you to the correct option. Review: **continuous positive airway pressure (CPAP).**
Reference(s): Potter et al (2013), pp. 848-849.

277. The nurse is caring for a client scheduled to undergo a cardiac catheterization for the first time. Which information should the nurse share with the client?

1. "The procedure is performed in the operating room."
2. "The initial catheter insertion is quite painful; after that, there is little or no pain."
3. "You may feel fatigue and have various aches because it is necessary to lie quietly on a hard x-ray table for about 4 hours."
4. "You may feel certain sensations at various points during the procedure, such as a fluttery feeling, flushed warm feeling, desire to cough, or palpitations."

Level of Cognitive Ability: Applying
Client Needs: Physiological Integrity
Integrated Process: Nursing Process/Implementation
Content Area: Adult Health: Cardiovascular
Priority Concepts: Client Education; Perfusion

Answer: 4
Rationale: Cardiac catheterization is an invasive test that involves the insertion of a catheter and the injection of dye into the heart and surrounding vessels to obtain information about the structure and function of the heart chambers and valves and the coronary circulation. Access is made by the insertion of a needle in either side of the groin into an artery and the catheter is advanced up to the heart through the abdomen and chest. Preprocedure teaching points include that the procedure is done in a darkened cardiac catheterization room and that ECG leads are attached to the client. A local anesthetic is used so there is little to no pain with catheter insertion. The x-ray table is hard and may be tilted periodically. The procedure may take up to 2 hours, and the client may feel various sensations with catheter passage and dye injection.
Priority Nursing Tip: Monitor the postcardiac catheterization client closely. If the client complains of numbness or tingling of the affected extremity; the extremity becomes cool, pale, or cyanotic; or loss of peripheral pulses occurs, notify the health care provider immediately.
Test-Taking Strategy: Focus on the subject, cardiac catheterization. The location (operating room) eliminates option 1. The duration of the procedure, 4 hours, eliminates option 3. From the remaining options, noting the words "quite painful" in option 2 will assist in eliminating this option. Review: client preparation for **cardiac catheterization.**
Reference(s): Pagana, Pagana (2013), p. 220.

❖ **278.** The nurse hangs an intravenous (IV) bag of 1000 mL of 5% dextrose in water (D_5W) at 3 PM and sets the flow rate to infuse at 75 mL/hour. At 11 PM, the nurse should expect the fluid remaining in the IV bag to be at approximately which level? **Fill in the blank and round to the nearest whole number.**
Answer: _____ mL

Level of Cognitive Ability: Understanding
Client Needs: Physiological Integrity
Integrated Process: Nursing Process/Assessment
Content Area: Fundamental Skills: Medications/ IV Calculations
Priority Concepts: Clinical Judgment; Safety

Answer: 400 mL
Rationale: In an 8-hour period, 600 mL would infuse if an IV is set to infuse at 75 mL/hour. Therefore, 400 mL would remain in the IV bag.
Priority Nursing Tip: If a solution of 5% dextrose in water (D_5W) is prescribed for a client with diabetes mellitus, confirm the prescription because the solution can increase the client's blood glucose level.
Test-Taking Strategy: Focus on the subject, IV calculations. Review the data in the question and use simple math to determine that in an 8-hour period (3 PM to 11 PM), 600 mL would infuse (8 hours × 75 mL/hour = 600 mL). This means that 400 mL would remain. Perform the calculation and then verify your answer using a calculator. Review: **IV infusions calculation.**
Reference(s): Potter et al (2013), pp. 925-926.

279. The nurse admits a client with myocardial infarction (MI) to the coronary care unit (CCU). What should the nurse plan to do in delivering care to this client?
1. Begin thrombolytic therapy.
2. Place the client on continuous cardiac monitoring.
3. Infuse intravenous (IV) fluid at a rate of 150 mL per hour.
4. Administer oxygen at a rate of 6 L per minute by nasal cannula.

Level of Cognitive Ability: Applying
Client Needs: Physiological Integrity
Integrated Process: Nursing Process/Planning
Content Area: Critical Care: Emergency Situations
Priority Concepts: Perfusion; Safety

Answer: 2
Rationale: Standard interventions upon admittance to the CCU as they relate to this question include continuous cardiac monitoring. Thrombolytic therapy may or may not be prescribed by the health care provider. Thrombolytic agents are most effective if administered within the first 6 hours of the coronary event. The nurse should ensure there is an adequate IV line insertion of an intermittent lock. If an IV infusion is administered, it is maintained at a keep-vein-open rate to prevent fluid overload and heart failure. Oxygen should be administered at a rate of 2 to 4 liters per minute unless otherwise prescribed.
Priority Nursing Tip: Not all clients experience the classic symptoms of myocardial infarction. Women may experience atypical discomfort, shortness of breath, or fatigue, and often present with NSTEMI (non-ST elevation myocardial infarction) or T-wave inversion.
Test-Taking Strategy: Focus on the subject, myocardial infarction care. Eliminate options 3 and 4 because the values related to the rates of IV fluid and oxygen are high. From the remaining options, note the relationship between the client's diagnosis and option 2. Review: care of the client following **myocardial infarction (MI)**.
Reference(s): Dolan, Holt (2013), pp. 297, 396; Ignatavicius, Workman (2013), p. 836.

280. The nurse is analyzing an electrocardiogram (ECG) rhythm strip on an assigned client. The nurse notes that there are three small boxes from the beginning of the "P" wave to "R" wave. What should the nurse record as the client's PR interval?
1. 0.12 second
2. 0.20 second
3. 0.24 second
4. 0.40 second

Level of Cognitive Ability: Understanding
Client Needs: Physiological Integrity
Integrated Process: Nursing Process/Implementation
Content Area: Adult Health: Cardiovascular
Priority Concepts: Clinical Judgment; Perfusion

Answer: 1
Rationale: Standard ECG graph paper measurements are 0.04 second for each small box on the horizontal axis (measuring time) and 1 mm (measuring voltage) for each small box on the vertical axis.
Priority Nursing Tip: Inform the client that an electrical shock will not occur when performing an electrocardiogram test.
Test-Taking Strategy: Focus on the subject, electrocardiogram (ECG). Knowledge regarding ECG basics is necessary to answer this question. Knowing that each small box is equal to 0.04 second and that there are three small boxes will direct you to the correct option. Review: **electrocardiogram (ECG)**.
Reference(s): Pagana, Pagana (2013), p. 365.

281. The nurse is applying electrocardiogram (ECG) electrodes to a diaphoretic client. Which intervention should the nurse take to keep the electrodes from coming loose?
1. Secure the electrodes with adhesive tape
2. Place clear, transparent dressings over the electrodes
3. Apply lanolin to the skin before applying the electrodes
4. Cleanse the skin with alcohol before applying the electrodes

Level of Cognitive Ability: Applying
Client Needs: Physiological Integrity
Integrated Process: Nursing Process/Implementation
Content Area: Adult Health: Cardiovascular
Priority Concepts: Clinical Judgment; Perfusion

Answer: 4
Rationale: Alcohol defats the skin and helps the electrodes adhere to the skin. Placing adhesive tape or a clear dressing over the electrodes will not help the adhesive gel of the actual electrode make better contact with the diaphoretic skin. Lanolin or any other lotion makes the skin slippery and prevents good initial adherence.
Priority Nursing Tip: To obtain an accurate reading when performing an electrocardiogram, instruct the client to lie still, breathe normally, and refrain from talking during the test.
Test-Taking Strategy: Focus on the subject, electrocardiogram (ECG). Note that options 1 and 2 are comparable or alike in that they both provide an external form of providing security of the electrodes. From the remaining options, note that option 4 addresses cleansing the skin. Review: **electrocardiogram (ECG)**.
Reference(s): Ignatavicius, Workman (2013), p. 714; Pagana, Pagana (2013), p. 367.

282. The nurse has developed a plan of care for a client with a diagnosis of anterior cord syndrome. Which intervention should the nurse include in the plan of care?
1. Change the client's positions slowly.
2. Assess the client for decreased sensation to touch.
3. Assess the client for decreased sensation to vibration.
4. Teach the client about loss of motor function and decreased pain sensation.

Level of Cognitive Ability: Applying
Client Needs: Physiological Integrity
Integrated Process: Nursing Process/Planning
Content Area: Adult Health: Neurological
Priority Concepts: Mobility; Intracranial Regulation

Answer: 4
Rationale: Anterior cord syndrome is caused by damage to the anterior portion of the gray and white matter. Clinical findings related to anterior cord syndrome include loss of motor function, temperature sensation, and pain sensation below the level of injury. The syndrome does not affect sensations of fine touch, position, and vibration.
Priority Nursing Tip: The level of the spinal cord injury is determined by assessing for the lowest spinal cord segment with intact motor and sensory function.
Test-Taking Strategy: Focus on the subject, anterior cord syndrome. Specific knowledge of anterior cord syndrome is necessary to answer this question. Eliminate option 1 first, knowing that position is not affected below the level of injury. Eliminate options 2 and 3, knowing that in anterior cord syndrome sensations of touch and vibration remain intact. Remember that this type of injury involves complete motor function loss and decreased temperature and pain sensation, directing you to the correct option. Review: **anterior cord syndrome.**
Reference(s): Hammond, Zimmermann (2013), pp. 403-404.

283. The nurse is caring for a client with a thoracic spinal cord injury. As part of the nursing care plan, the nurse monitors for spinal shock. In the event that spinal shock occurs, which intravenous (IV) fluid should the nurse anticipate being prescribed?
1. Dextran
2. 0.9% normal saline
3. 5% dextrose in water
4. 5% dextrose in 0.9% normal saline

Level of Cognitive Ability: Understanding
Client Needs: Physiological Integrity
Integrated Process: Nursing Process/Planning
Content Area: Adult Health: Neurological
Priority Concepts: Intracranial Regulation; Perfusion

Answer: 2
Rationale: Normal saline 0.9% is an isotonic solution that primarily remains in the intravascular space, increasing intravascular volume. This IV fluid would increase the client's blood pressure. Dextran is rarely used in spinal shock because isotonic fluid administration is usually sufficient. Additionally, Dextran has potential adverse effects. Dextrose 5% in water is a hypotonic solution that pulls fluid out of the intravascular space and is not indicated for shock. Dextrose 5% in normal saline 0.9% is hypertonic and may be indicated for shock resulting from hemorrhage or burns.
Priority Nursing Tip: Spinal shock occurs within the first hour of spinal cord injury and can last days to months.
Test-Taking Strategy: Focus on the subject, spinal shock. Thinking about the manifestations of shock and using knowledge of the treatment for spinal shock and the purpose of the various IV fluids will direct you to the correct option. Also, remember that normal saline 0.9% is an isotonic solution that primarily remains in the intravascular space, increasing intravascular volume. Review: **spinal shock.**
Reference(s): Hammond, Zimmermann (2013), p. 397; Perry, Potter, Ostendorf (2014), p. 694.

284. The nurse prepares to teach a client to ambulate with a cane. Before teaching cane-assisted ambulation, what should the nurse check for as the **priority**?
1. A high level of stamina and energy
2. Self-consciousness about using a cane
3. Full range of motion in lower extremities
4. Balance, muscle strength, and confidence

Level of Cognitive Ability: Applying
Client Needs: Physiological Integrity
Integrated Process: Nursing Process/Assessment
Content Area: Adult Health: Musculoskeletal
Priority Concepts: Functional Ability; Mobility

Answer: 4
Rationale: Assessing the client's balance, strength, and confidence helps determine if the cane is a suitable assistive device for the client. A high level of stamina and full range of motion are not needed for walking with a cane. Although body image (self-consciousness) is a component of the assessment, it is not the priority.
Priority Nursing Tip: Safety is a priority concern when the client uses an assistive device such as a cane.
Test-Taking Strategy: Note the strategic word, priority. Eliminate options 1 and 2 first because they are not required for the use of a cane. Use Maslow's Hierarchy of Needs theory to assist in directing you to the correct option. Review: teaching points related to the use of a **cane.**
Reference(s): Perry, Potter, Ostendorf (2014), p. 240.

❖ **285.** A health care provider prescribes 1000 mL of normal saline to infuse at 100 mL/hour. The drop factor is 10 drops/mL. The nurse should set the flow rate at how many drops per minute? **Fill in the blank and round your answer to the nearest whole number.**

Answer: _____ drops per minute

Level of Cognitive Ability: Applying
Client Needs: Physiological Integrity
Integrated Process: Nursing Process/Implementation
Content Area: Fundamental Skills: Medications/IV Calculations
Priority Concepts: Clinical Judgment; Safety

Answer: **17 drops per minute**
Rationale: It will take 10 hours for 1000 mL to infuse at 100 mL/hour (1000 mL ÷ 100 mL = 10 hour × 60 min = 600 min). Next, use the intravenous (IV) flow rate formula.
Formula:

$$\frac{\text{Total volume} \times \text{Drop factor}}{\text{Time in minutes}} = \text{Drops/minute}$$

$$\frac{1000\,\text{mL} \times 10\,\text{Drops/mL}}{600\,\text{min}} = \frac{10,000}{600} = 16.6, \text{or}\,17\,\text{Drops/minute}$$

Priority Nursing Tip: The nurse should never increase the rate of an intravenous (IV) solution to catch up if the infusion is running behind schedule.
Test-Taking Strategy: Focus on the subject, IV calculations. First, determine how many hours that it will take for 1000 mL to infuse at 100 mL/hour. Next use the formula for calculating IV flow rates and verify the answer using a calculator. Remember to round the answer to the nearest whole number. Review: **IV infusion rates.**
Reference(s): Potter et al (2013), pp. 925-926.

286. The nurse is assessing a client with cardiac disease at the 30-week gestation antenatal visit. The nurse assesses lung sounds in the lower lobes after a routine blood pressure screening. The nurse performs this assessment to elicit what information?
1. Identify mitral valve prolapse.
2. Identify cardiac dysrhythmias.
3. Rule out the possibility of pneumonia.
4. Assess for early signs of heart failure (HF).

Level of Cognitive Ability: Analyzing
Client Needs: Physiological Integrity
Integrated Process: Nursing Process/Assessment
Content Area: Maternity: Antepartum
Priority Concepts: Perfusion; Reproduction

Answer: **4**
Rationale: Fluid volume during pregnancy peaks between 18 and 32 weeks' gestation. During this period, it is essential to observe and record maternal data that would indicate further signs of cardiac decompensation or HF in the pregnant client with cardiac disease. By assessing lung sounds, the nurse may identify early symptoms of diminished oxygen exchange and potential HF. Options 1, 2, and 3 are not related to the data in the question.
Priority Nursing Tip: Monitor the client with cardiac disease for manifestations of cardiac stress and decompensation, such as cough, fatigue, dyspnea, chest pain, and tachycardia.
Test-Taking Strategy: Focus on the subject, a pregnant client with cardiac disease. Note the relationship between cardiac disease and lung sounds in the question and the words "heart failure" in the correct option. Review: **pregnancy and cardiac disease.**
Reference(s): McKinney et al (2013), pp. 616-617.

❖ **287.** The nurse is caring for a client receiving digoxin (Lanoxin). Which manifestations correlate with a digoxin level of 2.3 ng/dL? **Select all that apply.**
☐ 1. Nausea
☐ 2. Drowsiness
☐ 3. Photophobia
☐ 4. Increased appetite
☐ 5. Increased energy level
☐ 6. Seeing halos around bright objects

Level of Cognitive Ability: Analyzing
Client Needs: Physiological Integrity
Integrated Process: Nursing Process/Assessment
Content Area: Pharmacology: Cardiovascular Medications
Priority Concepts: Clinical Judgment; Safety

Answer: **1, 2, 3, 6**
Rationale: Digoxin is a cardiac glycoside used to manage and treat heart failure, control ventricular rate in clients with atrial fibrillation, and treat and prevent recurrent paroxysmal atrial tachycardia. The therapeutic range is 0.5 to 2.0 ng/dL. Signs of toxicity include gastrointestinal disturbances, including anorexia, nausea, and vomiting; neurological abnormalities such as fatigue, headache, depression, weakness, drowsiness, confusion, and nightmares; facial pain; personality changes; and ocular disturbances such as photophobia, halos around bright lights, and yellow or green color perception.
Priority Nursing Tip: The nurse needs to check the client's apical pulse rate for 1 full minute before administering digoxin (Lanoxin). If it is lower than 60 beats per minute, the medication is withheld and the health care provider is notified.
Test-Taking Strategy: Focus on the subject, a digoxin level of 2.3 ng/dL. Recalling that signs of digoxin toxicity include gastrointestinal disturbances, neurological abnormalities, and ocular disturbances will assist in answering the question correctly. Review: **digoxin (Lanoxin).**
Reference(s): Hodgson, Kizior (2014), pp. 351-353; Lehne (2013), pp. 566-567.

288. Which interventions should the emergency department nurse prepare for in the care of a child with epiglottitis? **Select all that apply.**
- ❑ 1. Obtaining a chest x-ray
- ❑ 2. Obtaining a throat culture
- ❑ 3. Monitoring pulse oximetry
- ❑ 4. Maintaining a patent airway
- ❑ 5. Providing humidified oxygen
- ❑ 6. Administering antipyretics and antibiotics

Level of Cognitive Ability: Analyzing
Client Needs: Physiological Integrity
Integrated Process: Nursing Process/Implementation
Content Area: Critical Care: Emergency Situations
Priority Concepts: Clinical Judgment; Inflammation

Answer: 1, 3, 4, 5, 6
Rationale: Epiglottitis is an acute inflammation and swelling of the epiglottis and surrounding tissue. It is a life-threatening, rapidly progressive condition that may cause complete airway obstruction within a few hours of onset. The most reliable diagnostic sign is an edematous, cherry-red epiglottis. Some interventions include obtaining a chest x-ray film, monitoring pulse oximetry, maintaining a patent airway, providing humidified oxygen, and administering antipyretics and antibiotics. The child may also require intubation and mechanical ventilation. The primary concern in a child with epiglottis is the development of complete airway obstruction. Therefore, the child's throat is not examined or cultured because any stimulation with a tongue depressor or culture swab could trigger complete airway obstruction.
Priority Nursing Tip: Epiglottitis is considered an emergency situation because it can progress rapidly to severe respiratory distress.
Test-Taking Strategy: Focus on the subject, epiglottitis. Focus on ABCs—airway, breathing, and circulation. Remember that the primary concern is the development of complete airway obstruction and that any stimulation with a tongue depressor or culture swab could trigger complete airway obstruction. This will assist in eliminating the only incorrect option, option 2. Review: **epiglottitis.**
Reference(s): McKinney et al (2013), p. 1163.

289. A child with rheumatic fever is admitted to the hospital. The nurse reviews the child's record and expects to note which clinical manifestations documented in the record? **Select all that apply.**
- ❑ 1. Cardiac murmur
- ❑ 2. Cardiac enlargement
- ❑ 3. Cool pale skin over the joints
- ❑ 4. White painful skin lesions on the trunk
- ❑ 5. Small nontender lumps on bony prominences
- ❑ 6. Purposeless jerky movements of the extremities and face

Level of Cognitive Ability: Analyzing
Client Needs: Physiological Integrity
Integrated Process: Nursing Process/Assessment
Content Area: Child Health: Cardiovascular
Priority Concepts: Clinical Judgment; Inflammation

Answer: 1, 2, 5, 6
Rationale: Rheumatic fever is a systemic inflammatory disease that may develop as a delayed reaction to an inadequately treated infection of the upper respiratory tract by group A beta-hemolytic streptococci. Clinical manifestations of rheumatic fever are related to the inflammatory response. Major manifestations include carditis manifested as inflammation of the endocardium, including the valves, myocardium, and pericardium; cardiac murmur and cardiac enlargement; subcutaneous nodules, manifested as small nontender lumps on joints and bony prominences; chorea, manifested as involuntary, purposeless jerky movements of the legs, arms, and face with speech impairment; arthritis manifested as tender, warm erythematous skin over the joints; and erythema marginatum, manifested as red, painless skin lesions usually over the trunk.
Priority Nursing Tip: Initiate seizure precautions if the child with rheumatic fever exhibits manifestations of chorea (involuntary, purposeless jerky movements of the legs, arms, and face with speech impairment).
Test-Taking Strategy: Focus on the subject, rheumatic fever. Recalling that rheumatic fever is a systemic inflammatory disease and noting the words cool in option 3 and white in option 4 will assist in answering this question. Remember that the client will exhibit tender, warm, erythematous skin over the joints and red, painless skin lesions usually over the trunk. Review: **rheumatic fever.**
Reference(s): McKinney et al (2013), p. 1229.

290. A client is hospitalized with a diagnosis of thrombophlebitis and is being treated with heparin infusion therapy. About 24 hours after the infusion has begun, the nurse notes that the client's partial thromboplastin time (PTT) is 65 seconds with a control of 30 seconds. What is the appropriate nursing action?
1. Discontinue the heparin infusion.
2. Prepare to administer protamine sulfate.
3. Notify the health care provider of the laboratory results.
4. Do nothing because the client is adequately anticoagulated.

Level of Cognitive Ability: Applying
Client Needs: Physiological Integrity
Integrated Process: Nursing Process/Implementation
Content Area: Pharmacology: Hematological Medications
Priority Concepts: Clotting; Safety

Answer: 4
Rationale: The effectiveness of heparin therapy is monitored by the results of the PTT. Desired range for therapeutic anticoagulation is 1.5 to 2.5 times the control. A PTT of 65 seconds is within the therapeutic range. Therefore options 1, 2, and 3 are incorrect actions.
Priority Nursing Tip: Heparin is an anticoagulant and the priority concern when a client is receiving an anticoagulant is bleeding.
Test-Taking Strategy: Focus on the subject, heparin infusion therapy. Remember that the desired range for therapeutic anticoagulation is 1.5 to 2.5 times the control. Noting that the control is 30 and that 1.5 to 2.5 times the control is a range of 45 to 75 will direct you to the correct option. Review: **heparin infusion** and **thrombophlebitis**.
Reference(s): Gahart, Nazareno (2012), pp. 700-701; Ignatavicius, Workman (2013), p. 667; Pagana, Pagana (2013), p. 698.

291. A man is brought to the emergency department complaining of chest pain. His vital signs are blood pressure (BP) 150/90 mm Hg, pulse (P) 88 beats per minute (BPM), and respirations (R) 20 breaths per minute. The nurse administers nitroglycerin 0.4 mg sublingually. To evaluate the **effectiveness** of this medication, the nurse assesses for the relief of chest pain and expects to note which changes in the vital signs?
1. BP 150/90 mm Hg, P 70 BPM, R 24 breaths per minute
2. BP 100/60 mm Hg, P 96 BPM, R 20 breaths per minute
3. BP 100/60 mm Hg, P 70 BPM, R 24 breaths per minute
4. BP 160/100 mm Hg, P 120 BPM, R 16 breaths per minute

Level of Cognitive Ability: Evaluating
Client Needs: Physiological Integrity
Integrated Process: Nursing Process/Evaluation
Content Area: Pharmacology: Cardiovascular Medications
Priority Concepts: Clinical Judgment; Perfusion

Answer: 2
Rationale: Nitroglycerin dilates both arteries and veins, causing blood to pool in the periphery. This causes a reduced preload and therefore a drop in cardiac output. This vasodilation causes the blood pressure to fall. The drop in cardiac output causes the sympathetic nervous system to respond and attempt to maintain cardiac output by increasing the pulse. Beta blockers, such as propranolol (Inderal), are often used in conjunction with nitroglycerin to prevent this rise in heart rate. If chest pain is reduced and cardiac workload is reduced, the client will be more comfortable; therefore, a rise in respirations should not be seen.
Priority Nursing Tip: Check the client's blood pressure before administering each dose of nitroglycerin. Nitroglycerin dilates the blood vessels and causes a drop in blood pressure.
Test-Taking Strategy: Focus on the subject, nitroglycerin administration. Note the strategic word, *effectiveness*. Knowing that nitroglycerin is a vasodilator and that it causes the BP to drop will assist in eliminating options 1 and 4. Next recall that if chest pain is reduced and cardiac workload is reduced, the client will be more comfortable; therefore, a rise in respirations should not be seen. This assists in eliminating option 3. Review: the physiological effects of **nitroglycerin**.
Reference(s): Dolan, Holt (2013), p. 396; Ignatavicius, Workman (2013), pp. 837, 843; Jarvis (2012), p. 135.

292. A client who has had an abdominal aortic aneurysm repair is 1 day postoperative. The nurse performs an abdominal assessment and notes the absence of bowel sounds. What action should the nurse take **next**?

1. Feed the client.
2. Remove the nasogastric (NG) tube.
3. Call the health care provider immediately.
4. Document the finding and continue to assess for bowel sounds.

Level of Cognitive Ability: Applying
Client Needs: Physiological Integrity
Integrated Process: Nursing Process/Implementation
Content Area: Fundamental Skills: Perioperative Care
Priority Concepts: Clinical Judgment; Elimination

Answer: 4
Rationale: Bowel sounds may be absent for 3 to 4 postoperative days because of bowel manipulation during surgery. The nurse should document the finding and continue to monitor the client. The NG tube should stay in place if present, and the client is kept NPO until after the onset of bowel sounds. Additionally, the nurse does not remove the tube without a prescription to do so. There is no need to call the health care provider immediately at this time.
Priority Nursing Tip: In the postoperative period, ask the client about the passage of flatus. This is the best initial indicator of the return of intestinal activity.
Test-Taking Strategy: Note the strategic word, *next*. Note the words "1 day postoperative." Eliminate option 2 because there are no data in the question regarding the presence of an NG tube. Additionally, an NG tube would not be removed and the client would not be fed (option 1) if bowel sounds were absent. Recalling that bowel sounds may not return for 3 to 4 postoperative days will direct you to the correct option from the remaining options. Review: **postoperative abdominal assessment.**
Reference(s): Ignatavicius, Workman (2013), p. 290.

293. The nurse is caring for a client with gestational hypertension who is in labor. The nurse monitors the client closely for which complication of gestational hypertension?

1. Seizures
2. Hallucinations
3. Placenta previa
4. Altered respiratory status

Level of Cognitive Ability: Analyzing
Client Needs: Physiological Integrity
Integrated Process: Nursing Process/Assessment
Content Area: Maternity: Intrapartum
Priority Concepts: Perfusion; Reproduction

Answer: 1
Rationale: Gestational hypertension can lead to preeclampsia and eclampsia; therefore, a major complication of gestational hypertension is seizures. Hallucinations, placenta previa, and altered respiratory status are not directly associated with gestational hypertension.
Priority Nursing Tip: Gestational hypertension refers to a condition in which blood pressure elevation is first detected after midpregnancy. Proteinuria is absent.
Test-Taking Strategy: Focus on the subject, complications of gestational hypertension. Remember that seizures are a concern with gestational hypertension to direct you to the correct option. Review: **gestational hypertension.**
Reference(s): McKinney et al (2013), p. 593.

❖ **294.** Which medication instructions should the nurse provide to a client who has been prescribed levothyroxine (Synthroid)? **Select all that apply.**

☐ 1. Monitor your own pulse rate.
☐ 2. Take the medication in the morning.
☐ 3. Take the medication at the same time each day.
☐ 4. Notify the health care provider if chest pain occurs.
☐ 5. Expect the pulse rate to be greater than 100 beats per min.
☐ 6. It may take 1 to 3 weeks for a full therapeutic effect to occur.

Level of Cognitive Ability: Applying
Client Needs: Physiological Integrity
Integrated Process: Teaching and Learning
Content Area: Pharmacology: Endocrine Medications
Priority Concepts: Client Education; Safety

Answer: 1, 2, 3, 4, 6
Rationale: Levothyroxine is a thyroid hormone. The client is instructed to monitor his or her own pulse rate. The client is also instructed to take the medication in the morning before breakfast to prevent insomnia and to take the medication at the same time each day to maintain hormone levels. The client is told not to discontinue the medication and that thyroid replacement is lifelong. Additional instructions include contacting the health care provider if the rate is greater than 100 beats per minute and notifying the health care provider if chest pain occurs, or if weight loss, nervousness and tremors, or insomnia develops. The client is also told that full therapeutic effect may take 1 to 3 weeks and that he or she needs to have follow-up thyroid blood studies to monitor therapy.
Priority Nursing Tip: Foods that can inhibit thyroid secretion include strawberries, peaches, pears, cabbage, turnips, spinach, kale, Brussels sprouts, cauliflower, radishes, and peas.
Test-Taking Strategy: Focus on the subject, levothyroxine (Synthroid). Think about the effects of the medication as you read each option. Noting the words "greater than 100 beats per minute" in option 5 will assist in eliminating this option. Review: **levothyroxine (Synthroid).**
Reference(s): Hodgson, Kizior (2014), pp. 685-687.

295. During an initial prenatal visit a hemoglobin level is obtained on a client in her first trimester of pregnancy. The nurse reviews the results and determines the findings to be abnormal and indicative of iron deficiency anemia. The nurse performs an assessment on the client expecting to note which finding in this type of anemia?
1. Pink mucous membranes
2. Increased vaginal secretions
3. Complaints of headaches and fatigue
4. Complaints of increased frequency of voiding

Level of Cognitive Ability: Understanding
Client Needs: Physiological Integrity
Integrated Process: Nursing Process/Assessment
Content Area: Maternity: Antepartum
Priority Concepts: Gas Exchange; Reproduction

Answer: 3
Rationale: Iron deficiency anemia is described as a hemoglobin blood concentration of less than 10.5 to 11.0 g/dL. Complaints of headaches and fatigue are abnormal findings and may reflect complications of this type of anemia caused by the decreased oxygen supply to vital organs. Options 1, 2, and 4 are normal findings in the first trimester of pregnancy.
Priority Nursing Tip: The hemoglobin and hematocrit levels decline during pregnancy as a result of increased plasma volume.
Test-Taking Strategy: Focus on the subject, iron-deficiency anemia, and note that the client is in her first trimester of pregnancy. Options 1, 2, and 4 are normal findings during the first trimester of pregnancy. Option 3 is abnormal and may reflect complications caused by the decreased oxygen supply to vital organs. Review: **iron-deficiency anemia.**
Reference(s): McKinney et al (2013), p. 621.

296. The nurse is caring for a client with multiple myeloma who is receiving intravenous hydration at 100 mL per hour. Which finding indicates a positive response to the treatment plan?
1. Creatinine of 1.0 mg/dL
2. Weight increase of 1 kilogram
3. Respirations of 18 breaths per minute
4. White blood cell count of 6000 cells/mm³

Level of Cognitive Ability: Evaluating
Client Needs: Physiological Integrity
Integrated Process: Nursing Process/Evaluation
Content Area: Adult Health: Oncology
Priority Concepts: Cellular Regulation; Fluid and Electrolyte Balance

Answer: 1
Rationale: Multiple myeloma is a malignant proliferation of plasma cells within the bone. Renal failure is a concern in the client with multiple myeloma. In multiple myeloma, hydration is essential to prevent renal damage resulting from precipitation of protein in the renal tubules and excessive calcium and uric acid in the blood. Creatinine is the most accurate measure of renal status. Options 3 and 4 are unrelated to the subject of hydration. Weight gain is not a positive sign when concerned with renal status.
Priority Nursing Tip: The client with multiple myeloma is at risk for pathological fractures.
Test-Taking Strategy: Focus on the subject, hydration and multiple myeloma. Recalling that kidney failure is a concern in multiple myeloma will direct you to the correct option. Additionally option 1 is the only choice that is related to hydration status. Review: care of the client with **multiple myeloma.**
Reference(s): Ignatavicius, Workman (2013), pp. 894-895; Pagana, Pagana (2013), p. 313.

297. The nurse provides discharge instructions to a client with testicular cancer who had testicular surgery. Which instruction should the nurse instruct the client to follow?
1. To avoid driving a car for at least 8 weeks
2. Not to be fitted for a prosthesis for at least 6 months
3. To avoid sitting for long periods for at least 6 months
4. To report any elevation in temperature to the health care provider

Level of Cognitive Ability: Applying
Client Needs: Physiological Integrity
Integrated Process: Teaching and Learning
Content Area: Adult Health: Oncology
Priority Concepts: Cellular Regulation; Client Education

Answer: 4
Rationale: For the client who has had testicular surgery, the nurse should emphasize the importance of notifying the health care provider if chills, fever, drainage, redness, or discharge occurs. These symptoms may indicate the presence of an infection. One week after testicular surgery, the client may drive. Often, a prosthesis is inserted during surgery. Sitting needs to be avoided with prostate surgery because of the risk of hemorrhage, but this risk is not as high with testicular surgery.
Priority Nursing Tip: Testicular self-examination needs to be performed monthly. A day of the month is selected, and the examination is performed on the same day each month.
Test-Taking Strategy: Use Maslow's Hierarchy of Needs theory and principles related to prioritizing. Infection is a priority. After any surgical procedure, elevation of temperature could signal an infection and should be reported. Also note the lengthy time periods in options 1, 2, and 3. These will assist in eliminating these options. Review: **testicular surgery.**
Reference(s): Ignatavicius, Workman (2013), p. 1646.

298. A multidisciplinary team is working with the spouse of a home care client who has end-stage liver failure and is teaching the spouse about pain management. Which statement by the spouse indicates the **need for further teaching**?

1. "My husband can use breathing exercises to control pain."
2. "I will help prevent constipation with increased fluids."
3. "If the pain increases, I will report it to the nurse promptly."
4. "The medication causes very deep sleep that my husband needs."

Level of Cognitive Ability: Evaluating
Client Needs: Physiological Integrity
Integrated Process: Teaching and Learning
Content Area: Adult Health: Gastrointestinal
Priority Concepts: Pain; Safety

Answer: 4
Rationale: In the client with liver disease, the ability to metabolize medication is affected. A decreased level of consciousness is a potential clinical indicator of medication overdose, as well as fluid, electrolyte, and oxygenation deficiencies; thus, the nurse teaches the client's spouse about the differences between sleep related to pain relief and a deteriorating change in neurological status. Options 1, 2, and 3 all indicate an understanding of suitable steps to be taken in pain management.
Priority Nursing Tip: The administration of opioids, sedatives, barbiturates, and any hepatotoxic medications is avoided in the client with liver disease.
Test-Taking Strategy: Note the strategic words, *need for further teaching*. These words indicate a negative event query and the need to select the option that is an incorrect statement. Note that the client has end-stage liver disease, meaning that analgesics take longer to metabolize so the dosage is likely to have a greater and longer effect than a client without liver disease. Focusing on the subject, pain management in a client who has end-stage liver failure will direct you to the correct option. Review: **pain management** in the client with **liver disease**.
Reference(s): Ignatavicius, Workman (2013), p. 1304.

299. The nurse is reviewing the antenatal history of a client in early labor. The nurse recognizes which factor documented in the history as having the **most** potential for causing neonatal sepsis after delivery?

1. Adequate prenatal care
2. History of substance abuse during pregnancy
3. Appropriate maternal nutrition and weight gain
4. Spontaneous rupture of membranes 2 hours ago

Level of Cognitive Ability: Analyzing
Client Needs: Physiological Integrity
Integrated Process: Nursing Process/Assessment
Content Area: Maternity: Intrapartum
Priority Concepts: Development; Infection

Answer: 2
Rationale: Risk factors for neonatal sepsis can arise from maternal, intrapartal, or neonatal conditions. Maternal risk factors before delivery include a history of substance abuse during pregnancy, low socioeconomic status, and poor prenatal care and nutrition. Premature rupture of the membranes or prolonged rupture of membranes greater than 18 hours before birth is also a risk factor for neonatal acquisition of infection.
Priority Nursing Tip: If antibiotics are prescribed for a newborn, monitor the newborn carefully for toxicity because a newborn's liver and kidneys are immature.
Test-Taking Strategy: Focus on the subject, risk factor for neonatal sepsis. Note the strategic word, *most*. Options 1 and 3 are optimal findings and can be eliminated. From the remaining options, note the words "2 hours ago" to assist in eliminating option 4. Review: **neonatal sepsis**.
Reference(s): Lowdermilk, Perry, Cashion, Alden (2012), p. 844; McKinney et al (2013), pp. 724-726.

300. The nurse performs a prenatal assessment on a client in the first trimester of pregnancy and discovers that the client frequently consumes beverages containing alcohol. Why should the nurse initiate interventions to assist the client in avoiding alcohol consumption?

1. Reduce the potential for fetal growth restriction in utero.
2. Promote the normal psychosocial adaptation of the mother to pregnancy.
3. Minimize the potential for placental abruptions during the intrapartum period.
4. Reduce the risk of teratogenic effects to developing fetal organs, tissues, and structures.

Level of Cognitive Ability: Applying
Client Needs: Physiological Integrity
Integrated Process: Teaching and Learning
Content Area: Maternity: Antepartum
Priority Concepts: Reproduction; Safety

Answer: 4
Rationale: The first trimester, "organogenesis," is characterized by the differentiation and development of fetal organs, systems, and structures. The effects of alcohol on the developing fetus during this critical period depend not only on the amount of alcohol consumed, but also on the interaction of quantity, frequency, type of alcohol, and other drugs that may be abused during this period by the pregnant woman. Eliminating consumption of alcohol during this time may promote normal fetal organ development. Although options 1, 2, and 3 may be concerns, they are not specifically associated with the first trimester of pregnancy.
Priority Nursing Tip: Fetal alcohol syndrome is caused by maternal alcohol use during pregnancy and causes physical and mental retardation.
Test-Taking Strategy: Focus on the subject, effects of alcohol on the fetus, and note the client is in the first trimester of pregnancy. Recall that during this trimester, development of fetal organs, tissues, and structures take place. Review: effects of **alcohol on a fetus**.
Reference(s): McKinney et al (2013), pp. 258, 559.

301. The nurse is admitting a client with a diagnosis of hypothyroidism to the hospital. What action should the nurse perform to obtain data related to this diagnosis?
1. Inspect facial features
2. Auscultate lung sounds
3. Percuss the thyroid gland
4. Assess the client's ability to ambulate

Level of Cognitive Ability: Applying
Client Needs: Physiological Integrity
Integrated Process: Nursing Process/Assessment
Content Area: Adult Health: Endocrine
Priority Concepts: Clinical Judgment; Thermoregulation

Answer: 1
Rationale: Inspection of facial features will reveal the characteristic coarse features, presence of edema around the eyes and face, and the blank expression that are characteristic of hypothyroidism. The assessment techniques in options 2, 3, and 4 will not reveal information related to the diagnosis of hypothyroidism.
Priority Nursing Tip: Hypothyroidism is characterized by a decreased rate of metabolism. Assessment findings relate to this characteristic.
Test-Taking Strategy: Focus on the **subject,** hypothyroidism. Eliminate options 2 and 4 because they do not relate to the thyroid gland. From the remaining options, recall that palpation, rather than percussion, of the thyroid is the assessment technique used to evaluate the thyroid gland. Review: **hypothyroidism.**
Reference(s): Ignatavicius, Workman (2013), pp. 1401-1402.

302. The nurse is teaching a client with chronic obstructive pulmonary disease (COPD) how to do pursed-lip breathing. Evaluation of understanding is evident if the client performs which action?
1. Breathes in and then holds the breath for 30 seconds
2. Loosens the abdominal muscles while breathing out
3. Inhales with pursed lips and exhales with the mouth open wide
4. Breathes so that expiration is two to three times as long as inspiration

Level of Cognitive Ability: Evaluating
Client Needs: Physiological Integrity
Integrated Process: Nursing Process/Evaluation
Content Area: Adult Health: Respiratory
Priority Concepts: Client Education; Gas Exchange

Answer: 4
Rationale: Chronic obstructive pulmonary disease is a disease state characterized by airflow obstruction. Prolonging expiration time reduces air trapping caused by airway narrowing that occurs in COPD. The client is not instructed to breathe in and hold the breath for 30 seconds; this action has no useful purpose for the client with COPD. Tightening (not loosening) the abdominal muscles aids in expelling air. Exhaling through pursed lips (not with the mouth wide open) increases the intraluminal pressure and prevents the airways from collapsing.
Priority Nursing Tip: For the client with chronic obstructive pulmonary disease, the stimulus to breathe is a low arterial P_{O_2} instead of an increased P_{CO_2}.
Test-Taking Strategy: Focus on the subject, pursed-lip breathing in a client with chronic obstructive pulmonary disease (COPD). Visualize each of the actions in the options. Recalling that a major purpose of pursed-lip breathing is to prevent air trapping during exhalation will direct you to the correct option. Review: the principles of **pursed-lip breathing** and **chronic obstructive pulmonary disease (COPD).**
Reference(s): Ignatavicius, Workman (2013), p. 619; Potter et al (2013), p. 854.

❖ **303.** While providing care to a client with a head injury, the nurse notes that a client exhibits this posture (**refer to figure**). What should the nurse document that the client is exhibiting?

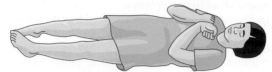

Figure from Ignatavicius D, Workman M: *Medical-surgical nursing: patient-centered collaborative care*, ed 7, Philadelphia, 2013, Saunders.

1. Flaccidity
2. Decorticate posturing
3. Decerebrate posturing
4. Rigidity in the upper extremities

Level of Cognitive Ability: Analyzing
Client Needs: Physiological Integrity
Integrated Process: Nursing Process/Assessment
Content Area: Adult Health: Neurological
Priority Concepts: Clinical Judgment; Intracranial Regulation

Answer: 2
Rationale: Decortication is abnormal posturing seen in the client with lesions that interrupt the corticospinal pathways. In this posturing, the client's arms, wrists, and fingers are flexed with internal rotation and plantar flexion of the feet and legs extended. Flaccidity indicates weak, soft, and flabby muscles that lack normal muscle tone. Decerebration is abnormal posturing and rigidity characterized by extension of the arms and legs, pronation of the arms, plantar flexion, and opisthotonos. Decerebration is usually associated with dysfunction in the brainstem area. Rigidity indicates hardness, stiffness, or inflexibility. Decerebrate posturing is associated with rigidity.
Priority Nursing Tip: Decorticate posturing is also known as flexor posturing and decerebrate posturing is also known as extensor posturing.
Test-Taking Strategy: Focus on the subject, posturing. Review the figure and use knowledge regarding the characteristics of posturing to answer the question. First eliminate options 3 and 4 because they are comparable or alike in that decerebrate posturing is associated with rigidity. Next, recalling that flaccidity indicates weak, soft, and flabby muscles that lack normal muscle tone will assist in eliminating option 1. Review: the characteristics of **posturing**.
Reference(s): Ignatavicius, Workman (2013), pp. 918-919.

304. A client is taking lithium carbonate (Lithobid) for the treatment of bipolar disorder. Which assessment question should the nurse ask the client to determine signs of **early** lithium toxicity?
1. "Do you have frequent headaches?"
2. "Have you noted excessive urination?"
3. "Have you been experiencing leg aches over the past few days?"
4. "Have you been experiencing any nausea, vomiting, or diarrhea?"

Level of Cognitive Ability: Analyzing
Client Needs: Physiological Integrity
Integrated Process: Nursing Process/Assessment
Content Area: Pharmacology: Psychiatric Medications
Priority Concepts: Clinical Judgment; Safety

Answer: 4
Rationale: One of the most common early signs of lithium toxicity is gastrointestinal (GI) disturbances such as nausea, vomiting, or diarrhea. The assessment questions in options 1, 2, and 3 are unrelated to the findings in lithium toxicity.
Priority Nursing Tip: Instruct the client taking lithium carbonate (Lithobid) to drink six to eight glasses of water daily and to maintain an adequate intake of salt to prevent lithium toxicity.
Test-Taking Strategy: Focus on the subject, early signs of lithium toxicity and note the strategic word, *early*. Recalling that GI disturbances are early manifestations will direct you to the correct option. Review: **lithium carbonate (Lithobid) toxicity**.
Reference(s): Hodgson, Kizior (2014), pp. 700-701.

305. A postpartum nurse is caring for a client who delivered a viable newborn infant 2 hours ago. The nurse palpates the fundus and notes the character of the lochia. Which characteristic of the lochia should the nurse expect to note at this time?
1. Pink-colored lochia
2. White-colored lochia
3. Serosanguineous lochia
4. Dark red-colored lochia

Level of Cognitive Ability: Applying
Client Needs: Physiological Integrity
Integrated Process: Nursing Process/Assessment
Content Area: Maternity: Antepartum
Priority Concepts: Health Promotion; Reproduction

Answer: 4
Rationale: When checking the perineum, the lochia is monitored for amount, color, and the presence of clots. The color of the lochia during the fourth stage of labor (the first 1 to 4 hours after birth) is a dark red color. Options 1, 2, and 3 are not the expected characteristics of lochia at this time period.
Priority Nursing Tip: Lochia discharge should smell like normal menstrual flow. If it has a foul-smelling odor, infection should be suspected.
Test-Taking Strategy: Focus on the subject, lochia assessment postpartum. Noting that the question refers to a client who delivered 2 hours ago will direct you to the correct option. Review: **postpartum assessments**.
Reference(s): McKinney et al (2013), pp. 434-435, 441.

306. The nurse is performing a prenatal examination on a client in the third trimester. The
nurse begins an abdominal examination
and performs Leopold maneuvers. What
should the nurse determine after performing the first maneuver?
1. Fetal descent
2. Placenta previa
3. Fetal lie and presentation
4. Strength of uterine contractions

Level of Cognitive Ability: Analyzing
Client Needs: Physiological Integrity
Integrated Process: Nursing Process/Assessment
Content Area: Maternity: Antepartum
Priority Concepts: Health Promotion; Reproduction

Answer: 3
Rationale: The first maneuver, the fundal grip, determines the contents (size, consistency, shape and mobility) of the fundus (either
the fetal head or breech) and thereby the fetal lie. Fetal descent is
determined with the fourth maneuver. Placenta previa is diagnosed
by ultrasound and not by palpation. Leopold maneuvers are not performed during a contraction.
Priority Nursing Tip: Before performing Leopold maneuvers, the
nurse should assist the client in emptying her bladder.
Test-Taking Strategy: Focus on the subject, Leopold maneuvers, and
this will assist in eliminating options 2 and 4. From the remaining
options, it is necessary to know that the first maneuver determines
fetal lie. Review: **Leopold maneuvers.**
Reference(s): McKinney et al (2013), pp. 251, 342-343.

307. The nurse is caring for a client with a spinal cord injury who is in spinal shock. The
nurse performs an assessment on the client,
knowing that which assessment will provide
the **best** information about recovery from
spinal shock?
1. Reflexes
2. Pulse rate
3. Temperature
4. Blood pressure

Level of Cognitive Ability: Analyzing
Client Needs: Physiological Integrity
Integrated Process: Nursing Process/Assessment
Content Area: Adult Health: Neurological
Priority Concepts: Mobility; Intracranial Regulation

Answer: 1
Rationale: Areflexia characterizes spinal shock; therefore, reflexes
would provide the best information about recovery. Vital sign changes
(options 2, 3, and 4) are not consistently affected by spinal shock.
Because vital signs are affected by many factors, they do not give reliable information about spinal shock recovery. Blood pressure would
provide good information about recovery from other types of shock,
but not spinal shock.
Priority Nursing Tip: Spinal shock can occur following a spinal cord
injury and ends when the reflexes are regained.
Test-Taking Strategy: Focus on the subject, recovery from spinal
shock. Note the strategic word, *best.* Note that options 2, 3, and 4 are
comparable or alike and are all vital signs. Therefore, eliminate these
options. Review: the characteristics of **spinal shock.**
Reference(s): Ignatavicius, Workman (2013), p. 969.

308. A client is admitted to the hospital for repair
of an unruptured cerebral aneurysm. Before
surgery, the nurse performs frequent assessments on the client. Which assessment finding would be noted **first** if the aneurysm
ruptures?
1. Widened pulse pressure
2. Unilateral motor weakness
3. Unilateral slowing of pupil response
4. A decline in the level of consciousness

Level of Cognitive Ability: Analyzing
Client Needs: Physiological Integrity
Integrated Process: Nursing Process/Assessment
Content Area: Adult Health: Neurological
Priority Concepts: Clinical Judgment; Intracranial
Regulation

Answer: 4
Rationale: Rupture of a cerebral aneurysm usually results in increased
intracranial pressure (ICP). The first sign of pressure in the brain is
a change in the level of consciousness. This change in consciousness can be as subtle as drowsiness or restlessness. Because centers
that control blood pressure are located lower in the brain than those
that control consciousness, blood pressure alteration is a later sign.
Slowing of pupil response and motor weakness are also late signs.
Priority Nursing Tip: The level of consciousness is the most sensitive
and earliest indicator of a change in the neurological status.
Test-Taking Strategy: Note the strategic word, *first.* Remember that
changes in level of consciousness are the first indication of increased
ICP. Review: **cerebral aneurysm.**
Reference(s): Hammond, Zimmermann (2013), pp. 263-264;
Ignatavicius, Workman (2013), p. 1014.

309. An emergency department staff member calls the mental health unit and tells the nurse that a severely depressed client is being transported to the unit. The nurse in the mental health unit expects to note which finding on assessment of this client?
1. Reports of weight gain, hypersomnia, and a blunted affect
2. Reports of crying spells, normal weight and sleep patterns
3. Reports of a reluctance to participate in activities, but a normal affect
4. Reports of substantial weight loss, insomnia, and decreased crying spells

Level of Cognitive Ability: Analyzing
Client Needs: Physiological Integrity
Integrated Process: Nursing Process/Assessment
Content Area: Mental Health
Priority Concepts: Clinical Judgment; Mood and Affect

Answer: 4
Rationale: In the severely depressed client, loss of weight is typical, while the mildly depressed client may experience a gain in weight. Sleep is generally affected in a similar way, with hypersomnia in the mildly depressed client and insomnia in the severely depressed client. The severely depressed client may report that no tears are left for crying.
Priority Nursing Tip: If the client has depression, always assess the client's risk of harm to self or others.
Test-Taking Strategy: Focus on the subject, a severely depressed client. Options 2 and 3 identify some degree of normalcy and can be eliminated. From the remaining options, focusing on the subject will direct you to the correct option. Review: **severe depression.**
Reference(s): Hammond, Zimmermann (2013), pp. 509-510; Varcarolis (2013), pp. 255-256.

❖ **310.** A client admitted to the hospital is suspected of having Guillain-Barré syndrome and the nurse performs an assessment. The nurse next reviews the client's medical record, expecting to note documentation of which manifestations of this disorder? **Select all that apply.**
☐ 1. Dysphagia
☐ 2. Paresthesia
☐ 3. Facial weakness
☐ 4. Difficulty speaking
☐ 5. Hyperactive deep tendon reflexes
☐ 6. Descending symmetrical muscle weakness

Level of Cognitive Ability: Analyzing
Client Needs: Physiological Integrity
Integrated Process: Nursing Process/Assessment
Content Area: Adult Health: Neurological
Priority Concepts: Clinical Judgment; Mobility

Answer: 1, 2, 3, 4
Rationale: Guillain-Barré syndrome is an acute autoimmune disorder characterized by varying degrees of motor weakness and paralysis. Motor manifestations include ascending symmetrical muscle weakness that leads to flaccid paralysis without muscle atrophy, decreased or absent deep tendon reflexes, respiratory compromise and respiratory failure, and loss of bladder and bowel control. Sensory manifestations include pain (cramping) and paresthesia. Cranial nerve manifestations include facial weakness, dysphagia, diplopia, and difficulty speaking. Autonomic manifestations include labile blood pressure, dysrhythmias, and tachycardia.
Priority Nursing Tip: To remember that an ascending progression of paralysis occurs in Guillain-Barré syndrome, think about G to B (Guillain-Barré), from the Ground to the Brain.
Test-Taking Strategy: Focus on the subject, Guillain-Barré syndrome and note that it is an acute autoimmune disorder characterized by varying degrees of motor weakness and paralysis. This will assist in determining that options 1, 2, 3, and 4 are correct. Review: **Guillain-Barré syndrome.**
Reference(s): Ignatavicius, Workman (2013), p. 987.

311. A home care nurse finds a client in the bedroom, unconscious, with a pill bottle in hand. The pill bottle had contained the selective serotonin reuptake inhibitor, sertraline (Zoloft). The nurse should **immediately** assess which item?
1. Pulse
2. Respirations
3. Blood pressure
4. Urinary output

Level of Cognitive Ability: Analyzing
Client Needs: Physiological Integrity
Integrated Process: Nursing Process/Assessment
Content Area: Critical Care: Emergency Situations
Priority Concepts: Clinical Judgment; Safety

Answer: 2
Rationale: In an emergency situation, the nurse should determine breathlessness first, then pulselessness. Blood pressure would be assessed after these assessments were determined. Urinary output is also important but is not the priority at this time.
Priority Nursing Tip: Selective serotonin reuptake inhibitors (SSRIs) can interact with numerous medications. Therefore, it is important to check the client's prescribed medications to determine the potential for an adverse interaction.
Test-Taking Strategy: Note the strategic word, *immediately.* Use the ABCs—airway, breathing, and circulation—as the guide for answering this question. Respirations specifically relate to airway and breathing. Review: **selective serotonin reuptake inhibitors.**
Reference(s): Dolan, Holt (2013), pp. 224-225; Hammond, Zimmermann (2013), p. 516.

312. The nurse checks a unit of blood received from the blood bank and notes the presence of gas bubbles in the bag. What should the nurse do?
1. Return the bag to the blood bank.
2. Infuse the blood using filter tubing.
3. Add 10 mL normal saline to the bag.
4. Agitate the bag to mix contents gently.

Level of Cognitive Ability: Applying
Client Needs: Physiological Integrity
Integrated Process: Nursing Process/Implementation
Content Area: Critical Care: Blood Administration
Priority Concepts: Clinical Judgment; Safety

Answer: 1
Rationale: The nurse should return the unit of blood to the blood bank because the gas bubbles in the bag indicate possible contamination. If the nurse were going to administer the blood, the nurse would use filter tubing to trap particulate matter. Although normal saline can be infused concurrently with the blood, normal saline or any other substance should never be added to the blood in a blood bag. The bag should not be agitated because this can harm red blood cells.
Priority Nursing Tip: The blood for infusion is always checked for leaks, abnormal color, clots, and bubbles before administration. If any of these are noted, it is not administered and is returned to the blood bank.
Test-Taking Strategy: Focus on the subject, blood administration. Recalling that the presence of gas bubbles indicates potential bacterial growth directs you to the correct option. Remember that, when in doubt, consult with the blood bank. Review: **blood transfusion.**
Reference(s): Ignatavicius, Workman (2013), p. 898; Potter et al (2013), p. 912.

313. The nurse checks the gauge of the client's intravenous catheter. Which is the smallest gauge catheter that the nurse can use to administer blood?
1. 12-Gauge
2. 20-Gauge
3. 22-Gauge
4. 24-Gauge

Level of Cognitive Ability: Applying
Client Needs: Physiological Integrity
Integrated Process: Nursing Process/Implementation
Content Area: Critical Care: Blood Administration
Priority Concepts: Clinical Judgment; Safety

Answer: 2
Rationale: An intravenous catheter used to infuse blood should be at least 20-gauge or larger to help prevent additional hemolysis of red blood cells and to allow infusion of the blood without occluding the IV catheter.
Priority Nursing Tip: Ensure that the client has an adequate and functioning intravenous catheter inserted before obtaining the blood for administration from the blood bank.
Test-Taking Strategy: Focus on the subject, the smallest gauge catheter that the nurse can use for infusion of blood. This focus will assist in eliminating options 3 and 4. From the remaining options, think about the gauge of IV catheters to direct you to the correct option. Review: **IV catheter sizes and blood transfusions.**
Reference(s): Ignatavicius, Workman (2013), p. 898; Perry, Potter, Ostendorf (2014), p. 744.

314. A client began receiving an intravenous (IV) infusion of packed red blood cells 30 minutes ago. The client complains of difficulty breathing, itching, and a tight sensation in the chest. Which is the **first** action of the nurse?
1. Stop the transfusion.
2. Call the health care provider.
3. Check the client's temperature.
4. Recheck the unit of blood for compatibility.

Level of Cognitive Ability: Analyzing
Client Needs: Physiological Integrity
Integrated Process: Nursing Process/Implementation
Content Area: Critical Care: Blood Administration
Priority Concepts: Clinical Judgment; Safety

Answer: 1
Rationale: The symptoms reported by the client indicate that the client is experiencing a transfusion reaction. The first action of the nurse when a transfusion reaction is observed is to discontinue the transfusion. The IV of normal saline with new IV tubing is started and the health care provider is notified. The nurse then checks the client's vital signs: temperature, pulse, and respirations and then rechecks the unit of blood as appropriate for infusion into the client. Depending on agency protocol, the nurse may also obtain a urinalysis, draw a sample of blood, and return the unit of blood and tubing to the blood bank. The nurse also institutes supportive care for the client, which may include administration of antihistamines, crystalloids, epinephrine steroids or vasopressors as prescribed.
Priority Nursing Tip: If a blood transfusion reaction occurs, do not leave the client alone and continuously monitor the client for any life-threatening symptoms.
Test-Taking Strategy: Focus on the subject, the action to take if a transfusion reaction occurs. Noting the strategic word, *first,* will direct you to the correct option. Remember that the first action of the nurse when a transfusion reaction is observed is to discontinue the transfusion. Review: **transfusion reaction.**
Reference(s): Ignatavicius, Workman (2013), pp. 900-901; Perry, Potter, Ostendorf (2014), p. 751.

315. A client has not eaten or had anything to drink for 4 hours following two episodes of nausea and vomiting. Which item would be **best** to offer the client who is ready to try resuming oral intake?
1. Toast
2. Gelatin
3. Dry cereal
4. Ginger ale

Level of Cognitive Ability: Applying
Client Needs: Physiological Integrity
Integrated Process: Nursing Process/Implementation
Content Area: Adult Health: Gastrointestinal
Priority Concepts: Clinical Judgment; Nutrition

Answer: 4
Rationale: Clear liquids are best tolerated first after episodes of nausea and vomiting. If the client tolerates sips (20 to 30 mL at a time) of clear liquids, such as water or ginger ale (with the carbonation removed if better tolerated), then the amounts may be increased and gelatin, tea, and broth may be added. Once these are tolerated, solid foods such as toast, cereal, chicken, and other easily digested foods may be tried.
Priority Nursing Tip: Vomiting places the client at risk for dehydration and metabolic alkalosis.
Test-Taking Strategy: Focus on the subject, nausea and vomiting and the strategic word, *best.* Begin to answer this question by eliminating options 1 and 3, which identify solid foods and are less well tolerated than liquids. Choose ginger ale over gelatin because it is a liquid at all temperatures. Review: care of the client with **nausea** and **vomiting.**
Reference(s): Nix (2013), p. 481; Perry, Potter, Ostendorf (2014), p. 765.

316. A client has just undergone an upper gastrointestinal (GI) series. Upon the client's return to the unit, what health care provider's prescriptions does the nurse expect to note as a part of routine postprocedure care?
1. Bland diet
2. NPO status
3. Mild laxative
4. Decreased fluids

Level of Cognitive Ability: Applying
Client Needs: Physiological Integrity
Integrated Process: Nursing Process/Implementation
Content Area: Fundamental Skills: Diagnostic Tests
Priority Concepts: Clinical Judgment; Elimination

Answer: 3
Rationale: Barium sulfate, which is used as a contrast material during an upper GI series, is constipating. If it is not eliminated from the GI tract, it can cause obstruction. Therefore, laxatives or cathartics are administered as part of routine postprocedure care. Increased (not decreased) fluids are also helpful but do not act in the same way as a laxative to eliminate the barium. Options 1 and 2 are not routine postprocedure measures.
Priority Nursing Tip: Following an upper gastrointestinal (GI) series, instruct the client to increase oral fluid intake to help pass the barium.
Test-Taking Strategy: Focus on the subject, upper GI series and the words "routine postprocedure." Recalling that barium is used in this diagnostic test will direct you to the correct option. Review: postprocedure care following an **upper GI series.**
Reference(s): Ignatavicius, Workman (2013), p. 1187.

317. The nurse prepares the client for the removal of a nasogastric tube. During the tube removal, the nurse instructs the client to take which action?

1. Inhale deeply.
2. Exhale slowly.
3. Hold in a deep breath.
4. Pause between breaths.

Level of Cognitive Ability: Applying
Client Needs: Physiological Integrity
Integrated Process: Nursing Process/Implementation
Content Area: Fundamental Skills: Safety
Priority Concepts: Clinical Judgment; Safety

Answer: 3
Rationale: Just before removing the tube, the client is asked to take a deep breath and hold it because breath-holding minimizes the risk of aspirating gastric contents spilled from the tube during removal. The maneuver partially occludes the airway during tube removal; afterward, the client exhales as soon as the tube is out and thus avoids drawing the gastric contents into the trachea. The nurse pulls the tube out steadily and smoothly while the client holds the breath. The remaining options are incorrect because options 1 and 2 increase the risk of aspiration, and option 4 is ineffective.
Priority Nursing Tip: Following removal of a nasogastric tube, monitor the client for abdominal distention and signs of aspiration.
Test-Taking Strategy: Focus on the subject, nasogastric tube removal. Visualize this procedure. Recalling that the airway is partially occluded during tube removal and that the risk of aspiration is present will direct you to the correct option. Review: the procedure for removal of a nasogastric tube.
Reference(s): Perry, Potter, Ostendorf (2014), p. 862; Potter et al (2013), p. 1120.

318. The nurse is caring for a client who is receiving total parenteral nutrition and has a prescription for an intravenous intralipid infusion. What should the nurse implement before hanging the intralipid infusion?

1. Refrigerate the bottle of solution.
2. Add 100 mL normal saline to the infusion bottle.
3. Place an in-line filter on the administration tubing.
4. Check the solution for separation or an oily residue.

Level of Cognitive Ability: Applying
Client Needs: Physiological Integrity
Integrated Process: Nursing Process/Implementation
Content Area: Fundamental Skills: Nutrition
Priority Concepts: Nutrition; Safety

Answer: 4
Rationale: Intralipids provide nonprotein calories and prevent or correct fatty acid deficiency. The nurse checks the solution for separation or an oily appearance because this can indicate a spoiled or contaminated solution. Refrigeration renders the intralipid solution too thick to administer. Because they can affect the stability of the solution, the nurse avoids injecting additives into the intralipid infusion. Furthermore, an in-line filter is not used because it can disrupt the flow of solution by becoming clogged.
Priority Nursing Tip: Fat emulsions (lipids) should not be given to a client with an egg allergy because lipids contain egg yolk phospholipids.
Test-Taking Strategy: Focus on the subject, actions to take before administering intralipids. Think about the consistency of this solution to direct you to the correct option. Review: infusing intralipid solutions.
Reference(s): Gahart, Nazareno (2012), p. 594; Perry, Potter, Ostendorf (2014), p. 802.

❖ **319.** The nurse develops a discharge plan for a client with diabetes mellitus who has peripheral neuropathy of the lower extremities. Which instructions should the nurse include in the plan? **Select all that apply.**
❑ 1. Wear support or elastic stockings.
❑ 2. Wear well-fitted shoes and walk barefoot only when at home.
❑ 3. Wear dark-colored stockings or socks and change them daily.
❑ 4. Use a heating pad set at low setting on the feet if they feel cold.
❑ 5. Apply lanolin or lubricating lotion to the legs and feet once or twice daily.
❑ 6. Wash the feet and legs with mild soap and water and rinse and dry them well.

Level of Cognitive Ability: Analyzing
Client Needs: Physiological Integrity
Integrated Process: Teaching and Learning
Content Area: Adult Health: Neurological
Priority Concepts: Client Education; Glucose Regulation

Answer: 1, 5, 6
Rationale: Peripheral neuropathy is any functional or organic disorder of the peripheral nervous system. Clinical manifestations can include muscle weakness, stabbing pain, paresthesia or loss of sensation, impaired reflexes, and autonomic manifestations. Home care instructions include wearing support or elastic stockings for dependent edema, applying lanolin or lubricating lotion to the legs and feet once or twice daily, washing the feet and legs with mild soap and water and rinsing and drying them well, inspecting the legs and feet daily and reporting any skin changes or open areas to the health care provider, wearing white or colorfast stockings or socks and changing them daily, checking the temperature of the bath water with a thermometer before putting the feet into the water, avoiding the use of heat (hot foot soaks, heating pad, hot water bottle) on the feet because of the risk of burning, avoiding the use of sharp devices to cut nails, and wearing well-fitted shoes and avoiding going barefoot.
Priority Nursing Tip: A complication of diabetes mellitus is peripheral neuropathy. The client experiences decreased sensation and must be cautious about exposure to extreme temperatures and potential injuries.
Test-Taking Strategy: Focus on the subject, peripheral neuropathy. This client will experience paresthesia or loss of sensation. This will assist in eliminating option 4. Next eliminate option 2 because of the closed-ended word *only*. Finally eliminate option 3 because the client must wear white or colorfast stockings or socks. Review: home care instructions for a client with **peripheral neuropathy.**
Reference(s): Ignatavicius, Workman (2013), p. 999.

320. A health care provider is inserting a chest tube. Which materials should the nurse select to be used as the first layer of the dressing at the chest tube insertion site?
1. Petrolatum jelly gauze
2. Sterile 4×4 gauze pad
3. Absorbent gauze dressing
4. Gauze impregnated with povidone-iodine

Level of Cognitive Ability: Applying
Client Needs: Physiological Integrity
Integrated Process: Nursing Process/Implementation
Content Area: Adult Health: Respiratory
Priority Concepts: Gas Exchange; Safety

Answer: 1
Rationale: The first layer of the chest tube dressing is petrolatum gauze, which allows for an occlusive seal at the chest tube insertion site. Additional layers of gauze cover this layer, and the dressing is secured with a strong adhesive tape or Elastoplast tape. The items in the remaining options would not be selected as the first protective layer.
Priority Nursing Tip: An occlusive sterile dressing is maintained at the chest tube insertion site to prevent an air leak.
Test-Taking Strategy: Focus on the subject, the first layer of the dressing at the chest tube insertion site. Recall that an occlusive seal at the site is needed and think about which dressing material will help achieve this seal. Review: care of the client requiring **chest tube** insertion.
Reference(s): Perry, Potter, Ostendorf (2014), p. 660.

321. A client being seen in the health care provider's office for follow-up 2 weeks after pneumonectomy complains of numbness and tenderness at the surgical site. Which statement should the nurse make to the client?
1. "This is not likely to be permanent, but may last for some months."
2. "You are having a severe problem and will probably be rehospitalized"
3. "This is probably caused by permanent nerve damage as a result of surgery."
4. "This is often the first sign of a wound infection, and I will check your temperature."

Level of Cognitive Ability: Applying
Client Needs: Physiological Integrity
Integrated Process: Nursing Process/Implementation
Content Area: Fundamental Skills: Perioperative Care
Priority Concepts: Gas Exchange; Tissue Integrity

Answer: 1
Rationale: Clients who undergo pneumonectomy or other surgical procedures may experience numbness, altered sensation, or tenderness in the area that surrounds the incision. These sensations may last for months. It is not considered to be a severe problem and is not indicative of a wound infection.
Priority Nursing Tip: After pneumonectomy, check the health care provider's prescription regarding client positioning. Avoid complete lateral turning of the client.
Test-Taking Strategy: Focus on the subject, numbness and tenderness at the surgical site after pneumonectomy. Eliminate option 2 because of the word "severe." Eliminate option 3 because of the word "permanent." Eliminate option 4 because numbness and tenderness are not signs of infection. Review: postoperative expectations after pneumonectomy.
Reference(s): Ignatavicius, Workman (2013), p. 638.

322. A client scheduled for pneumonectomy tells the nurse that a friend of his had lung surgery and had chest tubes. The client asks the nurse about how long his chest tubes will be in place after surgery. Which statement indicates the **best** response by the nurse?
1. "They will be removed after 3 to 4 days."
2. "They will be in place for 24 to 48 hours."
3. "They usually remain in place for a full week after surgery."
4. "Most likely, there will be no chest tubes in place after surgery."

Level of Cognitive Ability: Analyzing
Client Needs: Physiological Integrity
Integrated Process: Nursing Process/Implementation
Content Area: Adult Health: Respiratory
Priority Concepts: Client Education; Gas Exchange

Answer: 4
Rationale: Pneumonectomy involves removal of the entire lung, usually caused by extensive disease such as bronchogenic carcinoma, unilateral tuberculosis, or lung abscess. Chest tubes are not inserted because the cavity is left to fill with serosanguineous fluid, which later solidifies. Therefore options 1, 2, and 3 are incorrect.
Priority Nursing Tip: After pneumonectomy, serous fluid accumulates in the empty thoracic cavity and eventually consolidates, preventing shifts of the mediastinum, heart, and remaining lung.
Test-Taking Strategy: Focus on the subject, postoperative expectations following pneumonectomy. Note the strategic word, best. Recall that the entire lung is removed with this procedure. This would guide you to reason that chest tubes are unnecessary because there is no lung remaining to reinflate to fill the pleural space (option 4). Review: care of the client after pneumonectomy.
Reference(s): Ignatavicius, Workman (2013), p. 638.

❖ **323.** The nurse is developing a plan of care for a client with a dissecting abdominal aortic aneurysm. Which interventions should be included in the plan of care? **Select all that apply.**
☐ 1. Assess peripheral circulation.
☐ 2. Monitor for abdominal distention.
☐ 3. Tell the client that abdominal pain is expected.
☐ 4. Turn the client to the side to look for ecchymoses on the lower back.
☐ 5. Perform deep palpation of the abdomen to assess the size of the aneurysm.

Level of Cognitive Ability: Analyzing
Client Needs: Physiological Integrity
Integrated Process: Nursing Process/Planning
Content Area: Critical Care: Emergency Situations
Priority Concepts: Clinical Judgment; Perfusion

Answer: 1, 2, 4
Rationale: If the client has an abdominal aortic aneurysm, the nurse is concerned about rupture and monitors the client closely. The nurse should assess peripheral circulation and monitor for abdominal distention. The nurse also looks for ecchymoses on the lower back to determine if the aneurysm is leaking. The nurse tells the client to report abdominal pain, or back pain, which may radiate to the groin, buttocks, or legs because this is a sign of rupture. The nurse also avoids deep palpation in the client in whom a dissecting abdominal aortic aneurysm is known or suspected. Doing so could place the client at risk for rupture.
Priority Nursing Tip: Systolic bruit heard over the abdominal aorta is a manifestation of an abdominal aortic aneurysm.
Test-Taking Strategy: Focus on the subject, care for a client with a dissecting abdominal aortic aneurysm. Eliminate options 3 and 5 because the presence of abdominal pain is a sign of rupture and deep palpation places the aneurysm at risk for rupture. Review: care of the client with a dissecting abdominal aortic aneurysm.
Reference(s): Ignatavicius, Workman (2013), p. 794.

324. A client has undergone angioplasty of the iliac artery. Which technique should the nurse perform to **best** detect bleeding from the angioplasty in the region of the iliac artery?
1. Palpate the pedal pulses.
2. Measure the abdominal girth.
3. Ask the client about mild pain in the area.
4. Auscultate over the iliac area with a Doppler device.

Level of Cognitive Ability: Analyzing
Client Needs: Physiological Integrity
Integrated Process: Nursing Process/Assessment
Content Area: Adult Health: Cardiovascular
Priority Concepts: Clinical Judgment; Perfusion

Answer: 2
Rationale: Bleeding after iliac artery angioplasty causes blood to accumulate in the retroperitoneal area. This can most directly be detected by measuring abdominal girth. Palpation and auscultation of pulses determine patency. Assessment of pain is routinely done, and mild regional discomfort is expected.
Priority Nursing Tip: After angioplasty, assess the insertion site frequently for the presence of bloody drainage or hematoma formation.
Test-Taking Strategy: Note the strategic word, *best*. Focus on the subject of bleeding from the angioplasty in the region of the iliac artery. Select the option that addresses an abdominal assessment because the iliac arteries are located in the peritoneal cavity. This will direct you to the correct option. Review: care of the client who underwent **angioplasty of the iliac artery.**
Reference(s): Ignatavicius, Workman (2013), p. 1298; Perry, Potter, Ostendorf (2014), p. 147.

❖ **325.** A client comes into the health care clinic stating that she thinks she has restless leg syndrome. The nurse assesses the client and determines that which data are characteristics of this disorder? **Select all that apply.**
❑ 1. A heavy feeling in the legs
❑ 2. Burning sensations in the limbs
❑ 3. Symptom relief when lying down
❑ 4. Decreased ability to move the legs
❑ 5. Symptoms that are worse in the morning
❑ 6. Feeling the need to move the limbs repeatedly

Level of Cognitive Ability: Analyzing
Client Needs: Physiological Integrity
Integrated Process: Nursing Process/Assessment
Content Area: Adult Health: Neurological
Priority Concepts: Clinical Judgment; Mobility

Answer: 2, 6
Rationale: Restless leg syndrome is characterized by leg paresthesia associated with an irresistible urge to move. The client complains of intense burning or "crawling-type" sensations in the limbs and subsequently feels the need to move the limbs repeatedly to relieve the symptoms. The symptoms are worse in the evening and night when the client is still.
Priority Nursing Tip: Some nonpharmacological measures to relieve the symptoms of restless leg syndrome include walking, stretching, moderate exercise, or a warm bath.
Test-Taking Strategy: Focus on the subject, manifestations of restless leg syndrome. This will assist in eliminating options 1, 3, and 4. Next recall that the symptoms of this disorder are worse in the evening and night when the client is still. Review: the characteristics of **restless leg syndrome.**
Reference(s): Ignatavicius, Workman (2013), p. 999.

326. A client who underwent peripheral arterial bypass surgery 16 hours ago complains of increasing pain in the leg at rest, which worsens with movement and is accompanied by paresthesias. Based on this data, which action should the nurse take?
1. Call the health care provider.
2. Administer an opioid analgesic.
3. Apply warm moist heat for comfort.
4. Apply ice to minimize any developing swelling.

Level of Cognitive Ability: Analyzing
Client Needs: Physiological Integrity
Integrated Process: Nursing Process/Implementation
Content Area: Adult Health: Cardiovascular
Priority Concepts: Clinical Judgment; Perfusion

Answer: 1
Rationale: Compartment syndrome is characterized by increased pressure within a muscle compartment caused by bleeding or excessive edema. It compresses the nerves in the area and can cause vascular compromise. The classic signs of compartment syndrome are pain at rest that intensifies with movement and the development of paresthesias. Compartment syndrome is an emergency, and the health care provider is notified immediately because the client could require an emergency fasciotomy to relieve the pressure and restore perfusion. Options 2, 3, and 4 are incorrect actions.
Priority Nursing Tip: After arterial bypass surgery, warmth, redness, and edema of the affected extremity are expected occurrences because of the increased blood flow to the area.
Test-Taking Strategy: Focus on the subject, a postoperative client who had peripheral arterial bypass surgery. Note the words "increasing pain." Also note that the surgery was 16 hours ago. The signs and symptoms described indicate a new problem. These factors should indicate that the health care provider needs to be notified. Review: the complications of **arterial bypass surgery.**
Reference(s): Ignatavicius, Workman (2013), p. 792.

327. The nurse in an ambulatory care clinic takes a client's blood pressure (BP) in the left arm; it is 200/118 mm Hg. Which action should the nurse implement **next**?
1. Notify the health care provider.
2. Inquire about the presence of kidney disorders.
3. Check the client's blood pressure in the right arm.
4. Recheck the pressure in the same arm within 30 seconds.

Level of Cognitive Ability: Analyzing
Client Needs: Physiological Integrity
Integrated Process: Nursing Process/Implementation
Content Area: Adult Health: Cardiovascular
Priority Concepts: Clinical Judgment; Perfusion

Answer: 3
Rationale: When a high BP reading is noted, the nurse takes the pressure in the opposite arm to see if the blood pressure is elevated in one extremity only. The nurse would also recheck the blood pressure in the same arm but would wait at least 2 minutes between readings. The nurse would inquire about the presence of kidney disorders that could contribute to the elevated blood pressure. The nurse would notify the health care provider because immediate treatment may be required, but this would not be done without obtaining verification of the elevation.
Priority Nursing Tip: Hypertension is a major risk factor for coronary, cerebral, renal, and peripheral vascular disease.
Test-Taking Strategy: Focus on the subject, hypertension. Note the strategic word, *next*. Eliminate option 4 first because of the time frame, 30 seconds. From the remaining options, select the correct option because it provides verification of the initial reading. Review: the procedures for **blood pressure (BP) measurement**.
Reference(s): Potter et al (2013), p. 484.

328. A new prenatal client is 6 months pregnant. On the first prenatal visit, the nurse notes that the client is gravida 4, para 0, aborta 3. The client is 5′ 6″ tall, weighs 130 pounds, and is 25 years old. The client states, "I get really tired after working all day, and I can't keep up with my housework." Which factor in the above data would lead the nurse to suspect gestational diabetes?
1. Fatigue
2. Obesity
3. Maternal age
4. Previous fetal demise

Level of Cognitive Ability: Analyzing
Client Needs: Physiological Integrity
Integrated Process: Nursing Process/Analysis
Content Area: Maternity: Antepartum
Priority Concepts: Glucose Regulation; Reproduction

Answer: 4
Rationale: A previous history of unexplained stillbirths or miscarriages puts the client at high risk for gestational diabetes. Fatigue is a normal occurrence during pregnancy. The client's height (5′ 6″ tall) and weight (130 pounds) do not meet the criteria of 20% over ideal weight. Therefore, the client is not obese. To be at high risk for gestational diabetes, the maternal age should be greater than 25 years.
Priority Nursing Tip: Pregnant women should be screened for gestational diabetes between 24 and 28 weeks of pregnancy.
Test-Taking Strategy: Focus on the subject, gestational diabetes. Option 1 can be eliminated because fatigue is a normal occurrence during pregnancy. Recalling the risk factors associated with gestational diabetes will indicate that options 2 and 3 do not apply to this client. Review: gestational diabetes.
Reference(s): McKinney et al (2013), p. 613.

329. The nurse is caring for a client with preeclampsia. If the client's condition progresses from preeclampsia to eclampsia, what should the nurse's **first** action be?
1. Maintain an open airway.
2. Administer oxygen by face mask.
3. Assess the maternal blood pressure and fetal heart tones.
4. Administer an intravenous infusion of magnesium sulfate.

Level of Cognitive Ability: Applying
Client Needs: Physiological Integrity
Integrated Process: Nursing Process/Implementation
Content Area: Leadership/Management: Prioritizing
Priority Concepts: Perfusion; Reproduction

Answer: 1
Rationale: Eclampsia is characterized by the occurrence of seizures. If the client experiences seizures, it is important as a first action to establish and maintain an open airway and prevent injuries to the client. Options 2, 3, and 4 are all interventions that should be done but not initially.
Priority Nursing Tip: The nurse would never leave the client who is having a seizure. The nurse stays with the client, maintaining an open airway and calling for help.
Test-Taking Strategy: Note the strategic word, *first*. Use the ABCs—airway, breathing, and circulation—to direct you to the correct option. Review: **preeclampsia** and **eclampsia**.
Reference(s): Lowdermilk, Perry, Cashion, Alden (2012), p. 667.

330. The nurse in the emergency department admits a client who is bleeding freely from a scalp laceration obtained during a fall from a stepladder when the client was doing outdoor home repair. The nurse should take which action **first** in the care of this wound?

1. Prepare for suturing the area.
2. Administer a prophylactic antibiotic.
3. Cleanse the wound with sterile normal saline.
4. Apply direct pressure to the laceration to stop the bleeding.

Level of Cognitive Ability: Applying
Client Needs: Physiological Integrity
Integrated Process: Nursing Process/Implementation
Content Area: Critical Care: Emergency Situations
Priority Concepts: Clotting; Tissue Integrity

Answer: 4

Rationale: The initial nursing action is to stop the bleeding, and direct pressure is applied. The nurse will then cleanse the wound thoroughly with sterile normal saline. This action removes dirt or foreign matter in the wound and allows visualization of the size of the wound. If suturing is necessary, the surrounding hair may be shaved. Prophylactic antibiotics are often prescribed. The date of the client's last tetanus shot is determined, and prophylaxis is given if needed.

Priority Nursing Tip: The nurse must ask the client who sustains a laceration about the date of the last tetanus immunization because the client may need a tetanus injection.

Test-Taking Strategy: Note the strategic word, *first*, which implies that more than one or all of the options may be partially or totally correct. Focus on ABCs—airway, breathing, circulation. This will direct you to the correct option. Review: care of the client with a laceration.

Reference(s): Dolan, Holt (2013), pp. 339-340; Ignatavicius, Workman (2013), p. 1021.

331. A client was admitted to the nursing unit with a closed head injury 6 hours ago. During initial assessment, the nurse finds that the client has vomited, is confused, and complains of dizziness and headache. Based on these data, which is the **most important** nursing action?

1. Administer an antiemetic.
2. Notify the health care provider.
3. Reorient the client to surroundings.
4. Change the client's gown and bed linens.

Level of Cognitive Ability: Analyzing
Client Needs: Physiological Integrity
Integrated Process: Nursing Process/Implementation
Content Area: Critical Care: Emergency Situations
Priority Concepts: Clinical Judgment; Intracranial Regulation

Answer: 2

Rationale: The client with a closed head injury is at risk of developing increased intracranial pressure (ICP). Increased ICP is evidenced by signs and symptoms such as headache, dizziness, confusion, weakness, and vomiting. Because of the implications of the client's manifestations, the most important nursing action is to notify the health care provider. Other nursing actions that are appropriate include physical care of the client and reorientation to surroundings.

Priority Nursing Tip: The head of the bed of the client with increased intracranial pressure should be elevated 30 to 40 degrees.

Test-Taking Strategy: Note the strategic words, *most important*. This directs you to prioritize the possible nursing actions. Considering the client's diagnosis, a closed head injury, and the signs and symptoms, the nurse should suspect increased ICP. The health care provider needs to be notified. Review: care of a client with a **head injury**.

Reference(s): Hammond, Zimmermann (2013), p. 382.

332. A client is being brought into the emergency department after suffering a head injury. Which should the nurse assess **first**?
1. Level of consciousness
2. Pulse and blood pressure
3. Respiratory rate and depth
4. Ability to move extremities

Level of Cognitive Ability: Applying
Client Needs: Physiological Integrity
Integrated Process: Nursing Process/Implementation
Content Area: Critical Care: Emergency Situations
Priority Concepts: Clinical Judgment; Intracranial Regulation

Answer: 3
Rationale: The first action of the nurse is to ensure that the client has an adequate airway and respiratory status. In rapid sequence, the client's circulatory status is evaluated (option 2), followed by evaluation of the neurological status (options 1 and 4).
Priority Nursing Tip: Complications of a head injury include cerebral bleeding, hematomas, uncontrolled increased intracranial pressure, infections, and seizures.
Test-Taking Strategy: Note the strategic word, *first*. Use the ABCs—airway, breathing, and circulation. The correct option will most often be the one that deals with the client's airway. Respiratory rate and depth support this action. Review: **head injury.**
Reference(s): Hammond, Zimmermann (2013), p. 383.

333. A client with a spinal cord injury is at risk of developing footdrop. What should the nurse use as the **effective** preventive measure?
1. Foot board
2. Heel protectors
3. Posterior splints
4. Pneumatic boots

Level of Cognitive Ability: Applying
Client Needs: Physiological Integrity
Integrated Process: Nursing Process/Implementation
Content Area: Adult Health: Neurological
Priority Concepts: Clinical Judgment; Mobility

Answer: 3
Rationale: The effective means of preventing footdrop is the use of posterior splints or high-top sneakers. A foot board prevents plantar flexion but also places the client more at risk for developing pressure ulcers of the feet. Heel protectors protect the skin but do not prevent footdrop. Pneumatic boots prevent deep vein thrombosis but not footdrop.
Priority Nursing Tip: Footdrop is preventable and the nurse needs to be alert to clients at risk for developing footdrop, such as immobile and bedridden clients, and initiate measures to prevent it.
Test-Taking Strategy: Note the strategic word, *effective*. Focus on the subject, preventing footdrop. This guides you to select the option that immobilizes the foot in a functional position while protecting the skin of the extremities. Review: **footdrop.**
Reference(s): Ignatavicius, Workman (2013), p. 281; Potter et al (2013), pp. 1131, 1134.

334. After a cervical spine fracture, this device **(refer to figure)** is placed on the client. The nurse develops a discharge plan for the client to ensure safety and includes which measures? **Select all that apply.**

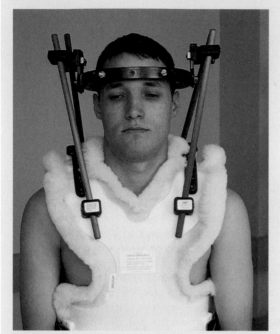

Figure from Ignatavicius D, Workman M: *Medical-surgical nursing: patient-centered collaborative care*, ed 7, Philadelphia, 2013, Saunders.

☐ 1. Teach the client how to ambulate with a walker.
☐ 2. Instruct the client to bend at the waist to pick up needed items.
☐ 3. Demonstrate the procedure for scanning the environment for vision.
☐ 4. Inform the client about the importance of wearing rubber-soled shoes.
☐ 5. Teach the spouse to use the metal frame to assist the client to turn in bed.

Level of Cognitive Ability: Analyzing
Client Needs: Physiological Integrity
Integrated Process: Nursing Process/Planning
Content Area: Adult Health: Neurological
Priority Concepts: Clinical Judgment; Safety

Answer: 1, 3, 4
Rationale: The client with a halo fixation device should be taught that the use of a walker and rubber-soled shoes may help prevent falls and injury and are therefore also helpful. It is helpful for the client to scan the environment visually because the client's peripheral vision is diminished from keeping the neck in a stationary position. The client with a halo fixation device should avoid bending at the waist because the halo vest is heavy, and the client's trunk is limited in flexibility. The nurse instructs the client and family that the metal frame on the device is never used to move or lift the client because this will disrupt the attachment to the client's skull, which is stabilizing the fracture.
Priority Nursing Tip: The weight of the halo fixation device can alter the client's balance, and the nurse must teach the client measures that will ensure safety.
Test-Taking Strategy: Focus on the subject, client instructions for a halo fixation device. Visualize the actions in the options to assist in identifying how injury could be prevented. This will assist in eliminating options 2 and 5. Review: **halo fixation device.**
Reference(s): Ignatavicius, Workman (2013), p. 972; Perry, Potter, Ostendorf (2014), pp. 264, 266-267.

335. The nurse is caring for a client who has undergone transsphenoidal resection of a pituitary adenoma. What should the nurse measure to detect occurrence of a common complication of this type of surgery?

1. Pulse rate
2. Temperature
3. Urine output
4. Oxygen saturation

Level of Cognitive Ability: Analyzing
Client Needs: Physiological Integrity
Integrated Process: Nursing Process/Assessment
Content Area: Adult Health: Neurological
Priority Concepts: Clinical Judgment; Fluid and Electrolyte Balance

Answer: 3
Rationale: A common complication of surgery on the pituitary gland is temporary diabetes insipidus. This results from a deficiency in antidiuretic hormone (ADH) secretion as a result of surgical trauma. The nurse measures the client's urine output to determine whether this complication is occurring. Polyuria of 4 to 24 liters per day is characteristic of this complication. Options 1, 2, and 4 are not specifically related to a common complication after this surgery.
Priority Nursing Tip: Following transsphenoidal resection of a pituitary adenoma, monitor the client for postnasal or nasal drainage, which might indicate leakage of cerebrospinal fluid.
Test-Taking Strategy: Focus on the subject, transsphenoidal resection of a pituitary adenoma. Recalling that the pituitary gland is responsible for the production of ADH and a deficiency results in diabetes insipidus will direct you to the correct option. Review: the complications of transsphenoidal resection of a **pituitary adenoma.**
Reference(s): Ignatavicius, Workman (2013), pp. 1377-1378.

336. The nurse is preparing to check the fetal heart rate of a pregnant woman who is at gestational week 16. Which piece of equipment will the nurse appropriately use to check the fetal heart rate?

1. Fetal heart monitor
2. An adult stethoscope
3. Bell of a stethoscope
4. Ultrasound fetoscope

Level of Cognitive Ability: Applying
Client Needs: Physiological Integrity
Integrated Process: Nursing Process/Assessment
Content Area: Maternity: Antepartum
Priority Concepts: Development; Perfusion

Answer: 4
Rationale: Toward the end of the first trimester, the fetal heart tones can be heard with an ultrasound fetoscope. Options 2 and 3 will not adequately assess the fetal heart rate. A fetal heart monitor is used during labor or in other situations when the fetal heart rate needs continuous monitoring.
Priority Nursing Tip: The normal fetal heart rate is 120 to 160 beats per minute.
Test-Taking Strategy: Focus on the subject, fetal heart assessment. Eliminate options 2 and 3 first because they are comparable or alike. Recalling that a fetal heart monitor is used for continuous monitoring will direct you to the correct option. Review: **fetal heart assessment.**
Reference(s): McKinney et al (2013), pp. 371, 386.

337. The nurse is developing a discharge plan for a postoperative client who had one adrenal gland removed. What should the nurse include in the plan?

1. Teaching the client to maintain a diabetic diet
2. Teaching proper application of an ostomy pouch
3. Providing a list of the early signs of a wound infection
4. Explaining the need for lifelong replacement of all adrenal hormones

Level of Cognitive Ability: Analyzing
Client Needs: Physiological Integrity
Integrated Process: Nursing Process/Planning
Content Area: Adult Health: Endocrine
Priority Concepts: Client Education; Infection

Answer: 3
Rationale: A client who had a unilateral adrenalectomy will be placed on corticosteroids temporarily to avoid a cortisol deficiency; lifelong replacement is not necessary. Corticosteroids will be gradually weaned in the postoperative period until they are discontinued. Also, because of the anti-inflammatory properties of corticosteroids produced by the adrenals, clients who undergo an adrenalectomy are at increased risk of developing wound infections. Because of this increased risk of infection, it is important for the client to know measures to prevent infection, early signs of infection, and what to do if an infection seems to be present. The client does not need to maintain a diabetic diet, and the client will not have an ostomy after this surgery.
Priority Nursing Tip: After adrenalectomy, monitor the client closely for bleeding because the adrenal glands are highly vascular.
Test-Taking Strategy: Focus on the subject, unilateral adrenalectomy. Recalling that the hormones from the adrenal glands are needed for proper immune system function will eliminate options 1 and 2. From the remaining options, recalling that one gland can take over the function of two adrenal glands will direct you to the correct option. Review: care of the client after a **unilateral adrenalectomy.**
Reference(s): Ignatavicius, Workman (2013), pp. 1388-1389.

338. The nurse is caring for a client who has undergone transsphenoidal surgery for a pituitary adenoma. In the postoperative period, which action should the nurse teach the client to take?

1. Cough and deep breathe hourly.
2. Remove the nasal packing after 48 hours.
3. Report frequent swallowing or postnasal drip.
4. Take acetaminophen (Tylenol) for severe headache.

Level of Cognitive Ability: Applying
Client Needs: Physiological Integrity
Integrated Process: Teaching and Learning
Content Area: Adult Health: Neurological
Priority Concepts: Client Education; Intracranial Regulation

Answer: 3
Rationale: The client should report frequent swallowing or postnasal drip or nasal drainage after transsphenoidal surgery because it could indicate cerebrospinal fluid (CSF) leakage. The client should deep breathe, but coughing is contraindicated because it could cause increased intracranial pressure. The surgeon removes the nasal packing placed during surgery, usually after 24 hours. The client should also report severe headache because it could indicate increased intracranial pressure.
Priority Nursing Tip: After transsphenoidal surgery for a pituitary adenoma, assess nasal drainage for quantity, quality, and the presence of glucose, which indicates that the drainage is cerebrospinal fluid.
Test-Taking Strategy: Focus on the subject, transsphenoidal surgery. Think about the anatomical location of this surgical procedure. Recalling that the concern is increased intracranial pressure and CSF leakage will direct you to the correct option. Review: care of the client after **transsphenoidal surgery.**
Reference(s): Ignatavicius, Workman (2013), p. 1377.

339. A client is receiving desmopressin (DDAVP) intranasally for management of diabetes insipidus. Which assessment parameters should the nurse check to determine the **effectiveness** of this medication?

1. Daily weight
2. Temperature
3. Apical heart rate
4. Pupillary response

Level of Cognitive Ability: Evaluating
Client Needs: Physiological Integrity
Integrated Process: Nursing Process/Evaluation
Content Area: Pharmacology: Endocrine Medications
Priority Concepts: Fluid and Electrolyte Balance; Safety

Answer: 1
Rationale: DDAVP is an analog of vasopressin (antidiuretic hormone). It is used in the management of diabetes insipidus. The nurse monitors the client's fluid balance to determine the effectiveness of the medication. Fluid status can be evaluated by noting intake and urine output, daily weight, and the presence of edema. The measurements in options 2, 3, and 4 are not related to this medication.
Priority Nursing Tip: Monitor the client taking desmopressin (DDAVP) for signs of water intoxication (drowsiness, listlessness, shortness of breath, headache), indicating the need to decrease the dosage.
Test-Taking Strategy: Focus on the subject, desmopressin (DDAVP). Note the strategic word, *effectiveness.* Noting the client's diagnosis and recalling the pathophysiology associated with this diagnosis will direct you to the correct option. Review: **desmopressin (DDAVP).**
Reference(s): Hodgson, Kizior (2014), pp. 330-331; Ignatavicius, Workman (2013), p. 1379.

340. As the nurse brings the 10:00 AM doses of furosemide (Lasix) and nifedipine (Procardia) into the room of an assigned client, the client asks the nurse for a dose of aluminum hydroxide (AlternaGEL), which is prescribed on a PRN basis for dyspepsia. Which action by the nurse would be **best**?

1. Assess the client's need for the antacid.
2. Administer all three medications at the same time.
3. Administer the nifedipine and aluminum hydroxide, then the furosemide 1 hour later.
4. Administer the furosemide and aluminum hydroxide, then the nifedipine 1 hour later.

Level of Cognitive Ability: Applying
Client Needs: Physiological Integrity
Integrated Process: Nursing Process/Implementation
Content Area: Pharmacology: Cardiovascular Medications
Priority Concepts: Clinical Judgment; Safety

Answer: 1
Rationale: Antacids such as aluminum hydroxide often interfere with the absorption of other medications. For this reason, antacids should be separated from other medications by at least 1 hour. Because of the diuretic action of the furosemide and the antihypertensive action of the nifedipine, it is important to administer them on time if the client can tolerate waiting for the aluminum hydroxide. The nurse should assess the client to determine the need for the antacid. Therefore, options 2, 3, and 4 are incorrect.
Priority Nursing Tip: Always check medication interactions before administering medications. Generally the client should not take an antacid with medication because it will affect the absorption of the medication.
Test-Taking Strategy: Note the strategic word, *best.* Recalling that antacids interfere with absorption of other medications will assist in eliminating options 2, 3, and 4. Also recalling that the diuretic and antihypertensive medication should be administered on time will assist in directing you to the correct option. Additionally, option 1 addresses the first step of the nursing process, assessment. Review: **aluminum hydroxide (AlternaGEL).**
Reference(s): Kee, Hayes, McCuistion (2012), p. 720; Lehne (2013), p. 996.

341. The nurse monitors the client taking amitriptyline (Elavil) for which common side
effect of this medication?
1. Diarrhea
2. Drowsiness
3. Hypertension
4. Increased salivation

Level of Cognitive Ability: Analyzing
Client Needs: Physiological Integrity
Integrated Process: Nursing Process/Assessment
Content Area: Pharmacology: Psychiatric Medi-
cations
Priority Concepts: Clinical Judgment; Safety

Answer: 2
Rationale: Common side effects of amitriptyline (a tricyclic antidepressant) include the central nervous system effects of drowsiness,
fatigue, lethargy, and sedation. Other common side effects include
dry mouth or eyes, blurred vision, hypotension, and constipation.
The nurse monitors the client for these side effects.
Priority Nursing Tip: If a tricyclic antidepressant is prescribed,
instruct the client to avoid driving or other activities requiring alertness until the response to the medication is known.
Test-Taking Strategy: Focus on the subject, side effect of amitriptyline (Elavil). Recalling that amitriptyline is an antidepressant will
lead you to the correct option. Review: **amitriptyline (Elavil).**
Reference(s): Hodgson, Kizior (2014), p. 54.

342. A client has been admitted to the mental
health unit on a voluntary basis. The client
has reported a history of depression over the
past 5 years. Which question by the nurse
would elicit the **most** thorough assessment
data regarding the client's recent sleeping
patterns?
1. "Are you sleeping well at home?"
2. "Did you get much sleep last night?"
3. "Tell me about your sleeping patterns."
4. "You look as if you could use some sleep."

Level of Cognitive Ability: Analyzing
Client Needs: Physiological Integrity
Integrated Process: Nursing Process/Assessment
Content Area: Mental Health
Priority Concepts: Clinical Judgment; Commu-
nication

Answer: 3
Rationale: Option 3 is an open-ended question and provides the client the opportunity to express thoughts and feelings. Options 1 and
2 could lead to a one-word answer that would not provide thorough
assessment data. Additionally, one night of sleep may not tell the
nurse how the pattern has been over time. Anyone may or may not
sleep well for one night, and that sleep or loss of sleep does not indicate a problem. Option 4 could be interpreted by the depressed person as a negative statement and could block communication needed
for a thorough assessment.
Priority Nursing Tip: Adequate sleep is essential for the client with
depression because fatigue can worsen the feelings associated with
depression.
Test-Taking Strategy: Focus on the subject, therapeutic communication during a sleeping pattern assessment. Note the strategic word,
most. Use the therapeutic communication techniques. Select the
option that is open-ended and allows the client to take the lead in
the conversation. This will direct you to the correct option. Review:
therapeutic communication techniques.
Reference(s): Fortinash, Holoday-Worret (2012), pp. 71-74; Stuart
(2013), pp. 294, 300-301.

343. A client is admitted to the emergency department with drug-induced anxiety related to
overingestion of prescribed antipsychotic
medication. The **most important** piece of
information the nurse should obtain **initially** would be which data?
1. Name of the nearest relative and his or her
phone number
2. Name of the ingested medication and the
amount ingested
3. Cause of the attempt and if the client plans
another attempt
4. Length of time on the medication and any
noted side effects

Level of Cognitive Ability: Analyzing
Client Needs: Physiological Integrity
Integrated Process: Nursing Process/Assessment
Content Area: Critical Care: Emergency Situations
Priority Concepts: Clinical Judgment; Safety

Answer: 2
Rationale: In an emergency, lifesaving facts are obtained first. The
name of and the amount of medication ingested is of utmost importance in treating this potentially life-threatening situation. The relatives and the reason for the suicide attempt are not the most important
initial assessment information. The length of time on the medication
is also not the priority in this situation.
Priority Nursing Tip: Extrapyramidal side effects can occur in the client taking an antipsychotic medication.
Test-Taking Strategy: Note the strategic words, *most important* and
initially. Lifesaving treatment cannot begin until the medication and
amount are identified. Review: care of the client with a **drug overdose.**
Reference(s): Dolan, Holt (2013), p. 52; Fortinash, Holoday-Worret
(2012), pp. 347, 349-350.

344. The nurse determines that a client understands the purpose of a phytonadione (vitamin K) injection for her newborn if the client states that vitamin K is administered for which purpose?
1. Newborns lack vitamins.
2. Newborns have low blood levels.
3. Newborns lack intestinal bacteria.
4. Newborns cannot produce vitamin K in the liver.

Level of Cognitive Ability: Evaluating
Client Needs: Physiological Integrity
Integrated Process: Nursing Process/Evaluation
Content Area: Maternity: Newborn
Priority Concepts: Clotting; Development

Answer: 3
Rationale: The absence of normal flora needed to synthesize vitamin K in the normal newborn gut results in low levels of vitamin K and creates a transient blood coagulation deficiency between the second and fifth day of life. From a low point at about 2 to 3 days after birth, these coagulation factors rise slowly, but do not approach normal adult levels until 9 months of age or later. Increasing levels of these vitamin K–dependent factors indicate a response to dietary intake and bacterial colonization of the intestines. An injection is administered prophylactically on the day of birth to combat the deficiency. Options 1, 2, and 4 are incorrect.
Priority Nursing Tip: In the newborn, vitamin K (phytonadione) is administered in the lateral aspect of the middle third of the vastus lateralis muscle of the thigh.
Test-Taking Strategy: Focus on the subject, the purpose of administering vitamin K (phytonadione) injection to a newborn. Recalling the physiology associated with the synthesis of vitamin K in the newborn will direct you to the correct option. Review: the purpose of administering **vitamin K to the newborn.**
Reference(s): McKinney et al (2013), p. 509.

345. The nurse is assigned to give a child a tepid tub bath to treat hyperthermia. After the bath, which action should the nurse take?
1. Leave the child uncovered for 15 minutes.
2. Assist the child to put on a cotton sleep shirt.
3. Take the child's axillary temperature in 2 hours.
4. Place the child in bed and cover the child with a blanket.

Level of Cognitive Ability: Applying
Client Needs: Physiological Integrity
Integrated Process: Nursing Process/Implementation
Content Area: Child Health: Metabolic/Endocrine
Priority Concepts: Clinical Judgment; Thermoregulation

Answer: 2
Rationale: Cotton is a lightweight material that will protect the child from becoming chilled after the bath. Option 1 is incorrect because the child should not be left uncovered. Option 3 is incorrect because the child's temperature should be reassessed a half hour after the bath. Option 4 is incorrect because a blanket is heavy and may increase the child's body temperature and further increase metabolism.
Priority Nursing Tip: Aspirin (acetylsalicylic acid) should not be administered to a child unless specifically prescribed because of the risk of Reye's syndrome.
Test-Taking Strategy: Focus on the subject, to treat hyperthermia. Eliminate option 1 because of the word "uncovered." Eliminate option 3 because of the time frame. Eliminate option 4 because of the word "blanket." Review: care of a child with **hyperthermia.**
Reference(s): Hockenberry, Wilson (2013), p. 651.

346. The nurse is caring for an infant who has diarrhea. The nurse should monitor the infant for which **early** sign of dehydration?
1. Cool extremities
2. Gray, mottled skin
3. Capillary refill of 3 seconds
4. Apical pulse rate of 200 beats per minute

Level of Cognitive Ability: Analyzing
Client Needs: Physiological Integrity
Integrated Process: Nursing Process/Assessment
Content Area: Child Health: Metabolic/Endocrine
Priority Concepts: Development; Fluid and Electrolyte Balance

Answer: 4
Rationale: Dehydration causes interstitial fluid to shift to the vascular compartment in an attempt to maintain fluid volume. When the body is unable to compensate for fluid lost, circulatory failure occurs. The blood pressure will decrease and the pulse rate will increase. This will be followed by peripheral symptoms. Options 1, 2, and 3 are not early signs, and these assessment findings relate to peripheral circulatory status.
Priority Nursing Tip: Acute diarrhea is a cause of dehydration, particularly in children younger than 5 years.
Test-Taking Strategy: Note the strategic word, *early,* and think about the physiology that occurs in dehydration. Also note that options 1, 2, and 3 are comparable or alike and relate directly to peripheral circulatory status. Review: the early signs of **dehydration** in an infant
Reference(s): Hockenberry, Wilson (2013), p. 771; McKinney et al (2013), p. 808; Potter et al (2013), p. 457.

347. Acetylsalicylic acid (aspirin) is prescribed for a client with coronary artery disease before a percutaneous transluminal coronary angioplasty (PTCA). The nurse administers the medication, understanding that it is prescribed for what purpose?
1. Relieve postprocedure pain
2. Prevent thrombus formation
3. Prevent postprocedure hyperthermia
4. Prevent inflammation of the puncture site

Level of Cognitive Ability: Applying
Client Needs: Physiological Integrity
Integrated Process: Nursing Process/Implementation
Content Area: Adult Health: Cardiovascular
Priority Concepts: Clotting; Perfusion

Answer: 2
Rationale: Before PTCA, the client is usually given an anticoagulant, commonly aspirin, to help reduce the risk of occlusion of the artery during the procedure because the aspirin inhibits platelet aggregation. Options 1, 3, and 4 are unrelated to the purpose of administering aspirin to this client.
Priority Nursing Tip: A daily dose of acetylsalicylic acid (aspirin) may be prescribed after percutaneous transluminal coronary angioplasty because of its antiplatelet aggregation properties.
Test-Taking Strategy: Focus on the **subject**, aspirin prescribed to a client before percutaneous transluminal coronary angioplasty (PTCA). Think about the potential complications of a PTCA and the action and properties of aspirin to direct you to the correct option. Review: **aspirin and the percutaneous transluminal coronary angioplasty (PTCA).**
Reference(s): Hodgson, Kizior (2014), pp. 83-85; Ignatavicius, Workman (2013), pp. 844-845.

348. The nurse reviews a health care provider's prescriptions and notes that a topical nitrate is prescribed. The nurse notes that acetaminophen (Tylenol) is also prescribed to be administered before the nitrate. The nurse implements the prescription, with which understanding about why acetaminophen is prescribed?
1. Headache is a common side effect of nitrates.
2. Fever usually accompanies myocardial infarction.
3. Acetaminophen potentiates the therapeutic effect of nitrates.
4. Acetaminophen does not interfere with platelet action as acetylsalicylic acid (aspirin) does.

Level of Cognitive Ability: Applying
Client Needs: Physiological Integrity
Integrated Process: Nursing Process/Implementation
Content Area: Pharmacology: Cardiovascular Medications
Priority Concepts: Clinical Judgment; Safety

Answer: 1
Rationale: Headache occurs as a side effect of nitrates in many clients. Acetaminophen may be administered before nitrates to prevent headaches or minimize the discomfort from the headaches. Options 2, 3, and 4 are incorrect.
Priority Nursing Tip: Nitrates produce vasodilation, which can cause a headache. Although headaches are a common side effect of nitrates, they may become less frequent with continued use.
Test-Taking Strategy: Focus on the **subject**, nitrate administration. Eliminate option 3 first because this is an incorrect statement. Whereas options 2 and 4 are true statements, they do not address the **subject** of the question. Also recalling that headache is a common side effect of nitrates will direct you to the correct option. Review: the side effects of **nitrates** and the purpose of administering **acetaminophen (Tylenol)** before these medications.
Reference(s): Dolan, Holt (2013), p. 298; Hodgson, Kizior (2014), pp. 845-847.

❖ **349.** The nurse performs an assessment on a client newly diagnosed with rheumatoid arthritis. The nurse expects to note which **early** manifestations of the disease? **Select all that apply.**
❑ 1. Fatigue
❑ 2. Anorexia
❑ 3. Weakness
❑ 4. Low-grade fever
❑ 5. Joint deformities
❑ 6. Joint inflammation

Level of Cognitive Ability: Analyzing
Client Needs: Physiological Integrity
Integrated Process: Nursing Process/Assessment
Content Area: Adult Health: Musculoskeletal
Priority Concepts: Functional Ability; Mobility

Answer: 1, 2, 3, 4, 6
Rationale: Rheumatoid arthritis is a chronic, progressive, systemic inflammatory autoimmune disease process that primarily affects the synovial joints. It also affects other joints and body tissues. Early manifestations include fatigue, anorexia, weakness, joint inflammation, low-grade fever and paresthesia. Joint deformities are late manifestations.
Priority Nursing Tip: For rheumatoid arthritis, the earlier treatment is begun, the slower the progression of the disease. Treatment includes exercise, physical therapy, medications, and possibly surgery.
Test-Taking Strategy: Focus on the **subject**, manifestations of rheumatoid arthritis and note the **strategic word**, *early*. Keeping this word in mind will assist in eliminating option 5, because joint deformities are late manifestations. Review: the early and late manifestations of **rheumatoid arthritis.**
Reference(s): Ignatavicius, Workman (2013), p. 334.

350. A client taking warfarin sodium (Coumadin) has been instructed to limit the intake of foods high in vitamin K. The nurse determines that the client understands the instructions if the client indicates that which food items need to be avoided? **Select all that apply.**
- ☐ 1. Tea
- ☐ 2. Turnips
- ☐ 3. Oranges
- ☐ 4. Cabbage
- ☐ 5. Broccoli
- ☐ 6. Strawberries

Level of Cognitive Ability: Evaluating
Client Needs: Physiological Integrity
Integrated Process: Nursing Process/Evaluation
Content Area: Pharmacology: Hematological Medications
Priority Concepts: Clotting; Nutrition

Answer: 1, 2, 4, 5
Rationale: Warfarin sodium is an anticoagulant that interferes with the hepatic synthesis of vitamin K–dependent clotting factors. The client is instructed to limit the intake of foods high in vitamin K while taking this medication. These foods include coffee or tea (caffeine), turnips, cabbage, broccoli, greens, fish, and liver. Oranges and strawberries are high in vitamin C.
Priority Nursing Tip: Warfarin sodium (Coumadin) is an anticoagulant and bleeding is a concern when this medication is administered.
Test-Taking Strategy: Focus on the subject, foods high in vitamin K. Knowledge regarding the foods high in vitamin K is needed to answer correctly. However, note that options 3 and 6 are comparable or alike in that they are both fruits. Review: the foods high in vitamin K.
Reference(s): Hodgson, Kizior (2014), pp. 1262-1263; Ignatavicius, Workman (2013), p. 803; Nix (2013), p. 105.

351. The nurse is caring for a newly delivered breast-feeding infant. Which intervention performed by the nurse would **best** prevent jaundice in this infant?
1. Placing the infant under phototherapy
2. Keeping the infant NPO until the second period of reactivity
3. Encouraging the mother to breast-feed the infant every 2 to 3 hours
4. Encouraging the mother to offer a formula supplement after each breast-feeding session

Level of Cognitive Ability: Applying
Client Needs: Physiological Integrity
Integrated Process: Nursing Process/Implementation
Content Area: Maternity: Newborn
Priority Concepts: Development; Safety

Answer: 3
Rationale: To help prevent jaundice, the mother should feed the infant frequently in the immediate birth period because colostrum is a natural laxative and helps promote the passage of meconium. Breast-feeding should begin as soon as possible after birth while the infant is in the first period of reactivity. Delaying breast-feeding decreases the production of prolactin, which decreases the mother's milk production. Phototherapy requires a health care provider's prescription and is not implemented until bilirubin levels are 12 mg/dL or higher in the healthy term infant. Offering the infant a formula supplement will cause nipple confusion and decrease the amount of milk produced by the mother.
Priority Nursing Tip: The appearance of jaundice in the first 24 hours of life is abnormal and must be reported to the health care provider.
Test-Taking Strategy: Focus on the subject, newborn jaundice. Recalling the physiology associated with jaundice and noting the strategic word, *best*, will assist in eliminating options 1 and 2. From the remaining options, select the correct option based on the fact that offering a formula supplement will cause nipple confusion. Review: the interventions to prevent jaundice.
Reference(s): Lowdermilk, Perry, Cashion, Alden (2012), p. 621; McKinney et al (2013), p. 540.

352. The nurse develops a postoperative plan of care for a client undergoing an arthroscopy. The nurse should include which **priority** action in the plan?
1. Monitor intake and output.
2. Assess the tissue at the surgical site.
3. Monitor the area for numbness or tingling.
4. Assess the complete blood cell count results.

Level of Cognitive Ability: Applying
Client Needs: Physiological Integrity
Integrated Process: Nursing Process/Planning
Content Area: Adult Health: Musculoskeletal
Priority Concepts: Perfusion; Safety

Answer: 3
Rationale: Arthroscopy provides an endoscopic examination of the joint and is used to diagnose and treat acute and chronic disorders of the joint. The priority nursing action is to monitor the affected area for numbness or tingling. Options 1, 2, and 4 are also components of postoperative care, but from the options presented, are not the initial priorities.
Priority Nursing Tip: Assessment of neurovascular status of an extremity includes checking distal pulses, capillary refill, warmth, presence of pain, color, movement, and sensation.
Test-Taking Strategy: Note the strategic word, *priority.* Use the ABCs—airway, breathing, and circulation—to answer the question. The correct option relates to circulation. Review: nursing care following **arthroscopy.**
Reference(s): Ignatavicius, Workman (2013), pp. 1116-1117.

353. The nurse is caring for a client with active tuberculosis who has started medication therapy that includes rifampin (Rifadin). The nurse instructs the client to expect which side effect of this medication?
1. Bilious urine
2. Yellow sclera
3. Orange secretions
4. Clay-colored stools

Level of Cognitive Ability: Applying
Client Needs: Physiological Integrity
Integrated Process: Teaching and Learning
Content Area: Pharmacology: Respiratory Medications
Priority Concepts: Client Education; Safety

Answer: 3
Rationale: Rifampin (Rifadin) is an antituberculosis medication. Secretions will become orange in color as a result of the rifampin. The client should be instructed that this side effect will likely occur and should be told that soft contact lenses, if used by the client, will become permanently discolored. Options 1, 2, and 4 are not expected effects.
Priority Nursing Tip: Rifampin (Rifadin) is hepatotoxic and the client needs to notify the health care provider if jaundice (yellow eyes or skin) occurs.
Test-Taking Strategy: Focus on the subject, Rifampin (Rifadin) to answer this question. Eliminate options 1, 2, and 4 because they are comparable or alike in that they are all symptoms of intrahepatic obstruction as seen in viral hepatitis. Review: the side effects of **rifampin (Rifadin).**
Reference(s): Hodgson, Kizior (2014), p. 1038.

354. The nurse sends a sputum specimen to the laboratory for culture from a client with suspected active tuberculosis (TB). The results report that *Mycobacterium tuberculosis* is cultured. How should the nurse correctly analyze these results?
1. The results are positive for active tuberculosis.
2. The results indicate a less virulent strain of tuberculosis.
3. The results are inconclusive until a repeat sputum specimen is sent.
4. The results are unreliable unless the client has also had a positive Mantoux test.

Level of Cognitive Ability: Analyzing
Client Needs: Physiological Integrity
Integrated Process: Nursing Process/Analysis
Content Area: Adult Health: Respiratory
Priority Concepts: Clinical Judgment; Infection

Answer: 1
Rationale: Culture of *Mycobacterium tuberculosis* from sputum or other body secretions or tissue confirms the diagnosis of active tuberculosis. Options 2 and 3 are incorrect statements. The Mantoux test is performed to assist in diagnosing TB but does not confirm active disease.
Priority Nursing Tip: The client with active tuberculosis is placed in respiratory isolation precautions in a negative-pressure room.
Test-Taking Strategy: Focus on the subject, tuberculosis. Recall that culture of the bacteria from sputum confirms the diagnosis. Because tuberculosis affects the respiratory system, it would make sense that the bacteria would be found in the sputum if the client had active disease, thereby confirming the diagnosis. Review: the diagnostic tests associated with **active tuberculosis (TB).**
Reference(s): Ignatavicius, Workman (2013), p. 653.

355. A coronary care unit (CCU) nurse is caring for a client admitted with acute myocardial infarction (MI). The nurse should monitor the client for which **most** common complication of MI?
1. Heart failure
2. Cardiogenic shock
3. Cardiac dysrhythmias
4. Recurrent myocardial infarction

Level of Cognitive Ability: Analyzing
Client Needs: Physiological Integrity
Integrated Process: Nursing Process/Assessment
Content Area: Critical Care: Emergency Situations
Priority Concepts: Clinical Judgment; Perfusion

Answer: 3
Rationale: Dysrhythmias are the most common complication and cause of death after an MI. Heart failure, cardiogenic shock, and recurrent MI are also complications but occur less frequently.
Priority Nursing Tip: Administering morphine sulfate as prescribed is a priority in managing pain in the client having a myocardial infarction. Pain relief increases oxygen supply to the myocardium.
Test-Taking Strategy: Note the strategic word, *most*. Think about the pathophysiology associated with MI and the complications of MI to direct you to the correct option. Review: the complications of myocardial infarction (MI).
Reference(s): Ignatavicius, Workman (2013), p. 835.

356. The nurse in the newborn nursery is planning for the admission of a large for gestational age (LGA) infant. In preparing to care for this infant, the nurse should obtain equipment to perform which diagnostic test?
1. Serum insulin level
2. Heel stick blood glucose
3. Rh and ABO blood typing
4. Indirect and direct bilirubin levels

Level of Cognitive Ability: Applying
Client Needs: Physiological Integrity
Integrated Process: Nursing Process/Planning
Content Area: Maternity: Newborn
Priority Concepts: Development; Glucose Regulation

Answer: 2
Rationale: After birth, the most common problem in the LGA infant is hypoglycemia, especially if the mother is diabetic. At delivery when the umbilical cord is clamped and cut, maternal blood glucose supply is lost. The newborn continues to produce large amounts of insulin, which depletes the infant's blood glucose within the first hours after birth. If immediate identification and treatment of hypoglycemia are not performed, the newborn may suffer central nervous system damage caused by inadequate circulation of glucose to the brain. Serum insulin levels are not helpful because there is no intervention to decrease these levels to prevent hypoglycemia. There is no rationale for prescribing an Rh and ABO blood type unless the maternal blood type is O or Rh negative. Indirect and direct bilirubin levels are usually prescribed after the first 24 hours because jaundice is usually seen at 48 to 72 hours after birth.
Priority Nursing Tip: Feedings should be provided to the large for gestational age (LGA) newborn soon after birth because of the risk for hypoglycemia in the infant.
Test-Taking Strategy: Focus on the subject, an LGA infant. Recalling that hypoglycemia is the concern will direct you to the correct option. Review: care of the large for gestational age (LGA) infant.
Reference(s): McKinney et al (2013), pp. 494, 712, 728-729.

❖ **357.** The nurse caring for a client receiving intravenous therapy monitors for which signs of infiltration of an intravenous (IV) infusion? **Select all that apply.**
❑ 1. Slowing of the IV rate
❑ 2. Tenderness at the insertion site
❑ 3. Edema around the insertion site
❑ 4. Skin tightness at the insertion site
❑ 5. Warmth of skin at the insertion site
❑ 6. Fluid leaking from the insertion site

Level of Cognitive Ability: Analyzing
Client Needs: Physiological Integrity
Integrated Process: Nursing Process/Assessment
Content Area: Critical Care: Medications and Intravenous Therapy
Priority Concepts: Tissue Integrity; Safety

Answer: 1, 2, 3, 4, 6
Rationale: Infiltration is the leakage of an IV solution into the extravascular tissue. Manifestations include slowing of the IV rate; burning, tenderness, or general discomfort at the insertion site; increasing edema in or around the catheter insertion site; complaints of skin tightness; blanching or coolness of the skin; and fluid leaking from the insertion site.
Priority Nursing Tip: Infiltration at an intravenous site produces coolness of the skin, whereas phlebitis at an intravenous site produces warmth of the skin.
Test-Taking Strategy: Focus on the subject, IV infiltration. Read each option, thinking about the characteristics of infiltration. Recalling that infiltration is the leakage of an IV solution into the extravascular tissue will assist in eliminating option 5. Remember that fluid infusing into tissue will result in coolness, not warmth. Review: the manifestations of **infiltration**.
Reference(s): Ignatavicius, Workman (2013), p. 228.

358. A client receiving total parenteral nutrition (TPN) through a subclavian catheter suddenly develops dyspnea, tachycardia, cyanosis, and decreased level of consciousness. Based on these findings, which is the **best** intervention for the nurse to implement for the client?
1. Obtain a stat oxygen saturation level.
2. Examine the insertion site for redness.
3. Perform a stat finger-stick glucose level.
4. Turn the client to the left side in Trendelenburg's position.

Level of Cognitive Ability: Analyzing
Client Needs: Physiological Integrity
Integrated Process: Nursing Process/Analysis
Content Area: Critical Care: Emergency Situations
Priority Concepts: Gas Exchange; Perfusion

Answer: 4
Rationale: Clinical indicators of air embolism include chest pain, tachycardia, dyspnea, anxiety, feelings of impending doom, cyanosis, and hypotension. Positioning the client in Trendelenburg's and on the left side helps isolate the air embolism in the right atrium and prevents a thromboembolic event in a vital organ. Monitoring the oxygen saturation is a reasonable nursing response to the client's condition; however, acting to prevent deterioration in the client's condition is more important than obtaining additional client data. Options 2 and 3 are unrelated to the symptoms identified in the question.
Priority Nursing Tip: Measures that prevent air embolism from an intravenous (IV) infusion include priming the tubing with fluid before use, securing all connections, and replacing the IV fluid before the container is empty.
Test-Taking Strategy: Focus on the subject, air embolism, and note the strategic word, *best*. Note the assessment findings in the question and recall that the signs of air embolism are similar to those experienced with pulmonary embolism. Then analyze the options to determine the one that is the best in this situation, which will direct you to the correct option. Review: the signs of **air embolism** and the immediate nursing interventions.
Reference(s): Ignatavicius, Workman (2013), p. 231.

359. A client has a total serum calcium level of 7.5 mg/dL. Which clinical manifestations should the nurse expect to note on assessment of the client? **Select all that apply.**
☐ 1. Constipation
☐ 2. Muscle twitches
☐ 3. Hypoactive bowel sounds
☐ 4. Hyperactive deep tendon reflexes
☐ 5. Positive Trousseau's sign and positive Chvostek's sign
☐ 6. Prolonged ST interval and QT interval on electrocardiogram (ECG)

Level of Cognitive Ability: Analyzing
Client Needs: Physiological Integrity
Integrated Process: Nursing Process/Assessment
Content Area: Fundamental Skills: Fluids & Electrolytes
Priority Concepts: Clinical Judgment; Fluid and Electrolyte Balance

Answer: 2, 4, 5, 6
Rationale: Hypocalcemia is a total serum calcium level less than 8.6 mg/dL. Clinical manifestations of hypocalcemia include decreased heart rate, diminished peripheral pulses, hypotension, and prolonged ST interval and QT interval on ECG. Neuromuscular manifestations include anxiety and irritability; paresthesia followed by numbness; muscle twitches, cramps, tetany, and seizures; hyperactive deep tendon reflexes; and positive Trousseau's and Chvostek's signs. Gastrointestinal manifestations include increased gastric motility, hyperactive bowel sounds, abdominal cramping, and diarrhea.
Priority Nursing Tip: Calcium gluconate 10% may be prescribed to treat acute calcium deficit.
Test-Taking Strategy: Focus on the subject, hypocalcemia. Note the data in the question and the calcium level. First determine that the level is low and the client is experiencing hypocalcemia. Next think about the manifestations associated with hypocalcemia. Remember that hyperactive bowel sounds and diarrhea occur in hypocalcemia. Review: the manifestations of **hypocalcemia**.
Reference(s): Ignatavicius, Workman (2013), pp. 188-189.

360. A client is experiencing acute cardiac and cerebral symptoms as a result of an excess fluid volume. Which measures should the nurse implement to increase the client's comfort until specific therapy is prescribed by the health care provider?
1. Measure urine output on an hourly basis.
2. Measure intravenous and oral fluid intake.
3. Elevate the client's head to at least 45 degrees.
4. Administer oxygen at 4 liters per minute by nasal cannula.

Level of Cognitive Ability: Applying
Client Needs: Physiological Integrity
Integrated Process: Nursing Process/Implementation
Content Area: Critical Care: Emergency Situations
Priority Concepts: Caregiving; Perfusion

Answer: 3
Rationale: Elevating the head of the bed to 45 degrees decreases venous return to the heart from the lower body, thus reducing the volume of blood that has to be pumped by the heart. It also promotes venous drainage from the brain, reducing cerebral symptoms. Intake and output should be monitored and recorded to provide current information about the client's volume status but this measure will not increase the client's comfort. Oxygen is a medication and is not administered without a prescription to do so. Options 1, 2, and 4 are important measures, although they do not improve the client's comfort.
Priority Nursing Tip: A client with kidney failure is at high risk for fluid volume excess.
Test-Taking Strategy: Focus on the subject, measures to increase the client's comfort. This tells you that the correct option is one that directly involves care delivery to the client. With this in mind, eliminate options 1 and 2 because they are assessment measures and will not improve the condition of the client. From the remaining options, note that the correct option identifies the nursing measure. Review: care of the client with **excess fluid volume.**
Reference(s): Ignatavicius, Workman (2013), p. 179; Potter et al (2013), p. 1022.

361. The nurse develops a discharge plan for a client who had a total abdominal hysterectomy. Which activity instructions should the nurse include in the plan? **Select all that apply.**
❑ 1. Avoid heavy lifting.
❑ 2. Sit as much as possible.
❑ 3. Take baths rather than showers.
❑ 4. Limit stair climbing to five times a day.
❑ 5. Gradually increase walking as exercise but stop before becoming fatigued.
❑ 6. Avoid jogging, aerobic exercises, sports, or any strenuous exercise for 6 weeks.

Level of Cognitive Ability: Analyzing
Client Needs: Physiological Integrity
Integrated Process: Nursing Process/Planning
Content Area: Fundamental Skills: Perioperative Care
Priority Concepts: Client Education; Safety

Answer: 1, 4, 5, 6
Rationale: After a total abdominal hysterectomy, the client should avoiding lifting anything that is heavy and limit stair climbing to five times a day. The client should walk indoors for the first week and then gradually increase walking as exercise, but stop before becoming fatigued. The client should avoiding jogging, aerobic exercises, sports, or any strenuous exercise for 6 weeks. The client is also told to avoid the sitting position for extended periods, to take showers rather than tub baths, avoid crossing the legs at the knees, and avoid driving for at least 4 weeks or until the surgeon has given permission to do so.
Priority Nursing Tip: Monitor vaginal bleeding after hysterectomy. More than one saturated pad per hour may indicate excessive bleeding.
Test-Taking Strategy: Focus on the subject, activity instructions following abdominal hysterectomy. Read each option carefully, focusing on the type and location of the surgery and the importance of protecting the surgical area. This will assist in eliminating options 2 and 3. Review: activity instructions after **total abdominal hysterectomy.**
Reference(s): Ignatavicius, Workman (2013), p. 1620.

362. The nurse has a prescription to ambulate a client with a nephrostomy tube in the hall four times a day. The nurse determines that the safest way to accomplish this while maintaining the integrity of the nephrostomy tube is to carry out which intervention?

1. Change the drainage bag to a leg collection bag.
2. Tie the drainage bag to the client's waist while ambulating.
3. Use a walker to hang the drainage bag from while ambulating.
4. Tell the client to hold the drainage bag higher than the level of the bladder.

Level of Cognitive Ability: Analyzing
Client Needs: Physiological Integrity
Integrated Process: Nursing Process/Planning
Content Area: Adult Health: Renal and Urinary
Priority Concepts: Elimination; Safety

Answer: 1
Rationale: The safest approach to protect the integrity and safety of the nephrostomy tube with a mobile client is to attach the tube to a leg collection bag. This allows for greater freedom of movement, while preventing accidental disconnection or dislodgment. The drainage bag is kept below the level of the bladder. Option 3 presents the risk of tension or pulling on the nephrostomy tube by the client during ambulation.
Priority Nursing Tip: The total bladder capacity for an adult is 600 to 800 mL, and the normal urine output is 1500 to 2000 mL a day.
Test-Taking Strategy: Focus on the subject, safety in regard to a nephrostomy tube. Note that options 2, 3, and 4 are comparable or alike because they all indicate placing the drainage bag above the level of the bladder. Review: care of the client with a **nephrostomy tube.**
Reference(s): Potter et al (2013), pp. 1063, 1065.

363. A client newly diagnosed with polycystic kidney disease has just finished speaking with the health care provider about the disorder. The client asks the nurse to explain again what the **most** serious complication of the disorder might be. In formulating a response, the nurse indicates that which is the **most** serious complication?

1. Diabetes insipidus
2. End-stage renal disease (ESRD)
3. Chronic urinary tract infection (UTI)
4. Syndrome of inappropriate antidiuretic hormone secretion (SIADH)

Level of Cognitive Ability: Applying
Client Needs: Physiological Integrity
Integrated Process: Nursing Process/Implementation
Content Area: Adult Health: Renal and Urinary
Priority Concepts: Client Education; Elimination

Answer: 2
Rationale: In polycystic kidney disease, cystic formation and hypertrophy of the kidneys occur. The most serious complication of polycystic kidney disease is ESRD, which is managed with dialysis or transplant. There is no reliable way to predict who will ultimately progress to ESRD. Chronic UTIs are the most common complication because of the altered anatomy of the kidney and from development of resistant strains of bacteria. Diabetes insipidus and SIADH secretion are unrelated disorders.
Priority Nursing Tip: The nurse should discuss the importance of seeking genetic counseling with the client diagnosed with polycystic kidney disease because the disease is hereditary.
Test-Taking Strategy: Note the strategic word, *most.* Also noting the words "end-stage" and recalling that ESRD is life threatening and requires dialysis for treatment will direct you to the correct option. Review: the complications of **polycystic kidney disease.**
Reference(s): Ignatavicius, Workman (2013), pp. 1518, 1521-1522.

❖ **364.** The nurse is developing a plan of care for a client who has returned to the nursing unit after left nephrectomy. Which assessments should the nurse include in the plan of care? **Select all that apply.**
- ❑ 1. Pain level
- ❑ 2. Vital signs
- ❑ 3. Hourly urine output
- ❑ 4. Tolerance for sips of clear liquids
- ❑ 5. Ability to cough and deep breathe

Level of Cognitive Ability: Analyzing
Client Needs: Physiological Integrity
Integrated Process: Nursing Process/Assessment
Content Area: Adult Health: Renal and Urinary
Priority Concepts: Clinical Judgment; Elimination

Answer: 1, 2, 3, 5
Rationale: After nephrectomy, it is imperative to measure the urine output on an hourly basis. This is done to monitor the effectiveness of the remaining kidney and detect renal failure early, if it should occur. The client may also experience significant pain after this surgery, which could affect the client's ability to reposition, cough, and deep breathe. Therefore, the next most important measurements are vital signs, pain level, and ability to cough and deep breathe. Clear liquids are not given until the client has bowel sounds.
Priority Nursing Tip: After nephrectomy, monitor for a urinary output of 30 to 50 mL per hour.
Test-Taking Strategy: Focus on the subject, assessment following nephrectomy. Note the relationship between "nephrectomy" in the question and "urine output" option 3. Remember that the client may also experience significant pain after surgery, which could affect the client's ability to cough, and deep breathe. Therefore options 1, 2, and 5, vital signs, pain level, and ability to cough and deep breathe are necessary assessments after left nephrectomy. Review: care of the client after nephrectomy.
Reference(s): Ignatavicius, Workman (2013), pp. 299-300, 1510.

❖ **365.** The nurse instructs a mother of a child who had a plaster cast applied to the arm about measures that will help the cast dry. Which instructions should the nurse provide to the mother? **Select all that apply.**
- ❑ 1. Lift the cast using the fingertips.
- ❑ 2. Place the child on a firm mattress.
- ❑ 3. Direct a fan toward the cast to facilitate drying.
- ❑ 4. Support the cast and adjacent joints with pillows.
- ❑ 5. Place the extremity with the cast in a dependent position.
- ❑ 6. Reposition the extremity with the cast every 2 to 4 hours.

Level of Cognitive Ability: Applying
Client Needs: Physiological Integrity
Integrated Process: Teaching and Learning
Content Area: Child Health: Musculoskeletal
Priority Concepts: Client Education; Mobility

Answer: 2, 3, 4, 6
Rationale: To help the cast dry, the child should be placed on a firm mattress. A fan may be directed toward the cast to facilitate drying. Once the cast is dry, the cast should sound hollow and be cool to touch. The cast and adjacent joints should be elevated and supported with pillows. To ensure thorough drying, the extremity with the cast should be repositioned every 2 to 4 hours. The cast is lifted by using the palms of the hands (not the fingertips) to prevent indentation in the wet cast surface. Indentations could possibly cause pressure on the skin under the cast.
Priority Nursing Tip: Monitor the extremity with a cast for signs of circulatory impairment. If these occur, notify the health care provider immediately and prepare for bivalving and cutting the cast.
Test-Taking Strategy: Focus on the subject, measures that will help the cast dry. Eliminate option 1 because of the word "fingertips" and option 5 because of the word "dependent." Review: measures that will help a cast dry.
Reference(s): McKinney et al (2013), p. 1346.

366. A client with cancer is receiving cisplatin. On assessment of the client, which findings indicate that the client is experiencing an adverse effect of the medication?
1. Tinnitus
2. Increased appetite
3. Excessive urination
4. Yellow halos in front of the eyes

Level of Cognitive Ability: Analyzing
Client Needs: Physiological Integrity
Integrated Process: Nursing Process/Assessment
Content Area: Pharmacology: Oncological Medications
Priority Concepts: Cellular Regulation; Safety

Answer: 1
Rationale: Cisplatin is an antineoplastic medication. An adverse effect related to the administration of cisplatin is ototoxicity with hearing loss. The nurse should assess for this adverse reaction when administering this medication. Options 2, 3, and 4 are not adverse effects of this medication.
Priority Nursing Tip: Cisplatin, an antineoplastic medication, is a platinum compound and can cause ototoxicity, tinnitus, hypokalemia, hypocalcemia, hypomagnesemia, and nephrotoxicity.
Test-Taking Strategy: Focus on the subject, an adverse effect of cisplatin. Recalling that ototoxicity is an adverse effect will direct you to the correct option, the only option that relates to the ear. Review: cisplatin.
Reference(s): Hodgson, Kizior (2014), p. 205.

❖ **367.** A child is admitted to the hospital with a diagnosis of nephrotic syndrome. The nurse reads the child's medical record and expects to note documentation of which manifestations of this disorder? **Select all that apply.**
☐ 1. Edema
☐ 2. Proteinuria
☐ 3. Hypertension
☐ 4. Abdominal pain
☐ 5. Increased weight
☐ 6. Hypoalbuminemia

Level of Cognitive Ability: Analyzing
Client Needs: Physiological Integrity
Integrated Process: Nursing Process/Assessment
Content Area: Child Health: Renal and Urinary
Priority Concepts: Clinical Judgment; Elimination

Answer: 1, 2, 4, 5, 6
Rationale: Nephrotic syndrome refers to a kidney disorder characterized by edema, proteinuria, and hypoalbuminemia. The child also experiences anorexia, fatigue, abdominal pain, respiratory infection, and increased weight. The child's blood pressure is usually normal or slightly decreased.
Priority Nursing Tip: For the client with nephrotic syndrome, a regular diet without added salt may be prescribed if the child is in remission; sodium and fluids may be restricted during periods of massive edema.
Test-Taking Strategy: Focus on the subject, nephrotic syndrome. Recalling that nephrotic syndrome is characterized by proteinuria, hypoalbuminemia, and edema will assist in determining the correct options. Also remember that the blood pressure is usually normal in this condition. Review: the manifestations of **nephrotic syndrome.**
Reference(s): McKinney et al (2013), pp. 1131-1132.

368. It has been 12 hours since the client's delivery of a newborn. The nurse assesses the client for the process of involution and documents that it is progressing normally when palpation of the client's fundus is at which level?
1. At the level of the umbilicus
2. One finger breadth below the umbilicus
3. Two finger breadths below the umbilicus
4. Midway between the umbilicus and the symphysis pubis

Level of Cognitive Ability: Analyzing
Client Needs: Physiological Integrity
Integrated Process: Nursing Process/Assessment
Content Area: Maternity: Postpartum
Priority Concepts: Clinical Judgment; Reproduction

Answer: 1
Rationale: The term "involution" is used to describe the rapid reduction in size and the return of the uterus to a normal condition similar to its nonpregnant state. Immediately after the delivery of the placenta, the uterus contracts to the size of a large grapefruit. The fundus is situated in the midline between the symphysis pubis and the umbilicus. Within 6 to 12 hours after birth, the fundus of the uterus rises to the level of the umbilicus. The top of the fundus remains at the level of the umbilicus for about a day and then descends into the pelvis approximately one finger breadth on each succeeding day.
Priority Nursing Tip: By approximately 10 days postpartum, the uterus cannot be palpated abdominally.
Test-Taking Strategy: Focus on the subject, 12 hours after birth. Visualize the process of assessment of involution and the expected finding at this time to answer the question. Review: the process of involution.
Reference(s): Lowdermilk, Perry, Cashion, Alden (2012), pp. 478-479.

369. A client with a gastric tumor is scheduled for a subtotal gastrectomy (Billroth II procedure). The nurse explains the procedure to the client and tells the client that the procedure will entail which surgical tasks?
1. Proximal end of the distal stomach is anastomosed to the duodenum
2. Entire stomach is removed and the esophagus is anastomosed to the duodenum
3. Lower portion of the stomach is removed and the remainder is anastomosed to the jejunum
4. Antrum of the stomach is removed and the remaining portion is anastomosed to the duodenum

Level of Cognitive Ability: Applying
Client Needs: Physiological Integrity
Integrated Process: Nursing Process/Implementation
Content Area: Adult Health: Gastrointestinal
Priority Concepts: Client Education; Safety

Answer: 3
Rationale: In the Billroth II procedure, the lower portion of the stomach is removed and the remainder is anastomosed to the jejunum. The duodenal stump is preserved to permit bile flow to the jejunum. Options 1, 2, and 4 are incorrect descriptions.
Priority Nursing Tip: Postoperative complications after gastrectomy procedures include hemorrhage, dumping syndrome, diarrhea, hypoglycemia, and vitamin B$_{12}$ deficiency.
Test-Taking Strategy: Focus on the subject, gastrectomy (Billroth II procedure), which indicates removal of the stomach. This should assist in eliminating option 1. From the remaining options, note the word "subtotal" in the question which indicates "lower and a part of." This should direct you to the correct option. Review: the **subtotal gastrectomy (Billroth II procedure).**
Reference(s): Ignatavicius, Workman (2013), p. 1331.

370. A client with diabetes mellitus receives Humulin R regular insulin 8 units subcutaneously at 7:30 AM. The nurse should be **most** alert to signs of hypoglycemia at what time during the day?
1. 9:30 AM to 11:30 AM
2. 11:30 AM to 1:30 PM
3. 1:30 PM to 3:30 PM
4. 3:30 PM to 5:30 PM

Level of Cognitive Ability: Analyzing
Client Needs: Physiological Integrity
Integrated Process: Nursing Process/Assessment
Content Area: Pharmacology: Endocrine Medications
Priority Concepts: Clinical Judgment; Glucose Regulation

Answer: 1
Rationale: Humulin R regular insulin is a short-acting insulin. Its onset of action occurs in a half hour and peaks in 2 to 4 hours. Its duration of action is 4 to 6 hours. A hypoglycemic reaction will most likely occur at peak time, which in this situation is between 9:30 AM and 11:30 AM.
Priority Nursing Tip: Not all types of insulin can be administered by the intravenous route. Regular insulin is one type of insulin that can be administered intravenously.
Test-Taking Strategy: Note the strategic word, *most*. Recall knowledge regarding the onset, peak, and duration of action of Humulin R regular insulin to answer this question. Recalling that Humulin regular insulin is a short-acting insulin will direct you to the correct option. Review: **Humulin R regular insulin.**
Reference(s): Hodgson, Kizior (2014), pp. 613-614.

371. The nurse develops a postoperative plan of care for a client scheduled for hypophysectomy. Which interventions should be included in the plan of care? **Select all that apply.**
1. Obtain daily weights.
2. Monitor intake and output.
3. Elevate the head of the bed.
4. Use a soft toothbrush for mouth care.
5. Encourage coughing and deep breathing.

Level of Cognitive Ability: Analyzing
Client Needs: Physiological Integrity
Integrated Process: Nursing Process/Planning
Content Area: Adult Health: Endocrine
Priority Concepts: Intracranial Regulation; Safety

Answer: 1, 2, 3
Rationale: A hypophysectomy is done to remove a pituitary tumor. Because temporary diabetes insipidus or syndrome of inappropriate antidiuretic hormone can develop after this surgery, obtaining daily weights and monitoring intake and output are important interventions. The head of the bed is elevated to assist in preventing increased intracranial pressure. Toothbrushing, sneezing, coughing, nose blowing, and bending are activities that should be avoided postoperatively in the client who underwent a hypophysectomy because of the risk of increasing intracranial pressure. These activities interfere with the healing of the incision and can disrupt the graft.
Priority Nursing Tip: Increased intracranial pressure is a complication of hypophysectomy.
Test-Taking Strategy: Focus on the subject, postoperative care following hypophysectomy. Consider the anatomical location of the surgical procedure and associated complications. Although coughing and deep breathing are usually a normal component of postoperative care, in this situation, coughing is contraindicated. Additionally toothbrushing can interfere with healing. Review: care after a **hypophysectomy.**
Reference(s): Ignatavicius, Workman (2013), pp. 1376-1377.

372. A client undergoes a thyroidectomy, and the nurse monitors the client for signs of damage to the parathyroid glands postoperatively. Which findings indicate damage to the parathyroid glands?
  1. Fever
  2. Neck pain
  3. Hoarseness
  4. Tingling around the mouth

Level of Cognitive Ability: Analyzing
Client Needs: Physiological Integrity
Integrated Process: Nursing Process/Assessment
Content Area: Adult Health: Endocrine
Priority Concepts: Clinical Judgment; Fluid and Electrolyte Balance

Answer: 4
Rationale: The parathyroid glands can be damaged or their blood supply impaired during thyroid surgery. Hypocalcemia and tetany result when parathyroid hormone (PTH) levels decrease. The nurse monitors for complaints of tingling around the mouth or of the toes or fingers and muscular twitching because these are signs of calcium deficiency. Additional later signs of hypocalcemia are positive Chvostek's and Trousseau's signs. Fever may be expected in the immediate postoperative period but is not an indication of damage to the parathyroid glands. However, if a fever persists the health care provider is notified. Neck pain and hoarseness are expected findings postoperatively.
Priority Nursing Tip: After thyroidectomy, maintain the client in a semi-Fowler's position to reduce swelling at the operative site.
Test-Taking Strategy: Focus on the subject, damage to the parathyroid glands and consider the anatomical location of the surgical procedure. Recalling that neck pain and hoarseness are expected findings postoperatively will assist in eliminating options 1 and 2. From the remaining options, focusing on the subject will assist in eliminating option 3. Also, recalling that hypocalcemia results when PTH levels decrease will assist in directing you to the correct option. Review: postoperative care after **thyroidectomy** and the signs of **parathyroid damage.**
Reference(s): Ignatavicius, Workman (2013), p. 1399.

373. The nurse is performing an admission assessment for a client admitted to the hospital with a diagnosis of Raynaud's disease. The nurse assesses for the symptoms associated with Raynaud's disease by performing which actions?
  1. Checking for a rash on the digits
  2. Observing for softening of the nails or nail beds
  3. Palpating for a rapid or irregular peripheral pulse
  4. Palpating for diminished or absent peripheral pulses

Level of Cognitive Ability: Analyzing
Client Needs: Physiological Integrity
Integrated Process: Nursing Process/Assessment
Content Area: Adult Health: Cardiovascular
Priority Concepts: Clinical Judgment; Perfusion

Answer: 4
Rationale: Raynaud's disease is vasospasm of the arterioles and arteries of the upper and lower extremities. It produces closure of the small arteries in the distal extremities in response to cold, vibration, or external stimuli. Palpation for diminished or absent peripheral pulses checks for interruption of circulation. Skin changes include hair loss, thinning or tightening of the skin, and delayed healing of cuts or injuries. A rash on the digits is not a characteristic of this disorder. The nails grow slowly, become brittle or deformed, and heal poorly around the nail beds when infected. Although palpation of peripheral pulses is correct, a rapid or irregular pulse would not be noted.
Priority Nursing Tip: Teach the client with Raynaud's disease to avoid smoking; wear warm clothing, socks, and gloves in cold weather; and avoid injuries to the fingers and hands.
Test-Taking Strategy: Focus on the subject, assessment for Raynaud's disease. Recall the physiological occurrences in Raynaud's disease. Palpation for diminished or absent peripheral pulses checks for interruption of circulation. Review: **Raynaud's disease.**
Reference(s): Ignatavicius, Workman (2013), p. 798.

374. The nurse teaches a postpartum client about observation of lochia. The nurse determines the client's understanding when the client says that on the second day postpartum, the lochia should be which color?
1. Red
2. Pink
3. White
4. Yellow

Level of Cognitive Ability: Evaluating
Client Needs: Physiological Integrity
Integrated Process: Nursing Process/Evaluation
Content Area: Maternity: Postpartum
Priority Concepts: Client Education; Reproduction

Answer: 1
Rationale: The uterus rids itself of the debris that remains after birth through a discharge called lochia, which is classified according to its appearance and contents. Lochia rubra is dark red in color. It occurs from delivery to 3 days postpartum and contains epithelial cells, erythrocytes, leukocytes, shreds of decidua, and occasionally fetal meconium, lanugo, and vernix caseosa. Lochia serosa is a brownish pink discharge that occurs from days 4 to 10. Lochia alba is a white discharge that occurs from days 10 to 14. Lochia should not be yellow in color or contain large clots; if it does, the cause should be investigated without delay.
Priority Nursing Tip: The amount of lochial discharge may increase with ambulation.
Test-Taking Strategy: Focus on the subject, lochia. Noting the words "second day postpartum" will direct you to the correct option. Review: the normal postpartum assessment findings for **lochia discharge**.
Reference(s): McKinney et al (2013), pp. 360, 434-435.

❖ **375.** The nurse develops a care plan for a client receiving hemodialysis who has an arteriovenous (AV) fistula in the right arm. The nurse includes which interventions in the plan to protect the AV fistula? **Select all that apply.**
☐ 1. Assess pulses and circulation proximal to the fistula.
☐ 2. Palpate for thrills and auscultate for a bruit every 4 hours.
☐ 3. Check for bleeding and infection at hemodialysis needle insertion sites.
☐ 4. Avoid taking blood pressure or performing venipunctures in the extremity.
☐ 5. Instruct the client not to carry heavy objects or anything that compresses the extremity.
☐ 6. Instruct the client not to sleep in a position that places his or her body weight on top of the extremity.

Level of Cognitive Ability: Analyzing
Client Needs: Physiological Integrity
Integrated Process: Nursing Process/Planning
Content Area: Adult Health: Renal and Urinary
Priority Concepts: Perfusion; Safety

Answer: 2, 3, 4, 5, 6
Rationale: An AV fistula is an internal anastomosis of an artery to a vein and is used as an access for hemodialysis. The nurse should implement the following to protect the fistula: palpate for thrills and auscultate for a bruit every 4 hours, check for bleeding and infection at hemodialysis needle insertion sites, avoid taking blood pressures or performing venipunctures in the extremity, instruct the client not to carry heavy objects or anything that compresses the extremity, instruct the client not to sleep in a position that places his or her body weight on top of the extremity, and the nurse should assess pulses and circulation distal to the fistula.
Priority Nursing Tip: Arterial steal syndrome can develop in a client with an arteriovenous fistula. In this condition, too much blood is diverted to the vein and arterial perfusion to the hand is compromised.
Test-Taking Strategy: Focus on the subject, protecting the AV fistula. Visualize this vascular access device and read each option carefully. Noting the word *proximal* in option 1 will assist in eliminating this option. Review: measures to protect an **arteriovenous (AV) fistula**.
Reference(s): Ignatavicius, Workman (2013), p. 1562; Swearingen (2012), p. 210.

376. The nurse is performing an admission assessment on a newborn admitted to the nursery with the diagnosis of subdural hematoma after a difficult vaginal delivery. Which intervention should the nurse do to assess for the **primary** symptom associated with subdural hematoma?
1. Monitor the urine for blood.
2. Monitor the urinary output pattern.
3. Test for contractures of the extremities.
4. Test for equality of extremities when stimulating reflexes.

Level of Cognitive Ability: Analyzing
Client Needs: Physiological Integrity
Integrated Process: Nursing Process/Assessment
Content Area: Maternity: Newborn
Priority Concepts: Development; Intracranial Regulation

Answer: 4
Rationale: A subdural hematoma can cause pressure on a specific area of the cerebral tissue. This can cause changes in the stimuli responses in the extremities on the opposite side of the body, especially if the newborn is actively bleeding. Options 1 and 2 are incorrect. After delivery, a newborn would normally be incontinent of urine. Blood in the urine would indicate abdominal trauma and would not be a result of the hematoma. Option 3 is incorrect because contractures would not occur this soon after delivery.
Priority Nursing Tip: A subdural hematoma results from a venous bleed. An epidural hematoma results from arterial bleeding.
Test-Taking Strategy: Note the strategic word, *primary*. Eliminate options 1 and 2 because they are comparable or alike and are similar assessments. Remember that the method of assessing for complications and active bleeding into the cranial cavity is a neurological assessment. Checking newborn reflexes is a neurological assessment. Although contractures of extremities could occur as residual effects, this would not occur immediately. Review: the signs of **subdural hematoma** in the newborn.
Reference(s): Lowdermilk, Perry, Cashion, Alden (2012), p. 841.

377. A client has received atropine sulfate preoperatively. The nurse monitors the client for which effect of the medication in the immediate postoperative period?
1. Diarrhea
2. Bradycardia
3. Urinary retention
4. Excessive salivation

Level of Cognitive Ability: Analyzing
Client Needs: Physiological Integrity
Integrated Process: Nursing Process/Assessment
Content Area: Pharmacology: Neurological Medications
Priority Concepts: Clinical Judgment; Safety

Answer: 3
Rationale: Atropine sulfate is an anticholinergic medication that causes tachycardia, drowsiness, blurred vision, dry mouth, constipation, and urinary retention. The nurse should monitor the client for any of these effects in the immediate postoperative period.
Priority Nursing Tip: Anticholinergic medications are contraindicated in the client with glaucoma.
Test-Taking Strategy: Focus on the subject, effects of atropine sulfate. Recalling that atropine sulfate is an anticholinergic and recalling the effects of an anticholinergic will direct you to the correct option. Review: the side effects of **atropine sulfate**.
Reference(s): Hodgson, Kizior (2014), p. 95.

❖ **378.** A client with calcium oxalate renal calculi is told to limit dietary intake of oxalate. The nurse provides the client with a list of foods high in oxalate and places which items on the list? **Select all that apply.**
☐ 1. Beets
☐ 2. Spinach
☐ 3. Rhubarb
☐ 4. Black tea
☐ 5. Cantaloupe
☐ 6. Watermelon

Level of Cognitive Ability: Applying
Client Needs: Physiological Integrity
Integrated Process: Teaching and Learning
Content Area: Adult Health: Renal and Urinary
Priority Concepts: Client Education; Nutrition

Answer: 1, 2, 3, 4
Rationale: Food items that are high in oxalate include beets, spinach, rhubarb, black tea, Swiss chard, cocoa, wheat germ, cashews, almonds, pecans, peanuts, okra, chocolate, and lime peel.
Priority Nursing Tip: Encourage the client with renal calculi to increase fluid intake up to 3000 mL a day, unless contraindicated, to facilitate the passage of the stone and prevent infection.
Test-Taking Strategy: Focus on the subject, food high in oxalate. Knowledge regarding food items high in oxalate is needed to answer this question. Remembering that fruits are generally not sources of dietary oxalate will assist in answering questions similar to this one. Review: the foods high in **oxalate**.
Reference(s): Ignatavicius, Workman (2013), pp. 1511-1512; Nix (2013), p. 443.

379. The nurse is conducting a health history on a client with hyperparathyroidism. Which question asked of the client would elicit information about this condition?
1. "Do you have tremors in your hands?"
2. "Are you experiencing pain in your joints?"
3. "Have you had problems with diarrhea lately?"
4. "Do you notice any swelling in your legs at night?"

Level of Cognitive Ability: Analyzing
Client Needs: Physiological Integrity
Integrated Process: Nursing Process/Assessment
Content Area: Adult Health: Endocrine
Priority Concepts: Clinical Judgment; Fluid and Electrolyte Balance

Answer: **2**
Rationale: Hyperparathyroidism causes an oversecretion of parathyroid hormone (PTH), which causes excessive osteoblast growth and activity within the bones. When bone reabsorption is increased, calcium is released from the bones into the blood, causing hypercalcemia. The bones suffer demineralization as a result of calcium loss, leading to bone and joint pain and pathological fractures. Options 1 and 3 relate to assessment of hypoparathyroidism. Option 4 is unrelated to hyperparathyroidism.
Priority Nursing Tip: Safety is a priority in the care of the client with hyperparathyroidism. Move the client slowly and carefully because the client is at risk for pathological fractures.
Test-Taking Strategy: Focus on the subject, hyperparathyroidism. Knowledge regarding the pathophysiology associated with hyperparathyroidism is required to answer the question. Eliminate options 1 and 3 first because these options provide information about hypoparathyroidism. From the remaining options, it is necessary to know the relationship among hyperparathyroidism, PTH, and joint pain to direct you to the correct option. Review: the characteristics of **hyperparathyroidism**.
Reference(s): Ignatavicius, Workman (2013), p. 1407.

380. An 18-year-old client seeks medical attention for intermittent episodes in which the fingers of both hands become cold, pale, and numb, followed by redness and swelling and throbbing, achy pain. Raynaud's disease is suspected. The nurse should assess the client to see if these episodes occur with which events?
1. Exposure to heat
2. Being in a relaxed environment
3. Ingestion of coffee or chocolate
4. Prolonged episodes of inactivity

Level of Cognitive Ability: Analyzing
Client Needs: Physiological Integrity
Integrated Process: Nursing Process/Assessment
Content Area: Adult Health: Cardiovascular
Priority Concepts: Clinical Judgment; Perfusion

Answer: **3**
Rationale: Raynaud's disease is vasospasm of the arterioles and arteries of the upper and lower extremities. It produces closure of the small arteries in the distal extremities in response to cold, vibration, or external stimuli. Episodes are characterized by pallor, cold, numbness, and possible cyanosis of the fingers, followed by erythema, tingling, and aching pain. Attacks are triggered by exposure to cold, nicotine, caffeine, trauma to the fingertips, and stress. Prolonged episodes of inactivity are unrelated to these episodes.
Priority Nursing Tip: Because stress can trigger vasospasm, the nurse should teach the client with Raynaud's disease stress management techniques.
Test-Taking Strategy: Focus on the subject, precipitating factors for Raynaud's disease. Recalling that symptoms occur with vasoconstriction will assist in eliminating options 1, 2, and 4 because these events are unlikely to cause vasoconstriction. Review: the characteristics associated with **Raynaud's disease**.
Reference(s): Ignatavicius, Workman (2013), p. 798.

❖ **381.** The nurse provides information to a client with diabetes mellitus who is taking insulin about the manifestations of hypoglycemia. Which manifestations should the nurse include in the information? **Select all that apply.**
❑ 1. Hunger
❑ 2. Sweating
❑ 3. Weakness
❑ 4. Nervousness
❑ 5. Cool clammy skin
❑ 6. Increased urinary output

Level of Cognitive Ability: Analyzing
Client Needs: Physiological Integrity
Integrated Process: Teaching and Learning
Content Area: Adult Health: Endocrine
Priority Concepts: Clinical Judgment; Glucose Regulation

Answer: **1, 2, 3, 4, 5**
Rationale: Hypoglycemia is characterized by a blood glucose level less than 70 mg/dL. Clinical manifestations of hypoglycemia include hunger, sweating, weakness, nervousness, cool clammy skin, blurred vision or double vision, tachycardia, and palpitations. Increased urinary output is a manifestation of hyperglycemia.
Priority Nursing Tip: If the client exhibits signs of a hypoglycemic reaction, perform a finger stick and check the client's glucose level. If hypoglycemia is confirmed, give the client a 10- to 15-g carbohydrate item such as a ½ cup of fruit juice to drink.
Test-Taking Strategy: Focus on the subject, the manifestations of hypoglycemia. Recall that hypoglycemia is characterized by a blood glucose level lower than 70 mg/dL. Next think about the manifestations that occur when the blood glucose level is low. Also recalling the "3 P's" associated with hyperglycemia—polyuria, polydipsia, and polyphagia—will assist in eliminating option 6. Review: **hypoglycemia**.
Reference(s): Ignatavicius, Workman (2013), pp. 1451-1452.

382. The ambulatory care nurse is assessing a client with chronic sinusitis. The nurse determines that which manifestations reported by the client are related to this problem? **Select all that apply.**
- ❏ 1. Anosmia
- ❏ 2. Chronic cough
- ❏ 3. Nasal stuffiness
- ❏ 4. Purulent nasal discharge
- ❏ 5. Headache that worsens in the evening

Level of Cognitive Ability: Analyzing
Client Needs: Physiological Integrity
Integrated Process: Nursing Process/Assessment
Content Area: Adult Health: Respiratory
Priority Concepts: Clinical Judgment; Inflammation

Answer: 1, 2, 3, 4
Rationale: Chronic sinusitis is characterized by anosmia (loss of smell), a chronic cough resulting from nasal discharge, nasal stuffiness, persistent purulent nasal discharge, and headache that is worse upon arising after sleep.
Priority Nursing Tip: Inhaling steam may be a helpful measure to treat sinusitis, but the nurse must teach the client the safe method to do so because of the risk associated with burns from the steam.
Test-Taking Strategy: Focus on the subject, chronic sinusitis. Think about the pathophysiology associated with this disorder. This will assist in determining the signs and symptoms and will direct you to the correct option. Remember that headache is worse upon arising after sleep. Review: the manifestations of chronic sinusitis.
Reference(s): Ignatavicius, Workman (2013), p. 642.

383. A client is diagnosed with hypothyroidism. The nurse performs an assessment on the client, expecting to note which findings? **Select all that apply.**
- ❏ 1. Weight loss
- ❏ 2. Bradycardia
- ❏ 3. Hypotension
- ❏ 4. Dry, scaly skin
- ❏ 5. Heat intolerance
- ❏ 6. Decreased body temperature

Level of Cognitive Ability: Analyzing
Client Needs: Physiological Integrity
Integrated Process: Nursing Process/Assessment
Content Area: Adult Health: Endocrine
Priority Concepts: Clinical Judgment; Thermoregulation

Answer: 2, 3, 4, 6
Rationale: The manifestations of hypothyroidism are the result of decreased metabolism from low levels of thyroid hormones. Some of these manifestations are bradycardia; hypotension; cool, dry, scaly skin; decreased body temperature; dry, coarse, brittle hair; decreased hair growth; cold intolerance; slowing of intellectual functioning; lethargy; weight gain; and constipation.
Priority Nursing Tip: A severe complication of hypothyroidism is myxedema coma, a rare but serious disorder that results from persistently low thyroid production. It can be caused by acute illness, anesthesia and surgery, hypothermia, and the use of sedatives and opioids.
Test-Taking Strategy: Focus on the subject, hypothyroidism. Recall that it occurs as the result of decreased metabolism from low levels of thyroid hormones. Correlate *hypo*thyroidism with *decreased* body functioning to assist in answering the question. Weight loss and heat intolerance occur in hyperthyroidism. Review: the manifestations of hypothyroidism.
Reference(s): Ignatavicius, Workman (2013), p. 1401.

384. A client is diagnosed with diabetes insipidus. The nurse performs an assessment on the client and expects to note which manifestations? **Select all that apply.**
- ❏ 1. Bradycardia
- ❏ 2. Hypertension
- ❏ 3. Poor skin turgor
- ❏ 4. Increased urinary output
- ❏ 5. Dry mucous membranes
- ❏ 6. Decreased pulse pressure

Level of Cognitive Ability: Analyzing
Client Needs: Physiological Integrity
Integrated Process: Nursing Process/Assessment
Content Area: Adult Health: Endocrine
Priority Concepts: Clinical Judgment; Fluid and Electrolyte Balance

Answer: 3, 4, 5, 6
Rationale: Diabetes insipidus is a water metabolism problem caused by an antidiuretic hormone (ADH) deficiency (either a decrease in ADH synthesis or an inability of the kidneys to respond to ADH). Clinical manifestations include poor skin turgor, increased urinary output, dry mucous membranes, decreased pulse pressure, tachycardia, hypotension, weak peripheral pulses, and increased thirst.
Priority Nursing Tip: Monitor for an electrolyte imbalance and signs of dehydration in the client with diabetes insipidus. If the condition is untreated, the client experiences a urine output of 4 to 24 liters a day.
Test-Taking Strategy: Focus on the subject, diabetes insipidus. Think about the pathophysiology of this disorder and recall that diabetes insipidus is caused by an ADH deficiency. This will assist in eliminating options 1 and 2. Review: the manifestations of diabetes insipidus.
Reference(s): Ignatavicius, Workman (2013), p. 1378.

385. A client with pneumonia has anorexia caused by the effort required for eating while dyspneic and decreased taste sensation. Which action by the nurse would be **most** helpful in increasing the client's appetite?
1. Keep fresh water at the bedside.
2. Provide three large meals daily.
3. Provide mouth care before meals.
4. Encourage drinking fluids up to 3 liters per day.

Level of Cognitive Ability: Applying
Client Needs: Physiological Integrity
Integrated Process: Nursing Process/Implementation
Content Area: Adult Health: Respiratory
Priority Concepts: Gas Exchange; Nutrition

Answer: **3**
Rationale: The client with pneumonia may experience decreased taste sensation as a result of sputum expectoration. To minimize this adverse effect, the nurse should provide oral hygiene before meals. The client should also have small, frequent meals because of dyspnea. Increased oral fluids and keeping water at the bedside are good measures to prevent fluid deficit associated with pneumonia, but they do nothing to alleviate anorexia.
Priority Nursing Tip: Unless contraindicated, encourage the client with pneumonia to consume fluids, up to 3 liters per day, to thin secretions.
Test-Taking Strategy: Focus on the **subject**, anorexia and increasing the client's appetite. Note the **strategic word**, *most*. Eliminate options 1 and 4 because they are **comparable or alike** and will not increase the client's appetite. From the remaining options, focusing on the **subject** will direct you to the correct option. Additionally, as a general measure, small frequent meals are better tolerated than large meals. Review: **anorexia** and **pneumonia**.
Reference(s): Ignatavicius, Workman (2013), p. 648.

❖ **386.** The clinic nurse notes that a large number of clients whose chief complaint is the presence of flulike symptoms are being seen in the clinic. Which recommendations should the nurse provide to these clients? **Select all that apply.**
☐ 1. Get plenty of rest.
☐ 2. Increase intake of liquids.
☐ 3. Get a flu shot immediately.
☐ 4. Take antipyretics for fever.
☐ 5. Eat a well-balanced diet with nutritious foods.

Level of Cognitive Ability: Analyzing
Client Needs: Physiological Integrity
Integrated Process: Teaching and Learning
Content Area: Adult Health: Respiratory
Priority Concepts: Client Education; Infection

Answer: **1, 2, 4, 5**
Rationale: Treatment for the flu includes getting rest, drinking fluids, and taking in nutritious foods and beverages. Medications such as antipyretics and analgesics may also be used for symptom management. Immunizations against influenza are a prophylactic measure and are not used to treat flu symptoms.
Priority Nursing Tip: Because the strain of influenza virus is different every year, annual vaccination is recommended.
Test-Taking Strategy: Focus on the **subject**, interventions for influenza. Recalling that a flu shot is a prophylactic measure will assist in directing you to the correct option. Review: measures for the client with **flulike symptoms**.
Reference(s): Ignatavicius, Workman (2013), p. 645.

❖ **387.** The nurse instructs a client with chronic pancreatitis about measures to prevent its exacerbation and provides which information to the client? **Select all that apply.**
☐ 1. Eat bland foods.
☐ 2. Avoid alcohol ingestion.
☐ 3. Avoid cigarette smoking.
☐ 4. Avoid caffeinated beverages.
☐ 5. Eat small meals and snacks high in calories.
☐ 6. Eat high-fat, low-protein, high-carbohydrate meals.

Level of Cognitive Ability: Analyzing
Client Needs: Physiological Integrity
Integrated Process: Teaching and Learning
Content Area: Adult Health: Gastrointestinal
Priority Concepts: Nutrition; Inflammation

Answer: **1, 2, 3, 4, 5**
Rationale: Chronic pancreatitis is a progressive, destructive disease of the pancreas, characterized by remissions and exacerbations (recurrence). Measures to prevent an exacerbation include eating bland, low-fat, high-protein, moderate-carbohydrate meals; avoiding alcohol ingestion, nicotine and caffeinated beverages; eating small meals and snacks high in calories; and avoiding gastric stimulants such as spices.
Priority Nursing Tip: The pain that is associated with acute pancreatitis is aggravated if the client lies in a recumbent position.
Test-Taking Strategy: Focus on the **subject**, measures to prevent an exacerbation of chronic pancreatitis. Thinking about the pathophysiology associated with pancreatitis and noting the **strategic words**, *high-fat*, in option 6 will direct you to eliminate this option. Review: the measures to prevent an exacerbation of **pancreatitis**.
Reference(s): Ignatavicius, Workman (2013), p. 1328.

392. The nurse is monitoring a client diagnosed with a ruptured appendix for signs of peritonitis. The nurse should assess for which manifestations of this complication? **Select all that apply.**
- ❏ 1. Bradycardia
- ❏ 2. Distended abdomen
- ❏ 3. Subnormal temperature
- ❏ 4. Rigid, boardlike abdomen
- ❏ 5. Diminished bowel sounds
- ❏ 6. Inability to pass flatus or feces

Level of Cognitive Ability: Analyzing
Client Needs: Physiological Integrity
Integrated Process: Nursing Process/Assessment
Content Area: Adult Health: Gastrointestinal
Priority Concepts: Clinical Judgment; Inflammation

Answer: 2, 4, 5, 6
Rationale: Peritonitis is an acute inflammation of the visceral and parietal peritoneum, the endothelial lining of the abdominal cavity. Clinical manifestations include distended abdomen; a rigid, board-like abdomen; diminished bowel sounds; inability to pass flatus or feces; abdominal pain (localized, poorly localized, or referred to the shoulder or thorax); anorexia, nausea, and vomiting; rebound tenderness in the abdomen; high fever; tachycardia; dehydration from the high fever; decreased urinary output; hiccups; and possible compromise in respiratory status.
Priority Nursing Tip: Avoid the application of heat to the abdomen of a client with appendicitis because heat can cause rupture of the appendix leading to peritonitis.
Test-Taking Strategy: Focus on the subject, signs of peritonitis. Remember that the suffix -*itis* indicates inflammation or infection. This will assist in determining that options 1 and 3 are incorrect. In inflammation, the client would experience an elevated temperature, and tachycardia is a physiological bodily response to fever. Review: the signs of peritonitis.
Reference(s): Ignatavicius, Workman (2013), p. 1268.

393. The nurse prepares to administer an intravenous (IV) medication when the nurse notes that the medication is incompatible with the IV solution. Which is the **best** intervention for the nurse to implement for safe medication administration?
1. Ask the provider to prescribe a compatible IV solution.
2. Start a new IV catheter for the incompatible medication.
3. Collaborate with the provider for a new administration route.
4. Flush tubing before and after administering the medication with normal saline.

Level of Cognitive Ability: Applying
Client Needs: Physiological Integrity
Integrated Process: Nursing Process/Implementation
Content Area: Fundamental Skills: Safety
Priority Concepts: Clinical Judgment; Safety

Answer: 4
Rationale: When giving a medication intravenously, if the medication is incompatible with the IV solution, the tubing is flushed before and after the medication with infusions of normal saline to prevent in-line precipitation of the incompatible agents. Starting a new IV, changing the solution, or changing the administration route is unnecessary because a simpler, less risky, viable option exists.
Priority Nursing Tip: Normal saline is physiologically similar to body fluid and is generally the solution of choice to flush an intravenous line.
Test-Taking Strategy: Note the strategic word, *best*. Focus on the subject, intravenous medication administration. You can eliminate options 1, 2, and 3 because they are unnecessary; in addition, option 2 increases the risk of infection and is likely to cause the client discomfort. Review: the procedures for administering IV medications.
Reference(s): Perry, Potter, Ostendorf (2014), pp. 571-573.

394. The nurse is preparing to administer eardrops to an infant. The nurse should plan to proceed by taking which step?
1. Pull down and back on the auricle, and direct the solution onto the eardrum.
2. Pull up and back on the earlobe, and direct the solution toward the wall of the ear canal.
3. Pull up and back on the auricle, and direct the solution toward the wall of the ear canal.
4. Pull down and back on the auricle, and direct the solution toward the wall of the ear canal.

Level of Cognitive Ability: Applying
Client Needs: Physiological Integrity
Integrated Process: Nursing Process/Implementation
Content Area: Pharmacology: Eye and Ear Medications
Priority Concepts: Development; Safety

Answer: 4
Rationale: The infant should be turned on the side with the affected ear uppermost. With the nondominant hand, the nurse pulls down and back on the auricle. The wrist of the dominant hand is rested on the infant's head. The medication is administered by aiming it at the wall of the ear canal rather than directly onto the eardrum. The infant should be held or positioned with the affected ear uppermost for 10 to 15 minutes to retain the solution. In the adult, the auricle is pulled up and back to straighten the auditory canal.
Priority Nursing Tip: For an infant or child younger than 3 years, pull the auricle down and back to administer ear medications. For a child older than 3 years, pull the auricle up and back.
Test-Taking Strategy: Focus on the subject, administering ear medications. Basic safety principles related to the administration of ear medications should assist in eliminating option 1. Option 3 is eliminated because it is the adult procedure. It would be difficult to pull up and back on an earlobe; therefore, eliminate option 2. Review: the procedure for administering ear medications in an infant.
Reference(s): McKinney et al (2013), p. 960.

395. A client seeks treatment in an ambulatory clinic for a complaint of hoarseness that has persisted for 8 weeks. Based on the symptom, the nurse interprets that the client is at risk of being diagnosed with which disorder?
1. Thyroid cancer
2. Acute laryngitis
3. Laryngeal cancer
4. Bronchogenic cancer

Level of Cognitive Ability: Analyzing
Client Needs: Physiological Integrity
Integrated Process: Nursing Process/Analysis
Content Area: Adult Health: Respiratory
Priority Concepts: Clinical Judgment; Cellular Regulation

Answer: 3
Rationale: Hoarseness is a common early sign of laryngeal cancer, but not of thyroid or bronchogenic cancer. Hoarseness that persists for 8 weeks is not associated with an acute problem, such as laryngitis.
Priority Nursing Tip: Risk factors for laryngeal cancer include smoking, heavy alcohol use, exposure to environmental pollutants such as asbestos or wood dust, and exposure to radiation.
Test-Taking Strategy: Focus on the subject, persistent hoarseness. Begin to answer this question by eliminating option 2, because an acute problem would not generally last for 8 weeks. From the remaining options, recall that the vocal cords are in the larynx when selecting the correct option. Review: the signs of laryngeal cancer.
Reference(s): Ignatavicius, Workman (2013), pp. 590-591.

396. A client is admitted to the cardiac intensive care unit after coronary artery bypass graft surgery (CABG). The nurse notes that in the first hour after admission, the mediastinal chest tube drainage was 75 mL. During the second hour, the drainage has dropped to 5 mL. The nurse interprets that which may be the reason?

1. This is normal.
2. The tube may be occluded.
3. The lung has fully reexpanded.
4. The client needs to cough and deep breathe.

Level of Cognitive Ability: Analyzing
Client Needs: Physiological Integrity
Integrated Process: Nursing Process/Analysis
Content Area: Critical Care: Emergency Situations
Priority Concepts: Clinical Judgment; Safety

Answer: 2
Rationale: After coronary artery bypass graft surgery, chest tube drainage should not exceed 100 to 150 mL per hour during the first 2 hours postoperatively, and approximately 500 mL of drainage is expected in the first 24 hours after coronary artery bypass graft surgery. The sudden drop in drainage between the first and second hour indicates that the tube is possibly occluded and requires further assessment by the nurse. Options 1, 3, and 4 are incorrect interpretations.
Priority Nursing Tip: After coronary artery bypass graft surgery, monitor the client for hypotension and hypertension. Hypotension can cause collapse of a vein graft. Hypertension causes increased pressure and can promote leakage from the suture line and bleeding.
Test-Taking Strategy: Focus on the subject, chest tube drainage. Eliminate option 3 first because the mediastinal chest tubes remove fluid from the mediastinum and are unrelated to restoration of negative pleural pressure. Needing to cough and deep breathe is a response that is unrelated to the client's problem, so option 4 is eliminated next. From the remaining options, knowing that the drainage would not drop so radically in 1 hour in the immediate postoperative period directs you to the correct option. Review: the concepts related to chest tube drainage systems in the postoperative coronary artery bypass graft surgery client.
Reference(s): Ignatavicius, Workman (2013), pp. 847-848.

397. The nurse is auscultating the chest of a client who was diagnosed with pleurisy 48 hours ago. The client does not currently have a pleural friction rub, which was auscultated the previous day. After verifying these data in the client's health record, the nurse interprets that this **most likely** occurred because of which result?

1. Effectiveness of medication therapy
2. Deep breaths that the client is taking
3. Decreased inflammatory reaction at the site
4. Accumulation of pleural fluid in the inflamed area

Level of Cognitive Ability: Analyzing
Client Needs: Physiological Integrity
Integrated Process: Nursing Process/Analysis
Content Area: Adult Health: Respiratory
Priority Concepts: Clinical Judgment; Gas Exchange

Answer: 4
Rationale: Pleurisy is the inflammation of the visceral and parietal membranes. These membranes rub together during respiration and cause pain. Pleural friction rub is auscultated early in the course of pleurisy, before pleural fluid accumulates. Once fluid accumulates in the inflamed area, there is less friction between the visceral and parietal lung surfaces, and the pleural friction rub disappears. Options 1, 2, and 3 are incorrect interpretations.
Priority Nursing Tip: Instruct the client with pleurisy to lie on the affected side to splint the chest. This will ease the pain when coughing and deep breathing.
Test-Taking Strategy: Focus on the subject, pleurisy and pleural friction rub. Note the strategic words, *most likely*. Options 1 and 3 are comparable or alike, and because the question states that the problem was diagnosed 48 hours ago, these options should be eliminated. Eliminate option 2 because deep breaths would intensify the pain. Remember that fluid accumulation in the area provides a buffer between the lung and chest wall surfaces, which resolves the friction rub. Review: assessment findings in the client with pleurisy.
Reference(s): Dolan, Holt (2013), p. 296; Ignatavicius, Workman (2013), p. 335.

❖ **398.** The nurse provides information to a client with a colostomy about the foods that will help prevent odor from the colostomy and tells the client to consume which foods? **Select all that apply.**
- ❑ 1. Parsley
- ❑ 2. Yogurt
- ❑ 3. Buttermilk
- ❑ 4. Cucumbers
- ❑ 5. Cauliflower
- ❑ 6. Cranberry juice

Level of Cognitive Ability: Applying
Client Needs: Physiological Integrity
Integrated Process: Teaching and Learning
Content Area: Adult Health: Gastrointestinal
Priority Concepts: Nutrition; Elimination

Answer: 1, 2, 3, 6
Rationale: The nurse should provide information about foods and measures that will prevent odor from a colostomy. Parsley, yogurt, buttermilk, and cranberry juice will prevent odor. Charcoal filters, pouch deodorizers, or placement of a breath mint in the pouch will also eliminate odors. Foods that cause flatus and thus odor, including broccoli, Brussels sprouts, cabbage, cauliflower, cucumbers, mushrooms, and peas, should be avoided.
Priority Nursing Tip: Body image is a concern for a client with a colostomy, and the nurse needs to be sensitive to the client when discussing this concern with the client.
Test-Taking Strategy: Focus on the subject, foods to control odor. Eliminate options 4 and 5 using basic knowledge regarding nutrition because these foods cause flatus. Review: the foods to control odor in a client with a colostomy.
Reference(s): Ignatavicius, Workman (2013), p. 1253.

❖ **399.** A client has frequent runs of ventricular tachycardia, and the health care provider prescribes flecainide (Tambocor). Because of the effects of the medication, what should the nurse do?
- ❑ 1. Monitor the client's urinary output.
- ❑ 2. Assess the client for neurological problems.
- ❑ 3. Ensure that the bed rails remain in the up position.
- ❑ 4. Monitor the client's vital signs and electrocardiogram (ECG) frequently.

Level of Cognitive Ability: Analyzing
Client Needs: Physiological Integrity
Integrated Process: Nursing Process/Implementation
Content Area: Pharmacology: Cardiovascular Medications
Priority Concepts: Perfusion; Safety

Answer: 4
Rationale: Flecainide is an antidysrhythmic medication that slows conduction and decreases excitability, conduction velocity, and automaticity. However, the nurse must monitor for the development of a new or worsening dysrhythmia. Options 1, 2, and 3 are components of standard care but are not specific to this medication.
Priority Nursing Tip: Monitor the client receiving flecainide (Tambocor) for an increase and severity of dysrhythmias. This adverse effect may warrant a decrease in dosage or discontinuation of the medication.
Test-Taking Strategy: Focus on the subject, flecainide (Tambocor). Note the relation of the information in the question (the client has a dysrhythmia) and the nursing action in the correct option. Select the option that relates to cardiac status monitoring. Review: the effects of flecainide (Tambocor).
Reference(s): Ignatavicius, Workman (2013), p. 723; Lehne (2013), p. 579.

❖ **400.** The nurse provides information to a client with gastroesophageal reflux disease (GERD) about the factors that contribute to decreased lower esophageal sphincter (LES) pressure and worsen the condition. The nurse should tell the client that which factors contribute to decreased LES pressure? **Select all that apply.**

❑ 1. Alcohol
❑ 2. Fatty foods
❑ 3. Citrus fruits
❑ 4. Baked potatoes
❑ 5. Caffeinated beverages
❑ 6. Tomatoes and tomato products

Level of Cognitive Ability: Applying
Client Needs: Physiological Integrity
Integrated Process: Nursing Process/Implementation
Content Area: Adult Health: Gastrointestinal
Priority Concepts: Client Education; Nutrition

Answer: 1, 2, 3, 5, 6

Rationale: GERD occurs as a result of the backward flow (reflux) of gastrointestinal contents into the esophagus. The most common cause of GERD is inappropriate relaxation of the LES, which allows the reflux of gastric contents into the esophagus and exposes the esophageal mucosa to gastric contents. Factors that influence the tone and contractility of the LES and lower LES pressure include alcohol; fatty foods; citrus fruits; caffeinated beverages such as coffee, tea, and cola; tomatoes and tomato products; chocolate; nicotine in cigarette smoke; calcium channel blockers; nitrates; anticholinergics; high levels of estrogen and progesterone; peppermint and spearmint; and nasogastric tube placement.

Priority Nursing Tip: Teach the client with gastroesophageal reflux disease (GERD) to avoid lying down with a full stomach and avoid eating within 2 to 3 hours of bedtime; to avoid wearing tight-fitting clothing, particularly around the waist; and to sleep with the head of the bed raised at least 6 to 8 inches.

Test-Taking Strategy: Note the client's diagnosis of gastroesophageal reflux disease (GERD) and focus on the subject, factors that contribute to decreased lower esophageal sphincter (LES) pressure. Read each option and consider whether the item will aggravate the client's condition. The only item that will not is option 4, baked potatoes. Review: gastroesophageal reflux disease (GERD) and decreased lower esophageal sphincter (LES) pressure.

Reference(s): Ignatavicius, Workman (2013), p. 1204.

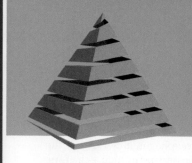

Test 2

Safe and Effective Care Environment

❖ **401.** The nurse is developing an educational session on client advocacy for the nursing staff. The nurse should plan to tell the nursing staff that which interventions are examples of the nurse acting as a client advocate? **Select all that apply.**
  ❏ 1. Obtaining an informed consent for a surgical procedure
  ❏ 2. Providing information necessary for a client to make informed decisions
  ❏ 3. Providing assistance in asserting the client's human and legal rights if the need arises
  ❏ 4. Ignoring the client's religious or cultural beliefs when assisting the client in making an informed decision
  ❏ 5. Defending the client's rights by speaking out against policies or actions that might endanger the client's well-being

Level of Cognitive Ability: Applying
Client Needs: Safe and Effective Care Environment
Integrated Process: Caring
Content Area: Leadership/Management: Ethical/Legal
Priority Concepts: Ethics; Leadership

Answer: 2, 3, 5
Rationale: In the role of client advocate, the nurse protects the client's human and legal rights and provides assistance in asserting those rights if the need arises. The nurse advocates for the client by providing information needed so that the client can make an informed decision. The nurse also defends clients' rights in a general way by speaking out against policies or actions that might endanger the client's well-being or conflict with his or her rights. Informed consent is part of the health care provider–client relationship; in most situations, obtaining the client's informed consent does not fall within the nursing duty. Even though the nurse assumes the responsibility for witnessing the client's signature on the consent form, the nurse does not legally assume the duty of obtaining informed consent. The nurse needs to consider the client's religion and culture when functioning as an advocate and when providing care. The nurse would not ignore the client's religious or cultural beliefs in discussions about treatment plans, so that an informed decision can be made.
Priority Nursing Tip: The nurse is a care provider who spends a significant amount of time with the client, and therefore is in a critical position to act as a client advocate.
Test-Taking Strategy: Focus on the subject, examples of the nurse acting as a client advocate. Read each option carefully and recall the definition of a client advocate. Remembering that in this role the nurse protects the client's human and legal rights and provides assistance in asserting those rights if the need arises will assist in selecting the correct examples. Review: the nurse's role as a client advocate.
Reference(s): Potter et al (2013), pp. 7, 36.

402. The registered nurse (RN) is creating a plan for the assignments for the day and is leading a team composed of a licensed practical nurse (LPN) and an unlicensed assistive personnel (UAP). Based on licensure, which client is **most appropriate** to assign to the LPN?
1. A client with dementia
2. A 1-day postoperative mastectomy client
3. A client who requires some assistance with bathing
4. A client who requires some assistance with ambulation

Level of Cognitive Ability: Creating
Client Needs: Safe and Effective Care Environment
Integrated Process: Nursing Process/Planning
Content Area: Leadership/Management: Delegating
Priority Concepts: Care Coordination; Leadership

Answer: **2**
Rationale: Assignment of tasks must be implemented based on the job description of the LPN and UAP, the level of education and clinical competence, and state law. The 1-day postoperative mastectomy client will need care that requires the skill of a licensed nurse. The UAP has the skills to care for a client requiring noninvasive care such as a client with dementia, a client who requires some assistance with bathing, and a client who requires some assistance with ambulation.
Priority Nursing Tip: Do not delegate an activity to anyone who has never performed the task. Perform the activity with the individual and teach them about the procedure for performing it; this ensures client safety. Clients who are potentially unstable or complicated need to be assigned to licensed staff.
Test-Taking Strategy: Note the strategic words, *most appropriate*. Also, focus on the subject, client assignments for the LPN and UAP. Think about the needs of each client to assist in determining the assignment. Remember that the LPN will be performing at a higher skill level than the UAP. Review: the principles associated with **delegating and assignment making**.
Reference(s): Huber (2014), pp. 147-148; Potter et al (2013), pp. 262, 282-283.

❖ **403.** The nurse is creating a plan for delegating unit activities for the day. Which activities should the nurse delegate to the unlicensed assistive personnel (UAP)? **Select all that apply.**
❑ 1. Deliver fresh water to clients.
❑ 2. Empty urine out of Foley bags.
❑ 3. Take temperatures, pulses, respirations, and blood pressures.
❑ 4. Count the substance control medications in the opioid medication supply.
❑ 5. Check the crash cart (cardiopulmonary resuscitation cart) for necessary supplies using a checklist.
❑ 6. Check all intravenous (IV) solution bags on clients receiving IV therapy for the remaining amounts of solution in the bags.

Level of Cognitive Ability: Analyzing
Client Needs: Safe and Effective Care Environment
Integrated Process: Nursing Process/Planning
Content Area: Leadership/Management: Delegating
Priority Concepts: Care Coordination; Leadership

Answer: **1, 2, 3**
Rationale: Delegation is the transfer of responsibility for the performance of an activity or task while retaining accountability for the outcome. When delegating an activity, the nurse must consider the educational preparation and experience of the individual. UAP are trained to perform noninvasive tasks and those that meet basic client needs. The UAP is also trained to take vital signs. Therefore, the appropriate activities to assign to the UAP would be to deliver fresh water to clients; empty urine out of Foley bags; and take temperatures, pulses, respirations, and blood pressures. Although UAP are trained in performing cardiopulmonary resuscitation, the UAP is not trained to check a crash cart, and this activity must be assigned to a licensed nurse. Any activities related to medications and IV therapy must be delegated to a licensed nurse.
Priority Nursing Tip: To ensure client safety, it is very important for the nurse to delegate appropriately to the unlicensed assistive personnel (UAP). Most tasks that are noninvasive can be assigned to the UAP.
Test-Taking Strategy: Focus on the subject, activities to be delegated to a UAP. Recalling that a UAP is trained to perform noninvasive tasks and that medication and IV therapy and any activity that requires critical thinking skills must be delegated to a licensed nurse will assist in answering this question. Review: principles related to **delegation**.
Reference(s): Huber (2014), pp. 148-150; Potter et al (2013), pp. 262, 282-283.

404. The nurse is in the process of giving a client a bed bath. In the middle of the procedure, the unit secretary calls the nurse on the intercom to tell the nurse that there is an emergency phone call. Which appropriate action should the nurse take?
1. Finish the bath before answering the phone call.
2. Immediately walk out of the client's room and answer the phone call.
3. Cover the client, place the call light within reach, and answer the phone call.
4. Leave the client's door open so the client can be monitored and the nurse can answer the phone call.

Level of Cognitive Ability: Applying
Client Needs: Safe and Effective Care Environment
Integrated Process: Nursing Process/Implementation
Content Area: Fundamental Skills: Safety
Priority Concepts: Clinical Judgment; Safety

Answer: 3
Rationale: Because the telephone call is an emergency, the nurse may need to answer it. The other appropriate action is to ask another nurse to accept the call. This, however, is not one of the options. To maintain privacy and safety, the nurse covers the client and places the call light within the client's reach. Additionally, the client's door should be closed or the room curtains pulled around the bathing area.
Priority Nursing Tip: If it is necessary to leave the client's bedside, return the bed to low position, elevate side rails as appropriate per state and agency policies, place the call light in the client's reach, and ensure that the client knows how to use it.
Test-Taking Strategy: Focus on the subject, the need for the nurse to respond to an emergency call. Eliminate option 1 because this delays the nurse responding. Eliminate option 2 because this action does not provide client safety. From the remaining options, recalling the rights of the client and the principles related to safety will assist in eliminating option 4. Review: guidelines for maintaining safety while bathing a client.
Reference(s): Potter et al (2013), p. 784.

405. The nurse manager is reviewing with the nursing staff the purposes for applying wrist and ankle restraints to a client. The nurse manager determines that **further education is necessary** when a nursing staff member states that which is an indication for the use of a restraint?
1. Limit movement of a limb.
2. Keep the client in bed at night.
3. Prevent the violent client from injuring self and others.
4. Prevent the client from pulling out intravenous lines and catheters.

Level of Cognitive Ability: Evaluating
Client Needs: Safe and Effective Care Environment
Integrated Process: Teaching and Learning
Content Area: Leadership/Management: Ethical/Legal
Priority Concepts: Health Care Law; Safety

Answer: 2
Rationale: Wrist and ankle restraints are devices used to limit the client's movement in situations when it is necessary to immobilize a limb. Restraints are not applied to keep a client in bed at night and should never be used as a form of punishment. Restraints are applied to prevent the client from injuring self or others; pulling out intravenous lines, catheters, or tubes; or removing dressings. Restraints also may be used to keep children still and from injuring themselves during treatments and diagnostic procedures. A health care provider's prescription is required for the use of restraints, and state and agency procedures are always followed when restraints are used.
Priority Nursing Tip: Assess the client with restraints applied continuously to determine if the restraints remain necessary.
Test-Taking Strategy: Note the strategic words, *further education is necessary*. These words indicate a negative event query and the need to select the option that identifies an inaccurate use for restraints. Eliminate options 1 and 4 first because they are comparable or alike. From the remaining options, read each option carefully. Recalling the guidelines for the use of restraints will direct you to the correct option. Review: guidelines for the use of restraints.
Reference(s): Potter et al (2013), pp. 300, 388.

406. A client has a prescription to receive valproic acid (Depakene) 250 mg once daily. To maximize the client's safety, at which time should the nurse schedule administration of the medication?
1. With lunch
2. With breakfast
3. Before breakfast
4. At bedtime with a snack

Level of Cognitive Ability: Applying
Client Needs: Safe and Effective Care Environment
Integrated Process: Nursing Process/Implementation
Content Area: Pharmacology: Neurological Medications
Priority Concepts: Clinical Judgment; Safety

Answer: 4
Rationale: Valproic acid is an anticonvulsant that causes central nervous system (CNS) depression. For this reason, the side/adverse effects include sedation, dizziness, ataxia, and confusion. When the client is taking this medication as a single daily dose, administering it at bedtime negates the risk of injury from sedation and enhances client safety. Otherwise, it may be given after meals to avoid gastrointestinal upset.
Priority Nursing Tip: If the client is taking a central nervous system depressant, inform the client that sedation can occur and of the measures that ensure safety.
Test-Taking Strategy: Recalling that this medication is an anticonvulsant with CNS depressant properties and that sedation can occur will direct you to option 4. Administration at bedtime allows the sedative effects of the medication to occur at a time when the client is sleeping. Also note that options 1, 2, and 3 are comparable or alike in that they indicate administering the medication with meals. Review: valproic acid (Depakene).
Reference(s): Lehne (2013), p. 250; Lilley et al (2014), p. 240.

❖ **407.** The nurse is reading the history and physical examination of an older client admitted to the hospital. Which findings documented in the history should require the nurse to implement an accident prevention protocol? **Select all that apply.**
❑ 1. Range of motion is limited.
❑ 2. Peripheral vision is decreased.
❑ 3. Transmission of hot impulses is delayed.
❑ 4. The client denies complaints of nocturia.
❑ 5. High-frequency hearing tones are perceptible.
❑ 6. Voluntary and autonomic reflexes are slowed.

Level of Cognitive Ability: Analyzing
Client Needs: Safe and Effective Care Environment
Integrated Process: Nursing Process/Assessment
Content Area: Fundamental Skills: Safety
Priority Concepts: Development; Safety

Answer: 1, 2, 3, 6
Rationale: The physiologic changes that occur during the aging process increase the client's risk for accidents. Musculoskeletal changes include a decrease in muscle strength and function, lessened joint mobility, and limited range of motion. Sensory changes include a decrease in peripheral vision and lens accommodation, delayed transmission of hot and cold impulses, and impaired hearing as high-frequency tones become less perceptible. Nervous system changes include slowed voluntary and autonomic reflexes. Genitourinary changes may include nocturia.
Priority Nursing Tip: Age-related changes occur on an individual basis, and one client may experience an age-related change to a lesser extent than another client. The nurse must gather baseline data and then assess for changes and determine the appropriate course of action to compensate to promote client safety.
Test-Taking Strategy: Focus on the subject, accident prevention in an older client. Reading each option carefully and keeping in mind the factors that affect client safety will assist in answering the question. Review: the factors that place a client at risk for accidents.
Reference(s): Potter et al (2013), pp. 184-185.

408. The nurse has a prescription to obtain a sputum culture from a client admitted to the hospital with a diagnosis of pneumonia. Which actions should the nurse take when obtaining the specimen? **Select all that apply.**

- ❑ 1. Explain the procedure to the client.
- ❑ 2. Obtain the specimen early in the morning.
- ❑ 3. Have the client brush his teeth before expectoration.
- ❑ 4. Instruct the client to take deep breaths before coughing.
- ❑ 5. Place the lid of the culture container face down on the bedside table.

Level of Cognitive Ability: Applying
Client Needs: Safe and Effective Care Environment
Integrated Process: Nursing Process/Implementation
Content Area: Fundamental Skills: Infection Control
Priority Concepts: Clinical Judgment; Infection

Answer: 1, 2, 3, 4
Rationale: The nurse always explains a procedure to a client. The specimen is obtained early in the morning whenever possible because increased amounts of sputum collect in the airways during sleep. The client should rinse the mouth or brush the teeth before specimen collection to avoid contaminating the specimen. The client should take deep breaths before expectoration for best sputum production. Placing the lid face down on the bedside table contaminates the lid and could result in inaccurate findings.
Priority Nursing Tip: Any specimen for culture needs to be collected via sterile technique because contamination of the specimen invalidates the results.
Test-Taking Strategy: Focus on the subject, a sputum culture. Read each option carefully. Visualizing the procedures for using the basic principles of aseptic technique will direct you to eliminate option 5. Review: the procedure for **sputum collection**.
Reference(s): Pagana, Pagana (2013), pp. 861-862.

409. The nurse should plan to wear this protective device when caring for hospitalized clients with which disorders? **(Refer to the figure.)** Select all that apply.

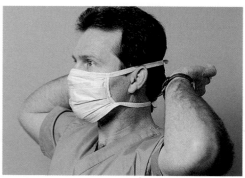

(From Potter P, Perry A, Stockert P, Hall A: *Fundamentals of nursing*, ed 8, St. Louis, 2013, Mosby.)

- ❑ 1. Scabies
- ❑ 2. Tuberculosis
- ❑ 3. Hepatitis A virus
- ❑ 4. Pharyngeal diphtheria
- ❑ 5. Streptococcal pharyngitis
- ❑ 6. Meningococcal pneumonia

Level of Cognitive Ability: Applying
Client Needs: Safe and Effective Care Environment
Integrated Process: Nursing Process/Implementation
Content Area: Fundamental Skills: Infection Control
Priority Concepts: Infection; Safety

Answer: 4, 5, 6
Rationale: A standard mask is used as part of droplet precautions to protect the nurse from acquiring the client's infection. Droplet precautions refer to precautions used for organisms that can spread through the air but are unable to remain in the air farther than 3 feet. Many respiratory viral infections such as respiratory viral influenza require the use of a standard mask when caring for the client. Some other disorders requiring the use of a standard mask include pharyngeal diphtheria; rubella; streptococcal pharyngitis; pertussis; mumps; pneumonia, including meningococcal pneumonia; and the pneumonic plague. Scabies and hepatitis A are transmitted by direct contact with an infected person and require the use of contact precautions for protection. Tuberculosis requires the use of airborne precautions and the use of an individually fitted particulate filter mask. A standard mask would not protect the nurse from *Mycobacterium tuberculosis*.
Priority Nursing Tip: Infection control is very important to implement when caring for clients. Nosocomial, or hospital-acquired infections, can be prevented if these practices are properly implemented. In-service educational sessions are effective ways to remind health care workers of proper precautionary procedures.
Test-Taking Strategy: Focus on the subject, use of a standard mask. This indicates the need for the nurse to protect himself or herself from inhaling an organism. You can eliminate option 2 by recalling that tuberculosis requires the use of an individually fitted particulate filter mask. Next eliminate options 1 and 3 by recalling that these infections are not transmitted by the respiratory route. Noting that options 4, 5, and 6 are respiratory disorders will assist in answering correctly. Review: the indications for the use of a **standard mask**.
Reference(s): Potter et al (2013), pp. 416, 419-420.

410. The nurse is developing a hospital policy on guidelines for telephone and verbal prescriptions. Which guidelines should the nurse include in the policy? **Select all that apply.**
- ❏ 1. Clarify any questions with the health care provider
- ❏ 2. Repeat the prescribed prescriptions back to the health care provider
- ❏ 3. Avoid using abbreviations such as TO (telephone order) because they are never acceptable.
- ❏ 4. Remember that verbal prescriptions are never acceptable; the health care provider must document the prescription.
- ❏ 5. Cosigning the prescription by the health care provider is not necessary if the nurse repeats the prescription for verification.
- ❏ 6. Documentation of the name of the health care provider giving the prescription is not necessary if the health care provider is the client's primary health care provider.

Level of Cognitive Ability: Applying
Client Needs: Safe and Effective Care Environment
Integrated Process: Nursing Process/Implementation
Content Area: Leadership/Management: Ethical/Legal
Priority Concepts: Communication; Safety

Answer: 1, 2
Rationale: A telephone order (TO) involves a health care provider (HCP) stating a prescribed therapy over the phone to the nurse. Telephone orders are frequently given at night or during an emergency and need to be given only when absolutely necessary. Likewise, a verbal order (VO) is acceptable when there is no opportunity for the HCP to write the prescription such as in an emergency situation. To avoid misunderstandings, the nurse would always clarify a telephone or verbal order with the HCP if he or she had any questions about the prescription and would repeat any prescribed prescriptions back to the HCP. Additional guidelines for telephone and verbal prescriptions include the following: clearly determine the client's name, room number, and diagnosis; write TO (telephone order) or VO (verbal order), including the date and time, name of the client, complete prescription, name of the HCP giving the prescription, and nurse taking the prescription; and have the HCP cosign the prescription within the time frame designated by the health care agency (usually 24 hours).
Priority Nursing Tip: The nurse plays a vital role in maintaining the safety of the client. The nurse is considered the "last line of defense" for a client in terms of noting a prescription that may be harmful to him or her.
Test-Taking Strategy: Focus on the subject, guidelines for taking telephone and verbal orders. You can easily eliminate options 3 and 4 because of the closed-ended word "never" in these options. Next eliminate option 5 because of the words *not necessary* and option 6 because the prescription must indicate the prescribing HCP. Also, reading each option carefully and thinking about the legal issues related to health care providers' prescriptions will assist you in answering correctly. Review: the guidelines for **telephone orders** and **verbal orders**.
Reference(s): Potter et al (2013), p. 358.

411. The nurse employed in a preschool agency is planning a staff education program to prevent the spread of an outbreak of an intestinal parasitic disease. Which prevention measure should the nurse include in the educational session?
1. All food will be cooked before eating.
2. Only bottled water will be used for drinking.
3. All toileting areas will be cleansed daily with soap and water.
4. Standard precautions will be used when changing diapers and assisting children with toileting.

Level of Cognitive Ability: Applying
Client Needs: Safe and Effective Care Environment
Integrated Process: Teaching and Learning
Content Area: Fundamental Skills: Infection Control
Priority Concepts: Infection; Safety

Answer: 4
Rationale: The fecal-oral route is the mode of transmission of an intestinal parasitic disease. Standard precautions prevent the transmission of infection. Some fresh foods do not need to be cooked as long as they are washed well and were not grown in soil contaminated with human feces. Water and fresh foods can be vehicles for transmission, but municipal water sources are usually safe. Cleaning with soap and water is not as effective as the use of bleach.
Priority Nursing Tip: Regardless of the infectious agent, infection control measures are essential to protect health care providers and clients.
Test-Taking Strategy: Focus on the subject, preventing the spread of an intestinal parasitic infection. Option 4 addresses the subject of the question and is the umbrella option, addressing standard precautions. Also, note that options 1, 2, and 3 contain the closed-ended words "all" and "only." Review: measures that will prevent the spread of an intestinal **parasitic infection**.
Reference(s): Hockenberry, Wilson (2013), pp. 653-654; McKinney et al (2013), p. 1032.

412. A client has arrived at the labor and delivery unit in active labor. The nursing assessment reveals a history of recurrent genital herpes and the presence of lesions in the genital tract. Which intervention should the nurse initiate?

1. Prepare the client for a cesarean delivery.
2. Limit visitors and maintain reverse isolation.
3. Prepare the client for a spontaneous vaginal delivery.
4. Rupture the membranes artificially, looking for meconium-stained fluid.

Level of Cognitive Ability: Applying
Client Needs: Safe and Effective Care Environment
Integrated Process: Nursing Process/Implementation
Content Area: Maternity: Intrapartum
Priority Concepts: Infection; Reproduction

Answer: 1
Rationale: A cesarean delivery can reduce the risk of neonatal infection with a mother in labor who has herpetic genital tract lesions. There is no need to limit visitors or maintain isolation, although standard precautions should be maintained. A vaginal delivery presents a risk of transmitting the disease to the neonate. Intact membranes provide another barrier to transmitting the disease to the neonate.
Priority Nursing Tip: No vaginal examinations are performed on a pregnant woman who has active vaginal herpetic lesions.
Test-Taking Strategy: Focus on the subject, the presence of genital herpes lesions. Eliminate options 3 and 4 first because they are comparable or alike and would place the neonate in contact with the lesions. From the remaining options, consider the risks to the neonate to direct you to the correct option. Review: labor and genital herpes.
Reference(s): McKinney et al (2013), pp. 424-425, 799.

---

413. The nurse prepares to insert an indwelling Foley catheter into a client. To maintain the integrity of the Foley catheter and client safety, which interventions should the nurse perform? **Select all that apply.**

☐ 1. Use strict aseptic technique.
☐ 2. Place the drainage bag lower than the bladder level.
☐ 3. Advance the catheter after urine appears in the tubing.
☐ 4. Inflate the balloon with 4 to 5 mL beyond its capacity.
☐ 5. Test the balloon for patency before catheter insertion.

Level of Cognitive Ability: Applying
Client Needs: Safe and Effective Care Environment
Integrated Process: Nursing Process/Implementation
Content Area: Fundamental Skills: Safety
Priority Concepts: Clinical Judgment; Safety

Answer: 1, 2, 3
Rationale: The nurse would use strict aseptic technique to insert the catheter. The drainage bag is placed lower than bladder level to ensure drainage, prevent retrograde flow of urine, and reduce the risk of infection. Advancing the catheter 1 to 2 inches beyond the point where the flow of urine is first noted is also good practice because this ensures that the catheter balloon is completely in the bladder before it is inflated. Testing the balloon before catheter insertion is not done because this may distort and stretch it leading to damage and trauma on insertion. The nurse risks rupturing the catheter's balloon by overinflating it; therefore, the nurse inflates the balloon with the specified volume for the catheter because inflating the balloon with 4 to 5 mL beyond its capacity is unsafe.
Priority Nursing Tip: When preparing to insert a Foley catheter, it is advisable to bring an extra Foley catheter, an extra pair of gloves, and a flashlight along with the regular Foley catheter insertion equipment to the client's room.
Test-Taking Strategy: Focus on the subject, the procedure for inserting a Foley catheter, visualizing the procedure to answer correctly. Also, noting the words *beyond its capacity* in option 4 will assist in eliminating this option. Review: the procedure for inserting a Foley catheter.
Reference(s): Perry, Potter, Elkin (2012), pp. 437-439; Potter et al (2013), pp. 1068, 1077-1078.

414. A moderately depressed client who was admitted to the mental health unit 2 days ago suddenly begins smiling and reporting that the crisis is over. The client says to the nurse, "Call the doctor. I'm finally cured." Which modification to the treatment plan should occur based on the behavioral cues of the client?
1. Allowing off-unit privileges PRN
2. Suggesting a reduction of medication
3. Allowing increased "in-room" activities
4. Increasing the level of suicide precautions

Level of Cognitive Ability: Analyzing
Client Needs: Safe and Effective Care Environment
Integrated Process: Nursing Process/Planning
Content Area: Mental Health
Priority Concepts: Mood and Affect; Safety

Answer: 4
Rationale: A client who is moderately depressed and has only been hospitalized 2 days is unlikely to have such a dramatic cure. When a mood suddenly lifts, it is likely that the client may have made the decision to cause self-harm. Suicide precautions are necessary to keep the client safe. Options 1 and 2 are incorrect because they support a "quick" cure. In-room activities do not encourage social interaction; social interaction would be a desired outcome for a moderately depressed client.
Priority Nursing Tip: When a depressed client at risk for suicide displays increased alertness and energy, suicide precautions should be continued. These observations are an indication that the client has the energy to perform the act of suicide.
Test-Taking Strategy: Focus on the subject, moderately depressed client, and recall that depression does not resolve in 2 days. Options 1 and 2 support the client's notion that a cure has occurred. Option 3 allows the client to increase isolation. Recalling that safety is of the utmost importance will direct you to option 4. Review: **depression and suicide.**
Reference(s): Varcarolis (2013), p. 255.

415. The nurse is planning care for a suicidal client. At which time should the nurse implement additional precautions?
1. During the day shift
2. On weekday evenings
3. Between 8 AM and 10 AM
4. During the unit shift change

Level of Cognitive Ability: Applying
Client Needs: Safe and Effective Care Environment
Integrated Process: Nursing Process/Implementation
Content Area: Mental Health
Priority Concepts: Mood and Affect; Safety

Answer: 4
Rationale: At shift change, there is often less availability of staff. The psychiatric nurse and staff should increase precautions for suicidal clients at that time. The night shift also presents a high-risk time, as do weekends, not weekdays.
Priority Nursing Tip: Provide one-on-one supervision at all times for a client at risk for suicide.
Test-Taking Strategy: Options 1, 2, and 3 are comparable or alike and can be eliminated. Remember that the nurse should anticipate that times with less supervision of the client could be times of increased risks. Review: care of the **suicidal client.**
Reference(s): Varcarolis (2013), p. 453.

416. The nurse assists with the transfer of a client from the operating room table to a stretcher. Which interventions should the nurse perform to ensure client safety? **Select all that apply.**
☐ 1. Check the client's level of consciousness
☐ 2. Check wheel locks of the operating room table
☐ 3. Complete the client transfer as quickly as possible
☐ 4. Tell the client to move self from the table to the stretcher
☐ 5. Raise side rails after the client is positioned on the stretcher per agency policy

Level of Cognitive Ability: Applying
Client Needs: Safe and Effective Care Environment
Integrated Process: Nursing Process/Implementation
Content Area: Fundamental Skills: Safety
Priority Concepts: Clinical Judgment; Safety

Answer: 1, 2, 5
Rationale: As part of the safe transfer of a client after a surgical procedure, the nurse should assess the client's level of consciousness, and if appropriate, let the client know that she will be transferred from the operating room table to the stretcher. The nurse checks the wheel locks of the table and the stretcher to prevent any movement during the transfer. In addition, the nurse raises the side rails per agency policy to prevent the client from falling off the stretcher. This is important because the client is likely to be sedated or disoriented and unable to protect herself from falling. Personnel avoid hurried movements and rapid changes in position because hurried movements predispose the client to hypotension; moreover, secure, deliberate movement increases the security of the client. Because the client remains affected by anesthesia, the client should not move herself.
Priority Nursing Tip: The nurse should always obtain additional nursing staff assistance when moving a client or transferring a client from a bed to a stretcher or other location.
Test-Taking Strategy: Focus on the subject, safety during client transfer. Option 4 is unsuitable because of the residual effects of anesthesia. Also, options 3 and 4 are likely to increase the risk of client injury. Review: care of the **postoperative client.**
Reference(s): Potter et al (2013), p. 1277.

417. The nurse is planning care for a hallucinating and delusional client who has been
rescued from a suicide attempt. Which
intervention should the nurse incorporate
into the nursing care plan?
1. Check the client's location every 15 minutes.
2. Begin suicide precautions with 30-minute
checks.
3. Initiate one-to-one suicide precautions immediately.
4. Ask the client to report suicidal thoughts
immediately.

Level of Cognitive Ability: Applying
Client Needs: Safe and Effective Care Environment
Integrated Process: Nursing Process/Planning
Content Area: Mental Health
Priority Concepts: Mood and Affect, Safety

Answer: 3
Rationale: One-to-one suicide precautions are required for the client rescued from a suicide attempt. In this situation, additional significant information is that the client is delusional and hallucinating.
Both of these factors increase the risk of unpredictable behavior, compromised judgment, and the risk of suicide. Options 1, 2, and 4 do
not provide the constant supervision necessary for this client.
Priority Nursing Tip: Never leave a client at risk for suicide alone.
Test-Taking Strategy: Focusing on the subject, suicide attempt with
hallucinations and delusions will direct you to option 3, the intervention that will provide the most supervision. Review: **suicide
precautions.**
Reference(s): Varcarolis (2013), pp. 320-321, 453.

418. The nurse is developing a plan of care for a
client receiving anticoagulant agents. What
should the nurse identify as a potential
problem for this client?
1. Injury
2. Fatigue
3. Infection
4. Dehydration

Level of Cognitive Ability: Analyzing
Client Needs: Safe and Effective Care Environment
Integrated Process: Nursing Process/Planning
Content Area: Pharmacology: Cardiovascular Med-
ications
Priority Concepts: Clotting; Safety

Answer: 1
Rationale: Anticoagulant therapy predisposes the client to injury
because of the agent's inhibitory effects on the body's normal blood-
clotting mechanism. Bruising, bleeding, and hemorrhage may occur
in the course of activities of daily living and with other activities.
Options 2, 3, and 4 are unrelated to this form of therapy.
Priority Nursing Tip: Teach the client taking warfarin sodium
(Coumadin) to avoid consuming green, leafy vegetables and foods
high in vitamin K because they interact with the action of the
medication.
Test-Taking Strategy: Focus on the subject, risks associated with
anticoagulant therapy. Recalling that anticoagulants present a risk for
bleeding will assist in directing you to option 1. Review: the effects of
anticoagulants.
Reference(s): Ignatavicius, Workman (2013), p. 863; Lewis et al
(2014), p. 854.

419. A client seen in the emergency department
with complaints of abdominal pain has a
diagnosis of acute abdominal syndrome
and the cause has not been determined.
Which prescription should the nurse question at this time?
1. Clear liquid diet only
2. Insertion of a nasogastric tube
3. Administration of an analgesic
4. Insertion of an intravenous (IV) line

Level of Cognitive Ability: Analyzing
Client Needs: Safe and Effective Care Environment
Integrated Process: Nursing Process/Implementation
Content Area: Adult Health: Gastrointestinal
Priority Concepts: Collaboration; Safety

Answer: 1
Rationale: Until the cause of the acute abdominal syndrome is determined and a decision about the need for surgery is made, the nurse
would question a prescription to give a clear liquid diet. The nurse
can expect the client to be placed on NPO status and to have an IV
line inserted. Insertion of a nasogastric tube may be helpful to provide decompression of the stomach. Pain management with medications that do not alter level of consciousness can decrease diffuse
abdominal pain and rigidity, help with localizing the pain, and lead
to more prompt diagnosis and treatment.
Priority Nursing Tip: Signs of perforation and peritonitis include
restlessness, guarding of the abdomen, distention and a rigid abdomen, increased fever, chills, tachycardia, and tachypnea.
Test-Taking Strategy: Focus on the subject, undetermined abdominal pain and the prescription that the nurse would question. Think
about the client's diagnosis. Recalling that surgery may be a necessary
intervention should direct you to the correct option. Review: interventions for the client with **acute abdominal syndrome.**
Reference(s): Lewis et al (2014), pp. 974-975.

420. A family friend telephones the home health nurse to inquire if there is anything she can do, as a friend, to assist her neighbors, the parents of a newborn with congenital tracheoesophageal fistula. The parents had expressed nervousness about giving enteral feedings. What should be the **best** nursing action at this time?

1. Inform the friend to directly contact the family and offer assistance to them.
2. Request that the friend come to the client's home, to be taught to administer the feedings.
3. Report the friend's telephone call to the nurse manager for referral to the client's social worker.
4. Inform the friend that the family has no need for assistance because the nurse is making daily visits.

Level of Cognitive Ability: Applying
Client Needs: Safe and Effective Care Environment
Integrated Process: Caring
Content Area: Leadership/Management: Ethical/Legal
Priority Concepts: Ethics; Health Care Law

Answer: 1
Rationale: The nurse must uphold the client's rights and does not give any information regarding a client's care needs to anyone who is not directly involved in the client's care. To request that the friend come for teaching is a direct violation of the client's right to privacy. There is no information in the question to indicate that the family desires assistance from the friend. To refer the call to the nurse manager and social worker again assumes that the friend's assistance and involvement are desired by the family. Informing the friend that the nurse is visiting daily is providing information that is considered confidential. Option 1 directly refers the friend to the family.
Priority Nursing Tip: The nurse must protect client confidentiality at all times.
Test-Taking Strategy: Note the strategic word, *best*. Focus on the subject, confidentiality and the client's right to privacy. Option 1 is the only option that upholds the client's rights. Review: **confidentiality** and **client rights.**
Reference(s): Potter et al (2013), pp. 299-300.

---

421. The nurse has been assigned to care for a client recovering at home from a disabling lung infection. While obtaining a nursing history, the nurse learns that the infection is probably the result of human immunodeficiency virus (HIV) contracted through homosexual activity. The nurse is morally opposed to homosexuality and cannot care for the client. The nurse then leaves the client's home. Which is acceptable regarding the nurse's actions? **Select all that apply.**

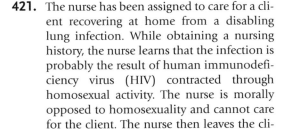

1. The nurse has the moral right to leave the client's home at any time.
2. The nurse has a legal right to inform the client of any barriers to providing care.
3. The nurse has a duty to protect self from client care situations that are morally repellent.
4. The nurse has a duty to provide competent care to assigned clients in a nondiscriminatory manner.
5. The nurse has the right to refuse to care for any client on religious grounds if competent care coverage is arranged.

Level of Cognitive Ability: Analyzing
Client Needs: Safe and Effective Care Environment
Integrated Process: Caring
Content Area: Leadership/Management: Ethical/Legal
Priority Concepts: Ethics; Health Care Law

Answer: 4, 5
Rationale: The nurse has a duty to provide care to all clients in a nondiscriminatory manner. Personal autonomy does not apply if it interferes with the rights of the client. Refusal to provide care may be acceptable if that refusal does not put the client's safety at risk and the refusal is primarily associated with religious objections, not personal objection to lifestyle or medical diagnosis. There is no legal obligation to inform the client of the nurse's personal objections to the client. The nurse also has an obligation to observe the principle of nonmaleficence (neither causing nor allowing harm to befall the client).
Priority Nursing Tip: The client always has the right to considerate and respectful care.
Test-Taking Strategy: Focus on the subject, client's rights and the nurse's ethical and legal responsibilities. Recognize that refusal to care for a client on religious grounds is permitted if client coverage is arranged. Note the words *competent care* and *nondiscriminatory* in the correct choices. The remaining options are incorrect related to the client's rights and the nurse's moral and legal obligations. Review: **client rights.**
Reference(s): Potter et al (2013), pp. 4, 287.

422. The nurse is preparing to administer heparin sodium 5000 units subcutaneously. Which action should the nurse take to safely administer the medication?
1. Inject via an infusion device.
2. Inject within 1 inch of the umbilicus.
3. Massage the injection site after administration for a full minute.
4. Change the needle on the syringe after withdrawing the medication from the vial.

Level of Cognitive Ability: Applying
Client Needs: Safe and Effective Care Environment
Integrated Process: Nursing Process/Implementation
Content Area: Fundamental Skills: Safety
Priority Concepts: Clinical Judgment; Safety

Answer: 4
Rationale: After withdrawal of heparin from the vial, the needle is changed before injection to prevent leakage of medication along the needle tract. Heparin administered subcutaneously does not require an infusion device. The injection site is located in the abdominal fat layer. It is not injected within 2 inches of the umbilicus or into any scar tissue. The needle is withdrawn rapidly, pressure is applied, and the area is not massaged. Injection sites are rotated.
Priority Nursing Tip: Monitor the client receiving an anticoagulant for bleeding, such as bleeding gums, bruises, nosebleeds, hematuria, hematemesis, petechiae, and occult blood in the stool.
Test-Taking Strategy: Focus on the subject, heparin administration. Noting that the heparin is to be administered subcutaneously will assist in eliminating option 1. From the remaining options, recall that heparin is an anticoagulant. This will assist in eliminating options 2 and 3. Review: the procedure for administering subcutaneous heparin.
Reference(s): Hodgson, Kizior (2014), p. 561.

423. A client asks the nurse to act as a witness for an advance directive. Which is the **best** intervention for the nurse to implement?
1. Decline the client's request politely.
2. Agree to sign the document as a witness.
3. Notify the provider of the client's request.
4. Help the client find an unrelated third party.

Level of Cognitive Ability: Applying
Client Needs: Safe and Effective Care Environment
Integrated Process: Nursing Process/Implementation
Content Area: Leadership/Management: Ethical/Legal
Priority Concepts: Ethics; Health Care Law

Answer: 4
Rationale: An advance directive addresses the withdrawal or withholding of life-sustaining interventions that can prolong life and identifies the person who will make care decisions if the client becomes incompetent. Two people unrelated to the client witness the client's signature and then sign the document signifying that the client signed the advance directive authentically. Nurses or employees of a facility in which the client is receiving care and beneficiaries of the client should not serve as a witness because of conflict of interest concerns. There is no reason to call the provider unless the absence of the advance directive interferes with client care.
Priority Nursing Tip: If the client signs an advance directive at the time of hospital admission, it must be documented in the client's medical record.
Test-Taking Strategy: Note the strategic word, *best*. Focus on the subject, witness for a legal document. Eliminate option 1 because it demonstrates lack of client advocacy. Examine the remaining options and recall the nurse's role as a witness of a legal document. Review: the concepts surrounding an **advance directive**.
Reference(s): Ignatavicius, Workman (2013), p. 108; Lewis et al (2014), p. 146; Potter et al (2013), pp. 298-299.

424. The nurse provides home care instructions to the mother of a child with chickenpox about preventing the transmission of the virus. Which instruction should the nurse include?

1. Isolate the child until the skin vesicles have dried and crusted.
2. Ensure that the child uses a separate bathroom for elimination.
3. Bring all household members to the clinic immediately for a varicella vaccine.
4. Ask the health care provider for a prescription for antibiotics for all household members.

Level of Cognitive Ability: Applying
Client Needs: Safe and Effective Care Environment
Integrated Process: Teaching and Learning
Content Area: Child Health: Infectious and Communicable Diseases
Priority Concepts: Client Education; Infection

Answer: 1
Rationale: Chickenpox is caused by the varicella-zoster virus. The communicable period is from 1 to 2 days before the onset of the rash to 6 days after the first crop of vesicles, when crusts have formed. Transmission occurs by direct contact with secretions from the vesicles or contaminated objects, and via respiratory tract secretions. It is not transmitted via urine or feces. The recommended preventative schedule for receiving the varicella vaccine is at 12 to 15 months of age (first dose) and 4 to 6 years of age (second dose). It is not administered at the time of exposure to the virus. Antibiotics are not used to treat a viral infection. Rather, they are used for treating bacterial infections.
Priority Nursing Tip: The skin is the first line of defense against infection. Altered skin integrity can lead to a skin or systemic infection.
Test-Taking Strategy: Focus on the subject, preventing the transmission of chickenpox. Eliminate option 4 first recalling that antibiotics are not used to treat a viral infection. Eliminate option 3 because of the word "immediately" in this option and recalling that recommended schedule for the administration of the varicella vaccine. Next, eliminate option 2 recalling the mode of transmission of the virus. Review: home care measures for the child with **chickenpox**.
Reference(s): Hockenberry, Wilson (2013), p. 424.

425. An older adult client has been identified as a victim of physical abuse. Which is the **priority** nursing intervention?

1. Obtaining treatment for the abusing family member
2. Adhering to federal mandatory abuse reporting laws
3. Notifying the case worker to intervene in the family situation
4. Removing the client from any situation that presents immediate danger

Level of Cognitive Ability: Applying
Client Needs: Safe and Effective Care Environment
Integrated Process: Nursing Process/Planning
Content Area: Mental Health
Priority Concepts: Interpersonal Violence; Safety

Answer: 4
Rationale: The priority nursing intervention is to remove the abused victim from the abusive environment. Options 1, 2, and 3 may be appropriate interventions but are not the priority.
Priority Nursing Tip: Older clients most at risk for abuse include individuals who are dependent because of illness, immobility, or altered mental status.
Test-Taking Strategy: Note the strategic word *priority*. Use Maslow's Hierarchy of Needs theory, remembering that if a physiological need is not present, then safety is the priority. Option 4 is the only option that directly addresses immediate client safety. Review: care of the **abused older client**.
Reference(s): Stuart (2013), p. 746.

426. A client diagnosed with leukemia asks the nurse questions about preparing a living will. Which recommendation from the nurse should be the **best** method of preparing this document?
1. Talk to the hospital chaplain.
2. Obtain advice from an attorney.
3. Consult the American Cancer Society.
4. Discuss the request with the health care provider (HCP).

Level of Cognitive Ability: Applying
Client Needs: Safe and Effective Care Environment
Integrated Process: Nursing Process/Implementation
Content Area: Leadership/Management: Ethical/Legal
Priority Concepts: Ethics; Health Care Law

Answer: 4
Rationale: Living wills are legal documents known as advance directives wherein the client delineates the withdrawal or withholding of treatment when the client is incompetent. Living wills should not be confused with a will that bequeaths personal property and specifies other actions at the time of the client's death. The client starts the process of writing a living will by discussing treatment options and other related issues with the HCP. In addition, the client should discuss this issue with the family. Although options 1 and 2 may be helpful, contacting them is not the initial step because both professionals lack the medical information the client needs to make an informed decision; however, the lawyer may be involved after discussion with the HCP and family. The American Cancer Society may have pertinent information on living wills; however, the information is not individualized to the client's needs.
Priority Nursing Tip: A living will lists the medical treatment that a client chooses to omit or refuse if the client becomes unable to make decisions and is terminally ill.
Test-Taking Strategy: Note the strategic word, *best*. This indicates an initial step. Remembering that the HCP is the primary care person will assist in directing you to the correct option. Contacts addressed in options 1, 2, and 3 may follow the discussion with the provider. Review: the concepts related to **living wills**.
Reference(s): Lewis et al (2014), p. 146; Potter et al (2013), pp. 298-299.

427. The nurse identifies which clinical situation as slander?
1. The health care provider tells a client that the nurse "does not know anything."
2. The nurse tells a client that a nasogastric tube will be inserted if the client continues to refuse to eat.
3. The nurse restrains a client at bedtime because the client gets up during the night and wanders around.
4. The laboratory technician restrains the arm of a client refusing to have blood drawn so that the specimen can be obtained.

Level of Cognitive Ability: Applying
Client Needs: Safe and Effective Care Environment
Integrated Process: Nursing Process/Implementation
Content Area: Leadership/Management: Ethical/Legal
Priority Concepts: Ethics; Health Care Law

Answer: 1
Rationale: Defamation takes place when a falsehood is said (slander) or written (libel) about a person that results in injury to that person's good name and reputation. Battery involves offensive touching or the use of force by a perpetrator without the permission of the victim. An assault occurs when a person puts another person in fear of a harmful or offensive act.
Priority Nursing Tip: A tort is a civil wrong, other than a breach in contract, in which the law allows an injured person to seek damages from a person who caused the injury.
Test-Taking Strategy: Focus on the subject, the situation that constitutes slander. Read the situation presented in each option carefully. Recalling that slander constitutes verbal defamation will direct you to the correct option. Review: **slander.**
Reference(s): Potter et al (2013), p. 302.

428. A client with a subarachnoid hemorrhage secondary to ruptured cerebral aneurysm has been placed on aneurysm precautions. To provide a safe environment, the nurse should ensure that which item is provided to the client?
1. Bright lights
2. Enemas as needed
3. Television and radio
4. Daily stool softeners

Level of Cognitive Ability: Applying
Client Needs: Safe and Effective Care Environment
Integrated Process: Nursing Process/Implementation
Content Area: Adult Health: Neurological
Priority Concepts: Intracranial Regulation; Safety

Answer: 4
Rationale: Aneurysm precautions include a variety of measures designed to decrease stimuli that could increase the client's intracranial pressure. These include instituting dim lighting and reducing environmental noise and stimuli. Enemas should be avoided, but stool softeners should be provided. Straining at stool is contraindicated because it increases intracranial pressure.
Priority Nursing Tip: An early sign of increased intracranial pressure is a change in the level of consciousness.
Test-Taking Strategy: Focus on the subject, ruptured cerebral aneurysm with subarachnoid hemorrhage. With this condition, there is a need to reduce environmental stimuli and prevent increased intracranial pressure. Options 1 and 3 can be eliminated first because these items will stimulate the client. From the remaining options, eliminate option 2 because administration of an enema will increase intracranial pressure. Review: the nursing interventions for the client with a **subarachnoid hemorrhage and cerebral aneurysm.**
Reference(s): Ignatavicius, Workman (2013), pp. 1014-1015.

429. The nurse is about to administer an intravenous dose of tobramycin (Tobrex) when the client complains of vertigo and ringing in the ears. What action should the nurse take next?
1. Check the client's pupillary responses.
2. Hang the dose of medication immediately.
3. Give a dose of droperidol with the tobramycin.
4. Hold the dose and call the health care provider (HCP).

Level of Cognitive Ability: Applying
Client Needs: Safe and Effective Care Environment
Integrated Process: Nursing Process/Implementation
Content Area: Pharmacology: Immune Medications
Priority Concepts: Clinical Judgment; Safety

Answer: 4
Rationale: Tobramycin (Tobrex) is an antibiotic (aminoglycoside). Ringing in the ears and vertigo are two symptoms that may indicate dysfunction of the eighth cranial nerve. Ototoxicity is a toxic effect of therapy with aminoglycosides and could result in permanent hearing loss. The nurse should hold the dose and notify the HCP. There is no need to check the pupillary response. Administering the dose would be an unsafe response.
Priority Nursing Tip: The client with vertigo is at risk for injury; therefore, safety is a priority.
Test-Taking Strategy: Note the strategic word, *next*. Focus on the client's complaints and recall that ototoxicity can occur with this medication. Recalling that the HCP is notified if toxicity is suspected will direct you to option 4. Review: side/adverse effects of **tobramycin (Tobrex).**
Reference(s): Gahart, Nazareno (2012), pp. 1318-1319; Hodgson, Kizior (2014), p. 1179.

430. The nurse is preparing to administer amiodarone (Cordarone) intravenously. To provide a safe environment, the nurse should ensure that which specific item is in place for the client before administering the medication?
1. Oxygen therapy
2. Oxygen saturation monitor
3. Continuous cardiac monitoring
4. Noninvasive blood pressure cuff

Level of Cognitive Ability: Applying
Client Needs: Safe and Effective Care Environment
Integrated Process: Nursing Process/Implementation
Content Area: Critical Care: Medications and Intravenous Therapy
Priority Concepts: Caregiving; Safety

Answer: 3
Rationale: Amiodarone is an antidysrhythmic used to treat life-threatening ventricular dysrhythmias. The client should have continuous cardiac monitoring in place, and the medication should be infused by intravenous pump. Although options 1, 2, and 4 may be in place for the client, they are not specific items needed for the administration of this medication.
Priority Nursing Tip: Electrolyte and mineral imbalances can cause cardiac electrical instability that can result in life-threatening dysrhythmias.
Test-Taking Strategy: Focus on the subject, care to the client receiving amiodarone (Cordarone). Recalling that this medication is an antidysrhythmic will direct you to continuous cardiac monitoring. Review: the classification of **amiodarone (Cordarone)** and the nursing considerations when administering this medication.
Reference(s): Hodgson, Kizior (2014), p. 52.

431. During the admission process of a client who is admitted to the hospital for surgery to remove a tumor, the client asks the nurse if a living will, prepared 3 years ago, remains in effect. Which response should the nurse provide to the client?

1. "Yes, a living will never expires."
2. "You need to speak with an attorney."
3. "I will call someone to answer your question."
4. "It requires renewal yearly with your health care provider."

Level of Cognitive Ability: Applying
Client Needs: Safe and Effective Care Environment
Integrated Process: Nursing Process/Implementation
Content Area: Leadership/Management: Ethical/Legal
Priority Concepts: Ethics; Health Care Law

Answer: 4
Rationale: The client should discuss the living will with the health care provider (HCP) on a regular basis (at least annually) to ensure that it contains the client's current wishes and desires based on the client's current health status. Option 1 is incorrect. Although the client consults an attorney if the living will must be changed, the accurate nursing response is to tell the client that a living will should be reviewed. Option 3 is not at all helpful to the client and is, in fact, a communication block and places the client's question on hold.
Priority Nursing Tip: On admission to a health care facility, the nurse should determine whether an advance directive exists and ensure that it is part of the client's medical record.
Test-Taking Strategy: Eliminate options 1 and 3 first because they are nontherapeutic and place the client's question on hold. Also note the closed-ended word "never" in option 1. From the remaining options, it is necessary to know that the document is reviewed on a regular basis with the HCP. Review: the concepts related to **living wills**.
Reference(s): Ignatavicius, Workman (2013), p. 108; Potter et al (2013), pp. 298-299.

432. The nurse reviews wound culture results and learns that an assigned client has methicillin-resistant *Staphylococcus aureus* (MRSA) in a wound bed. Which type of transmission-based precautions does the nurse institute for this client?

1. Enteric precautions
2. Droplet precautions
3. Contact precautions
4. Airborne precautions

Level of Cognitive Ability: Applying
Client Needs: Safe and Effective Care Environment
Integrated Process: Nursing Process/Implementation
Content Area: Fundamental Skills: Infection Control
Priority Concepts: Infection; Safety

Answer: 3
Rationale: Contact precautions include standard precautions and require the use of barrier precautions such as gloves and goggles. Contact precautions are used for clients who have diarrhea, draining wounds, or methicillin-resistant infections. The goal of these precautions is to eliminate disease transmission resulting either from direct contact with the client or from indirect contact through inanimate objects or surfaces that the pathogen has contaminated, such as instruments, linens, dressing materials, or hands. Enteric precautions are initiated if the organism is transmitted via the gastrointestinal tract. Droplet and airborne precautions are used if the organism is transmitted via the respiratory tract.
Priority Nursing Tip: Handle all blood and body fluids from all clients as if they were contaminated.
Test-Taking Strategy: Focus on the subject, the client's diagnosis (MRSA), which can be transmitted by contact with the infecting organism. Note the location of the pathogen to decide how its transmission can be prevented to assist in answering the question. Recall that *enteric* refers to the gastrointestinal tract and eliminate option 1. Eliminate options 2 and 4 because they are comparable or alike and unrelated to a wound bed. Review: **contact precautions**.
Reference(s): Ignatavicius, Workman (2013), pp. 440-442; Potter et al (2013), pp. 414-415.

433. The nurse is caring for a client immediately after a bronchoscopy. The client received intravenous sedation and a topical anesthetic for the procedure. Which nursing intervention should the nurse perform to provide a safe environment for the client at this time?

1. Place pads on the side rails in case of a seizure.
2. Connect the client to a bedside ECG to monitor for dysrhythmias.
3. Place a water-seal chest drainage set at the bedside in case of a pneumothorax.
4. Check the bedside to ensure that no food or fluid is within the client's reach to prevent aspiration.

Level of Cognitive Ability: Applying
Client Needs: Safe and Effective Care Environment
Integrated Process: Nursing Process/Implementation
Content Area: Adult Health: Respiratory
Priority Concepts: Gas Exchange; Safety

Answer: 4
Rationale: After this procedure, the client remains NPO until the cough, gag, and swallow reflexes have returned, which is usually in 1 to 2 hours. Once the client can swallow and the gag reflex has returned, oral intake may begin with ice chips and small sips of water. No information in the question suggests that the client is at risk for a seizure. Even though the client is monitored for signs of any distress, seizures would not be anticipated. No data are given to support that the client is at increased risk for cardiac dysrhythmias. A pneumothorax is a possible complication of this procedure, and the nurse should monitor the client for signs of distress. However, a water-seal chest drainage set would not be placed routinely at the bedside.
Priority Nursing Tip: Complications after bronchoscopy include bronchospasm or bronchial perforation indicated by facial or neck crepitus, dysrhythmias, hemorrhage, hypoxemia, and pneumothorax.
Test-Taking Strategy: Consider that this client is sedated and has received a topical anesthetic. Use the ABCs—airway, breathing, and circulation—to direct you to the correct option. Review: postprocedure care for **bronchoscopy.**
Reference(s): Pagana, Pagana (2013), p. 196.

434. A client with a history of silicosis is admitted to the hospital with respiratory distress and impending respiratory failure. The nurse should plan to have which item readily available at the client's bedside to ensure a safe environment?

1. Code cart
2. Intubation tray
3. Thoracentesis tray
4. Chest tube and drainage system

Level of Cognitive Ability: Applying
Client Needs: Safe and Effective Care Environment
Integrated Process: Nursing Process/Planning
Content Area: Critical Care: Emergency Situations
Priority Concepts: Gas Exchange; Safety

Answer: 2
Rationale: Respiratory failure occurs when insufficient oxygen is transported to the blood or inadequate carbon dioxide is removed from the lungs and the client's compensatory mechanisms fail. The client with impending respiratory failure may need intubation and mechanical ventilation. The nurse ensures that an intubation tray is readily available. The other items are not needed at the client's bedside. A code cart is used for resuscitation. A thoracentesis tray contains the necessary items for performing a thoracentesis. A chest tube drainage system is used to treat a pneumothorax.
Priority Nursing Tip: For the client with respiratory failure, mechanical ventilation is needed if supplemental oxygen cannot maintain acceptable Pao_2 and $Paco_2$ levels.
Test-Taking Strategy: Focus on the subject, impending respiratory failure. Use the ABCs—airway, breathing, and circulation—to direct you to the correct option. Review: care of the client with impending **respiratory failure.**
Reference(s): Ignatavicius, Workman (2013), pp. 671, 674-675.

435. The nurse is preparing to administer a first dose of pentamidine isethionate (Pentam 300) intravenously to a client. Before administering the dose, which safety measure should the nurse consider for this client?

1. Assign to a private room
2. Establish a supine position
3. Place on respiratory precautions
4. Assist to a semi-Fowler's position

Level of Cognitive Ability: Applying
Client Needs: Safe and Effective Care Environment
Integrated Process: Nursing Process/Implementation
Content Area: Pharmacology: Immune Medications
Priority Concepts: Clinical Judgment; Safety

Answer: 2
Rationale: Pentamidine isethionate is an anti-infective medication and can cause severe and sudden hypotension, even with administration of a single dose. The client should be lying down during administration of this medication. The blood pressure is monitored frequently during administration. Assigning to a private room, instituting respiratory precautions, or assisting to a semi-Fowler position are all unnecessary interventions.
Priority Nursing Tip: Pentamidine isethionate (Pentam 300) may be prescribed to treat opportunistic infections such as *Pneumocystis jiroveci* pneumonia.
Test-Taking Strategy: Focus on the subject, an adverse effect of pentamidine isethionate. It is necessary to know these adverse effects to answer correctly. Recalling that the medication causes hypotension will direct you to the correct option. Review: the nursing considerations related to **pentamidine isethionate (Pentam 300).**
Reference(s): Hodgson, Kizior (2014), pp. 931-932.

436. The nurse is administering a dose of intravenous hydralazine (Apresoline) to a client. To provide a safe environment, the nurse should ensure that which item is in place before injecting the medication?

1. Central line
2. Thermometer
3. Foley catheter
4. Blood pressure cuff

Level of Cognitive Ability: Applying
Client Needs: Safe and Effective Care Environment
Integrated Process: Nursing Process/Implementation
Content Area: Pharmacology: Cardiovascular Medications
Priority Concepts: Clinical Judgment; Safety

Answer: 4
Rationale: Hydralazine is an antihypertensive medication used in the management of moderate to severe hypertension. The blood pressure and pulse should be monitored frequently after administration, so a blood pressure cuff is the item to have in place. Although intravenous access is needed, a central line is unnecessary. The other options are also unnecessary and are unrelated to the administration of this medication.
Priority Nursing Tip: Safety is a priority when an antihypertensive medication is administered because of the risk for hypotension after administration.
Test-Taking Strategy: Focus on the subject, hydralazine (Apresoline). The name of the medication *Apre*soline may provide you with the clue that the medication is used to lower the blood pressure. Also, use of the ABCs—airway, breathing, and circulation—will direct you to the correct option. Review: the action of **hydralazine (Apresoline)**.
Reference(s): Gahart, Nazareno (2012), p. 711; Hodgson, Kizior (2014), pp. 563-564.

❖ **437.** A hospitalized client is found lying on the floor next to the bed. Once the client is cared for, the nurse completes an incident report. Which written statements exemplify correct documentation on the report? (**Refer to exhibit.**) **Select all that apply.**

INCIDENT REPORT

❑ **1.** The client fell out of bed.
❑ **2.** No bruises or injuries are noted on the client.
❑ **3.** The client apparently climbed over the side rails when the nurse was out of the room.
❑ **4.** The health care provider was notified that the client was found lying on the floor next to the bed.
❑ **5.** The client is alert and oriented and stated that he needed to "go to the bathroom and didn't want to bother the nurse."
❑ **6.** Vital signs are temperature: 98.6°F; pulse 78 beats per minute and regular; respirations 16 breaths per minute and regular; blood pressure 188/78 mm Hg.

Level of Cognitive Ability: Applying
Client Needs: Safe and Effective Care Environment
Integrated Process: Communication and Documentation
Content Area: Fundamental Skills: Safety
Priority Concepts: Communication; Safety

Answer: 2, 4, 5, 6
Rationale: An incident report is a tool used by health care facilities to document situations that have caused harm or have the potential to cause harm to clients, employees, or visitors. The nurse who identifies the situation initiates the report. The report identifies the people involved in the incident, including witnesses; describes the event; and records the date, time, location, factual findings, actions taken, and any other relevant information. The health care provider is notified of the incident and completes the report after examining the client. Documentation on the report should always be as factual as possible and needs to avoid accusations. Because the client was found lying on the floor, it is unknown whether the client actually fell out of bed. Additionally, the nurse does not know that the client climbed over the side rails when the nurse was out of the room.
Priority Nursing Tip: An incident (unusual occurrence) report is considered a legal document and should not be placed in the client's chart after completion. It should be maintained and filed in a designated area as determined by agency procedure.
Test-Taking Strategy: Focus on the subject, correct documentation on the incident report. Recalling that documentation on the report should always be as factual as possible and must avoid accusations will assist in answering this question. Review: **documentation** and **incident report**.
Reference(s): Huber (2014), pp. 318-319; Potter et al (2013), pp. 305, 358.

❖ **438.** A home care nurse is visiting an older client who has been recovering from a mild stroke affecting the left side. The client lives alone but receives regular assistance from her daughter and son, who both live within 10 miles. To assess for risk factors related to safety, which actions should the nurse take? **Select all that apply.**
❑ 1. Assess the client's visual acuity.
❑ 2. Observe the client's gait and posture.
❑ 3. Evaluate the client's muscle strength.
❑ 4. Look for any hazards in the home care environment.
❑ 5. Ask a family member to move in with the client until recovery is complete.
❑ 6. Request that the client transfer to an assisted living environment for at least 1 month.

Level of Cognitive Ability: Analyzing
Client Needs: Safe and Effective Care Environment
Integrated Process: Nursing Process/Assessment
Content Area: Fundamental Skills: Safety
Priority Concepts: Intracranial Regulation; Safety

Answer: 1, 2, 3, 4
Rationale: To conduct a thorough client assessment, the nurse assesses for possible risk factors related to safety. The assessment should include assessing visual acuity, gait and posture, and muscle strength because alterations in these areas place the client at risk for falls and injury. The nurse should also assess the home environment, looking for any hazards or obstacles that would affect safety. Asking a family member to move in with the client until recovery is complete and requesting that the client transfer to an assisted living environment for at least 1 month are not assessment activities. Additionally, nothing in the question indicates that these actions are necessary; therefore, these options are unrealistic and unreasonable.
Priority Nursing Tip: Age-related changes occur on an individual basis, and one client may experience an age-related change to a lesser extent than another client. The older client who has suffered a stroke will be at a higher risk for injury related to age-related changes.
Test-Taking Strategy: Focus on the subject, assessing for risk factors related to safety after a stroke. Note that options 5 and 6 are unrelated to the subject of the question. Review: the items that should be included in a **safety assessment** and **stroke**.
Reference(s): Ignatavicius, Workman (2013), pp. 1019-1020; Potter et al (2013), p. 374.

❖ **439.** Which medical asepsis actions should the nurse take to reduce and prevent the spread of microorganisms? **Select all that apply.**
❑ 1. Practicing hand hygiene
❑ 2. Reapplying a sterile dressing
❑ 3. Sterilizing contaminated items
❑ 4. Applying a sterile gown and gloves
❑ 5. Routinely cleaning the hospital environment
❑ 6. Wearing clean gloves to prevent direct contact with blood or body fluids

Level of Cognitive Ability: Analyzing
Client Needs: Safe and Effective Care Environment
Integrated Process: Nursing Process/Implementation
Content Area: Fundamental Skills: Infection Control
Priority Concepts: Infection; Safety

Answer: 1, 5, 6
Rationale: Medical asepsis, or clean technique, includes procedures to reduce and prevent the spread of microorganisms. Practicing hand hygiene, routinely cleaning the hospital environment, and wearing clean gloves to prevent direct contact with blood or body fluids are examples of medical asepsis. Surgical asepsis involves the use of sterile technique. Examples of surgical asepsis include reapplying a sterile dressing, sterilization of contaminated items, and applying a sterile gown and gloves.
Priority Nursing Tip: Medical asepsis is intended to reduce and prevent the spread of microorganisms, whereas surgical asepsis aims to eliminate all microorganisms in a particular environment.
Test-Taking Strategy: Focus on the subject, medical asepsis. Recalling the definition of medical asepsis and that it involves clean techniques will assist in answering this question. Also note the words *sterile* in options 2 and 4 and the word *sterilizing* in option 3. These words indicate surgical asepsis. Review: the difference between **medical asepsis and surgical asepsis**.
Reference(s): Potter et al (2013), pp. 410-412, 421.

440. The nurse is caring for a hospitalized client who is having a prescribed dosage of clonazepam (Klonopin) adjusted. Because of the adjustment in the medication administration, which activity should the nurse plan to perform?
1. Weigh the client daily.
2. Assess for ecchymoses.
3. Institute seizure precautions.
4. Monitor blood glucose levels.

Level of Cognitive Ability: Analyzing
Client Needs: Safe and Effective Care Environment
Integrated Process: Nursing Process/Planning
Content Area: Pharmacology: Neurological Medications
Priority Concepts: Clinical Judgment; Safety

Answer: 3
Rationale: Clonazepam is a benzodiazepine that is used as an anticonvulsant. During initial therapy and periods of dosage adjustment, the nurse should initiate seizure precautions for the client. This medication does not cause weight gain or loss, bleeding or bruising, or fluctuations in blood glucose levels.
Priority Nursing Tip: Flumazenil (Romazicon) reverses the effects of benzodiazepines.
Test-Taking Strategy: Focus on the subject, clonazepam and think about its classification. Recalling that this medication is an anticonvulsant will direct you to the correct option. Review: the nursing considerations related to **clonazepam (Klonopin)**.
Reference(s): Hodgson, Kizior (2014), p. 265; Ignatavicius, Workman (2013), pp. 934-935.

441. The nurse is planning to obtain an arterial blood gas (ABG) from the radial artery of a client with chronic obstructive pulmonary disease (COPD). To prevent bleeding after the procedure, which activity should the nurse plan time for after the arterial blood is drawn?
1. Holding a warm compress over the puncture site for 5 minutes
2. Encouraging the client to open and close the hand rapidly for 2 minutes
3. Applying pressure to the puncture site by applying a 2×2 gauze for 5 minutes
4. Having the client keep the radial pulse puncture site in a dependent position for 5 minutes

Level of Cognitive Ability: Applying
Client Needs: Safe and Effective Care Environment
Integrated Process: Nursing Process/Planning
Content Area: Fundamental Skills: Acid-Base
Priority Concepts: Clotting; Safety

Answer: 3
Rationale: Applying pressure over the puncture site for 5 to 10 minutes reduces the risk of hematoma formation and damage to the artery. A cold compress would aid in limiting blood flow; a warm compress would increase blood flow. Keeping the extremity still and out of a dependent position will aid in the formation of a clot at the puncture site.
Priority Nursing Tip: Before drawing blood for an arterial blood gas analysis, perform the Allen's test to determine the presence of collateral circulation.
Test-Taking Strategy: Focus on the subject, preventing bleeding following an arterial blood gas draw. Eliminate options 1, 2, and 4 because these activities promote bleeding. Option 3, applying pressure, aids in the prevention of bleeding into the surrounding tissues. Review: nursing responsibilities after drawing an **arterial blood gas (ABG)**.
Reference(s): Pagana, Pagana (2013), p. 117.

442. The nurse is admitting to the nursing unit a client who has an arteriovenous (AV) fistula in the right arm for hemodialysis. Which strategy should the nurse plan to implement to **best** prevent injury to the site?

1. Applying an allergy bracelet to the right arm
2. Placing an alert bracelet per agency procedure on the client's right arm
3. Putting a large note about the access site on the front of the medical record
4. Telling the client to inform all caregivers who enter the room about the presence of the access site.

Level of Cognitive Ability: Applying
Client Needs: Safe and Effective Care Environment
Integrated Process: Nursing Process/Planning
Content Area: Fundamental Skills: Safety
Priority Concepts: Clinical Judgment; Safety

Answer: 2
Rationale: There should be no venipunctures or blood pressure measurements in the extremity with a hemodialysis access device. This is commonly communicated to all caregivers by placing an alert bracelet on the arm that needs to be protected. This alert bracelet prompts the health care provider to investigate the need for the bracelet. The use of an alert wrist bracelet (rather than a visibly posted note or sign) also maintains client confidentiality. Agency procedure is always followed. An allergy bracelet is placed on the client with an allergy. Placing a note on the front of the medical record does not ensure that everyone caring for the client is aware of the access device. The client should not be responsible for informing the caregivers.
Priority Nursing Tip: To assess for patency of the arteriovenous (AV) fistula, feel for a thrill and listen for a bruit. The health care provider is notified immediately if disruption of patency is suspected.
Test-Taking Strategy: Note the strategic word, *best*. Eliminate option 1 because an allergy bracelet is used for a client with an allergy. Eliminate option 3 because placing a note on the client chart does not ensure all caregivers will have access to this information in a timely manner. Eliminate option 4 next because this responsibility should not be placed on the client. Option 2 best informs those caring for the client of the presence of the fistula. Review: care of the client with an AV fistula.
Reference(s): Ignatavicius, Workman (2013), p. 1562; Lewis et al (2014), pp. 1120-1121.

443. Regular insulin by continuous intravenous (IV) infusion is prescribed for a client with a blood glucose level of 700 mg/dL. How should the nurse administer this medication?

1. Mix the solution in 5% dextrose.
2. Change the solution every 6 hours.
3. Infuse the medication via an electronic infusion pump.
4. Titrate the infusion according to the client's urine glucose levels.

Level of Cognitive Ability: Applying
Client Needs: Safe and Effective Care Environment
Integrated Process: Nursing Process/Implementation
Content Area: Critical Care: Medications and Intravenous Therapy
Priority Concepts: Glucose Regulation; Safety

Answer: 3
Rationale: Insulin is administered via an infusion pump to prevent inadvertent overdose and subsequent hypoglycemia. Dextrose is added to the IV infusion once the serum glucose level reaches 250 mg/dL to prevent the occurrence of hypoglycemia. Administering dextrose to a client with a serum glucose level of 700 mg/dL would counteract the beneficial effects of insulin in reducing the glucose level. There is no reason to change the solution every 6 hours. Glycosuria is not a reliable indicator of the actual serum glucose levels because many factors affect the renal threshold for glucose loss in the urine.
Priority Nursing Tip: Regular insulin is a type of insulin that can be given by the intravenous route. When administering intravenous insulin, monitor the blood glucose level and the potassium levels closely.
Test-Taking Strategy: Focus on the subject, administration of IV insulin to the client with severe blood glucose elevation. Eliminate option 1, knowing that dextrose would not be administered to a client with a blood glucose of 700 mg/dL. Eliminate option 2 because there is no need to change the solution every 6 hours. Eliminate option 4, knowing that urine glucose levels do not provide an accurate indication of the client's status. Insulin should be administered with an electronic infusion pump. Review: nursing care of a client with a continuous IV infusion of insulin.
Reference(s): Lewis et al (2014), pp. 1161-1162, 1168; Potter et al (2013), pp. 906-907.

444. Which situation demonstrates the use of a situational leadership style?
1. The nurse manager delegates tasks to each team member
2. The nurse manager allows team members to work without supervision
3. The nurse manager invites team members to provide input about a unit problem
4. The nurse manager quickly delegates activities to team members during an emergency situation

Level of Cognitive Ability: Applying
Client Needs: Safe and Effective Care Environment
Integrated Process: Nursing Process/Implementation
Content Area: Leadership/Management: Delegating
Priority Concepts: Leadership; Professionalism

Answer: 4
Rationale: The situational leadership style uses a style depending on the situation and events. This type of leadership style is used in emergency situations when the nurse manager needs to quickly delegate activities to achieve a successful outcome for the situation. A laissez-faire leader abdicates leadership and responsibilities, allowing staff to work without assistance, direction, or supervision. Participative leadership demonstrates an "in-between" style, neither authoritarian nor democratic. In participative leadership, the manager presents an analysis of problems and proposals for actions to team members, inviting critique and comments. The participative leader then analyzes the comments and makes the final decision. The autocratic style of leadership is task oriented and directive.
Priority Nursing Tip: The nurse is always responsible for his/her actions when providing care to a client.
Test-Taking Strategy: Focus on the subject, style of leadership, noting the words *situational leadership*. Recalling that a situational leadership style uses a style depending on the situation and events will direct you to the correct option. Review: the various types of **leadership styles**.
Reference(s): Huber (2014), p. 48.

445. The clinic nurse wants to develop a teaching program for clients with diabetes mellitus. Which strategy should the nurse initiate **first** in order to meet the clients' needs?
1. Assess the clients' functional abilities.
2. Ensure that insurance will pay for participation in the program.
3. Discuss the focus of the program with the multidisciplinary team.
4. Include everyone who comes into the clinic in the teaching sessions.

Level of Cognitive Ability: Applying
Client Needs: Safe and Effective Care Environment
Integrated Process: Teaching and Learning
Content Area: Leadership/Management: Prioritizing
Priority Concepts: Client Education; Health Promotion

Answer: 1
Rationale: Nurse-managed clinics focus on individualized disease prevention and health promotion and maintenance. Therefore, the nurse must first assess the clients and their needs to effectively plan the program. Options 2, 3, and 4 do not address the clients' needs.
Priority Nursing Tip: When determining priorities for client teaching, identify the client's immediate learning needs, as well as what the client perceives as important.
Test-Taking Strategy: Note the strategic word, *first*. Use the steps of the nursing process. Remember that the first step is assessment. Option 1 reflects assessment. Review: **teaching and learning principles**.
Reference(s): Potter et al (2013), pp. 73, 329-330.

446. The nurse notes that a postoperative client has not been obtaining relief from pain with the prescribed opioid analgesics when a particular licensed coworker is assigned to the client. Which action is **most appropriate** for the nurse to take?

1. Reassign the coworker to the care of clients not receiving opioids.
2. Notify the health care provider that the client needs an increase in opioid dosage.
3. Review the client's medication administration record immediately and discuss the observations with the nursing supervisor.
4. Confront the coworker with the information about the client having pain control problems and ask if the coworker is using the opioids personally.

Level of Cognitive Ability: Applying
Client Needs: Safe and Effective Care Environment
Integrated Process: Nursing Process/Implementation
Content Area: Leadership/Management: Ethical/Legal
Priority Concepts: Ethics; Professionalism

Answer: 3
Rationale: In this situation, the nurse has noted an unusual occurrence, but before deciding what action to take next, the nurse needs more data than just suspicion. This can be obtained by reviewing the client's record. State and federal labor and opioid regulations, as well as institutional policies and procedures, must be followed. It is therefore most appropriate that the nurse discuss the situation with the nursing supervisor before taking further action. To reassign the coworker to clients not receiving opioids ignores the issue. The client does not need an increase in opioids. A confrontation is not the most advisable action because it could result in an argumentative situation.
Priority Nursing Tip: If the nurse suspects that a coworker is abusing chemicals and potentially jeopardizing a client's safety, the nurse must report the individual to nursing administration in a confidential manner.
Test-Taking Strategy: Focus on the subject, suspicion of substance abuse in another nurse. Note the strategic words, *most appropriate*. Recall knowledge regarding the roles and responsibilities of the nurse in a situation where another nurse may be abusing the client's medication and the organizational channels of communication that should be used. Option 3 is the only option that includes consultation with an authority figure, the nursing supervisor. Review: the nurse's role when **substance abuse** in another nurse is suspected.
Reference(s): Potter et al (2013), p. 300.

447. The medication nurse is supervising a newly hired licensed practical nurse (LPN) during the administration of oral pyridostigmine bromide (Mestinon) to a client with myasthenia gravis. Which observation by the medication nurse indicates safe practice by the LPN?

1. Asking the client to take sips of water
2. Asking the client to lie down on his right side
3. Asking the client to look up at the ceiling for 30 seconds
4. Instructing the client to void before taking the medication

Level of Cognitive Ability: Evaluating
Client Needs: Safe and Effective Care Environment
Integrated Process: Nursing Process/Evaluation
Content Area: Pharmacology: Neurological Medications
Priority Concepts: Clinical Judgment; Safety

Answer: 1
Rationale: Myasthenia gravis can affect the client's ability to swallow. The primary assessment is to determine the client's ability to handle oral medications or any oral substance. Options 2 and 3 are not appropriate. Option 2 could result in aspiration, and option 3 has no useful purpose. There is no specific reason for the client to void before taking this medication.
Priority Nursing Tip: To assess the client's ability to swallow, elevate the head of the bed to high Fowler's and ask the client to sit up straight in bed before swallowing.
Test-Taking Strategy: Focus on the subject, myasthenia gravis. Recalling that myasthenia gravis affects the client's ability to swallow will direct you to the correct option, assessing for the ability to swallow oral medication. Also, note the relation between the words *oral* in the question and *sips of water* in the correct option. Review: nursing care of the client with **myasthenia gravis.**
Reference(s): Hodgson, Kizior (2014), pp. 1004-1006; Ignatavicius, Workman (2013), p. 995.

448. The nurse does not intervene when a client becomes hypotensive after surgery. The client requires emergency surgery to stop postoperative bleeding later that night. The nurse could potentially face which types of prosecution for failing to act? **Select all that apply.**

- ❑ 1. Felony
- ❑ 2. Tort law
- ❑ 3. Malpractice
- ❑ 4. Statutory law
- ❑ 5. Misdemeanor

Level of Cognitive Ability: Applying
Client Needs: Safe and Effective Care Environment
Integrated Process: Nursing Process/Implementation
Content Area: Leadership/Management: Ethical/Legal
Priority Concepts: Ethics; Health Care Law

Answer: 2, 3
Rationale: Tort law deals with wrongful acts intentionally or unintentionally committed against a person or the person's property. The nurse commits a tort offense by failing to act when the client became hypotensive. Malpractice occurs when a duty to the client is established and the nurse neglects to act responsibly. Options 1 and 5 are offenses under criminal law. Option 4 describes laws enacted by state, federal, or local governments.
Priority Nursing Tip: Malpractice is negligence on the part of the nurse. The nurse who does not meet appropriate standards of care may be held liable.
Test-Taking Strategy: Focus on the subject, laws applying to failure to meet standards of care. Recalling that both a tort and malpractice refer to wrongful acts will direct you to option 2 and 3. Review: **Tort Law** and **malpractice**.
Reference(s): Huber (2014), p. 97; Potter et al (2013), pp. 301-302.

449. An individual from the community is admitted to the hospital with a diagnosis of Parkinson's disease. The nurse gives medical information regarding the client's condition to a person who is assumed to be a family member. Later the nurse discovers that this person is not a family member and realizes that this violated which legal concepts of the nurse–client relationship? **Select all that apply.**

- ❑ 1. Duty to provide care
- ❑ 2. Client's right to privacy
- ❑ 3. Nurse's lack of experience
- ❑ 4. Client's right to confidentiality
- ❑ 5. Failure to communicate to the health care provider

Level of Cognitive Ability: Applying
Client Needs: Safe and Effective Care Environment
Integrated Process: Nursing Process/Implementation
Content Area: Leadership/Management: Ethical/Legal
Priority Concepts: Ethics; Health Care Law

Answer: 2, 4
Rationale: Discussing a client's condition without client permission violates a client's rights to privacy and confidentiality and places the nurse in legal jeopardy. This action by the nurse is both an invasion of privacy and affects the confidentiality issue with client rights. Options 1, 3, and 5 do not represent violation of the situation presented.
Priority Nursing Tip: Leaving the curtains or room door open while a treatment or procedure is being performed constitutes an invasion of client privacy.
Test-Taking Strategy: Focus on the subject, sharing of client information. Sharing information constitutes an invasion of privacy and violates maintenance of confidentiality. Review **client rights** and **invasion of privacy** and **confidentiality**.
Reference(s): Huber (2014), p. 103; Potter et al (2013), pp. 301-302.

450. In which situation is the nurse utilizing autocratic leadership style?
1. The nurse manager provides the solution for a unit problem.
2. The nurse manager allows the staff to solve their own unit problem.
3. The nurse manager proposes several alternatives and has the unit staff vote on the best proposal.
4. The nurse manager arranges for a staff meeting where all unit employees can share proposals to solve a problem.

Level of Cognitive Ability: Analyzing
Client Needs: Safe and Effective Care Environment
Integrated Process: Nursing Process/Implementation
Content Area: Leadership/Management: Delegating
Priority Concepts: Leadership; Professionalism

Answer: 1
Rationale: The autocratic style of leadership is task oriented and directive. The leader uses his or her power and position in an authoritarian manner to set and implement organizational goals or solutions. Decisions are made without input from the staff. The situational leadership style uses a style depending on the situation and events. Democratic styles best empower staff toward excellence because this style of leadership allows nurses to provide input regarding the decision-making process and an opportunity to grow professionally. Participatory leadership encourages input from the staff.
Priority Nursing Tip: Leadership is an interpersonal process that involves influencing others (followers) to achieve goals.
Test-Taking Strategy: Focus on the subject, autocratic leadership. Recall the definition of this style of leadership to answer correctly. Also note that options 2, 3, and 4 are comparable or alike in that they all deal with staff input. Review: the various **leadership styles.**
Reference(s): Huber (2014), p. 133.

451. The nurse performing an initial admission assessment notes that a client has been taking metoclopramide (Reglan) for a prolonged period. The nurse should **immediately** call the health care provider if which signs/symptoms were then noted by the nurse?
1. Anxiety or irritability
2. Excessive drowsiness
3. Uncontrolled rhythmic movements of the face or limbs
4. Dry mouth relieved with the use of sugar-free hard candy

Level of Cognitive Ability: Analyzing
Client Needs: Safe and Effective Care Environment
Integrated Process: Nursing Process/Implementation
Content Area: Pharmacology: Gastrointestinal Medications
Priority Concepts: Clinical Judgment; Safety

Answer: 3
Rationale: If the client experiences tardive dyskinesia (rhythmic movements of the face or limbs), the nurse should call the health care provider because these adverse effects may be irreversible. The medication would be discontinued, and no further doses should be given by the nurse. Anxiety, irritability, and dry mouth are mild side effects that do not harm the client.
Priority Nursing Tip: Metoclopramide (Reglan) stimulates the motility of the upper gastrointestinal tract and is contraindicated in clients with mechanical obstruction, perforation, or gastrointestinal hemorrhage.
Test-Taking Strategy: Note that the question contains the strategic word, *immediately*, which guides you to select the most harmful option. Recalling that this medication causes tardive dyskinesia will direct you to option 3. Review: the side/adverse effects of **metoclopramide (Reglan)** and the signs of **tardive dyskinesia.**
Reference(s): Hodgson, Kizior (2014), p. 765.

452. Which clinical situation should be viewed as assault?
1. The nurse threatens to apply restraints to a client who is exhibiting aggressive behavior.
2. The client requests a medical discharge, but the nurse physically forces the client to stay.
3. The charge nurse sends an email to a staff member which includes a poor performance evaluation about another person.
4. The nurse overhears the health care provider making derogatory remarks to the client about the nurse's level of competency.

Level of Cognitive Ability: Applying
Client Needs: Safe and Effective Care Environment
Integrated Process: Nursing Process/Implementation
Content Area: Leadership/Management: Ethical/Legal
Priority Concepts: Ethics; Health Care Law

Answer: 1
Rationale: An assault occurs when a person puts another person in fear of a harmful or offensive act. Battery involves offensive touching or the use of force by a perpetrator without the permission of the victim. Defamation takes place when a falsehood is said (slander) or written (libel) about a person that results in injury to that person's good name and reputation.
Priority Nursing Tip: False imprisonment occurs when a client is not allowed to leave a health care facility when there is no legal justification to detain the client.
Test-Taking Strategy: Focus on the subject, an assault. Eliminate option 2 noting the words, *physically forces;* this constitutes battery. Next eliminate options 3 and 4 because they address written and verbal information that can be harmful to another. Review: assault.
Reference(s): Potter et al (2013), p. 302.

453. The nurse finds the client sitting on the floor, ensures the client's safety, completes an incident report, and notifies the health care provider of the incident. What should the nurse implement **next**?
1. Staple the incident report in the client's medical record.
2. Document the client events and follow-up nursing actions.
3. Provide a copy of the incident report to the provider and family.
4. Document in the client's medical record that the nurse sent a copy of the report to risk management.

Level of Cognitive Ability: Applying
Client Needs: Safe and Effective Care Environment
Integrated Process: Nursing Process/Implementation
Content Area: Leadership/Management: Ethical/Legal
Priority Concepts: Communication; Health Care Law

Answer: 2
Rationale: The nurse documents the incident completely and objectively in the client's record to communicate client data to the health care team. The incident report is a confidential, privileged, and internal document used to improve client safety and quality of care and therefore should not be copied, stapled, or placed in the chart. Furthermore, the nurse avoids referring to the incident report in the client's record, such as recording that the incident report has been sent to another department. These actions are necessary because any mention of an incident report in the medical record allows the plaintiff's attorney access to the document through discovery.
Priority Nursing Tip: An incident report is used as a means of identifying risk situations and improving client care.
Test-Taking Strategy: Note the strategic word, *next.* Focus on the subject, an incident report. Eliminate options 1 and 4 first because incident reports are neither stapled nor referred to in the medical record. From the remaining options, recall that an incident report is an internal, confidential document that is not intended for the family and is never copied to eliminate option 3. Review: nursing responsibilities related to incident reports.
Reference(s): Huber (2014), pp. 318-319; Potter et al (2013), pp. 305, 358.

454. A client had a colon resection. A nasogastric tube was in place when a regular diet was brought to the client's room. The client did not want to eat solid food and asked that the health care provider be called. The nurse insisted that the solid food was the correct diet. The client ate and subsequently had additional surgery as a result of complications. The determination of negligence is based on which premise?
1. The nurse's persistence
2. A duty existed and it was breached
3. Not notifying the health care provider
4. The dietary department sending the wrong food

Level of Cognitive Ability: Applying
Client Needs: Safe and Effective Care Environment
Integrated Process: Nursing Process/Implementation
Content Area: Leadership/Management: Ethical/ Legal
Priority Concepts: Ethics; Health Care Law

Answer: 2
Rationale: For negligence to be proved, there must be a duty, and then a breach of duty; the breach of duty must cause the injury, and damages or injury must be experienced. Options 1, 3, and 4 do not fall under the criteria for negligence. Option 2 is the only option that fits the criteria of negligence.
Priority Nursing Tip: Negligence is conduct that falls below the standard of care.
Test-Taking Strategy: Focus on the subject, negligence. Options 1, 3, and 4 do not directly support the subject of negligence because it would be difficult to determine that these elements caused injury. The focus relates to what the nurse is responsible for. Review the legal elements of nursing practice and criteria for **negligence.**
Reference(s): Potter et al (2013), p. 302.

455. The nurse is caring for a child with intussusception. During care, the child passes a normal brown stool. Which action should the nurse take at this time?
1. Note the child's physical symptoms.
2. Prepare the child for hydrostatic reduction.
3. Prepare the child and parents for the possibility of surgery.
4. Report the passage of a normal brown stool to the health care provider.

Level of Cognitive Ability: Applying
Client Needs: Safe and Effective Care Environment
Integrated Process: Nursing Process/Implementation
Content Area: Child Health: Gastrointestinal
Priority Concepts: Collaboration; Elimination

Answer: 4
Rationale: Intussusception is the telescoping of one portion of the bowel into another portion. Passage of a normal brown stool usually indicates that the intussusception has reduced itself. This is immediately reported to the health care provider, who may choose to alter the diagnostic or therapeutic plan of care. Although the nurse would note the child's physical symptoms, based on the data in the question, option 4 is the appropriate action. Hydrostatic reduction and surgery may not be necessary.
Priority Nursing Tip: Currant jellylike stools that contain blood and mucus are characteristic of intussusception.
Test-Taking Strategy: Focus on the subject, intussusception. Note the similarity between the information in the question and the correct option. Also, recalling the physiology associated with intussusception will direct you to the correct option. Review: care of the child with **intussusception.**
Reference(s): Hockenberry, Wilson (2013), p. 810.

456. The nurse caring for a client with end-stage kidney failure is asked by a family member about advance directives. Which statements should the nurse include when discussing advance directives with the client's family member? **Select all that apply.**

☐ 1. A health care proxy can write a living will for a client if the client becomes incompetent and unable to do so.

☐ 2. Two witnesses, either a relative or health care provider (HCP), are needed when the client signs a living will.

☐ 3. The determination of decisional capacity of a client is usually made by the health care provider and family.

☐ 4. Living wills are written documents that direct treatment in accordance with a client's wishes in the event of a terminal illness or condition.

☐ 5. Under the Patient Self-Determination Act (PSDA), it must be documented in the client's record whether the client has signed an advance directive.

☐ 6. For advance directives to be enforceable, the client must be legally incompetent or lack decisional capacity to make decisions regarding health care treatment.

Level of Cognitive Ability: Applying
Client Needs: Safe and Effective Care Environment
Integrated Process: Nursing Process/Implementation
Content Area: Leadership/Management: Ethical/Legal
Priority Concepts: Ethics; Health Care Law

Answer: 3, 4, 5, 6

Rationale: The two basic advance directives are living wills and durable powers of attorney for health care. Under the PSDA, it must be documented in the client's record whether the client has signed an advance directive. For living wills or durable powers of attorney for health care to be enforceable, the client must be legally incompetent or lack decisional capacity to make decisions regarding health care treatment. The determination of decisional capacity is usually made by the HCP and family, whereas the determination of legal competency is made by a judge. Living wills are written documents that direct treatment in accordance with a client's wishes in the event of a terminal illness or condition. Generally, two witnesses, neither of whom can be a relative or HCP, are needed when the client signs the document. A durable power of attorney for health care designates an agent, surrogate, or proxy to make health care decisions if and when the client is no longer able to make decisions on his or her own behalf; however, a health care proxy cannot legally write a living will for a client.

Priority Nursing Tip: Advance directives are used so that health care professionals can make decisions that are based on the client's wishes if the client is unable to make them. They clearly delineate end-of-life care decisions ahead of time so that appropriate action can be taken.

Test-Taking Strategy: Focus on the subject, the characteristics of advance directives. Read each option carefully. Recalling that these are legal documents based on the client's wishes will assist in determining the correct options. Review: the characteristics of **advance directives**.

Reference(s): Dolan, Holt (2013), p. 208; Potter et al (2013), pp. 298-299.

457. A client asks the nurse how to become an organ donor. What should the nurse include in the discussion?

1. The client can donate by written consent.
2. A family member must witness the consent.
3. The donor must be older than 21 years of age.
4. A family member must be present when a client consents to organ donation.

Level of Cognitive Ability: Applying
Client Needs: Safe and Effective Care Environment
Integrated Process: Nursing Process/Implementation
Content Area: Leadership/Management: Ethical/Legal
Priority Concepts: Health Policy; Health Care Law

Answer: 1

Rationale: The client has the right to donate her or his own organs for transplantation, and any person who is 18 years of age or older may become an organ donor by written consent without the permission or presence of the family. In the absence of suitable documentation, a family member or legal guardian can authorize donation of the decedent's organs.

Priority Nursing Tip: Requests to the deceased's family for organ donation usually are done by the health care provider or nurse or designated person specially trained for making such requests.

Test-Taking Strategy: Focus on the subject, organ donation and issues related to client rights. This will direct you to the correct option. Also note the closed-ended word "must" in all of the incorrect options. Review the procedure for **organ donation**.

Reference(s): Dolan, Holt (2013), p. 207; Potter et al (2013), p. 299.

458. A registered nurse (RN) is providing post-mortem care for a deceased client whose eyes will be donated. Which measure should the nurse anticipate will **most likely** be prescribed that will provide sound care of the client's body?
1. Closing the eyes and placing the bed flat
2. Maintaining the client in a supine position
3. Placing gauze pads wet with saline covered by a small ice pack on the eyes
4. Placing the client in a lateral recumbent position rotating right and left sides

Level of Cognitive Ability: Applying
Client Needs: Safe and Effective Care Environment
Integrated Process: Nursing Process/Implementation
Content Area: Critical Care: Emergency Situations
Priority Concepts: Safety; Tissue Integrity

Answer: 3
Rationale: When a corneal donor dies, the eyes are closed and usually the health care provider prescribes placing gauze pads wet with saline over them with a small ice pack. Within 2 to 4 hours the eyes are enucleated, and the corneas are usually transplanted within 24 to 48 hours. The head of the bed should be elevated. With the head of the bed elevated, the eyes will likely remain closed.
Priority Nursing Tip: Donor eyes are obtained from cadavers and must be enucleated soon after death because of rapid endothelial cell death.
Test-Taking Strategy: Focus on the subject, donation of the eyes. Also note the strategic words, *most likely,* in the question. These words indicate that a procedure specific to eye harvesting is necessary to preserve the cornea. Visualize each option and think about the subject of preserving the eyes. This will direct you to option 3. Also note that the positions identified in the incorrect options are comparable or alike. Review: **corneal transplantation.**
Reference(s): Ignatavicius, Workman (2013), p. 1059.

459. A clinical nurse manager conducts an in-service educational session for the staff nurses about case management. Which premise, if stated by the staff nurse, regarding case management, should necessitate a **need for further teaching?**
1. Manages client care by managing the client care environment
2. Maximizes hospital revenues while providing for optimal client care
3. Represents a primary health prevention focus managed by a single case manager
4. Is designed to promote appropriate use of hospital personnel and material resources

Level of Cognitive Ability: Evaluating
Client Needs: Safe and Effective Care Environment
Integrated Process: Teaching and Learning
Content Area: Leadership/Management: Delegating
Priority Concepts: Care Coordination; Professionalism

Answer: 3
Rationale: Case management represents an interdisciplinary health care delivery system to promote appropriate use of hospital personnel and material resources to maximize hospital revenues while providing for optimal client care. It manages client care by managing the client care environment and includes assessment and development of a plan of care, coordination of all services, referral, and follow-up.
Priority Nursing Tip: Case management involves consultation and collaboration with an interprofessional health care team.
Test-Taking Strategy: Note the strategic words, *need for further teaching.* These words indicate a negative event query and the need to select the option that is an incorrect characteristic of case management. Noting the word *single* in option 3 will direct you to this option. Review: the characteristics of **case management.**
Reference(s): Ignatavicius, Workman (2013), p. 4; Potter et al (2013), pp. 276, 355.

460. A registered nurse is delegating activities to the nursing staff. Which activities can be safely assigned to the unlicensed assistive personnel (UAP)? **Select all that apply.**
  ❑ 1. Collecting a urine specimen from a client
  ❑ 2. Obtaining frequent oral temperatures on a client
  ❑ 3. Assessing a client who returned from the recovery room 6 hours ago
  ❑ 4. Assisting a postcardiac catheterization client who needs to lie flat to eat lunch
  ❑ 5. Accompanying a client being discharged to meet his spouse at the hospital exit door

Level of Cognitive Ability: Applying
Client Needs: Safe and Effective Care Environment
Integrated Process: Nursing Process/Implementation
Content Area: Leadership/Management: Delegating
Priority Concepts: Leadership; Safety

Answer: 1, 2, 5
Rationale: Work that is delegated to others must be consistent with the individual's level of expertise and licensure, if any. Options 1, 2 and 5 do not include situations that indicate that these activities carry foreseeable risk. The least appropriate activities for unlicensed assistive personnel would be assessing a client and assisting the post-cardiac catheterization client. The UAP is not trained or educated to safely and accurately perform an assessment on a client. Since the postcardiac catheterization client needs to eat while lying flat, the client is at risk for aspiration.
Priority Nursing Tip: Generally, noninvasive interventions, such as skin care, range-of-motion exercises, ambulation, grooming, and hygiene measures, can be assigned to unlicensed assistive personnel (UAP).
Test-Taking Strategy: Focus on the subject, delegation to UAP. Use the ABCs—airway, breathing, and circulation—to assist in eliminating option 4. Next note the word *assessing* in option 3 and recall that the UAP is not educated to assess a client. Review: the principles of assignments and delegation.
Reference(s): Ignatavicius, Workman (2013), p. 5; Potter et al (2013), pp. 262, 281-283.

461. The nurse manager is reviewing the critical paths of the clients on the nursing unit. The nurse manager collaborates with each nurse assigned to the clients and performs a variance analysis. Which finding should indicate the **need for further action and analysis?**
  1. A client is performing his own colostomy care.
  2. A 1-day postoperative client has a temperature of 98.8° F.
  3. A 2-day post–abdominal hysterectomy client has drainage noted from the incision.
  4. A client newly diagnosed with diabetes mellitus is preparing his own insulin for injection.

Level of Cognitive Ability: Evaluating
Client Needs: Safe and Effective Care Environment
Integrated Process: Nursing Process/Evaluation
Content Area: Leadership/Management: Ethical/Legal
Priority Concepts: Health Care Quality; Leadership

Answer: 3
Rationale: Variances are actual deviations or detours from the critical paths. Variances can be either positive or negative, or avoidable or unavoidable, and can be caused by a variety of things. Positive variance occurs when the client achieves maximum benefit and is discharged earlier than anticipated. Negative variance occurs when untoward events prevent a timely discharge. Variance analysis occurs continually to anticipate and recognize negative variance early so that appropriate action can be taken. Option 3 is the only option that identifies the need for further action.
Priority Nursing Tip: Variation analysis is a continuous process that the case manager and other caregivers conduct by comparing the specific client outcomes with expected outcomes.
Test-Taking Strategy: Note the strategic words, *need for further action and analysis.* These words indicate a negative event query and the need to identify the negative variance. Options 1, 2, and 4 identify positive outcomes. Option 3 identifies a negative outcome. Review: the purpose of **variance analysis.**
Reference(s): Huber (2014), p. 324; Potter et al (2013), p. 355.

462. The nurse is planning the client assignments for the shift. Which client should the nurse assign to the unlicensed assistive personnel (UAP)?
  1. A client requiring dressing changes
  2. A client requiring frequent ambulation
  3. A client on a bowel management program requiring rectal suppositories and a daily enema
  4. A client with diabetes mellitus requiring daily insulin and reinforcement of dietary measures

Level of Cognitive Ability: Applying
Client Needs: Safe and Effective Care Environment
Integrated Process: Nursing Process/Planning
Content Area: Leadership/Management: Delegating
Priority Concepts: Leadership; Safety

Answer: 2
Rationale: Assignment of tasks to UAP needs to be made based on job description, level of clinical competence, and state law. The client described in option 2 has needs that can be met by UAP. Options 1, 3, and 4 involve care that requires the skill of a licensed nurse.
Priority Nursing Tip: Client safety is the priority when determining which tasks can be delegated and to whom.
Test-Taking Strategy: Focus on the subject, the assignment to UAP. Think about the tasks that UAP can safely perform and match the client's needs with these tasks. Eliminate options 1, 3, and 4 because these clients require care that needs to be provided by a licensed nurse. Remember that UAP can perform noninvasive tasks. Review: the guidelines regarding assignment making and delegating.
Reference(s): Huber (2014), pp. 147-148; Potter et al (2013), pp. 281-282.

463. A psychotic client on an acute care psychiatric unit is pacing, agitated, and presenting with aggressive gestures. The client's speech pattern is rapid, and the client's affect is belligerent. Which **priority** nursing intervention should the nurse implement based on these objective data?
  1. Provide safety for the client and other clients on the unit.
  2. Bring the client to a less stimulated area to regain control.
  3. Provide the clients on the unit with a sense of comfort and safety.
  4. Assist the staff in caring for the client in a controlled environment.

Level of Cognitive Ability: Applying
Client Needs: Safe and Effective Care Environment
Integrated Process: Nursing Process/Implementation
Content Area: Mental Health
Priority Concepts: Clinical Judgment; Safety

Answer: 1
Rationale: If a client is exhibiting signs that indicate loss of control, the nurse's immediate priority is to ensure safety for all clients. Option 1 is the only option that addresses the client's and other clients' safety needs. Option 2 addresses the client's needs. Option 3 addresses other clients' needs. Option 4 is not client centered.
Priority Nursing Tip: Encourage the client who is agitated to talk out instead of acting out feelings of frustration and aggression.
Test-Taking Strategy: Focus on the data in the question. Note the subject of the question, safety. Note the strategic word, priority. Option 1 is an umbrella option and addresses the safety of all. Review: nursing care for the client who is agitated.
Reference(s): Varcarolis (2013), pp. 571-572.

❖ **464.** The nurse manager is developing an educational session for nursing staff on the components of informed consent and the information to be shared with a client to obtain informed consent. Which information should the nurse manager include in the session? **Select all that apply.**
- ❑ 1. The client needs to be informed of the prognosis if the test, procedure, or treatment is refused.
- ❑ 2. The client cannot refuse a test, procedure, or treatment once the test, procedure, or treatment is started.
- ❑ 3. The name(s) of the persons performing the test or procedure or providing treatment should be documented on the informed consent form.
- ❑ 4. A description of the complications and risks of the test, procedure, or treatment, as well as anticipated pain or discomfort, needs to be explained to the client.
- ❑ 5. The nurse is responsible for obtaining the client's signature on an informed consent form even if the client has questions about the test, procedure, or treatment to be performed.

Level of Cognitive Ability: Applying
Client Needs: Safe and Effective Care Environment
Integrated Process: Teaching and Learning
Content Area: Leadership/Management: Ethical/Legal
Priority Concepts: Health Care Law, Health Policy

Answer: 1, 3, 4
Rationale: Informed consent is a person's agreement to allow something to happen based on full disclosure of risks, benefits, alternatives, and consequences of refusal. The health care provider (HCP) is responsible for conveying information and obtaining the informed consent. The nurse may be the person who actually ensures that the client signs the informed consent form; however, the nurse does this only after the HCP has instructed the client, and it has been determined that the client has understood the information. The following factors are required for informed consent: a brief, complete explanation of the test, procedure, or treatment; names and qualifications of persons performing and assisting in the test, procedure, or treatment; a description of the complications and risks, as well as anticipated pain or discomfort; an explanation of alternative therapies to the proposed test, procedure, or treatment, as well as the risks of doing nothing; and his or her right to refuse the test, procedure, or treatment even after it has been started.
Priority Nursing Tip: An informed consent is a legal document. The client needs to be a participant in decisions regarding health care and can withdraw consent at any time.
Test-Taking Strategy: Focus on the subject, informed consent. To answer this question correctly, there are two primary factors to bear in mind. The first factor is that the HCP is responsible for conveying information and obtaining the informed consent. The second factor is that the client has the right to be fully informed. Bearing these factors in mind will assist in answering this question and other questions related to informed consent. Review: the issues surrounding informed consent.
Reference(s): Potter et al (2013), pp. 60, 302-303.

❖ **465.** Wrist restraints have been prescribed for a client who is continuously pulling at his gastrostomy tube. The nurse develops a care plan and should determine that which findings are unexpected outcomes related to the use of restraints? **Select all that apply.**
- ❑ 1. The client is agitated.
- ❑ 2. The client's left hand is pale and cold.
- ❑ 3. The client's skin under the restraint is red.
- ❑ 4. The client verbalizes the reason for the restraints.
- ❑ 5. The client is unable to reach the gastrostomy tube with his hands.
- ❑ 6. The client slips his hand out of the restraint and pulls at his gastrostomy tube.

Level of Cognitive Ability: Evaluating
Client Needs: Safe and Effective Care Environment
Integrated Process: Nursing Process/Evaluation
Content Area: Fundamental Skills: Safety
Priority Concepts: Health Care Law, Health Care Quality

Answer: 1, 2, 3, 6
Rationale: A physical restraint is a mechanical or physical device used to immobilize a client or extremity. The restraint restricts freedom of movement. Unexpected outcomes in the use of restraints include signs of impaired skin integrity such as redness or skin breakdown; altered neurovascular status such as cyanosis, pallor, coldness of the skin, or complaints of tingling, numbness, or pain; increased confusion, disorientation, or agitation; or escape from the restraint device resulting in a fall or injury. Client verbalization of the reason for the restraints and the client's inability to reach the gastrostomy tube with his hands are expected outcomes.
Priority Nursing Tip: If the restraints are placed on a client during a period in which the behavior cannot be controlled, or in an emergency situation, a health care provider's prescription for the restraints must be obtained in a timely manner. Additionally, the continued need for restraints needs to be assessed regularly according to agency policy.
Test-Taking Strategy: Focus on the subject, use of restraints. Recognize that the word *unexpected* asks you to select the options that indicate undesirable effects of the use of the restraints. Focusing on the data in the question and recalling the nursing responsibilities related to care of a client in restraints will assist in answering the question. Review: the expected and unexpected outcomes related to the use of restraints.
Reference(s): Potter et al (2013), pp. 300, 388-389.

466. The nurse is discussing accident prevention with the family of an older client who is being discharged from the hospital after having hip surgery. Which physical factors place the client at risk for injury in the home? **Select all that apply.**
- ❑ 1. A night-light in the bathroom
- ❑ 2. Elevated toilet seat with armrests
- ❑ 3. Cooking equipment such as a stove
- ❑ 4. Smoke and carbon monoxide detectors
- ❑ 5. A low thermostat setting on the water heater
- ❑ 6. Common household objects such as a doormat

Level of Cognitive Ability: Analyzing
Client Needs: Safe and Effective Care Environment
Integrated Process: Nursing Process/Assessment
Content Area: Fundamental Skills: Safety
Priority Concepts: Client Education; Safety

Answer: 3, 6
Rationale: Physical hazards in the environment place the client at risk for accidental injury and death. Injuries in the home frequently result from tripping over or coming into contact with common household objects such as a doormat, small rugs on the floor or stairs, or clutter around the house. Adequate lighting such as night-lights in dark hallways and bathrooms reduces the physical hazard by illuminating areas in which a person moves about. An elevated toilet seat with armrests and nonslip strips on the floor in front of the toilet are useful in reducing falls in the bathroom. Cooking equipment and appliances, particularly stoves, can be a main source for in-home fires and fire injuries. Smoke and carbon monoxide detectors should be placed throughout the home to alert members of the household of a potential danger. A low thermostat setting on the water heater reduces the risk of burns during water use such as bathing or showering.
Priority Nursing Tip: A client with peripheral neuropathy (decreased sensation in the extremities), such as the client with diabetes mellitus, is at a high risk for injury, such as falls, cuts, or burns because of the inability to sense objects or high temperatures.
Test-Taking Strategy: Focus on the subject, the physical factors that place the client at risk for injury at home. Next think about whether the factor is safe or presents a potential for injury; this will assist in answering the question. Review: the physical factors that place clients at risk for injury.
Reference(s): Lewis et al (2014), p. 73; Potter et al (2013), p. 374.

467. The nurse is caring for a client receiving total parenteral nutrition (TPN). Which action should the nurse implement to decrease the risk of infection?
1. Assess vital signs at 4-hour intervals.
2. Administer prophylactic antimicrobial agents.
3. Check the solution's label against the prescription.
4. Use aseptic technique in handling the TPN solution.

Level of Cognitive Ability: Applying
Client Needs: Safe and Effective Care Environment
Integrated Process: Nursing Process/Implementation
Content Area: Fundamental Skills: Infection Control
Priority Concepts: Infection; Safety

Answer: 4
Rationale: Clients receiving TPN are at high risk for developing infection because the concentrated glucose solutions are an excellent medium for bacterial growth. The nurse reduces the client's risk of infection by using aseptic technique when handling all equipment and solutions related to the TPN infusion. Option 1 is a reasonable intervention for early detection of infection but does not prevent infection. Prophylactic antibiotics are not indicated for TPN infusions and can contribute to the development of secondary infections. The nurse implements option 3 to ensure that the client receives the correct infusion but is not relevant to decreasing the risk of infection.
Priority Nursing Tip: Total parenteral nutrition is the least desirable form of providing nutrition and is used when there is no other nutritional alternative.
Test-Taking Strategy: Focus on the subject, TPN and decreasing the risk for infection. Option 1 relates to early detection of infection, option 2 is not indicated, and option 3 does not relate to the subject. Remember that aseptic technique is critical to prevent infection. Review: care of the client receiving **total parenteral nutrition (TPN)** and infection prevention.
Reference(s): Lewis et al (2014), pp. 230, 901-902.

468. The home care nurse is assisting a client in managing cancer pain. To ensure that the client has adequate and safe pain control, which plan should the nurse implement?

1. Rely totally on prescription and over-the-counter medications to relieve pain.
2. Keep a baseline level of pain so that the client does not become sedated or addicted.
3. Try multiple medication modalities for pain relief to get the maximum pain relief effect.
4. Start with low doses of medication and gradually increase to a safe dose that relieves pain.

Level of Cognitive Ability: Applying
Client Needs: Safe and Effective Care Environment
Integrated Process: Caring
Content Area: Adult Health: Oncology
Priority Concepts: Cellular Regulation; Pain

Answer: 4
Rationale: Safe pain control includes starting with low doses and working up to a dose of medication that relieves the pain. Option 1 does not take into account other nursing interventions that may relieve pain, such as massage, therapeutic touch, or music. Maintaining a baseline level of pain to avoid sedation or addiction is not appropriate practice, unless the client requests this, and this information has not been provided in the case situation. Interventions using multiple medication modalities can be unsafe and ineffective.
Priority Nursing Tip: Pain is what the client describes or says that it is. Do not undermedicate the cancer client who is in pain.
Test-Taking Strategy: Focus on the subject, safe and effective pain management for the cancer client. Option 1 uses the word *totally*, and does not allow for any alternative interventions. Option 3 uses the word *multiple*, which is not appropriate in this instance. Mixing of multiple medications may be unsafe. Option 2 can be eliminated because it is inaccurate information. Option 4 is the only safe, effective approach. Review: safe **pain control** management.
Reference(s): Lewis et al (2014), p. 279; Potter et al (2013), pp. 986, 988.

469. The home care nurse provides medication instructions to a client. To ensure that the client self-administers medications safely in the home, which plan should the nurse implement?

1. Perform a pill count of each prescription bottle at every home visit
2. Instruct the client to double up on a medication when a dose is missed
3. Demonstrate the proper procedure for self-administration of medications
4. Ask the client to explain and demonstrate self-administration procedures

Level of Cognitive Ability: Applying
Client Needs: Safe and Effective Care Environment
Integrated Process: Teaching and Learning
Content Area: Fundamental Skills: Safety
Priority Concepts: Client Education; Safety

Answer: 4
Rationale: To ensure safe administration of medication, the nurse asks the client to explain and demonstrate correct self-administration of medication procedures because demonstrating the proper procedure for the client does not ensure that the client can safely perform any procedure. Usually it is not acceptable to double up on missed medication and conducting a pill count on each visit is unrealistic and disrespectful.
Priority Nursing Tip: Determine the client's readiness to learn before implementing a teaching plan. If the client is not ready to learn, learning will not take place.
Test-Taking Strategy: Focus on the subject, safe administration of medication. Eliminate options 1, 2, and 3 because these are unlikely to ensure correct client practices. Option 4 is the only client-centered choice. Review: **teaching and learning principles** and the methods of ensuring safe administration of medication.
Reference(s): Potter et al (2013), pp. 329-330.

470. A client remains in atrial fibrillation with rapid ventricular response despite pharmacological intervention. Synchronous cardioversion is scheduled to convert the rapid rhythm. What action should the nurse plan to take to ensure safety and prevent complications of this procedure?

1. Cardiovert the client at 360 joules.
2. Sedate the client before cardioversion.
3. Ensure that emergency equipment is available.
4. Check that the defibrillator is set on the synchronous mode.

Level of Cognitive Ability: Applying
Client Needs: Safe and Effective Care Environment
Integrated Process: Nursing Process/Implementation
Content Area: Critical Care: Emergency Situations
Priority Concepts: Perfusion; Safety

Answer: 4
Rationale: Cardioversion is similar to defibrillation with two major exceptions: the countershock is synchronized to occur during ventricular depolarization (QRS complex), and less energy is used for the countershock. The rationale for delivering the shock during the QRS complex is to prevent the shock from being delivered during repolarization (T wave), often termed the "vulnerable period." If the shock is delivered during this period, the resulting complication is ventricular fibrillation. It is crucial that the defibrillator is set on the "synchronous" mode for a successful cardioversion. Cardioversion usually begins with 50 to 100 joules. Options 2 and 3 will not prevent complications.
Priority Nursing Tip: Indicators of a successful response to cardioversion include conversion of the dysrhythmia to sinus rhythm, strong peripheral pulses, an adequate blood pressure, and an adequate urine output.
Test-Taking Strategy: Focus on the subject, ensuring safety and preventing complications with synchronous cardioversion. Note that the question denotes *synchronous* cardioversion and its relationship to the information in option 4. Review: the procedure for performing **cardioversion**.
Reference(s): Ignatavicius, Workman (2013), p. 737.

471. A client with a diagnosis of thrombophlebitis is being treated with heparin sodium therapy. In planning a safe environment, the nurse should ensure that which medication is available if the client develops a significant bleeding problem?
1. Protamine sulfate
2. Fresh frozen plasma
3. Retavase (Reteplase)
4. Phytonadione (vitamin K)

Level of Cognitive Ability: Applying
Client Needs: Safe and Effective Care Environment
Integrated Process: Nursing Process/Planning
Content Area: Pharmacology: Hematological Medications
Priority Concepts: Clotting; Safety

Answer: 1
Rationale: Protamine sulfate is the antidote for heparin sodium. Fresh frozen plasma may be used for bleeding related to warfarin (Coumadin) therapy. Retavase is a thrombolytic agent used to dissolve blood clots. Phytonadione is the antidote for warfarin (Coumadin).
Priority Nursing Tip: To maintain a therapeutic level of anticoagulation when a client is receiving a continuous infusion of heparin sodium, the activated partial thromboplastin time (aPTT) should be 1.5 to 2.5 times the normal value.
Test-Taking Strategy: Focus on the subject, planning a safe environment for the client receiving heparin. It is necessary to recall that the antidote for heparin sodium is protamine sulfate to answer correctly. Review: the antidote for **heparin sodium.**
Reference(s): Hodgson, Kizior (2014), p. 561; Ignatavicius, Workman (2013), p. 667.

472. The nurse is teaching a client with cardiomyopathy about home care safety measures. Which **most important** instruction should the nurse provide?
1. Reporting pain
2. Taking vasodilators
3. Avoiding over-the-counter medications
4. Moving slowly from a sitting to a standing position

Level of Cognitive Ability: Applying
Client Needs: Safe and Effective Care Environment
Integrated Process: Teaching and Learning
Content Area: Adult Health: Cardiovascular
Priority Concepts: Perfusion; Safety

Answer: 4
Rationale: Orthostatic changes can occur in the client with cardiomyopathy as a result of venous return obstruction. Sudden changes in blood pressure may lead to falls. Reporting pain, while important, is not directly related to the issue of safety. Vasodilators are not normally prescribed for the client with cardiomyopathy. Option 3, although important, is not directly related to the issue of safety.
Priority Nursing Tip: Treatment for cardiomyopathy is palliative, not curative, and the client needs to deal with numerous lifestyle changes and a shortened life span.
Test-Taking Strategy: Focus on the subject, to ensure client safety at home, and note the strategic words *most important.* Recalling that blood pressure changes occur in cardiomyopathy will direct you to option 4. Review: client teaching related to **cardiomyopathy.**
Reference(s): Ignatavicius, Workman (2013), pp. 769-770.

473. The nurse instructs a client with a diagnosis of atrial fibrillation to use an electric razor for shaving. Which premise supports the rationale for this instruction?
1. Cuts need to be avoided.
2. Any cut may cause infection.
3. Electric razors can be disinfected.
4. All straight razors contain bacteria.

Level of Cognitive Ability: Applying
Client Needs: Safe and Effective Care Environment
Integrated Process: Teaching and Learning
Content Area: Adult Health: Cardiovascular
Priority Concepts: Clotting; Safety

Answer: 1
Rationale: Clients with atrial fibrillation are placed on anticoagulants to prevent thrombus formation and possible stroke. Therefore, measures to prevent bleeding need to be taught to the client. The importance of use of an electric razor is to prevent cuts and possible bleeding. Not all cuts cause infection. Electric razors can be cleaned but usually cannot be disinfected. Not all straight razors contain bacteria. Additionally, options 2, 3, and 4 are all unrelated to the subject of bleeding; rather, they relate to infection.
Priority Nursing Tip: In atrial fibrillation, usually no definitive P wave can be observed, only fibrillatory waves before each QRS.
Test-Taking Strategy: Recalling that the client with atrial fibrillation will be prescribed anticoagulants will assist in answering the question. Note that options 2, 3, and 4 are comparable or alike and relate to infection. Additionally options 2 and 4 can be eliminated because of the words "any" and "all," which are closed-ended words. Option 1 relates to bleeding. Review: care of the client with **atrial fibrillation.**
Reference(s): Ignatavicius, Workman (2013), p. 727.

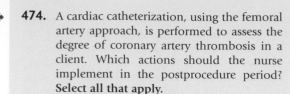

474. A cardiac catheterization, using the femoral artery approach, is performed to assess the degree of coronary artery thrombosis in a client. Which actions should the nurse implement in the postprocedure period? **Select all that apply.**
- ❑ 1. Restricting visitors
- ❑ 2. Checking the client's groin for bleeding
- ❑ 3. Encouraging the client to increase fluid intake
- ❑ 4. Placing the client's bed in the high-Fowler's position
- ❑ 5. Instructing the client to move the toes when checking circulation, motion, and sensation

Level of Cognitive Ability: Applying
Client Needs: Safe and Effective Care Environment
Integrated Process: Nursing Process/Implementation
Content Area: Adult Health: Cardiovascular
Priority Concepts: Perfusion; Safety

Answer: 2, 3, 5
Rationale: Immediately after a cardiac catheterization with the femoral artery approach, the client should not flex or hyperextend the affected leg to avoid blood vessel occlusion or hemorrhage. The groin is checked for bleeding, and if any occurs, the nurse immediately places pressure on the site and asks another staff member to contact the health care provider. Fluids are encouraged to assist in removing the contrast medium from the body. Asking the client to move the toes is done to assess motion, which could be impaired if a hematoma or thrombus was developing. There is no need to restrict visitors. Placing the client in the high-Fowler's position (flexion) increases the risk of occlusion or hemorrhage.
Priority Nursing Tip: Inform the client undergoing a cardiac catheterization that he or she may experience a fluttery feeling as the catheter is passed through the heart, a flushed warm feeling when the dye is injected, a desire to cough, and palpitations caused by heart irritability.
Test-Taking Strategy: Focus on the subject, cardiac catheterization. Also note the words *femoral artery approach*. Recalling that flexion or hyperextension is avoided after this procedure will assist in determining that option 4 is incorrect. There is no useful or helpful reason for restricting visitors, so eliminate option 1. Review: **post–cardiac catheterization** care.
Reference(s): Ignatavicius, Workman (2013), p. 705.

475. The nurse is reviewing general injury prevention information with the staff of the pediatric department in the hospital. Which interventions aimed at promoting safety specifically for infants and toddlers should the nurse review with the staff? **Select all that apply.**
- ❑ 1. Ensure that crib sides are up.
- ❑ 2. Place large, soft pillows in the crib.
- ❑ 3. Use large, soft toys without small parts.
- ❑ 4. Attach a pacifier to a stretchable piece of ribbon and pin to the infant's clothing.
- ❑ 5. Allow a toddler who is toilet training to stay in the bathroom alone to provide privacy.
- ❑ 6. Ensure that an infant or toddler is never left unattended while lying on a changing table.

Level of Cognitive Ability: Applying
Client Needs: Safe and Effective Care Environment
Integrated Process: Teaching and Learning
Content Area: Fundamental Skills: Safety
Priority Concepts: Health Promotion; Safety

Answer: 1, 3, 6
Rationale: To promote safety for infants and toddlers, crib sides should never be left down because the child could roll and fall. Large, soft toys without small parts should be used because small parts can become dislodged and choking and aspiration may occur. For this same reason, an infant or toddler is never left unattended while lying on a changing table. Pillows, stuffed toys, comforters, or other objects should not be placed in the crib because the child can become entwined in these items and suffocate. Pacifiers should not be attached to string or ribbon because of the risk associated with choking. The child is never left alone in the bathroom, in the tub, or near any other water source because of the risk of drowning.
Priority Nursing Tip: The nurse needs to educate the parents about baby-proofing the home.
Test-Taking Strategy: Focus on the subject, safety measures specific for infants and toddlers. Read each option carefully, thinking about the subject of the question and how the intervention may present a risk to the child. This will assist in answering correctly. Review: interventions to ensure **safety for infants and toddlers.**
Reference(s): Hockenberry, Wilson (2013), pp. 345, 397-398.

❖ **476.** Which scenarios demonstrate the participative style of leadership? **Select all that apply.**

❑ 1. The nurse manager presents a problem to the staff and tells the staff to solve the problem.

❑ 2. The nurse manager arranges unit meetings for all shifts to deal with an identified problem.

❑ 3. The nurse manager assesses a problem and informs the staff of the solution to be implemented.

❑ 4. The nurse manager proposes several methods of dealing with a problem and invites team input.

❑ 5. The nurse manager proposes several solutions to a problem and has the unit staff vote on the best option.

❑ 6. The nurse manager considers staff input related to a problem but makes the final decision on implementation of the solution.

Level of Cognitive Ability: Analyzing
Client Needs: Safe and Effective Care Environment
Integrated Process: Nursing Process/Implementation
Content Area: Leadership/Management: Delegating
Priority Concepts: Leadership; Professionalism

Answer: 2, 4, 6
Rationale: Participative leadership demonstrates an "in-between" style, neither authoritarian nor democratic. In participative leadership, the manager presents an analysis of problems and proposals for actions to team members, inviting critique and comments. The participative leader then analyzes the comments and makes the final decision. The autocratic style of leadership is task oriented and directive. A laissez-faire leader abdicates leadership and responsibilities, allowing staff to work without assistance, direction, or supervision. The democratic style of leadership involves a majority rule.
Priority Nursing Tip: The nurse is always responsible for his/her actions when providing care to a client.
Test-Taking Strategy: Focus on the subject, participatory leadership. Options 2, 4, and 6 involve staff input to the nurse manager. The remaining options reflect other forms of leadership that do not seek staff input. Review: the various types of **leadership styles.**
Reference(s): Huber (2014), p. 48.

❖ **477.** A health care provider prescribes 1000 mL of 0.45% normal saline solution to run over 8 hours. The drop factor is 15 drops/mL. The nurse plans to adjust the flow rate to how many drops per minute to safely administer this intravenous (IV) solution? **Fill in the blank and round answer to the nearest whole number.**

_____ drops/min

Level of Cognitive Ability: Applying
Client Needs: Safe and Effective Care Environment
Integrated Process: Nursing Process/Implementation
Content Area: Fundamental Skills: Medication/IV Calculations
Priority Concepts: Clinical Judgment; Safety

Answer: 31
Rationale: The prescribed 1000 mL is to be infused over 8 hours. Follow the formula for calculating IV flow rates and multiply 1000 mL by 15 (drop factor). Then divide the result by 480 minutes (8 hours × 60 minutes). The infusion is to run at 31.2 or 31 drops/min.

Formula:

$$\frac{\text{Total volume in mL} \times \text{drop factor}}{\text{Time in minutes}} = \text{Flow rate in drops/min}$$

$$\frac{1000\,\text{mL} \times 15\,\text{drops per mL}}{480\,\text{minutes}} = \frac{15,000}{480} = 31.2, \text{ or } 31\,\text{drops/min}$$

Priority Nursing Tip: Most intravenous flow rate calculations involve changing the time for infusion from hours to minutes.
Test-Taking Strategy: Focus on the subject, IV flow rate calculation. Recall the formula for calculating the infusion rate for an IV and be certain to change 8 hours to 480 minutes. After you have performed the calculation, verify your answer using a calculator. Review: the formula for safely **calculating infusion rates.**
Reference(s): Potter et al (2013), pp. 925-926.

478. A client asks the home care nurse to witness the client's signature on a living will with the client's attorney in attendance. Which action should the nurse implement?
1. Decline to witness the signature on the living will.
2. Sign the living will as a witness to the signature only.
3. Notify the supervisor that a living will is being witnessed.
4. Sign the living will with identifying credentials and employment agency.

Level of Cognitive Ability: Applying
Client Needs: Safe and Effective Care Environment
Integrated Process: Nursing Process/Implementation
Content Area: Leadership/Management: Ethical/Legal
Priority Concepts: Ethics; Health Care Law

Answer: 1
Rationale: Living wills are written documents and need to be signed by the client. The client's signature either must be witnessed by non-agency individuals or notarized; thus, the nurse should decline to sign the will to avoid a conflict of interest. There is no need to contact the supervisor or sign the living will with or without credentials because the nurse cannot sign this document as a witness. Therefore, options 2, 3, and 4 are incorrect.
Priority Nursing Tip: A living will is a type of advance directive and all health care workers must follow the directions of an advance directive to ensure that the client's wishes are implemented and to be safe from liability.
Test-Taking Strategy: Eliminate options 2, 3, and 4 because they are comparable or alike and indicate that the nurse will sign the will as a witness. Review: legal implications associated with **living wills**.
Reference(s): Ignatavicius, Workman (2013), p. 108.

479. The nurse notes old and new ecchymotic areas on an older adult client's arms and buttocks upon admission. The client tells the nurse in confidence that her family members frequently hit her. Which statement should the nurse use in response?
1. "I have a legal obligation to report this type of abuse."
2. "Let's get these treated, and I will maintain confidence."
3. "Let's talk about ways to prevent someone from hitting you."
4. "If this happens again, you must call the emergency department."

Level of Cognitive Ability: Applying
Client Needs: Safe and Effective Care Environment
Integrated Process: Nursing Process/Implementation
Content Area: Leadership/Management: Ethical/Legal
Priority Concepts: Interpersonal Violence; Safety

Answer: 1
Rationale: The nurse should inform the client that nurses cannot maintain confidence about alleged abusive behavior and that the nurse must report situations related to abuse. The nurse avoids bargaining with the client about treatment to maintain a confidence that the nurse is legally bound to report. Options 3 and 4 delay protective action and place the client at risk for future abuse.
Priority Nursing Tip: Victims of abuse may attempt to dismiss injuries as accidental, and abusers may prevent victims from receiving proper medical care to avoid discovery.
Test-Taking Strategy: Focus on the subject, elder abuse. The nurse is legally obligated to report the occurrence of elder abuse. Option 2 can be eliminated first because this action does not protect the client from injury. Options 3 and 4 should be eliminated next because they place the client at risk for future abuse. Review: the nursing responsibilities related to **reporting obligations** and **elder abuse**.
Reference(s): Ignatavicius, Workman (2013), p. 25.

480. At the scene of a train crash, the nurse triages the victims. Which clients should be coded for triage as **most** urgent or the **first priority?** Refer to chart. Select all that apply.

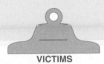

VICTIMS

- ☐ 1. Is dead
- ☐ 2. Has chest pain
- ☐ 3. Has a leg sprain
- ☐ 4. Has a chest wound
- ☐ 5. Has multiple fractures
- ☐ 6. Has full-thickness burns over 30% of the body

Level of Cognitive Ability: Analyzing
Client Needs: Safe and Effective Care Environment
Integrated Process: Nursing Process/Assessment
Content Area: Leadership/Management: Triage
Priority Concepts: Clinical Judgment; Safety

Answer: 2, 4, 6
Rationale: In a disaster situation, saving the greatest number of lives is the most important goal. During a disaster the nurse would triage the victims to maximize the number of survivors and sort the treatable from the untreatable victims. Prioritizing victims can be done in many ways, and many communities use a color coding system. First priority victims (most urgent and coded red) have life-threatening injuries and are experiencing hypoxia or near hypoxia. Examples of injuries in this category are shock, chest wounds, internal hemorrhage, head injuries producing loss of consciousness, partial- or full-thickness burns over 20% of the body surface, and chest pain. Second priority victims (urgent and coded yellow) have injuries with systemic effects but are not yet hypoxic or in shock and can withstand a 2-hour wait without immediate risk (e.g., a victim with multiple fractures). Third priority victims (coded green) have minimal injuries unaccompanied by systemic complications and can wait for more than 2 hours for treatment without risk (leg sprain). Dying or dead victims have catastrophic injuries, and the dying victims would not survive under the best of circumstances (coded black).
Priority Nursing Tip: As a first responder to the scene of a disaster, think survivability. The priority victim is the one whose life can be saved.
Test-Taking Strategy: Note the strategic words, *most* and *first priority.* Focus on the subject, the victims of a disaster that are most urgent or the first priority. Read each option carefully and recall that in a disaster situation, saving the greatest number of lives is the most important goal and that the nurse would triage the victims to maximize the number of survivors. Also, use of the ABCs—airway, breathing, and circulation—will direct you to the correct options. Review: **triage** systems for **disasters**.
Reference(s): Ignatavicius, Workman (2013), pp. 157-158.

481. A client tells the home care nurse of a personal decision to refuse external cardiac resuscitation measures. Which is the **most appropriate initial** nursing action?
1. Discuss the client's request with the client's family.
2. Notify the health care provider (HCP) of the client's request.
3. Document the client's request in the home care nursing care plan.
4. Conduct a client conference with the home care staff to share the client's request.

Level of Cognitive Ability: Applying
Client Needs: Safe and Effective Care Environment
Integrated Process: Nursing Process/Implementation
Content Area: Leadership/Management: Ethical/Legal
Priority Concepts: Health Care Law; Palliation

Answer: 2
Rationale: External cardiac resuscitation is a life-saving treatment that a client may refuse. The most appropriate initial nursing action is to notify the HCP because a written "do not resuscitate" (DNR) prescription from the HCP is needed to ensure that the client's wishes are followed. The DNR prescription must be reviewed or renewed on a regular basis per agency policy. Although options 1, 3, and 4 may be appropriate, remember that obtaining a written health care provider's DNR prescription must be completed first.
Priority Nursing Tip: All health care personnel must know whether a client has a *do not resuscitate* (DNR) prescription.
Test-Taking Strategy: Note the strategic words *most appropriate initial.* The strategic words indicate that more than one option may be correct, but there is only one initial action. Although options 1, 3, and 4 may be appropriate, remember that first a written health care provider's prescription is necessary. Review: **DNR procedures.**
Reference(s): Ignatavicius, Workman (2013), pp. 107-108, 278.

482. The nurse prepares a client for discharge who needs intermittent antibiotic infusions through a peripherally inserted central catheter (PICC) line. What should the nurse include in client teaching about daily infusion care in the home?

1. Keep the affected arm immobilized.
2. Aspirate 3 mL of blood from the PICC line.
3. Maintain a continuous intravenous infusion.
4. Check the insertion site for redness and swelling.

Level of Cognitive Ability: Applying
Client Needs: Safe and Effective Care Environment
Integrated Process: Nursing Process/Planning
Content Area: Fundamental Skills: Safety
Priority Concepts: Client Education; Safety

Answer: 4

Rationale: A PICC is designed for long-term intravenous infusions and, usually, is inserted into the median cubital vein with the terminal end of the catheter in the superior vena cava. Although the risk of infection is less with a PICC line than with a central venous catheter, it is possible for phlebitis or infection to develop. Clients must inspect the insertion site and affected arm daily and report any discharge, redness, swelling, or pain to the nurse or provider immediately. A PICC line does not require the affected arm to be immobilized. Although a PICC line can be used to obtain a blood specimen, the risk of occlusion from aspirating blood as part of the related daily care is greater than any potential benefit. The PICC line can be used for intermittent or continuous fluid infusion.

Priority Nursing Tip: A small amount of bleeding may occur at the time of insertion of a peripherally inserted central catheter (PICC) line and may continue for 24 hours, but bleeding thereafter is not expected.

Test-Taking Strategy: Focus on the subject, daily infusion care for a PICC line. Basic principles of infection control lead you to choose option 4. Additionally, option 4 represents the first step of the nursing process, assessment. Eliminate option 1 because this action can be appropriate for a short-length peripheral intravenous catheter if placed in a movable or vulnerable spot (such as the wrist). Eliminate option 2 because it is contraindicated; the risks of aspirating blood from the catheter are greater than the potential benefit, and this practice is not recommended as routine care. Because the nature of a PICC line allows for either continuous or intermittent infusions, option 3 is also incorrect. Review: home care instructions for a client with a **peripherally inserted central catheter (PICC) line.**

Reference(s): Ignatavicius, Workman (2013), pp. 217, 224-225.

483. The nurse is preparing the client assignment for the day and needs to assign clients to a licensed practical nurse (LPN) and an unlicensed assistive personnel (UAP). Which clients should the nurse assign to the LPN because of client needs that cannot be met by UAP? **Select all that apply.**

❑ 1. A client requiring frequent suctioning
❑ 2. A client requiring a dressing change to the foot
❑ 3. A client requiring range-of-motion exercises twice daily
❑ 4. A client requiring reinforcement of teaching about a diabetic diet
❑ 5. A client on bed rest requiring vital sign measurement every 4 hours
❑ 6. A client requiring collection of a urine specimen for urinalysis testing

Level of Cognitive Ability: Analyzing
Client Needs: Safe and Effective Care Environment
Integrated Process: Nursing Process/Planning
Content Area: Leadership/Management: Delegating
Priority Concepts: Care Coordination; Leadership

Answer: 1, 2, 4

Rationale: Delegation is the transferring to a competent individual the authority to perform a nursing task. When the nurse plans client assignments, he or she needs to consider the educational level and experience of the individual and the needs of the client. The LPN is trained to perform all the tasks indicated in the options; the clients who have needs that cannot be met by the UAP are those requiring suctioning, a dressing change, and reinforcement of teaching about a diabetic diet. UAP are trained to perform range-of-motion exercises, measure vital signs, and collect a urine specimen.

Priority Nursing Tip: The safety of the client is always the nurse's primary concern when delegating nursing tasks.

Test-Taking Strategy: Focus on the subject, client needs that cannot be met by the UAP. Read each option carefully and consider the needs of the client. Recalling that the UAP can be assigned activities that are noninvasive will assist in answering the question. Review: the principles related to **delegation.**

Reference(s): Ignatavicius, Workman (2013), p. 5; Potter et al (2013), pp. 281-282.

484. A charge nurse observes that a staff nurse is not able to meet client needs in a reasonable time frame, does not problem-solve situations, and does not prioritize nursing care. Based on responsibility, which strategy should the charge nurse employ?
1. Ask other staff members to help the staff nurse get the work done.
2. Supervise the staff nurse more closely so that tasks are completed.
3. Provide support and identify the underlying cause of the staff nurse's problem.
4. Report the staff nurse to the supervisor so that something is done to resolve the problem.

Level of Cognitive Ability: Applying
Client Needs: Safe and Effective Care Environment
Integrated Process: Nursing Process/Implementation
Content Area: Leadership/Management: Prioritizing
Priority Concepts: Leadership; Professionalism

Answer: 3
Rationale: Option 3 empowers the charge nurse to assist the staff nurse while trying to identify and reduce the behaviors that make it difficult for the staff nurse to function. Options 1, 2, and 4 are punitive actions, shift the burden to other workers, and do not solve the problem.
Priority Nursing Tip: Problem-solving involves obtaining information and using it to reach an acceptable solution to a problem.
Test-Taking Strategy: Remember that assessment is the first step of the nursing process. The charge nurse needs to gather information before making any decisions or deciding on a course of action. Identifying the underlying cause of the problem is a process of assessment. Review: the **leadership** role of the nurse with regard to **supervising** nursing staff.
Reference(s): Potter et al (2013), p. 282.

485. A registered nurse is a preceptor for a new nursing graduate and is observing the new nursing graduate organize the client assignment and prioritize daily tasks. The registered nurse should intervene if the new nursing graduate performs which action?
1. Provides time for unexpected tasks
2. Lists the supplies needed for a task
3. Prioritizes client needs and daily tasks
4. Plans to document task completion at the end of the day

Level of Cognitive Ability: Evaluating
Client Needs: Safe and Effective Care Environment
Integrated Process: Teaching and Learning
Content Area: Leadership/Management: Prioritizing
Priority Concepts: Leadership; Professionalism

Answer: 4
Rationale: The nurse should document task completion continuously throughout the day. Options 1, 2, and 3 identify accurate components of time management.
Priority Nursing Tip: Time management involves efficiency in completing tasks safely as quickly as possible and effectiveness in deciding on the most important task to do (prioritizing) and doing it correctly.
Test-Taking Strategy: Note the word, *intervene*, and focus on the subject, the incorrect component of time management. Recalling that the nurse needs to document client data and task completion continuously throughout the day will direct you to option 4. Review: **time management** principles and the principles related to **documentation**.
Reference(s): Potter et al (2013), p. 360.

486. A registered nurse is a preceptor for a new nursing graduate and is describing critical paths and variance analysis to the new graduate. The registered nurse instructs the new nursing graduate that a variance analysis is performed on all clients with respect to which time frame?
1. Continuously
2. Daily during hospitalization
3. Every third day of hospitalization
4. Every other day of hospitalization

Level of Cognitive Ability: Applying
Client Needs: Safe and Effective Care Environment
Integrated Process: Teaching and Learning
Content Area: Leadership/Management: Ethical/Legal
Priority Concepts: Health Care Quality; Leadership

Answer: 1
Rationale: Variance analysis occurs continually as the case manager and other caregivers monitor client outcomes against critical paths. The goal of critical paths is to anticipate and recognize negative variance early so that appropriate action can be taken. A negative variance occurs when untoward events preclude a timely discharge and the length of stay is longer than planned for a client on a specific critical path. Options 2, 3, and 4 are incorrect.
Priority Nursing Tip: Variance analysis is a continuous process that the case manager and other caregivers conduct by comparing the specific client outcomes with the expected outcomes described on the critical pathway.
Test-Taking Strategy: Focus on the subject, critical paths and variance analysis. Recall that the goal of critical paths is to recognize negative variance early. This will direct you to option 1. Remember that it is best to monitor a client continuously. Review: the characteristics of **critical paths** and **variance analysis**.
Reference(s): Potter et al (2013), p. 355.

487. When the nurse manager encourages staff to provide input in the decision-making process, which type of leadership style is the nurse manager demonstrating?
1. Autocratic
2. Situational
3. Democratic
4. Laissez-faire

Level of Cognitive Ability: Applying
Client Needs: Safe and Effective Care Environment
Integrated Process: Nursing Process/Implementation
Content Area: Leadership/Management: Delegating
Priority Concepts: Leadership; Professionalism

Answer: 3
Rationale: The democratic style of leadership best empowers staff toward excellence because this style of leadership allows nurses to provide input regarding the decision-making process and an opportunity to grow professionally. The autocratic style of leadership is task oriented and directive. The leader uses his or her power and position in an authoritarian manner to set and implement organizational goals. Decisions are made without input from the staff. The situational leadership style uses a style depending on the situation and events. The laissez-faire style allows staff to work without assistance, direction, or supervision.
Priority Nursing Tip: A democratic leader acts primarily as a facilitator and resource person and is concerned about the ideas and input that each member of the group offers. This style is based on the belief that every group member should have input into the development of goals and problem solving.
Test-Taking Strategy: Focus on the subject, the type of leadership employed. Note the words, *encourages staff to provide input*. This will assist in directing you to the correct option. Review: the various **leadership styles**.
Reference(s): Huber (2014), p. 133.

488. A hospital administrator has implemented a change in the method of assigning nurses to client care units. Nurses will now be required to work in other nursing departments and will not be specifically assigned to a client care unit. A group of registered nurses is resistant to the change, and the nursing administrator anticipates that the nurses will not facilitate the process of change. Which approach should the administrator take in dealing with the resistance?
1. Ignore the resistance.
2. Exert coercion with the nurses.
3. Manipulate the nurses to participate in the change.
4. Encourage the nurses to verbalize feelings regarding resistance to change.

Level of Cognitive Ability: Applying
Client Needs: Safe and Effective Care Environment
Integrated Process: Nursing Process/Implementation
Content Area: Leadership/Management: Prioritizing
Priority Concepts: Collaboration; Leadership

Answer: 4
Rationale: Face-to-face meetings to address the issue at hand will allow verbalization of feelings, identification of problems and issues, and the development of strategies to solve the problem. Option 1 will not address the problem. Option 2 may produce additional resistance. Option 3 may provide a temporary solution to the resistance but will not specifically address the concern.
Priority Nursing Tip: Resistance to change by staff occurs when an individual(s) rejects proposed new ideas without critically thinking about the proposal. The nurse leader should describe the proposed new idea and focus on the benefits of the idea in relation to improvement in client care.
Test-Taking Strategy: Focus on the subject, resistance to change. Options 1 and 2 can be easily eliminated first because these actions do not address the problem and may produce additional resistance. From the remaining options, select option 4 because this option specifically addresses the subject and would provide problem-solving measures. Review: the strategies associated with dealing with resistance to change.
Reference(s): Huber (2014), pp. 174-176; Potter et al (2013), p. 322.

489. Which situation represents the primary nursing care delivery model?

1. The registered nurse (RN) performs all tasks needed by the individual client to optimize health.
2. The RN provides care to 4 clients while the unlicensed assistive personnel (UAP) is assigned to care for 2 clients.
3. The RN develops a plan of care for each client and collaborates with other staff members assigned to the same group of clients.
4. The UAP is assigned to make beds and fill water pitchers. The RN is assigned to administer medications.

Level of Cognitive Ability: Applying
Client Needs: Safe and Effective Care Environment
Integrated Process: Nursing Process/Implementation
Content Area: Leadership/Management: Delegating
Priority Concepts: Clinical Judgment; Leadership

Answer: 1
Rationale: In primary nursing, option 1, concern is with keeping the nurse at the bedside actively involved in care, providing goal-directed and individualized client care. Option 2 does not follow the guidelines for any specific type of nursing care delivery approach. Team nursing, option 3 is characterized by a high degree of communication and collaboration among members. The team is generally led by a registered nurse, who is responsible for assessing, developing nursing diagnoses, planning, and evaluating each client's plan of care. The functional model of care involves an assembly-line approach to client care, with major tasks being delegated by the charge nurse to individual staff members.
Priority Nursing Tip: The functional model of nursing care delivery focuses on the delegated task rather than the total client. This can result in fragmentation of care and lack of accountability by the health care member.
Test-Taking Strategy: Focus on the subject, primary nursing care delivery model. Read each option carefully and note the words *individual client* in the correct option. Review: **primary nursing care.**
Reference(s): Huber (2014), pp. 263, 265.

490. The nurse receives a client from the post-anesthesia care unit (PACU) following an above-the-knee amputation. Which action should the nurse take to safely position the client?

1. Elevate the foot of the bed.
2. Put the bed in reverse Trendelenburg.
3. Position the residual limb flat on the bed.
4. Keep the residual limb flat with the client lying on the operative side.

Level of Cognitive Ability: Applying
Client Needs: Safe and Effective Care Environment
Integrated Process: Nursing Process/Implementation
Content Area: Adult Health: Musculoskeletal
Priority Concepts: Mobility; Tissue Integrity

Answer: 1
Rationale: Edema of the residual limb is controlled by elevating the foot of the bed for the first 24 hours only after surgery. After the first 24 hours, the residual limb is usually placed flat on the bed (as prescribed) to reduce hip contracture. Edema is also controlled by residual limb wrapping techniques. Reverse Trendelenburg does not provide direct limb elevation.
Priority Nursing Tip: After amputation, assess the client for phantom limb sensation and pain. Explain these feelings of sensation and pain to the client, and medicate the client as prescribed.
Test-Taking Strategy: Eliminate options 3 and 4 first because they are comparable or alike positions. To select from the remaining options, note that the client has just returned from surgery. Using basic principles related to immediate postoperative care and preventing postoperative edema will assist in directing you to option 1. Review: postoperative positioning after **amputation.**
Reference(s): Ignatavicius, Workman (2013), p. 1166.

❖ **491.** An emergency department nurse is a member of an All-Hazards Disaster Preparedness planning group. The group is developing a specific emergency response plan in the event that a client with smallpox arrives in the emergency department. Which interventions should be included in the plan? **Select all that apply.**
- ❏ 1. Isolate the client.
- ❏ 2. Don protective equipment immediately.
- ❏ 3. Notify infectious disease specialists, public health officials, and the police.
- ❏ 4. Lock down the emergency department and the entire hospital immediately.
- ❏ 5. Identify all client contacts, including transport services to the emergency department and clients in the waiting room.
- ❏ 6. Administer smallpox vaccines to all hospital staff, client contacts, and clients sitting in the emergency department waiting room immediately.

Level of Cognitive Ability: Analyzing
Client Needs: Safe and Effective Care Environment
Integrated Process: Nursing Process/Planning
Content Area: Leadership/Management: Disasters
Priority Concepts: Infection; Safety

Answer: 1, 2, 3, 5
Rationale: An All-Hazards Disaster Preparedness group is a multifaceted internal and external disaster preparedness group that establishes action plans for every type of disaster or combination of disaster events. In the event of emergency department exposure to a communicable disease such as smallpox, the client would be isolated immediately and the staff would immediately don protective equipment. The emergency department would be locked down immediately. Locking down the entire hospital may not be necessary and infectious disease specialists and public health officials will determine whether it is necessary to take this action. Infectious disease specialists, public health officials, and the police are notified. All client contacts (name, addresses, telephone numbers), including transport services to the emergency department and clients in the waiting room, would be identified so that the public health department can follow through on notifying and treating these individuals appropriately. Although getting the vaccine within 3 days after exposure will help prevent the disease or make it less severe, it is unreasonable and unnecessary to administer smallpox vaccines to all hospital staff, client contacts, and clients sitting in the emergency department waiting room.
Priority Nursing Tip: Smallpox is transmitted in air droplets and by handling contaminated materials and is highly contagious.
Test-Taking Strategy: Focus on the subject, a client with smallpox in the emergency department. Next read each option carefully, noting that the client is in the emergency department. Eliminate option 4 because of the words *entire hospital* and option 6 because of the words *all hospital staff*. Review: **disaster preparedness** guidelines and **small pox**.
Reference(s): Potter et al (2013), pp. 387, 416-417.

492. A pregnant client tests positive for the hepatitis B virus. The client asks the nurse if she will be able to breast-feed the baby as planned after delivery. Which response should the nurse make to the client?
1. "You will not be able to breast-feed the baby until 6 months after delivery."
2. "Breast-feeding is not advised, and you should seriously consider bottle-feeding the baby."
3. "Breast-feeding is not a problem, and you will be able to breast-feed immediately after delivery."
4. "Breast-feeding is allowed if the baby receives prophylaxis at birth and remains on the scheduled immunization timeline."

Level of Cognitive Ability: Applying
Client Needs: Safe and Effective Care Environment
Integrated Process: Nursing Process/Implementation
Content Area: Maternity: Antepartum
Priority Concepts: Client Education; Infection

Answer: 4
Rationale: The pregnant client who tests positive for hepatitis B virus should be reassured that breast-feeding is not contraindicated if the infant receives prophylaxis at birth and remains on the schedule for immunizations. Therefore, options 1, 2, and 3 are incorrect.
Priority Nursing Tip: Hepatitis is transmitted through blood, saliva, vaginal secretions, semen, breast milk, and across the placental barrier.
Test-Taking Strategy: Eliminate options 1, 2, and 3 because of the closed-ended word "not" in these options. Also, use therapeutic communication techniques to direct you to option 4. Review: the management of **hepatitis B virus** in the pregnant client and her newborn.
Reference(s): McKinney et al (2013), p. 628.

493. The nurse manager is planning to implement a change in the method of the documentation system for the nursing unit. Many problems have occurred as a result of the present documentation system, and the nurse manager determines that a change is required. What should be the **initial** step in the process of change for the nurse manager?
1. Plan strategies to implement the change.
2. Set goals and priorities regarding the change process.
3. Identify the inefficiency that needs improvement or correction.
4. Identify potential solutions and strategies for the change process.

Level of Cognitive Ability: Applying
Client Needs: Safe and Effective Care Environment
Integrated Process: Nursing Process/Planning
Content Area: Leadership/Management: Prioritizing
Priority Concepts: Leadership; Professionalism

Answer: 3
Rationale: When beginning the change process, the nurse should identify and define the problem that needs improvement or correction. This important first step can prevent many future problems because, if the problem is not correctly identified, a plan for change may be aimed at the wrong problem. This is followed by goal setting, prioritizing, and identifying potential solutions and strategies to implement the change.
Priority Nursing Tip: When implementing change, evaluate the change process on an ongoing basis, and keep everyone involved in the process informed of the progress.
Test-Taking Strategy: Note the strategic word, *initial.* Eliminate options 1 and 4 because they are comparable or alike. Next use the steps of the nursing process and knowledge regarding the change process to answer this question. This will direct you to the correct option. Review: the steps of the **change process.**
Reference(s): Huber (2014), pp. 45-47.

494. A delivery room nurse is preparing a client for a cesarean delivery. Which position will promote maximum uteroplacental perfusion during this surgery?
1. Prone position
2. Semi-Fowler's position
3. Trendelenburg's position
4. Supine position with a wedge under the right hip

Level of Cognitive Ability: Applying
Client Needs: Safe and Effective Care Environment
Integrated Process: Nursing Process/Implementation
Content Area: Maternity: Intrapartum
Priority Concepts: Perfusion; Reproduction

Answer: 4
Rationale: Vena cava and descending aorta compression by the pregnant uterus impedes blood return from the lower trunk and extremities, thereby decreasing cardiac return, cardiac output, and blood flow to the uterus and subsequently the fetus. The best position to prevent this would be side-lying with the uterus displaced off the abdominal vessels. Positioning for abdominal surgery necessitates a supine position, so a wedge placed under the right hip provides displacement of the uterus off of the vena cava. A semi-Fowler's or prone position is not practical for this type of abdominal surgery. Trendelenburg positioning places pressure from the pregnant uterus on the diaphragm and lungs, decreasing respiratory capacity and oxygenation.
Priority Nursing Tip: Vena cava syndrome, also known as supine hypotension, occurs when the venous return to the heart is impaired by the weight of the pregnant uterus on the vena cava.
Test-Taking Strategy: Focus on the subject, positioning for a cesarean delivery. Visualize each of the positions in the options. Recalling the concern in the pregnant client related to vena cava and descending aorta compression will direct you to the correct option. Review: **vena cava syndrome** and positioning principles for the pregnant client.
Reference(s): McKinney et al (2013), p. 426.

495. The nurse in the day care center is told that a child with autism will be attending the center. The nurse collaborates with the staff of the day care center and plans activities that will meet the child's needs. Which **priority** consideration should the nurse incorporate in planning activities for this child?

1. Safety with activities
2. That activities provide verbal stimulation
3. Social interactions with other children in the same age group
4. Familiarity with all activities and providing orientation throughout the activities

Level of Cognitive Ability: Applying
Client Needs: Safe and Effective Care Environment
Integrated Process: Nursing Process/Planning
Content Area: Fundamental Skills: Safety
Priority Concepts: Functional Ability; Safety

Answer: 1
Rationale: The child with autism is unable to anticipate danger, has a tendency for self-mutilation, and has sensory perceptual deficits. Safety with activities is a priority in planning activities with the child. Although verbal communications, social interactions, and providing familiarity and orientation are also appropriate interventions, the priority is safety.
Priority Nursing Tip: For a child with autism, the nurse should plan care so that disruption in the child's normal routines does not occur. A child with autism is usually unable to tolerate even the slightest change in routine and may withdraw or become self-abusive or violent if his or her routine is altered.
Test-Taking Strategy: Note the strategic word, *priority*. Use Maslow's Hierarchy of Needs theory to answer this question. Physiological needs take priority. When a physiological need does not exist, safety needs are the priority. None of the options addresses a physiological need. Option 1 addresses the safety need. Options 2, 3, and 4 address psychosocial needs. Review: care of the child with **autism**.
Reference(s): McKinney et al (2013), p. 1498.

496. The registered nurse (RN) is reviewing a plan of care developed by a nursing student for a child who is being admitted to the pediatric unit with a diagnosis of seizures. The RN determines that the student nurse **needs further teaching** and should revise the plan of care if which incorrect intervention is documented?

1. Maintain the bed in a low position.
2. Restrain the child if a seizure occurs.
3. Place pads on the side rails of the bed.
4. Place the child in a side-lying lateral position if a seizure occurs.

Level of Cognitive Ability: Evaluating
Client Needs: Safe and Effective Care Environment
Integrated Process: Teaching and Learning
Content Area: Child Health: Neurological
Priority Concepts: Intracranial Regulation; Safety

Answer: 2
Rationale: Restraints are not to be applied to a child with a seizure because they could cause injury to the child. The bed is maintained in low position to provide safety in the event that the child has a seizure. The side rails of the bed are padded to prevent injury. Positioning the child on his or her side will prevent aspiration as the saliva drains out of the child's mouth during the seizure.
Priority Nursing Tip: If a child is experiencing a seizure, do not restrain the child, place anything in the child's mouth, or give any foods or liquids to the child.
Test-Taking Strategy: Note the strategic words, *needs further teaching* and the words *revise* and *incorrect* in the question. These indicate a negative event query and the need to select the incorrect intervention. Focus on safety to eliminate the appropriate interventions and recall that restraints are not to be used. Review: safety measures related to the child with **seizures**.
Reference(s): McKinney et al (2013), pp. 1435-1437.

❖ **497.** A deceased client with multiple gunshot wounds arrives by ambulance to the emergency department. The nurse is caring for the client's personal belongings, which may be needed as legal evidence. Which actions should the nurse take to properly secure and handle legal evidence? **Select all that apply.**

❑ 1. Place paper bags on the hands and feet.

❑ 2. Give the clothing and wallet to the family.

❑ 3. Cut clothing along the seams, avoiding bullet holes.

❑ 4. Collect all personal items, including items from clothing pockets.

❑ 5. Place wet clothing and personal belongings in a labeled, sealed plastic bag.

❑ 6. Do not allow family members, significant others, or friends to be alone with the client.

Level of Cognitive Ability: Applying
Client Needs: Safe and Effective Care Environment
Integrated Process: Nursing Process/Implementation
Content Area: Critical Care: Emergency Situations
Priority Concepts: Evidence; Health Care Law

Answer: 1, 3, 4, 6
Rationale: Basic rules for securing and handling evidence include minimally handling the body of a deceased person; placing paper bags on the hands and feet and possibly over the head of a deceased person (protects trace evidence and residue); placing clothing and personal items in paper bags (plastic bags can destroy items because items can sweat in plastic); cutting clothes along seams, avoiding areas where there are obvious holes or tears; and collecting all personal items, including items from clothing pockets. Evidence is never released to the family to take home, and family members, significant others, or friends are not allowed to be alone with the client because of the possibility of jeopardizing any existing legal evidence.
Priority Nursing Tip: Nurses are required to report certain communicable diseases or criminal activities such as child or elder abuse or domestic violence; a dog bite or other animal bite; gunshot or stab wounds, assaults, or homicides; and suicides to the appropriate authorities.
Test-Taking Strategy: Focus on the subject, proper securing and handling of legal evidence. Read each option carefully and visualize and think about how the action may or may not preserve evidence. This strategy will direct you to the correct actions. Review: the basic rules for securing and handling **legal evidence.**
Reference(s): Hammond, Zimmermann (2013), pp. 8, 56-58.

---

498. The nurse receives a telephone call from the emergency department and is told that a child with a diagnosis of tonic-clonic seizures will be admitted to the pediatric unit. The nurse prepares for the admission of the child and instructs the unlicensed assistive personnel to place which items at the bedside?

1. A tracheotomy set and oxygen
2. Suction apparatus and oxygen
3. An endotracheal tube and an airway
4. An emergency cart and laryngoscope

Level of Cognitive Ability: Applying
Client Needs: Safe and Effective Care Environment
Integrated Process: Nursing Process/Planning
Content Area: Leadership/Management: Delegating
Priority Concepts: Intracranial Regulation; Safety

Answer: 2
Rationale: Tonic-clonic seizures cause tightening of all body muscles followed by tremors. Obstructed airway and increased oral secretions are the major complications during and after a seizure. Suction is helpful to prevent choking and oxygen is helpful to prevent cyanosis. Options 1 and 3 are incorrect because inserting an endotracheal tube or a tracheostomy is not performed. It is not necessary to have an emergency cart (which contains a laryngoscope) at the bedside, but a cart should be available in the treatment room or on the nursing unit.
Priority Nursing Tip: If a child is experiencing a seizure, the priority is to ensure a patent airway.
Test-Taking Strategy: Focus on the subject, tonic-clonic seizures. Recalling that tonic-clonic seizures produce excessive oral secretions and airway obstruction will assist in selecting the correct option. Review: the plan of care associated with **seizure precautions.**
Reference(s): Hockenberry, Wilson (2013), pp. 963-965; McKinney et al (2013), p. 1436.

499. The nurse is admitting a 56-year-old client with exacerbation of chronic obstructive pulmonary disease (COPD) to the hospital and questions the client as to whether he has received previous immunization for pneumococcal pneumonia. The client replies that he received the vaccine 6 years ago. Which consideration is essential to include in the plan of care during the client's hospital admission?

1. Offer revaccination to the client.
2. Document the previous immunization on the client record.
3. Instruct the client that this vaccine provides lifelong immunity.
4. Explain to the client that he can only be revaccinated during the fall months.

Level of Cognitive Ability: Applying
Client Needs: Safe and Effective Care Environment
Integrated Process: Nursing Process/Planning
Content Area: Adult Health: Respiratory
Priority Concepts: Gas Exchange; Health Promotion

Answer: 1
Rationale: During the history-taking of a client with a respiratory disorder, the nurse should ask if the client had been previously vaccinated for influenza (flu) and had received pneumococcal pneumonia vaccine (Pneumovax). Revaccination with pneumococcal pneumonia vaccine is currently advised in a client with COPD if the client received the vaccine more than 5 years previously and if the client was younger than 65 years of age at the time of vaccination. Although documentation would be done, this is not the essential action at this time. This vaccine does not provide lifelong immunity in a 56-year-old client who received the vaccine 6 years ago. The pneumococcal pneumonia vaccine is administered any time during the year.
Priority Nursing Tip: Because the strain of the influenza virus is different every year, annual vaccination is recommended (usually in October or November).
Test-Taking Strategy: Focus on the subject, pneumococcal pneumonia vaccination. Recognize that this client does not have lifelong immunity and some type of intervention besides documentation is needed. Eliminate options 3 and 4, knowing that pneumococcal pneumonia vaccine can be administered any time of the year and does not provide lifelong immunity to this client. Review: criteria for immunization with **pneumococcal pneumonia vaccine** and **chronic obstructive pulmonary disease (COPD)**.
Reference(s): Lewis et al (2014), pp. 504, 526, 588.

500. The nurse in a well-baby clinic is providing safety instructions to the mother of a 1-month-old infant. Which safety instructions are **most appropriate** at this age? **Select all that apply.**
❑ 1. Lock up all poisons.
❑ 2. Cover electrical outlets.
❑ 3. Never shake the infant's head.
❑ 4. Place the infant on the back to sleep.
❑ 5. Remove hazardous objects from low places.

Level of Cognitive Ability: Applying
Client Needs: Safe and Effective Care Environment
Integrated Process: Teaching and Learning
Content Area: Developmental Stages: Infancy to Adolescence
Priority Concepts: Health Promotion; Safety

Answer: 3, 4
Rationale: The age-appropriate instructions that are most important are to instruct the mother not to shake or vigorously jiggle the baby's head and to place the infant on his back to sleep. Options 1, 2, and 5 are important instructions to provide to the mother as the child reaches the age of 6 months and begins to explore the environment.
Priority Nursing Tip: Shaken baby syndrome is caused by the violent shaking of an infant younger than 1 year and results in intracranial (usually subdural hemorrhage) trauma; this can lead to cerebral edema and death.
Test-Taking Strategy: Focus on the subject, safety and the 1-month-old infant. A 1-month-old is not at a developmental level to explore the environment, which will assist in eliminating options 1, 2, and 5. Review: **age-appropriate safety measures.**
Reference(s): Hockenberry, Wilson (2013), p. 446; McKinney et al (2013), p. 103.

501. A registered nurse (RN) in charge of the client care unit is preparing the assignments for the day. The RN assigns unlicensed assistive personnel (UAP) to make beds and bathe one of the clients on the unit and assigns additional UAP to fill the water pitchers and serve juice to all of the clients. Another RN is assigned to administer all medications. Based on the assignments designed by the RN in charge, which type of nursing care is being implemented?
1. Team nursing
2. Primary nursing
3. Functional nursing
4. Exemplary nursing

Level of Cognitive Ability: Applying
Client Needs: Safe and Effective Care Environment
Integrated Process: Nursing Process/Implementation
Content Area: Leadership/Management: Delegating
Priority Concepts: Clinical Judgment; Leadership

Answer: 3
Rationale: The functional model of care involves an assembly-line approach to client care, with major tasks being delegated by the charge nurse to individual staff members. Team nursing is characterized by a high degree of communication and collaboration among members. The team is generally led by a registered nurse, who is responsible for assessing, developing nursing diagnoses, planning, and evaluating each client's plan of care. In primary nursing, concern is with keeping the nurse at the bedside actively involved in care, providing goal-directed and individualized client care. In an exemplary model of team nursing, each staff member works fully within the realm of educational and clinical experience in an effort to provide comprehensive individualized client care. Each staff member is accountable for client care and outcomes of care.
Priority Nursing Tip: The functional model of nursing care delivery focuses on the delegated task rather than the total client. This can result in fragmentation of care and lack of accountability by the health care member.
Test-Taking Strategy: Focus on the subject, nursing care delivery systems. Noting that each staff member is assigned a specific task will direct you to option 3. Review: the various **nursing care delivery systems.**
Reference(s): Huber (2014), pp. 263, 265.

502. A client who is immunosuppressed is being admitted to the hospital on neutropenic precautions. Which nursing interventions should be implemented to protect the client from infection? **Select all that apply.**
❑ 1. Restrict all visitors.
❑ 2. Admit the client to a semiprivate room.
❑ 3. Place a mask on the client if the client leaves the room.
❑ 4. Use strict aseptic technique for all invasive procedures.
❑ 5. Place a "See the Nurse before Entering" sign on the door to the room.
❑ 6. Remove a vase with fresh flowers in the room that was left by a previous client.

Level of Cognitive Ability: Analyzing
Client Needs: Safe and Effective Care Environment
Integrated Process: Nursing Process/Implementation
Content Area: Fundamental Skills: Infection Control
Priority Concepts: Infection; Safety

Answer: 3, 4, 5, 6
Rationale: The client should wear a mask for protection from exposure to microorganisms whenever he or she leaves the room. The use of strict aseptic technique is necessary with all invasive procedures to prevent infection. A sign indicating "See the Nurse before Entering" should be placed on the door to the client's room, so the nurse can ensure that neutropenic precautions are implemented by anyone entering the room. Sources of standing water and fresh flowers should be removed to decrease the microorganism count. Not all visitors must be restricted; however, visitors need to be restricted to healthy adults and must perform strict hand-washing procedures and don a mask before entering the client's room. The client who is on neutropenic precautions is immunosuppressed and therefore is admitted to a single room on the nursing unit.
Priority Nursing Tip: Neutropenia can be caused by chemotherapy and places the cancer client at risk for a life-threatening infection. White blood cell counts and differentials are monitored closely, and the client is placed on neutropenic precautions if the counts decrease.
Test-Taking Strategy: Focus on the subject, an immunosuppressed client and neutropenic precautions. Read each option carefully and recall that the client is at risk for contracting infection. Select the options that protect the client from infection. Review: **neutropenic precautions.**
Reference(s): Ignatavicius, Workman (2013), pp. 420-421.

503. A home care nurse is providing instructions to the mother of a toddler regarding safety measures in the home to prevent an accidental burn injury. Which statement by the mother indicates a **need for further instruction**?

1. "I need to use the back burners for cooking."
2. "I need to remain in the kitchen when I prepare meals."
3. "I need to be sure to place my cup of coffee on the counter."
4. "I need to turn pot handles inward and to the middle of the stove."

Level of Cognitive Ability: Evaluating
Client Needs: Safe and Effective Care Environment
Integrated Process: Teaching and Learning
Content Area: Developmental Stages: Infancy to Adolescence
Priority Concepts: Client Education; Safety

Answer: 3
Rationale: Toddlers, with their increased mobility and developing motor skills, can reach hot water or hot objects placed on counters and open fires or burners on stoves above their eye level. The mother's statement in option 3 does not indicate an adequate understanding of the principles of safety. Hot liquids should never be left unattended, and the toddler should always be supervised. Parents should be encouraged to use the back burners on the stove, remain in the kitchen when preparing a meal, and turn pot handles inward and toward the middle of the stove.
Priority Nursing Tip: Toddlers are eager to explore the environment around them, and they need to be supervised at all times to ensure safety.
Test-Taking Strategy: Note the strategic words, *need for further instruction*. These words indicate a negative event query and the need to select the option that identifies an incorrect statement by the mother. Options 1, 2, and 4 can be eliminated because they identify basic safety principles. Also recalling that the toddler is in the stage of developing motor skills will assist in directing you to option 3. Review: the **safety principles for toddlers**.
Reference(s): Hockenberry, Wilson (2013), p. 397; McKinney et al (2013), p. 133.

504. The nurse prepares a client who has a right pleural effusion for a thoracentesis; however, the client experiences severe dizziness when sitting upright. Which alternate position should the nurse assist the client into to maintain safety during the procedure?

1. Right side-lying with the head of the bed flat
2. Prone with the head turned toward the affected side
3. Sims' position with the head of the bed elevated 45 degrees
4. Left side-lying with the head of the bed elevated 45 degrees

Level of Cognitive Ability: Applying
Client Needs: Safe and Effective Care Environment
Integrated Process: Nursing Process/Implementation
Content Area: Fundamental Skills: Diagnostic Tests
Priority Concepts: Gas Exchange; Safety

Answer: 4
Rationale: A thoracentesis is a procedure in which fluid or air is removed from the pleural space via a transthoracic aspiration. Positioning can help isolate the fluid in a pleural effusion; generally, the client sits at the edge of the bed, leaning over the bedside table, allowing the fluid to collect in a dependent body area. If the client is unable to sit up, the nurse turns the client to the unaffected side and elevates the head of the bed 30 to 45 degrees. Turning to the affected side, the prone, and the Sims' positions are unsuitable positions for this procedure because these do not facilitate fluid removal.
Priority Nursing Tip: After a thoracentesis, monitor the client for signs of pneumothorax, air embolism, and pulmonary edema.
Test-Taking Strategy: Focus on the subject, alternate position for thoracentesis procedure. Eliminate option 1 because lying on the affected side makes it difficult to perform the procedure. Eliminate option 2 because prone positioning does not facilitate fluid removal, and eliminate option 3 because the Sims' position is used for rectal enemas or irrigations primarily. Review: the procedure for a **thoracentesis**.
Reference(s): Chernecky, Berger (2013), pp. 1068-1069; Pagana, Pagana (2013), p. 889.

505. A health care provider has written a prescription to administer methylergonovine maleate (Methergine) to a postpartum client with uterine atony. The nurse should contact the health care provider to verify the prescription if which condition is present in the mother?
1. Hypertension
2. Excessive lochia
3. Difficulty locating the uterine fundus
4. Excessive bleeding and saturation of more than one peripad per hour

Level of Cognitive Ability: Analyzing
Client Needs: Safe and Effective Care Environment
Integrated Process: Nursing Process/Implementation
Content Area: Pharmacology: Reproductive/Maternity/Newborn Medications
Priority Concepts: Clinical Judgment; Safety

Answer: 1
Rationale: Methylergonovine maleate (Methergine) is an ergot alkaloid. It is contraindicated for the hypertensive woman, individuals with severe hepatic or renal disease, and during the third stage of labor. Excessive lochia, a uterine fundus that is difficult to locate, and excessive bleeding are clinical manifestations of uterine atony indicating the need for methylergonovine.
Priority Nursing Tip: Methylergonovine maleate (Methergine) is an ergot alkaloid that produces vasoconstriction. The client's blood pressure needs to be monitored closely, and if an increase is noted, the medication is withheld and the health care provider is notified.
Test-Taking Strategy: Eliminate options 2, 3, and 4 because they are comparable or alike in that they are clinical manifestations of uterine atony. Review: **methylergonovine (Methergine).**
Reference(s): Hodgson, Kizior (2014), pp. 756-757; McKinney et al (2013), p. 668.

506. After receiving detailed information about a colonoscopy from the health care provider (HCP), the nurse asks the client to sign the informed consent form and discovers that the client cannot write. Which is the **best** intervention for the nurse to implement?
1. Contact the provider to obtain informed consent.
2. Obtain a verbal informed consent from the client.
3. Have two nurses witness the client sign with an X.
4. Clarify information to the client with another nurse.

Level of Cognitive Ability: Applying
Client Needs: Safe and Effective Care Environment
Integrated Process: Nursing Process/Implementation
Content Area: Leadership/Management: Ethical/Legal
Priority Concepts: Ethics; Health Care Law

Answer: 3
Rationale: Nurses are responsible to make sure that the signed informed consent form is in the client's medical record before a procedure and for clarifying facts that have already been presented by the HCP. Nonetheless, the person performing the procedure obtains informed consent and provides the explanations to the client. Informed consent can be obtained verbally, but that is also the responsibility of the HCP. Clients who cannot write may sign an informed consent with an X in the presence of two witnesses. Nurses can serve as a witness to the client's signature but not to the fact that the client is informed.
Priority Nursing Tip: A client who has been medicated with sedating medications or any other medications that can affect the client's cognitive abilities should not be asked to sign an informed consent.
Test-Taking Strategy: Note the strategic word, *best*. Focus on the subject, inability to sign an informed consent form. Eliminate options 1, 2, and 4 because they are unnecessary, and the HCP has already provided detailed information to the client. Review: the principles related to **informed consent.**
Reference(s): Ignatavicius, Workman (2013), pp. 250, 252.

507. A child with a brain tumor is admitted to the hospital for removal of the tumor. The nurse should include which action in the plan of care to ensure a safe environment for the child?
1. Initiating seizure precautions
2. Using a wheelchair for out-of-bed activities
3. Assisting the child with ambulation at all times
4. Avoiding contact with other children on the nursing unit

Level of Cognitive Ability: Applying
Client Needs: Safe and Effective Care Environment
Integrated Process: Nursing Process/Planning
Content Area: Child Health: Neurological
Priority Concepts: Intracranial Regulation; Safety

Answer: 1
Rationale: Seizure precautions should be implemented for any child with a brain tumor, both preoperatively and postoperatively. Options 2 and 3 are not required unless functional deficits exist. Based on the child's diagnosis, option 4 is not necessary.
Priority Nursing Tip: Monitor the child with a brain tumor or a child who has had a craniotomy for signs of increased intracranial pressure (ICP). If signs of increased ICP occur, notify the health care provider immediately.
Test-Taking Strategy: Focus on the subject, safe environment for a child with a brain tumor. Eliminate options 2 and 3 first because they are comparable or alike. Additionally, note the closed-ended word "all" in option 3. From the remaining options, eliminate option 4 because there is no reason for the child to avoid contact with other children. Review: nursing interventions related to the **child with a brain tumor.**
Reference(s): McKinney et al (2013), p. 1282.

508. The nurse caring for a chronically ill client with a poor prognosis shows an understanding of the basic values that guide the implementation of a living will by asking which question? **Select all that apply.**
☐ 1. "Are you planning to become an organ donor?"
☐ 2. "Do you feel the need to discuss your end-of-life decisions with your family?"
☐ 3. "Did you have the discussion with your son about being your health care surrogate?"
☐ 4. "Can we discuss what will happen if you decide to refuse antibiotics if you get an infection?"
☐ 5. "Have you given thought to whether you want cardiopulmonary resuscitation (CPR) measures if your condition worsens?"

Level of Cognitive Ability: Analyzing
Client Needs: Safe and Effective Care Environment
Integrated Process: Nursing Process/Assessment
Content Area: Developmental Stages: End-of-Life Care
Priority Concepts: Health Care Law; Palliation

Answer: 2, 4, 5
Rationale: A living will lists the treatment that a client chooses to omit or refuse if the client becomes unable to make decisions and is terminally ill. The client may want to discuss his or her decisions with the family. Although both the living will and durable powers of attorney for health care are based on values of informed consent, autonomy over end-of-life decisions, and control over the dying process, living wills do not involve health care surrogates or the decision to donate organs.
Priority Nursing Tip: A living will is based on the client's decisions regarding end-of-life wishes related to health care.
Test-Taking Strategy: Focus on the subject, living will. Understanding the purpose and components of a living will direct you to the correct options 2, 4, and 5. Remember that living wills do not involve health care surrogates or the decision to donate organs. Review: the issues related to a living will.
Reference(s): Lewis et al (2014), p. 146. Potter et al (2013), pp. 298-299.

509. The nurse is reviewing the results of the rubella screening (titer) with a pregnant 24-year-old client. The test results are positive, and the client asks if it is safe for her toddler to receive the vaccine. Which response by the nurse is most appropriate?
1. "Most children do not receive the vaccine until they are 5 years of age."
2. "You are still susceptible to rubella, so your toddler should receive the vaccine."
3. "It is not advised for children of pregnant women to be vaccinated during their mother's pregnancy."
4. "Your titer supports your immunity to rubella, and it is safe for your toddler to receive the vaccine at this time."

Level of Cognitive Ability: Applying
Client Needs: Safe and Effective Care Environment
Integrated Process: Nursing Process/Implementation
Content Area: Maternity: Antepartum
Priority Concepts: Immunity; Safety

Answer: 4
Rationale: All pregnant women should be screened for prior rubella exposure. A positive maternal titer indicates that a significant antibody titer has developed in response to a prior exposure to the *Rubivirus*. All children of pregnant women should receive their immunizations according to schedule. Additionally, no definitive evidence suggests that the rubella vaccine virus is transmitted from person to person.
Priority Nursing Tip: Rubella vaccine is not administered to a pregnant woman because the live attenuated virus may cross the placenta and present a risk to the developing fetus.
Test-Taking Strategy: Focus on the subject, administration of rubella vaccine to a toddler who has a pregnant mother. Recalling that a positive titer indicates immunity will direct you to option 4. Review: candidates for **rubella immunization** and the meaning of the results of the **rubella screening (titer)**.
Reference(s): McKinney et al (2013), p. 249.

510. After delivery, the postpartum nurse instructs the client with known cardiac disease to call for the nurse when she needs to get out of bed or when she plans to care for her newborn infant. Which rationale is the basis for these instructions?
1. Help the mother assume the parenting role.
2. Minimize the potential of postpartum hemorrhage.
3. Provide an opportunity for the nurse to teach newborn infant care techniques.
4. Avoid maternal or infant injury caused by the potential for syncope or overexertion.

Level of Cognitive Ability: Applying
Client Needs: Safe and Effective Care Environment
Integrated Process: Teaching and Learning
Content Area: Maternity: Postpartum
Priority Concepts: Client Education; Safety

Answer: 4
Rationale: The immediate postpartum period is associated with increased risks for the cardiac client. Hormonal changes and fluid shifts from extravascular tissues to the circulatory system cause additional stress on cardiac functioning. Although options 1, 2, and 3 are appropriate nursing concerns during the postpartum period, the primary concern for the cardiac client is to maintain a safe environment because of the potential for cardiac compromise.
Priority Nursing Tip: Monitor the postpartum client with cardiac disease closely for signs and symptoms of cardiac stress and decompensation. These include cough, fatigue, dyspnea, chest pain, and tachycardia.
Test-Taking Strategy: Focus on the subject, safety for the postpartum mother with cardiac disease. Option 4 is the only option that relates directly to the subject of safety. Review: the physiological manifestations that occur in a **postpartum cardiac client** and the need to implement safety precautions.
Reference(s): McKinney et al (2013), pp. 620-621.

511. The nurse is assessing a client who has just been measured and fitted for crutches. How will the nurse determine if the client's crutches are fitted correctly?
1. The top of the crutch is even with the axilla.
2. The elbow is straight when the hand is on the handgrip.
3. The client's axilla is resting on the crutch pad during ambulation.
4. The elbow is at a 30-degree angle when the hand is on the handgrip.

Level of Cognitive Ability: Evaluating
Client Needs: Safe and Effective Care Environment
Integrated Process: Nursing Process/Evaluation
Content Area: Adult Health: Musculoskeletal
Priority Concepts: Mobility; Safety

Answer: 4
Rationale: When using crutches, for optimal upper extremity leverage, the elbow should be at approximately 30 degrees of flexion when the hand is resting on the handgrip. The top of the crutch needs to be two to three finger widths lower than the axilla. When crutch walking, all weight needs to be on the hands to prevent nerve palsy from pressure on the axilla. Therefore, options 1, 2, and 3 are incorrect.
Priority Nursing Tip: An accurate measurement of the client for crutches is important because an incorrect measurement could damage the brachial plexus.
Test-Taking Strategy: Options 1 and 3 are comparable or alike and can be eliminated first. Visualize the mechanics of crutch walking to assist in selecting from the remaining options. If the weight should be resting on the hands, then there needs to be some flexion to push off from during ambulation. Review: **crutch walking.**
Reference(s): Potter et al (2013), pp. 760-761.

512. When assessing the client with a wrist restraint at the beginning of the day shift, which observation by the charge nurse should indicate that the nurse who placed the restraint on the client failed to follow safety guidelines?
1. A safety knot was used to secure the restraint.
2. The call light was placed within reach of the client.
3. The restraint was applied tightly around the client's wrist.
4. The client's record indicates that the restraint was released every 2 hours.

Level of Cognitive Ability: Evaluating
Client Needs: Safe and Effective Care Environment
Integrated Process: Nursing Process/Evaluation
Content Area: Fundamental Skills: Safety
Priority Concepts: Clinical Judgment; Safety

Answer: 3
Rationale: A restraint should never be applied tightly because it could impair circulation. A safety knot may be used on the client because it can easily be released in an emergency. The call light must always be within the client's reach in case the client needs assistance. The restraint needs to be released every 2 hours (or per agency policy) to provide movement.
Priority Nursing Tip: A health care provider's prescription for the use of a restraint (security device) is needed.
Test-Taking Strategy: Focus on the subject, safety with the use of restraints. The words *failed to follow safety guidelines* indicates the need to select the unsafe action performed by the nurse. Noting the word *tightly* in option 3 will direct you to this option. Review: the principles regarding the safe use of **restraints.**
Reference(s): Potter et al (2013), pp. 391-392.

513. The nurse documents a written entry regarding client care in the client's medical record. When checking the entry, the nurse notices that she documented some incorrect information. Which approach should the nurse implement?

1. Obliterate the incorrect information with a black marker
2. Use correction fluid to cover up the incorrect information.
3. Erase the error completely and write in the correct information.
4. Draw a line through the incorrect information and initial the change.

Level of Cognitive Ability: Applying
Client Needs: Safe and Effective Care Environment
Integrated Process: Communication and Documentation
Content Area: Leadership/Management: Ethical/Legal
Priority Concepts: Communication; Health Care Law

Answer: 4
Rationale: To correct a written error documented in a medical record, the nurse draws one line through the incorrect information and then initials the error. The information remains visible and properly labeled as incorrect. Errors are never erased, and correction fluid or black markers are never used on a legal document such as the medical record.
Priority Nursing Tip: Documentation in a client's medical record is legally required by accrediting agencies, state licensing laws, and state nurse and medical practice acts.
Test-Taking Strategy: Focus on the subject, correcting a written error documented in a medical record. Note that options 1, 2, and 3 are comparable or alike in that they indicate completely covering up or eliminating the incorrect information. Review: the principles of documentation.
Reference(s): Potter et al (2013), p. 351.

514. A client receiving chemotherapy has an extremely low white blood cell count and is immediately placed on neutropenic precautions that include a low-bacteria diet. Which food items is the client allowed to consume? **Select all that apply.**
☐ 1. Raw celery
☐ 2. Fresh apple
☐ 3. Italian bread
☐ 4. Tossed salad
☐ 5. Baked chicken
☐ 6. Well-cooked cheeseburger

Level of Cognitive Ability: Applying
Client Needs: Safe and Effective Care Environment
Integrated Process: Nursing Process/Implementation
Content Area: Fundamental Skills: Infection Control
Priority Concepts: Infection; Safety

Answer: 3, 5, 6
Rationale: An extremely low white blood cell count places the client at risk for infection. In the immunocompromised client, a low-bacteria diet is implemented. Italian bread, baked chicken, and a well-done cheeseburger are acceptable to consume because all products are thoroughly cooked. The client avoids eating fresh fruits and vegetables. Fresh fruits and vegetables harbor organisms and place the client at risk for infection.
Priority Nursing Tip: Most antineoplastic medications cause neutropenia and thrombocytopenia. Monitor the white blood cell count and the platelet count closely for indications of these adverse effects.
Test-Taking Strategy: Focus on the subject, a low-bacteria diet. Read each option carefully and think about the food items that harbor bacteria. Recalling that fresh fruits and vegetables are restricted from a low-bacteria diet will assist in selecting the correct items. Review: interventions for the client on a **low-bacteria diet** and **neutropenic precautions.**
Reference(s): Ignatavicius, Workman (2013), p. 420.

❖ **515.** When teaching a competent postoperative client about a patient controlled analgesia (PCA) pump, the nurse should provide which instructions to the client? **Select all that apply.**
- ❑ 1. Report the inability to void.
- ❑ 2. Report any nausea and vomiting.
- ❑ 3. Push the button before the pain becomes too great.
- ❑ 4. Inform the nurse about the pain levels being experienced.
- ❑ 5. Ask the family to push the button every 6 minutes, if the client decides to take a nap.

Level of Cognitive Ability: Analyzing
Client Needs: Safe and Effective Care Environment
Integrated Process: Teaching and Learning
Content Area: Fundamental Skills: Pain
Priority Concepts: Client Education; Pain

Answer: 1, 2, 3, 4
Rationale: PCA pumps have opioid medications infusing. Opioids can have an effect on the parasympathetic nervous system causing nausea, vomiting, and an inability to void and defecate; these occurrences need to be reported. The nurse must be kept informed about the pain relief achieved by the client and if there is any breakthrough pain. The client needs to be instructed to push the button before the pain becomes too great. Because the client is competent and there is a basal dose being administered, there is no need for the family to push the buttons for pain relief. In addition, no one other than the client should touch the pump unless instructed to do so.
Priority Nursing Tip: Patient controlled analgesia (PCA) pumps are very effective in controlling client pain. A basal dose is given continuously, so that if a client falls asleep or naps they do not wake in excruciating pain. When a PCA pump administers a basal rate, it is imperative that the nurse monitor the client's vital signs; especially respiratory rate. The demand rate is just that, it is the dose the client receives when they press the button on the PCA pump. Both the basal and demand rates are set by the health care provider to prevent overdose.
Test-Taking Strategy: Focus on the subject, teaching regarding a PCA pump. A PCA pump is designed for a client to administer their own dose of pain medication within the parameters set by the health care provider. Use these guidelines to assist in answering. Also, note that the incorrect option addresses the family not the client. Review: **PCA pumps.**
Reference(s): Ignatavicius, Workman (2013), p. 54.

516. The nurse observes that a postoperative client has episodes of extreme agitation. Which is the **best** nursing measure to implement to prevent escalating the agitation?
1. Gently hold the client's hand while speaking.
2. Wait until the client's agitation has subsided.
3. Speak while moving slowly toward the client.
4. Speak to the client from the entrance to the room.

Level of Cognitive Ability: Applying
Client Needs: Safe and Effective Care Environment
Integrated Process: Nursing Process/Implementation
Content Area: Fundamental Skills: Safety
Priority Concepts: Mood and Affect; Safety

Answer: 3
Rationale: Speaking and moving slowly toward the client will prevent the client from becoming further agitated because any sudden moves or speaking too quickly may cause the client to have a violent episode. Holding the client's hand can be misinterpreted by a client to mean restraint. If the client's agitation is not addressed, it is likely to increase; therefore, waiting for the agitation to subside is not a suitable option. Remaining at the entrance of the room can make the client feel alienated.
Priority Nursing Tip: Client safety is always the priority. Protect the client and remove any objects in the environment that could be potentially harmful to the client.
Test-Taking Strategy: Note the strategic word, *best*. Focus on the subject, agitated client. Remember that one of the most basic principles in preventing episodes of agitation or violent episodes is to avoid further agitation. Remember to be empathetic to the client while avoiding actions that potentially startle the client. These principles will direct you to the correct option. Review: nursing interventions for the **agitated client.**
Reference(s): Lewis et al (2014), pp. 357-358.

517. A 17-year-old client is discharged home with her newborn baby, and the nurse provides information to the client about home safety for children. Which statement by the client should alert the nurse that **further teaching is required** regarding home safety?

1. "I can keep my aluminum pots and pans in my lower cabinets."
2. "I will not use the microwave oven to heat my baby's formula."
3. "I have locks on all my cabinets that contain my cleaning supplies."
4. "I have a car seat that I will put in the front seat to keep my baby safe."

Level of Cognitive Ability: Evaluating
Client Needs: Safe and Effective Care Environment
Integrated Process: Teaching and Learning
Content Area: Fundamental Skills: Safety
Priority Concepts: Client Education; Safety

Answer: 4
Rationale: A baby car seat should never be placed in the front seat because of the potential for life-threatening injury on impact. It is perfectly safe to leave pots and pans in the lower cabinets for a child to investigate, as long as they are not made of glass, which would harm the baby if broken. Microwave ovens should never be used to heat formula because the formula heats unevenly, and it could burn and even scald the baby's mouth. Even though the bottle may feel warm, it could contain hot spots that could severely damage the baby's mouth. Any cabinets that contain dangerous items that a baby or child could swallow should be locked.
Priority Nursing Tip: Teach parents that when traveling with a child, always lock the car doors. Four-door cars should be equipped with child safety locks on the back doors.
Test-Taking Strategy: Note the strategic words, *further teaching is required*. These words indicate a negative event query and the need to select the incorrect client statement. Remember that a baby car seat should never be placed in the front seat because of the potential for injury on impact. Review: **car safety for children.**
Reference(s): Hockenberry, Wilson (2013), pp. 344, 346; McKinney et al (2013), pp. 107-108.

518. The nurse has administered an injection to a client. After the injection, the nurse accidentally drops the syringe on the floor. Which nursing action is appropriate in this situation?

1. Obtain a dust pan and mop to sweep up the syringe.
2. Call the housekeeping department to pick up the syringe.
3. Carefully pick up the syringe from the floor and gently recap the needle.
4. Carefully pick up the syringe from the floor and dispose of it in a sharps container.

Level of Cognitive Ability: Applying
Client Needs: Safe and Effective Care Environment
Integrated Process: Nursing Process/Implementation
Content Area: Fundamental Skills: Safety
Priority Concepts: Clinical Judgment; Safety

Answer: 4
Rationale: Used syringes should always be placed in a sharps container immediately after use to avoid individuals from becoming injured. A syringe should not be swept up because this action poses an additional risk for getting pricked. It is not the responsibility of the housekeeping department to pick up the syringe. Syringes should never be recapped under any circumstances because of the risk of getting pricked with a contaminated needle.
Priority Nursing Tip: Sharps, such as needles, are disposed of immediately after use in closed, puncture-resistant disposal containers that are leakproof and labeled or color-coded.
Test-Taking Strategy: Focus on the subject, procedure for disposal of a used needle. Recall basic principles related to the safe disposal of syringes to answer the question. Remember that recapping a needle places the nurse at risk for injury and that the needle is always disposed of in a sharps container. Review: safety principles related to **disposal of needles.**
Reference(s): Potter et al (2013), pp. 608-609.

519. The nurse is assigned to care for a client who is in traction. How can the nurse ensure a safe environment for the client?

1. Making sure that the knots are at the pulleys
2. Checking the weights to be sure that they are off the floor
3. Making sure that the head of the bed is kept at a 90-degree angle
4. Monitoring the weights to be sure that they are resting on a firm surface

Level of Cognitive Ability: Applying
Client Needs: Safe and Effective Care Environment
Integrated Process: Nursing Process/Implementation
Content Area: Adult Health: Musculoskeletal
Priority Concepts: Mobility; Safety

Answer: 2
Rationale: To achieve proper traction, weights need to be free-hanging, with knots kept away from the pulleys. The head of the bed is usually kept low to provide countertraction. Weights are not to be kept resting on a firm surface.
Priority Nursing Tip: For a client in traction, the nurse needs to frequently monitor color, motion, and sensation of the affected extremity.
Test-Taking Strategy: Focus on the subject, traction. Visualize the traction, recalling that there must be weight to exert the pull from the traction setup. This concept will assist in eliminating options 1 and 4. Recalling that countertraction is needed will assist in eliminating option 3. Review: care of the client in **traction.**
Reference(s): Ignatavicius, Workman (2013), p. 1154.

520. The nurse is observing a client using a walker. How should the nurse determine if the client is using the walker correctly?

1. Puts weight on the hand pieces, slides the walker forward, and then walks into it
2. Puts weight on the hand pieces, moves the walker forward, and then walks into it
3. Puts all four points of the walker flat on the floor, puts weight on the hand pieces, and then walks into it
4. Walks into the walker, puts weight on the hand pieces, and then puts all four points of the walker flat on the floor

Level of Cognitive Ability: Evaluating
Client Needs: Safe and Effective Care Environment
Integrated Process: Nursing Process/Evaluation
Content Area: Fundamental Skills: Safety
Priority Concepts: Mobility; Safety

Answer: 3
Rationale: When the client uses a walker, the nurse stands adjacent to the affected side. The client is instructed to put all four points of the walker 2 feet forward flat on the floor before putting weight on the hand pieces. This will ensure client safety and prevent stress cracks in the walker. The client is then instructed to move the walker forward and walk into it. Therefore, options 1, 2, and 4 are incorrect procedures for using a walker.
Priority Nursing Tip: Safety is a priority concern when the client uses an assistive device for ambulating. Be certain that the client can demonstrate correct use of the device.
Test-Taking Strategy: Focus on the subject, correct use of a walker. Visualize each of the options. Options 1 and 2 can be eliminated because putting weight on the hand pieces initially would cause an unsafe situation. From the remaining options, recalling that the walker is placed on all four points first will direct you to option 3. Review: the procedure for teaching a client to use a walker.
Reference(s): Potter et al (2013), p. 760.

521. A client is admitted to the labor and delivery unit for a labor induction. The health care provider has prescribed oxytocin (Pitocin) to be initiated by piggyback at an initial rate of 2 milliunits/min and increased by a rate of 2 milliunits/min every 30 minutes until contractions are 2 to 3 minutes apart, lasting 80 to 90 seconds. How many mL/hr will the nurse initially set the infusion pump if the dilution of the oxytocin is 10 units of oxytocin in 1000 mL of 0.225% normal saline? **Fill in the blank.**
Answer: _____ mL/hr

Level of Cognitive Ability: Applying
Client Needs: Safe and Effective Care Environment
Integrated Process: Nursing Process/Implementation
Content Area: Maternity: Intrapartum
Priority Concepts: Clinical Judgment; Safety

Answer: 12
Rationale: Use the medication calculation formula to calculate the correct dose.
Formula:
10 units of oxytocin in 1000 mL of 0.225% normal saline = 10,000 milliunits per 1000 mL or 10 milliunits per 1 mL. Solve by the ratio proportion method.
10 milliunits : 1 mL :: 2 milliunits : x mL/min =
$10x = 2$
$x = 2$ divided by 10
$x = 0.2$ mL/min

Multiply by 60 minutes to get the amount infused per hour
$0.2 \times 60 = 12$ mL/hr

Priority Nursing Tip: Oxytocin stimulates the smooth muscle of the uterus and increases the force, frequency, and duration of uterine contractions.
Test-Taking Strategy: Focus on the subject, a medication calculation. Use ratio and proportion method to perform the calculation. Follow the formula for the calculation of the correct dose. Once you have performed the calculation, verify your answer using a calculator and make sure that the answer is reasonable. Review: the formula for calculating medication doses.
Reference(s): McKinney et al (2013), p. 952.

522. The nurse is caring for an adolescent client with conjunctivitis. Which instruction is **most appropriate** to relate to the adolescent?

1. Avoid using all eye makeup to prevent possible reinfection.
2. Apply hot compresses to decrease pain and lessen irritation.
3. Obtain a new set of contact lenses for use after the infection clears.
4. Stay home for 3 days after starting antibiotic eye drops to avoid the spread of infection.

Level of Cognitive Ability: Applying
Client Needs: Safe and Effective Care Environment
Integrated Process: Teaching and Learning
Content Area: Child Health: Eye/Ear
Priority Concepts: Client Education; Infection

Answer: 3
Rationale: Conjunctivitis is inflammation of the conjunctiva. A new set of contact lenses should be obtained. If the client has conjunctivitis, eye makeup should be replaced but can still be worn. Cool compresses decrease pain and irritation. Isolation for 24 hours after antibiotics are initiated is necessary.
Priority Nursing Tip: Chlamydial conjunctivitis is rare in older children. If diagnosed in a child who is not sexually active, the child should be assessed for possible sexual abuse.
Test-Taking Strategy: Focus on the strategic words, *most appropriate*. Eliminate option 1 because of the closed-ended word, "all." Recalling the principles related to the effectiveness of antibiotics will assist in eliminating option 4. From the remaining options, noting the word *hot* in option 2 will assist in eliminating this option. Review: home care instructions for the client with **conjunctivitis**.
Reference(s): McKinney et al (2013), p. 1509.

❖ **523.** A client who has experienced a stroke has partial hemiplegia of the left leg. The straight-leg cane formerly used by the client is not sufficient to provide support. The nurse determines that the client could benefit from the somewhat greater support, stability, and safety provided by which devices? **Select all that apply**.
   ❑ 1. Walker
   ❑ 2. Wheelchair
   ❑ 3. Tripod cane
   ❑ 4. Wooden crutch
   ❑ 5. Quadripod cane
   ❑ 6. Lofstrand crutch

Level of Cognitive Ability: Analyzing
Client Needs: Safe and Effective Care Environment
Integrated Process: Nursing Process/Assessment
Content Area: Adult Health: Neurological
Priority Concepts: Mobility; Safety

Answer: 1, 3, 5
Rationale: A tripod or quadripod cane may be prescribed for the client who requires greater support and stability than is provided by a straight-leg cane. The tripod or quad-cane provides multiple points of support and is indicated for use by clients with partial or complete hemiplegia. A walker may potentially be needed by this client, if only for a short duration, and still encourages some client mobility. Neither wheelchair nor crutches are indicated for use with a client such as described in this question. A Lofstrand crutch is useful for clients with bilateral weakness.
Priority Nursing Tip: A quadripod cane provides more security to the client than a single-tipped cane.
Test-Taking Strategy: Focus on the subject, support device for the client with hemiplegia. Providing a wheelchair to a client with partial hemiplegia is excessive and is eliminated first. Wooden crutches are not indicated because there is no restriction in weight bearing. Lofstrand crutches (forearm crutches) are useful for bilateral weakness. Review: the use of various **assistive devices for ambulation**.
Reference(s): Potter et al (2013), p. 760.

524. A postoperative client begins to drain small amounts of bright red blood from the tracheostomy tube 24 hours after a laryngectomy. Which nursing action is **best** to implement?
1. Notify the surgeon.
2. Increase the frequency of suctioning.
3. Add moisture to the oxygen delivery system.
4. Document the character and amount of drainage.

Level of Cognitive Ability: Applying
Client Needs: Safe and Effective Care Environment
Integrated Process: Nursing Process/Implementation
Content Area: Critical Care: Emergency Situations
Priority Concepts: Clinical Judgment; Safety

Answer: 1
Rationale: Immediately after laryngectomy, a small amount of bleeding occurs from the tracheostomy that resolves within the first few hours. Otherwise, bleeding that is bright red may be a sign of impending rupture of a vessel. The bleeding in this instance represents a potential life-threatening situation, and the surgeon is notified to further evaluate the client and suture or repair the bleed. The other options do not address the urgency of the problem. Failure to notify the surgeon places the client at risk.
Priority Nursing Tip: The presence of bright red bleeding indicates active bleeding and is always a cause for concern, indicating the need to notify the surgeon.
Test-Taking Strategy: Note the strategic word, *best*. The additional information provided—*bright red blood* and *24 hours after the surgery*—should indicate that a potential complication exists and directs you to the correct option. Review: the complications after **laryngectomy**.
Reference(s): Ignatavicius, Workman (2013), pp. 591-592; Lewis et al (2014), p. 516.

❖ **525.** The nurse needs to withdraw 7000 units from the medication vial for administration. For a safe dose of medication how many milliliters should the nurse withdraw? **Refer to the figure.**

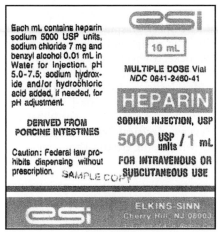

Each mL contains heparin sodium 5000 USP units, sodium chloride 7 mg and benzyl alcohol 0.01 mL in Water for Injection. pH 5.0-7.5; sodium hydroxide and/or hydrochloric acid added, if needed, for pH adjustment.

DERIVED FROM PORCINE INTESTINES

Caution: Federal law prohibits dispensing without prescription. SAMPLE COPY

esi

10 mL

MULTIPLE DOSE Vial
NDC 0641-2460-41

HEPARIN

SODIUM INJECTION, USP

5000 USP units / 1 mL

FOR INTRAVENOUS OR SUBCUTANEOUS USE

ELKINS-SINN
Cherry Hill NJ 08003

(Figure from Kee J, Marshall S: *Clinical calculations: with applications to general and specialty areas*, ed 7, St. Louis, 2013, Saunders.)

Answer: _____ mL

Level of Cognitive Ability: Applying
Client Needs: Safe and Effective Care Environment
Integrated Process: Nursing Process/Implementation
Content Area: Fundamental Skills: Medication/IV Calculations
Priority Concepts: Clinical Judgment; Safety

Answer: 1.4 mL
Rationale: Use the medication calculation formula.
Formula:

$$\frac{\text{Desired} \times \text{Volume}}{\text{Available}} = \text{mL/dose}$$

$$\frac{7000 \text{ units} \times 1 \text{ mL}}{5000 \text{ units}} = 1.4 \text{ mL/dose}$$

Priority Nursing Tip: It is important for the nurse to check the expiration date on a medication label. Medications that have expired lose their potency and may not be effective any longer.
Test-Taking Strategy: Focus on the subject, medication administration, and focus on the data on the medication label. Follow the formula for calculating the correct dose. Once you have performed the calculation, recheck your work with a calculator, and make certain that the answer makes sense. Review: **medication calculations.**
Reference(s): Potter et al (2013), pp. 574-577.

526. The nurse assists a postoperative client from a lying to a sitting position to prepare for ambulation. Which nursing action is **most appropriate** to maintain the safety of the client?

1. Assess the client for signs of dizziness and hypotension.
2. Allow the client to rise from the bed to a standing position unassisted.
3. Elevate the head of the bed quickly to assist the client to a sitting position.
4. Assist the client to move quickly from the lying position to the sitting position.

Level of Cognitive Ability: Applying
Client Needs: Safe and Effective Care Environment
Integrated Process: Nursing Process/Implementation
Content Area: Fundamental Skills: Safety
Priority Concepts: Clinical Judgment; Safety

Answer: 1
Rationale: Early ambulation should not exceed the client's tolerance. The client should be assessed before sitting. The client is assisted to rise from the lying position to the sitting position gradually until any evidence of dizziness, if present, has subsided. After sitting, the client may be assisted to a standing position. A sitting position can be achieved by raising the head of the bed slowly. The nurse should be at the client's side to provide physical support and encouragement.
Priority Nursing Tip: When moving a client from a lying to a sitting position, monitor for signs of orthostatic hypotension. If the client complains of dizziness, lightheadedness, or nausea, place the client back into the lying position and check the blood pressure and pulse.
Test-Taking Strategy: Focus on the strategic words, *most appropriate.* Eliminate options 3 and 4 because of the word *quickly* and option 2 because of the word *unassisted.* Additionally, option 1 is the only option that reflects assessment, the first step of the nursing process. Review: safety measures for **ambulation.**
Reference(s): Lewis et al (2014), pp. 356-357.

527. The nurse should implement which measures to prevent an electrical shock when using electrical equipment? **Select all that apply.**
  ❑ 1. Use a two-prong outlet.
  ❑ 2. Check the electrical cord for fraying.
  ❑ 3. Keep the electrical cord away from the sink.
  ❑ 4. Place the excess electrical cord under a small carpet.
  ❑ 5. Grasp the electrical cord when unplugging the equipment.
  ❑ 6. Disconnect the electrical cord from the wall socket when cleaning the equipment.

Level of Cognitive Ability: Applying
Client Needs: Safe and Effective Care Environment
Integrated Process: Nursing Process/Implementation
Content Area: Fundamental Skills: Safety
Priority Concepts: Clinical Judgment; Safety

Answer: 2, 3, 6
Rationale: The nurse needs to implement measures to prevent an electrical shock when using electrical equipment. These measures include using a three-prong plug that is grounded, checking the electrical cord for fraying or other damage, keeping the electrical cord away from the sink or other sources of water, using electrical tape to secure the excess electrical cord to the floor where it will not be stepped on (the cord should not be placed under carpet), grasping the plug (not the electrical cord) when unplugging the equipment, and disconnecting the electrical cord from the wall socket when cleaning the equipment.
Priority Nursing Tip: Any electrical equipment that a client brings into a health care facility should be inspected for safety before use.
Test-Taking Strategy: Focus on the subject, electrical safety. Read each option carefully and visualize how the measure may or may not prevent an electrical shock. Review: **electrical safety** measures that will prevent an **electrical shock** when using electrical equipment.
Reference(s): Potter et al (2013), p. 371.

528. Upon transfer from the postanesthesia care unit after spinal fusion with rod insertion, which technique should the nurse use to transfer the client from the stretcher to the bed?
  1. A bath blanket and the assistance of four people
  2. A bath blanket and the assistance of three people
  3. A transfer board and the assistance of two people
  4. A transfer board and the assistance of four people

Level of Cognitive Ability: Applying
Client Needs: Safe and Effective Care Environment
Integrated Process: Nursing Process/Implementation
Content Area: Fundamental Skills: Safety
Priority Concepts: Mobility; Safety

Answer: 4
Rationale: After spinal fusion, with or without instrumentation, the client is transferred from the stretcher to the bed using a transfer board and the assistance of four people. This permits optimal stabilization and support of the spine, while allowing the client to be moved smoothly and gently. Therefore, options 1, 2, and 3 are incorrect and unsafe.
Priority Nursing Tip: Physical stress for the health care provider can be decreased significantly by the use of a transfer board. In addition, the use of a transfer board prevents friction on the client's skin during the move.
Test-Taking Strategy: Focus on the subject, transfer of the client with spinal fusion. Think about the level of comfort and stability provided to the client's spine with the amounts of assistance given in each option. Using this approach will assist in eliminating options 1, 2, and 3. Review: care of the client after **spinal fusion.**
Reference(s): Potter et al (2013), pp. 749, 1161.

❖ **529.** Which actions should the nurse take in the event of an accidental poisoning? **Select all that apply.**
  ❑ 1. Save vomitus for laboratory analysis.
  ❑ 2. Place the client in a flat supine position.
  ❑ 3. Induce vomiting if a household cleaner was ingested.
  ❑ 4. Assess for airway patency, breathing, and circulation.
  ❑ 5. Determine the type and amount of substance ingested.
  ❑ 6. Remove any visible materials from the nose and mouth.

Level of Cognitive Ability: Applying
Client Needs: Safe and Effective Care Environment
Integrated Process: Nursing Process/Implementation
Content Area: Critical Care: Emergency Situations
Priority Concepts: Clinical Judgment; Safety

Answer: 1, 4, 5, 6
Rationale: In the event of accidental poisoning, the poison control center is called before attempting any interventions. Additional interventions in an accidental poisoning include saving vomitus for laboratory analysis, which may assist with further treatment; assessing for airway patency, breathing, and circulation; determining the type and amount of substance ingested if possible to identify an antidote; removing any visible materials from the nose and mouth to terminate exposure; and positioning the victim with the head to the side to prevent aspiration of vomitus and assist in keeping the airway open. Vomiting is never induced in an unconscious client or one who is experiencing seizures because of the risk of aspiration. Additionally, vomiting is not induced if lye, household cleaners, hair care products, grease or petroleum products, or furniture polish was ingested because of the risk of internal burns.
Priority Nursing Tip: In the event of a poisoning, the Poison Control Center is contacted immediately.
Test-Taking Strategy: Focus on the subject, accidental poisoning. Visualize each of the interventions and how they may be helpful in treating the poisoning. Use of the ABCs—airway, breathing, and circulation—will assist in determining the correct interventions. Also remember that any substances that are caustic can result in further injury to the client. Review: the interventions for treating a victim of accidental **poisoning.**
Reference(s): Potter et al (2013), p. 383.

530. The nurse inserts an indwelling urinary catheter into a client. As the catheter moves into the bladder, urine begins to flow into the tubing. Which action should the nurse implement **next**?
  1. Inflate the balloon with water.
  2. Secure the catheter to the client.
  3. Measure the initial urine output.
  4. Advance the catheter 2.5 to 5 cm.

Level of Cognitive Ability: Applying
Client Needs: Safe and Effective Care Environment
Integrated Process: Nursing Process/Implementation
Content Area: Fundamental Skills: Safety
Priority Concepts: Elimination; Safety

Answer: 4
Rationale: The balloon of a urinary catheter is behind the opening at the insertion tip, so the nurse inserts the catheter 2.5 to 5 cm further after urine begins to flow so as to provide sufficient space to inflate the balloon. The balloon is not inflated as soon as urine appears because the balloon could be located in the urethra. After the insertion procedure and inflation of the balloon, the nurse secures the catheter to the client's leg and then measures the initial urine output.
Priority Nursing Tip: Strict aseptic technique is required when inserting a urinary catheter into a client.
Test-Taking Strategy: Note the strategic word, *next*. Visualize the procedure described in the question and the effects of each description in the options to direct you to option 4. Review: the procedure for **urinary catheter insertion.**
Reference(s): Potter et al (2013), pp. 1074-1075.

531. The nurse is preparing to administer oxygen to a client who has chronic obstructive pulmonary disease (COPD) and is at risk for carbon dioxide narcosis. The nurse should check to see that the oxygen flow rate is prescribed at which rate?
1. 2 to 3 liters per minute
2. 4 to 5 liters per minute
3. 6 to 8 liters per minute
4. 8 to 10 liters per minute

Level of Cognitive Ability: Analyzing
Client Needs: Safe and Effective Care Environment
Integrated Process: Nursing Process/Implementation
Content Area: Adult Health: Respiratory
Priority Concepts: Clinical Judgment; Gas Exchange

Answer: 1
Rationale: In carbon dioxide narcosis, the central chemoreceptors lose their sensitivity to increased levels of carbon dioxide and no longer respond by increasing the rate and depth of respiration. For these clients, the stimulus to breathe is a decreased arterial oxygen concentration. In the client with COPD, a low arterial oxygen level is the client's primary drive for breathing. If high levels of oxygen are administered, the client loses the respiratory drive, and respiratory failure results. Thus the nurse checks the flow of oxygen to see that it does not exceed 2 to 3 liters per minute.
Priority Nursing Tip: The chest x-ray for a client with COPD typically reveals hyperinflation.
Test-Taking Strategy: Focus on the subject, COPD. Recalling the pathophysiology that occurs in COPD and that a low arterial oxygen level is the client's primary drive for breathing will direct you to option 1, the lowest oxygen liter flow. Review: **chronic obstructive pulmonary disease (COPD).**
Reference(s): Ignatavicius, Workman (2013), p. 619; Lewis et al (2014), pp. 589-590.

532. A client undergoes a subtotal thyroidectomy. The nurse ensures that which **priority** item is at the client's bedside upon arrival from the operating room?
1. An apnea monitor
2. A suction unit and oxygen
3. A blood transfusion warmer
4. An ampule of phytonadione (vitamin K)

Level of Cognitive Ability: Applying
Client Needs: Safe and Effective Care Environment
Integrated Process: Nursing Process/Implementation
Content Area: Adult Health: Endocrine
Priority Concepts: Gas Exchange; Safety

Answer: 2
Rationale: After thyroidectomy, respiratory distress can occur from tetany, tissue swelling, or hemorrhage. It is important to have oxygen and suction equipment readily available and in working order if such an emergency were to arise. Apnea is not a problem associated with thyroidectomy, unless the client experienced respiratory arrest. Blood transfusions can be administered without a warmer, if necessary. Vitamin K would not be administered for a client who is hemorrhaging, unless deficiencies in clotting factors warrant its administration.
Priority Nursing Tip: Following thyroidectomy, the client should be maintained in a semi-Fowler's position to prevent edema at the surgical site.
Test-Taking Strategy: Note the strategic word, *priority*. Recall the anatomic location of the thyroid gland and its proximity to the trachea. Use the ABCs—airway, breathing, and circulation—to direct you to the correct option. Review: postoperative care after **thyroidectomy.**
Reference(s): Lewis et al (2014), p. 1201.

533. The nurse places a hospitalized client with active tuberculosis in a private, well-ventilated isolation room. In addition, which action should the nurse take before entering the client's room?
1. Wash the hands.
2. Wash the hands and wear a gown and gloves.
3. Wash the hands and place a high-efficiency particulate air (HEPA) respirator over the nose and mouth.
4. The nurse needs no special precautions, but the client is instructed to cover his or her mouth and nose when coughing or sneezing.

Level of Cognitive Ability: Applying
Client Needs: Safe and Effective Care and Environment
Integrated Process: Nursing Process/Implementation
Content Area: Fundamental Skills: Infection Control
Priority Concepts: Infection; Safety

Answer: 3
Rationale: Tuberculosis is a highly communicable disease caused by *Mycobacterium tuberculosis*. The nurse wears a HEPA respirator when caring for a client with active tuberculosis. Hands are always thoroughly washed before and after caring for the client. Option 1 is an incomplete action. Option 2 is also inaccurate and incomplete. Gowning is only indicated when there is a possibility of contaminating clothing. Option 4 is an incorrect statement because special precautions are needed.
Priority Nursing Tip: A positive Mantoux skin test reaction does not mean that active tuberculosis is present, but it does indicate previous exposure to tuberculosis or the presence of inactive (dormant) disease.
Test-Taking Strategy: Focus on the subject, caring for the client with tuberculosis. Recalling the route of transmission and the need for airborne precautions will direct you to the correct option. Review: **airborne precautions** and **tuberculosis.**
Reference(s): Ignatavicius, Workman (2013), pp. 440, 442, 657.

534. The nurse is assigned to care for a hospitalized toddler. Which measure should the nurse plan to implement as the **highest priority** of care?
1. Providing a consistent caregiver
2. Protecting the toddler from injury
3. Adapting the toddler to the hospital routine
4. Allowing the toddler to participate in play and diversional activities

Level of Cognitive Ability: Applying
Client Needs: Safe and Effective Care Environment
Integrated Process: Nursing Process/Planning
Content Area: Developmental Stages: Infancy to Adolescence
Priority Concepts: Development; Safety

Answer: 2
Rationale: The toddler is at high risk for injury as a result of developmental abilities and an unfamiliar environment. Whereas consistency, adaptation, and diversion are important, protection from injury is the highest priority.
Priority Nursing Tip: Although safety is the highest priority, the nurse must remember that hospitalization, with its own set of rituals and routines, can severely disrupt the life of a toddler.
Test-Taking Strategy: Note the strategic words, *highest priority*. Use Maslow's Hierarchy of Needs theory. Physiological needs come first, followed by safety. Because no physiological needs are addressed, the safety option of preventing injury takes priority. Review: care of the **hospitalized toddler**.
Reference(s): McKinney et al (2013), pp. 883-884.

535. A client is to undergo pleural biopsy at the bedside. Knowing the potential complications of the procedure, what should the nurse plan to have available at the bedside?
1. Intubation tray
2. Morphine sulfate injection
3. Portable chest x-ray machine
4. Chest tube and drainage system

Level of Cognitive Ability: Applying
Client Needs: Safe and Effective Care Environment
Integrated Process: Nursing Process/Planning
Content Area: Fundamental Skills: Diagnostic Tests
Priority Concepts: Gas Exchange; Safety

Answer: 4
Rationale: Complications after pleural biopsy include hemothorax, pneumothorax, and temporary pain from intercostal nerve injury. The nurse has a chest tube and drainage system available at the bedside for use if hemothorax or pneumothorax develops. An intubation tray is not indicated. The client should be premedicated before the procedure, or a local anesthetic is used. A portable chest x-ray machine would be called for to verify placement of a chest tube if one was inserted, but it is unnecessary to have at the bedside before the procedure.
Priority Nursing Tip: Absent breath sounds on the affected side of the lungs is a manifestation of pneumothorax.
Test-Taking Strategy: Focus on the subject, pleural biopsy. Think about how this procedure is done. Recalling the complications of this procedure and noting the relation of this procedure to option 4 will direct you to this option. Review: **pleural biopsy**.
Reference(s): Ignatavicius, Workman (2013), pp. 560-561; Pagana, Pagana (2013), pp. 732-733.

536. The nurse manager of a hemodialysis unit observes a new nurse preparing hemodialysis on a client with chronic kidney disease. The nurse manager should note the new nurse **needs further teaching** and intervene if which action is carried out by the new nurse?
1. Uses sterile technique for needle insertion
2. Wears full protective clothing such as goggles, mask, gown, and gloves
3. Covers the connection site with a bath blanket to enhance extremity warmth
4. Puts on a mask and gives one to the client to wear during connection to the machine

Level of Cognitive Ability: Evaluating
Client Needs: Safe and Effective Care Environment
Integrated Process: Teaching and Learning
Content Area: Fundamental Skills: Infection Control
Priority Concepts: Infection; Safety

Answer: 3
Rationale: While the client is receiving hemodialysis, the connection site should not be covered, and it should be visible so that the nurse can assess for bleeding, ischemia, and infection at the site during the procedure. Infection is a major concern with hemodialysis. For that reason, the use of sterile technique and the application of a face mask for both the nurse and client are extremely important. It is also imperative that standard precautions be followed, which includes the use of goggles, mask, gloves, and a gown.
Priority Nursing Tip: The nurse should assess the client for fluid overload before hemodialysis and fluid volume deficit after hemodialysis.
Test-Taking Strategy: Note the strategic words, *needs further teaching* and the word *intervene*. These words indicate a negative event query and require you to select the option that indicates an incorrect nursing action. Eliminate options 1, 2, and 4 because they are comparable or alike in that they relate to infection control and standard precautions. Review: the basic procedure related to **hemodialysis**.
Reference(s): Ignatavicius, Workman (2013), p. 1562; Lewis et al (2014), p. 1124.

537. The nurse is going to suction an adult client with a tracheostomy who has copious amounts of respiratory secretions. Which intervention should the nurse take to perform this procedure safely?
1. Set the suction pressure range between 160 to 180 mm Hg.
2. Hyperoxygenate the client using a manual resuscitation bag.
3. Apply continuous suction in the airway for up to 20 seconds.
4. Occlude the Y-port of the suction catheter while advancing it into the tracheostomy.

Level of Cognitive Ability: Applying
Client Needs: Safe and Effective Care Environment
Integrated Process: Nursing Process/Implementation
Content Area: Adult Health: Respiratory
Priority Concepts: Gas Exchange; Safety

Answer: 2
Rationale: To perform suctioning, the nurse hyperoxygenates the client using a manual resuscitation bag or the sigh mechanism if the client is on a mechanical ventilator. The safe suction range for an adult is 100 to 120 mm Hg. The nurse uses intermittent suction in the airway for up to 10 to 15 seconds. The nurse advances the suction catheter into the tracheostomy without occluding the Y-port; suction is never applied while introducing the catheter because it would traumatize mucosa and remove oxygen from the respiratory tract.
Priority Nursing Tip: To perform suctioning, the client is assisted to a sitting upright position such as semi-Fowler's with the head hyperextended (unless contraindicated).
Test-Taking Strategy: Visualize this procedure. Recalling that suction is applied intermittently and on catheter withdrawal only will eliminate options 3 and 4. From the remaining options, use the ABCs—airway, breathing, and circulation—to direct you to the correct option. Review: the procedure for **suctioning.**
Reference(s): Ignatavicius, Workman (2013), pp. 574-575; Lewis et al (2014), p. 509.

538. The nurse is collecting a sputum specimen for culture and sensitivity testing from a client who has a productive cough. Which intervention should the nurse take to obtain the specimen?
1. Ask the client to obtain the specimen after breakfast.
2. Use a sterile plastic container for obtaining the specimen.
3. Provide tissues for expectoration and obtaining the specimen.
4. Ask the client to expectorate a small amount of sputum into the emesis basin.

Level of Cognitive Ability: Applying
Client Needs: Safe and Effective Care Environment
Integrated Process: Nursing Process/Implementation
Content Area: Fundamental Skills: Diagnostic Tests
Priority Concepts: Infection; Safety

Answer: 2
Rationale: Sputum specimens for culture and sensitivity testing need to be obtained using sterile techniques because the test is done to determine the presence of organisms. If the procedure for obtaining the specimen is not sterile, then the specimen would be contaminated and the results of the test would be invalid. A first-morning specimen is preferred because it represents overnight secretions of the tracheobronchial tree.
Priority Nursing Tip: Always collect a specimen for culture and sensitivity before prescribed antibiotics are initiated because the antibiotic may alter the testing by affecting the organism count.
Test-Taking Strategy: Focus on the subject, sputum specimen for culture and sensitivity. The words *culture and sensitivity* tell you that the test is being done to identify the presence of microorganisms. Recalling that microorganisms will multiply in the specimen and that accurate identification of organisms is needed to determine treatment will direct you to the correct option. Also, noting the word *sterile* in option 2 will direct you to this option. Review: the procedure for **sputum collection.**
Reference(s): Pagana, Pagana (2013), pp. 861-862.

539. The postmyocardial infarction client is scheduled for a technetium-99 m ventriculography (multigated acquisition [MUGA] scan). The nurse should ensure that which item is in place before the procedure?
1. A Foley catheter
2. Signed informed consent
3. A central venous pressure (CVP) line
4. Notation of allergies to iodine or shellfish

Level of Cognitive Ability: Applying
Client Needs: Safe and Effective Care Environment
Integrated Process: Nursing Process/Implementation
Content Area: Adult Health: Cardiovascular
Priority Concepts: Perfusion; Safety

Answer: 2
Rationale: MUGA is a radionuclide study used to detect myocardial infarction and decreased myocardial blood flow and to determine left ventricular function. A radioisotope is injected intravenously. Therefore, a signed informed consent is necessary. A Foley catheter and CVP line are not required. The procedure does not use radiopaque dye; therefore, allergy to iodine and shellfish is not a concern.
Priority Nursing Tip: The left ventricular ejection fraction (LVEF) should be above 55%.
Test-Taking Strategy: Focus on the subject, MUGA scan. Think about how the procedure is performed. Recalling that the procedure involves injection of a radioisotope will direct you to the correct option. Review: preparation for a **MUGA scan.**
Reference(s): Ignatavicius, Workman (2013), pp. 250, 252; Pagana, Pagana (2013), pp. 224-225.

540. Which interventions should the emergency department nurse use during the management of a client suspected of exposure to anthrax? **Select all that apply.**
- ❑ **1.** Handle clothing minimally.
- ❑ **2.** Store contaminated clothing in a labeled paper bag
- ❑ **3.** Instruct the client to remove contaminated clothing.
- ❑ **4.** Wear sterile gloves when handling contaminated items.
- ❑ **5.** Instruct the client to shower thoroughly using soap and water.
- ❑ **6.** Consult with the health care provider regarding postexposure prophylaxis with oral fluoroquinolones for the client.

Level of Cognitive Ability: Applying
Client Needs: Safe and Effective Care Environment
Integrated Process: Nursing Process/Implementation
Content Area: Leadership/Management: Disasters
Priority Concepts: Clinical Judgment; Safety

Answer: 1, 3, 5, 6
Rationale: An important aspect of care for a client who has a bioterrorism-related illness is postexposure management. Decontamination and exposure management of the client suspected of anthrax exposure include instructing the client to remove contaminated clothing and store contaminated clothing in a labeled plastic (not paper) bag; handling clothing minimally to avoid agitation; instructing the client to shower thoroughly using soap and water; and using Standard Precautions and wearing appropriate protective barriers when handling contaminated clothing or other items. Postexposure prophylaxis with oral fluoroquinolones for the client is also recommended. The use of sterile gloves is unnecessary.
Priority Nursing Tip: Anthrax is transmitted by direct contact with bacteria and spores and can be contracted through the digestive system, abrasions in the skin, or inhalation through the lungs.
Test-Taking Strategy: Focus on the subject, a client suspected of exposure to anthrax. Read each option carefully. Recalling that postexposure management involves decontamination will assist in selecting the correct interventions. Remember that preventing exposure is a critical intervention. Review: the interventions for postexposure management of **anthrax**.
Reference(s): Ignatavicius, Workman (2013), p. 448; Potter et al (2013), p. 374.

541. Which are the characteristics of case management? **Select all that apply.**
- ❑ **1.** A case manager usually does not provide direct care.
- ❑ **2.** Critical pathways and CareMaps are types of case management.
- ❑ **3.** A case manager does not need to be concerned with standards of cost management.
- ❑ **4.** A case manager collaborates with and supervises the care delivered by other staff members.
- ❑ **5.** The evaluation process involves continuous monitoring and analysis of the needs of the client and services provided.
- ❑ **6.** A case manager coordinates a hospitalized client's acute care and follows up with the client after discharge to home.

Level of Cognitive Ability: Applying
Client Needs: Safe and Effective Care Environment
Integrated Process: Nursing Process/Planning
Content Area: Leadership/Management: Delegating
Priority Concepts: Care Coordination; Health Care Quality

Answer: 1, 4, 5, 6
Rationale: Case management is a care management approach that coordinates health care services to clients and their families while maintaining quality of care and minimizing health care costs. Case managers usually do not provide direct care; instead they collaborate with and supervise the care delivered by other staff members and actively coordinate client discharge planning. A case manager is usually held accountable for some standard of cost management. A case manager coordinates a hospitalized client's acute care, follows up with the client after discharge to home, and is responsible and accountable for appraising the overall usefulness and effectiveness of the case managed services. This evaluation process involves continuous monitoring and analysis of the client's needs and services provided. Critical pathways or CareMaps are not types of case management; rather, they are multidisciplinary treatment plans used in a case management delivery system to implement timely interventions in a coordinated care plan.
Priority Nursing Tip: Case management requires the nurse to analyze a client's situation from a holistic perspective and determine his or her needs. The nurse then consults the appropriate disciplines to meet these needs.
Test-Taking Strategy: Focus on the subject, the characteristics of case management, and read each option carefully. Recall that case management is a care management approach that coordinates health care services to clients and their families while maintaining quality of care and keeping health care costs at a minimum. This will assist in selecting the correct options. Review: the characteristics of **case management**.
Reference(s): Huber (2014), pp. 208-209; Potter et al (2013), pp. 36, 276.

542. A client is being admitted to the hospital after receiving a radiation implant for cervical cancer. Which **priority** action should the nurse take in the care of this client?
1. Encourage the family to visit.
2. Admit the client to a private room.
3. Place the client on protective isolation.
4. Encourage the client to take frequent rest periods.

Level of Cognitive Ability: Applying
Client Needs: Safe and Effective Care Environment
Integrated Process: Nursing Process/Implementation
Content Area: Fundamental Skills: Safety
Priority Concepts: Clinical Judgment; Safety

Answer: 2
Rationale: The client who has a radiation implant is placed in a private room and has limited visitors. This reduces the exposure of others to the radiation. Protective isolation is unnecessary; rather, individuals other than the client need to be protected. Frequent rest periods are a helpful general intervention but are not a priority for the client in this situation.
Priority Nursing Tip: Pregnant women and any individual younger than 16 years of age are not allowed in the room of a client with a radiation implant.
Test-Taking Strategy: Note the strategic word, *priority* and focus on the subject, radiation implant. Recalling the concepts related to environmental safety and that other individuals should have limited exposure to clients with radiation implants will direct you to option 2. Review: care of the client with a **radiation implant.**
Reference(s): Ignatavicius, Workman (2013), p. 413.

543. A client is to undergo weekly intravesical chemotherapy for bladder cancer for the next 8 weeks. Which statement by the client should indicate to the nurse that the client understands how to manage urine as a biohazard?
1. Void into a bedpan and then empty the urine into the toilet.
2. Purchase extra bottles of scented disinfectant for daily bathroom cleansing.
3. Have one bathroom strictly set aside for the client's use for the next 8 weeks.
4. Disinfect the toilet with household bleach after voiding for 6 hours after a treatment.

Level of Cognitive Ability: Evaluating
Client Needs: Safe and Effective Care Environment
Integrated Process: Nursing Process/Evaluation
Content Area: Fundamental Skills: Safety
Priority Concepts: Clinical Judgment; Safety

Answer: 4
Rationale: Intravesical instillation involves instilling a chemotherapeutic agent into the bladder via a urethral catheter. This method of treatment provides a concentrated topical treatment with minimal systemic absorption. The client retains the medication for approximately 2 hours. After intravesical chemotherapy, the client treats the urine as a biohazard. This involves disinfecting the toilet after voiding with household bleach for 6 hours after a treatment. There is no value in using a bedpan for voiding. Scented disinfectants are of no particular use. The client does not need to have a separate bathroom for personal use.
Priority Nursing Tip: After intravesical instillation with a chemotherapeutic agent to treat bladder cancer, the client is instructed to increase fluid intake to flush the bladder.
Test-Taking Strategy: Focus on the subject, intravesical instillation with a chemotherapeutic agent. Option 1 has no value and is eliminated first. Because scented disinfectants also have no value, option 2 is eliminated next. Also, option 3 is unnecessary and may be unrealistic for many clients. Knowing that the urine and toilet need special treatment for 6 hours after intravesical chemotherapy directs you to option 4. Review: care of the client receiving **intravesical chemotherapy.**
Reference(s): Ignatavicius, Workman (2013), p. 420.

544. A client who is admitted to the hospital for an unrelated medical problem is diagnosed with urethritis caused by chlamydial infection. The unlicensed assistive personnel (UAP) assigned to the client asks the nurse what measures are necessary to prevent contraction of the infection during care. The nurse tells the UAP that which intervention is needed for infection control?
1. Enteric precautions should be instituted for the client.
2. Gloves and mask should be used when in the client's room.
3. Contact isolation should be initiated because the disease is highly contagious.
4. Standard precautions are sufficient because the disease is transmitted sexually.

Level of Cognitive Ability: Applying
Client Needs: Safe and Effective Care Environment
Integrated Process: Teaching and Learning
Content Area: Fundamental Skills: Infection Control
Priority Concepts: Infection; Safety

Answer: 4
Rationale: *Chlamydia* is a sexually transmitted infection. Caregivers cannot acquire the disease during administration of care, and standard precautions are the only measure that needs to be used. Therefore, options 1, 2, and 3 are incorrect.
Priority Nursing Tip: A pregnant client with a chlamydial infection can transmit the infection to the neonate during a vaginal birth. This occurrence can result in neonatal conjunctivitis or pneumonitis.
Test-Taking Strategy: Focus on the subject, infection control for a *Chlamydia* infection. Recall that this infection is sexually transmitted. Also, note that option 4 is the umbrella option. Review: transmission of a chlamydial infection and standard precautions.
Reference(s): Ignatavicius, Workman (2013), pp. 440, 1496-1497.

❖ **545.** The nurse manager is reviewing the principles of surgical asepsis with the nursing staff. In which situations should the nurse manager tell the staff that it is necessary to use the principles of surgical asepsis? **Select all that apply.**
☐ 1. Removing a dressing
☐ 2. Reapplying sterile dressings
☐ 3. Inserting an intravenous (IV) line
☐ 4. Inserting a urinary (Foley) catheter
☐ 5. Suctioning the tracheobronchial airway
☐ 6. Caring for an immunosuppressed client

Level of Cognitive Ability: Applying
Client Needs: Safe and Effective Care Environment
Integrated Process: Teaching and Learning
Content Area: Fundamental Skills: Infection Control
Priority Concepts: Infection; Safety

Answer: 2, 3, 4, 5
Rationale: Surgical asepsis involves the use of sterile technique. Some examples of procedures in which surgical asepsis is necessary include reapplying sterile dressings, inserting an IV or urinary catheter, and suctioning the tracheobronchial airway. Medical asepsis, or clean technique, includes procedures to reduce and prevent the spread of microorganisms. Removing a dressing can be done by clean technique using clean gloves (although reapplying the dressing requires surgical asepsis). Caring for an immunosuppressed client requires medical asepsis techniques.
Priority Nursing Tip: Medical and surgical asepsis are measures instituted to protect both the client and health care workers. Medical asepsis is intended to reduce and prevent the spread of microorganisms, whereas surgical asepsis aims to eliminate all microorganisms in a particular environment.
Test-Taking Strategy: Focus on the subject, surgical asepsis. Recalling the definitions of medical and surgical asepsis and thinking about the invasiveness of each activity in the options will assist in answering this question. Review: the difference between medical and surgical asepsis.
Reference(s): Potter et al (2013), pp. 421-422.

546. The nurse is preparing the client's morning NPH insulin dose and notices a clumpy precipitate inside the insulin vial. What should the nurse do?
1. Draw the dose from a new vial.
2. Draw up and administer the dose.
3. Shake the vial in an attempt to disperse the clumps.
4. Warm the bottle under running water to dissolve the clump.

Level of Cognitive Ability: Applying
Client Needs: Safe and Effective Care Environment
Integrated Process: Nursing Process/Implementation
Content Area: Pharmacology: Endocrine Medications
Priority Concepts: Glucose Regulation; Safety

Answer: 1
Rationale: The nurse should always inspect the vial of insulin before use for solution changes that may signify loss of potency. NPH insulin is normally uniformly cloudy. Clumping, frosting, and precipitates are signs of insulin damage. In this situation, because potency is questionable, it is safer to discard the vial and draw up the dose from a new vial.
Priority Nursing Tip: NPH insulin is an intermediate-acting insulin whose onset of action is 1.5 hours, peak time is 4 to 12 hours, and duration of action is approximately 16 to 24 hours.
Test-Taking Strategy: Focus on the subject, NPH insulin. Remember that NPH insulin is cloudy but not clumpy. This will direct you to option 1, the safest action. Remember that when in doubt, throw it out. Review: the characteristics of **NPH insulin**.
Reference(s): Lehne (2013), pp. 716, 733; Potter et al (2013), pp. 603-604.

547. The nurse is preparing the bedside for a postoperative parathyroidectomy client who is expected to return to the nursing unit from the recovery room in 1 hour. The nurse should ensure that which specific item is at the client's bedside?
1. Cardiac monitor
2. Tracheotomy set
3. Intermittent gastric suction
4. Underwater seal chest drainage system

Level of Cognitive Ability: Applying
Client Needs: Safe and Effective Care Environment
Integrated Process: Nursing Process/Planning
Content Area: Adult Health: Endocrine
Priority Concepts: Clinical Judgment; Safety

Answer: 2
Rationale: Respiratory distress caused by hemorrhage and swelling and compression of the trachea is a primary concern for the nurse managing the care of a postoperative parathyroidectomy client. An emergency tracheotomy set is always routinely placed at the bedside of the client with this type of surgery, in anticipation of this potential complication. Although a cardiac monitor may be attached to the client in the postoperative period, it is not specific to this type of surgery. Options 3 and 4 also are not specifically needed with the surgical procedure.
Priority Nursing Tip: After parathyroidectomy, monitor the client for hypocalcemic crisis, as evidenced by tingling and twitching in the extremities and face.
Test-Taking Strategy: Focus on the subject, specific equipment needed after parathyroidectomy. Think about the location of the surgical incision and what potential problems might occur from that location. This will direct you to option 2. Review: postoperative **parathyroidectomy** care.
Reference(s): Ignatavicius, Workman (2013), p. 1399.

548. The nurse has a prescription to administer foscarnet sodium intravenously to a client with acquired immunodeficiency syndrome (AIDS). Before administering this medication, which measure should the nurse implement?

1. Obtain a sputum culture.
2. Obtain folic acid (Folvite) as an antidote.
3. Place the solution on a controlled infusion pump.
4. Ensure that liver enzyme levels have been drawn as a baseline.

Level of Cognitive Ability: Applying
Client Needs: Safe and Effective Care Environment
Integrated Process: Nursing Process/Implementation
Content Area: Adult Health: Immune
Priority Concepts: Immunity; Safety

Answer: 3
Rationale: Foscarnet sodium is an antiviral agent used to treat cytomegalovirus (CMV) retinitis in clients with AIDS. Because of the potential toxicity of the medication, it is administered with the use of a controlled infusion device. A sputum culture is not necessary. Folic acid is not an antidote. Foscarnet sodium is highly toxic to the kidneys, and serum creatinine levels are measured frequently during therapy, not liver enzymes.
Priority Nursing Tip: The client with human immunodeficiency virus (HIV) or AIDS is at high risk for the development of opportunistic infections.
Test-Taking Strategy: Focus on the subject, administration of foscarnet sodium. Eliminate option 1 because the medication is usually indicated in the treatment of CMV retinitis, not respiratory infection. Additionally, no data in the question indicate the need for a sputum culture. Option 2 is eliminated next because folic acid is not an antidote. From the remaining options, it is necessary to know that the medication can be toxic and cannot be infused too quickly. This will direct you to option 3. Also, recalling that the medication is toxic to the kidneys, not the liver, will direct you to the correct option. Review: **foscarnet sodium.**
Reference(s): Gahart, Nazareno (2012), p. 646; Hodgson, Kizior (2014), p. 516.

549. An adult client who has a severe mental impairment is scheduled for gallbladder surgery. With regard to the informed consent, which should the nurse implement **first** to facilitate the scheduled surgery?

1. Check for the identity of the client's legal guardian.
2. Inform the legal guardian about advance directives.
3. Arrange for the surgeon to provide informed consent.
4. Ensure that the legal guardian signed the informed consent.

Level of Cognitive Ability: Applying
Client Needs: Safe and Effective Care Environment
Integrated Process: Nursing Process/Implementation
Content Area: Leadership/Management: Ethical/Legal
Priority Concepts: Ethics; Health Care Law

Answer: 1
Rationale: A mentally impaired client is not competent to sign an informed consent, so the nurse should first verify the identity of the client's legal guardian. This action fulfills part of the nurse's duty in informed consent, helps avoid improperly signed documents, and directs the surgeon to the legal representatives of the client's interests. The client and/or legal guardian is asked about the existence of an advance directive at the time of admission, so this should have already been done, making option 2 incorrect. The surgeon is responsible for obtaining the informed consent, but based on the options provided, option 3 is not the first nursing action. Likewise, option 4 is not the first action; the nurse checks identity of the legal guardian first.
Priority Nursing Tip: A mentally or emotionally incompetent client is an individual who has been declared incompetent, is unconscious, is under the influence of chemical agents such as alcohol or drugs, or has chronic dementia or another mental deficiency that impairs thought processes and the ability to make decisions.
Test-Taking Strategy: Note the strategic word, *first* and focus on the subject, obtaining permission for the surgical procedure for a client who is mentally impaired. To ensure safe, effective care, the nurse ensures the identity of the client's legal guardian before checking any other aspect of obtaining informed consent. Review: **the process of informed consent.**
Reference(s): Ignatavicius, Workman (2013), p. 252; Potter et al (2013), pp. 302-303.

550. A client with an acute respiratory infection is admitted to the hospital with a diagnosis of sinus tachycardia. The nurse should develop a plan of care for the client and include which intervention?
1. Limiting oral and intravenous fluids
2. Measuring the client's pulse once each shift
3. Providing the client with short, frequent walks
4. Eliminating sources of caffeine from meal trays

Level of Cognitive Ability: Applying
Client Needs: Safe and Effective Care Environment
Integrated Process: Nursing Process/Planning
Content Area: Adult Health: Cardiovascular
Priority Concepts: Perfusion; Safety

Answer: 4
Rationale: In sinus tachycardia, the heart rate is greater than 100 beats per minute. Sinus tachycardia is often caused by fever, physical and emotional stress, heart failure, hypovolemia, certain medications, nicotine, caffeine, and exercise. Fluid restriction and exercise will not alleviate tachycardia and could exacerbate the condition. Measuring the client's pulse during each shift will not decrease the heart rate. Additionally, the pulse should be taken more frequently than once each shift.
Priority Nursing Tip: If the client experiences sinus tachycardia, the health care provider is notified. The cause is identified, and the heart rate is decreased to normal by treating the underlying cause.
Test-Taking Strategy: Focus on the subject, sinus tachycardia. Recalling the causes of tachycardia will direct you to option 4. Remember that caffeine is a stimulant and will increase the heart rate. Review: care of the client with **tachycardia.**
Reference(s): Ignatavicius, Workman (2013), pp. 720-721.

551. Which action should the nurse implement to obtain a urine specimen for a urinalysis from a client with an indwelling urinary catheter?
1. Cleanse the perineum.
2. Detach the tubing of the drainage bag.
3. Use a sterile container for the specimen.
4. Aspirate the urine from the drainage bag port.

Level of Cognitive Ability: Applying
Client Needs: Safe and Effective Care Environment
Integrated Process: Nursing Process/Implementation
Content Area: Fundamental Skills: Diagnostic Tests
Priority Concepts: Elimination; Infection

Answer: 4
Rationale: A specimen for urinalysis does not need to be sterile; however, the indwelling urinary catheter system must remain sterile to reduce the risk of infection. Therefore, the nurse obtains the specimen using sterile technique and obtains a fresh specimen by aspirating urine from the drainage bag port after sanitizing the port and inserting a sterile needle. The nurse avoids breaking the integrity of the urinary collection system to prevent contamination. The nurse also avoids taking urine from the urinary drainage bag because the urine is less likely to reflect the current client status and because urine undergoes chemical changes and particulate matter settles over time. A sterile container is unnecessary for a urinalysis, and because the client has an indwelling catheter, perineal cleansing before obtaining a urine specimen is unnecessary.
Priority Nursing Tip: Specimens need to be labeled properly and placed in a biohazard bag for transport to the laboratory. Specific agency procedure is always followed.
Test-Taking Strategy: Focus on the subject of obtaining a urine specimen for urinalysis. Basic principles of asepsis direct you to eliminate options 2 and 3. Eliminate option 1 because the client has an indwelling catheter. Review: the procedure for obtaining a specimen for **urinalysis** from a client with an indwelling catheter.
Reference(s): Perry, Potter, Elkin (2012), pp. 167-168; Potter et al (2013), p. 1053.

552. An unlicensed assistive personnel (UAP) is caring for a client who has an indwelling urinary catheter. Which directions should the registered nurse provide to the UAP regarding urinary catheter care?
1. Loop the tubing under the client's leg
2. Place the tubing below the client's knee
3. Use soap and water to cleanse the perineal area
4. Keep the drainage bag above the level of the bladder

Level of Cognitive Ability: Applying
Client Needs: Safe and Effective Care Environment
Integrated Process: Teaching and Learning
Content Area: Leadership/Management: Delegating
Priority Concepts: Elimination; Leadership

Answer: 3
Rationale: Proper care of an indwelling urinary catheter is especially important to prevent infection. The perineal area is cleansed thoroughly using mild soap and water at least three times a day and after a bowel movement. The drainage tubing is not placed or looped under the client's leg because this would inhibit the flow of urine. The drainage bag is kept below the level of the bladder to prevent urine from being trapped in the bladder. The tubing must drain freely at all times.
Priority Nursing Tip: If permitted, the client with a urinary catheter should consume a daily fluid intake of 2000 to 2500 mL.
Test-Taking Strategy: Eliminate options 1 and 2 first because they are comparable or alike. From the remaining options, noting the word *above* in option 4 will assist in eliminating this option. Also, note that option 3 relates to preventing infection. Review: care of the client with an **indwelling urinary catheter**.
Reference(s): Potter et al (2013), pp. 1062, 1080.

553. The nurse is assigned to care for a client with preeclampsia. The nurse should plan to initiate which action to provide a safe environment?
1. Maintain fluid and sodium restrictions.
2. Take the client's vital signs every 4 hours.
3. Turn off the room lights and draw the window shades.
4. Encourage visits from family and friends for psychosocial support.

Level of Cognitive Ability: Applying
Client Needs: Safe and Effective Care Environment
Integrated Process: Nursing Process/Planning
Content Area: Maternity: Antepartum
Priority Concepts: Reproduction; Safety

Answer: 3
Rationale: Clients with preeclampsia are at risk of developing eclampsia (seizures). Bright lights and sudden loud noises may initiate seizures in this client. A woman with preeclampsia should be placed in a dimly lighted, quiet, private room. Clients with preeclampsia have decreased plasma volume, and adequate fluid and sodium intake are necessary to maintain fluid volume and tissue perfusion. Vital signs need to be monitored more frequently than every 4 hours when preeclampsia is present. Visitors should be limited to allow for rest and prevent overstimulation.
Priority Nursing Tip: The signs of preeclampsia are hypertension and proteinuria. Swelling (edema), particularly in the face and hands, often accompanies preeclampsia but is not considered a reliable sign of preeclampsia, however, because it also occurs in many normal pregnancies.
Test-Taking Strategy: Focus on the subject, preeclampsia. Eliminate option 4 because it is not a physiological need and provides too much stimulation for this client. Eliminate option 2 next because vital signs need to be monitored more frequently than every 4 hours. From the remaining options, knowing that seizures may be precipitated by sudden loud noises and bright lights will assist in directing you to the correct option. Review: care of the client with **preeclampsia**.
Reference(s): McKinney et al (2013), p. 594.

554. The client is scheduled for a bronchoscopy. Which **priority** measure should the nurse plan to implement?
1. Obtain informed consent
2. Ask the client about allergies to shellfish
3. Restrict the diet to clear liquids on the day of the test
4. Administer preprocedure antibiotics prophylactically

Level of Cognitive Ability: Applying
Client Needs: Safe and Effective Care Environment
Integrated Process: Nursing Process/Planning
Content Area: Fundamental Skills: Diagnostic Tests
Priority Concepts: Ethics; Health Care Law

Answer: 1
Rationale: Bronchoscopy is a procedure in which the health care provider uses a fiber-optic bronchoscope for direct visualization of the larynx, trachea, and bronchi. Because the procedure is invasive, it requires obtaining informed consent from the client. It is unnecessary to inquire about allergies to shellfish before this procedure because contrast dye is not injected. The client is kept NPO for at least 6 hours before the procedure. There is also no need for prophylactic antibiotics.
Priority Nursing Tip: Any procedure that is invasive requires an informed consent from the client.
Test-Taking Strategy: Note the strategic word, *priority*. Focus on the subject, bronchoscopy. Recalling that bronchoscopy is an invasive procedure and requires an informed consent will direct you to the correct option. Review: preprocedure preparation for **bronchoscopy**.
Reference(s): Pagana, Pagana (2013), p. 194.

❖ **555.** The nurse hangs a 1000-mL intravenous (IV) solution of D_5W (5% dextrose in water) at 9 AM and sets the infusion controller device to administer 100 gtt/min via microdrip infusion set (60 gtt = 1 mL). On assessment of the IV infusion, the nurse expects that the remaining amount of solution in the IV bag at 2 PM will be represented at which level? **Fill in the blank.**

Answer: ___ mL

Level of Cognitive Ability: Analyzing
Client Needs: Safe and Effective Care Environment
Integrated Process: Nursing Process/Assessment
Content Area: Fundamental Skills: Medication/IV Calculations
Priority Concepts: Clinical Judgment; Safety

Answer: **500 mL**
Rationale: The nurse hangs an IV solution at 9 AM and sets the IV solution to infuse at 100 gtt/min per microdrip. With a microdrip, gtt/min = mL/hr infused. Therefore, 100 mL/hr is being infused. A total of 500 mL will be infused in the 5 elapsed hours. At 2 PM the nurse would expect 500 mL of solution to be safely infused and 500 mL to be remaining.
Priority Nursing Tip: Monitor IV flow rates frequently (per agency policy) even if the IV solution is being administered via an electronic infusion device.
Test-Taking Strategy: Focus on the subject, infusion of an IV using a microdrip infusion setup. Use the formula gtt/min = mL/hr because a microdrip is being used. In a 5-hour period, 500 mL of fluid will infuse for a solution infusing at 100 gtt/min. Review: **intravenous flow rates.**
Reference(s): Potter et al (2013), pp. 925-926.

556. The nurse is planning care for a client with acute glomerulonephritis. Which action should the nurse instruct the unlicensed assistive personnel (UAP) to take in the care of the client?
1. Ambulate the client frequently.
2. Encourage a diet that is high in protein.
3. Monitor the temperature every 2 hours.
4. Remove the water pitcher from the bedside.

Level of Cognitive Ability: Applying
Client Needs: Safe and Effective Care Environment
Integrated Process: Teaching and Learning
Content Area: Leadership/Management: Delegating
Priority Concepts: Fluid and Electrolyte Balance; Leadership

Answer: **4**
Rationale: A client with acute glomerulonephritis commonly experiences fluid volume excess and fatigue. Interventions include fluid restriction, as well as monitoring weight and intake and output. The client may be placed on bed rest or at least encouraged to rest because a direct correlation exists among proteinuria, hematuria, edema, and increased activity levels. The diet is high in calories but low in protein. It is unnecessary to monitor the temperature as frequently as every 2 hours.
Priority Nursing Tip: A cause of glomerulonephritis is infection of the pharynx with group A beta-hemolytic streptococcus.
Test-Taking Strategy: Focus on the subject, acute glomerulonephritis. Knowing that the client needs rest eliminates option 1. The question provides no information about the client's actual temperature, so option 3 is eliminated next. From the remaining options, it is necessary to know either that fluid is restricted or protein is limited. Review: interventions related to **acute glomerulonephritis.**
Reference(s): Lewis et al (2014), p. 1074.

557. The nurse is caring for a client with a C-6 spinal cord injury during the spinal shock phase. What should the nurse implement when preparing the client to sit in a chair?
1. Apply knee splints to stabilize the joints during transfer
2. Teach the client to lock the knees during the pivoting stage of the transfer
3. Administer a vasodilator in order to improve circulation of the lower limbs
4. Raise the head of the bed slowly to decrease orthostatic hypotensive episodes

Level of Cognitive Ability: Applying
Client Needs: Safe and Effective Care Environment
Integrated Process: Nursing Process/Implementation
Content Area: Adult Health: Neurological
Priority Concepts: Mobility; Safety

Answer: **4**
Rationale: Spinal shock is a sudden depression of reflex activity in the spinal cord that occurs below the level of injury (areflexia). It is often accompanied by vasodilation in the lower limbs, which results in a fall in blood pressure upon rising. The client can have dizziness and feel faint. The nurse should provide for a gradual progression in head elevation while monitoring the blood pressure. The use of splints would impair the transfer. Clients with cervical cord injuries cannot lock their knees. A vasodilator would exacerbate the problem.
Priority Nursing Tip: Spinal shock is also called spinal shock syndrome. It occurs immediately as the cord's response to the injury. The client develops complete but temporary loss of motor, sensory, reflex, and autonomic function. This often lasts less than 48 hours but may continue for several weeks.
Test-Taking Strategy: Focusing on the subject, spinal cord injury during spinal shock phase will assist in eliminating options 1 and 2. From the remaining options, recalling that spinal shock is accompanied by vasodilation will direct you to option 4. Review: care of the client with **spinal shock.**
Reference(s): Ignatavicius, Workman (2013), pp. 698, 969; Lewis et al (2014), p. 1479.

558. The nurse notes that a client's lithium level is 3.9 mEq/L. Which **priority** intervention should the nurse implement?
1. Determining visual acuity
2. Assisting with ambulation
3. Monitoring intake and output
4. Instituting seizure precautions

Level of Cognitive Ability: Applying
Client Needs: Safe and Effective Care Environment
Integrated Process: Nursing Process/Implementation
Content Area: Pharmacology: Psychiatric Medications
Priority Concepts: Clinical Judgment; Safety

Answer: 4
Rationale: The lithium level must be monitored closely in a client taking lithium (Lithobid). A therapeutic regimen is designed to attain a serum lithium level of 1.0 to 1.5 mEq/L during acute mania, and levels of 0.6 to 1.4 mEq/L for maintenance treatment. A level of 3.9 mEq/L is in the toxic range, and seizures may occur at levels of 3.5 mEq/L and higher. Options 1, 2, and 3 are appropriate interventions but are not the priority.
Priority Nursing Tip: The nurse should instruct the client taking lithium (Lithobid) to maintain a fluid intake of six to eight glasses of water a day and an adequate salt intake to prevent lithium toxicity.
Test-Taking Strategy: Note the strategic word, *priority*. Focus on the medication name and recall that it can cause toxicity. Next, recall the manifestations that occur in a toxic lithium level. This will direct you to option 4. Review: toxicity related to **lithium**.
Reference(s): Kee, Hayes, McCuistion (2012), p. 404; Lehne (2013), pp. 388-389.

559. A hospitalized child develops exanthema (rash) that covers the trunk and extremities. The nurse reviews the child's health history and notes that the child was exposed to varicella 2 weeks ago. Which nursing intervention is **most appropriate** to implement?
1. Immediately admit the client to any available bed.
2. Place the child in a private room on strict isolation.
3. Assess the progression of the exanthema and report it to the health care provider.
4. Allow the child to play in the playroom until the health care provider can be contacted.

Level of Cognitive Ability: Applying
Client Needs: Safe and Effective Care Environment
Integrated Process: Nursing Process/Implementation
Content Area: Fundamental Skills: Infection Control
Priority Concepts: Infection; Safety

Answer: 2
Rationale: The child with undiagnosed exanthema needs to be placed on strict isolation. Varicella causes a profuse rash on the trunk with a sparse rash on the extremities. The incubation period is 14 to 21 days. It is important to prevent the spread of this communicable disease by placing the child in isolation until further diagnosis and treatment are made. Options 1 and 4 are inaccurate, and option 3 is not the most appropriate intervention.
Priority Nursing Tip: Varicella-zoster virus can be transmitted via direct contact, droplet (airborne) spread, or contaminated objects.
Test-Taking Strategy: Noting the strategic words *most appropriate* and the subject, exposure to varicella will direct you to option 2. This action will prevent exposure of this communicable disease to others. Review: care of the child with **varicella**.
Reference(s): Hockenberry, Wilson (2013), p. 424; Potter et al (2013), p. 414.

560. The experienced nurse watches a novice nurse performing hemodialysis on a client. The novice nurse is drinking coffee and eating a doughnut next to the hemodialysis machine while talking with the client about the client's week. Which action should the experienced nurse take?

1. Get a cup of coffee and join in on the conversation.
2. Determine whether or not the client would like a cup of coffee.
3. Admire the therapeutic relationship the novice nurse has with the client.
4. Ask the novice nurse to refrain from eating and drinking in the client area.

Level of Cognitive Ability: Applying
Client Needs: Safe and Effective Care Environment
Integrated Process: Nursing Process/Implementation
Content Area: Fundamental Skills: Infection Control
Priority Concepts: Infection; Safety

Answer: 4
Rationale: A potential complication of hemodialysis is the acquisition of dialysis-associated hepatitis B. This is a concern for clients (who may carry the virus), client families (at risk from contact with the client and with environmental surfaces), and staff (who may acquire the virus from contact with the client's blood). This risk is minimized by the use of standard precautions; appropriate hand-washing and sterilization procedures; and the prohibition of eating, drinking, or other hand-to-mouth activity in the hemodialysis unit. The first nurse should ask the second nurse to stop eating and drinking in the client area.
Priority Nursing Tip: The nurse should measure the client's weight before and after the hemodialysis procedure to determine the amount of fluid removed during the procedure.
Test-Taking Strategy: Focus on the subject, hemodialysis. Recall the complications associated with hemodialysis and principles related to standard precautions to direct you to the correct option. Review: infection control measures related to the client receiving **hemodialysis**.
Reference(s): Lewis et al (2014), pp. 1122-1123.

❖ **561.** A nursing student is learning the functions of the nurse manager in a nursing class. Which functions are responsibilities of the nurse manager? **Select all that apply.**

❑ 1. Recruit new employees.
❑ 2. Conduct regular staff meetings.
❑ 3. Assist staff in meeting annual goals.
❑ 4. Monitor professional standards of practice on the nursing unit.
❑ 5. Expect nursing staff to problem-solve all client or family complaints.
❑ 6. Write prescriptions for health care providers (HCP) when conducting rounds with the HCP.

Level of Cognitive Ability: Applying
Client Needs: Safe and Effective Care Environment
Integrated Process: Nursing Process/Implementation
Content Area: Leadership/Management: Ethical/Legal
Priority Concepts: Leadership; Professionalism

Answer: 1, 2, 3, 4
Rationale: Responsibilities of the nurse manager (middle manager) include recruiting new employees (interviewing and hiring), conducting regular staff meetings, assisting staff in meeting annual goals for the unit and systems needed to accomplish goals, monitoring professional standards of practice on the nursing unit, developing an ongoing staff development plan, conducting routine staff evaluations, acting as a role model, submitting staff schedules for the unit, conducting regular client rounds and problem-solving client and family complaints, establishing and implementing a unit quality improvement plan, and conducting rounds with health care providers. The nurse is not responsible for writing prescriptions for HCPs when conducting rounds; the HCP is responsible for writing prescriptions.
Priority Nursing Tip: An effective leader and manager is visible to employees, is flexible, and provides guidance, assistance, and feedback to employees.
Test-Taking Strategy: Focus on the subject, the responsibilities of the nurse manager. Recalling that a nurse manager functions in the role of a leader and facilitator and recalling the legal issues relating to health care providers' prescriptions will assist in answering the question. Also, option 5 can be eliminated because of the closed-ended word "all." Review: the responsibilities of the **nurse manager**.
Reference(s): Potter et al (2013), p. 277.

562. Which are characteristics of team nursing? **Select all that apply.**

❑ 1. A registered nurse leads a team of staff members.

❑ 2. Each nurse assumes responsibility for a specific task.

❑ 3. Team members provide direct care to groups of clients.

❑ 4. Unlicensed assistive personnel are given a client assignment.

❑ 5. The registered nurse assumes responsibility for a caseload of clients over time.

❑ 6. Team nursing maintains continuity of care across nursing shifts, days, and home care visits.

Level of Cognitive Ability: Applying
Client Needs: Safe and Effective Care Environment
Integrated Process: Nursing Process/Implementation
Content Area: Leadership/Management: Delegating
Priority Concepts: Caregiving; Leadership

Answer: 1, 3, 4
Rationale: In team nursing, a registered nurse (RN) leads a team that is composed of other RNs, licensed practical or licensed vocational nurses, and unlicensed assistive personnel and technicians. The team members provide direct client care to groups of clients under the direct supervision of the RN team leader. In this model, unlicensed assistive personnel are given client assignments rather than being assigned particular nursing tasks. In functional nursing, tasks are divided, with one nurse assuming responsibility for specific tasks. Primary nursing is a model in which the RN assumes responsibility for a caseload of clients over time. In primary nursing, continuity of care across nursing shifts, days, and home care visits is maintained.
Priority Nursing Tip: In team nursing, the team leader determines the work assignment. Each staff member works fully within the realm of his or her educational and clinical expertise and job description.
Test-Taking Strategy: Focus on the subject, the characteristics of team nursing. Thinking about the definition of and the concepts related to the word *team* will assist in answering the question. Review: the characteristics of **team nursing**.
Reference(s): Huber (2014), pp. 265-266.

563. The nurse is planning a discharge teaching plan for a client with a spinal cord injury. To provide for a safe environment regarding home care, which option should be the **priority** in the discharge teaching plan?

1. Assisting the client to deal with long-term care placement

2. Including the client's significant others in the teaching session

3. Follow-up laboratory and diagnostic tests that need to be done

4. What the health care provider has indicated needs to be taught

Level of Cognitive Ability: Analyzing
Client Needs: Safe and Effective Care Environment
Integrated Process: Nursing Process/Planning
Content Area: Adult Health: Neurological
Priority Concepts: Client Education; Safety

Answer: 2
Rationale: Involving the client's significant others in discharge teaching is a priority in planning for the client with a spinal cord injury. The client will need the support of the significant others. Knowledge and understanding of what to expect will help both the client and significant others deal with the client's limitations. Long-term placement is not the only option for a client with a spinal cord injury. Laboratory and diagnostic testing are not priority discharge instructions for this client. A health care provider's prescription is not necessary for discharge planning and teaching; this is an independent nursing action.
Priority Nursing Tip: Involving the client's significant others in discharge teaching will assist in ensuring support for the client. However, the client should be consulted about the inclusion of others in the teaching process before initiating the plan.
Test-Taking Strategy: Note the strategic word, *priority*. Focus on the subject, a safe home care environment for a client with a spinal cord injury. Eliminate option 4 because although the health care provider's prescriptions need to be addressed, teaching is an independent nursing action. Eliminate option 1 because long-term placement is not the only choice for a client with a spinal cord injury. There is no indication that laboratory or diagnostic tests have been imminently prescribed. Remember that home care and support will be needed. Review: care of the client with a **spinal cord injury**.
Reference(s): Ignatavicius, Workman (2013), p. 970.

564. The nurse observes a client wringing her hands and looking frightened. The client reports to the nurse that she "feels out of control." Which approach by the nurse is **most appropriate** to maintain a safe environment?

1. Administer a PRN antianxiety medication immediately.
2. Provide isolation for the client in the unit's "time-out" room.
3. Observe the client in an ongoing manner but do not intervene.
4. Encourage the client to talk about her feelings in a quiet setting.

Level of Cognitive Ability: Applying
Client Needs: Safe and Effective Care Environment
Integrated Process: Nursing Process/Implementation
Content Area: Mental Health
Priority Concepts: Anxiety; Communication

Answer: 4
Rationale: The anxiety symptoms demonstrated by this client require some form of intervention. Moving the client to a quiet setting decreases environmental stimuli. Talking provides the nurse an opportunity to assess the cause of the client's feelings and identify appropriate interventions. Medication is used only when other noninvasive approaches have been unsuccessful. Isolation is appropriate if a client is a danger to self or others.
Priority Nursing Tip: The nurse should not leave a client who feels "out of control." The nurse should be sure the client is in a quiet area, encourage the client to talk about his or her feelings, and determine what the client considers to be his or her needs.
Test-Taking Strategy: Use therapeutic communication techniques. Focus on the strategic words, *most appropriate.* Option 4 is the only choice that addresses the client's feelings. Remember that a client's feelings are most important. Review: **therapeutic communication techniques.**
Reference(s): Stuart (2013), p. 230; Varcarolis (2013), pp. 120-122.

565. A client with urolithiasis is scheduled for extracorporeal shock wave lithotripsy. Which information should the nurse provide to ensure that the client understands the procedure?

1. There is no discomfort at all involved with this procedure.
2. There are no side effects or complications associated with this procedure.
3. The stone granules are passed in the urine within a few days after the procedure.
4. The procedure involves breaking up the stone by a vibrating needle that is inserted into the urinary tract.

Level of Cognitive Ability: Applying
Client Needs: Safe and Effective Care Environment
Integrated Process: Nursing Process/Implementation
Content Area: Fundamental Skills: Diagnostic Tests
Priority Concepts: Client Education; Elimination

Answer: 3
Rationale: In extracorporeal shock wave lithotripsy, a noninvasive procedure, shock waves are administered that shatter the stone without damaging the surrounding tissues. The stone is broken into fine sand, which is secreted into the client's urine within a few days after the procedure. The client may feel some discomfort from the shock waves. Hematuria is common after the procedure. The presence of clots in the urine needs to be reported to the health care provider. Clots could indicate a complication such as a hematoma.
Priority Nursing Tip: After extracorporeal shock wave lithotripsy, the client is instructed to increase fluid intake to flush out stone fragments.
Test-Taking Strategy: Eliminate options 1 and 2 first because of the closed-ended word "no" in these options. From the remaining options, recalling that the procedure is noninvasive and is done via shock waves (not a vibrating needle) will direct you to option 3. Review: the procedure for extracorporeal **shock wave lithotripsy.**
Reference(s): Ignatavicius, Workman (2013), pp. 1509-1510.

566. Which clients require contact precautions? Refer to the chart. Select all that apply.

CLIENTS

- ❑ 1. A child with mumps
- ❑ 2. A client with scabies
- ❑ 3. A child with streptococcal pharyngitis
- ❑ 4. A client with pulmonary tuberculosis
- ❑ 5. A child with respiratory syncytial virus (RSV)
- ❑ 6. A client infected with a multidrug-resistant organism

Level of Cognitive Ability: Analyzing
Client Needs: Safe and Effective Care Environment
Integrated Process: Nursing Process/Implementation
Content Area: Fundamental Skills: Infection Control
Priority Concepts: Infection; Safety

Answer: 2, 5, 6
Rationale: Contact precautions are initiated when disease transmission occurs from direct contact with the client or his or her environment. Diseases that require the use of contact precautions include colonization or infection with multidrug-resistant organisms, respiratory syncytial virus, shigella and other enteric pathogens, wound infections, herpes simplex, scabies, and disseminated varicella zoster. Clients with mumps or streptococcal pharyngitis require droplet precautions. A client with pulmonary tuberculosis requires airborne precautions.
Priority Nursing Tip: Contact precautions require placing the client in a private room or with a cohort client.
Test-Taking Strategy: Focus on the subject, clients who require contact precautions. Read each client diagnosis. Determining the mode of transmission for each illness will assist in answering this question correctly. Review: the modes of transmission for **communicable diseases** and the diseases that require **contact precautions**.
Reference(s): Potter et al (2013), pp. 414-415.

567. The nurse is planning the discharge instructions from the emergency department for an adult client who is a victim of family violence. The nurse should understand that it is **most important** that which information is included in the discharge plans?

1. Instructions to call the police the next time the abuse occurs
2. Exploration of the pros and cons of remaining with the abusive family member
3. Specific information regarding "safe havens" or shelters in the client's neighborhood
4. Specific information about available opportunities to enroll in local self-defense classes

Level of Cognitive Ability: Applying
Client Needs: Safe and Effective Care Environment
Integrated Process: Nursing Process/Planning
Content Area: Mental Health
Priority Concepts: Interpersonal Violence; Safety

Answer: 3
Rationale: For the victim of family violence, any of the options might be included in the discharge plan at some point if long-term therapy or a long-term relationship with the nurse is established. The question refers to an emergency department setting. It is most important to assist victims of abuse with identifying a plan for how to remove self from harmful situations should they arise again. An abused person is usually reluctant to call the police. It is not the best time for the nurse to explore the pros and cons of remaining with the abusive family member; additionally, this action does not ensure safety for the victim. Teaching the victim to fight back (as in the use of self-defense) is not the best action when dealing with a violent person.
Priority Nursing Tip: In a victim of violence, self-esteem becomes diminished with chronic abuse. The victim may blame herself or himself for the violence and be unable to see a way out of the situation.
Test-Taking Strategy: Note the strategic words, *most important*. Use Maslow's Hierarchy of Needs theory. Remember that if a physiological need is not present, then safety is the priority. This will direct you to option 3. Review: care of the victim of **abuse**.
Reference(s): Varcarolis (2013), pp. 425-426.

568. During a code, a health care provider is about to defibrillate a client in ventricular fibrillation and says in a loud voice, "CLEAR!" Which action should the nurse **immediately** take?
1. Shut off the mechanical ventilator.
2. Shut off the intravenous infusion going into the client's arm.
3. Place the conductive gel pads for defibrillation on the client's chest.
4. Step away from the bed and make sure that all others have done the same.

Level of Cognitive Ability: Applying
Client Needs: Safe and Effective Care Environment
Integrated Process: Nursing Process/Implementation
Content Area: Critical Care: Emergency Situations
Priority Concepts: Perfusion; Safety

Answer: 4
Rationale: For the safety of all personnel, when the defibrillator paddles are being discharged, all personnel must stand back and be clear of all contact with the client or the client's bed. It is the primary responsibility of the person defibrillating to communicate the "clear" message loudly enough for all to hear and ensure their compliance. All personnel must immediately comply with this command. Stepping back from the bed prevents the nurse or others from being defibrillated along with the client. A ventilator is not in use during a code; rather an Ambu (resuscitation) bag is used. Shutting off the intravenous infusion has no useful purpose. The gel pads should have been placed on the client's chest before the defibrillator paddles were applied.
Priority Nursing Tip: To perform defibrillation, one paddle is placed at the third intercostal space to the right of the sternum; the other is placed at the fifth intercostal space on the left midaxillary line.
Test-Taking Strategy: Focus on the subject, the procedure for defibrillation. Note the strategic word, *immediately*. Recalling the risks associated with this procedure and noting the word *clear* in the question will direct you to the correct option. Review: the risks associated with **defibrillation**.
Reference(s): Ignatavicius, Workman (2013), p. 737.

569. A client with chronic kidney disease has an indwelling peritoneal catheter in the abdomen for peritoneal dialysis. While bathing, the client spills water on the abdominal dressing covering the abdomen. Which action should the nurse perform **immediately**?
1. Change the dressing.
2. Reinforce the dressing.
3. Flush the peritoneal dialysis catheter.
4. Scrub the catheter with povidone-iodine.

Level of Cognitive Ability: Applying
Client Needs: Safe and Effective Care Environment
Integrated Process: Nursing Process/Implementation
Content Area: Adult Health: Renal and Urinary
Priority Concepts: Clinical Judgment; Infection

Answer: 1
Rationale: Clients with peritoneal dialysis catheters are at high risk for infection. A dressing that is wet is a conduit for bacteria to reach the catheter insertion site. The nurse ensures that the dressing is kept dry at all times. Reinforcing the dressing is not a safe practice to prevent infection in this circumstance. Flushing the catheter is not indicated. Scrubbing the catheter with povidone-iodine is done at the time of connection or disconnection of peritoneal dialysis.
Priority Nursing Tip: If the outflow of the peritoneal dialysis solution is cloudy or opaque, the nurse should suspect peritonitis.
Test-Taking Strategy: Note the strategic word, *immediately*. Focus on the subject, a wet dressing to a peritoneal catheter. The correct option would focus on the dressing, not the catheter. Therefore, eliminate options 3 and 4. Knowing that it is better to change a wet dressing than reinforce it will direct you to option 1. Review: care of the client with a **peritoneal dialysis catheter**.
Reference(s): Ignatavicius, Workman (2013), p. 1567.

❖ **570.** The nurse manager is providing an educational session to the nursing staff in a skilled nursing facility on the guidelines for the safe use of physical restraints. Which are safe guidelines? **Select all that apply.**
- ❑ 1. A health care provider's prescription is required.
- ❑ 2. Restraints should be secured with a quick-release tie.
- ❑ 3. Restraints are secured to side rails so that they can be easily removed as necessary.
- ❑ 4. Restraints are used when other measures have failed to prevent self-injury or injury to others.
- ❑ 5. Restraints can be used as a usual part of treatment plans, as indicated by the client's condition or symptoms.
- ❑ 6. The use of restraints can be prescribed PRN (as needed) as long as the nurse performs a thorough assessment before applying them.

Level of Cognitive Ability: Applying
Client Needs: Safe and Effective Care Environment
Integrated Process: Teaching and Learning
Content Area: Leadership/Management: Ethical/Legal
Priority Concepts: Health Care Law; Safety

Answer: 1, 2, 4
Rationale: A physical restraint is a mechanical or physical device that is used to immobilize a client or extremity. It restricts the freedom of movement or normal access to a client's body. A health care provider's prescription is required for the use of restraints. Restraints should be secured with a quick-release tie so that they can be easily removed in an emergency. Restraints are considered for use only when other measures have failed to prevent self-injury or injury to others. Restraints are secured to the bed frame, not the side rails, because the client may be injured if the side rail is lowered. Restraints are not a usual part of treatment plans, indicated by the person's condition or symptoms, and are not prescribed on a PRN basis.
Priority Nursing Tip: The reason for using a restraint should be given to the client and the family, and their permission should be sought.
Test-Taking Strategy: Focus on the subject, guidelines for the safe use of physical restraints. Read each option and carefully think about two issues: client safety and the legalities related to the use of restraints. This will assist in answering the question. Review: the guidelines for the safe use of **restraints**.
Reference(s): Potter et al (2013), pp. 300, 388-389, 392.

571. The nurse is planning activities for a depressed client who was just admitted to the hospital. Which activity should be part of the nurse's plan?
1. Provide an activity that is quiet and solitary in nature.
2. Plan nothing until the client asks to participate in the milieu.
3. Offer the client a menu of activities and insist that the client participate in all of them.
4. Provide a structured daily program of activities and encourage the client to participate.

Level of Cognitive Ability: Applying
Client Needs: Safe and Effective Care Environment
Integrated Process: Nursing Process/Planning
Content Area: Mental Health
Priority Concepts: Functional Ability; Mood and Affect

Answer: 4
Rationale: A depressed person is often withdrawn. In addition, the person experiences difficulty concentrating, loss of interest or pleasure, low energy and fatigue, and feelings of worthlessness and poor self-esteem. The plan of care needs to provide stimulation in a structured environment. Options 1 and 2 are restrictive and offer little or no structure and stimulation. The nurse should not insist that a client participate in all activities.
Priority Nursing Tip: For the client with depression, the nurse should provide gentle encouragement to participate in activities of daily living and unit therapies.
Test-Taking Strategy: Focus on the subject, a depressed client. Eliminate option 3 first because of the word *insist* and the closed-ended word, "all." From the remaining options, noting the word *structured* in option 4 will direct you to this option. Review: care of the client with **depression**.
Reference(s): Stuart (2013), pp. 314-315; Varcarolis (2013), pp. 261-274.

572. A client who is 85 years old had an open reduction with internal fixation (ORIF) for a hip fracture 4 days ago. What should the nurse implement to provide safe care?
1. Provide ice chips instead of drinking water.
2. Instruct the client to call for help before getting up.
3. Minimize opioid administration to prevent dizziness.
4. Tell the client to roll to the affected side first before getting up.

Level of Cognitive Ability: Applying
Client Needs: Safe and Effective Care Environment
Integrated Process: Nursing Process/Implementation
Content Area: Fundamental Skills: Safety
Priority Concepts: Mobility; Safety

Answer: 2
Rationale: The nurse instructs the client to call for help before getting up because the client has multiple risk factors for falls, is of older age, has postoperative status, and may also be receiving opioid analgesia. Restricting fluid intake with ice chips is not indicated; besides, adequate hydration is important for maintaining cardiac output and renal function, for keeping respiratory secretions thin, and in preventing constipation. The nurse administers opioid analgesics as indicated and fulfills the nurse's duty owed to the client by acting to resolve pain. The nurse instructs the client to roll to the unaffected side to get up to prevent excessive stress on the fragile surgical wound.
Priority Nursing Tip: The nurse should assign a client at risk for falling to a room near the nurses' station.
Test-Taking Strategy: Focusing on the subject, preventing injury, will direct you to option 2. Restricting fluid, inadequate pain control, and inaccurate mobility instructions prevent the nurse from fulfilling the duty owed to the client to prevent safe and effective care. Review: **measures to prevent injury.**
Reference(s): Ignatavicius, Workman (2013), p. 1161.

573. The nurse is assisting in the care of a client who is to be cardioverted. The nurse should plan to set the monophasic defibrillator to which starting energy range levels, depending on the specific health care provider prescription?
1. 50 to 100 joules
2. 200 to 250 joules
3. 250 to 300 joules
4. 350 to 400 joules

Level of Cognitive Ability: Applying
Client Needs: Safe and Effective Care Environment
Integrated Process: Nursing Process/Planning
Content Area: Critical Care: Basic Life Support/ Cardiopulmonary Resuscitation
Priority Concepts: Perfusion; Safety

Answer: 1
Rationale: Cardioversion is synchronized countershock to convert an undesirable rhythm to a stable rhythm. When a client is cardioverted, the defibrillator is charged to the energy level prescribed by the health care provider. Cardioversion is usually started at 50 to 100 joules. Options 2, 3, and 4 are incorrect and identify energy levels that are too high for cardioversion.
Priority Nursing Tip: When cardioversion is performed, the defibrillator is synchronized to the client's R wave to avoid discharging the shock during the vulnerable period (T wave).
Test-Taking Strategy: Focus on the subject, cardioversion. Remember that in instances in which cardioversion is used, an underlying cardiac rhythm needs to be converted to a better rhythm; therefore, lower voltages are used. Review: the procedure for **cardioversion.**
Reference(s): Lewis et al (2014), p. 802.

574. The nurse has a prescription to get the client out of bed to a chair on the first postoperative day after total knee replacement. Which action should the nurse plan to do to protect the knee joint?
1. Apply a compression dressing and put ice on the knee while sitting.
2. Obtain a walker to minimize weight-bearing by the client on the affected leg.
3. Lift the client to the bedside chair, leaving the continuous passive motion (CPM) machine in place.
4. Apply a knee immobilizer before getting the client up and elevate the client's surgical leg while sitting.

Level of Cognitive Ability: Applying
Client Needs: Safe and Effective Care Environment
Integrated Process: Nursing Process/Planning
Content Area: Adult Health: Musculoskeletal
Priority Concepts: Mobility; Safety

Answer: 4
Rationale: After a total knee replacement, as prescribed, the nurse assists the client to get out of bed on the first postoperative day after putting a knee immobilizer on the affected joint to provide stability. The leg is elevated while the client is sitting in the chair to minimize edema. A compression dressing should already be in place on the wound. Ice is not used unless prescribed. The surgeon prescribes the weight-bearing limits on the affected leg. A CPM machine is used only while the client is in bed and is initiated when prescribed.
Priority Nursing Tip: The nurse instructs the client who has had a total knee replacement to avoid leg dangling.
Test-Taking Strategy: Focus on the subject, transfer of a client with a new total knee replacement. Note the relation between the subject, the words *protect the knee joint* in the question, and *knee immobilizer* in option 4. Review: postoperative care after **total knee replacement.**
Reference(s): Ignatavicius, Workman (2013), p. 330.

575. A client is admitted to the psychiatric unit after a suicide attempt by hanging. The nurse should plan which intervention as the **most important** aspect of care to maintain client safety?

1. Assign a staff member who will remain with the client at all times.
2. Request that the client's peers arrange to remain with the client continuously.
3. Remove the client's personal clothing and replace them with a hospital gown.
4. Place the client in a seclusion room where all dangerous articles are removed.

Level of Cognitive Ability: Applying
Client Needs: Safe and Effective Care Environment
Integrated Process: Nursing Process/Planning
Content Area: Mental Health
Priority Concepts: Mood and Affect; Safety

Answer: 1
Rationale: Hanging is a serious suicide attempt. The plan of care must reflect the action that will promote the client's safety. Constant observation by a staff member is necessary. It is not a peer's responsibility to safeguard a client. Removing one's clothing does not maximize all possible safety strategies. Placing the client in seclusion further isolates the client.
Priority Nursing Tip: The nurse who is caring for a client with a diagnosis of depression should always consider the client's risk for attempting suicide.
Test-Taking Strategy: Focus on the subject, attempted suicide. Note the strategic words, *most important*. Recalling that one-to-one supervision is necessary will direct you to the correct option. Review: suicide precautions.
Reference(s): Stuart (2013), p. 337; Varcarolis (2013), p. 108.

576. The nurse receives a telephone call from a client who states that he wants to kill himself and has a loaded gun on the table. Which is the **best** nursing intervention to employ at this time?

1. Keep the client talking while encouraging him to ventilate his feelings.
2. Tell the client that killing himself is not the way to deal with his problem.
3. Use therapeutic communication techniques, especially the reflection of feelings.
4. Keep the client talking while another staff member contacts the police so that appropriate help can be sent.

Level of Cognitive Ability: Applying
Client Needs: Safe and Effective Care Environment
Integrated Process: Nursing Process/Implementation
Content Area: Critical Care: Emergency Situations
Priority Concepts: Clinical Judgment; Safety

Answer: 4
Rationale: In a crisis, the nurse must take an authoritative, active role to promote the client's safety. A loaded gun in the home of the client who says that he wants to kill himself is a crisis. The client's safety is of prime concern. Keeping the client on the phone and getting help to the client is the best intervention. Option 1 lacks the authoritative action stance of securing the client's safety. Option 2 is not a helpful strategy and may block communication. Using therapeutic communication techniques is important, but overuse of reflection may sound uncaring or superficial and is lacking direction and a solution to the immediate problem of the client's safety.
Priority Nursing Tip: Assessment of the client at risk for suicide includes determining if the client has a plan, determining the lethality of the plan, and if the client has a means of carrying out the plan.
Test-Taking Strategy: Focus on the subject, the potential for suicide. Note the strategic word, *best*. Utilizing Maslow's Hierarchy of Needs theory, recognize that there is no physiological need and therefore safety becomes the priority. The only choice that will provide direct help is option 4. Review: crisis intervention for a client contemplating suicide.
Reference(s): Varcarolis (2013), p. 442.

577. The nurse must place a wrist restraint on a client. The client tells the nurse that he does not want to wear the restraint. Which is the **best** nursing action to implement at this time?
1. Sedate the client first.
2. Apply the wrist restraint.
3. Contact the client's family.
4. Reconsider alternative measures.

Level of Cognitive Ability: Applying
Client Needs: Safe and Effective Care Environment
Integrated Process: Nursing Process/Implementation
Content Area: Leadership/Management: Ethical/Legal
Priority Concepts: Health Care Law; Safety

Answer: 4
Rationale: Before applying restraints, the nurse must exhaust alternative measures to restraints such as a bed alarm, distraction, and a sitter. If the nurse determines that a restraint is necessary, its use is discussed with the client and family and a prescription is obtained from the health care provider. The nurse should explain carefully to the client and family the indications for the restraint, the type of restraint selected, and the anticipated duration for its use. Sedation can be considered as a chemical restraint. The nurse avoids applying the restraint on a client who refused it to prevent client coercion and future charges of battery.
Priority Nursing Tip: If a restraint is used on a client, it must not interfere with any treatments or affect the client's health problem.
Test-Taking Strategy: Focus on the subject, use of restraints. Note the strategic word, *best*. Recall principles and concepts related to ethical and legal issues. Eliminate option 1 because, potentially, it is another type of restraint. Eliminate option 2 because the client refused and the nurse does not have the right to coerce a client. Eliminate option 3, which is not the best action because it places responsibility on the family and alternative measures need to be implemented. Review: the legal implications related to the use of restraints.
Reference(s): Potter et al (2013), pp. 300, 385.

578. The nurse prepares a client who is being discharged from the hospital to receive oxygen therapy at home. Which should the nurse include in client teaching about oxygen safety?
1. Hold the oxygen tank on your lap when traveling.
2. Light candles a few feet away from the oxygen tank.
3. Check the oxygen level of the tank on a regular basis.
4. Report low oxygen levels in the tank to the health care provider (HCP).

Level of Cognitive Ability: Applying
Client Needs: Safe and Effective Care Environment
Integrated Process: Teaching and Learning
Content Area: Fundamental Skills: Safety
Priority Concepts: Client Education; Safety

Answer: 3
Rationale: The nurse instructs the client and family to check the oxygen level in the tank on a regular basis to prevent the oxygen from running out. When traveling, the oxygen tank should be secured in place to prevent tank damage and a potentially devastating injury from a moving tank. Oxygen is a highly combustible gas, and, although it will not spontaneously burn or cause an explosion, it contributes to a fire if it contacts a spark from a cigarette, burning candle, or electrical equipment. The nurse instructs the client to contact the oxygen supplier about low oxygen levels in the tank; contacting the HCP is likely to delay prompt replacement of the oxygen tank.
Priority Nursing Tip: An "Oxygen in Use" sign should be placed at the bedside of the client using the oxygen. For the client at home who uses oxygen, the sign should be placed in an area that is visible to all, such as the front window.
Test-Taking Strategy: Focus on the subject, safe administration of oxygen. Eliminate option 1 by visualizing travel with an oxygen tank. A heavy, metal tank can cause an injury if it is not secured in place. Recall that oxygen is a highly combustible gas to eliminate option 2, and recall that oxygen is not supplied by the HCP to eliminate option 4. Review client teaching points related to home care and oxygen therapy.
Reference(s): Potter et al (2013), p. 878.

579. What should the nurse implement to ensure electrical safety for a home care client who needs to receive intravenous (IV) therapy via an IV pump?
1. Keep the pump on at all times.
2. Use an extension cord during ambulation.
3. Obtain a three-pronged grounded plug adapter.
4. Keep the pump plugged in the wall at all times.

Level of Cognitive Ability: Applying
Client Needs: Safe and Effective Care Environment
Integrated Process: Nursing Process/Implementation
Content Area: Fundamental Skills: Safety
Priority Concepts: Clinical Judgment; Safety

Answer: 3
Rationale: Electrical equipment requires grounding to prevent static, sparks, and uninterrupted operation. Extension cords are never recommended; instead, the nurse suggests that the client sit close to a three-pronged outlet during therapy. The pump should not be left "on" at all times, and plugging into wall power at all times may be unnecessary because many pump batteries recharge during operation of the pump. Keeping the pump plugged into the wall also can create a trip hazard.
Priority Nursing Tip: Teach the client and family that electrical equipment should never be used near sinks, bathtubs, or other water sources.
Test-Taking Strategy: Read each option carefully. Focus on the subject, basic electrical safety, to direct you to the correct option. Remember that a three-pronged grounded plug adapter needs to be used. Review: **electrical safety principles**.
Reference(s): Potter et al (2013), p. 382.

580. The home care nurse assesses the client's environment for potential hazards. Which observation requires the nurse to counsel the client and family about the potential for injury?
1. Fluorescent light bulbs in every table lamp
2. Trash can next to the client's favorite chair
3. Stairway with a landing that leads to bedrooms
4. Extension cord tucked away between the seating area and wall

Level of Cognitive Ability: Evaluating
Client Needs: Safe and Effective Care Environment
Integrated Process: Nursing Process/Evaluation
Content Area: Fundamental Skills: Safety
Priority Concepts: Client Education; Safety

Answer: 3
Rationale: The stairway creates a potential hazard for the client because stairs are associated with an increased risk of falls. Options 1 and 2 do not represent potential hazards for the client. An extension cord tucked away from a traffic area is not a potential hazard as long as a suitable electrical demand is drawn on the cord, the cord is grounded properly, and the cord does not traverse a pathway.
Priority Nursing Tip: The nurse should inform the client and family of potential environmental hazards for falling, such as clutter and physical obstacles.
Test-Taking Strategy: Focus on the subject, potential environmental hazards. Recalling that stairs are associated with an increased risk of falls will direct you to option 3. Review: the safety principles for performing a **home assessment**.
Reference(s): Perry, Potter, Elkin (2012) p. 746; Potter et al (2013), p. 185.

581. A hospitalized client wants to leave the hospital before being discharged by the health care provider (HCP). Which is the **priority** nursing intervention?
1. Notify the nursing supervisor of the client's plans to leave.
2. Ask the client about transportation plans from the hospital.
3. Arrange medication prescriptions at the client's preferred pharmacy.
4. Discuss the potential consequences of the plans for leaving with the client.

Level of Cognitive Ability: Applying
Client Needs: Safe and Effective Care Environment
Integrated Process: Nursing Process/Implementation
Content Area: Leadership/Management: Ethical/ Legal
Priority Concepts: Ethics; Health Care Law

Answer: 1
Rationale: The nurse notifies the nursing supervisor of the client's plan to leave without the health care provider's approval to ensure client safety and to help the nurse manage the situation. This will help the nurse manage the situation in a thoughtful, comprehensive manner and complete nursing interventions that include asking about transportation, arranging medication prescriptions, and discussing the risks and benefits of leaving or remaining in the hospital. The HCP should be contacted and the client encouraged to remain until the HCP arrives. The nurse avoids coercion, restraint, or security measures meant to prohibit the client's exit to prevent claims of false imprisonment.
Priority Nursing Tip: False imprisonment occurs when a client is not allowed to leave a health care facility when there is no legal justification to detain the client.
Test-Taking Strategy: Note the strategic word, *priority*. This indicates that one intervention is most important. Review the options for the choice that offers the most potential for a positive outcome. Note that option 1 offers the nurse assistance in a difficult situation involving client safety. Review: the points related to **false imprisonment**.
Reference(s): Potter et al (2013), p. 301.

❖ **582.** The nurse is in the cafeteria and tells a physical therapist about a client who is physically abused. During the next visit to physical therapy, the client discovers that the nurse told the therapist about the abuse and is emotionally harmed. As a result of the events in the cafeteria, which legal ramification do the nurse and physical therapist potentially face? **Select all that apply.**

❏ 1. They can be charged with libel.
❏ 2. They can be charged with slander.
❏ 3. They can be charged with battery.
❏ 4. None; both can receive privileged client data.
❏ 5. They can be charged with a HIPAA (Health Insurance Portability and Accountability Act) violation.

Level of Cognitive Ability: Applying
Client Needs: Safe and Effective Care Environment
Integrated Process: Nursing Process/Implementation
Content Area: Leadership/Management: Ethical/Legal
Priority Concepts: Ethics; Health Care Law

Answer: 2, 5
Rationale: Defamation of a client occurs when information is communicated to a third party that causes damage to the client's reputation either verbally (slander) or in writing (libel). In addition, this situation violates the client's right to confidentiality as defined by HIPAA. Common examples of slander are discussing information about a client in public areas or speaking negatively about coworkers. Both the nurse and the therapist can receive privileged information about the client but not in this manner because communicating aspects of the medical record should not occur in a public setting. The nurse and therapist do not know with certainty that the conversation was not overheard by another person.
Priority Nursing Tip: The nurse is bound to protect client confidentiality. Disclosure of confidential information exposes the nurse to liability.
Test-Taking Strategy: Focus on the subject, client rights and confidentiality, and the health care team's responsibilities with privileged information. Recall that slander constitutes verbal discussion regarding a client and that client information is protected under HIPAA. Eliminate libel and battery because they do not apply to the given situation. Although both parties are eligible to receive confidential information, eliminate option 4 because the exchange of information occurred in a public place. Review: **client rights** and **confidentiality**.
Reference(s): Potter et al (2013), p. 302.

583. A registered nurse (RN) asks a licensed practical nurse (LPN) to change the colostomy bag on a client. The LPN tells the RN that although attendance at the hospital in-service was completed regarding this procedure, the LPN has never performed a colostomy bag change on a client. Which is the **most appropriate** action by the RN to implement?

1. Perform the procedure with the LPN.
2. Request that the LPN observe another LPN perform the procedure.
3. Ask the LPN to review the materials from the in-service before performing the procedure.
4. Instruct the LPN to review the procedure in the hospital manual and take the written procedure into the client's room for reference.

Level of Cognitive Ability: Applying
Client Needs: Safe and Effective Care Environment
Integrated Process: Teaching and Learning
Content Area: Leadership/Management: Delegating
Priority Concepts: Leadership; Safety

Answer: 1
Rationale: The RN must remember that, even though a task may be delegated to someone, the nurse who delegates maintains accountability for the overall nursing care of the client. Only the task, not the ultimate accountability, may be delegated to another. The RN is responsible for ensuring that competent and accurate care is delivered to the client. Because colostomy bag change is a new procedure for this LPN, the RN should accompany the LPN, provide guidance, and answer questions following the procedure. Requesting that the LPN observe another LPN perform the procedure does not ensure that the procedure will be done correctly. Although it is appropriate to review the in-service materials and the hospital procedure manual, it is best for the RN to accompany the LPN to perform the procedure.
Priority Nursing Tip: The five rights to delegation include the right task, right circumstances, right person, right direction/communication, and right supervision/evaluation.
Test-Taking Strategy: Focus on the subject, delegation. Note the strategic words, *most appropriate*. Eliminate options 3 and 4 first. Although it may be important for the LPN to review in-service materials and the hospital procedure manual, these options are not complete. From the remaining options, select option 1 because option 2 does not ensure that another LPN will perform this procedure appropriately. Additionally, it is the RN's responsibility to educate. Review: the principles related to **delegating**.
Reference(s): Huber (2014), p. 154; Potter et al (2013), pp. 281-283.

584. The nurse has applied the patch electrodes of an automatic external defibrillator (AED) to the chest of a client who is pulseless. The defibrillator has interpreted the rhythm to be ventricular fibrillation. Which action should the nurse prepare to perform **next**?
1. Administer rescue breathing during the defibrillation
2. Perform cardiopulmonary resuscitation (CPR) for 1 minute before defibrillating
3. Charge the machine and immediately pushes the "discharge" buttons on the console
4. Order any personnel away from the client, charge the machine, and defibrillate through the console

Level of Cognitive Ability: Applying
Client Needs: Safe and Effective Care Environment
Integrated Process: Nursing Process/Implementation
Content Area: Critical Care: Emergency Situations
Priority Concepts: Clinical Judgment; Safety

Answer: 4
Rationale: If the AED advises to defibrillate, the nurse or rescuer orders all persons away from the client, charges the machine, and pushes both of the "discharge" buttons on the console at the same time. The charge is delivered through the patch electrodes, and this method is known as "hands-off" defibrillation, which is safest for the rescuer. The sequence of charges is similar to that of conventional defibrillation. Option 1 is contraindicated for the safety of any rescuer. Performing CPR delays the defibrillation attempt.
Priority Nursing Tip: An automatic external defibrillator (AED) is used by laypersons and emergency medical technicians for prehospital cardiac arrest situations.
Test-Taking Strategy: Focus on the subject, defibrillation and recall the guidelines related to defibrillation using an AED. Recalling the need to avoid contact with the client during this procedure will direct you to option 4. Review: the procedure for **defibrillation.**
Reference(s): Ignatavicius, Workman (2013), p. 737.

❖ **585.** The nurse is planning care for a client diagnosed with deep vein thrombosis (DVT) of the left leg who is experiencing severe edema and pain in the affected extremity. Which interventions should the nurse plan to include in the care of this client? **Select all that apply.**
❑ 1. Elevate the left leg.
❑ 2. Apply moist heat to the left leg.
❑ 3. Administer acetaminophen (Tylenol).
❑ 4. Ambulate in the hall three times per shift.
❑ 5. Administer anticoagulation as prescribed.

Level of Cognitive Ability: Analyzing
Client Needs: Safe and Effective Care Environment
Integrated Process: Nursing Process/Planning
Content Area: Adult Health: Cardiovascular
Priority Concepts: Clinical Judgment; Clotting

Answer: 1, 2, 3, 5
Rationale: Management of the client with DVT who is experiencing severe edema and pain includes bed rest; limb elevation; relief of discomfort with warm, moist heat and analgesics as needed; anticoagulant therapy; and monitoring for signs of pulmonary embolism. In current practice, activity restriction may not be prescribed if the client is receiving low-molecular-weight anticoagulation; however, some health care providers may still prefer bed rest for the client.
Priority Nursing Tip: The client with deep vein thrombosis is at risk for pulmonary embolism.
Test-Taking Strategy: Focus on the subject, deep vein thrombosis (DVT). Noting that the client is experiencing severe edema and pain and recalling the complications associated with DVT will direct you to the correct options. Review: care of the client with **deep vein thrombosis (DVT).**
Reference(s): Ignatavicius, Workman (2013), pp. 799-800.

586. The nurse is caring for a pregnant client who is receiving an intravenous (IV) infusion of magnesium sulfate. To provide a safe environment, the nurse should ensure that which **priority** item is available?
1. Tongue blade
2. Percussion hammer
3. Calcium gluconate injection
4. Potassium chloride injection

Level of Cognitive Ability: Applying
Client Needs: Safe and Effective Care Environment
Integrated Process: Nursing Process/Implementation
Content Area: Critical Care: Emergency Situations
Priority Concepts: Clinical Judgment; Safety

Answer: 3
Rationale: Magnesium sulfate is a central nervous system depressant and relaxes smooth muscle. Toxic effects of magnesium sulfate may cause loss of deep tendon reflexes, heart block, respiratory paralysis, and cardiac arrest. The antidote for magnesium sulfate is calcium gluconate and should be available. An airway rather than a tongue blade is also an appropriate item. A percussion hammer may be important to assess reflexes but is not the priority item. Potassium chloride is not related to the administration of magnesium sulfate.
Priority Nursing Tip: An intravenous controller device is always used when administering magnesium sulfate. Respiratory depression is a concern with the administration of magnesium sulfate, and the health care provider is notified if respirations are less than 12 breaths per minute.
Test-Taking Strategy: Note the strategic word, *priority*. This indicates that more than one or all of the options may be correct but that you need to identify the most important one. Remember that the percussion hammer would identify the decrease in deep tendon reflexes, but the calcium gluconate is required to treat the life-threatening condition that can occur. Review: care of the client receiving IV **magnesium sulfate**.
Reference(s): McKinney et al (2013), p. 595.

587. The nurse administers digoxin (Lanoxin) 0.25 mg by mouth rather than the prescribed dose of 0.125 mg to the client. Which should the nurse implement **first**?
1. Write an incident report.
2. Tell the client about the medication error.
3. Administer digoxin immune Fab (Digibind).
4. Tell the client about the adverse effects of digoxin.

Level of Cognitive Ability: Applying
Client Needs: Safe and Effective Care Environment
Integrated Process: Nursing Process/Implementation
Content Area: Leadership/Management: Ethical/Legal
Priority Concepts: Clinical Judgment; Safety

Answer: 1
Rationale: According to agency policy, the nurse should file an incident report when a medication error occurs to accurately document the facts. The nurse should assess the client first and then contact the health care provider (HCP) because in this situation the client received too much medication. The client should be informed of the error and the adverse effects in a professional manner to avoid alarm and concern. However, in many situations, the HCP prefers to discuss this with the client. Digoxin immune Fab is reserved for extreme toxicity and requires a prescription and may be prescribed depending on the client's response and the serum digoxin level.
Priority Nursing Tip: The nurse always counts the client's apical heart rate for 1 full minute before administering digoxin (Lanoxin) to an adult client. If the rate is less than 60 beats per minute for an adult, the digoxin is withheld and the health care provider is notified.
Test-Taking Strategy: Note the strategic word, *first*. Eliminate options 2 and 4 because the HCP usually prefers to inform the client of the error. Eliminate option 3 because a HCP's prescription is needed for its administration. Remember after assessing the client and notifying the HCP, complete an incident report when an error occurs. Review: the principles related to **incident reports**.
Reference(s): Potter et al (2013), pp. 305, 358.

588. When planning the discharge of a client with chronic anxiety, the nurse develops goals to promote a safe environment at home. Which area should the appropriate maintenance goal for the client focus on?
1. Identifying anxiety-producing situations
2. Maintaining contact with a crisis counselor
3. Techniques for ignoring feelings of anxiety
4. Eliminating all anxiety from daily situations

Level of Cognitive Ability: Analyzing
Client Needs: Safe and Effective Care Environment
Integrated Process: Nursing Process/Planning
Content Area: Mental Health
Priority Concepts: Anxiety; Safety

Answer: 1
Rationale: Recognizing situations that produce anxiety allows the client to prepare to cope with anxiety or avoid a specific stimulus. Counselors will not be available for all anxiety-producing situations. Additionally, this option does not encourage the development of internal strengths. Ignoring feelings will not resolve anxiety. It is impossible to eliminate all anxiety from life.
Priority Nursing Tip: The immediate nursing action for a client with anxiety is to decrease stimuli in the environment and provide a calm and quiet environment.
Test-Taking Strategy: Focus on the subject, the client experiencing anxiety. Eliminate option 4 first because of the closed-ended word "all." Eliminate option 3 next because feelings should not be ignored. From the remaining choices, select option 1 because it is more client-centered and provides preparation for the client to deal with anxiety if it occurs. Review: goals of care for the client with anxiety.
Reference(s): Varcarolis (2013), pp. 182-183.

589. The nurse is planning to instruct a client with chronic vertigo about safety measures to prevent exacerbation of symptoms or injury. Which instruction is **most important** for the nurse to incorporate in a teaching plan?
1. Turn the head slowly when spoken to.
2. Remove throw rugs and clutter in the home.
3. Drive at times when the client does not feel dizzy.
4. Walk to the bedroom and lie down when vertigo is experienced.

Level of Cognitive Ability: Applying
Client Needs: Safe and Effective Care Environment
Integrated Process: Teaching and Learning
Content Area: Adult Health: Ear
Priority Concepts: Safety; Sensory Perception

Answer: 2
Rationale: The client should maintain the home in a clutter-free state and have throw rugs removed because the effort of trying to regain balance after slipping could trigger the onset of vertigo. To further prevent vertigo attacks, the client should change position slowly and should turn the entire body, not just the head, when spoken to. The client with chronic vertigo should avoid driving and using public transportation. The sudden movements involved in each could precipitate an attack. If vertigo does occur, the client should immediately sit down or lie down (rather than walking to the bedroom) or grasp the nearest piece of furniture.
Priority Nursing Tip: The inner ear contains the sensory receptors for sound and equilibrium. Provide safety measures for the client with an inner ear disorder because the client may experience vertigo.
Test-Taking Strategy: Focus on the subject, chronic vertigo and preventing injury. Note the strategic words, *most important.* Eliminate options 3 and 4 first because they put the client at greatest risk of injury secondary to vertigo. From the remaining options, recalling that the client is taught to turn the entire body, not just the head, will direct you to option 2. Review: safety measures for the client with **chronic vertigo.**
Reference(s): Ignatavicius, Workman (2013), p. 1095; Perry, Potter, Elkin (2012), p. 746.

590. A client receiving heparin therapy for acute myocardial infarction has an activated partial thromboplastin time (aPTT) value of 100 seconds. Before reporting the results to the health care provider, the nurse verifies that which medication is available for use if prescribed?
1. Methylene blue
2. Protamine sulfate
3. Phytonadione (vitamin K)
4. Cyanocobalamin (vitamin B₁₂)

Level of Cognitive Ability: Applying
Client Needs: Safe and Effective Care Environment
Integrated Process: Nursing Process/Implementation
Content Area: Pharmacology: Hematological Medications
Priority Concepts: Clotting; Safety

Answer: 2
Rationale: Heparin is an anticoagulant. Therapeutic values of the aPTT for clients on heparin range between 60 and 70 seconds, depending on the control value. A value of 100 seconds indicates that the client has received too much heparin and is at risk for bleeding. The antidote for heparin overdosage is protamine sulfate and may be prescribed. Vitamin K is the antidote for warfarin sodium (Coumadin) overdosage. Methylene blue is an antidote for cyanide poisoning. Vitamin B₁₂ is used to treat clients with pernicious anemia.
Priority Nursing Tip: For a client receiving heparin therapy, as prescribed, if the activated partial thromboplastin time (aPTT) value is too long, longer than 80 seconds, the heparin dosage should be lowered. If the aPTT is too short, less than 60 seconds, the dosage should be increased.
Test-Taking Strategy: Focus on the subject, heparin therapy and aPTT results. Recalling that protamine sulfate is the antidote for heparin will direct you to the correct option. Review: the normal aPTT and the antidote for **heparin.**
Reference(s): Lehne (2013), p. 659.

591. A suicidal client is being discharged home with family. Which statement by a family member might constitute criteria for delaying discharge?
1. The client's wife asks, "Does he know that I've already moved out and filed for a divorce?"
2. The client's daughter states, "I've decided to postpone my wedding until Dad's feeling better."
3. The client's son states, "One of his friends visited last week to tell us Dad's union is out on strike."
4. The client's brother asks, "Will my brother be able to continue as executor of our parent's trust?"

Level of Cognitive Ability: Analyzing
Client Needs: Safe and Effective Care Environment
Integrated Process: Nursing Process/Assessment
Content Area: Mental Health
Priority Concepts: Mood and Affect; Safety

Answer: 1
Rationale: Single, divorced, and widowed clients have suicide rates that are greater than those who are married. Although the client might feel responsible for his daughter's postponement of the wedding, if presented as an action to include him, the client will feel loved and cared for. Although the situation of the strike is stressful, the client will probably receive a portion of his wages and can derive hope and a sense of belonging from being a member of the union. Although being suicidal may reduce the ability to concentrate, if the client perceives the executorship positively, taking the role away reinforces the client's low self-esteem and self-worth. This statement by the client's brother also indicates a need for the client's brother to be educated about depressive illness.
Priority Nursing Tip: One clue that the client is suicidal is when the client at risk gives away personal, special, and prized possessions.
Test-Taking Strategy: Focus on the subject, delaying discharge in a suicidal client. Read each option carefully. Recalling the risks associated with suicidal intention will direct you to option 1. Review: the risks associated with **suicide.**
Reference(s): Varcarolis (2013), p. 441.

592. The nurse is preparing to ambulate a client with Parkinson's disease who has recently been started on levodopa. The nurse should assess which **most important** item before ambulating the client?
  1. The client's history of falls
  2. Assistive devices used by the client
  3. The client's postural (orthostatic) vital signs
  4. The degree of intention tremors exhibited by the client

Level of Cognitive Ability: Analyzing
Client Needs: Safe and Effective Care Environment
Integrated Process: Nursing Process/Assessment
Content Area: Pharmacology: Neurological Medications
Priority Concepts: Clinical Judgment; Safety

Answer: 3
Rationale: Clients with Parkinson's disease are at risk for postural (orthostatic) hypotension from the disease. This problem is exacerbated with the introduction of levodopa, which can also cause postural hypotension. Although knowledge of the client's risk for falls and the client's use of assistive devices are helpful, it is not the most important piece of assessment data, based on the wording of this question. Clients with Parkinson's disease generally have resting, not intention, tremors.
Priority Nursing Tip: Foods high in vitamin B_6 must be avoided with the use of some antiparkinsonian medications, such as levodopa because the vitamin blocks the effects of the medications.
Test-Taking Strategy: Focus on the strategic words, *most important.* Postural hypotension presents the greatest safety risk to the client. Also, use of the ABCs—airway, breathing, and circulation—will direct you to the correct option. Checking postural vital signs is one way to assess circulation. Review: the complications associated with **Parkinson's disease** and the effects of **levodopa.**
Reference(s): Lehne (2013), p. 199.

593. The nurse prepares to transfer a client who has right-sided weakness from the bed to the wheelchair. With the client dangling on the side of the bed, where should the nurse position the wheelchair?
  1. Directly in front of the client
  2. At a right angle to the client's left leg
  3. Ninety degrees to the client's right leg
  4. At a right angle to the client's right leg

Level of Cognitive Ability: Applying
Client Needs: Safe and Effective Care Environment
Integrated Process: Nursing Process/Implementation
Content Area: Fundamental Skills: Safety
Priority Concepts: Mobility; Safety

Answer: 2
Rationale: When a client has a weakened lower extremity, movement should occur toward the client's unaffected (strong) side, the left side. This wheelchair position allows the client to use the unaffected leg effectively and safely to stand, pivot, and sit in the wheelchair. Placing the wheelchair in front of the client directly increases the risk to the client because the client must pivot 180 degrees to the wheelchair in this position.
Priority Nursing Tip: Safety is the priority concern when transferring a client from the bed to a chair. Always obtain ample assistance to transfer the client, especially if the client's ability to participate in the transfer is unknown.
Test-Taking Strategy: Focus on the subject, a safe transfer technique with right-sided weakness. Visualize each option to direct you to option 2. Positioning the wheelchair next to the client's unaffected leg allows the client to use the stronger leg more effectively for a safe transfer. Also, eliminate options 3 and 4 because they are comparable or alike. Review: **transfer techniques.**
Reference(s): Perry, Potter, Elkin (2012), pp. 359-361; Potter et al (2013), pp. 1155, 1157.

594. The nurse is caring for a client diagnosed with brain death who is a potential organ donor. Before approaching the family to discuss organ donation, the nurse reviews the client's medical record for potential contraindications to organ donation. Which finding is a contraindication to organ donation?
  1. Allergy to penicillin
  2. Hepatitis B infection
  3. Older than 20 years old
  4. History of foreign travel

Level of Cognitive Ability: Analyzing
Client Needs: Safe and Effective Care Environment
Integrated Process: Nursing Process/Assessment
Content Area: Developmental Stages: End-of-Life Care
Priority Concepts: Ethics; Health Care Law

Answer: 2
Rationale: A decedent who had a hepatitis B infection cannot donate organs because the organ recipient may contract the infection. Contraindications to organ donation do not include penicillin allergies or foreign travel. Although foreign travel increases the risk of contracting certain communicable diseases, foreign travel alone does not constitute a contraindication. Age may or may not be a contraindication depending on the organ involved.
Priority Nursing Tip: An individual who is at least 18 years old may indicate a wish to become a donor on his or her driver's license (state-specific) or in an advance directive.
Test-Taking Strategy: Focus on the subject, contraindications to organ donations. Noting the word *infection* in option 2 will direct you to this option. Review: the contraindications for **organ donation.**
Reference(s): Ignatavicius, Workman (2013), p. 1568; Lewis et al (2014), pp. 1007-1008.

595. The nurse monitors a client who has been diagnosed with brain death and is a potential organ donor. Which client assessment data indicate to the nurse that the standard of care as an organ donor has been maintained?
1. Urine output: 100 mL/hr
2. pH of arterial blood: 7.32
3. Capillary refill: 5 seconds
4. Blood pressure: 90/48 mm Hg

Level of Cognitive Ability: Evaluating
Client Needs: Safe and Effective Care Environment
Integrated Process: Nursing Process/Evaluation
Content Area: Developmental Stages: End-of-Life Care
Priority Concepts: Clinical Judgment; Palliation

Answer: 1
Rationale: Urine output at 100 mL per hour indicates adequate renal perfusion and indicates that care standards as an organ donor are maintained. Clinical indicators of care below the standard include a pH of 7.32, indicating acidosis; capillary refill at 5 seconds, which is too slow; and hypotension, indicating an inadequate cardiac output. Guidelines that may be used and are helpful in determining organ viability are the "rules of 100s" in which the systolic blood pressure is maintained at 100 mm Hg, urine output at 100 mL per hour, heart rate at 100 beats per minute, and Pao$_2$ at 100 mm Hg.
Priority Nursing Tip: A client has a right to decide to become an organ donor and a right to refuse organ transplantation as a treatment option.
Test-Taking Strategy: Focus on the subject, organ donation. Eliminate options 2, 3, and 4 because they are comparable or alike and because the listed criteria are below optimal values. Review: normal values for physical assessment measurements and the criteria related to organ donation.
Reference(s): Ignatavicius, Workman (2013), p. 1568; Potter et al (2013), pp. 1043, 1052.

596. A client diagnosed with brain death had received vigorous treatment to control cerebral edema. Which intervention should the nurse plan to implement as a **priority** to maintain viability of the kidneys before organ donation?
1. Screen the donor for infection.
2. Administer intravenous (IV) fluids.
3. Maintain ventilation and oxygenation.
4. Administer vasopressors intravenously.

Level of Cognitive Ability: Analyzing
Client Needs: Safe and Effective Care Environment
Integrated Process: Nursing Process/Planning
Content Area: Developmental Stages: End-of-Life Care
Priority Concepts: Palliation; Perfusion

Answer: 2
Rationale: The kidneys require a minimum perfusion pressure of 80 mm Hg to produce urine and maintain renal function, and because of the aggressive treatment for cerebral edema, the client is likely to have a fluid volume deficiency. Therefore, the nurse restores the intravascular blood volume to maintain the blood pressure and renal perfusion pressure. The nurse screens the donor for infections because diseases such as hepatitis B and human immunodeficiency virus contraindicate organ donation; however, this option is unrelated to viability of the kidneys. Ventilation and oxygenation are important factors in tissue viability; however, the organ must be perfused adequately, first, to deliver any blood. The nurse administers vasopressors with caution to help maintain the donor's blood pressure; however, vasopressors potentially contribute to tissue destruction.
Priority Nursing Tip: The most desirable source of kidneys for transplantation is living related donors whose tissues closely match the client.
Test-Taking Strategy: Note the strategic word, *priority.* Focus on the subject, maintenance of kidney viability before organ donation. Note that this client has had *treatment to control cerebral edema*, which may impact the level of hydration. Next, note the relation between the subject and option 2. Review: the concepts related to organ donation of the kidneys.
Reference(s): Ignatavicius, Workman (2013), pp. 1568-1569.

597. The nurse is working in the emergency department of a small local hospital when a client with multiple stab wounds arrives by ambulance. Which action by the nurse is contraindicated when handling legal evidence?

1. Initiate a chain of custody log.
2. Give clothing and wallet to the family.
3. Cut clothing along seams, avoiding stab holes.
4. Place personal belongings in a labeled, sealed paper bag.

Level of Cognitive Ability: Applying
Client Needs: Safe and Effective Care Environment
Integrated Process: Nursing Process/Implementation
Content Area: Leadership/Management: Ethical/Legal
Priority Concepts: Ethics; Health Care Law

Answer: 2
Rationale: Potential evidence is never released to the family to take home. Basic rules for handling evidence include initiating a chain of custody log to track handling and movement of evidence, limiting the number of people with access to the evidence, and carefully removing clothing and placing personal belongings in a labeled, sealed paper bag to avoid destroying evidence. This also usually includes cutting clothes along seams, while avoiding areas where there are obvious holes or tears.
Priority Nursing Tip: Family members, significant others, or friends of a client who is the victim of a crime, such as a stabbing or gunshot incident, are not allowed to be alone with the client because of the possibility of jeopardizing any existing legal evidence.
Test-Taking Strategy: Focus on the subject, client with multiple stab wounds. Note the word *contraindicated*; this requires you to select the option that identifies an incorrect nursing action. Use knowledge of basic emergency care principles related to a potential crime to eliminate each of the incorrect options. Remember that giving the client's belongings to the family may be giving up evidence. Review: legal evidence.
Reference(s): Hammond, Zimmermann (2013), pp. 8, 56-58.

598. The nurse working on a medical nursing unit during an external disaster is called to assist with care for clients coming into the emergency department. Using principles of triage, the nurse should initiate **immediate** care for a client with which injury?

1. Fractured tibia
2. Penetrating abdominal injury
3. Bright red bleeding from a neck wound
4. Open massive head injury, resulting in deep coma

Level of Cognitive Ability: Applying
Client Needs: Safe and Effective Care Environment
Integrated Process: Nursing Process/Implementation
Content Area: Leadership/Management: Triage
Priority Concepts: Clinical Judgment; Safety

Answer: 3
Rationale: The client with bright red (arterial) bleeding from a neck wound is in "immediate" need of treatment to save the client's life. This client is classified as an emergent (life-threatening) client and would wear a color tag of red from the triage process. A green or "minimal" (nonurgent) designation would be given to the client with a fractured tibia, who requires intervention but who can provide self-care if needed. The client with a penetrating abdominal injury would be tagged yellow and classified as "urgent," requiring intervention within 60 to 120 minutes. A designation of "expectant" would be applied to the client with massive injuries and minimal chance of survival. This client would be color-coded "black" in the triage process. The client who is color-coded "black" is given supportive care and pain management but is given definitive treatment last.
Priority Nursing Tip: The purpose of primary assessment for triage in an emergency department is to identify any client problems that pose an immediate or potential threat to life.
Test-Taking Strategy: Focus on the strategic word, *immediate*. Use the principles of triage and prioritize. Noting the words *bright red* in option 3 will direct you to this option. Review: **disaster** planning and the principles of **triage**.
Reference(s): Ignatavicius, Workman (2013), p. 158.

599. The nurse working on an adult nursing unit is told to review the client census to determine which clients could be discharged if there are a large number of admissions from a newly declared disaster. The nurse determines that the clients with which problems would need to remain hospitalized? **Select all that apply.**

❑ 1. Laparoscopic cholecystectomy
❑ 2. Fractured hip, pinned 5 days ago
❑ 3. Diabetes mellitus with blood glucose at 180 mg/dL
❑ 4. Ongoing ventricular dysrhythmias while receiving procainamide
❑ 5. Newly delivered postpartal client with a blood pressure of 146/94 and 2+ proteinuria.

Level of Cognitive Ability: Analyzing
Client Needs: Safe and Effective Care Environment
Integrated Process: Nursing Process/Analysis
Content Area: Leadership/Management: Triage
Priority Concepts: Clinical Judgment; Safety

Answer: 4, 5
Rationale: The client with ongoing ventricular dysrhythmias requires ongoing medical evaluation and treatment because of potentially lethal complications of the problem. The newly delivered postpartal client is showing classic signs for mild preeclampsia. This condition would need to be reversed before discharge. Each of the other problems listed may be managed at home with appropriate agency referrals for home care services and support from the family at home.
Priority Nursing Tip: The nurse should use the ABCs—airway, breathing, and circulation—as a guide in assessing a client's needs and their severity.
Test-Taking Strategy: Use the principles of triage. Severity of illness usually guides the determination of who requires ongoing monitoring and care. The use of the ABCs—airway, breathing, and circulation—will direct you to option 4. Use of the steps of the nursing process, indicate that the newly delivered postpartal client has not been stabilized and requires further assessment. Review: the principles of **triage** and **prioritizing.**
Reference(s): Ignatavicius, Workman (2013), pp. 160-161.

600. A registered nurse (RN) is orienting an unlicensed assistive personnel (UAP) to the clinical nursing unit. The RN determines that the UAP **needs further teaching** if which procedure is performed by the UAP during a routine handwashing procedure?

1. Keeps hands lower than elbows
2. Dries from forearm down to fingers
3. Washes continuously for 10 to 15 seconds
4. Uses 3 to 5 mL of soap from the dispenser

Level of Cognitive Ability: Evaluating
Client Needs: Safe and Effective Care Environment
Integrated Process: Teaching and Learning
Content Area: Fundamental Skills: Infection Control
Priority Concepts: Leadership; Safety

Answer: 2
Rationale: Proper handwashing procedure involves wetting the hands and wrists and keeping the hands lower than the forearms so that water flows toward the fingertips. The nurse uses 3 to 5 mL of soap and scrubs for 10 to 15 seconds, using rubbing and circular motions. The hands are rinsed and then dried, moving from the fingers to the forearms. The paper towel is then discarded, and a second one is used to turn off the faucet to avoid hand contamination.
Priority Nursing Tip: The nurse is a supervisor and educator, and a primary responsibility is to ensure client safety. If the nurse observes a health care worker performing a procedure incorrectly, he or she must intervene and teach the health care worker how to perform the procedure correctly and safely.
Test-Taking Strategy: Note the strategic words *needs further teaching.* These words indicate a negative event query and require you to select the option that identifies an incorrect action by the UAP. Use basic principles of medical asepsis and visualize each of the actions in the options to assist in directing you to option 2. Review: the nursing procedure for **handwashing.**
Reference(s): Ignatavicius, Workman (2013), p. 435; Potter et al (2013), pp. 410, 425-427.

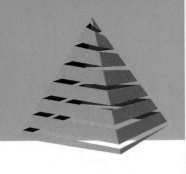
Health Promotion and Maintenance

❖ **601.** The nurse caring for a client in labor should plan to assess the fetal heart rate (FHR) at which specific times? **Select all that apply.**
   ❑ 1. Before voiding
   ❑ 2. Before ambulation
   ❑ 3. After vaginal examination
   ❑ 4. After rupture of the membranes
   ❑ 5. Before turning the client on her side
   ❑ 6. Before the administration of oxytocin (Pitocin)

Level of Cognitive Ability: Analyzing
Client Needs: Health Promotion and Maintenance
Integrated Process: Nursing Process/Planning
Content Area: Maternity: Intrapartum
Priority Concepts: Perfusion; Reproduction

Answer: 2, 3, 4, 6
Rationale: Assessment of the mother and fetus is continuous during the process of labor. However, for all clients, the FHR needs to be assessed before ambulation; immediately after vaginal examinations; rupture of the membranes, or any other invasive procedure; and before the administration of oxytocin because these activities or situations can cause alterations in the FHR. The FHR is also assessed in between contractions, during the contraction, and for at least 30 seconds after the contraction. It is not necessary to assess the FHR before voiding or before turning the client to her side.
Priority Nursing Tip: Electronic fetal heart monitoring is performed during labor to monitor the well-being of the fetus. The normal fetal heart rate at term is 120 to 160 beats/minute.
Test-Taking Strategy: Note that the subject of the question relates to the times at which FHR monitoring is necessary. Read each option and think about the effect that the activity or situation has on the FHR. Eliminate options 1 (before voiding) and option 5 (before turning the client on her side) because these activities will not affect the FHR. Review: care of the client in **labor**.
Reference(s): McKinney et al (2013), pp. 384-385.

❖ **602.** A mother of a 3-year-old child asks the nurse what personal and social developmental milestones she can expect to see in her child. The nurse should tell the mother to expect which findings? **Select all that apply.**
   - ❑ 1. Begins problem solving
   - ❑ 2. Exhibits sexual curiosity
   - ❑ 3. May begin to masturbate
   - ❑ 4. Notices gender differences
   - ❑ 5. Develops a sense of initiative
   - ❑ 6. Develops positive self-esteem through skill acquisition

Level of Cognitive Ability: Analyzing
Client Needs: Health Promotion and Maintenance
Integrated Process: Nursing Process/Implementation
Content Area: Developmental Stages: Infancy to Adolescence
Priority Concepts: Development; Health Promotion

Answer: 2, 3, 4
Rationale: Personal and social developmental milestones of the 3-year-old include exhibiting sexual curiosity; possibly beginning to masturbate; noticing gender differences and identifying with children of like gender; putting on articles of clothing; brushing teeth with help; washing and drying hands using soap and water; knowing own name; and understanding the need to take turns and share with others, but perhaps not being ready to do so. Developmental milestones for the 4- and 5-year-old child include developing a sense of initiative and beginning to problem solve. Developing positive self-esteem through skill acquisition and task completion is characteristic of a 6- to 8-year-old child.
Priority Nursing Tip: A major socializing mechanism of a toddler is parallel play; therapeutic play can also begin at this age.
Test-Taking Strategy: Focus on the subject, the developmental milestones of a 3-year-old. Read each option carefully, thinking about what can be expected of a child at this age. This will assist in eliminating options 1, 5, and 6 because they are higher-level abilities. Review: the developmental milestones of a 3-year-old child.
Reference(s): McKinney et al (2013), p. 136.

603. The nurse has taught a client with a below-the-knee amputation about home care and about monitoring for and preventing complications related to prosthesis and residual limb care. The nurse determines that the client has understood the instructions if the client stated that which action should be taken?
   1. Wear a clean nylon sock over the residual limb every day.
   2. Use a mirror to inspect all areas of the residual limb each day.
   3. Toughen the skin of the residual limb by rubbing it with alcohol.
   4. Prevent cracking of the skin of the residual limb by applying lotion daily.

Level of Cognitive Ability: Evaluating
Client Needs: Health Promotion and Maintenance
Integrated Process: Nursing Process/Evaluation
Content Area: Adult Health: Musculoskeletal
Priority Concepts: Client Education; Tissue Integrity

Answer: 2
Rationale: The client should inspect all surfaces of the residual limb daily for irritation, blisters, and breakdown. The client should wear a clean woolen (not nylon) sock each day. The residual limb is cleansed daily with a gentle soap and water and dried carefully. Alcohol is avoided because it could cause drying or cracking of the skin. Oils and creams are also avoided because they are too softening to the skin for safe prosthesis use.
Priority Nursing Tip: Encourage the client who underwent an amputation to verbalize feelings regarding the loss of the body part and assist the client to identify coping mechanisms to deal with the loss.
Test-Taking Strategy: Focus on the subject, prosthesis and residual limb care. Recall that nylon is a synthetic material that does not allow for the best air circulation and holds in moisture; therefore, option 1 is incorrect. Alcohol and lotion can interfere with the natural condition of the skin, thus increasing the likelihood of breakdown either from drying or excess moisture; therefore, eliminate options 3 and 4. Review: the client teaching points related to residual limb care after amputation.
Reference(s): Ignatavicius, Workman (2013), pp. 1166-1168.

604. The nurse is teaching a client with a right-leg fracture who has a prescription for partial weight-bearing status how to ambulate with crutches. The nurse determines that the client demonstrates compliance with this restriction to prevent complications of the fracture if the client follows which direction?
1. Allows the right foot to only touch the floor
2. Does not bear any weight on the right leg/foot
3. Puts 30% to 50% of the weight on the right leg/foot
4. Puts 60% to 80% of the weight on the right leg/foot

Level of Cognitive Ability: Evaluating
Client Needs: Health Promotion and Maintenance
Integrated Process: Nursing Process/Evaluation
Content Area: Adult Health: Musculoskeletal
Priority Concepts: Mobility; Safety

Answer: 3
Rationale: The client who has partial weight-bearing status is allowed to place 30% to 50% of the body weight on the affected limb. Touchdown weight-bearing allows the client to let the limb touch the floor but not to bear weight. Non–weight-bearing status does not allow the client to let the limb touch the floor. There is no classification for 60% to 80% weight-bearing status. Full weight-bearing status involves placing full weight on the limb.
Priority Nursing Tip: Instruct the client with crutches never to rest the axillae on the axillary bars because of the risk of damaging the brachial plexus.
Test-Taking Strategy: Strategy: Focus on the subject, partial weight-bearing status. Think about the description of what partial weight-bearing means. Option 3 is the only choice that fits this description. Review: the categories related to **weight-bearing**.
Reference(s): Lewis et al (2014), p. 1521; Potter et al (2013), p. 762.

605. To promote self-care, the nurse is planning to teach a client in skeletal leg traction about measures to increase bed mobility. Which item would be **most** helpful for this client?
1. Fracture bedpan
2. Overhead trapeze
3. Isometric exercises
4. Range-of-motion exercises

Level of Cognitive Ability: Applying
Client Needs: Health Promotion and Maintenance
Integrated Process: Nursing Process/Planning
Content Area: Adult Health: Musculoskeletal
Priority Concepts: Mobility; Safety

Answer: 2
Rationale: The use of an overhead trapeze is extremely helpful for assisting a client with moving about in bed and getting on and off the bedpan. This device has the greatest value for increasing overall bed mobility. A fracture bedpan is useful for reducing discomfort with elimination. Isometric exercises will not increase bed mobility and could be harmful for a client in skeletal traction. Range-of-motion exercises can also be harmful to a client in skeletal traction and should not be initiated unless there are specific prescriptions to do so.
Priority Nursing Tip: Monitor the color, motion, and sensation of the affected extremity for a client in traction. If the client is in skeletal traction, also monitor insertion sites for redness, swelling, drainage, or increased pain.
Test-Taking Strategy: Note the strategic word, *most,* and focus on the subject, promoting self-care and increased bed mobility. Eliminate options 3 and 4 first because they can be harmful to a client in skeletal traction. To select from the remaining options, note that the only one that helps with bed mobility is the trapeze. Review: the care of the client in **traction**.
Reference(s): Ignatavicius, Workman (2013), p. 1154; Potter et al (2013), p. 1153.

❖ **606.** The nurse at a community health care clinic is teaching parents about measures to take to prevent and manage obesity in children. The nurse determines that the parents **need additional teaching** if they indicate that they will implement which measures? **Select all that apply.**

1. Use foods as a reward.
2. Offer options of healthy foods.
3. Avoid eating at fast-food restaurants.
4. Keep unhealthy food out of the house.
5. Allow eating in between meals and snack times.
6. Establish consistent times for meals and snacks.

Level of Cognitive Ability: Evaluating
Client Needs: Health Promotion and Maintenance
Integrated Process: Teaching and Learning
Content Area: Fundamental Skills: Nutrition
Priority Concepts: Client Education; Health Promotion

Answer: 1, 5
Rationale: Parents can implement several measures to prevent and manage obesity in their children. These measures include not using food as a reward; establishing consistent times for meals and snacks, and not allowing eating in-between; offering only healthy food options; minimizing trips to fast-food restaurants; keeping unhealthy food out of the house; acting as a role model for children; encouraging the child to do fun, physical activities with the family; and praising the child for making appropriate food choices and increasing physical activity levels.
Priority Nursing Tip: Obesity places a client at risk for hypertension, hyperlipidemia, myocardial infarction, stroke, diabetes mellitus, cancer, and other health conditions.
Test-Taking Strategy: Note the strategic words, *need additional teaching.* These words indicate a negative event query and ask you to select the options that are incorrect statements. Read each option and think about its effect on preventing and managing obesity; this will direct you to the correct options. Review: the measures to manage childhood obesity.
Reference(s): Hockenberry, Wilson (2013), pp. 520-522; McKinney et al (2013), p. 159.

❖ **607.** The nurse is percussing the anterior thorax and the abdomen for tones and expects to note dullness in which anatomic location? **Refer to figure.**

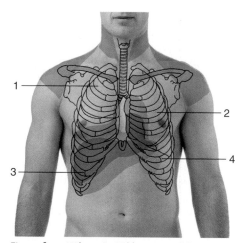

Figure from Wilson S, Giddens J: *Health assessment for nursing practice,* ed 5, St. Louis, 2013, Mosby.

Level of Cognitive Ability: Applying
Client Needs: Health Promotion and Maintenance
Integrated Process: Nursing Process/Assessment
Content Area: Developmental Stages: Health Assessment/Physical Exam
Priority Concepts: Clinical Judgment; Health Promotion

Answer: 3
Rationale: Percussion involves tapping the body with the fingertips to set the underlying structures in motion and thus produce a sound. Dullness will be noted over the liver, located in the upper right quadrant of the abdomen and beneath the lower ribs on the right side. Tympany is the most common percussion tone heard in the abdomen and is caused by the presence of gas. Resonance is the percussion tone heard between the ribs.
Priority Nursing Tip: The presence of a mass produces dullness on percussion and is an abnormal finding.
Test-Taking Strategy: Focus on the subject, the anatomic location in which dullness would be percussed. Look at the figure. Recalling that dullness on percussion indicates the presence of an organ will assist in answering the question. Review: the technique of percussion and the expected findings.
Reference(s): Jarvis (2012), pp. 116-117.

608. The home-care nurse visits an older client with arthritis. The client complains of difficulty instilling glaucoma eye drops because of shaking hands caused by the arthritis. Which instruction should the nurse plan to provide to the client to alleviate this problem?

1. Tilt the head back to instill the eye drops.
2. Have a family member instill the eye drops.
3. Lie down on a bed or sofa to instill the eye drops.
4. Keep the eye drops in the refrigerator so that they will thicken and be easier to instill.

Level of Cognitive Ability: Applying
Client Needs: Health Promotion and Maintenance
Integrated Process: Teaching and Learning
Content Area: Adult Health: Eye
Priority Concepts: Client Education; Safety

Answer: 3
Rationale: Older clients with arthritis or shaking hands have difficulty instilling their own eye drops. The older client is instructed to lie down on a bed or sofa to instill the eye drops. Tilting the head back can lead to a loss of balance. Eye drop regimens for glaucoma require accurate timing, and it is unreasonable to expect a family member to instill the eye drops. Additionally, this discourages client independence. Placing the eye drops in the refrigerator should not be done unless specifically prescribed.
Priority Nursing Tip: If both an eye drop and eye ointment are scheduled to be administered at the same time, administer the eye drop first.
Test-Taking Strategy: Focus on the subject, safety when administering eye medications. Eliminate option 4 first because eye medication should not be refrigerated unless specifically prescribed. Considering the need to promote client independence and the fact that the question does not provide data regarding the client's family, eliminate option 2. From the remaining choices, select option 3 because it provides greater safety for the older client. Review: the procedures for instilling eye drops.
Reference(s): Ignatavicius, Workman (2013), p. 1062; Potter et al (2013), pp. 596, 616-619.

❖ **609.** A client at the family planning clinic requests a prescription for oral contraceptives from the nurse who is performing an assessment. After reviewing the client's chart, the nurse determines that oral contraceptives are contraindicated because of which documented item? **Refer to chart.**

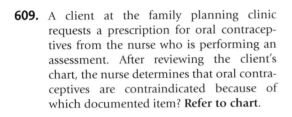

CLIENT'S CHART

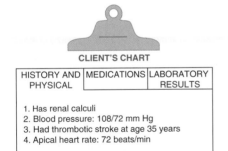

HISTORY AND PHYSICAL	MEDICATIONS	LABORATORY RESULTS
1. Has renal calculi		
2. Blood pressure: 108/72 mm Hg		
3. Had thrombotic stroke at age 35 years		
4. Apical heart rate: 72 beats/min		

Level of Cognitive Ability: Analyzing
Client Needs: Health Promotion and Maintenance
Integrated Process: Nursing Process/Analysis
Content Area: Developmental Stages: Health Assessment/Physical Exam
Priority Concepts: Reproduction; Safety

Answer: 3
Rationale: Oral contraceptives are contraindicated in women with a history of thrombophlebitis and thromboembolic disorders; cardiovascular or cerebrovascular diseases (including stroke); any estrogen-dependent cancer or breast cancer, or benign or malignant liver tumors; impaired liver function; hypertension; or diabetes mellitus with vascular involvement. Adverse effects of oral contraceptives include increased risk of superficial and deep vein thrombosis, pulmonary embolism, thrombotic stroke (or other types of strokes), myocardial infarction, and accelerations of preexisting breast tumors.
Priority Nursing Tip: Antibiotics may decrease the absorption and effectiveness of contraceptives.
Test-Taking Strategy: Focus on the subject, the item that is a contraindication to the use of oral contraceptives. Eliminate items 2 and 4 because these are normal findings. To select from the remaining choices, remember that oral contraceptives are contraindicated in cardiovascular or cerebrovascular disorders. Review: the contraindications to the use of **oral contraceptives**.
Reference(s): Ignatavicius, Workman (2013), p. 694; Lehne (2013), pp. 788-790, 803.

610. The nurse provides dietary instruction to the parents of a child with a diagnosis of cystic fibrosis. The nurse should tell the parents that which diet plan should be followed?
1. Fat free
2. Low in protein
3. Low in sodium
4. High in calories

Level of Cognitive Ability: Applying
Client Needs: Health Promotion and Maintenance
Integrated Process: Teaching and Learning
Content Area: Fundamental Skills: Nutrition
Priority Concepts: Client Education; Nutrition

Answer: 4
Rationale: Children with cystic fibrosis are managed with a high-calorie, high-protein diet; pancreatic enzyme replacement therapy; fat-soluble vitamin supplements; and if nutritional problems are severe, nighttime gastrostomy feedings or parental nutrition. Fats are not restricted unless steatorrhea cannot be controlled by increased pancreatic enzymes. Sodium intake is unrelated to this disorder.
Priority Nursing Tip: The child with cystic fibrosis needs to be monitored closely for signs/symptoms of failure to thrive.
Test-Taking Strategy: Focus on the subject, diet for the child with cystic fibrosis. Think about the pathophysiology associated with cystic fibrosis. Select option 4 because children require calories for growth and development and because this choice is the umbrella option. Review: the dietary measures for the child with cystic fibrosis.
Reference(s): McKinney et al (2013), p. 1190.

611. A clinic nurse provides home care instructions to an adolescent with iron deficiency anemia about the administration of oral iron preparations. The nurse should tell the adolescent that it is **best** to take the iron with which liquid?
1. Cola
2. Soda
3. Water
4. Tomato juice

Level of Cognitive Ability: Applying
Client Needs: Health Promotion and Maintenance
Integrated Process: Teaching and Learning
Content Area: Pharmacology: Hematological Medications
Priority Concepts: Client Education; Health Promotion

Answer: 4
Rationale: Iron should be administered with vitamin C–rich fluids because vitamin C enhances the absorption of the iron preparation. Tomato juice has a high ascorbic acid (vitamin C) content, whereas cola, soda, and water do not contain vitamin C.
Priority Nursing Tip: Liquid iron preparations stain the teeth. Teach the child and parents that liquid iron should be taken through a straw, and the teeth should be brushed after administration.
Test-Taking Strategy: Note the strategic word, *best*. Eliminate options 1 and 2 first because they are comparable or alike. From the remaining choices, recall that vitamin C increases the absorption of iron to direct you to option 4. Review: the administration of **oral iron**.
Reference(s): McKinney et al (2013), p. 1243.

❖ **612.** The nurse is performing an assessment on an older client. Which signs/symptoms are age-related changes in the eye? **Select all that apply.**
❑ 1. Clear sclera
❑ 2. Blurred vision
❑ 3. Protruding cornea
❑ 4. Increased tear production
❑ 5. Diminished pupillary adaptation to darkness
❑ 6. Increased ability to discriminate among colors

Level of Cognitive Ability: Analyzing
Client Needs: Health Promotion and Maintenance
Integrated Process: Nursing Process/Assessment
Content Area: Developmental Stages: Early Adulthood to Later Adulthood
Priority Concepts: Development; Sensory Perception

Answer: 2, 5
Rationale: Age-related changes in the eye include flattening of the cornea, which causes blurred vision; poor pupillary adaptation to darkness; yellowing sclera; a sunken appearance; diminished tear production; diminished ability to discriminate among colors; and reduced ocular muscle strength.
Priority Nursing Tip: The client experiencing age-related changes in the eye is at risk for injury; therefore, it is important for the nurse to teach the client about ways to compensate for these changes.
Test-Taking Strategy: Focus on the subject, age-related changes in the eye. Eliminate options 4 and 6 because of the word *increased*. Noting the word *blurred* in option 2 and *diminished* in option 5 will direct you to these choices. Review: **age-related eye changes**.
Reference(s): Ignatavicius, Workman (2013), p. 1043; Potter et al (2013), p. 176.

613. The nurse has given the client with a nephrostomy tube instructions to follow after hospital discharge to prevent complications. The nurse determines that the client understands the instructions if the client verbalizes the need to drink how many glasses of water per day?
1. 1 to 3
2. 6 to 8
3. 10 to 12
4. 14 to 16

Level of Cognitive Ability: Evaluating
Client Needs: Health Promotion and Maintenance
Integrated Process: Nursing Process/Evaluation
Content Area: Adult Health: Renal and Urinary
Priority Concepts: Client Education; Elimination

Answer: 2
Rationale: The client with a nephrostomy tube needs to have adequate fluid intake to dilute urinary particles that could cause calculus and provide good mechanical flushing of the kidney and the tube. The nurse encourages the client to take in 2000 mL of fluid per day, which is roughly equivalent to 6 to 8 glasses of water. Option 1 is an inadequate amount. Options 3 and 4 are amounts that could distend the renal pelvis.
Priority Nursing Tip: If the client has a ureteral or nephrostomy tube, monitor the output closely; urine output of less than 30 mL/hr or lack of output for more than 15 minutes should be reported to the health care provider immediately.
Test-Taking Strategy: Focus on the subject, fluid intake for a client with a nephrostomy tube. Recall that the client needs 2 L of fluid per day. This will direct you to option 2. Also, avoid options in the much higher range because these are unnecessary and could possibly place undue distention on the renal pelvis. Review: the care of the client with a **nephrostomy tube.**
Reference(s): Ignatavicius, Workman (2013), pp. 1511, 1525.

614. The nurse provides home care instructions to a female client who has recurrent trichomoniasis, and she then has the client explain the plan of care. The nurse determines the **need for follow-up** if the client indicates she should take which action?
1. Avoids sexual intercourse.
2. Performs good perineal hygiene.
3. Discontinues treatment during menstruation.
4. Uses the metronidazole (Flagyl) as prescribed.

Level of Cognitive Ability: Evaluating
Client Needs: Health Promotion and Maintenance
Integrated Process: Teaching and Learning
Content Area: Fundamental Skills: Infection Control
Priority Concepts: Client Education; Infection

Answer: 3
Rationale: Treatment for a recurrent vaginal trichomoniasis infection continues through the menstrual period because the vagina is more alkaline during menses, and a flare-up is more likely to occur. While the infection remains active, the client should refrain from sexual intercourse or instruct her partner to wear a condom. To help break the chain of infection, the nurse directs the client to perform perineal hygiene after each voiding and each bowel movement. Metronidazole (Flagyl) must be taken as prescribed.
Priority Nursing Tip: Trichomoniasis is a sexually transmitted infection and is associated with premature rupture of the membranes and postpartum endometritis.
Test-Taking Strategy: Note the strategic words, *need for follow-up*. These words indicate a negative event query and that the answer will be a client misunderstanding about self-care while treating this infection. Recall the basic principles related to infection control for vaginal fungal infections and medication administration to direct you to the correct option. Review: the treatment for **trichomoniasis.**
Reference(s): Hodgson, Kizior (2014), pp. 769-770; Ignatavicius, Workman (2013), pp. 1665-1666.

❖ **615.** Which problems might adoptive parents encounter? **Select all that apply.**
  ❑ 1. Set unrealistically high standard for themselves
  ❑ 2. Lack knowledge about the child's biological health history
  ❑ 3. Have difficulty assimilating if the child is adopted from another country
  ❑ 4. Have difficulty deciding when and how to tell the child about being adopted
  ❑ 5. Feel the need for more assistance and support in child-rearing than biological parents do
  ❑ 6. Face problems with child-rearing that are different from those encountered by natural parents

Level of Cognitive Ability: Analyzing
Client Needs: Health Promotion and Maintenance
Integrated Process: Nursing Process/Analysis
Content Area: Adult Health: Reproductive
Priority Concepts: Family Dynamics; Reproduction

Answer: 1, 2, 3, 4
Rationale: Adoptive parents may add pressure to themselves by setting unrealistically high standards for themselves as parents. Additional problems adoptive families may face include possible lack of knowledge about the child's biological health history, difficulty assimilating if the child is adopted from another country, and difficulty deciding when and how to tell the child about being adopted. Otherwise, most problems faced by adoptive parents are no different from those encountered by natural parents. All parents want to be good parents. Both adoptive parents and biological parents need information, support, and guidance to prepare them to care for their child.
Priority Nursing Tip: In adoption, all rights and responsibilities that belonged to the original parent or parents are legally transferred to the person(s) who becomes the new parent(s).
Test-Taking Strategy: Focus on the subject, problems that adoptive parents may encounter. Read each option and determine if the information distinctively relates to adoption. This will assist in answering the question. Review: problems encountered by **adoptive parents**.
Reference(s): Hockenberry, Wilson (2013), pp. 60-61; McKinney et al (2013), p. 39.

616. A client with a history of depression will be participating in cognitive therapy for health maintenance. The client asks the nurse, "How does this treatment work?" Which statement is **most appropriate** for the nurse to make to the client?
  1. "This treatment helps you relax and develop new coping skills."
  2. "This treatment helps you confront your fears by gradually exposing you to them."
  3. "This treatment helps you examine how your past life has contributed to your problems."
  4. "This treatment helps examine how your thoughts and feelings contribute to your difficulties."

Level of Cognitive Ability: Applying
Client Needs: Health Promotion and Maintenance
Integrated Process: Nursing Process/Implementation
Content Area: Mental Health
Priority Concepts: Health Promotion; Mood and Affect

Answer: 4
Rationale: Cognitive therapy is frequently used with clients who have depression. This type of therapy is based on exploring the client's personal experience. It includes examining the client's thoughts and feelings about situations and how these thoughts and feelings contribute to and perpetuate the client's difficulties and mood. Options 1, 2, and 3 are not characteristics of cognitive therapy.
Priority Nursing Tip: Cognitive therapy is based on the principle that how individuals feel and behave is determined by how they think about the world and their place in it.
Test-Taking Strategy: Note the strategic words, *most appropriate*, and focus on the subject, a description of cognitive therapy. Note the relationship between the word *cognitive* and option 4. Option 4 uses the word "thoughts" when describing the treatment. Review: cognitive therapy.
Reference(s): Varcarolis (2013), pp. 32-33, 260.

617. A client with acquired immunodeficiency syndrome (AIDS) has a problem with nutrition and has lost weight. The nurse has instructed the client regarding methods of maintaining and increasing weight. The nurse determines that the client **needs further instruction** if the client stated the need to implement which measure?

1. Eat low-calorie snacks between meals.
2. Eat small, frequent meals throughout the day.
3. Consume nutrient-dense foods and beverages.
4. Keep easy-to-prepare foods available in the home.

Level of Cognitive Ability: Evaluating
Client Needs: Health Promotion and Maintenance
Integrated Process: Teaching and Learning
Content Area: Adult Health: Immune
Priority Concepts: Client Education; Nutrition

Answer: 1

Rationale: The client who has a problem with nutrition and is losing weight should take in nutrient-dense and high-calorie meals and snacks. The client should also eat small, frequent meals throughout the day. The client is encouraged to eat favorite foods to keep intake up and plan meals that are easy to prepare. The client should also avoid taking fluids with meals to increase food intake before satiety occurs.

Priority Nursing Tip: Acquired immunodeficiency syndrome (AIDS) is manifested by opportunistic infections and neoplasms.

Test-Taking Strategy: Note the strategic words, *needs further instruction*. These words indicate a negative event query and ask you to select an option that is an incorrect statement. Also note the client has a problem with nutrition and is losing weight. Recalling that the client should choose snacks that are high in calories (rather than low in calories) will direct you to the correct option. Review: the care of the client with imbalanced **nutrition**.

Reference(s): Ignatavicius, Workman (2013), p. 376; Swearingen (2012), p. 508.

618. A school nurse is performing screening examinations for scoliosis. Which signs of scoliosis should the nurse assess for? **Select all that apply.**
☐ 1. Chest asymmetry
☐ 2. Equal waist angles
☐ 3. Unequal rib heights
☐ 4. Equal rib prominences
☐ 5. Equal shoulder heights
☐ 6. Lateral deviation and rotation of each vertebra

Level of Cognitive Ability: Analyzing
Client Needs: Health Promotion and Maintenance
Integrated Process: Nursing Process/Assessment
Content Area: Child Health: Musculoskeletal
Priority Concepts: Health Promotion; Mobility

Answer: 1, 3, 6

Rationale: Scoliosis is a lateral curvature of the spine. To ensure early detection and treatment, children ages 9 through 15 years should be screened for scoliosis; those at greatest risk are girls from 10 years of age through adolescence. The child should be unclothed or wearing only underpants so that the chest, back, and hips can be clearly seen. The child should stand with her or his weight equally on both feet, legs straight, and arms hanging loosely at the sides. The nurse then observes for the signs of scoliosis. These signs include nonpainful lateral curvature of the spine, a curve with one turn (C curve) or two compensating curves (S curve), lateral deviation and rotation of each vertebra, unequal shoulder heights, unequal waist angles, unequal rib prominences and chest asymmetry, and unequal rib heights.

Priority Nursing Tip: If scoliosis is suspected, radiographs will be done to confirm the diagnosis.

Test-Taking Strategy: Focus on the subject, the signs of scoliosis, and recall the definition of scoliosis, a lateral curvature of the spine. Visualize this disorder and note the word "equal" in options 2, 4, and 5, the incorrect choices. Review: the signs of **scoliosis**.

Reference(s): McKinney et al (2013), p. 832.

619. The nurse is teaching a client with histoplasmosis infection about the prevention of future exposure to infectious sources. The nurse determines that the client **needs further instruction** if the client states that which is a potential source of this infection?

1. Grape arbors
2. Bird droppings
3. Mushroom cellars
4. Floors of chicken houses

Level of Cognitive Ability: Evaluating
Client Needs: Health Promotion and Maintenance
Integrated Process: Teaching and Learning
Content Area: Fundamental Skills: Infection Control
Priority Concepts: Client Education; Infection

Answer: 1
Rationale: The client with histoplasmosis is taught to avoid exposure to potential sources of the fungus, including bird droppings (especially those of starlings and blackbirds), mushroom cellars, and the floors of chicken houses and bat caves.
Priority Nursing Tip: Transmission of histoplasmosis occurs by the inhalation of spores commonly found in contaminated soil.
Test-Taking Strategy: Note the strategic words, *needs further instruction*. These words indicate a negative event query and ask you to select an option that is an incorrect statement. Eliminate options 2 and 4 first because they are comparable or alike. Because histoplasmosis is a fungus, recall that there is increased exposure to areas in which the fungus thrives. Therefore, the least likely option is the grape arbor, which is above ground and is not in a dark and damp area. Review: the sources and causes of **histoplasmosis** infection.
Reference(s): Ignatavicius, Workman (2013), pp. 366, 550; Lewis et al (2014), pp. 229-230.

620. Which factors increase the risk for hypothermia in an older client? **Select all that apply.**

☐ 1. Burns
☐ 2. Anemia
☐ 3. Alcohol abuse
☐ 4. Hypoglycemia
☐ 5. Hyperthyroidism
☐ 6. Ability to sense cold temperatures

Level of Cognitive Ability: Analyzing
Client Needs: Health Promotion and Maintenance
Integrated Process: Nursing Process/Analysis
Content Area: Developmental Stages: Early Adulthood to Later Adulthood
Priority Concepts: Development; Thermoregulation

Answer: 1, 2, 3, 4
Rationale: The median oral temperature of an older client is 96.8° F (36° C). Environmental temperatures below 65° F (18° C) may cause a serious drop in core body temperature to 95° F (35° C) or less in the older client. Numerous factors increase the risk of hypothermia in the older client, including conditions that increase heat loss (e.g., burns); conditions that decrease heat production such as hypothyroidism, hypoglycemia, or anemia; medications or substances that interfere with thermoregulation, such as alcohol; or thermoregulatory impairment (failure to sense cold).
Priority Nursing Tip: Hypothermia can lead to hypoxia and subsequently insufficient circulation, which can be fatal. Early signs include shivering and mental confusion.
Test-Taking Strategy: Focus on the subject, the risks associated with hypothermia. Recall that hypothermia is an abnormally dangerous and low body temperature. Next think about the pathophysiology or effects of each item in the options to answer correctly. Review: risk factors for **hypothermia** in an older client.
Reference(s): Dolan, Holt (2013), pp. 308-309; Ignatavicius, Workman (2013), p. 148.

621. The nurse is assigned to care for a client being admitted to the hospital with a diagnosis of cirrhosis and ascites. Which dietary measure should the nurse expect to be prescribed for the client?

1. Sodium restriction
2. Increased fat intake
3. Decreased carbohydrates
4. Calorie restriction of 1500 daily

Level of Cognitive Ability: Analyzing
Client Needs: Physiological Integrity
Integrated Process: Nursing Process/Planning
Content Area: Adult Health: Gastrointestinal
Priority Concepts: Fluid and Electrolyte Balance; Nutrition

Answer: 1
Rationale: If the client has ascites, sodium and possibly fluids would be restricted in the diet. Fat restriction is not necessary, and the client should maintain a normal amount of fat intake. The diet should supply sufficient carbohydrates to maintain weight and spare protein. The total daily calories should range between 2000 and 3000. The diet should provide ample protein to rebuild tissue but not an amount that will precipitate hepatic encephalopathy.
Priority Nursing Tip: For the client with cirrhosis, protein may not be restricted in the diet if ascites and edema are absent, and the client does not exhibit signs of impending coma.
Test-Taking Strategy: Focus on the subject, cirrhosis and ascites. Recalling that ascites refers to the accumulation of body fluid will direct you to the correct option. Review: dietary measures for the client with **cirrhosis and ascites**.
Reference(s): Ignatavicius, Workman (2013), p. 1300.

❖ **622.** The nurse reviews the pattern of a non-stress test performed on a pregnant client and interprets the finding as which result? **Refer to figure.**

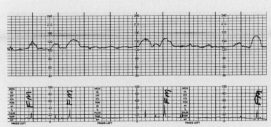

Figure from McKinney E, James S, Murray S, et al: *Maternal-child nursing*, ed 4, St. Louis, 2013, Saunders.

1. Reactive
2. Abnormal
3. Nonreactive
4. Nonreassuring

Level of Cognitive Ability: Analyzing
Client Needs: Health Promotion and Maintenance
Integrated Process: Nursing Process/Analysis
Content Area: Maternity: Antepartum
Priority Concepts: Health Promotion; Reproduction

Answer: 1
Rationale: A non-stress test assesses fetal well-being and evaluates the ability of the fetal heart to accelerate, often in association with fetal movement. Accelerations of the fetal heart rate are associated with adequate oxygenation, a healthy neural pathway, and the fetal heart's ability to respond to stimuli. A reactive test is described as at least two fetal heart rate accelerations, with or without fetal movement, occurring within a 20-minute period and peaking at least 15 beats/minute above the baseline and lasting 15 seconds from baseline to baseline. This recording (see figure) identifies a reactive non-stress test. The fetal heart rate acceleration peaks at least 15 beats/minute and lasts for at least 15 seconds in response to fetal movement. A nonreactive test is an abnormal or nonreassuring test. In a nonreactive test, the recording does not demonstrate the required characteristics of a reactive test within a 40-minute period.
Priority Nursing Tip: A non-stress test is a noninvasive measure of fetal well-being. A contraction stress test is performed if the non-stress test is abnormal and involves exposing the fetus to the stress of contractions using a dilute dose of oxytocin (Pitocin).
Test-Taking Strategy: Note the accelerations identified in the figure. Also note that options 2, 3, and 4 are comparable or alike in that they all indicate a nonreactive test result. Review: interpretation of non-stress test.
Reference(s): McKinney et al (2013), pp. 309-310.

❖ **623.** A client has hyperphosphatemia. To prevent worsening of the condition, the nurse should instruct the client to avoid which food selections? **Select all that apply.**
- ❑ 1. Fish
- ❑ 2. Eggs
- ❑ 3. Coffee
- ❑ 4. Grapes
- ❑ 5. Bananas
- ❑ 6. Whole grain breads

Level of Cognitive Ability: Applying
Client Needs: Health Promotion and Maintenance
Integrated Process: Teaching and Learning
Content Area: Fundamental Skills: Nutrition
Priority Concepts: Health Promotion; Nutrition

Answer: 1, 2, 6
Rationale: Food items and liquids that are naturally high in phosphates include fish, eggs, milk products, whole grains, vegetables, and carbonated beverages, and they should be avoided by the client with hyperphosphatemia. The food items in options 3, 4, and 5 are acceptable for this client to consume.
Priority Nursing Tip: The normal phosphorus level is 2.7 to 4.5 mg/dL.
Test-Taking Strategy: Focus on the subject, hyperphosphatemia, and the items to avoid because they will worsen the condition. Eliminate options 4 and 5 because they are comparable or alike and are fruits. For the remaining options, recalling the phosphate content of foods and fluids will assist in answering correctly. Review: the dietary measures for the client with hyperphosphatemia.
Reference(s): Ignatavicius, Workman (2013), p. 190; Nix (2013), p. 135.

624. The community health nurse provides an educational session regarding the risk factors for cervical cancer to women in the local community. The nurse determines that **further teaching is needed** if a woman attending the session identifies which as a risk factor for this type of cancer?
1. Smoking tobacco
2. Single sex partner
3. Early first intercourse
4. Human papillomavirus (HPV) infection

Level of Cognitive Ability: Evaluating
Client Needs: Health Promotion and Maintenance
Integrated Process: Teaching and Learning
Content Area: Adult Health: Oncology
Priority Concepts: Client Education; Health Promotion

Answer: 2
Rationale: Some risk factors for cervical cancer include having multiple sexual partners or a partner who had multiple sexual partners, smoking tobacco, early age of first intercourse, and HPV infection.
Priority Nursing Tip: Premalignant changes for cervical cancer are described on a continuum from dysplasia, which is the earliest premalignancy change, to carcinoma in situ, the most advanced premalignant change.
Test-Taking Strategy: Note the strategic words, *further teaching is needed*. These words indicate a negative event query and ask you to select an option that is an incorrect risk factor. Noting the word "single" in option 2 will direct you to this option. Review: risk factors for cervical cancer.
Reference(s): Ignatavicius, Workman (2013), p. 1622; Lewis et al (2014), pp. 1292-1293.

625. The high school nurse teaches the female students how to prevent pelvic inflammatory disease (PID). What instructions should the nurse include?
1. To douche monthly
2. To avoid single sexual partners
3. To avoid unprotected intercourse
4. To consult with a gynecologist regarding the placement of an intrauterine device (IUD)

Level of Cognitive Ability: Applying
Client Needs: Health Promotion and Maintenance
Integrated Process: Teaching and Learning
Content Area: Fundamental Skills: Infection Control
Priority Concepts: Client Education; Health Promotion

Answer: 3
Rationale: Pelvic inflammatory disease is an infection of the pelvis. The primary prevention of pelvic inflammatory disease includes avoiding unprotected intercourse, douching, multiple sexual partners, and the use of an IUD.
Priority Nursing Tip: Pelvic inflammatory disease occurs when organisms from the lower genital tract invade the uterine cavity and the fallopian tubes.
Test-Taking Strategy: Focus on the subject, preventing PID. Recall the principle of the exposure of the pelvic area to factors that cause infection. With this concept in mind, eliminate options 1, 2, and 4. Review: the preventive measures for pelvic inflammatory disease.
Reference(s): Ignatavicius, Workman (2013), p. 1665.

626. The nurse provides discharge teaching to a client after a vasectomy. Which statement by the client would indicate the **need for further teaching**?
1. "I can use a scrotal support if I need to."
2. "I don't need to practice birth control any longer."
3. "I can resume sexual intercourse whenever I want."
4. "If I have pain or swelling, I can use an ice bag and take Tylenol."

Level of Cognitive Ability: Evaluating
Client Needs: Health Promotion and Maintenance
Integrated Process: Teaching and Learning
Content Area: Adult Health: Reproduction
Priority Concepts: Client Education; Reproduction

Answer: 2
Rationale: After vasectomy, the client must continue to practice a method of birth control until the follow-up semen analysis shows azoospermia. Live sperm may be present in the vas deferens after this procedure. Options 1, 3, and 4 are appropriate client statements.
Priority Nursing Tip: A vasectomy is a surgical procedure performed to prevent the release of sperm when a man ejaculates. It is a method of birth control.
Test-Taking Strategy: Note the strategic words, *need for further teaching*. These words indicate a negative event query and ask you to select an option that is an incorrect statement. Options 1 and 4 can be eliminated because these measures assist with alleviating discomfort and swelling after the procedure. Option 3 can be eliminated because there would be no reason to avoid sexual intercourse unless the client was experiencing discomfort. Thinking about the purpose of a vasectomy will direct you to the correct option. Review: the client teaching points after a vasectomy.
Reference(s): Lewis et al (2014), p. 1326.

627. A nursing instructor asks a student to identify risk factors for and methods of preventing prostate cancer. Which statement by the student indicates the **need for further teaching?**

1. "Smoking increases the risk for this type of cancer."
2. "A high-fat diet will assist in preventing this type of cancer."
3. "A history of a sexually transmitted infection is a risk for this disease."
4. "Men more than 50 years old should be monitored with a yearly digital rectal exam"

Level of Cognitive Ability: Evaluating
Client Needs: Health Promotion and Maintenance
Integrated Process: Teaching and Learning
Content Area: Adult Health: Oncology
Priority Concepts: Client Education; Health Promotion

Answer: 2
Rationale: Prostate cancer is a slow-growing malignancy of the prostate gland. A high intake of dietary fat is a risk factor for prostate cancer. Options 1, 3, and 4 are accurate statements regarding the risks and prevention measures related to this type of cancer.
Priority Nursing Tip: The risk of prostate cancer increases in men with each decade after the age of 50.
Test-Taking Strategy: Note the strategic words, *the need for further teaching*. These words indicate a negative event query and ask you to select an option that is an incorrect statement. Recalling the general principles related to cancer prevention will direct you to option 2. Review: **Prostate cancer.**
Reference(s): Ignatavicius, Workman (2013), p. 1637.

628. A clinic nurse provides information to a married couple regarding measures to prevent infertility. Which statement made by the husband indicates the **need for further education?**

1. "We need to eat a nutritious diet."
2. "We need to avoid the excessive intake of alcohol."
3. "We need to decrease exposure to environmental hazards."
4. "I need to maintain warmth to my scrotum by taking hot baths frequently."

Level of Cognitive Ability: Evaluating
Client Needs: Health Promotion and Maintenance
Integrated Process: Teaching and Learning
Content Area: Adult Health: Reproduction
Priority Concepts: Client Education; Reproduction

Answer: 4
Rationale: Keeping the testes cool by avoiding hot baths and tight clothing appears to improve the sperm count. Avoiding factors that depress spermatogenesis (such as the use of drugs, alcohol, and marijuana), maintaining good nutrition, and limiting exposure to occupational and environmental hazards are vital components of preventing infertility.
Priority Nursing Tip: Infertility is the involuntary inability to conceive when desired. Several diagnostic tests are available to determine the probable cause of infertility, and the therapy recommended may depend on the cause.
Test-Taking Strategy: Note the strategic words, *need for further education*. These words indicate a negative event query and ask you to select an option that is an incorrect statement. Eliminate option 1 first because the maintenance of a nutritious diet is important in all situations. From the remaining options, recalling that heat decreases the motility of sperm will assist with directing you to the correct option. Review: the measures that prevent **infertility.**
Reference(s): McKinney et al (2013), pp. 754-755.

629. The nurse is teaching a client who is preparing for discharge from the hospital after a total hip replacement. Which statement by the client would indicate the **need for further teaching?**
1. "I cannot drive a car for probably 6 weeks."
2. "I should not sit in one position for more than 4 hours."
3. "I need to wear a support stocking on my unaffected leg."
4. "I need to place a pillow between my knees when I lie down."

Level of Cognitive Ability: Evaluating
Client Needs: Health Promotion and Maintenance
Integrated Process: Teaching and Learning
Content Area: Adult Health: Musculoskeletal
Priority Concepts: Client Education; Health Promotion

Answer: 2
Rationale: The client needs to be instructed to not sit continuously for more than 1 hour. The client should be instructed to stand, stretch, and take a few steps periodically. The client cannot drive a car for 6 weeks after surgery unless allowed to do so by a health care provider. A support stocking should be worn on the unaffected leg (as prescribed), and an Ace bandage usually is prescribed to be placed on the affected leg until there is no swelling in the legs and feet and until full activities are resumed. The legs are abducted by placing a pillow between them when the client lies down.
Priority Nursing Tip: In the postoperative period after total hip replacement, an important nursing intervention is to perform frequent neurovascular assessments of the affected extremity checking color, pulses, capillary refill, movement, and sensation.
Test-Taking Strategy: Note the strategic words, *need for further teaching*. These words indicate a negative event query and ask you to select an option that is an incorrect statement. Recalling standard measures related to the postoperative period will assist you in eliminating option 1. Knowing that leg abduction is maintained postoperatively during hospitalization will assist you in eliminating option 4. From the remaining options, note the time frame of 4 hours given in option 2. This is a lengthy time period for the client to remain in one position. Review: the client teaching points after **total hip replacement**.
Reference(s): Ignatavicius, Workman (2013), pp. 327-328.

630. The nurse is working at an osteoporosis screening clinic and is interviewing and performing physical assessments on women. Which clients are at greatest risk for developing osteoporosis? **Select all that apply.**
☐ 1. An Asian woman
☐ 2. A large-boned, dark-skinned woman
☐ 3. A client who started menopause early
☐ 4. A client with a family history of the disease
☐ 5. A client who has a physically active lifestyle
☐ 6. A client with an inadequate intake of calcium and vitamin D

Level of Cognitive Ability: Analyzing
Client Needs: Health Promotion and Maintenance
Integrated Process: Nursing Process/Assessment
Content Area: Developmental Stages: Health Assessment/Physical Exam
Priority Concepts: Health Promotion; Mobility

Answer: 1, 3, 4, 6
Rationale: Osteoporosis is a disorder characterized by abnormal loss of bone density and deterioration of bone tissue, with an increased fracture risk. Asian, white, small-boned, and fair-skinned women are at greatest risk for osteoporosis. Other risk factors include early menopause, a family history of the disease, and a sedentary lifestyle. Inadequate intake of calcium and vitamin D is a major risk factor because it results in abnormal loss of bone density and deterioration of bone tissue. Women who smoke, drink alcohol, or take corticosteroids or anticonvulsants, as well as those who consume excessive amounts of caffeine, also have increased risk for osteoporosis.
Priority Nursing Tip: A client with osteoporosis is at risk for pathological fractures.
Test-Taking Strategy: Focus on the subject, the risk factors for osteoporosis. Recalling that osteoporosis is characterized by an abnormal loss of bone density and deterioration of bone tissue will assist in identifying the risk factors. Also remember that small-boned, fair-skinned, white and Asian women are at greatest risk for osteoporosis. Review: osteoporosis risk factors.
Reference(s): Ignatavicius, Workman (2013), p. 1120; Lewis et al (2014), p. 1554.

631. The clinic nurse instructs a client with diabetes mellitus about how to prevent diabetic ketoacidosis on days when the client is feeling ill. Which statement by the client indicates the **need for further teaching**?

1. "I need to stop my insulin if I am vomiting."
2. "I need to eat 10 to 15 g of carbohydrates every 1 to 2 hours."
3. "I need to drink small quantities of fluid every 15 to 30 minutes."
4. "I need to call my health care provider if I am ill for more than 24 hours."

Level of Cognitive Ability: Evaluating
Client Needs: Health Promotion and Maintenance
Integrated Process: Teaching and Learning
Content Area: Adult Health: Endocrine
Priority Concepts: Client Education; Glucose Regulation

Answer: 1
Rationale: Diabetic ketoacidosis is a life-threatening complication of type 1 diabetes mellitus that develops when a severe insulin deficiency occurs. The client needs to be instructed to take insulin, even if he or she is vomiting and unable to eat. It is important to self-monitor blood glucose more frequently during illness (every 2 to 4 hours). If the premeal blood glucose is more than 250 mg/dL, the client should test for urine ketones and contact the health care provider. Options 2, 3, and 4 are accurate interventions.
Priority Nursing Tip: The primary clinical manifestations of diabetic ketoacidosis include hyperglycemia, dehydration, ketosis, and acidosis. The client will have a "fruity" breath odor.
Test-Taking Strategy: Note the strategic words, *need for further teaching.* These words indicate a negative event query and ask you to select an option that is an incorrect statement. Recalling that insulin must be taken every day will assist with directing you to the correct option. Review: the sick-day rules for the client with **diabetes mellitus.**
Reference(s): Ignatavicius, Workman (2013), p. 1456.

632. The nurse is instructing a client with diabetes mellitus regarding hypoglycemia. Which statement by the client indicates the **need for further teaching**?

1. "Hypoglycemia can occur at any time of the day or night."
2. "I can drink 6 to 8 ounces of milk if hypoglycemia occurs."
3. "If I feel sweaty or shaky, I might be experiencing hypoglycemia."
4. "If hypoglycemia occurs, I need to take my regular insulin as prescribed."

Level of Cognitive Ability: Evaluating
Client Needs: Health Promotion and Maintenance
Integrated Process: Teaching and Learning
Content Area: Adult Health: Endocrine
Priority Concepts: Client Education; Glucose Regulation

Answer: 4
Rationale: Hypoglycemia occurs when the blood glucose level falls below 70 mg/dL. Insulin is not taken as a treatment for hypoglycemia because the insulin will lower the blood glucose level. Hypoglycemic reactions can occur at any time of the day or night. If a hypoglycemic reaction occurs, the client will need to consume 10 to 15 g of carbohydrate; 6 to 8 ounces of milk for example, contain this amount of carbohydrate. Tremors and diaphoresis are signs of mild hypoglycemia.
Priority Nursing Tip: Never attempt to administer food or fluids to a client experiencing a severe hypoglycemic reaction who is semiconscious or unconscious and is unable to swallow because the client is at risk for aspiration.
Test-Taking Strategy: Note the strategic words, *need for further teaching.* These words indicate a negative event query and ask you to select an option that is an incorrect statement. Remember that the blood glucose level is lowered in clients with hypoglycemia. Insulin also lowers blood glucose; therefore, it would seem reasonable that insulin is not a treatment for this condition. Review: the signs/symptoms of **hypoglycemia** and the appropriate interventions.
Reference(s): Ignatavicius, Workman (2013), p. 1453.

633. A client with nephrolithiasis arrives at the clinic for a follow-up visit. The laboratory analysis of the stone that the client passed 1 week ago indicates that the stone is composed of calcium oxalate. On the basis of this analysis, the nurse should tell the client that it is **best** to avoid which food to minimize the risk of recurrence?

1. Pasta
2. Lentils
3. Lettuce
4. Spinach

Level of Cognitive Ability: Applying
Client Needs: Health Promotion and Maintenance
Integrated Process: Teaching and Learning
Content Area: Adult Health: Renal and Urinary
Priority Concepts: Client Education; Health Promotion

Answer: 4
Rationale: Many kidney stones are composed of calcium oxalate. Foods that raise urinary oxalate excretion include spinach, rhubarb, strawberries, chocolate, wheat bran, nuts, beets, almonds, cashews, rhubarb, and tea. Therefore, the client should avoid spinach.
Priority Nursing Tip: Renal colic originates in the lumbar region and radiates around the side and down to the testicles in men and to the bladder in women. Ureteral colic radiates toward the genitalia and thighs.
Test-Taking Strategy: Note the strategic word, *best,* and the subject, "the food to avoid," and focus on the type of stone and that it is composed of calcium oxalate. Recalling that foods such as spinach raise urinary oxalate excretion will direct you to the correct option. Review: the foods that raise **urinary oxalate** excretion.
Reference(s): Ignatavicius, Workman (2013), p. 1511; Nix (2013), p. 443.

634. The nurse provides instructions to a new mother who is about to breast-feed her newborn infant. The nurse observes the new mother as she breast-feeds for the first time and determines the mother **needs further teaching** if the new mother applies which technique?

1. Turns the newborn infant on his side, facing the mother
2. Tilts up the nipple or squeezes the areola, pushing it into the newborn's mouth
3. Draws the newborn the rest of the way onto the breast when the newborn opens his mouth
4. Places a clean finger in the side of the newborn's mouth to break the suction before removing the newborn from the breast

Level of Cognitive Ability: Evaluating
Client Needs: Health Promotion and Maintenance
Integrated Process: Teaching and Learning
Content Area: Maternity: Postpartum
Priority Concepts: Client Education; Health Promotion

Answer: 2
Rationale: The mother is instructed to avoid tilting up the nipple or squeezing the areola and pushing it into the newborn's mouth; doing so does not facilitate the breast-feeding process or the flow of milk. Options 1, 3, and 4 are correct procedures for breast-feeding.
Priority Nursing Tip: A breast-fed infant's stools are usually light yellow, seedy, watery, and frequent.
Test-Taking Strategy: Note the strategic words, *needs further teaching*. This creates a negative event query and asks you to select the incorrect client action. Visualize the descriptions in each of the options. This will eliminate options 1, 3, and 4. Also, carefully reading option 2 and noting the word *pushing*, which suggests force or resistance, should assist with directing you to this option. Review: the procedure for breast-feeding.
Reference(s): McKinney et al (2013), pp. 536-537.

635. The clinic nurse provides home care instructions to a mother regarding the care of her child who is diagnosed with croup. Which statement by the mother indicates the **need for further instructions?**

1. "I will give Tylenol for the fever."
2. "I will give cough syrup every night at bedtime."
3. "Sips of warm fluids during a croup attack will help."
4. "I will place a cool-mist humidifier next to my child's bed."

Level of Cognitive Ability: Evaluating
Client Needs: Health Promotion and Maintenance
Integrated Process: Teaching and Learning
Content Area: Child Health: Throat/Respiratory
Priority Concepts: Client Education; Health Promotion

Answer: 2
Rationale: The mother needs to be instructed that cough syrup and cold medicines should not be administered because they may dry and thicken secretions. Acetaminophen (Tylenol) will reduce the fever. Sips of warm fluid will relax the vocal cords and thin the mucus. A cool-mist humidifier rather than a steam vaporizer is recommended because of the danger of the child pulling the machine over and causing a burn.
Priority Nursing Tip: Monitor the child with croup for signs/symptoms of respiratory distress, including nasal flaring, sternal retraction, and inspiratory stridor.
Test-Taking Strategy: Note the strategic words, *need for further instructions*. These words indicate a negative event query and ask you to select an option that is an incorrect statement. Option 1 can be eliminated first, recalling that acetaminophen (Tylenol) is normally prescribed to reduce a fever. Recalling that warm fluids will thin secretions will assist you in eliminating option 3. From the remaining options, recalling that cough syrup will dry secretions will assist with directing you to the correct option. Review: the home care instructions for the child with croup.
Reference(s): McKinney et al (2013), pp. 1161-1162.

636. A client with anxiety disorder is taking buspirone (BuSpar) orally. The client tells the nurse that it is difficult to swallow the tablets. The nurse provides which instruction to the client to promote compliance?
1. Crush the tablets before taking them.
2. Mix the tablet uncrushed in applesauce.
3. Purchase the liquid preparation with the next refill.
4. Call the health care provider for a change in medication.

Level of Cognitive Ability: Applying
Client Needs: Health Promotion and Maintenance
Integrated Process: Nursing Process/Implementation
Content Area: Pharmacology: Psychiatric Medications
Priority Concepts: Adherence; Client Education

Answer: 1
Rationale: Buspirone (BuSpar) may be administered without regard to meals, and the tablets may be crushed. Mixing the tablet uncrushed in applesauce will not ensure ease of swallowing. It is premature to advise the client to call the health care provider for a change in medication without first trying alternative interventions. This medication is not available in liquid form.
Priority Nursing Tip: Most tablets can be crushed if needed to facilitate administration. Enteric-coated and sustained-released tablets are not to be crushed. Additionally, capsules are not to be crushed.
Test-Taking Strategy: Focus on the subject, buspirone (BuSpar). Eliminate option 4 first because, in most situations, a nursing intervention can be instituted before calling the health care provider. Next, eliminate option 2 because this instruction will not ensure ease of swallowing. From the remaining options, it is necessary to know that this medication is not available in liquid form. Review: buspirone (BuSpar).
Reference(s): Hodgson, Kizior (2014), pp. 160-161.

637. The nurse caring for a child with heart failure who will be discharged to home provides instructions to the parents regarding the administration of digoxin (Lanoxin). Which statement by the mother indicates a **need for further teaching**?
1. "I will mix the medication with food."
2. "I will check my child's pulse before giving the medication."
3. "If my child vomits after I give the medication, I will not repeat the dose."
4. "I will check the dose of medication with my husband before I give the medication."

Level of Cognitive Ability: Evaluating
Client Needs: Health Promotion and Maintenance
Integrated Process: Teaching and Learning
Content Area: Pharmacology: Cardiovascular Medications
Priority Concepts: Client Education; Safety

Answer: 1
Rationale: Digoxin (Lanoxin) is a cardiac glycoside. The medication should not be mixed with food or formula because this method would not ensure that the child receives the entire dose of medication. Options 2, 3, and 4 are correct. Additionally, if a dosage is missed and this is not identified until 4 or more hours later, the dose is not administered. If more than one consecutive dose is missed, the health care provider needs to be notified.
Priority Nursing Tip: Signs of digoxin (Lanoxin) toxicity in an infant include poor feeding and vomiting.
Test-Taking Strategy: Note the strategic words, *need for further teaching*. These words indicate a negative event query and ask you to select an option that is an incorrect statement. General principles regarding medication administration to children should assist with directing you to the correct option. Mixing medications with formula or food may alter the effectiveness of the medication. More important, if the child does not consume all of the formula or food, the total dosage may not be administered. Review: the parental instructions regarding the administration of **digoxin (Lanoxin)**.
Reference(s): Hockenberry, Wilson (2013), p. 839; McKinney et al (2013), p. 1207.

638. The nurse provides discharge instructions to the mother of a child who was hospitalized for heart surgery. Which instruction should the nurse provide to the mother?

1. The child can play outside for short periods of time.
2. After bathing, rub lotion and sprinkle powder on the incision.
3. The child may return to school 1 week after hospital discharge.
4. The health care provider is to be notified if the child develops a fever of more than 100.5° F.

Level of Cognitive Ability: Applying
Client Needs: Health Promotion and Maintenance
Integrated Process: Teaching and Learning
Content Area: Child Health: Cardiovascular
Priority Concepts: Client Education; Safety

Answer: 4
Rationale: After heart surgery, the health care provider must be notified if the child develops a fever of more than 100.5° F. The mother is instructed to not allow the child to play outside for several weeks. No creams, lotions, or powders should be placed on the incision until it is completely healed and without scabs. The child should not return to school until 3 weeks after hospital discharge, at which time the child should go to school for half days for the first few days.
Priority Nursing Tip: Immunizations, dental visits, and invasive procedures must be avoided for 2 months in the child who had cardiac surgery.
Test-Taking Strategy: Note the subject, a child who was hospitalized for heart surgery. Keep in mind the potential for infection in this child. Eliminate option 1 because outside play can expose the child to infection and the risk of injury. Eliminate option 3 because of the time frame of 1 week. Basic principles related to incision care should assist you in eliminating option 2. Review: the home care instructions for the child after **heart surgery**.
Reference(s): McKinney et al (2013), p. 1224.

639. The clinic nurse provides instructions to a client who will begin taking oral contraceptives. Which statement by the client indicates **the need for further teaching**?

1. "I will take one pill daily at the same time every day."
2. "If I miss a pill, I must take it as soon as I remember."
3. "I will not need to use an additional birth control method after I start these pills."
4. "If I miss two pills, I will take them both as soon as I remember, and I will take two pills the next day also."

Level of Cognitive Ability: Evaluating
Client Needs: Health Promotion and Maintenance
Integrated Process: Teaching and Learning
Content Area: Adult Health: Reproductive
Priority Concepts: Client Education; Reproduction

Answer: 3
Rationale: The client must be instructed to use a second birth control method during the first pill cycle of contraceptives. Options 1, 2, and 4 are correct. Additionally, the client must be instructed that, if she misses three pills, she will need to discontinue pill use for that cycle and use another birth control method.
Priority Nursing Tip: Contraceptives provide reversible prevention of pregnancy.
Test-Taking Strategy: Note the strategic words, *need for further teaching*. These words indicate a negative event query and ask you to select an option that is an incorrect statement. It would seem reasonable that, during the first pill cycle, a second birth control method would need to be used to prevent conception. Review: guidelines for **oral contraceptive** administration.
Reference(s): Kee, Hayes, McCuistion (2012), p. 877; Lehne (2013), p. 794.

640. The nurse is providing home care dietary instructions to a client who has been hospitalized for pancreatitis. Which food should the nurse instruct the client to avoid to prevent recurrence?

1. Chili
2. Bagels
3. Lentil soup
4. Watermelon

Level of Cognitive Ability: Applying
Client Needs: Health Promotion and Maintenance
Integrated Process: Teaching and Learning
Content Area: Adult Health: Gastrointestinal
Priority Concepts: Client Education; Inflammation

Answer: 1
Rationale: Pancreatitis is the acute or chronic inflammation of the pancreas with the associated escape of pancreatic enzymes into surrounding tissue. The client must avoid spicy foods, alcohol, coffee, tea, and heavy meals because they stimulate pancreatic secretions and produce attacks of pancreatitis. The client is instructed regarding the benefit of eating small, frequent meals that are high in protein, low in fat, and moderate to high in carbohydrates.
Priority Nursing Tip: Cullen's sign is the discoloration of the abdomen and periumbilical area. Turner's sign is the bluish coloration of the flanks. Both are signs indicative of pancreatitis.
Test-Taking Strategy: Focus on the subject, the food item to avoid. Note that options 2, 3, and 4 are foods that are moderately bland. Option 1 is different in that chili is a spicy food. Review: the dietary measures for the client with **pancreatitis**.
Reference(s): Ignatavicius, Workman (2013), p. 1328; Lewis et al (2014), p. 1032.

641. The home care nurse visits a client who was recently diagnosed with cirrhosis and provides home care management instructions to the client. Which statement by the client indicates the **need for further teaching**?
1. "I will obtain adequate rest."
2. "I should monitor my weight regularly."
3. "I should include sufficient carbohydrates in my diet."
4. "I will take acetaminophen (Tylenol) if I get a headache."

Level of Cognitive Ability: Evaluating
Client Needs: Health Promotion and Maintenance
Integrated Process: Teaching and Learning
Content Area: Adult Health: Gastrointestinal
Priority Concepts: Client Education; Safety

Answer: 4
Rationale: Cirrhosis is a chronic progressive disease of the liver characterized by diffuse degeneration and destruction of hepatocytes. Acetaminophen (Tylenol) is avoided because it can cause fatal liver damage in the client with cirrhosis. Adequate rest and nutrition are important. The client's weight should be monitored regularly. The diet should supply sufficient carbohydrates with a total daily intake of 2000 to 3000 calories.
Priority Nursing Tip: In cirrhosis, the repeated destruction of hepatic cells causes the formation of scar tissue.
Test-Taking Strategy: Note the strategic words, *need for further teaching*. These words indicate a negative event query and ask you to select an option that is an incorrect statement. Recalling that acetaminophen (Tylenol) is a hepatotoxic agent will assist with directing you to option 4. Review: the medications that are restricted or avoided in clients with cirrhosis.
Reference(s): Ignatavicius, Workman (2013), p. 1304.

642. A client has a history of urolithiasis related to hyperuricemia. To prevent the formation of future stones, the nurse instructs the client to avoid which food?
1. Liver
2. Carrots
3. White rice
4. Skim milk

Level of Cognitive Ability: Applying
Client Needs: Health Promotion and Maintenance
Integrated Process: Teaching and Learning
Content Area: Adult Health: Renal and Urinary
Priority Concepts: Client Education; Health Promotion

Answer: 1
Rationale: Because the client has a high level of uric acid in the blood and a history of kidney stones from crystallized uric acid in the renal pelvis, the nurse instructs the client to avoid foods that contain high amounts of purines because these foods contain a high concentration of uric acid. This includes limiting or avoiding organ meats, such as liver, brain, heart, and kidney. Other foods to avoid include sweetbreads, herring, sardines, anchovies, meat extracts, consommés, and gravies. Foods that are low in purines include all fruits, many vegetables, milk, cheese, eggs, refined cereals, coffee, tea, chocolate, and carbonated beverages.
Priority Nursing Tip: Allopurinol (Zyloprim) is a medication that may be prescribed to lower uric acid levels.
Test-Taking Strategy: Focus on the subject, the client's diagnosis of urolithiasis related to hyperuricemia. Also note the word *avoid*. Because purines are end products of protein metabolism, eliminate options 2 and 3 first. From the remaining options, recall that organ meats such as liver provide a greater quantity of protein than milk does. Review: the dietary instructions for the client with uric acid stones.
Reference(s): Ignatavicius, Workman (2013), p. 1511; Nix (2013), pp. 443-444.

643. A client tells the nurse that he gets dizzy and lightheaded with each use of the incentive spirometer. The nurse asks the client to demonstrate the use of the device. Which action should the nurse expect to be a contributing factor in this client's symptoms?
1. Inhaling too slowly
2. Exhaling too slowly
3. Not resting adequately between breaths
4. Not forming a tight seal around the mouthpiece

Level of Cognitive Ability: Evaluating
Client Needs: Health Promotion and Maintenance
Integrated Process: Nursing Process/Evaluation
Content Area: Adult Health: Respiratory
Priority Concepts: Client Education; Gas Exchange

Answer: 3
Rationale: Hyperventilation is the most common cause of respiratory alkalosis, which is characterized by lightheadedness and dizziness. If the client does not breathe normally between incentive spirometer breaths, hyperventilation and fatigue can result.
Priority Nursing Tip: Instruct the client to assume a sitting or upright position when using an incentive spirometer.
Test-Taking Strategy: Focus on the subject, the cause of the lightheadedness and dizziness when using an incentive spirometer. Think about each of the actions described in the options to direct you to option 3. Options 1, 2, and 4 would result in ineffective use but would not cause dizziness and lightheadedness. Review: the procedure for the use of the incentive spirometer.
Reference(s): Ignatavicius, Workman (2013), p. 256; Potter et al (2013), pp. 848, 1288-1289.

644. The nurse is conducting a health screening clinic. The nurse interprets that which client participating in the screening is the **highest priority** client to provide instruction to lower the risk of developing respiratory disease?
1. A 36-year-old who works with pesticides
2. A 40-year-old smoker who works in a hospital
3. A 25-year-old who does woodworking as a hobby
4. A 50-year-old smoker who has cracked asbestos lining on the basement pipes in her home

Level of Cognitive Ability: Analyzing
Client Needs: Health Promotion and Maintenance
Integrated Process: Nursing Process/Assessment
Content Area: Adult Health: Respiratory
Priority Concepts: Clinical Judgment; Gas Exchange

Answer: 4
Rationale: Smoking greatly enhances the client's risk of developing some form of respiratory disease. Other risk factors include exposure to harmful chemicals, airborne toxins, and dust or fumes. For the options provided, the client who is at the greatest risk has two identified risk factors, one of which is smoking.
Priority Nursing Tip: Risk factors for respiratory disorders include smoking and the use of chewing tobacco, allergies, crowded living conditions, exposure to chemicals and environmental pollutants, family history of infectious diseases, frequent respiratory illnesses and viral syndromes, surgery, and travel to foreign countries.
Test-Taking Strategy: Note the strategic words, *highest priority.* Eliminate options 1 and 3 first because the most harmful risk factor for the respiratory system is smoking. From the remaining options, select option 4 because asbestos is toxic to the lungs if its particles are inhaled. In addition, two risk factors are identified in option 4, which makes this client at greater risk than the others, who have only one factor identified. Review: the risk factors associated with **respiratory disease.**
Reference(s): Ignatavicius, Workman (2013), pp. 549-550.

645. The nurse has conducted teaching with a client who experienced pulmonary embolism about methods to prevent recurrence after discharge from the hospital. Which client statement shows understanding of the teaching?
1. "I will limit the intake of fluids."
2. "I will sit down whenever possible."
3. "I am planning to continue to wear supportive hose."
4. "I will cross my legs only at the ankle and not at the knees."

Level of Cognitive Ability: Evaluating
Client Needs: Health Promotion and Maintenance
Integrated Process: Nursing Process/Evaluation
Content Area: Adult Health: Respiratory
Priority Concepts: Client Education; Gas Exchange

Answer: 3
Rationale: The recurrence of pulmonary embolism can be minimized with the wearing of elastic or supportive hose because these hose enhance venous return. The client should take in sufficient fluids to prevent hemoconcentration and hypercoagulability. The client also enhances venous return by interspersing periods of sitting with walking, avoiding crossing the legs at the knees or ankles and doing active foot and ankle exercises.
Priority Nursing Tip: Pulmonary embolism occurs when a thrombus forms (most commonly in a deep vein), detaches, travels to the right side of the heart, and then lodges in a branch of the pulmonary artery.
Test-Taking Strategy: Note the subject of preventing reoccurrence of pulmonary embolism. Recalling that promoting venous return will prevent pulmonary embolism will direct you to the correct option. Review: the measures that will prevent the recurrence of **pulmonary embolism.**
Reference(s): Ignatavicius, Workman (2013), p. 663.

646. A female client is being discharged from the hospital to home with an indwelling urinary catheter after the surgical repair of the bladder after trauma. The nurse determines that the client understands the principles of catheter management to prevent complications if the client states that she will follow which instruction?
1. Cleanse the perineal area with soap and water once a day.
2. Keep the drainage bag lower than the level of the bladder.
3. Limit fluid intake so that the bag will not become full so quickly.
4. Coil the tubing and place it under the thigh when sitting to avoid tugging on the bladder.

Level of Cognitive Ability: Evaluating
Client Needs: Health Promotion and Maintenance
Integrated Process: Nursing Process/Evaluation
Content Area: Adult Health: Renal and Urinary
Priority Concepts: Client Education; Elimination

Answer: 2
Rationale: The drainage bag of an indwelling urinary catheter should be lower than the level of the bladder and the tubing should be free of kinks and compression. The perineal area should be cleansed twice daily and after each bowel movement with soap and water. Adequate fluid intake is necessary to prevent infection and provide natural irrigation of the catheter from increased urine flow. Coiling the tubing and placing it under the thigh can compress the tube.
Priority Nursing Tip: The total bladder capacity is 1 L. The normal adult urine output is 1500 mL/day.
Test-Taking Strategy: Note the subject, a client with an indwelling urinary catheter. Option 4 is eliminated first because sitting on coiled tubing could cause compression and obstruct drainage. Option 3 is eliminated next because increased fluids are important. From the remaining options, noting the words *once a day* in option 1 will assist you in eliminating this option. Review: the principles related to **urinary catheter care.**
Reference(s): Perry, Potter, Ostendorf (2014), p. 821; Potter et al (2013), pp. 1063, 1077-1078.

647. A 24-year-old woman with a family history of heart disease presents to the health care provider's office asking to begin oral contraceptive therapy for birth control. What important topic should the nurse ask the client about **next?**
1. Smoking
2. Regular exercise
3. A low-cholesterol diet
4. Alternative birth control methods

Level of Cognitive Ability: Analyzing
Client Needs: Health Promotion and Maintenance
Integrated Process: Nursing Process/Assessment
Content Area: Adult Health: Reproductive
Priority Concepts: Health Promotion; Reproduction

Answer: 1
Rationale: Oral contraceptive use is a risk factor for heart disease, particularly when it is combined with cigarette smoking. Regular exercise and keeping total cholesterol levels less than 200 mg/dL are general measures to decrease cardiovascular risk.
Priority Nursing Tip: Oral contraceptives are usually taken for 21 consecutive days and stopped for 7 days; the administration cycle is then repeated.
Test-Taking Strategy: Note the strategic word, *next*. Remember that smoking is the item that is linked to oral contraceptive use to make it a risk factor for cardiovascular disease. This will direct you to option 1. Review: the risks associated with the use of **oral contraceptives.**
Reference(s): Kee, Hayes, McCuistion (2012), pp. 875, 877; Lehne (2013), p. 789.

648. The nurse is teaching a client with atrial fibrillation about the need to begin long-term anticoagulant therapy. Which explanation should the nurse use to best describe the reasoning for this therapy?
1. "Because of this dysrhythmia, blood backs up in the legs and puts you at risk for blood clots."
2. "This dysrhythmia decreases the volume of blood flowing from the heart, which can lead to blood clots forming in the brain."
3. "The antidysrhythmic medications you are taking cause blood clots as a side effect, so you need this medication to prevent them."
4. "Because the atria are quivering, blood flows sluggishly through them, and clots can form along the heart wall, which could then loosen and travel to the lungs or brain."

Level of Cognitive Ability: Applying
Client Needs: Health Promotion and Maintenance
Integrated Process: Nursing Process/Implementation
Content Area: Adult Health: Cardiovascular
Priority Concepts: Client Education; Perfusion

Answer: 4
Rationale: A severe complication of atrial fibrillation is the development of mural thrombi. The blood stagnates in the "quivering" atria because of the loss of organized atrial muscle contraction and "atrial kick." The blood that pools in the atria can then clot, which increases the risk of pulmonary and cerebral emboli. Options 1, 2, and 3 do not provide accurate descriptions of the purpose for anticoagulant therapy.
Priority Nursing Tip: On a cardiac monitor, atrial fibrillation can be easily recognized because usually there is no definitive P wave; fibrillatory waves before each QRS are noted.
Test-Taking Strategy: Note the subject, a client with atrial fibrillation beginning long-term anticoagulant therapy. Note the relationship between the client's diagnosis of atrial fibrillation and the words *atria are quivering* in option 4. Review: the pathophysiology of **atrial fibrillation**.
Reference(s): Ignatavicius, Workman (2013), pp. 722, 727.

649. The clinic nurse is providing instructions to a client in the third trimester of pregnancy regarding relief measures for heartburn. Which instruction should the nurse provide to the client?
1. Sip on milk or hot tea.
2. Use antacids that contain sodium.
3. Eat fatty foods once a day in the morning only.
4. Eat three large meals a day rather than small, frequent meals.

Level of Cognitive Ability: Applying
Client Needs: Health Promotion and Maintenance
Integrated Process: Nursing Process/Implementation
Content Area: Maternity: Antepartum
Priority Concepts: Client Education; Health Promotion

Answer: 1
Rationale: Measures to provide relief of heartburn include frequent sips of milk or hot tea; avoiding fatty and fried foods, coffee, and cigarettes; and eating small, frequent meals. Mild antacids can be used if they do not contain aspirin or sodium.
Priority Nursing Tip: In pregnancy, heartburn most often occurs in the second and third trimesters and results from increased progesterone levels, decreased gastrointestinal motility, esophageal reflux, and displacement of the stomach by the enlarging uterus.
Test-Taking Strategy: Note the subject, teaching a pregnant client how to avoid heartburn. Eliminate option 2 first because sodium will lead to edema, and edema should be avoided, especially during pregnancy. Eliminate option 3 next on the basis of basic nutritional principles that fatty and fried foods should be avoided. From the remaining options, recalling that milk and hot tea can be soothing to the gastrointestinal tract will assist you in eliminating option 4. Review: the measures that relieve **heartburn**.
Reference(s): Lowdermilk, Perry, Cashion, Alden (2012), p. 354; McKinney et al (2013), p. 252.

650. The nurse provides instructions regarding home care to a parent of a 3-year-old child who has been hospitalized with hemophilia. Which statement by the parent indicates the **need for further teaching**?

1. "I should not leave my child unattended."
2. "I need to pad table corners in my home."
3. "My child should not have any immunizations."
4. "I need to remove household items that can tip over."

Level of Cognitive Ability: Evaluating
Client Needs: Health Promotion and Maintenance
Integrated Process: Teaching and Learning
Content Area: Child Health: Hematological
Priority Concepts: Client Education; Clotting

Answer: 3
Rationale: Hemophilia refers to a group of bleeding disorders resulting from a deficiency of specific coagulation proteins. The nurse must stress the importance of immunizations, dental hygiene, and routine well-child care. Options 1, 2, and 4 are appropriate. The parent should also be instructed regarding measures to implement if blunt trauma occurs (especially trauma involving the joints) and how to apply prolonged pressure to superficial wounds until the bleeding has stopped.
Priority Nursing Tip: Bleeding is a primary concern for the child with hemophilia. Teach the parents about safety measures to implement to prevent injury such as wearing protective devices (helmets and knee and elbow pads) when participating in sports such as bicycling.
Test-Taking Strategy: Note the strategic words, *need for further teaching.* These words indicate a negative event query and ask you to select an option that is an incorrect statement. Recalling that bleeding is a concern in clients with this disorder will assist you in eliminating options 1, 2, and 4, which include measures of protection and safety for the child. Recalling the importance of immunizations will direct you to the correct option. Review: the care of the child with hemophilia.
Reference(s): McKinney et al (2013), p. 1255.

651. The nurse provides instructions to the client taking clorazepate (Tranxene) for the management of an anxiety disorder. What information related to this medication should the nurse provide to the client?

1. Dizziness is a side effect.
2. If drowsiness occurs, call the health care provider.
3. Smoking increases the effectiveness of the medication.
4. If gastrointestinal disturbances occur, discontinue the medication.

Level of Cognitive Ability: Applying
Client Needs: Health Promotion and Maintenance
Integrated Process: Teaching and Learning
Content Area: Pharmacology: Psychiatric Medications
Priority Concepts: Client Education; Safety

Answer: 1
Rationale: Dizziness is a side effect of this medication. The client should be instructed that if dizziness occurs, he or she should change positions slowly from lying to sitting to standing. Drowsiness is also a side effect that diminishes with continued therapy and does not warrant the need to contact the health care provider. Smoking reduces medication effectiveness. Gastrointestinal disturbance is an occasional side effect, and the medication can be given with food if this occurs.
Priority Nursing Tip: Clorazepate (Tranxene) is a benzodiazepine. Abrupt withdrawal of benzodiazepines can be potentially life-threatening, and withdrawal should occur only under medical supervision.
Test-Taking Strategy: Note the subject, clorazepate (Tranxene). Eliminate option 4 first because the client should not be instructed to discontinue the medication. Eliminate option 2 because episodes of drowsiness commonly occur with antianxiety medications. Eliminate option 3 next because smoking reduces medication effectiveness. Review: the client teaching points related to **clorazepate (Tranxene).**
Reference(s): Hodgson, Kizior (2014), pp. 269-271.

652. The client with prostatitis asks the nurse, "Why do I need to take a stool softener? The problem is with my urine, not my bowels!" Which response should the nurse make to the client?

1. "This is a standard medication prescription for anyone with a urine problem."
2. "This will keep the bowel free of feces, which helps decrease the swelling inside."
3. "Being constipated puts you at more risk for developing complications of prostatitis."
4. "This will help you prevent constipation because straining is painful with prostatitis."

Level of Cognitive Ability: Applying
Client Needs: Health Promotion and Maintenance
Integrated Process: Nursing Process/Implementation
Content Area: Adult Health: Renal and Urinary
Priority Concepts: Client Education; Inflammation

Answer: 4
Rationale: Prostatitis is an inflammation of the prostate gland. Stool softeners are prescribed for the client with prostatitis to prevent constipation, which can be painful. Stool softeners are not a standard prescription for "anyone with a urine problem." Stool softeners have no direct effect on decreasing swelling. Constipation does not cause complications of prostatitis.
Priority Nursing Tip: Bacterial prostatitis occurs as a result of an organism reaching the prostate via the urethra, bladder, bloodstream, or lymphatic channels. The bacterial type usually occurs after a viral illness or a decrease in sexual activity.
Test-Taking Strategy: Note the subject, a client with prostatitis taking a stool softener. Recalling the purpose and use of stool softeners to prevent constipation will direct you to option 4. Review: the care of the client with **prostatitis**.
Reference(s): Ignatavicius, Workman (2013), p. 1649.

653. A client with Parkinson's disease has begun therapy with levodopa (Dopar). The nurse determines that the client understands the action of the medication if the client verbalizes that results may not be apparent for what period of time?

1. 1 week
2. 24 hours
3. 5 to 7 days
4. 2 to 3 weeks

Level of Cognitive Ability: Evaluating
Client Needs: Health Promotion and Maintenance
Integrated Process: Nursing Process/Evaluation
Content Area: Pharmacology: Neurological Medications
Priority Concepts: Client Education; Safety

Answer: 4
Rationale: Parkinson's disease is a degenerative illness caused by the depletion of dopamine. Signs and symptoms of Parkinson's disease usually begin to resolve within 2 to 3 weeks after starting therapy, although in some clients marked improvement may not be seen for up to 6 months. Clients must understand this concept to aid in their compliance with medication therapy.
Priority Nursing Tip: Levodopa taken with a monoamine oxidase inhibitor antidepressant can cause a hypertensive crisis.
Test-Taking Strategy: Note the subject, levodopa (Dopar) and recall knowledge regarding this medication. Eliminate options 1 and 3 because they involve similar time frames. From the remaining options, eliminate option 2 because it is unlikely that results would be noted in 24 hours. Review the initial therapeutic range of **levodopa (Dopar)**.
Reference(s): Lewis et al (2014), p. 1435.

❖ **654.** The nurse provides information to a client about performing a breast self-examination (BSE). The nurse determines that the client **needs additional teaching** if the client makes which statements? **Select all that apply.**
- ❑ 1. "The BSE must be done monthly."
- ❑ 2. "Lumps in my armpit area are normal."
- ❑ 3. "I can palpate my breasts with soapy water while showering."
- ❑ 4. "I should perform the examination on the day that I start my period."
- ❑ 5. "When I squeeze my nipples, I should expect to note some discharge."
- ❑ 6. "I should stand before a mirror and inspect each breast for anything unusual."

Level of Cognitive Ability: Evaluating
Client Needs: Health Promotion and Maintenance
Integrated Process: Teaching and Learning
Content Area: Adult Health: Oncology
Priority Concepts: Client Education; Health Promotion

Answer: 2, 4, 5
Rationale: Any lumps (including lumps in the armpit) and nipple discharge are abnormal and must be reported to the health care provider immediately. The examination is performed 2 or 3 days after menstruation ends, when the breasts are least likely to be tender and swollen. The client is taught that BSE should be done once a month, so that the client becomes familiar with the usual feel and appearance of the breasts. The client is taught to palpate each breast and axillary area; this part of the examination can be performed in the shower using soap, which allows the fingers to glide easily over the skin. The client is taught to also stand before a mirror and inspect each breast for anything unusual.
Priority Nursing Tip: Postmenopausal clients or clients who have had a hysterectomy should select a specific day of the month and perform breast self-examination (BSE) monthly on that day.
Test-Taking Strategy: Note the strategic words, *needs additional teaching*. These words indicate a negative event query and ask you to select the options that are incorrect statements. Read each option carefully, and remember that the examination is performed 2 or 3 days after menstruation ends, when the breasts are least likely to be tender and swollen. Also, recalling that any lumps (including lumps in the armpit) and nipple discharge are abnormal will assist in answering correctly. Review: the procedure for **breast self-examination (BSE)**.
Reference(s): Potter et al (2013), pp. 538-540.

655. A client is being discharged to home after prostatectomy. Which point should the nurse plan to teach the client as part of the discharge teaching?
1. Mowing the lawn is allowed after 1 week.
2. Avoid lifting more than 50 pounds for 4 to 6 weeks after surgery.
3. Drink at least 15 glasses of water a day to minimize clot formation.
4. Notify the health care provider if fever, increased pain, or an inability to void occurs.

Level of Cognitive Ability: Applying
Client Needs: Health Promotion and Maintenance
Integrated Process: Teaching and Learning
Content Area: Adult Health: Renal and Urinary
Priority Concepts: Client Education; Health Promotion

Answer: 4
Rationale: The client should notify the health care provider if there are any signs/symptoms of infection, bleeding, increased pain, or urinary obstruction. Strenuous activities that could increase intra-abdominal tension are restricted, such as mowing the lawn. Lifting more than 20 pounds is prohibited for 4 to 6 weeks after surgery. The client should take in 6 to 8 glasses of water or nonalcoholic beverages per day to minimize the risk of clot formation (15 glasses a day is excessive).
Priority Nursing Tip: Sterility is a possible occurrence after prostatectomy.
Test-Taking Strategy: Focus on the subject, discharge teaching for a client after prostatectomy. Eliminate option 3 first as an excessive fluid intake. Noting that the activities identified in options 1 and 2 are also excessive will assist you in eliminating these options. Review: the home care measures after **prostatectomy**.
Reference(s): Ignatavicius, Workman (2013), pp. 1639, 1641.

656. The nurse is teaching a client with acute kidney injury to include proteins in the diet that are considered high quality or complete proteins. The nurse determines that the client **needs further teaching** if he indicates that which food item is considered high quality?
1. Fish
2. Eggs
3. Chicken
4. Broccoli

Level of Cognitive Ability: Evaluating
Client Needs: Health Promotion and Maintenance
Integrated Process: Teaching and Learning
Content Area: Adult Health: Renal and Urinary
Priority Concepts: Client Education; Nutrition

Answer: 4
Rationale: High-quality or complete proteins come from animal sources and include such foods as eggs, chicken, meat, and fish. Low-quality or incomplete proteins are derived from plant sources and include vegetables and foods made from grains. Because the renal diet is limited in protein, it is important that the proteins ingested are of high quality.
Priority Nursing Tip: High-quality proteins or complete proteins contain adequate amounts of essential amino acids.
Test-Taking Strategy: Note the strategic words, *needs further teaching*. These words indicate a negative event query and the need to select the food that is low-quality protein. When comparing the choices, note that option 4 is the only item that does not derive from an animal source. Fish, eggs, and chicken derive from animal sources, whereas broccoli is a plant. Review: the food items that are high- and low-quality proteins.
Reference(s): Nix (2013), pp. 60-61.

657. The home care nurse visits a client who had a stroke with resultant unilateral neglect who was recently discharged from the hospital. Which instruction should the nurse provide to the family regarding care?
1. Assist the client from the affected side.
2. Place personal items directly in front of the client.
3. Discourage the client from scanning the environment.
4. Assist the client with grooming the unaffected side first.

Level of Cognitive Ability: Applying
Client Needs: Health Promotion and Maintenance
Integrated Process: Teaching and Learning
Content Area: Adult Health: Neurological
Priority Concepts: Client Education; Safety

Answer: 1
Rationale: Unilateral neglect is a pattern of a lack of awareness of body parts such as paralyzed arms or legs. Initially the environment is adapted to the deficit by focusing on the client's unaffected side, and the client's personal items are placed on the unaffected side; gradually the client's attention is focused on the affected side. Therefore, the family is taught to assist the client from the affected side, and the client grooms the affected side first. The client needs to scan the entire environment.
Priority Nursing Tip: Cerebral anoxia lasting longer than 10 minutes causes cerebral infarction with irreversible change.
Test-Taking Strategy: Note the client's diagnosis of unilateral neglect and the subject, home care instructions. Recalling the physiological alteration that occurs with unilateral neglect and that it involves a pattern of a lack of awareness of body parts will direct you to option 1. Review: the interventions associated with unilateral neglect.
Reference(s): Ignatavicius, Workman (2013), pp. 1011, 1019.

658. The nurse has completed discharge teaching with a client who has had surgery for lung cancer. The nurse determines that the client **needs additional teaching** about the elements of home management if the client verbalizes the need to follow which instruction?
1. Avoid exposure to crowds.
2. Deal with any increases in pain independently.
3. Sit up and lean forward to breathe more easily.
4. Call the health care provider in case of increased temperature or shortness of breath.

Level of Cognitive Ability: Evaluating
Client Needs: Health Promotion and Maintenance
Integrated Process: Teaching and Learning
Content Area: Adult Health: Oncology
Priority Concepts: Client Education; Health Promotion

Answer: 2
Rationale: The client who just had surgery for lung cancer should not be expected to deal with increases in pain independently. Health teaching includes avoiding exposure to crowds or persons with respiratory infections and reporting signs and symptoms of respiratory infection or increases in pain. The client should also use positions that facilitate respiration, such as sitting up and leaning forward.
Priority Nursing Tip: Pain is a very individualized experience. It is what the client describes or says it is.
Test-Taking Strategy: Note the strategic words, *needs additional teaching*. These words indicate a negative event query and ask you to select an option that is an incorrect statement. Focusing on the client's diagnosis of lung cancer will direct you to option 2. Review: the home care measures for the client who has had surgery for lung cancer.
Reference(s): Ignatavicius, Workman (2013), p. 637; Potter et al (2013), pp. 743, 977.

659. A client weighs 165 pounds at admission. During hospitalization, the nurse determines that the client is maintaining adequate nutritional status if the client's weight is how many pounds?
1. 153 pounds
2. 155 pounds
3. 157 pounds
4. 160 pounds

Level of Cognitive Ability: Evaluating
Client Needs: Health Promotion and Maintenance
Integrated Process: Nursing Process/Evaluation
Content Area: Fundamental Skills: Nutrition
Priority Concepts: Health Promotion; Nutrition

Answer: 4
Rationale: The nurse determines that the client has maintained adequate nutritional status if the client maintains the baseline body weight or loses less than 5 pounds. The client's baseline weight is 165 pounds, so the acceptable range for the client's postoperative weight is 160 to 165 pounds.
Priority Nursing Tip: To obtain the most accurate weight, the client should be weighed in the morning at the same time of day as previous weights have been measured and with the same amount of clothing. The client should also void before the weight measurement.
Test-Taking Strategy: Focus on the subject, maintaining adequate nutritional status. In this situation, it is best to select the option that identifies the least amount of weight loss; this will direct you to the correct option. Review: adequate nutrition in the hospitalized client.
Reference(s): Ignatavicius, Workman (2013), pp. 1337, 1339; Potter et al (2013), pp. 1012, 1014.

---

660. The nurse has given the client with a non-plaster (fiberglass) leg cast instructions regarding cast care at home. The nurse determines that the client **needs further teaching** if the client makes which statement?
1. "I should avoid walking on wet, slippery floors."
2. "I'm not supposed to scratch the skin underneath the cast."
3. "It's all right to wipe dirt off of the top of the cast with a damp cloth."
4. "If the cast gets wet, I can dry it with a hair dryer turned to the hot setting."

Level of Cognitive Ability: Evaluating
Client Needs: Health Promotion and Maintenance
Integrated Process: Teaching and Learning
Content Area: Adult Health: Musculoskeletal
Priority Concepts: Client Education; Mobility

Answer: 4
Rationale: If the cast gets wet, it can be dried with a hair dryer set to a cool setting. The client is instructed to avoid walking on wet, slippery floors to prevent falls. If the skin under the cast itches, cool air from a hair dryer may be used to relieve it. The client should never scratch under the cast because of the risk of skin breakdown and infection. Surface soil on a cast may be removed with a damp cloth.
Priority Nursing Tip: Monitor a casted extremity for circulatory impairment such as pain, swelling, discoloration, tingling, numbness, coolness, or diminished pulse.
Test-Taking Strategy: Note the strategic words, *needs further teaching*. These words indicate a negative event query and ask you to select an option that is an incorrect statement. Noting the word *hot* in option 4 will direct you to this option. Review: the home care instructions for a client with a cast.
Reference(s): Perry, Potter, Ostendorf (2014), p. 256.

---

661. A child is seen in the health care clinic, and testing for human immunodeficiency virus (HIV) is performed because of the child's exposure to HIV infection. Which home care instruction should the nurse provide to the parents of the child?
1. Avoid sharing toothbrushes.
2. Avoid all immunizations until the diagnosis is established.
3. Wipe up any blood spills with a rag, and allow them to air dry.
4. Wash your hands with half-strength bleach if they come in contact with the child's blood.

Level of Cognitive Ability: Applying
Client Needs: Health Promotion and Maintenance
Integrated Process: Teaching and Learning
Content Area: Child Health: Infectious and Communicable Diseases
Priority Concepts: Client Education; Infection

Answer: 1
Rationale: Parents are instructed that toothbrushes are not to be shared. Immunizations must be kept up to date. Blood spills are wiped up with a paper towel; the area is then washed with soap and water, rinsed with bleach and water, and allowed to air dry. Hands are washed with soap and water if they come in contact with blood.
Priority Nursing Tip: Human immunodeficiency virus (HIV) infects CD4+ T cells. A gradual decrease in the count occurs, and this results in a progressive immunodeficiency. The risk for opportunistic infections is present.
Test-Taking Strategy: Note the subject, a child exposed to HIV infection. Eliminate option 2 first because of the closed-ended word "all." Eliminate option 3 next on the basis of the knowledge that blood spills must be cleaned with a bleach solution. Eliminate option 4 because bleach would be irritating and caustic to the skin. Review: the home care instructions for the child exposed to **human immunodeficiency virus (HIV)**.
Reference(s): McKinney et al (2013), p. 1053.

662. The nurse prepares a postoperative client who is ready for discharge for care at home. The client must receive continued intravenous (IV) therapy, so the nurse provides the client with instructions on caring for the IV site. Which is the **best** method of evaluating the client's ability to care for the IV site?
1. Have the client role-play an IV dressing change.
2. Invite the client to change the IV dressing unaided.
3. Direct the client to explain IV site care completely.
4. Ask the client to provide self-care before being discharged.

Level of Cognitive Ability: Evaluating
Client Needs: Health Promotion and Maintenance
Integrated Process: Nursing Process/Evaluation
Content Area: Fundamental Skills: Perioperative Care
Priority Concepts: Client Education; Safety

Answer: 2
Rationale: The best method for the nurse to use to evaluate the client's acquisition of psychomotor skills is to observe the client performing the skill; in this case, it is an IV dressing change. Role-playing is a suitable method of rehearsing a skill. Explanations are suitable to evaluate client knowledge of a skill, but they will not draw attention to the client's physical inability to perform the psychomotor function. If the nurse was evaluating client self-care, having the client function independently before discharge is suitable; however, the question is asking about IV site care.
Priority Nursing Tip: Aseptic technique must be used when performing intravenous (IV) therapy procedures.
Test-Taking Strategy: Use teaching and learning principles to answer the question, and note the strategic word, *best*. This means that all options may be correct, but you must choose the option that is the best choice. The correct option must identify some type of active client participation. This concept will direct you to option 2. Review **teaching and learning principles**.
Reference(s): Potter et al (2013), pp. 261, 329-330.

663. The nurse provides home care instructions to a client with cancer who has an implanted vascular access port. Which statement by the client indicates the **need for further teaching**?
1. "I should keep the site clean and dry."
2. "I should pump the port daily to maintain patency."
3. "If the site becomes red, I will notify my health care provider."
4. "The port will need to be flushed with saline to maintain patency."

Level of Cognitive Ability: Evaluating
Client Needs: Health Promotion and Maintenance
Integrated Process: Teaching and Learning
Content Area: Adult Health: Oncology
Priority Concepts: Client Education; Safety

Answer: 2
Rationale: An implanted vascular access port does not need to be pumped to maintain patency. The site will need to be kept clean and dry, and the health care provider would need to be notified about signs and symptoms of infection. Saline is usually used to flush the site to maintain patency; however, agency procedures should always be followed (some agencies use heparin as the flush solution).
Priority Nursing Tip: For accessing an implanted vascular access port, the port requires palpation and injection through the skin into the self-sealing port with a noncoring needle such as a Huber-point needle.
Test-Taking Strategy: Note the strategic words, *need for further teaching*. These words indicate a negative event query and ask you to select an option that is an incorrect statement. Using the principles related to vascular access ports and care of an intravenous line will direct you to option 2. Review: care of the client with an **implanted vascular access port**.
Reference(s): Ignatavicius, Workman (2013), pp. 218-220; Perry, Potter, Ostendorf (2014), pp. 724-725.

664. The nurse is caring for a client who is a survivor of a disaster event. The client begins to display behaviors not demonstrated before. Which manifestations would indicate to the nurse that the client may be experiencing posttraumatic stress disorder (PTSD)? **Select all that apply.**
- ❑ 1. Irritability and sleep disturbances
- ❑ 2. Flashbacks or recollections of the disaster
- ❑ 3. Regression to an earlier developmental stage
- ❑ 4. A feeling of estrangement or detachment from others
- ❑ 5. Consistent discussion and rationalizing as to why the disaster occurred
- ❑ 6. Repression or the inability to remember an important aspect associated with the disaster

Level of Cognitive Ability: Analyzing
Client Needs: Health Promotion and Maintenance
Integrated Process: Nursing Process/Assessment
Content Area: Mental Health
Priority Concepts: Anxiety; Mood and Affect

Answer: 1, 2, 4, 6
Rationale: PTSD is characterized by a sustained maladaptive response to a traumatic event. In this condition, the client experiences recurrent and intrusive recollections of the event (flashbacks), has recurrent dreams of the event, acts or feels as though the event were recurring, and experiences psychological distress when internal or external cues resemble the event. The individual avoids stimuli associated with the trauma or event (thoughts, feelings, conversations about the event, and persons or places that evoke memories of the event). The individual also is unable to remember an important aspect of the event (repression) and experiences somatic symptoms such as irritability and sleep disturbances. Regression to an earlier developmental stage and consistent discussion and rationalizing as to why the disaster occurred are not characteristics of PTSD.
Priority Nursing Tip: In posttraumatic stress disorder, the individual is prone to re-experience the traumatic event and have recurrent and intrusive dreams or flashbacks.
Test-Taking Strategy: Focus on the subject of PTSD and recall that PTSD is a condition characterized by a sustained maladaptive response to a traumatic event. Read each option and associate the manifestation with the description of the disorder to answer correctly. Review: manifestations indicative of posttraumatic stress disorder (PTSD).
Reference(s): Stuart, (2013), p. 228; Varcarolis (2013), p. 159.

665. The nurse has completed instructions regarding diet and fluid restriction for the client with chronic kidney disease. The nurse determines that the client understands the information presented if the client selected which dessert from the dietary menu?
1. Jell-O
2. Sherbet
3. Ice cream
4. Angel food cake

Level of Cognitive Ability: Evaluating
Client Needs: Health Promotion and Maintenance
Integrated Process: Nursing Process/Evaluation
Content Area: Adult Health: Renal and Urinary
Priority Concepts: Client Education; Fluid and Electrolyte Balance

Answer: 4
Rationale: For clients on a fluid-restricted diet, it is helpful to avoid "hidden" fluids to whatever extent possible. This allows the client to take in more fluid by drinking, which can help alleviate thirst. Dietary fluid includes anything that is liquid at room temperature. This includes items such as Jell-O, sherbet, and ice cream.
Priority Nursing Tip: Acute kidney injury is the rapid loss of kidney function from renal cell damage. Chronic kidney disease is a slow, progressive, irreversible loss in kidney function.
Test-Taking Strategy: Note the subject of a client with chronic kidney disease and the words *fluid restriction*. Recalling that dietary fluid includes anything that is liquid at room temperature will direct you to option 4. Review: this type of **dietary fluid restriction**.
Reference(s): Ignatavicius, Workman (2013), pp. 1555-1556; Perry, Potter, Ostendorf (2014), p. 765.

666. The nurse has given instructions to the client with chronic kidney disease about reducing pruritus from uremia. The nurse determines that the client **needs further teaching** if the client states the intention to use which item for skin care?
1. Mild soap
2. Oil in the bath water
3. Lanolin-based lotion
4. Alcohol cleansing pads

Level of Cognitive Ability: Evaluating
Client Needs: Health Promotion and Maintenance
Integrated Process: Teaching and Learning
Content Area: Adult Health: Renal and Urinary
Priority Concepts: Client Education; Tissue Integrity

Answer: 4
Rationale: The client with chronic kidney disease often has dry skin that is accompanied by itching (pruritus) from uremia. Products that contain perfumes or alcohol increase skin dryness and pruritus and these should be avoided. The client should use mild soaps, bath oils, and lotions to reduce dryness without increasing skin irritation.
Priority Nursing Tip: Uremic syndrome is the accumulation of nitrogenous waste products in the blood caused by the kidneys' inability to filter out these waste products.
Test-Taking Strategy: Focus on the subject of reducing pruritus, and note the strategic words, *needs further teaching*. These words indicate a negative event query and ask you to select an incorrect statement. Eliminate options 2 and 3 first because they are comparable or alike. From the remaining options, eliminate option 1, knowing that the client should avoid putting irritating products such as alcohol on the skin. Review: the measures for the treatment of **pruritus**.
Reference(s): Ignatavicius, Workman (2013), pp. 471, 1475, 1552.

❖ **667.** A battered woman seen in the emergency department requires tertiary intervention because of repeated abuse. Which nursing interventions are appropriate? **Select all that apply.**
❑ 1. Report the abuse to the police.
❑ 2. Provide medications to relieve pain and anxiety.
❑ 3. Explore family and friends as support possibilities.
❑ 4. Focus on the woman's strengths, endurance, and abilities.
❑ 5. Avoid discussing the implications of pressing charges against the batterer.
❑ 6. Discourage the woman from discussing the events leading to past and present abuse situations.

Level of Cognitive Ability: Applying
Client Needs: Health Promotion and Maintenance
Integrated Process: Nursing Process/Implementation
Content Area: Mental Health
Priority Concepts: Clinical Judgment; Interpersonal Violence

Answer: 1, 2, 3, 4
Rationale: Tertiary prevention is necessary when a woman has been repeatedly abused. The focus is on helping the abused woman overcome the physical and psychological effects of the abuse and preventing future abuse. Some of the interventions include reporting the abuse to the police to provide for safety; providing medications to relieve pain and anxiety; exploring family and friends as support possibilities to increase the woman's awareness of potential support; focusing on the woman's strengths, endurance, and abilities to increase her self-esteem; discussing the implications of pressing charges against the batterer to increase her awareness of abuse implications; and encouraging the woman to discuss the events leading to past and present abuse situations (this helps reduce guilt and shame).
Priority Nursing Tip: A victim of abuse may feel trapped in the situation, dependent, helpless, and powerless.
Test-Taking Strategy: Focus on the subject, tertiary intervention for abuse. Recall that the focus of tertiary prevention is on helping the abused woman overcome the physical and psychological effects of the abuse and preventing future abuse. Next read and visualize each intervention and relate it to the focus of tertiary intervention to select correctly. Review: **tertiary interventions** for the **battered woman.**
Reference(s): Varcarolis (2013), pp. 414-415.

668. The nurse provides information to a client who is scheduled for the implantation of an implantable cardioverter defibrillator (ICD) regarding care after implantation. The nurse tells the client that there is a need to keep a diary. What information should the nurse provide concerning the **primary** purpose of the diary?

1. Analyze which activities to avoid.
2. Document events that precipitate a countershock.
3. Provide a count of the number of shocks delivered.
4. Record a variety of data that are useful for the health care provider during medical management.

Level of Cognitive Ability: Applying
Client Needs: Health Promotion and Maintenance
Integrated Process: Teaching and Learning
Content Area: Adult Health: Cardiovascular
Priority Concepts: Client Education; Perfusion

Answer: 4
Rationale: The client with an ICD maintains a log or diary of a variety of data. This includes recording the date and time of the shock, any activity that took place before the shock, any symptoms experienced, the number of shocks delivered, and how the client felt after the shock. The information is used by the health care provider to adjust the medical regimen and especially the medication therapy, which must be maintained after ICD insertion.
Priority Nursing Tip: The client with an implantable cardioverter defibrillator (ICD) should be taught to wear loose-fitting clothing over the ICD generator site and avoid contact sports to prevent trauma to the ICD generator and lead wires.
Test-Taking Strategy: Note the strategic word, *primary.* Each of the incorrect options lists one of the items that should be logged in the diary, but the correct option is the only one that could be considered a "primary" purpose. Option 4 is also the umbrella option. Review: the home care instructions for the client with an **implantable cardioverter defibrillator (ICD).**
Reference(s): Ignatavicius, Workman (2013), p. 741.

669. The nurse is evaluating a hypertensive client's understanding of dietary modifications to control the disease process. The nurse determines that the client's understanding is satisfactory if the client made which meal selections?

1. Corned beef, fresh carrots, boiled potato
2. Hot dog on a bun, sauerkraut, baked beans
3. Turkey, baked potato, salad with oil and vinegar
4. Scallops, French fries, salad with bleu cheese dressing

Level of Cognitive Ability: Evaluating
Client Needs: Health Promotion and Maintenance
Integrated Process: Nursing Process/Evaluation
Content Area: Adult Health: Cardiovascular
Priority Concepts: Health Promotion; Perfusion

Answer: 3
Rationale: The client with hypertension should avoid foods that are high in sodium. Foods from the meat group that are higher in sodium include bacon, hot dogs, luncheon meat, chipped or corned beef, Kosher meat, smoked or salted meat or fish, peanut butter, and a variety of shellfish. Processed foods are also high in sodium.
Priority Nursing Tip: In addition to limiting sodium intake, the client with hypertension should reduce fat intake to prevent the development of atherosclerosis.
Test-Taking Strategy: Note the subject of a hypertensive client making dietary modifications. Eliminate options 1 and 2 because they are highly processed meats that would be high in sodium. From the remaining options, recalling that shellfish and commercial salad dressing are high in sodium will assist you in eliminating option 4. Review: foods that are high in **sodium** and **hypertension**
Reference(s): Ignatavicius, Workman (2013), p. 784; Nix (2013), p. 389.

670. The nurse has completed instructions with a client who will be taking warfarin sodium (Coumadin) indefinitely. Which statement by the client indicates the **need for further teaching?**
1. "I must use a soft toothbrush."
2. "I must use a straight razor for shaving."
3. "I must avoid drinking alcohol while taking this medication."
4. "I must carry identification regarding the medication being taken."

Level of Cognitive Ability: Evaluating
Client Needs: Health Promotion and Maintenance
Integrated Process: Teaching and Learning
Content Area: Pharmacology: Hematological Medications
Priority Concepts: Clotting; Safety

Answer: 2
Rationale: Client instructions for oral anticoagulant therapy include reporting any signs/symptoms of bleeding and implementing measures to prevent bleeding, taking the medication only as prescribed and at the same time each day, avoiding other medications (including over-the-counter medications) without health care provider approval, avoiding alcohol, notifying all caregivers about the medication, carrying a Medic-Alert bracelet or card, and adhering to the schedule for follow-up blood work.
Priority Nursing Tip: The antidote for warfarin sodium is vitamin K.
Test-Taking Strategy: Note the strategic words, *need for further teaching.* These words indicate a negative event query and ask you to select an option that is an incorrect statement. Recalling that warfarin sodium is an anticoagulant and the client is at risk for bleeding will direct you to option 2. Review: the home care instructions for the client taking **warfarin sodium (Coumadin).**
Reference(s): Hodgson, Kizior (2014), pp. 1262-1263.

671. The home care nurse has given instructions to a client who was recently discharged from the hospital regarding the care of an arterial ischemic leg ulcer. The nurse determines that there is a **need for further teaching** if the client makes which statement?
1. "I should inspect my feet daily."
2. "I should wear shoes and socks."
3. "I should cut my toenails straight across."
4. "I should raise my legs above the level of my heart periodically."

Level of Cognitive Ability: Evaluating
Client Needs: Health Promotion and Maintenance
Integrated Process: Teaching and Learning
Content Area: Adult Health: Cardiovascular
Priority Concepts: Client Education; Perfusion

Answer: 4
Rationale: Foot care instructions for the client with peripheral arterial ischemia are the same instructions given to the client with diabetes mellitus. The client with arterial disease, however, should avoid raising the legs above heart level unless instructed to do so as part of an exercise program (such as Buerger's postural exercises) or venous stasis is also present. Options 1, 2, and 3 are accurate client statements.
Priority Nursing Tip: A manifestation of peripheral arterial disease is intermittent claudication (pain in the muscles resulting from an inadequate blood supply).
Test-Taking Strategy: Note the strategic words, *need for further teaching.* These words indicate a negative event query and ask you to select an option that is an incorrect statement. Note that the client has an arterial disorder. Recalling the anatomy of the blood vessels and the pattern of blood flow in the arteries will direct you to option 4. Review: the home care instructions for the client with an **arterial ischemic leg ulcer.**
Reference(s): Ignatavicius, Workman (2013), p. 791.

672. A client with chronic kidney disease is about to begin hemodialysis therapy. The client asks the nurse about the frequency and scheduling of hemodialysis treatments. What information should the nurse supply to the client regarding the typical hemodialysis schedule?
1. It is 2 hours of treatment 6 days per week
2. It is 5 hours of treatment 2 days per week
3. It is 2 to 3 hours of treatment 5 days per week
4. It is 3 to 4 hours of treatment 3 days per week

Level of Cognitive Ability: Applying
Client Needs: Health Promotion and Maintenance
Integrated Process: Nursing Process/Implementation
Content Area: Adult Health: Renal and Urinary
Priority Concepts: Client Education; Fluid and Electrolyte Balance

Answer: 4
Rationale: The typical schedule for hemodialysis is 3 to 4 hours of treatment 3 days per week. Individual adjustments may be made according to certain variables, such as the size of the client, the type of dialyzer, the rate of blood flow, and personal client preferences.
Priority Nursing Tip: Monitor the client's vital signs before, during, and after dialysis. The client's temperature may elevate because of slight warming of the blood from the dialysis machine. However, the health care provider should be notified if temperature elevations are excessive because this could indicate sepsis.
Test-Taking Strategy: Focus on the subject, the "typical" hemodialysis schedule. Recalling that the client receives dialysis 3 days per week will direct you to option 4. Review: the typical **hemodialysis** schedule.
Reference(s): Ignatavicius, Workman (2013), pp. 1559-1560.

673. The nurse prepares a client for discharge from the hospital with a peripheral intravenous (IV) site for home IV therapy. Which should the nurse teach the client to help prevent phlebitis and infiltration?
1. Massage the IV site daily.
2. Immobilize the extremity.
3. Stabilize the cannula with tape.
4. Cleanse the site daily with alcohol.

Level of Cognitive Ability: Applying
Client Needs: Health Promotion and Maintenance
Integrated Process: Teaching and Learning
Content Area: Fundamental Skills: Safety
Priority Concepts: Client Education; Safety

Answer: 3
Rationale: Providing IV therapy at home involves the same principles as are used in the hospital. Protecting the IV site and securing it with tape are extremely important to ensure that the IV site remains immobile to reduce the risk of phlebitis and infiltration; however, the extremity does not need to be immobilized. Massaging the site potentially contributes to catheter movement and tissue damage. Immobilization devices such as arm boards are used if a site is near a joint and the IV flow rate is affected by joint movement. Alcohol skin preparation is used during the catheter insertion; because of the potential for excessive drying and client discomfort, alcohol is not used in IV site care.
Priority Nursing Tip: Signs/symptoms of phlebitis include a sluggish intravenous infusion and heat, redness, and tenderness at the intravenous site. The area is not usually swollen or hard.
Test-Taking Strategy: Focus on the subject, preventing phlebitis and infiltration. Eliminate options 1, 2, and 4 because of the words *massage, immobilize,* and *alcohol,* respectively. Review: the interventions related to the prevention of **phlebitis** and **infiltration.**
Reference(s): Potter et al (2013), p. 910.

674. The nurse is teaching a client how to stand on crutches. What information should the nurse give the client related to placement of the crutches?
1. Place the crutches 3 inches to the front and side of the toes
2. Place the crutches 6 inches to the front and side of the toes
3. Place the crutches 15 inches to the front and side of the toes
4. Place the crutches 20 inches to the front and side of the toes

Level of Cognitive Ability: Applying
Client Needs: Health Promotion and Maintenance
Integrated Process: Nursing Process/Implementation
Content Area: Adult Health: Musculoskeletal
Priority Concepts: Client Education; Safety

Answer: 2
Rationale: The classic tripod position is taught to the client before instructions regarding gait are given. The crutches are placed anywhere from 6 to 10 inches in front of and to the side of the client's toes, depending on the client's body size. This provides a wide enough base of support for the client and improves balance. Therefore, the other options are incorrect.
Priority Nursing Tip: The nurse should instruct the client using crutches to look up and outward when ambulating.
Test-Taking Strategy: Note the subject, teaching a client how to stand on crutches. Three inches (option 1) and 20 inches (option 4) seem excessively short and long, respectively, and these options should be eliminated first. From the remaining options, visualize this procedure. Six inches seems more in keeping with the normal length of a stride than 15 inches. Review the proper use of **crutches.**
Reference(s): Potter et al (2013), p. 761.

675. The nurse is giving instructions to a client who is beginning therapy with digoxin (Lanoxin). To detect **early** complications of therapy, which action should the nurse teach the client to perform?
1. Take the pulse daily.
2. Have electrolyte levels drawn weekly.
3. Monitor the blood pressure once a week.
4. Measure the weight each morning before breakfast.

Level of Cognitive Ability: Applying
Client Needs: Health Promotion and Maintenance
Integrated Process: Teaching and Learning
Content Area: Pharmacology: Cardiovascular Medications
Priority Concepts: Client Education; Safety

Answer: 1
Rationale: Digoxin (Lanoxin) is a cardiac glycoside. Clients taking digoxin should take the pulse each day and notify the health care provider if the heart rate is less than 60 beats/min or more than 100 beats/min. Options 2, 3, and 4 are not necessary interventions for the client taking digoxin.
Priority Nursing Tip: Before administering digoxin (Lanoxin) to a client, the nurse should count the client's apical heart rate for 1 full minute.
Test-Taking Strategy: Note the strategic word, *early.* Focus on the medication identified in the question. Recalling that digoxin is a cardiac medication will direct you to the correct option. Review: the client instructions regarding **digoxin (Lanoxin).**
Reference(s): Hodgson, Kizior (2014), p. 353.

676. The nurse has completed client teaching with a hemodialysis client regarding the self-monitoring of the fluid status between hemodialysis treatments. The nurse determines that the client understands the information given if the client states the need to record which item(s) on a daily basis?
1. Activity
2. Pulse and respiratory rate
3. Intake, output, and weight
4. Blood urea nitrogen and creatinine levels

Level of Cognitive Ability: Evaluating
Client Needs: Health Promotion and Maintenance
Integrated Process: Nursing Process/Evaluation
Content Area: Adult Health: Renal and Urinary
Priority Concepts: Client Education; Fluid and Electrolyte Balance

Answer: 3
Rationale: The client receiving hemodialysis should monitor fluid status between hemodialysis treatments. This can be done by recording intake and output and measuring weight on a daily basis. Ideally the hemodialysis client should not gain more than 0.5 kg of weight per day. Options 1, 2, and 4 are not necessary.
Priority Nursing Tip: The nurse should weigh the client receiving hemodialysis before and after the treatment to determine fluid loss that occurred.
Test-Taking Strategy: Immediately eliminate option 4 because it would not be the client's responsibility to obtain or record this information. Next note the words *daily basis*. Focusing on these words and the subject of a hemodialysis client self-monitoring fluid status will direct you to option 3. Review the self-care instructions for the hemodialysis client.
Reference(s): Lewis et al (2014), pp. 1121-1122.

677. Diltiazem hydrochloride (Cardizem) is prescribed for the client with Prinzmetal angina. The nurse provides instructions to the client regarding this medication. Which statement by the client indicates the **need for further teaching?**
1. "I will take the medication after meals."
2. "I will rise slowly when getting out of bed in the morning."
3. "I will call the health care provider if shortness of breath occurs."
4. "I will avoid activities that require alertness until my body gets used to the medication."

Level of Cognitive Ability: Evaluating
Client Needs: Health Promotion and Maintenance
Integrated Process: Teaching and Learning
Content Area: Pharmacology: Cardiovascular Medications
Priority Concepts: Client Education; Safety

Answer: 1
Rationale: Diltiazem hydrochloride (Cardizem) is a calcium channel blocker. It is administered before meals and at bedtime, as prescribed. Hypotension can occur, and the client is instructed to rise slowly. The client should call the health care provider if an irregular heartbeat, shortness of breath, pronounced dizziness, nausea, or constipation occurs. The client should avoid tasks that require alertness until a response to the medication is established.
Priority Nursing Tip: Calcium channel blockers promote vasodilation of the coronary and peripheral vessels and are used to treat angina, certain dysrhythmias, or hypertension. They should be used with caution in clients with heart failure, bradycardia, or atrioventricular block.
Test-Taking Strategy: Note the strategic words, *need for further teaching*. These words indicate a negative event query and ask you to select an option that is an incorrect statement. Focusing on the client's diagnosis of Prinzmetal angina will assist you in eliminating options 2, 3, and 4. Review: the home care instructions regarding diltiazem hydrochloride (Cardizem).
Reference(s): Hodgson, Kizior (2014), p. 357.

678. The nurse has provided instructions to a client being discharged from the hospital to home after an abdominal aortic aneurysm (AAA) resection. The nurse determines that the client understands the instructions if the client states that which would be an appropriate activity?
1. Mowing the lawn
2. Playing a game of 18-hole golf
3. Lifting objects up to 30 pounds
4. Walking as tolerated, including outdoors

Level of Cognitive Ability: Evaluating
Client Needs: Health Promotion and Maintenance
Integrated Process: Nursing Process/Evaluation
Content Area: Adult Health: Cardiovascular
Priority Concepts: Perfusion; Safety

Answer: 4
Rationale: The client can walk as tolerated after the repair or resection of an AAA, including walking outdoors. The client should not engage in any activities that involve pushing, pulling, or straining, and the client should not lift objects that weigh more than 15 to 20 pounds for 6 to 12 weeks. Driving is also prohibited for several weeks.
Priority Nursing Tip: An abdominal aortic aneurysm resection is the surgical resection of the aneurysm. The excised section is replaced with a graft that is sewn end-to-end. In the postoperative period, graft occlusion is a concern, so it is important for the nurse to monitor peripheral pulses distal to the graft.
Test-Taking Strategy: Note the subject of a client being discharged after AAA resection and the words *understands the instructions*. Evaluate each option in terms of the strain that it could put on the sutured graft. This will direct you to option 4. Review: the discharge instructions after abdominal aortic aneurysm (AAA).
Reference(s): Ignatavicius, Workman (2013), pp. 795-796.

679. The nurse is planning dietary counseling for the client taking triamterene (Dyrenium). The nurse plans to include which item in a list of foods that are acceptable?

1. Bananas
2. Oranges
3. Baked potato
4. Canned pears

Level of Cognitive Ability: Applying
Client Needs: Health Promotion and Maintenance
Integrated Process: Teaching and Learning
Content Area: Pharmacology: Cardiovascular Medications
Priority Concepts: Client Education; Nutrition

Answer: 4
Rationale: Triamterene is a potassium-retaining diuretic, and clients taking this medication should be cautioned against eating foods that are high in potassium, including many vegetables, fruits, and fresh meats. Because potassium is very soluble in water, foods that are prepared in cans are often lower in potassium.
Priority Nursing Tip: Instruct the client taking a potassium-retaining diuretic to avoid using salt substitutes because they contain potassium.
Test-Taking Strategy: Focus on the subject, triamterene (Dyrenium) and note the words *foods that are acceptable.* Recall that triamterene is a potassium-retaining diuretic. Next, review the options, identifying the food item that is lowest in potassium. Review: **high-potassium foods** and **triamterene (Dyrenium).**
Reference(s): Hodgson, Kizior (2014), pp. 1210-1211; Nix (2013), p. 138.

680. Cyclophosphamide is prescribed for the client with breast cancer, and the nurse provides instructions to the client regarding the medication. Which statement by the client indicates the **need for further teaching?**

1. "If I lose my hair, it will grow back."
2. "I need to limit my fluid intake while taking this medication."
3. "If I develop a sore throat, I should notify the health care provider."
4. "I need to avoid contact with anyone who recently received a live virus vaccine."

Level of Cognitive Ability: Evaluating
Client Needs: Health Promotion and Maintenance
Integrated Process: Teaching and Learning
Content Area: Pharmacology: Oncology Medications
Priority Concepts: Client Education; Safety

Answer: 2
Rationale: Hemorrhagic cystitis is an adverse reaction associated with cyclophosphamide. The client needs to be instructed to consume copious amounts of fluid during therapy. The client's hair will grow back, although it may have a different color and texture. A sore throat may be an indication of an infection, and it must be reported to the health care provider. Avoiding contact with anyone who recently received a live virus vaccine is important because cyclophosphamide produces immunosuppression, thus placing the client at risk for infection.
Priority Nursing Tip: The client taking cyclophosphamide must be encouraged to consume 2 to 3 liters of fluid per day (unless contraindicated) to prevent hemorrhagic cystitis.
Test-Taking Strategy: Note the strategic words, *need for further teaching.* These words indicate a negative event query and ask you to select an option that is an incorrect statement. Eliminate options 3 and 4 because they are comparable or alike in that they both relate to the risk of infection. From the remaining options, recalling that hemorrhagic cystitis is an adverse effect of cyclophosphamide will direct you to the correct option. Review: the adverse effects of cyclophosphamide.
Reference(s): Lehne (2013), p. 1276.

681. The community health nurse has reviewed information about the population of a local community and has determined that there are groups in the population that are at high risk for infection with tuberculosis (TB). The nurse targets which high-risk group for screening?

1. French Canadians
2. White, Anglo-Saxon Americans
3. Older clients in long-term care facilities
4. Adolescents between the ages of 13 and 17 years

Level of Cognitive Ability: Analyzing
Client Needs: Health Promotion and Maintenance
Integrated Process: Nursing Process/Assessment
Content Area: Adult Health: Respiratory
Priority Concepts: Health Promotion; Infection

Answer: 3
Rationale: Older clients, particularly those in long-term care facilities, are at high risk for infection with TB. Other people at risk include children who are 5 years old and younger, the malnourished, the immunosuppressed, the economically disadvantaged, foreign-born persons, and persons of a minority race who formerly lived in a place where TB is common, such as Asia or the Pacific islands. Therefore, options 1, 2, and 4 are incorrect.
Priority Nursing Tip: Improper or noncompliant use of treatment programs for tuberculosis may cause the development of mutations in the tubercle bacilli, resulting in a multidrug-resistant strain of tuberculosis (MDR-TB).
Test-Taking Strategy: Focus on the subject, those at risk for tuberculosis. Recalling these risk factors will direct you to option 3. Remember that the very young and the very old often fall into high-risk categories. Review: the risk factors associated with **tuberculosis (TB).**
Reference(s): Ignatavicius, Workman (2013), p. 654.

682. A toddler with suspected conjunctivitis is crying and refuses to sit still during the eye examination. Which is the **most appropriate** statement for the nurse to make to the child?
1. "Would you like to see my flashlight?"
2. "Don't be scared, the light won't hurt you."
3. "If you will sit still, the exam will be over soon."
4. "I know you are upset. We can do this exam later."

Level of Cognitive Ability: Applying
Client Needs: Health Promotion and Maintenance
Integrated Process: Communication and Documentation
Content Area: Developmental Stages: Infancy to Adolescence
Priority Concepts: Development; Health Promotion

Answer: 1
Rationale: Fears in this age group can be decreased by getting the child actively involved in the examination. Option 2 tells the toddler how to feel. Option 3 ignores the toddler's feelings. Although option 4 acknowledges the toddler's feelings, it falsely puts off the inevitable.
Priority Nursing Tip: When approaching the toddler, the examiner should learn the words the toddler uses for common items and use them in conversations. The examiner should also use short, concrete terms, and use play for demonstrations.
Test-Taking Strategy: Note the strategic words, *most appropriate*. Use knowledge regarding the stages of growth and development, noting that the child is a toddler. The use of therapeutic communication techniques will direct you to the correct option. Review: the growth and development related to the toddler
Reference(s): Hockenberry, Wilson (2013), p. 107; McKinney et al (2013), pp. 879, 978.

683. The mother of a teenage client with an anxiety disorder is concerned about her daughter's progress after discharge. She states that her daughter "stashes food, eats all the wrong things that make her hyperactive," and "hangs out with the wrong crowd." To assist the mother with preparing for her daughter's discharge, the nurse advises the mother to implement which action in order to promote optimal health?
1. Restrict the daughter's socializing time with her school friends.
2. Consider taking time off to help her daughter readjust to the home environment.
3. Limit the amount of chocolate and caffeine products that are available in the home.
4. Keep her daughter out of school until she proves that she can adjust to the school environment.

Level of Cognitive Ability: Applying
Client Needs: Health Promotion and Maintenance
Integrated Process: Teaching and Learning
Content Area: Mental Health
Priority Concepts: Anxiety; Client Education

Answer: 3
Rationale: Clients with anxiety disorders are advised to limit their intake of caffeine, chocolate, and alcohol because these products have the potential to increase anxiety. Options 1 and 4 are unreasonable and involve unhealthy approaches. In addition, it may not be realistic for a family member to take time off from work.
Priority Nursing Tip: The immediate nursing action for a client experiencing anxiety is to decrease stimuli in the environment and provide a calm and quiet environment.
Test-Taking Strategy: Note the daughter's diagnosis of anxiety, and focus on the subject, to promote health. Options 1, 2, and 4 are comparable or alike, and they are concerned with monitoring or curtailing the daughter's physical activities, whereas option 3 focuses on the subject. Review: the health promotion measures for the client with an anxiety disorder.
Reference(s): Stuart, (2013), p. 222; Varcarolis (2013), p. 182.

684. The nurse assesses a client with hepatic encephalopathy for the presence of asterixis. What should the nurse do to appropriately test for asterixis?
1. Examine the client's handwriting movements
2. Check the stool for clay-colored pigmentation
3. Ask the client to extend the wrist and the fingers
4. Check the serum bilirubin and liver enzyme levels

Level of Cognitive Ability: Applying
Client Needs: Health Promotion and Maintenance
Integrated Process: Nursing Process/Assessment
Content Area: Developmental Stages: Health Assessment/Physical Exam
Priority Concepts: Clinical Judgment; Health Promotion

Answer: 3
Rationale: Asterixis is a rapid, nonrhythmic, abnormal muscle tremor of the wrists and fingers that is commonly associated with hepatic encephalopathy and referred to as "liver flap." Handwriting is a non-specific and insensitive test of motor function, so the nurse avoids using this to assess for asterixis. Clients with hepatic encephalopathy can experience changes in bowel habits and flatulence. The nurse expects the liver function studies of a client with hepatic encephalopathy to have above-normal results.
Priority Nursing Tip: The nurse should monitor the client with cirrhosis for signs associated with hepatic encephalopathy such as asterixis (rapid, nonrhythmic, abnormal muscle tremor of the wrists and fingers) and fetor hepaticus (fruity and musty breath odor).
Test-Taking Strategy: Focus on the subject of asterixis. Specific knowledge of the definition and manifestations of asterixis is needed to answer this question. Also recalling the signs and symptoms of hepatic encephalopathy will direct you to the correct option. Review the technique for assessment for asterixis.
Reference(s): Ignatavicius, Workman (2013), p. 1298.

685. The nurse assesses the cranial nerve XII in the client who sustained a stroke. To assess this cranial nerve, which action should the nurse ask the client to perform?
1. Extend the arms.
2. Extend the tongue.
3. Turn the head toward the nurse's arm.
4. Focus the eyes on an object held by the nurse.

Level of Cognitive Ability: Applying
Client Needs: Health Promotion and Maintenance
Integrated Process: Nursing Process/Assessment
Content Area: Developmental Stages: Health Assessment/Physical Exam
Priority Concepts: Health Promotion; Intracranial Regulation

Answer: 2
Rationale: Impairment of cranial nerve XII can occur with a stroke. To assess the function of cranial nerve XII (hypoglossal), the nurse would assess the client's ability to extend the tongue. Options 1, 3, and 4 do not test the function of the twelfth cranial nerve.
Priority Nursing Tip: The hypoglossal nerve (cranial nerve XII) controls the tongue movements involved with swallowing and speech. If the function of this nerve is affected, the client could have difficulty speaking and difficulty swallowing food and fluids, placing him or her at risk for aspiration.
Test-Taking Strategy: Focus on the subject, the procedure for checking cranial nerve XII. Recalling that cranial nerve XII is the hypoglossal nerve will direct you to option 2. Review: the cranial nerves and the methods of testing these nerves.
Reference(s): Jarvis (2012), p. 636.

686. A client with type 2 diabetes mellitus is being discharged from the hospital after an occurrence of hyperglycemic hyperosmolar state (HHS). The nurse develops a discharge teaching plan for the client and identifies which as a **priority**?
1. Exercise routines
2. Controlling dietary intake
3. Keeping follow-up appointments
4. Monitoring for signs/symptoms of dehydration

Level of Cognitive Ability: Analyzing
Client Needs: Health Promotion and Maintenance
Integrated Process: Teaching and Learning
Content Area: Leadership/Management: Prioritizing
Priority Concepts: Client Education; Glucose Regulation

Answer: 4
Rationale: Clients at risk for HHS should immediately report signs and symptoms of dehydration to health care providers. Dehydration can be severe, and it may progress rapidly. Although options 1, 2, and 3 are components of the teaching plan, for the client with HHS, dehydration is the priority.
Priority Nursing Tip: Hyperglycemic hyperosmolar state (HHS) most often occurs in individuals with type 2 diabetes mellitus. The major difference between HHS and diabetic ketoacidosis is that ketosis and acidosis do not occur with HHS.
Test-Taking Strategy: Note the strategic word, priority. Look at each option in terms of its seriousness, and recall that dehydration can rapidly progress to HHS. Review: diabetes mellitus and hyperglycemic hyperosmolar state (HHS).
Reference(s): Ignatavicius, Workman (2013), pp. 1455, 1458.

687. The nurse develops a plan of care for an older client with diabetes mellitus. It is important that the nurse plans to complete which action **first**?
1. Structure menus for adherence to diet.
2. Teach with videotapes showing insulin administration to ensure competence.
3. Encourage dependence on others to prepare the client for the chronicity of the disease.
4. Assess the client's ability to read label markings on syringes and blood glucose monitoring equipment.

Level of Cognitive Ability: Analyzing
Client Needs: Health Promotion and Maintenance
Integrated Process: Nursing Process/Planning
Content Area: Adult Health: Endocrine
Priority Concepts: Development; Glucose Regulation

Answer: 4
Rationale: The nurse first assesses the client's ability for self-care. Independence should be encouraged. Structuring menus for the client promotes dependence. Allowing the client to have hands-on experience rather than teaching with videos is more effective.
Priority Nursing Tip: There are several components to a teaching plan for a client with diabetes mellitus including diet, exercise, and medication. Before implementing the plan, it is important for the nurse to perform an assessment to determine the client's specific learning needs.
Test-Taking Strategy: Note the strategic word, *first*. Use the steps of the nursing process. Option 4 reflects assessment, which is the first step of the nursing process. Review **teaching and learning principles** and **diabetes mellitus**.
Reference(s): Potter et al (2013), p. 331.

688. The nurse is conducting a health screening on a client with a family history of hypertension. Which assessment finding would alert the nurse to the **need for further teaching** related to stroke prevention?
1. Eats two bowls of high-fiber grain cereal with skim milk for breakfast
2. Has a blood pressure of 118/78 mm Hg and has lost 10 pounds recently
3. Uses condoms for pregnancy and disease prevention and jogs 2 miles daily
4. Uses oral contraceptives for pregnancy prevention and works as a manager of a busy medical-surgical unit.

Level of Cognitive Ability: Analyzing
Client Needs: Health Promotion and Maintenance
Integrated Process: Nursing Process/Assessment
Content Area: Developmental Stages: Health Assessment/Physical Exam
Priority Concepts: Client Education; Health Promotion

Answer: 4
Rationale: Oral contraceptive use is discouraged in some clients because of the side effect of clot formation. The use of oral contraceptives, obesity, hypertension, hypercholesterolemia, and smoking are all modifiable risk factors for stroke. Low-fat diet and stress-reduction methods are encouraged and identified in options 1 and 3. In option 2, the client has a normal blood pressure and has lost weight.
Priority Nursing Tip: A transient ischemic attack may be a warning sign of a stroke (brain attack).
Test-Taking Strategy: Note the strategic words, *need for further teaching*. These words indicate a negative event query and ask you to select the option that is a risk factor for stroke. Noting the words *oral contraceptives* in option 4 will direct you to this option. Review: the risk factors related to **stroke**.
Reference(s): Ignatavicius, Workman (2013), p. 1007.

689. The nurse is reviewing the assessment data of a client. Which finding would be **most important** for the client to modify to lessen the risk for coronary artery disease (CAD)?
1. Elevated triglyceride levels
2. Elevated serum lipase levels
3. Elevated low-density lipoprotein (LDL) levels
4. Elevated high-density lipoprotein (HDL) levels

Level of Cognitive Ability: Analyzing
Client Needs: Health Promotion and Maintenance
Integrated Process: Nursing Process/Assessment
Content Area: Adult Health: Cardiovascular
Priority Concepts: Health Promotion; Perfusion

Answer: 3
Rationale: LDLs are more directly associated with CAD than are other lipoproteins. LDL levels, along with levels of cholesterol, have a higher predictive association with CAD than levels of triglycerides. Additionally, HDL is inversely associated with the risk of CAD. Lipase is a digestive enzyme that breaks down ingested fats in the gastrointestinal tract.
Priority Nursing Tip: Coronary artery narrowing is significant if the lumen diameter of the left main artery is reduced at least 50%, or if any major branch is reduced at least 75%.
Test-Taking Strategy: Note the strategic words, *most important*. Focus on the subject, the risk factor related to CAD. Recalling that LDL is the "bad" cholesterol will direct you to the correct option. Review: the risk factors associated with **coronary artery disease (CAD)**.
Reference(s): Ignatavicius, Workman (2013), p. 832.

690. The nurse is taking a history from a client who is suspected of having testicular cancer. Which data will be **most** helpful for determining the client's risk factors for this type of cancer?
1. Age and race
2. Marital status
3. Number of children
4. Number of sexual partners

Level of Cognitive Ability: Analyzing
Client Needs: Health Promotion and Maintenance
Integrated Process: Nursing Process/Assessment
Content Area: Adult Health: Oncology
Priority Concepts: Cellular Regulation; Health Promotion

Answer: 1
Rationale: Two basic but important risk factors for testicular cancer are age and race. The incidence of testicular cancer is four times higher among white males than black males. It is the most common type of cancer to occur in males between the ages of 15 and 34 years. Other risk factors include a history of an undescended testis and a family history of testicular cancer. Marital status and the number of children are not risk factors for testicular cancer.
Priority Nursing Tip: Monthly testicular self-examination is the method of early detection of testicular cancer. The nurse needs to teach the client the procedure for performing this self-examination.
Test-Taking Strategy: Note the strategic word, *most*. Use your knowledge of the risk factors associated with this type of cancer to answer the question. Recalling that testicular cancer most often occurs in males between the ages of 15 and 34 years will direct you to the correct option. Review: the risk factors related to **testicular cancer**.
Reference(s): Ignatavicius, Workman (2013), p. 1643.

691. The nurse instructs a perinatal client about measures to prevent urinary tract infections. Which statement by the client would indicate an understanding of these measures?
1. "I can wear my tight-fitting jeans."
2. "I should always use scented toilet paper."
3. "I should choose underwear with a cotton panel liner."
4. "I can take a bubble bath as long as the soap doesn't contain any oils."

Level of Cognitive Ability: Evaluating
Client Needs: Health Promotion and Maintenance
Integrated Process: Nursing Process/Evaluation
Content Area: Maternity: Antepartum
Priority Concepts: Client Education; Infection

Answer: 3
Rationale: Wearing items with a cotton panel liner allows for air movement in and around the genital area. Wearing tight clothes irritates the genital area and does not allow for air circulation. Harsh, scented, or printed toilet paper may cause irritation. Bubble bath or other bath oils should be avoided because these may be irritating to the urethra.
Priority Nursing Tip: Cystitis is more common in women because women have a shorter urethra than men and the urethra in women is located close to the rectum.
Test-Taking Strategy: Note the words *indicate an understanding*. Eliminate option 2 because of the closed-ended word "always" and option 1 because of the words *tight-fitting*. From the remaining options, recall that bubble baths need to be avoided. Review: the measures to prevent **urinary tract infections**.
Reference(s): McKinney et al (2013), p. 680.

692. The nurse instructs a client with mild pre-eclampsia about home care measures. What statement by the client indicates to the nurse that the teaching has been **effective** concerning the assessment of complications for preeclampsia?
1. "I need to check my weight every day at different times during the day."
2. "I need to take my blood pressure each morning and alternate arms each time."
3. "I need to check my urine with a dipstick every day for protein and call the health care provider if it is 2+ or more."
4. "As long as the home care nurse is visiting me daily, I do not have to keep my next health care provider's appointment."

Level of Cognitive Ability: Evaluating
Client Needs: Health Promotion and Maintenance
Integrated Process: Nursing Process/Evaluation
Content Area: Maternity: Antepartum
Priority Concepts: Client Education; Reproduction

Answer: 3
Rationale: The client with preeclampsia needs to be instructed to report any increases in blood pressure, 2+ proteinuria, weight gain of more than 1 pound per week, the presence of edema, and decreased fetal activity to the health care provider immediately to prevent worsening of the preeclamptic condition. The weight needs to be checked at the same time each day, after voiding, before breakfast, and with the client wearing the same clothes in order to obtain reliable weight readings. Blood pressure measurements need to be taken in the same arm every day in a sitting position to obtain consistent and accurate readings. It is important to keep health care provider appointments even if the client is receiving visits from a home care nurse.
Priority Nursing Tip: Predisposing conditions for the development of gestational hypertension include primigravida, women younger than 19 years or older than 40 years, chronic kidney disease, chronic hypertension, diabetes mellitus, Rh incompatibility, and history or family history of gestational hypertension.
Test-Taking Strategy: Note the strategic word, *effective*. Basic principles related to health care teaching and focusing on the specific subject of the question, mild preeclampsia, will assist with directing you to option 3. Review: the home care teaching points for the client with **preeclampsia**.
Reference(s): McKinney et al (2013), p. 594.

693. The nurse is providing instructions to a client and family regarding home care after left-eye cataract removal. The nurse tells the client and family about assuming which position during the postoperative period?
1. Sleep only on the left side.
2. Sleep on the right side or the back.
3. Bend below the waist as often as you are able.
4. Lower the head between the knees three times a day.

Level of Cognitive Ability: Applying
Client Needs: Health Promotion and Maintenance
Integrated Process: Teaching and Learning
Content Area: Adult Health: Eye
Priority Concepts: Client Education; Safety

Answer: 2
Rationale: After cataract surgery, the client should not sleep on the operative side to prevent the development of edema. The client should also avoid bending below the level of the waist or lowering the head because these actions will increase intraocular pressure.
Priority Nursing Tip: Blurred vision and decreased color perception are early signs/symptoms of a cataract.
Test-Taking Strategy: Eliminate options 3 and 4 first because they are comparable or alike and indicate that lowering the head below waist level is acceptable. From the remaining options, remembering that the client needs to be instructed to remain off of the operative side will direct you to option 2. Review: the postoperative instructions for the client after cataract surgery.
Reference(s): Lewis et al (2014), p. 395.

694. The nurse has provided instructions to a new mother with a urinary tract infection regarding foods and fluids to consume that will acidify the urine. The nurse determines that **further teaching is needed** if the mother indicates that which fluid will acidify the urine?
1. Prune juice
2. Apricot juice
3. Cranberry juice
4. Carbonated drinks

Level of Cognitive Ability: Evaluating
Client Needs: Health Promotion and Maintenance
Integrated Process: Teaching and Learning
Content Area: Maternity: Postpartum
Priority Concepts: Client Education; Infection

Answer: 4
Rationale: Acidification of the urine inhibits the multiplication of bacteria. Carbonated drinks should be avoided because they increase urine alkalinity. Fluids that acidify the urine include prune, apricot, and cranberry juice.
Priority Nursing Tip: In addition to apricots, prunes, and cranberries, other foods that acidify the urine include tomatoes, meat, fish, oysters, poultry, corn, legumes, cheese, eggs, and whole grains.
Test-Taking Strategy: Note the strategic words, *further teaching is needed.* These words indicate a negative event query and ask you to select the fluid item that will not acidify the urine. Note the similarity between options 1, 2, and 3 in that these items are fruit juices. This will assist with directing you to the correct option. Review: the foods and fluids that cause urine acidification.
Reference(s): McKinney et al (2013), p. 680.

695. A postpartum nurse has instructed a new mother regarding how to bathe her newborn. The nurse demonstrates the procedure to the mother and, on the following day, asks the mother to perform the procedure. Which observation by the nurse indicates that the mother is performing the procedure correctly?
1. The mother cleans the ears and then moves to the eyes and the face.
2. The mother begins to wash the newborn infant by starting with the eyes and face.
3. The mother washes the arms, chest, and back followed by the neck, arms, and face.
4. The mother washes the entire newborn infant's body and then washes the eyes, face, and scalp.

Level of Cognitive Ability: Evaluating
Client Needs: Health Promotion and Maintenance
Integrated Process: Nursing Process/Evaluation
Content Area: Maternity: Newborn
Priority Concepts: Development; Safety

Answer: 2
Rationale: Bathing should start at the eyes and face and with the cleanest area first. Next, the external ears and behind the ears are cleaned. The newborn infant's neck should be washed because formula, lint, and breast milk will often accumulate in the folds of the neck. The hands and arms are then washed. The newborn infant's legs are washed next, with the diaper area being washed last.
Priority Nursing Tip: Teach the mother to gather all of the necessary equipment needed for the bath before bathing the infant. The infant or child should never be left alone during bathing.
Test-Taking Strategy: Note the subject, bathing a newborn. Use the basic techniques and principles of bathing a client to answer this question. Remember to always start with the cleanest area of the body and proceed to the dirtiest area. This principle will direct you to the correct option. Review: the home care measures related to the care of the newborn.
Reference(s): Lowdermilk, Perry, Cashion, Alden (2012), p. 596; McKinney et al (2013), pp. 515, 522.

696. The nurse is teaching umbilical cord care to a new mother. What information should the nurse provide to the mother related to cord care?
1. Alcohol is the only agent to use to clean the cord.
2. Cord care is done only at birth to control bleeding.
3. It takes at least 21 days for the cord to dry up and fall off.
4. The process of keeping the cord clean and dry will decrease bacterial growth.

Level of Cognitive Ability: Applying
Client Needs: Health Promotion and Maintenance
Integrated Process: Teaching and Learning
Content Area: Maternity: Newborn
Priority Concepts: Client Education; Infection

Answer: 4
Rationale: The cord should be kept clean and dry to decrease bacterial growth. It should be cleansed two to three times a day with a prescribed agent. Usually the cord is cleansed with soap and water around base of the cord where it joins the skin. The health care provider is notified of any odor, discharge, or skin inflammation. The diaper should not cover the cord because a wet or soiled diaper will slow or prevent drying of the cord and foster infection. Cord care is required until the cord dries up and falls off between 7 and 14 days after birth.
Priority Nursing Tip: Note any bleeding or drainage from the cord. If symptoms of infection occur, notify the health care provider and use antibiotic prescription as prescribed.
Test-Taking Strategy: Eliminate options 1 and 2 first because of the closed-ended word "only." From the remaining options, recalling the purpose of cord care will direct you to the correct option. Review: the concepts related to cord care.
Reference(s): McKinney et al (2013), pp. 515, 522.

❖ **697.** Which would the nurse identify as a situational crisis? **Select all that apply.**
☐ 1. Divorce
☐ 2. Retirement
☐ 3. Loss of a job
☐ 4. An earthquake
☐ 5. The birth of a child
☐ 6. Death of a loved one

Level of Cognitive Ability: Analyzing
Client Needs: Health Promotion and Maintenance
Integrated Process: Nursing Process/Assessment
Content Area: Mental Health
Priority Concepts: Anxiety; Clinical Judgment

Answer: 1, 3, 6
Rationale: A situational crisis arises from an external rather than an internal source and often is unanticipated. Examples of external situations that can precipitate a situational crisis include divorce, the loss of a job, the death of a loved one, an abortion, a change in job, a change in financial status, and severe physical or mental illness. A maturational crisis occurs at a developmental stage; examples include marriage, the birth of a child, and retirement. An adventitious crisis, or crisis of disaster, is not a part of everyday life and is unplanned or accidental. This type of crisis can result from a natural disaster (flood, fire, earthquake), a national disaster (acts of terrorism, war, riots, airplane crashes), or a crime of violence (rape, assault, murder, bombing, spousal or child abuse).
Priority Nursing Tip: For crisis management, treatment is immediate, supportive, and directly responsive to the immediate crisis.
Test-Taking Strategy: Focus on the subject, a situational crisis. Read each option and recall that a situational crisis arises from an external rather than an internal source and often is unanticipated. This will assist in selecting the correct answers. Review: examples of situational crises.
Reference(s): Varcarolis (2013), p. 400.

---

698. The nurse prepares a teaching plan regarding the administration of eardrops for the parents of a 6-year-old child. The nurse tells the parents that, when administering the drops, which action is appropriate?
1. Wear gloves.
2. Pull the ear up and back.
3. Hold the child in a sitting position.
4. Position the child so that the affected ear is facing downward.

Level of Cognitive Ability: Applying
Client Needs: Health Promotion and Maintenance
Integrated Process: Teaching and Learning
Content Area: Child Health: Eye/Ear
Priority Concepts: Client Education; Development

Answer: 2
Rationale: To administer eardrops in a child who is more than 3 years old, the ear is pulled upward and back. The ear is pulled down and back in children less than 3 years old. Gloves do not need to be worn by the parents, but hand washing before and after the procedure must be performed. The child needs to be in a side-lying position with the affected ear facing upward to facilitate the flow of medication down the ear canal with the help of gravity.
Priority Nursing Tip: When administering the eardrops, the child should remain lying down for 1 to 2 minutes so medication can be absorbed.
Test-Taking Strategy: Focus on the subject, the administration of eardrops to a 6-year-old child. Visualizing this procedure will assist you in eliminating options 1, 3, and 4. Also recalling the anatomy of the child's ear canal and noting the age of the child will direct you to the correct option. Review this procedure for instilling ear drops.
Reference(s): McKinney et al (2013), p. 959.

699. The nurse is providing discharge instructions to the mother of an 8-year-old child who had a tonsillectomy. The mother tells the nurse that the child loves tacos and asks when the child can safely eat one. To prevent complications of the surgical procedure, what should be the appropriate response to the mother?

1. "In 1 week."
2. "In 3 weeks."
3. "Six days after surgery."
4. "When the health care provider says it is okay."

Level of Cognitive Ability: Applying
Client Needs: Health Promotion and Maintenance
Integrated Process: Teaching and Learning
Content Area: Child Health: Throat/Respiratory
Priority Concepts: Client Education; Safety

Answer: 2
Rationale: Rough or scratchy foods, as well as spicy foods, are to be avoided for 3 weeks after a tonsillectomy. Citrus juices that irritate the throat need to be avoided for 10 days. Red liquids are avoided because they will give the appearance of blood if the child vomits. The mother is instructed to add full liquids on the second day and soft foods as the child tolerates them.
Priority Nursing Tip: Following tonsillectomy, position the child prone or side-lying to facilitate drainage.
Test-Taking Strategy: Eliminate options 1 and 3 first because they are comparable and alike and identify similar time frames. Eliminate option 4 because it places the mother's question on hold. Review: the dietary instructions after **tonsillectomy**.
Reference(s): McKinney et al (2013), p. 1158.

700. After a cleft lip repair, the nurse instructs the parents about cleaning of the lip repair site. The nurse should plan to use which solution when demonstrating this procedure to the parents?

1. Tap water
2. Sterile water
3. Full-strength hydrogen peroxide
4. Half-strength hydrogen peroxide

Level of Cognitive Ability: Applying
Client Needs: Health Promotion and Maintenance
Integrated Process: Teaching and Learning
Content Area: Child Health: Gastrointestinal
Priority Concepts: Client Education; Infection

Answer: 2
Rationale: Following cleft lip repair, the site is cleansed with sterile water using a cotton swab after feeding and as prescribed. Agency procedure should also be followed. The parents should be instructed to use a rolling motion starting at the suture line and rolling out. Tap water is not a sterile solution. Hydrogen peroxide may disrupt the integrity of the site.
Priority Nursing Tip: Following cleft lip repair, avoid positioning the infant on the side of the repair or in the prone position because these positions can cause rubbing of the surgical site on the mattress.
Test-Taking Strategy: Eliminate options 3 and 4 first because they are comparable or alike. From the remaining options, recall the importance of asepsis when treating a surgical site to direct you to the correct option. Review: postoperative care following **cleft lip repair**.
Reference(s): McKinney et al (2013), p. 1073.

701. A child with a diagnosis of umbilical hernia has been scheduled for surgical repair in 2 weeks. The clinic nurse instructs the parents about the signs/symptoms of possible hernia strangulation. The nurse tells the parents that which sign/symptom would require health care provider notification?

1. Fever
2. Diarrhea
3. Vomiting
4. Constipation

Level of Cognitive Ability: Applying
Client Needs: Health Promotion and Maintenance
Integrated Process: Teaching and Learning
Content Area: Child Health: Gastrointestinal
Priority Concepts: Client Education; Safety

Answer: 3
Rationale: The parents of a child with an umbilical hernia need to be instructed regarding the signs/symptoms of strangulation, which include vomiting, pain, and an irreducible mass at the umbilicus. The parents should be instructed to contact the health care provider immediately if strangulation is suspected.
Priority Nursing Tip: An umbilical hernia is a soft swelling or protrusion around the umbilicus that is usually reducible with the finger.
Test-Taking Strategy: Note the subject, hernia strangulation. Recall the definition of the word *strangulation* to assist you in eliminating options 1 and 2. From the remaining options, think about the anatomy of the body and the expected occurrence if strangulation developed to direct you to the correct option. Review: the signs/symptoms of **hernia strangulation**.
Reference(s): Hockenberry, Wilson (2013), pp. 806-807.

702. A client with a compound (open) fracture of the radius has a plaster cast applied in the emergency department. The nurse provides home care instructions and tells the client to seek medical attention if which finding occurs?

1. Numbness and tingling are felt in the fingers.
2. The cast feels heavy and damp after 24 hours of application.
3. The entire cast feels warm during the first 24 hours after application.
4. Slightly bloody drainage is noted on the cast during the first 6 hours after application.

Level of Cognitive Ability: Applying
Client Needs: Health Promotion and Maintenance
Integrated Process: Teaching and Learning
Content Area: Adult Health: Musculoskeletal
Priority Concepts: Perfusion; Safety

Answer: 1
Rationale: A limb encased in a cast is at risk for nerve damage and diminished circulation from increased pressure caused by edema. Signs/symptoms of increased pressure from the cast include numbness, tingling, and increased pain. A cast can take up to 48 hours to dry and generates heat while drying. Some drainage may occur initially with a compound (open) fracture.
Priority Nursing Tip: Monitor the client with a cast for signs/symptoms of infection under the cast, which include an increased temperature, hot spots on the cast, a foul odor, or changes in pain.
Test-Taking Strategy: Note the words *compound (open)* in the question. These words and the use of the ABCs—airway, breathing, and circulation—will direct you to the correct option. Review: the teaching points for the client with a plaster cast.
Reference(s): Ignatavicius, Workman (2013), pp. 1152-1153.

703. The mother of a child with celiac disease asks the nurse how long a special diet is necessary. The nurse provides which instruction to the mother to promote dietary compliance?

1. A gluten-free diet will need to be followed for life.
2. A lactose-free diet will need to be followed temporarily.
3. Adequate nutritional status will help prevent celiac crisis.
4. Supplemental vitamins, iron, and folate will prevent complications.

Level of Cognitive Ability: Applying
Client Needs: Health Promotion and Maintenance
Integrated Process: Teaching and Learning
Content Area: Child Health: Gastrointestinal
Priority Concepts: Adherence; Client Education

Answer: 1
Rationale: Celiac disease is characterized by intolerance to gluten, the protein component of wheat, barley, rye, and oats. The main nursing consideration with celiac disease is helping the child adhere to dietary management. The treatment of celiac disease consists primarily of dietary management with a gluten-free diet. Options 2, 3, and 4 are all true statements, but they do not answer the question that the client is asking. Children with untreated celiac disease may have lactose intolerance, which usually improves with gluten withdrawal. Nutritional deficiencies resulting from malabsorption are treated with appropriate supplements.
Priority Nursing Tip: For the client with celiac disease, strict dietary avoidance of gluten minimizes the risk of developing malignant lymphoma of the small intestine and other gastrointestinal malignancies.
Test-Taking Strategy: Focus on the subject, the length of time that a special diet is necessary. Options 2, 3, and 4 are all true about celiac disease, but they do not answer the question that the client is asking. Option 1 relates directly to this subject. Review: the dietary requirements for celiac disease.
Reference(s): McKinney et al (2013), pp. 1104-1105.

704. The nurse teaches the mother of a newly circumcised infant about postcircumcision care. Which statement by the mother indicates an understanding of the care required?
　1. "I need to clean the penis every hour with baby wipes."
　2. "I need to check for bleeding every hour for the first 12 hours."
　3. "My baby will not urinate for the next 24 hours because of swelling."
　4. "I need to wrap the penis completely in dry sterile gauze, making sure that it is dry when I change his diaper."

Level of Cognitive Ability: Evaluating
Client Needs: Health Promotion and Maintenance
Integrated Process: Nursing Process/Evaluation
Content Area: Maternity: Newborn
Priority Concepts: Client Education; Infection

Answer: **2**
Rationale: Following circumcision, the mother needs to be taught to observe for bleeding and assess the site hourly for 8 to 12 hours. Water is used for cleaning because soap or baby wipes may irritate the area and cause discomfort. Voiding needs to be assessed. The mother should call the health care provider if the baby has not urinated within 24 hours because swelling or damage may obstruct urine output. When the diaper is changed, Vaseline gauze should be reapplied (if prescribed). Frequent diaper changing prevents contamination of the site.
Priority Nursing Tip: The nurse should inform the parents that a milky covering over the glans penis is normal and should not be disrupted.
Test-Taking Strategy: Focus on the subject, circumcision care. Eliminate option 1 because baby wipes will cause stinging of the newly circumcised penis. Eliminate option 3 because penile swelling that prevents voiding needs to be reported to the health care provider. Eliminate option 4 because gauze will stick to the penis if it is completely dry. Review: **circumcision** care.
Reference(s): McKinney et al (2013), pp. 520, 523.

705. The nurse is developing a teaching plan for a client who will be receiving phenelzine sulfate (Nardil). The nurse should tell the client to avoid which item(s) while taking this medication?
　1. Vasodilators
　2. Aged cheeses
　3. Digitalis preparations
　4. Cherries and blueberries

Level of Cognitive Ability: Applying
Client Needs: Health Promotion and Maintenance
Integrated Process: Teaching and Learning
Content Area: Pharmacology: Psychiatric Medications
Priority Concepts: Client Education; Safety

Answer: **2**
Rationale: Phenelzine sulfate is in the monoamine oxidase inhibitor (MAOI) class of antidepressant medications. An individual taking an MAOI must avoid aged cheeses, alcoholic beverages, avocados, bananas, and caffeine drinks. There are also other food items to avoid including chocolate, meat tenderizers, pickled herring, raisins, sour cream, yogurt, and soy sauce. Medications that should be avoided include amphetamines, antiasthmatics, and certain antidepressants. The client should also avoid vasoconstrictors because their concurrent use can cause hypertensive crisis.
Priority Nursing Tip: The client taking a monoamine oxidase inhibitor (MAOI) needs to avoid foods containing tyramine. Consuming tyramine-containing foods when taking an MAOI can cause hypertensive crisis.
Test-Taking Strategy: Focus on the subject, the food item to avoid. Recalling that phenelzine sulfate is an MAOI and recalling the foods that need to be avoided will direct you to the correct option. Review: **phenelzine sulfate (Nardil)**.
Reference(s): Hodgson, Kizior (2014), pp. 937-939; Lehne (2013), pp. 370, 378.

❖ **706.** A pregnant client, suspected of being physically abused by her husband, is brought to the emergency department by a neighbor after being found bleeding from her head. In evaluating the crisis situation, which questions should the nurse specifically ask to assess the client's perception of the precipitating event? **Select all that apply.**
- ❑ 1. Where do you go to worship?
- ❑ 2. Who is available to help you?
- ❑ 3. How does this situation affect your life?
- ❑ 4. Describe how you are feeling right now.
- ❑ 5. To whom do you talk when you are upset?
- ❑ 6. How do you see this event as affecting your future?

Level of Cognitive Ability: Analyzing
Client Needs: Health Promotion and Maintenance
Integrated Process: Nursing Process/Assessment
Content Area: Mental Health
Priority Concepts: Clinical Judgment; Interpersonal Violence

Answer: 3, 4, 6
Rationale: In a crisis situation, the nurse's initial task is to assess the individual or family and the problem. Assessing the client's perception of the precipitating event will assist in clearly defining the problem, which will result in identifying a more effective solution. Examples of some questions that the nurse can ask to assess the client's perception of the precipitating event include: How does this situation affect your life? Describe how you are feeling right now. How do you see this event as affecting your future? Has anything particularly upsetting happened to you within the past few days or weeks? What was happening in your life before you started to feel this way? What leads you to seek help now? What would need to be done to resolve this situation? The other questions listed—Where do you go to worship? Who is available to help you? To whom do you talk when you are upset?—assess situational supports, not the client's perception of the precipitating event.
Priority Nursing Tip: If the nurse suspects that a client is a victim of abuse, it is their responsibility to report the suspicion to the appropriate authorities. Additionally, the nurse must ensure confidentiality for the client and family as the appropriate procedures are carried out.
Test-Taking Strategy: Focus on the subject of a pregnant client suspected of being physically abused by her husband. The question is asking the client's perception of the precipitating event. This will assist in determining the correct questions to ask the client. The incorrect options assess situational supports, not the client's perception of the precipitating event. Review assessment of a client in crisis.
Reference(s): Varcarolis (2013), p. 388.

707. Which action by the client should lead the nurse to determine the **need for further teaching** regarding the use of the incentive spirometer?
1. Inhales slowly
2. Breathes through the nose
3. Removes the mouthpiece to exhale
4. Forms a tight seal around the mouthpiece with the lips

Level of Cognitive Ability: Evaluating
Client Needs: Health Promotion and Maintenance
Integrated Process: Teaching and Learning
Content Area: Adult Health: Respiratory
Priority Concepts: Client Education; Gas Exchange

Answer: 2
Rationale: Incentive spirometry is ineffective if the client breathes through the nose. The client should exhale, form a tight seal around the mouthpiece, inhale slowly, hold to the count of 5, and remove the mouthpiece to exhale. The client should repeat the exercise approximately 10 times every hour for best results.
Priority Nursing Tip: Use of an incentive spirometer will assist in preventing respiratory complications such as atelectasis in the postoperative client.
Test-Taking Strategy: Note the strategic words, *need for further teaching.* These words indicate a negative event query and ask you to select the option that identifies an incorrect client action. Visualizing the use of this device will direct you to the correct option. Review: the procedure for the use of the **incentive spirometer**.
Reference(s): Potter et al (2013), pp. 848, 1287-1289.

708. The nurse is giving a client with chronic obstructive pulmonary disease (COPD) information related to the positions used to breathe more easily. The nurse teaches the client to assume which position?

1. Sit bolt upright in bed with the arms crossed over the chest.
2. Lie on the side with the head of the bed at a 45-degree angle.
3. Sit in a reclining chair tilted slightly back with the feet elevated.
4. Sit on the edge of the bed with the arms leaning on an over-bed table.

Level of Cognitive Ability: Applying
Client Needs: Health Promotion and Maintenance
Integrated Process: Teaching and Learning
Content Area: Adult Health: Respiratory
Priority Concepts: Client Education; Gas Exchange

Answer: 4
Rationale: Proper positioning can decrease episodes of dyspnea in a client with COPD. Appropriate positions include sitting upright while leaning on an over-bed table, sitting upright in a chair with the arms resting on the knees, and leaning against a wall while standing. Option 1 restricts the movement of the anterior and posterior walls of the lung, and option 2 restricts the expansion of the lateral wall of the lung. Option 3 restricts posterior lung expansion.
Priority Nursing Tip: The arterial blood gas levels on a client with chronic obstructive pulmonary disease usually indicate respiratory acidosis and hypoxemia.
Test-Taking Strategy: Note the subject, a client with COPD. Visualize each of the positions described in the options, and think about how each position affects lung expansion to direct you to the correct option. Review: the positions that relieve dyspnea in the client with chronic obstructive pulmonary disease (COPD).
Reference(s): Ignatavicius, Workman (2013), pp. 614, 616.

709. The nurse has taught the client with pleurisy about measures to promote comfort during recuperation. The nurse determines that the client has understood the information if the client states the need to follow which instruction?

1. Try to take only small, shallow breaths.
2. Take as much pain medication as possible.
3. Lie as much as possible on the unaffected side.
4. Splint the chest wall during coughing and deep breathing.

Level of Cognitive Ability: Evaluating
Client Needs: Health Promotion and Maintenance
Integrated Process: Nursing Process/Evaluation
Content Area: Adult Health: Respiratory
Priority Concepts: Client Education; Gas Exchange

Answer: 4
Rationale: The client with pleurisy should splint the chest wall during coughing and deep breathing. The client may also lie on the affected side to minimize the movement of the affected chest wall. Taking small, shallow breaths promotes atelectasis. The client should take medication cautiously so that adequate coughing and deep breathing are performed and an adequate level of comfort is maintained.
Priority Nursing Tip: The client with pleurisy experiences a knife-like pain that is aggravated on deep-breathing and coughing. A pleural friction rub is heard on auscultation of the lungs.
Test-Taking Strategy: Focus on the subject, to promote comfort in a client with pleurisy. Eliminate option 1 because of the closed-ended word "only." From the remaining options, noting the word *splint* will direct you to this option. Review: the measures that will promote comfort in a client with pleurisy.
Reference(s): Lewis et al (2014), p. 550.

710. A client with a diagnosis of trigeminal neuralgia is started on a regimen of carbamazepine (Tegretol). The nurse provides instructions to the client about the medication. What statement by the client indicates that the client understands the instructions?

1. "I will report a fever or sore throat to my doctor."
2. "Some joint pain is expected and is nothing to worry about."
3. "I must brush my teeth frequently to avoid damage to my gums."
4. "My urine may turn red in color, but this is nothing to be concerned about."

Level of Cognitive Ability: Evaluating
Client Needs: Health Promotion and Maintenance
Integrated Process: Nursing Process/Evaluation
Content Area: Pharmacology: Neurological Medications
Priority Concepts: Client Education; Safety

Answer: 1
Rationale: Carbamazepine (Tegretol) is an anticonvulsant medication and one use is to alleviate the pain associated with trigeminal neuralgia. Agranulocytosis is an adverse effect of carbamazepine, and it places the client at risk for infection. If the client develops a fever or a sore throat, the health care provider should be notified. Unusual bruising and bleeding are also adverse effects of the medication, and they need to be reported to the health care provider if they occur.
Priority Nursing Tip: Trigeminal neuralgia is a sensory disorder of the trigeminal (fifth cranial) nerve that results in severe, recurrent, sharp facial pain along the trigeminal nerve.
Test-Taking Strategy: Eliminate option 3 because of the closed-ended word "must." Next, eliminate options 2 and 4 because both indicate that the development of an adverse effect is "nothing to be concerned about." Recalling that agranulocytosis is an adverse effect will direct you to the correct option. Review: carbamazepine (Tegretol).
Reference(s): Hodgson, Kizior (2014), p. 182.

711. The nurse teaches a preoperative client about the nasogastric (NG) tube that will be inserted in preparation for surgery. The nurse determines that the client understands when the tube will be removed during the postoperative period based on which statement by the client?

1. "When the doctor says so."
2. "When I can tolerate food without vomiting."
3. "When my gastrointestinal (GI) system is healed."
4. "When my bowels begin to function again and I begin to pass gas."

Level of Cognitive Ability: Evaluating
Client Needs: Health Promotion and Maintenance
Integrated Process: Nursing Process/Evaluation
Content Area: Adult Health: Gastrointestinal
Priority Concepts: Client Education; Health Promotion

Answer: 4
Rationale: NG tubes are discontinued when normal function returns to the GI tract. Although the health care provider determines when the NG tube will be removed, option 1 does not determine the effectiveness of teaching. Food would not be administered unless bowel function returns. The tube will be removed well before GI healing occurs.
Priority Nursing Tip: When removing a nasogastric tube, ask the client to take a deep breath and hold; then remove the tube slowly and evenly over the course of 3 to 6 seconds (coil the tube around the hand while removing it).
Test-Taking Strategy: Focus on the subject, the client's knowledge about NG tube removal. Option 1 can be easily eliminated first because it does not determine the effectiveness of teaching. Eliminate option 3 next, considering the time factor associated with the healing of the GI tract. From the remaining options, recalling that food would not be administered unless bowel function returns will assist you in eliminating option 2. Review: the use and care of the nasogastric (NG) tube in a postoperative client.
Reference(s): Ignatavicius, Workman (2013), p. 290.

712. A client is receiving lipids (fat emulsion) intravenously at home, and the client's spouse manages the infusion. The health care nurse makes a visit and discusses potential adverse reactions and the side effects of the therapy with the client and the spouse. After the discussion, the nurse expects the spouse to verbalize that, in case of a suspected adverse reaction, which action is the priority?

1. Stop the infusion.
2. Contact the nurse.
3. Take the client's blood pressure.
4. Contact the local area emergency response team.

Level of Cognitive Ability: Evaluating
Client Needs: Health Promotion and Maintenance
Integrated Process: Teaching and Learning
Content Area: Critical Care: Emergency Situations
Priority Concepts: Client Education; Safety

Answer: 1
Rationale: Signs/symptoms of an adverse reaction to lipids (fat emulsion) include chest and back pain, chills, vertigo, cyanosis, diaphoresis, dyspnea, fever, flushing, headache, nausea and vomiting, pressure over the eyes, and thrombophlebitis of the vein. The priority action is to stop the infusion to limit the adverse response. Although options 2, 3, and 4 are correct interventions, the priority is to stop the infusion.
Priority Nursing Tip: Usually a 1.2-um filter or larger should be used when administering lipids (fat emulsion).
Test-Taking Strategy: Note the strategic word, *priority*. Remembering that the priority action if an adverse reaction occurs when fat emulsion is infusing is to stop the infusion will direct you to the correct option. Review: lipid (fat emulsion) therapy.
Reference(s): Ignatavicius, Workman (2013), p. 1347.

713. The home care nurse suspects that a client's spouse is experiencing caregiver strain. Which action should the nurse take to assess for this condition?

1. Referring the family to a social services agency
2. Gathering data from the caregiver and the client
3. Waiting for the caregiver to talk about the stress
4. Obtaining feedback from the client about the caregiver

Level of Cognitive Ability: Analyzing
Client Needs: Health Promotion and Maintenance
Integrated Process: Caring
Content Area: Mental Health
Priority Concepts: Caregiving; Coping

Answer: 2
Rationale: Caregiver strain can occur when a client is significantly dependent on the caregiver for personal and health care needs. The nurse gathers data from the client and the caregiver to determine the caregiver's stressors and coping abilities and withholds making any referrals until the assessment is complete and the plan of care is in place. Because the nurse suspects caregiver strain, the nurse fulfills the duty to the client and family by approaching the family with the concern, gathering assessment data, and planning care. The nurse does not expect the client to assess the coping abilities of the caregiver because assessment is part of the nursing process and should not be delegated.
Priority Nursing Tip: The nurse should ensure that the client and family are familiar with the available support service in the community.
Test-Taking Strategy: Use the steps of the nursing process to eliminate options 1 and 4. From the remaining options, eliminate option 3 because it breaches the duty that the nurse owes to the family; however, the nurse begins to fulfill that duty by performing a comprehensive assessment that addresses both the client and the caregiver. Review: the concepts of **caregiver strain**.
Reference(s): Potter et al (2013), pp. 735, 739-740.

714. A client being discharged from the hospital will be taking warfarin sodium (Coumadin) at home on a daily basis. The nurse has provided instructions to the client about the medication and determines that **further teaching is needed** if the client makes which statement?

1. "I need to have a prothrombin time checked in 2 weeks."
2. "This medicine thins my blood and allows me to clot more slowly."
3. "I need to increase the intake of foods high in vitamin K in my diet."
4. "If I notice any increased bleeding or bruising, I need to call my doctor."

Level of Cognitive Ability: Evaluating
Client Needs: Health Promotion and Maintenance
Integrated Process: Teaching and Learning
Content Area: Pharmacology: Hematological Medications
Priority Concepts: Clotting; Safety

Answer: 3
Rationale: Warfarin sodium (Coumadin) is an oral anticoagulant that is used mainly to prevent thrombotic events, such as thrombophlebitis, pulmonary embolism, and embolism formation caused by atrial fibrillation or other disorders. Oral anticoagulants prolong the clotting time and are monitored by the prothrombin time and the international normalized ratio. Client education should include signs and symptoms of adverse effects and dietary restrictions such as limiting foods high in vitamin K (e.g., leafy green vegetables, liver, cheese, egg yolks) because these increase clotting times.
Priority Nursing Tip: The International Normalized Ratio (INR) is used to monitor warfarin therapy. The normal INR is 1.3 to 2.0. An INR of 2 to 3 is appropriate for most clients, although for some clients the target INR is 3 to 4.5.
Test-Taking Strategy: Note the strategic words, *further teaching is needed*. These words indicate a negative event query and ask you to select an option that is an incorrect statement. Recalling that warfarin sodium is an anticoagulant will assist you in eliminating options 1, 2, and 4. Also, remembering the role that vitamin K plays in the clotting mechanism will direct you to the correct option. Review: the client teaching points related to **warfarin sodium (Coumadin)**.
Reference(s): Hodgson, Kizior (2014), pp. 1262-1263; Lehne (2013), pp. 641-642.

715. A teenager returns to the gynecological clinic for a follow-up visit for a sexually transmitted infection (STI). Which statement by the teenager indicates the **need for further teaching?**
  1. "I know you won't tell my parents I'm sick."
  2. "I finished all of the antibiotics, just like you said."
  3. "I always make sure that my boyfriend uses a condom."
  4. "My boyfriend doesn't have to come in for treatment, does he?"

Level of Cognitive Ability: Evaluating
Client Needs: Health Promotion and Maintenance
Integrated Process: Teaching and Learning
Content Area: Fundamental Skills: Infection Control
Priority Concepts: Infection; Sexuality

Answer: 4
Rationale: When treating STIs, all sexual contacts must be contacted and treated with medication. The treatment of a teenager for an STI is confidential, and parents will not be contacted, even if the client is less than 18 years old. Clients should always finish the course of antibiotics prescribed by the health care provider. Clients should always use a condom with any sexual contact.
Priority Nursing Tip: Normally parental or guardian consent is needed before providing treatment to an adolescent. An exception is treatment of a minor for a sexually transmitted infection. In this situation, the minor can legally provide consent.
Test-Taking Strategy: Note the strategic words, *need for further teaching*. These words indicate a negative event query and ask you to select an option that is an incorrect statement. Recalling the concepts related to safe sex, the treatment of STIs in the teenager, and the principles related to antibiotic therapy will direct you to the correct option. Review: the content related to treating a teenager for a sexually transmitted infection.
Reference(s): McKinney et al (2013), p. 1036.

716. The nurse is teaching a client who had been newly diagnosed with diabetes mellitus about blood glucose monitoring. The nurse should teach the client to report glucose levels that consistently exceed which level?
  1. 150 mg/dL
  2. 200 mg/dL
  3. 250 mg/dL
  4. 350 mg/dL

Level of Cognitive Ability: Applying
Client Needs: Health Promotion and Maintenance
Integrated Process: Teaching and Learning
Content Area: Adult Health: Endocrine
Priority Concepts: Client Education; Glucose Regulation

Answer: 3
Rationale: The normal blood glucose level ranges from 70 to 110 mg/dL, or as designated and preferred by the health care provider. The client with diabetes mellitus should be taught to report blood glucose levels that exceed 250 mg/dL, unless otherwise instructed by the health care provider. Options 1 and 2 are high levels but do not require health care provider notification. Option 4 is a high value; the client should report an elevated level before it reaches this point.
Priority Nursing Tip: Self-monitoring of the blood glucose level for the client with diabetes mellitus provides the client with current information about the level and information that will assist in maintaining good glycemic control.
Test-Taking Strategy: Note the subject of glucose levels that need to be reported in a client with diabetes mellitus. Recalling the basic principles related to diabetic home care instructions for a client with diabetes mellitus will direct you to the correct option. Review: the principles related to blood glucose monitoring for clients with diabetes mellitus.
Reference(s): Chernecky, Berger (2013), p. 582; Ignatavicius, Workman (2013), p. 1421; Pagana, Pagana (2013), p. 478.

717. A client with gastritis asks the nurse at a screening clinic about analgesics that will not cause epigastric distress. The nurse should tell the client to take which medication?
  1. Aspirin (Ecotrin)
  2. Aspirin (Bufferin)
  3. Ibuprofen (Motrin)
  4. Acetaminophen (Tylenol)

Level of Cognitive Ability: Applying
Client Needs: Health Promotion and Maintenance
Integrated Process: Teaching and Learning
Content Area: Adult Health: Gastrointestinal
Priority Concepts: Client Education; Safety

Answer: 4
Rationale: The client should be advised to take analgesics that do not contain aspirin, such as acetaminophen (Tylenol). Aspirin is irritating to the gastrointestinal tract of the client with a history of gastritis. The medications listed in options 1 and 2 have aspirin in them. Other medications that are irritating to the gastrointestinal tract are the nonsteroidal anti-inflammatory drugs (option 3).
Priority Nursing Tip: The client with gastritis needs to avoid irritating foods, fluids, and other substances, such as spicy and highly seasoned foods, caffeine, alcohol, and nicotine.
Test-Taking Strategy: Note that options 1 and 2 are comparable or alike and that they are aspirin-containing medications. Next recall that nonsteroidal anti-inflammatory medications are very irritating to the gastrointestinal tract. Review: acetaminophen (Tylenol) and gastritis.
Reference(s): Ignatavicius, Workman (2013), p. 1228; Lewis et al (2014), p. 941.

718. A client is diagnosed with thromboangiitis obliterans (Buerger's disease). The nurse places **priority** on teaching the client about modifications of which risk factor related to this disorder?

1. Exposure to heat
2. Cigarette smoking
3. Diet low in vitamin C
4. Excessive water intake

Level of Cognitive Ability: Applying
Client Needs: Health Promotion and Maintenance
Integrated Process: Teaching and Learning
Content Area: Adult Health: Cardiovascular
Priority Concepts: Client Education; Perfusion

Answer: 2

Rationale: Buerger's disease is an occlusive disease of the median small arteries and veins. It occurs predominantly among men who are more than 40 years old who smoke cigarettes. A familial tendency is noted, but cigarette smoking is consistently a risk factor. Symptoms of the disease improve with smoking cessation. Options 1, 3, and 4 are not risk factors.

Priority Nursing Tip: The client with Buerger's disease is at risk for the development of ulcerations in the extremities.

Test-Taking Strategy: Note the strategic word *priority*. Recalling the pathophysiology related to this disorder will direct you to the correct option. Review: the risk factors for **Buerger's disease.**

Reference(s): Ignatavicius, Workman (2013), p. 797.

719. A client has a new prescription for timolol and the nurse provides medication instructions to the client. Which statement by the client indicates a **need for further teaching** regarding the instructions?

1. "I should change positions slowly."
2. "I need to report shortness of breath to the health care provider."
3. "I need to taper or discontinue the medication when I feel well."
4. "I have enough medication on hand to last through weekends and vacations."

Level of Cognitive Ability: Evaluating
Client Needs: Health Promotion and Maintenance
Integrated Process: Teaching and Learning
Content Area: Pharmacology: Cardiovascular Medications
Priority Concepts: Client Education; Safety

Answer: 3

Rationale: Timolol is a beta-adrenergic blocking agent. The client should not discontinue or change the medication dose. Common client teaching points about beta-adrenergic blocking agents include taking the pulse daily, holding it to a rate of less than 60 beats/min (and notifying the health care provider); changing positions slowly; and reporting shortness of breath. The client is also instructed to keep enough medication on hand, not take over-the-counter medications (especially decongestants, cough, and cold preparations) without consulting the health care provider, and carry medical identification that states that a beta-blocker is being taken.

Priority Nursing Tip: Monitor the client taking a beta-blocker for signs/symptoms of respiratory distress because these medications can cause bronchospasm.

Test-Taking Strategy: Note the strategic words, *need for further teaching.* These words indicate a negative event query and ask you to select an option that is an incorrect statement. Noting the word *discontinue* will direct you to this option. Review: the client teaching points related to **timolol.**

Reference(s): Hodgson, Kizior (2014), pp. 1169-1171.

720. The nurse has completed giving medication instructions to a client receiving benazepril (Lotensin) to treat hypertension. What statement made by the client indicates to the nurse that the client **needs further teaching?**

1. "Change positions slowly."
2. "Monitor the blood pressure every week."
3. "Use salt moderately in cooking and on foods."
4. "Report signs and symptoms of infection to the health care provider."

Level of Cognitive Ability: Evaluating
Client Needs: Health Promotion and Maintenance
Integrated Process: Teaching and Learning
Content Area: Pharmacology: Cardiovascular Medications
Priority Concepts: Client Education; Safety

Answer: 3

Rationale: Benazepril (Lotensin) is an angiotensin-converting enzyme (ACE) inhibitor. The client taking an angiotensin-converting enzyme inhibitor is instructed to avoid the use of salt. The medication needs to be taken exactly as prescribed. The client needs to change positions slowly to avoid orthostatic hypotension, monitor the blood pressure weekly, and continue with other lifestyle changes to control hypertension. The client should report fever, mouth sores, and sore throats to the health care provider (neutropenia).

Priority Nursing Tip: Hyperkalemia is a side effect of an angiotensin-converting enzyme (ACE) inhibitor. Therefore, the client taking an ACE inhibitor should avoid the use of potassium supplements and should not take potassium-sparing diuretics when taking an ACE inhibitor.

Test-Taking Strategy: Note the strategic words, *needs further teaching.* These words indicate a negative event query and ask you to select an option that is an incorrect statement. Noting that the medication is prescribed to treat hypertension will assist you in eliminating options 1, 2, and 4. Review: **benazepril (Lotensin).**

Reference(s): Hodgson, Kizior (2014), pp. 119-121; Lehne (2013), pp. 512-513.

721. The nurse has given medication instructions to a client receiving lovastatin (Mevacor). The nurse determines that the client understands the effects of the medication if the client stated the need to adhere to the periodic evaluation of which laboratory test?
1. Bleeding times
2. Creatinine levels
3. Blood glucose levels
4. Liver function studies

Level of Cognitive Ability: Evaluating
Client Needs: Health Promotion and Maintenance
Integrated Process: Nursing Process/Evaluation
Content Area: Pharmacology: Cardiovascular Medications
Priority Concepts: Client Education; Safety

Answer: 4
Rationale: Lovastatin is a HMG-CoA reductase inhibitor used to treat hyperlipidemia. It results in an increase in high-density lipoprotein cholesterol and a decrease in triglycerides and low-density lipoprotein cholesterol. This medication is converted by the liver to active metabolites and therefore is not used in clients with active hepatic disease or elevated transaminase levels. For this reason, it is recommended that clients have periodic liver function studies. Periodic cholesterol levels are also needed to monitor the effectiveness of therapy.
Priority Nursing Tip: Instruct the client taking an antilipemic medication to report any unexplained muscular pain to the health care provider.
Test-Taking Strategy: Focus on the subject, a client taking lovastatin (Mevacor). Recalling that medication names that end with the letters "-statin" are cholesterol-lowering medications and that cholesterol is synthesized in the liver will direct you to the correct option. Review: lovastatin (Mevacor).
Reference(s): Hodgson, Kizior (2014), pp. 715-717.

722. Clonazepam (Klonopin) has been prescribed for the client, and the nurse teaches the client about the medication. Which statement by the client indicates that **further teaching is necessary**?
1. "If I experience slurred speech, it will disappear in about 8 weeks."
2. "My drowsiness will decrease over time with continued treatment."
3. "I should take my medicine with food to decrease stomach problems."
4. "I can take my medicine at bedtime if it tends to make me feel drowsy."

Level of Cognitive Ability: Evaluating
Client Needs: Health Promotion and Maintenance
Integrated Process: Teaching and Learning
Content Area: Pharmacology: Psychiatric Medications
Priority Concepts: Client Education; Safety

Answer: 1
Rationale: Clonazepam (Klonopin) is a benzodiazepine. Clients who experience signs and symptoms of toxicity with the administration of clonazepam exhibit slurred speech, sedation, confusion, respiratory depression, hypotension, and eventually coma. Some drowsiness may occur, but it will decrease with continued use. The medication may be taken with food to decrease gastrointestinal irritation. Options 2, 3, and 4 are correct and show an accurate understanding of the medication.
Priority Nursing Tip: Benzodiazepines have anxiety-reducing, sedative-hypnotic, muscle-relaxing, and anticonvulsant actions.
Test-Taking Strategy: Note the strategic words, *further teaching is necessary*. These words indicate a negative event query and ask you to select an incorrect statement. Recalling the toxic effects that can occur with the use of this medication will direct you to the correct option. Review clonazepam (Klonopin).
Reference(s): Skidmore-Roth (2014), pp. 320-321.

723. Dipyridamole (Persantine) has been prescribed for the client who underwent a valve replacement, and the nurse has provided teaching to the client about the medication. Which statement indicates that the client understands the medication instructions?
1. "This medication will prevent a stroke."
2. "This medication will prevent a heart attack."
3. "This medicine will protect my artificial heart valve."
4. "This medication will help me keep my blood pressure down."

Level of Cognitive Ability: Evaluating
Client Needs: Health Promotion and Maintenance
Integrated Process: Nursing Process/Evaluation
Content Area: Pharmacology: Cardiovascular Medications
Priority Concepts: Client Education; Safety

Answer: 3
Rationale: Dipyridamole (Persantine) is an antiplatelet medication. It may be administered in combination with warfarin sodium to protect the client's artificial heart valves. Dipyridamole does not prevent strokes or heart attacks. It is an antiplatelet medication rather than an antihypertensive.
Priority Nursing Tip: Antiplatelet medications prolong the bleeding time and are contraindicated in those with bleeding disorders.
Test-Taking Strategy: Focus on the subject, client instructions about dipyridamole (Persantine). Recalling that this medication is an antiplatelet medication rather than an antihypertensive will assist you in eliminating option 4. Noting the word *prevent* in options 1 and 2 will assist you in eliminating these options. Review: the use of dipyridamole (Persantine).
Reference(s): Hodgson, Kizior (2014), pp. 365-366.

724. The nurse is preparing to care for the mother of a preterm infant. When should the nurse plan to begin discharge planning?
1. When the mother is in labor
2. When the discharge date is set
3. After stabilization of the infant during the early stages of hospitalization
4. When the parents feel comfortable with and can demonstrate adequate care of the infant

Level of Cognitive Ability: Applying
Client Needs: Health Promotion and Maintenance
Integrated Process: Nursing Process/Planning
Content Area: Maternity: Postpartum
Priority Concepts: Clinical Judgment; Collaboration

Answer: 3
Rationale: Discharge planning begins at admission. The determination of the services, needs, supplies, and equipment requirements should not be made on the day of discharge. Option 1 is incorrect because during labor, the outcome of the delivery is not known. Options 2 and 4 are incorrect because these times are much too late to make the plans that need to be made.
Priority Nursing Tip: A case manager is a nurse who assumes responsibility for coordinating the client's care at admission and after discharge.
Test-Taking Strategy: Note the subject, discharge planning for a mother of a preterm infant. Remember that discharge planning always begins at admission to the hospital. Noting the words *early stages of hospitalization* will direct you to the correct option. Review: the guidelines related to **discharge planning.**
Reference(s): McKinney et al (2013), p. 691.

725. The nurse is providing home care instructions to a client recovering from an acute inferior myocardial infarction (MI) with recurrent angina. What instruction should the nurse provide to this client?
1. Avoid sexual intercourse for at least 4 months.
2. Replace sublingual nitroglycerin tablets yearly.
3. Participate in an exercise program that includes overhead lifting and reaching.
4. Recognize the adverse effects of acetylsalicylic acid (aspirin), which include tinnitus and hearing loss.

Level of Cognitive Ability: Applying
Client Needs: Health Promotion and Maintenance
Integrated Process: Teaching and Learning
Content Area: Adult Health: Cardiovascular
Priority Concepts: Client Education; Safety

Answer: 4
Rationale: After an acute MI, many clients are instructed to take an aspirin daily. Adverse effects include tinnitus, hearing loss, epigastric distress, gastrointestinal bleeding, and nausea. Sexual intercourse usually can be resumed in 4 to 8 weeks after an acute MI if the health care provider agrees and if the client has been able to achieve traditional parameters such as climbing two flights of steps without chest pain or dyspnea. Clients should be advised to purchase a new supply of nitroglycerin tablets every 6 months. Expiration dates on the medication bottle should also be checked. Activities that include lifting and reaching over the head should be avoided because they reduce cardiac output.
Priority Nursing Tip: Acetylsalicylic acid (aspirin) is an antiplatelet medication that inhibits the aggregation of platelets in the clotting process, thereby prolonging the bleeding time.
Test-Taking Strategy: Focus on the subject, a client recovering from an acute inferior myocardial infarction (MI) with recurrent angina. Noting the time limits in options 1 and 2 ("4 months" and "yearly," respectively) will assist you in eliminating these options. From the remaining options, "overhead lifting and reaching" in option 3 should indicate that this is incorrect. Review: the client teaching points after a **myocardial infarction (MI).**
Reference(s): Hodgson, Kizior (2014), p. 85; Ignatavicius, Workman (2013), p. 837.

726. The nurse is reviewing home care instructions with an older client who has type 1 diabetes mellitus and a history of diabetic ketoacidosis (DKA). The client's spouse is present when the instructions are given. Which statement by the spouse indicates that **further teaching is necessary?**
1. "If he is vomiting, I shouldn't give him any insulin."
2. "If the grandchildren are sick, they probably shouldn't come to visit."
3. "I should bring him to the health care provider's office if he develops a fever."
4. "I should call the health care provider if he has nausea or abdominal pain lasting for more than 1 or 2 days."

Level of Cognitive Ability: Evaluating
Client Needs: Health Promotion and Maintenance
Integrated Process: Teaching and Learning
Content Area: Adult Health: Endocrine
Priority Concepts: Client Education; Glucose Regulation

Answer: 1
Rationale: Diabetic ketoacidosis (DKA) is a life-threatening complication of type 1 diabetes mellitus that develops when a severe insulin deficiency occurs. Infection and the stopping of insulin are precipitating factors for DKA. Nausea and abdominal pain that last more than 1 or 2 days need to be reported to the health care provider because these signs/symptoms may be indicative of DKA.
Priority Nursing Tip: Monitor the potassium level closely when the client with diabetic ketoacidosis (DKA) receives treatment for the dehydration and acidosis because the serum potassium level will decrease and potassium replacement may be required.
Test-Taking Strategy: Note the strategic words, *further teaching is necessary*. These words indicate a negative event query and ask you to select an option that is an incorrect statement. Eliminate options 2 and 3 first because both relate to infection. From the remaining options, recalling the causes of DKA will direct you to the correct option. Review: the precipitating factors associated with **diabetic ketoacidosis (DKA)**.
Reference(s): Ignatavicius, Workman (2013), pp. 1454-1455.

❖ **727.** The nurse is performing an assessment on a 34-year-old primigravida client who has been a marathon runner for several years. The client verbalizes concern because she is no longer able to run in marathons and is concerned about the brown discoloration on her face and her increasing size. Which statements by the nurse are therapeutic? **Select all that apply.**
❏ 1. "I can see you're disappointed at not being able to run."
❏ 2. "Tell me how you are feeling about the changes in your body."
❏ 3. "Don't worry. Your body will go back to normal after delivery."
❏ 4. "You need to ask your obstetrician about whether or not you can run."
❏ 5. "Wait and see. You will be back to marathon running after delivery before you know it."
❏ 6. "Some of the changes in pregnancy are permanent and that is the price that you have to pay for that bundle of joy."

Level of Cognitive Ability: Applying
Client Needs: Health Promotion and Maintenance
Integrated Process: Communication and Documentation
Content Area: Maternity: Antepartum
Priority Concepts: Communication; Reproduction

Answer: 1, 2
Rationale: The client is concerned about the body changes and life changes being experienced as a result of pregnancy. Therapeutic communication techniques include focusing on the client's feelings and concerns and acknowledging these concerns by the techniques of clarifying (option 1) and encouraging discussion of feelings (option 2). Telling a client "not to worry" (option 3), placing the client's feelings on hold (option 4), and avoiding discussion of the client's feelings (options 5 and 6) are nontherapeutic communication techniques.
Priority Nursing Tip: Chloasma (mask of pregnancy) is a blotchy brownish hyperpigmentation that occurs over the forehead, cheeks, and nose. It is a normal occurrence during pregnancy.
Test-Taking Strategy: Read each statement carefully. Use of therapeutic communication techniques will assist in determining the correct nursing statements. Review: **therapeutic communication techniques**.
Reference(s): McKinney et al (2013), pp. 30-31, 260.

❖ **728.** The nurse is performing a socioeconomic assessment of a Chinese client. Which questions would be appropriate for the nurse to ask? **Select all that apply.**
  □ 1. "What do you do for a living?"
  □ 2. "How much money do you make yearly?"
  □ 3. "Do you have a primary health care provider?"
  □ 4. "How many years of school did you complete?"
  □ 5. "How different is your life here from in your homeland?"
  □ 6. "What type of work did you do back in your homeland?"

Level of Cognitive Ability: Analyzing
Client Needs: Health Promotion and Maintenance
Integrated Process: Nursing Process/Assessment
Content Area: Fundamental Skills: Cultural Awareness
Priority Concepts: Culture; Health Promotion

Answer: 1, 3, 4, 5, 6
Rationale: Aspects to include in a cultural assessment include bio-cultural history and socioeconomic status (distinct health risks can be attributed to the ecological and socioeconomic context of the culture) and the client's country of origin. Other aspects to assess include religious and spiritual beliefs (to determine major influences in the client's worldview about health and illness, pain and suffering, and life and death), communication patterns (which reflect core cultural values of a society), time orientation (this information can be useful in planning a day of care, setting up appointments for procedures, and helping a client plan self-care activities in the home), caring beliefs and practices (to identify the central values of a culture), and previous experiences with professional health care (which may have implications for adherence to therapies and continuing access of services). Some specific questions to ask when performing a socioeconomic assessment are noted in the correct options. Asking the client about his or her yearly income is inappropriate, unnecessary, and unrelated to health care resources.
Priority Nursing Tip: Cultural assessment is a systematic and comprehensive examination of the cultural care values, beliefs, and practices of individuals, families, and communities and is important to the total care of any client.
Test-Taking Strategy: Focus on the subject, a socioeconomic assessment. Read each assessment question and think about its effect with regard to health risks, health care, and health care resources. This will assist in determining the correct assessment questions. Review: the components of a socioeconomic assessment.
Reference(s): Giger (2013), pp. 387-388, 392.

729. The nurse is developing a teaching plan for the client with Raynaud's disease. Which instruction should the nurse include?
  1. Daily cool baths will provide an analgesic effect.
  2. A high-protein diet will minimize tissue malnutrition.
  3. Vitamin K administration will prevent tendencies toward bleeding.
  4. Keeping the hands and feet warm and dry will prevent vasoconstriction.

Level of Cognitive Ability: Analyzing
Client Needs: Health Promotion and Maintenance
Integrated Process: Nursing Process/Planning
Content Area: Adult Health: Cardiovascular
Priority Concepts: Client Education; Perfusion

Answer: 4
Rationale: Raynaud's disease is a vasospasm of the arterioles and arteries of the upper and lower extremities. The use of measures to prevent vasoconstriction is helpful for the management of Raynaud's disease. The hands and feet should be kept dry. Gloves and warm fabrics should be worn in cold weather, and the client should avoid exposure to nicotine and caffeine. The avoidance of situations that trigger stress is also helpful. Options 1, 2, and 3 are not components of the treatment for this disorder.
Priority Nursing Tip: The attacks that occur in Raynaud's disease are intermittent, occur with exposure to cold or stress, and primarily affect the fingers, toes, ears, and cheeks.
Test-Taking Strategy: Focus on the subject, a teaching plan for the client with Raynaud's disease. Recalling the pathophysiology of the disorder and the need to promote vasodilation will direct you to the correct option. Review the teaching points related to Raynaud's disease.
Reference(s): Ignatavicius, Workman (2013), p. 798.

730. A client with peripheral arterial disease has received instructions from the nurse about how to limit the progression of the disease. The nurse determines that the client **needs further teaching** if which statement was made by the client?

1. "I need to eat a balanced diet."
2. "A heating pad on my leg will help soothe the leg pain."
3. "I need to take special care of my feet to prevent injury."
4. "I should walk daily to increase the circulation to my legs."

Level of Cognitive Ability: Evaluating
Client Needs: Health Promotion and Maintenance
Integrated Process: Teaching and Learning
Content Area: Adult Health: Cardiovascular
Priority Concepts: Perfusion; Safety

Answer: 2
Rationale: The application of heat directly to the extremity is contraindicated. The limb may have decreased sensitivity and be more at risk for burns. Additionally, the direct application of heat raises the oxygen and nutritional requirements of the tissue even further. The long-term management of peripheral arterial disease consists of measures that increase peripheral circulation (exercise), promote vasodilation (warmth), relieve pain, and maintain tissue integrity (foot care and nutrition).
Priority Nursing Tip: In severe cases of peripheral arterial disease, clients with edema may sleep with the affected limb hanging from the bed or they may sit upright (without leg elevation) in a chair for comfort.
Test-Taking Strategy: Focus on the client's diagnosis of peripheral arterial disease, and note the strategic words, *needs further teaching.* These words indicate a negative event query and ask you to select an option that is an incorrect statement. Noting the word *heating* in option 2 will direct you to the correct option. Review: the teaching points related to **peripheral arterial disease.**
Reference(s): Ignatavicius, Workman (2013), p. 788.

731. The nurse is teaching a client with hypertension about items that contain sodium and reviews a written list of items sent from the cardiac rehabilitation department. The nurse tells the client that which item is lowest in sodium content?

1. Antacids
2. Laxatives
3. Toothpaste
4. Demineralized water

Level of Cognitive Ability: Applying
Client Needs: Health Promotion and Maintenance
Integrated Process: Teaching and Learning
Content Area: Adult Health: Cardiovascular
Priority Concepts: Client Education; Health Promotion

Answer: 4
Rationale: Water that is bottled, distilled, deionized, or demineralized may be used for drinking and cooking. Clients are advised to read labels for sodium content. Sodium intake can be increased with the use of several types of products, including toothpaste and mouthwashes; over-the-counter medications such as analgesics, antacids, cough remedies, laxatives, and sedatives; and softened water, as well as some mineral waters.
Priority Nursing Tip: The normal sodium level is 135 to 145 mEq. A sodium imbalance is usually associated with a fluid volume imbalance.
Test-Taking Strategy: Focus on the subject, the item that is lowest in sodium. Noting the word *demineralized*, which means having the minerals taken out of, will direct you to option 4. Review: items that are low and high in sodium.
Reference(s): Ignatavicius, Workman (2013), pp. 180-181, 778; Nix (2013), pp. 389-390.

732. The school nurse provides teaching about the hazards of smoking to a group of high school students. Which comment by a student indicates the **need for additional teaching**?
1. "Chewing tobacco is much safer than is smoking tobacco."
2. "Smoking during pregnancy increases the risk of stillbirth."
3. "My health is at risk when my family smokes in the house."
4. "Inhaling smoke from other people is a public health issue."

Level of Cognitive Ability: Evaluating
Client Needs: Health Promotion and Maintenance
Integrated Process: Teaching and Learning
Content Area: Fundamental Skills: Safety
Priority Concepts: Client Education; Health Promotion

Answer: 1
Rationale: All forms of tobacco use including chewing tobacco are health hazards. Options 2, 3, and 4 are accurate regarding the health hazards of tobacco use.
Priority Nursing Tip: Cigarette smoking and exposure to passive smoke are causes of lung cancer.
Test-Taking Strategy: Note the strategic words, *need for additional teaching*. These words indicate a negative event query and ask you to select an option that is an incorrect statement. This should direct you to the correct option. Review the hazards of tobacco use
Reference(s): Lehne (2013), pp. 450-451.

733. The nurse is developing goals for the postpartum client who is at risk for uterine infection. Which goal would be **most appropriate** for this client?
1. The client will verbalize a reduction of pain.
2. The client will report how to treat an infection.
3. The client will be able to identify measures to prevent infection.
4. The client will identify the presence of Braxton Hicks contractions.

Level of Cognitive Ability: Analyzing
Client Needs: Health Promotion and Maintenance
Integrated Process: Nursing Process/Planning
Content Area: Maternity: Postpartum
Priority Concepts: Infection; Reproduction

Answer: 3
Rationale: The uterus is theoretically sterile during pregnancy until the membranes rupture. However, it is capable of being invaded by pathogens after membrane rupture. Options 1 and 4 are unrelated to the subject of infection. Option 2 indicates that an infection is present. Option 3 is a goal for the client who is at risk for infection.
Priority Nursing Tip: In the postpartum client, a temperature of 100.4° F or greater after 24 hours postpartum indicates infection.
Test-Taking Strategy: Focus on the strategic words, *most appropriate*. Noting the word *prevent* in option 3 will direct you to this option. Options 1 and 4 are unrelated to the subject of the question, a client at risk for uterine infection. Option 2 implies that an infection has been diagnosed. Review the goals for a client who is at risk for uterine infection.
Reference(s): McKinney et al (2013), pp. 682-683.

734. A neonatal intensive care unit (NICU) nurse teaches handwashing techniques to the parents of an infant who is receiving antibiotic treatment for a neonatal infection. The nurse determines that the parents understand the **primary** purpose of handwashing if which statement is made?
1. "It is primarily done to reduce their fears."
2. "It is primarily done to minimize the spread of infection to other siblings."
3. "It is primarily done to allow them an opportunity to communicate with each other and staff."
4. "It is primarily done to reduce the possibility of transmitting an environmental infection to the infant."

Level of Cognitive Ability: Evaluating
Client Needs: Health Promotion and Maintenance
Integrated Process: Nursing Process/Evaluation
Content Area: Maternity: Postpartum
Priority Concepts: Client Education; Infection

Answer: 4
Rationale: Appropriate handwashing by staff and parents has been effective for the prevention of nosocomial infections in nursery units. This action also promotes parents taking an active part in the care of their infant. Options 1 and 3 are not the primary reasons to perform handwashing. Because the infant has the infection and is in the NICU, option 2 is incorrect.
Priority Nursing Tip: Handwashing is the first line of defense against the spread of microorganisms.
Test-Taking Strategy: Note the strategic word, *primary*, to assist you in eliminating options 1 and 3. Noting that the infant is in the NICU will assist you in eliminating option 2. Review: the purposes of **handwashing**
Reference(s): McKinney et al (2013), p. 920.

735. The nurse monitors a client for brachial plexus compromise after shoulder arthroplasty and is checking the status of the ulnar nerve. Which technique should the nurse use to assess the status of this nerve?
1. Ask the client to raise the forearm above the head.
2. Have the client spread all of the fingers wide and resist pressure.
3. Ask the client to move the thumb toward the palm and then back to the neutral position.
4. Have the client grasp the nurse's hand, and note the strength of the client's first and second fingers.

Level of Cognitive Ability: Applying
Client Needs: Health Promotion and Maintenance
Integrated Process: Nursing Process/Assessment
Content Area: Developmental Stages: Health Assessment/Physical Exam
Priority Concepts: Clinical Judgment; Health Promotion

Answer: 2
Rationale: So that the nurse may assess the ulnar nerve status, the client is asked to spread all of the fingers wide and resist pressure. Weakness against pressure may indicate compromise of the ulnar nerve. Option 1 assesses the flexion of the biceps and determines the status of the cutaneous nerve. Option 3 describes the assessment of the status of the radial nerve. Option 4 describes the assessment of the status of the medial nerve.
Priority Nursing Tip: The ulnar nerve splits from the medial cord in the shoulder, descends along the medial aspect of the arm and along the forearm. It then enters the hand. The ulnar nerve is also responsible for the sensation that one feels when he or she "hits the funny bone," squashing the nerve.
Test-Taking Strategy: Focus on the subject, assessing the status of the ulnar nerve. Recalling the location and function of this nerve will direct you to the correct answer. Review: assessment technique and the **ulnar nerve.**
Reference(s): Perry, Potter, Elkin (2012), p. 144; Potter et al (2013), pp. 534-535.

736. A hospitalized client with active pulmonary tuberculosis has been receiving multidrug therapy for the past month and is being prepared for discharge. Which indicates that respiratory isolation is no longer required and that medication therapy has been **effective**?
1. Stools are clay colored.
2. The Mantoux test is negative.
3. Sputum cultures are negative.
4. Nausea and vomiting have stopped.

Level of Cognitive Ability: Evaluating
Client Needs: Health Promotion and Maintenance
Integrated Process: Nursing Process/Evaluation
Content Area: Adult Health: Respiratory
Priority Concepts: Clinical Judgment; Infection

Answer: 3
Rationale: The primary diagnostic tool for pulmonary tuberculosis is a sputum culture. A negative culture indicates the effectiveness of treatment. Nausea, vomiting, and clay-colored stools are side effects of the medication that is used to treat tuberculosis; their presence or absence does not measure the therapeutic effectiveness of the medication. The Mantoux test is a screening tool rather than a diagnostic test for tuberculosis. Because the Mantoux test indicates exposure to the organism but not active disease, the test results will remain positive.
Priority Nursing Tip: Tuberculosis has an insidious onset and many clients are not aware of symptoms until the disease is well advanced.
Test-Taking Strategy: Note the strategic word, *effective*. Remember that the absence of infectious organisms is a desired outcome in clients with communicable diseases. The sputum is the only diagnostic test that will determine the absence of infectious organisms. Review: **pulmonary tuberculosis.**
Reference(s): Ignatavicius, Workman (2013), p. 657.

737. The nurse has conducted a class for pregnant clients with diabetes mellitus about the signs and symptoms of potential complications. The nurse determines that the teaching was **effective** if a client makes which statement?
1. "I should not have ultrasounds done because I am diabetic."
2. "I'm glad I don't have to worry about developing hypoglycemia while I am pregnant."
3. "I need to watch my weight for any sudden gains because I could develop gestational hypertension."
4. "My insulin needs should decrease during the last 2 months because I will be using some of the baby's insulin supply."

Level of Cognitive Ability: Evaluating
Client Needs: Health Promotion and Maintenance
Integrated Process: Nursing Process/Evaluation
Content Area: Maternity: Antepartum
Priority Concepts: Glucose Regulation; Reproduction

Answer: 3
Rationale: A diabetic pregnant client has a higher incidence of developing gestational hypertension than the nondiabetic pregnant client does. Ultrasounds are done frequently during a diabetic pregnancy to check for congenital anomalies and to determine appropriate growth patterns. Hypoglycemia is a problem during pregnancy in the client with diabetes mellitus and needs to be assessed. Insulin needs will increase during the last trimester because of increased placenta degradation.
Priority Nursing Tip: Oral hypoglycemics are not usually prescribed for use during pregnancy.
Test-Taking Strategy: Note the strategic word, *effective*. Focus on the subject, a pregnant client with diabetes mellitus. Options 1 and 2 can be easily eliminated by recalling that hypoglycemia is a concern and that ultrasounds need to be performed. From the remaining options, remember that insulin needs will increase during the last trimester of pregnancy. This will assist you in eliminating option 4. Review: the complications associated with **diabetes mellitus** and **pregnancy.**
Reference(s): McKinney et al (2013), pp. 610-611.

738. A postpartum client recovering from disseminated intravascular coagulopathy is to be discharged on low dosages of an anticoagulant medication. What action should the nurse encourage the client to avoid?
1. Brushing her teeth
2. Taking acetylsalicylic acid (aspirin)
3. Walking long distances and climbing stairs
4. All activities because bruising injuries can occur

Level of Cognitive Ability: Applying
Client Needs: Health Promotion and Maintenance
Integrated Process: Teaching and Learning
Content Area: Pharmacology: Hematological Medications
Priority Concepts: Client Education; Clotting

Answer: 2
Rationale: Aspirin is an antiplatelet medication and can interact with the anticoagulant medication and increase the clotting time beyond therapeutic ranges, so avoiding aspirin is a priority. The client does not need to avoid brushing the teeth, but he or she should be instructed to use a soft toothbrush. Walking and climbing stairs are acceptable activities. Not all activities need to be avoided.
Priority Nursing Tip: Disseminated intravascular coagulopathy (DIC) is a maternal condition in which the clotting cascade is activated, resulting in the formation of clots in the microcirculation.
Test-Taking Strategy: Note the subject of a client recovering from disseminated intravascular coagulopathy. Also, note the word *avoid* in the question. This word indicates the need to select the harmful activity for the client. Recalling that bleeding is an adverse effect of anticoagulants will direct you to the correct option. Review: **disseminated intravascular coagulopathy** and **anticoagulants.**
Reference(s): McKinney et al (2013), pp. 619-620.

❖ **739.** The nurse teaches a client at risk for coronary artery disease about lifestyle changes needed to reduce his risks. The nurse determines that the client understands these necessary lifestyle changes if the client makes which statements? **Select all that apply.**
- ❏ 1. "I will cut down on my smoking habit."
- ❏ 2. "I will be sure to include some exercise such as walking in my daily activities."
- ❏ 3. "I will work at losing some weight so that my weight is at normal range for my age."
- ❏ 4. "I will limit my sodium intake every day and avoid eating high-sodium foods such as hot dogs."
- ❏ 5. "It is acceptable to eat red meat and cheese every day as I have been doing, as long as I cut down on the butter."
- ❏ 6. "I will schedule regular health care provider appointments for physical examinations and monitoring my blood pressure."

Level of Cognitive Ability: Evaluating
Client Needs: Health Promotion and Maintenance
Integrated Process: Nursing Process/Evaluation
Content Area: Adult Health: Cardiovascular
Priority Concepts: Client Education; Health Promotion

Answer: 2, 3, 4, 6
Rationale: Coronary artery disease affects the arteries that provide blood, oxygen, and nutrients to the myocardium. Modifiable risk factors include elevated serum cholesterol levels, cigarette smoking, hypertension, impaired glucose tolerance, obesity, physical inactivity, and stress. The client is instructed to stop smoking (not cut down), and the nurse should provide the client with resources to do so. The client is also instructed to maintain a normal weight and include physical activity in the daily schedule. The client is also instructed to limit sodium intake and foods high in cholesterol, including red meat and cheese. The client must follow up with regular health care provider appointments for physical examinations and monitoring blood pressure.
Priority Nursing Tip: Modifiable risk factors for coronary artery disease are those that can be changed to reduce the risk (e.g., smoking, diet intake). Nonmodifiable risk factors for coronary artery disease are those that cannot be changed (e.g., age, race).
Test-Taking Strategy: Focus on the subject, lifestyle changes to reduce the risk of coronary artery disease. Think about the pathophysiology associated with coronary artery disease. Read each option carefully and recall that coronary artery disease affects the arteries that provide blood, oxygen, and nutrients to the myocardium. This will assist in selecting the correct options. Review: the lifestyle changes to reduce the risk of coronary artery disease.
Reference(s): Ignatavicius, Workman (2013), pp. 832, 852.

❖ **740.** What factors should the nurse consider for teaching a child about his or her disease and related health care measures? **Select all that apply.**
- ❏ 1. A child rarely forms misconceptions.
- ❏ 2. The older the child, the shorter the attention span.
- ❏ 3. A child's imagination may create greater fear than the truth.
- ❏ 4. A child may regress developmentally in a situation of illness.
- ❏ 5. It is not necessary to assess the child's knowledge before teaching.
- ❏ 6. A child may better manage uncomfortable information through role-playing.

Level of Cognitive Ability: Analyzing
Client Needs: Health Promotion and Maintenance
Integrated Process: Teaching and Learning
Content Area: Developmental Stages: Infancy to Adolescence
Priority Concepts: Development; Health Promotion

Answer: 3, 4, 6
Rationale: For children, the teaching-learning process may be fundamentally different than that used for adults, and the nurse needs to adjust the complexity and volume of information based on the child's age and cognitive level. The factors that need to be addressed when teaching children include the following: Trust is essential to a therapeutic relationship; in general, the younger the child, the shorter the attention span; assessing the child's knowledge is important because children are exposed to various levels of information about health care; children form misconceptions easily, and a child's imagination may create greater fear than the truth; a child may regress developmentally in a situation of illness; and a child may better manage uncomfortable information through role-playing.
Priority Nursing Tip: Many factors need to be considered when determining the best teaching method. One factor is age. At a younger age, people tend to be visual and hands-on learners, thus presenting charts and pictures will enhance learning. Adults typically like to have control over their learning; thus, it is best to include them in planning the process.
Test-Taking Strategy: Focus on the subject, factors to consider for teaching a child. Read each option carefully and think about the concepts of growth and development. This will assist in selecting the correct options. Review: the factors that affect the teaching and learning process.
Reference(s): McKinney et al (2013), pp. 899-900.

❖ **741.** The nurse is caring for a client with end-stage renal disease. What areas are appropriate to assess to determine the client's wishes for end-of-life nursing care? **Select all that apply.**
- ❑ 1. Preferred place for death
- ❑ 2. Client expectations for nursing care
- ❑ 3. Financial responsibilities for the funeral
- ❑ 4. Where the funeral and burial will take place
- ❑ 5. Use of and the level of life-sustaining measures
- ❑ 6. Expectations regarding pain control and symptom management

Level of Cognitive Ability: Analyzing
Client Needs: Health Promotion and Maintenance
Integrated Process: Nursing Process/Assessment
Content Area: Developmental Stages: End-of-Life Care
Priority Concepts: Clinical Judgment; Palliation

Answer: 1, 2, 5, 6
Rationale: The nurse must assess the client's wishes for end-of-life nursing care because these can influence how the nurse sets priorities for planning and implementing care. End-of-life assessment related to nursing care should include the preferred place for death, client expectations for nursing care, the use of and the level of life-sustaining measures, and expectations regarding pain control and symptom management. Financial responsibilities for the funeral and where the funeral and burial will take place are issues that the client may want to discuss, but they are unrelated to nursing care.
Priority Nursing Tip: Each client's end-of-life experience will be unique, and the nurse needs to plan care based on the client's wishes.
Test-Taking Strategy: Focus on the subject, end-of-life nursing care. Read each option and select those that relate to nursing care. Financial responsibilities for the funeral and where the funeral and burial will take place are unrelated to nursing care. Review: **end-of-life** nursing care issues.
Reference(s): Potter et al (2013), pp. 720-722.

742. The school nurse teaches an athletic coach how to prevent dehydration among athletes practicing in the hot weather. What is the **best** advice for the nurse to give to the coach?
1. Drink plenty of fluids before and after practice.
2. Have the athletes take a salt tablet before practice.
3. Reschedule practice for before school and after sunset.
4. Provide a fluid break every 30 minutes during practice.

Level of Cognitive Ability: Applying
Client Needs: Health Promotion and Maintenance
Integrated Process: Teaching and Learning
Content Area: Fundamental Skills: Fluids & Electrolytes
Priority Concepts: Client Education; Fluid and Electrolyte Balance

Answer: 4
Rationale: Hot weather accelerates the body's loss of fluid and electrolytes during strenuous physical activity, so the nurse encourages the coach to schedule fluid breaks at 30-minute intervals, so that the athletes can periodically rest and restore body fluids. Drinking fluid before and after practice is a reasonable suggestion; however, because the hot weather accelerates fluid and electrolyte losses, body fluids must be periodically replenished to maintain the fluid and electrolyte balance. Although a sodium load increases fluid retention, the nurse avoids suggesting salt tablets for the athletes because the nurse needs approval from each athlete's health care provider before recommending the salt. Rescheduling practice times is unrealistic.
Priority Nursing Tip: Some causes of dehydration include decreased fluid intake, diaphoresis, vomiting, diarrhea, diabetic ketoacidosis, and extensive burns or other serious injuries.
Test-Taking Strategy: Focus on the subject of preventing dehydration. Note the strategic word, *best*; this indicates that each option may be a reasonable response for preventing dehydration. However, you must choose the option that is a better choice than the other three. Recall the principles of fluid and electrolyte balance and the causes of dehydration. Option 4 is the best answer because it is the most effective response that addresses fluid and electrolyte balance directly, and it is also the most practical choice. Review: the measures used to prevent **dehydration**.
Reference(s): Ignatavicius, Workman (2013), pp. 173, 176; Lewis et al (2014), p. 307.

743. The nurse instructs a client who is hospitalized and on a low-fat diet. Which menu does the nurse provide for the client?
1. Shrimp, avocado, and tomato salad
2. Calf's liver, potato salad, and sherbet
3. Lean steak, mashed potatoes, and gravy
4. Turkey breast, boiled rice, and strawberries

Level of Cognitive Ability: Applying
Client Needs: Health Promotion and Maintenance
Integrated Process: Nursing Process/Implementation
Content Area: Fundamental Skills: Nutrition
Priority Concepts: Client Education; Nutrition

Answer: 4
Rationale: Turkey breast without the skin, boiled rice, and strawberries offer the client nourishing foods that are low in fat. Some sources of fat include meats, avocado, salad dressing, mayonnaise, butter, cheese, and bacon. Options 1, 2, and 3 contain high-fat foods.
Priority Nursing Tip: A low-fat diet is indicated for disorders such as atherosclerosis, diabetes mellitus, hyperlipidemia, hypertension, and myocardial infarction.
Test-Taking Strategy: Focus on the subject, a low-fat diet. Eliminate options 1 and 2 first because avocado and liver have a very high fat content. Potato salad usually contains mayonnaise, which is high in fat. Next, eliminate option 3 because meat is high in fat and mashed potatoes are not very palatable without butter or gravy, and both are high in fat. Option 4 does not contain high-fat foods. Review the foods that contain fat.
Reference(s): Nix (2013), p. 38.

744. The camp nurse provides instructions regarding skin protection from the sun to the parents who are preparing their children for a camping adventure. Which statement by a parent indicates a **need for further instructions**?
1. "A protective sunscreen is best to prevent sunburn."
2. "My child won't need the sunscreen on cloudy, hazy days."
3. "I need to pack a hat, long-sleeved shirts, and long pants for my child to wear."
4. "My child should wear clothes that have a tightly woven material for greater protection from the sun's rays."

Level of Cognitive Ability: Evaluating
Client Needs: Health Promotion and Maintenance
Integrated Process: Teaching and Learning
Content Area: Child Health: Integumentary
Priority Concepts: Client Education; Tissue Integrity

Answer: 2
Rationale: The sun's rays are as damaging to the skin on cloudy, hazy days as they are on sunny days. Sunscreens are recommended and should be applied before exposure to the sun and reapplied frequently and liberally at least every 2 hours. A hat, long-sleeved shirt, and long pants should be worn when out in the sun. Tightly woven materials provide greater protection from the sun's rays.
Priority Nursing Tip: To prevent skin damage from the sun's rays, the client should be instructed to avoid sun exposure between the hours of 10 AM and 4 PM.
Test-Taking Strategy: Note the strategic words, *need for further instructions*. These words indicate a negative event query and ask you to select an option that is an incorrect statement. Eliminate options 1, 3, and 4 because these measures provide the greatest protection from the sun. Also recalling the concept that ultraviolet rays can be damaging regardless of cloudiness or haziness will assist in directing you to the correct option. Review: skin protection.
Reference(s): Hockenberry, Wilson (2013), pp. 1047-1048.

745. A client has urinary calculi that are composed of uric acid, and the nurse teaches the client dietary measures to prevent the further development of the calculi. The nurse determines that the client understands the dietary measures if the client states that it is necessary to avoid consuming what food products?
1. Milk
2. Dairy products
3. Spinach, chocolate, and tea
4. Fish with fine bones and organ meats

Level of Cognitive Ability: Evaluating
Client Needs: Health Promotion and Maintenance
Integrated Process: Nursing Process/Evaluation
Content Area: Adult Health: Renal and Urinary
Priority Concepts: Client Education; Health Promotion

Answer: 4
Rationale: The client with a uric acid stone should limit the intake of foods that are high in purines. Organ meats, sardines, herring, and other high-purine foods are eliminated from the diet. Foods with moderate levels of purines, such as red and white meats and some seafood, are also limited. Options 1, 2, and 3 are recommended dietary changes to prevent calculi that are composed of calcium phosphate or calcium oxalate.
Priority Nursing Tip: Uric acid stones are usually caused by excess dietary purine or gout.
Test-Taking Strategy: Note the subject, a client with urinary calculi that are composed of uric acid. Note the word *avoid*, which asks you to select the incorrect food choice. Remembering that organ meats are high in purines will direct you to the correct option. Also note that options 1, 2, and 3 are comparable or alike in that they are foods that are avoided if the client has calcium phosphate or calcium oxalate calculi. Review: the foods to avoid with uric acid calculi.
Reference(s): Ignatavicius, Workman (2013), p. 1511.

746. The nurse is teaching a mother with diabetes mellitus who delivered a large-for-gestational-age (LGA) infant about the care of the infant. The nurse tells the mother that LGA infants appear to be more mature because of their large size, but that, in reality, these infants frequently need to be aroused to facilitate nutritional intake and attachment. Which statement by the mother indicates the **need for additional teaching** about the care of the infant?

1. "I will talk to my baby when he is in a quiet, alert state."
2. "I will allow my baby to sleep through the night because he needs his rest."
3. "I will breast-feed my baby every 2½ to 3 hours and will use arousal techniques."
4. "I will watch my baby closely because I know that he may not be as mature in his motor development."

Level of Cognitive Ability: Evaluating
Client Needs: Health Promotion and Maintenance
Integrated Process: Teaching and Learning
Content Area: Maternity: Newborn
Priority Concepts: Client Education; Development

Answer: 2
Rationale: LGA infants tend to be more difficult to arouse and therefore must be aroused to facilitate nutritional intake and attachment opportunities. These infants also have problems maintaining a quiet, alert state. It is beneficial for the mother to interact with the infant during this time to enhance and lengthen the quiet, alert state. LGA infants need to be aroused for feedings, usually every 2½ to 3 hours for breast-feeding. Although the infant is large, motor function is not usually as mature as it is in the term infant.
Priority Nursing Tip: Monitor the large for gestational age newborn for signs of hypoglycemia. Initiate feedings early to prevent the occurrence of hypoglycemia.
Test-Taking Strategy: Note the strategic words, *need for additional teaching*. These words indicate a negative event query and ask you to select an option that is an incorrect statement. Focusing on the words *frequently need to be aroused* in the question will direct you to option 2. Options 1, 3, and 4 address observation and arousal, whereas option 2 does not. Review the care of the **large-for-gestational-age (LGA) infant**.
Reference(s): Lowdermilk, Perry, Cashion, Alden (2012), p. 926; McKinney et al (2013), pp. 712, 728-729.

747. A client has been experiencing muscle weakness for a period of several months. The health care provider suspects polymyositis, and the client asks the nurse about the disorder. The nurse explains to the client that which occurs in this disorder?

1. Increased fibers and tissue
2. Muscle fibers are inflamed
3. Muscle fibers are thickened
4. A decrease in elastic tissue

Level of Cognitive Ability: Applying
Client Needs: Health Promotion and Maintenance
Integrated Process: Teaching and Learning
Content Area: Adult Health: Musculoskeletal
Priority Concepts: Client Education; Inflammation

Answer: 2
Rationale: Polymyositis is a diffuse inflammatory disorder of skeletal (striated) muscle that is characterized by symmetrical weakness and atrophy. Option 1 refers to the increased fibrous tissue seen in clients with ankylosis. Option 3 describes the opposite of what is noted with this disorder. Option 4 is incorrect, but decreased elastic tissue in the aorta would be noted in a client with Marfan's syndrome.
Priority Nursing Tip: Using medical terminology skills will assist you with determining what an unfamiliar condition presented in a test question means. For example, *poly-* means many; *-myo-* refers to muscle; *-itis* indicates inflammation.
Test-Taking Strategy: Note the subject of the question, polymyositis. The ending, *-itis,* indicates inflammation. The only option that addresses inflammation is option 2. Review: the description of **polymyositis**.
Reference(s): Ignatavicius, Workman (2013), p. 351.

748. The nurse in an ambulatory clinic administers a tuberculin (Mantoux) skin test to a client on a Monday. When should the nurse tell the client to return to the clinic to have the results read?

1. Thursday or Friday
2. The following Monday
3. Tuesday or Wednesday
4. Wednesday or Thursday

Level of Cognitive Ability: Applying
Client Needs: Health Promotion and Maintenance
Integrated Process: Nursing Process/Implementation
Content Area: Adult Health: Respiratory
Priority Concepts: Health Promotion; Infection

Answer: 4
Rationale: The Mantoux skin test for tuberculosis is read in 48 to 72 hours; therefore, the client should return to the clinic on Wednesday or Thursday.
Priority Nursing Tip: For a Mantoux skin test, once the result is positive, it will be positive in any future tests.
Test-Taking Strategy: Focus on the subject, the time frame for reading a tuberculin skin test after it is administered. Recalling that this test is read within 48 to 72 hours will direct you to the correct option. Review: the procedure for the **Mantoux tuberculin skin test.**
Reference(s): Chernecky, Berger (2013), pp. 764-765; Potter et al (2013), p. 835.

749. A client with chronic obstructive pulmonary disease (COPD) is admitted to the hospital with an exacerbation. Which factor contributed **most** to the change in client status?

1. Decreased fat intake
2. Decreased fluid intake
3. Sleeping soundly during the night
4. Anxiety about the upcoming health care provider visit

Level of Cognitive Ability: Analyzing
Client Needs: Health Promotion and Maintenance
Integrated Process: Nursing Process/Assessment
Content Area: Adult Health: Respiratory
Priority Concepts: Gas Exchange; Health Promotion

Answer: 2
Rationale: The client with exacerbation of COPD has ineffective coughing and excess sputum in the airways. The nurse assesses the client for contributing factors such as dehydration and a lack of knowledge of proper coughing techniques. The reduction of these factors helps limit exacerbations of the disease. Options 1, 3, and 4 are not directly associated with this change in condition.
Priority Nursing Tip: The client with COPD should be instructed to avoid environmental irritants such as smoke from fireplaces, pets, feather pillows, and aerosol sprays.
Test-Taking Strategy: Note the strategic word, *most.* Also note the subject, exacerbation of COPD. This calls to mind the concept of sputum production and clearance. Evaluate each of the options in terms of the potential ability to inhibit sputum production or clearance. The fluid intake is the only factor that could affect the viscosity of secretions, thus affecting airway clearance. Review: **chronic obstructive pulmonary disease (COPD).**
Reference(s): Ignatavicius, Workman (2013), p. 620.

750. A client with acquired immunodeficiency syndrome (AIDS) gets recurrent *Candida* infections of the mouth (thrush). The nurse has given the client instructions to minimize the occurrence of thrush and determines that the client understands the instructions if which statement is made by the client?

1. "I should use warm saline or water to rinse my mouth."
2. "I should use a mouthwash at least once a week."
3. "I should brush my teeth and rinse my mouth once a day."
4. "Increasing the amount of red meat in my diet will keep this from recurring."

Level of Cognitive Ability: Evaluating
Client Needs: Health Promotion and Maintenance
Integrated Process: Nursing Process/Evaluation
Content Area: Adult Health: Immune
Priority Concepts: Immunity; Infection

Answer: 1
Rationale: When a client is in a state of immunosuppression or has decreased levels of some normal oral flora, an overgrowth of the normal flora *Candida* can occur. Careful routine mouth care is helpful to prevent the recurrence of *Candida* infections. The client should use a mouthwash that consists of warm saline or water. The time frames given for oral hygiene in options 2 and 3 are too infrequent. Red meat will not prevent thrush.
Priority Nursing Tip: A *Candida* infection of the mucous membranes of the mouth appears as red and whitish patches.
Test-Taking Strategy: Eliminate options 2 and 3 because they are comparable or alike and the time frames are too infrequent. From the remaining options, recalling that red meat is not likely to minimize the occurrence of thrush will direct you to the correct option. Review: the teaching points related to the prevention of *Candida* infections.
Reference(s): Ignatavicius, Workman (2013), pp. 376, 1194.

751. The nurse is teaching a client with acquired immunodeficiency syndrome (AIDS) how to avoid foodborne illnesses. The nurse instructs the client to prevent acquiring infection from food by avoiding which item?

1. Raw oysters
2. Bottled water
3. Pasteurized milk
4. Products with sorbitol

Level of Cognitive Ability: Applying
Client Needs: Health Promotion and Maintenance
Integrated Process: Teaching and Learning
Content Area: Adult Health: Immune
Priority Concepts: Client Education; Immunity

Answer: 1

Rationale: The client who is at risk for immunosuppression is taught to avoid raw or undercooked seafood, meat, poultry, and eggs. The client should also avoid unpasteurized milk and dairy products. Fruits that can be peeled, as well as bottled beverages, are safe. The client may be taught to avoid sorbitol, but this is to diminish diarrhea and has nothing to do with foodborne infections.

Priority Nursing Tip: Acquired immunodeficiency syndrome (AIDS) is considered to be a chronic illness. The disease has a long incubation period, sometimes 10 years or longer. Manifestations may not appear until late in the infection.

Test-Taking Strategy: Focus on the subject, foodborne illness. Sorbitol can cause diarrhea, but it is unrelated to foodborne illness, so option 4 is eliminated first. Eliminate option 3 next because products that are pasteurized are free of microbes. From the remaining options, noting the word *raw* in option 1 will direct you to this option. Review: **foodborne illnesses** and dietary teaching for the client with **acquired immunodeficiency syndrome (AIDS)**.

Reference(s): Ignatavicius, Workman (2013), p. 379.

752. A client with histoplasmosis has a prescription for ketoconazole (Nizoral). Which instruction should the nurse teach the client to follow while taking this medication?

1. Avoid exposure to sunlight.
2. Limit alcohol to 2 ounces per day.
3. Take the medication with an antacid.
4. Take the medication on an empty stomach.

Level of Cognitive Ability: Applying
Client Needs: Health Promotion and Maintenance
Integrated Process: Teaching and Learning
Content Area: Pharmacology: Immune Medications
Priority Concepts: Client Education; Safety

Answer: 1

Rationale: The client should be taught that ketoconazole is an antifungal medication. The client should avoid exposure to sunlight because the medication increases photosensitivity. The client should avoid the concurrent use of alcohol because the medication is hepatotoxic. Antacids should be avoided for 2 hours after it is taken because gastric acid is needed to activate the medication. This medication should be taken with food or milk.

Priority Nursing Tip: Ketoconazole (Nizoral), an antifungal medication, is hepatotoxic. Assess the client for a history of liver disorders and check the results of liver function blood tests.

Test-Taking Strategy: Focus on the subject, ketoconazole (Nizoral). Use general guidelines related to medication administration to eliminate options 2 and 3. From the remaining options, it is necessary to know that the medication causes photosensitivity reaction and should be taken with food or milk. Review: **ketoconazole (Nizoral)**.

Reference(s): Hodgson, Kizior (2014), pp. 647-649; Lehne (2013), p. 1141.

753. The nurse is planning to teach a teenage client about sexuality. What should the nurse do **first**?

1. Inform the teenager about the dangers of pregnancy.
2. Establish a relationship and determine prior knowledge.
3. Advise the teenager to maintain sexual abstinence until marriage.
4. Provide written information about sexually transmitted infections.

Level of Cognitive Ability: Applying
Client Needs: Health Promotion and Maintenance
Integrated Process: Teaching and Learning
Content Area: Adult Health: Reproductive
Priority Concepts: Development; Sexuality

Answer: 2

Rationale: The first step in effective communication is establishing a relationship. By exploring the client's interest and prior knowledge, rapport is established, and learning needs are assessed. The other options may or may not be later steps, depending on the data obtained.

Priority Nursing Tip: The nurse always needs to assess the client's readiness to learn before implementing a teaching plan.

Test-Taking Strategy: Note the strategic word, *first*. Use the steps of the nursing process, and select an assessment option. This will direct you to the correct option. When teaching, assessing motivation, interest, and level of knowledge is done before providing information. Review: the **principles of teaching and learning**.

Reference(s): McKinney et al (2013), pp. 61, 171.

754. The nurse provides home care instructions to a client with Cushing's syndrome. The nurse determines that the client understands the hospital discharge instructions if the client makes which statement?
1. "I need to eat foods low in potassium."
2. "I need to check the color of my stools."
3. "I need to check the temperature of my legs twice a day."
4. "I need to take aspirin rather than Tylenol for a headache."

Level of Cognitive Ability: Evaluating
Client Needs: Health Promotion and Maintenance
Integrated Process: Nursing Process/Evaluation
Content Area: Adult Health: Endocrine
Priority Concepts: Client Education; Health Promotion

Answer: 2
Rationale: Cushing's syndrome results in an increased secretion of cortisol. Cortisol stimulates the secretion of gastric acid, and this can result in the development of peptic ulcers and gastrointestinal bleeding. The client should be encouraged to eat potassium-rich foods to correct the hypokalemia that occurs with this disorder. Cushing's syndrome does not affect temperature changes in the lower extremities. Aspirin can increase the risk for gastric bleeding and skin bruising.
Priority Nursing Tip: Laboratory findings noted in Cushing's syndrome include hyperglycemia, hypernatremia, hypokalemia, and hypocalcemia.
Test-Taking Strategy: Focus on the subject, Cushing's syndrome. Recalling the pathophysiology of this disorder and that cortisol stimulates the secretion of gastric acid will direct you to the correct option. Review: **Cushing's syndrome.**
Reference(s): Ignatavicius, Workman (2013), pp. 1382, 1388.

755. A client with heart failure and secondary hyperaldosteronism is started on spironolactone (Aldactone) to manage this disorder. The nurse informs the client that the need for dosage adjustment may be necessary if which medication is also being taken?
1. Alprazolam (Xanax)
2. Warfarin sodium (Coumadin)
3. Potassium chloride (Klor-Con)
4. Verapamil hydrochloride (Calan SR)

Level of Cognitive Ability: Analyzing
Client Needs: Health Promotion and Maintenance
Integrated Process: Nursing Process/Implementation
Content Area: Pharmacology: Cardiovascular Medications
Priority Concepts: Client Education; Safety

Answer: 3
Rationale: Spironolactone (Aldactone) is a potassium-retaining diuretic. If the client is also taking potassium chloride or another potassium supplement, the risk for hyperkalemia exists. Potassium doses would need to be adjusted while the client is taking this medication. A dosage adjustment would not be necessary if the client was taking the medications identified in options 1, 2, or 4.
Priority Nursing Tip: Potassium-retaining diuretics act on the distal tubule to promote sodium and water excretion and potassium retention.
Test-Taking Strategy: Focus on the subject, dosage adjustment in a client taking spironolactone (Aldactone). Recalling that spironolactone is a potassium-retaining diuretic will direct you to the correct option. Review: **spironolactone (Aldactone).**
Reference(s): Hodgson, Kizior (2014), pp. 1102-1104.

756. The nurse is teaching health education classes to a group of expectant parents, and the topic is preventing mental retardation caused by congenital hypothyroidism. What should the nurse tell the parents is the **most effective** means of promoting early intervention?
1. Vitamin intake
2. Neonatal screening
3. Adequate protein intake
4. Limiting alcohol consumption

Level of Cognitive Ability: Applying
Client Needs: Health Promotion and Maintenance
Integrated Process: Nursing Process/Implementation
Content Area: Maternity: Antepartum
Priority Concepts: Client Education; Health Promotion

Answer: 2
Rationale: Congenital hypothyroidism is a common preventable cause of mental retardation. Neonatal screening is the only means of early diagnosis and the subsequent prevention of mental retardation. Newborn infants are screened for congenital hypothyroidism before discharge from the nursery and before 7 days of life. Treatment is begun immediately, if necessary. Adequate protein and vitamin intake will not specifically prevent this disorder. Alcohol consumption during pregnancy needs to be restricted rather than just limited.
Priority Nursing Tip: In mental retardation, a child manifests below average intellectual functioning along with deficits in adaptive skills.
Test-Taking Strategy: Note the strategic words, *most effective.* Focus on the subject, promoting early intervention. Options 1, 3, and 4 are measures to prevent all birth defects. In addition, note that neonatal screening is the umbrella option. Review: **congenital hypothyroidism.**
Reference(s): McKinney et al (2013), pp. 249-250, 1383.

757. The nurse in an outpatient diabetes clinic is monitoring a client with type 1 diabetes mellitus. Today's blood work reveals a glycosylated hemoglobin level of 10%. The nurse creates a teaching plan based on the understanding that this result indicates which finding?

1. A normal value that indicates that the client is managing blood glucose control well
2. A value that does not offer information regarding the client's management of the disease
3. A low value that indicates that the client is not managing blood glucose control very well
4. A high value that indicates that the client is not managing blood glucose control very well

Level of Cognitive Ability: Analyzing
Client Needs: Health Promotion and Maintenance
Integrated Process: Teaching and Learning
Content Area: Adult Health: Endocrine
Priority Concepts: Client Education; Glucose Regulation

Answer: 4
Rationale: Glycosylated hemoglobin is a measure of glucose control during the 6 to 8 weeks before the test. It is a reliable measure for determining the degree of glucose control in diabetic clients over a period of time, and it is not influenced by dietary management a day or two before the test is done. The glycosylated hemoglobin level should be 7.0% or less for a client with diabetes mellitus, with elevated levels indicating poor glucose control.
Priority Nursing Tip: Hyperglycemia in a client with diabetes mellitus is usually the cause of an increase in the HbA1c (glycosylated hemoglobin) level.
Test-Taking Strategy: Focus on the subject, an elevated glycosylated hemoglobin level. Specific knowledge regarding the normal values for this test will direct you to the correct option. Remember that the level should be 7.0% or less. Review: **glycosylated hemoglobin.**
Reference(s): Pagana, Pagana (2013), p. 489.

758. The nurse is instructing a client with type 1 diabetes mellitus about the management of hypoglycemic reactions. The nurse instructs the client that hypoglycemia **most likely** occurs during what time interval after insulin administration?

1. Peak
2. Onset
3. Duration
4. Anytime

Level of Cognitive Ability: Applying
Client Needs: Health Promotion and Maintenance
Integrated Process: Teaching and Learning
Content Area: Adult Health: Endocrine
Priority Concepts: Client Education; Glucose Regulation

Answer: 1
Rationale: Insulin reactions are most likely to occur during the peak time after insulin administration, when the medication is at its maximum action. Peak action depends on the type of insulin, the amount administered, the injection site, and other factors.
Priority Nursing Tip: Regular insulin peaks in 2 hours. NPH insulin peaks in 4 to 12 hours.
Test-Taking Strategy: Note the strategic words, *most likely.* Focus on the subject, hypoglycemia. Remember that insulin is a hypoglycemic agent. The word *peak* means the highest point. Remembering this should assist with directing you to the correct option. Review: the occurrence of **hypoglycemia** in a client with **type 1 diabetes mellitus.**
Reference(s): Ignatavicius, Workman (2013), p. 1431.

759. The nurse is caring for a client who is scheduled to have a thyroidectomy and provides instructions to the client about the surgical procedure. Which statement by the client would indicate an understanding of the nurse's instructions?

1. "I will definitely have to continue taking antithyroid medication after this surgery."
2. "I need to place my hands behind my neck when I have to cough or change positions."
3. "I need to turn my head and neck front, back, and side to side every hour for the first 12 hours after surgery."
4. "I will immediately report to the emergency room if I experience tingling of my toes, fingers, and lips after surgery."

Level of Cognitive Ability: Evaluating
Client Needs: Health Promotion and Maintenance
Integrated Process: Nursing Process/Evaluation
Content Area: Adult Health: Endocrine
Priority Concepts: Client Education; Safety

Answer: 2
Rationale: The client is taught that following thyroidectomy tension needs to be avoided on the suture line because hemorrhage may develop. One way of reducing incisional tension is to teach the client how to support the neck when coughing or being repositioned. Likewise, during the postoperative period, the client should avoid any unnecessary movement of the neck; that is why sandbags and pillows are frequently used to support the head and neck. The removal of the thyroid does not mean that the client will be taking antithyroid medications postoperatively. If a client experiences tingling in the fingers, toes, and lips, it is probably a result of injury to the parathyroid gland during surgery, resulting in hypocalcemia. These signs and symptoms need to be reported immediately.
Priority Nursing Tip: The nurse should ensure that a tracheostomy set, oxygen, and suction is at the bedside of a client following thyroidectomy.
Test-Taking Strategy: Focus on the subject, a client scheduled to have a thyroidectomy. Noting the anatomic location of the surgical procedure will assist you in eliminating options 1, 3, and 4. Review: postoperative care after thyroidectomy.
Reference(s): Ignatavicius, Workman (2013), p. 1399.

760. The nurse has been preparing a client with chronic obstructive pulmonary disease for discharge. Which statement by the client indicates the **need for further teaching** about nutrition?

1. "I will rest a few minutes before I eat."
2. "I will not eat as much cabbage as I once did."
3. "I will certainly try to drink 3 L of fluid every day."
4. "It's best to eat three large meals a day, so that I will get all my nutrients."

Level of Cognitive Ability: Evaluating
Client Needs: Health Promotion and Maintenance
Integrated Process: Teaching and Learning
Content Area: Adult Health: Respiratory
Priority Concepts: Client Education; Gas Exchange

Answer: 4
Rationale: Large meals distend the abdomen and elevate the diaphragm, which may interfere with breathing for the client with chronic obstructive pulmonary disease. Resting before eating may decrease the fatigue that is often associated with chronic obstructive pulmonary disease. Gas-forming foods may cause bloating, which interferes with normal diaphragmatic breathing. Adequate fluid intake helps liquefy pulmonary secretions.
Priority Nursing Tip: The client with chronic obstructive pulmonary disease should consume a high-calorie and high-protein diet with supplements.
Test-Taking Strategy: Note the strategic words, *need for further teaching.* These words indicate a negative event query and ask you to select an option that is an incorrect statement. Focusing on the client's diagnosis of chronic obstructive pulmonary disease and recalling the activities that produce dyspnea will direct you to the correct option. Review: nutrition and the client with chronic obstructive pulmonary disease.
Reference(s): Ignatavicius, Workman (2013), p. 621.

761. The nurse is preparing a client with pneumonia for discharge. Which statement by the client would alert the nurse to the fact that the client **needs further teaching** before being discharged?

1. "I will take all of my antibiotics, even if I do feel 100% better."
2. "You can toss out that incentive spirometer as soon as I leave for home."
3. "I realize that it may be weeks before my usual sense of well-being returns."
4. "It is a good idea for me to take a nap every afternoon for the next couple of weeks."

Level of Cognitive Ability: Evaluating
Client Needs: Health Promotion and Maintenance
Integrated Process: Teaching and Learning
Content Area: Adult Health: Respiratory
Priority Concepts: Client Education; Gas Exchange

Answer: 2
Rationale: Deep breathing and coughing exercises and the use of incentive spirometry should be practiced for 6 to 8 weeks after the client with pneumonia is discharged from the hospital to keep the alveoli expanded and promote the removal of lung secretions. If the entire regimen of antibiotics is not taken, the client may suffer a relapse. The period of convalescence with pneumonia is often lengthy, and it may be weeks before the client feels a sense of well-being. Adequate rest is needed to maintain progress toward recovery.
Priority Nursing Tip: The client with pneumonia should be placed in a semi-Fowler's position to facilitate breathing and lung expansion.
Test-Taking Strategy: Note the strategic words, *needs further teaching.* These words indicate a negative event query and ask you to select an option that is an incorrect statement. Focusing on the client's diagnosis of pneumonia and recalling the need to promote the removal of lung secretions will direct you to the correct option. Review: the teaching points for the client with pneumonia.
Reference(s): Ignatavicius, Workman (2013), p. 651; Potter et al (2013), pp. 1288-1289.

❖ **762.** The nurse employed in a well-baby clinic is preparing to administer the scheduled recommended immunizations to a 2-month-old infant. After consultation with the pediatrician, the nurse should prepare to administer which vaccines at this time? **Select all that apply.**
❑ **1.** Rotavirus (RV) (Rotarix)
❑ **2.** Inactivated poliovirus (IPV) (Ipol)
❑ **3.** Pneumococcal (PCV) (Pneumovax)
❑ **4.** Varicella; measles, mumps, and rubella (MMR)
❑ **5.** Haemophilus influenzae type b conjugate (Hib) (Hiberix)
❑ **6.** Diphtheria and tetanus toxoids and acellular pertussis (DTaP) (Adacel)

Level of Cognitive Ability: Applying
Client Needs: Health Promotion and Maintenance
Integrated Process: Nursing Process/Implementation
Content Area: Fundamental Skills: Infection Control
Priority Concepts: Development; Immunity

Answer: 1, 2, 3, 5, 6
Rationale: Rotavirus (RV) is administered at 2 months of age. IPV is administered at ages 2 and 4 months and then at age 4 to 6 years. PCV is administered at 2, 4, and 6 months of age and then between 12 and 15 months. Hib is administered at ages 2 and 4 months with a final dose administered at age 12 months or older. DTaP is administered at 2, 4, and 6 months of age; the fourth dose is administered as early as age 12 months as long as 6 months have elapsed since the third dose. Varicella vaccine is administered at age 12 months or older. MMR is administered at age 12 months with the second dose at age 4 to 6 years.
Priority Nursing Tip: Immunization produces active acquired immunity.
Test-Taking Strategy: Note the subject, the recommended childhood immunization schedule is needed to answer this question. Note that the infant is 2 months of age, and remember that a 2-month-old infant is scheduled for Rotavirus, PCV, IPV, Hib, and DTaP. Review: the recommended childhood immunization schedule.
Reference(s): Centers for Disease Control and Prevention (CDC): 2011 Child & Adolescent Immunization Schedules, retrieved June 2014, from http://www.cdc.gov/vaccines/schedules/index.html; Hockenberry, Wilson (2013), pp. 330-332; McKinney et al (2013), p. 84.

763. The nurse makes a home care visit to a client with Bell's palsy. Which statement by the client indicates a **need for further teaching**?
1. "I wear an eye patch at night."
2. "I am staying on a liquid diet."
3. "I wear dark glasses when I go out."
4. "I have been gently massaging my face."

Level of Cognitive Ability: Evaluating
Client Needs: Health Promotion and Maintenance
Integrated Process: Teaching and Learning
Content Area: Adult Health: Neurological
Priority Concepts: Client Education; Intracranial Regulation

Answer: 2
Rationale: Bell's palsy is caused by a lower motor neuron lesion of the seventh cranial nerve that may result from infection, trauma, hemorrhage, meningitis, or tumor. It is not necessary for a client with Bell's palsy to stay on a liquid diet. The client should be encouraged to chew on the unaffected side. Options 1, 3, and 4 identify accurate statements related to the management of Bell's palsy.
Priority Nursing Tip: Bell's palsy results in paralysis of one side of the face. Recovery usually occurs in a few weeks, without residual effects.
Test-Taking Strategy: Note the strategic words, *need for further teaching*. These words indicate a negative event query and ask you to select an option that is an incorrect statement. Recalling that Bell's palsy relates to the face will assist you in eliminating options 1, 3, and 4. Review: interventions associated with **Bell's palsy**.
Reference(s): Ignatavicius, Workman (2013), pp. 1001-1002.

764. The home care nurse is evaluating a client's understanding of the self-management of trigeminal neuralgia. Which client statement indicates that there is a **need for further teaching**?
1. "I should chew on my good side."
2. "An analgesic will relieve my pain."
3. "I should use warm mouthwash for oral hygiene."
4. "Taking my carbamazepine (Tegretol) will help control my pain."

Level of Cognitive Ability: Evaluating
Client Needs: Health Promotion and Maintenance
Integrated Process: Teaching and Learning
Content Area: Adult Health: Neurological
Priority Concepts: Client Education; Intracranial Regulation

Answer: 2
Rationale: Chronic irritation of cranial nerve V results in trigeminal neuralgia, and it is characterized by intermittent episodes of intense pain of sudden onset on the affected side of the face. The pain is rarely relieved by analgesics. It is recommended that clients chew on the unaffected side and use warm mouthwash for oral hygiene. Medications such as carbamazepine (Tegretol) help control the pain of trigeminal neuralgia.
Priority Nursing Tip: Situations that stimulate symptoms in the client with trigeminal neuralgia include cold, washing the face, chewing, or food or fluids of extreme temperatures.
Test-Taking Strategy: Note the strategic words, *need for further teaching*. These words indicate a negative event query and ask you to select an option that is an incorrect statement. Recalling that trigeminal neuralgia is characterized by intense pain will direct you to the correct option. Review: **trigeminal neuralgia**.
Reference(s): Ignatavicius, Workman (2013), p. 1001.

765. The nurse is caring for a client with type 1 diabetes mellitus. Because the client is at risk for hypoglycemia, which instructions should the nurse teach the client to follow?
1. Monitor the urine for acetone.
2. Report any feelings of drowsiness.
3. Keep glucose tablets and subcutaneous glucagon available.
4. Omit the evening dose of NPH insulin if the client has been exercising.

Level of Cognitive Ability: Applying
Client Needs: Health Promotion and Maintenance
Integrated Process: Teaching and Learning
Content Area: Adult Health: Endocrine
Priority Concepts: Client Education; Glucose Regulation

Answer: 3
Rationale: Glucose tablets are taken if a hypoglycemic reaction occurs. Glucagon (GlucaGen) is administered subcutaneously or intramuscularly if the client loses consciousness and is unable to take glucose by mouth. Glucagon releases glycogen stores and raises the blood glucose levels of hypoglycemic clients. Family members can be taught to administer this medication and possibly to prevent an emergency department visit. Acetone in the urine may indicate hyperglycemia. Although signs/symptoms of hypoglycemia need to be taught to the client, drowsiness is not the initial and key sign of this complication. The nurse would not instruct a client to omit insulin.
Priority Nursing Tip: Hypoglycemia in the client with diabetes mellitus is caused by too much insulin or oral hypoglycemic agents, too little food, or excessive activity.
Test-Taking Strategy: Focus on the subject, a client with type 1 diabetes mellitus who is at risk for hypoglycemia. Eliminate option 4 first because the nurse would not instruct a client to omit insulin doses. Options 1 and 2 can be eliminated next because they are not related to the subject of hypoglycemia. Review: Signs/symptoms of hypoglycemia and the appropriate interventions.
Reference(s): Ignatavicius, Workman (2013), p. 1453.

---

766. The nurse is caring for a client with a precipitous labor. What information should the nurse provide to the client regarding this type of labor?
1. Induction may be necessary.
2. The onset of contractions is gradual.
3. The labor may last less than 3 hours.
4. A lengthy period of pushing may be necessary.

Level of Cognitive Ability: Applying
Client Needs: Health Promotion and Maintenance
Integrated Process: Nursing Process/Implementation
Content Area: Maternity: Intrapartum
Priority Concepts: Client Education; Reproduction

Answer: 3
Rationale: Precipitous labor is defined as labor that lasts 3 hours or less for the entire labor and delivery. It usually has an abrupt rather than a gradual onset. Induction, particularly with an oxytocic agent, is contraindicated because of the enhanced stimulatory effects on the uterine muscle and an increased risk for fetal hypoxia.
Priority Nursing Tip: In the event of a precipitous labor, do not try to keep the fetus from being delivered.
Test-Taking Strategy: Focus on the subject, precipitous labor. The word *precipitous* should assist you with defining this condition. Note the relationship between this word and "less than 3 hours" in option 3. Review the information related to precipitate labor.
Reference(s): McKinney et al (2013), pp. 642-643.

---

767. The nurse is instructing a pregnant client regarding measures to prevent a recurrent episode of preterm labor. Which statement by the client indicates the **need for further teaching?**
1. "I will report any feeling of pelvic pressure."
2. "I will not engage in sexual intercourse at this time."
3. "I will adhere to the limitations in activity and stay off my feet."
4. "I will limit my fluid intake to three 8-ounce glasses of fluid per day."

Level of Cognitive Ability: Evaluating
Client Needs: Health Promotion and Maintenance
Integrated Process: Teaching and Learning
Content Area: Maternity: Antepartum
Priority Concepts: Client Education; Reproduction

Answer: 4
Rationale: Risks for preterm labor include dehydration. A client should not restrict fluids (except for those containing alcohol and caffeine). A sign of preterm labor may be pelvic pressure without the perception of a contraction. Mechanical stimulation of the cervix during intercourse can stimulate contractions. A decrease in activity and bed rest are often prescribed in an attempt to decrease pressure on the cervix and to increase uterine blood flow.
Priority Nursing Tip: Preterm labor occurs after the twentieth week but before the thirty-seventh week of gestation.
Test-Taking Strategy: Note the strategic words, *need for further teaching.* These words indicate a negative event query and ask you to select an option that is an incorrect statement. Focusing on the subject of the prevention of preterm labor will direct you to the correct option. Remember that it is generally not a good practice for the client to limit fluid intake to three 8-ounce glasses of fluid per day. Review: the measures to prevent preterm labor.
Reference(s): Lowdermilk, Perry, Cashion, Alden (2012), pp. 782-783; McKinney et al (2013), pp. 647-648.

768. The nurse has completed discharge teaching with the parents of a child with glomerulonephritis. Which statement by the parents indicates that **further teaching is necessary?**

1. "We'll check our child's blood pressure every day."
2. "We'll test our child's urine for albumin every week."
3. "It'll be so good to have our child back in tap-dancing classes next week."
4. "We'll be sure that our child eats a lot of vegetables and does not add extra salt to food."

Level of Cognitive Ability: Evaluating
Client Needs: Health Promotion and Maintenance
Integrated Process: Teaching and Learning
Content Area: Child Health: Renal and Urinary
Priority Concepts: Client Education; Safety

Answer: 3
Rationale: Glomerulonephritis results in destruction, inflammation, and sclerosis of the glomeruli of the kidneys. After discharge, parents should allow the child to return to his or her normal routine and activities, with adequate periods allowed for rest. Tap dancing classes 1 week after discharge would be unrealistic and involve a too rapid increase in activity. Options 1, 2, and 4 are appropriate home care measures.
Priority Nursing Tip: For the child with glomerulonephritis, foods high in potassium are restricted during periods of oliguria.
Test-Taking Strategy: Note the strategic words, *further teaching is necessary.* These words indicate a negative event query and ask you to select an option that is an incorrect statement. Select option 3 because tap dancing is an aggressive exercise. Review: the home care measures for **glomerulonephritis.**
Reference(s): McKinney et al (2013), pp. 1130-1131.

769. The nurse is planning discharge teaching for the parents of a child who sustained a head injury and who is now receiving tapering doses of dexamethasone. The nurse plans to make which statement to the parents?

1. "This medication decreases the chance of infection."
2. "This medication will be discontinued after two doses."
3. "If your child's face becomes puffy, the medication dose needs to be increased."
4. "This medication is tapered to decrease the chance of recurring swelling in the brain."

Level of Cognitive Ability: Applying
Client Needs: Health Promotion and Maintenance
Integrated Process: Teaching and Learning
Content Area: Pharmacology: Neurological Medications
Priority Concepts: Client Education; Safety

Answer: 4
Rationale: Dexamethasone sodium phosphate is a corticosteroid. The rebounding of cerebral edema is a side effect of dexamethasone sodium phosphate (Decadron) withdrawal if it is done abruptly. This medication decreases inflammation rather than infection. Facial edema is a common side effect that disappears when the medication is discontinued.
Priority Nursing Tip: Monitor the client receiving a corticosteroid for hypokalemia and hyperglycemia.
Test-Taking Strategy: Focus on the subject, a client taking dexamethasone sodium phosphate (Decadron). Recall that this medication is a corticosteroid. Remember that tapering is required with corticosteroids to prevent a rebound effect as a result of adrenal insufficiency. Review: **dexamethasone.**
Reference(s): Hodgson, Kizior (2014), p. 335; Lehne (2013), pp. 917-918.

770. The nurse has implemented a plan of care for a client with a cervical 5 (C5) spinal cord injury to promote health maintenance. Which client outcome would indicate the **effectiveness** of the plan?

1. Maintenance of intact skin
2. Regaining of bladder and bowel control
3. Performance of activities of daily living independently
4. Independent transfer of self to and from the wheelchair

Level of Cognitive Ability: Evaluating
Client Needs: Health Promotion and Maintenance
Integrated Process: Nursing Process/Evaluation
Content Area: Adult Health: Neurological
Priority Concepts: Clinical Judgment; Intracranial Regulation

Answer: 1
Rationale: A C5 spinal cord injury results in quadriplegia with no sensation below the clavicle, including most of the arms and hands. The client maintains the partial movement of the shoulders and elbows. Maintaining intact skin is an outcome for spinal cord injury clients. The remaining options are inappropriate for this client.
Priority Nursing Tip: The level of the spinal cord injury is assessed as the lowest spinal cord segment with intact motor and sensory function.
Test-Taking Strategy: Note the strategic word, *effectiveness.* Focus on the subject, a client with a C5 spinal cord injury. Eliminate options 3 and 4 first because they are comparable or alike. From the remaining options, recalling the effects of a C5 spinal cord injury will assist you in eliminating option 2 because it is unrealistic. Review: **spinal cord injuries.**
Reference(s): Ignatavicius, Workman (2013), p. 973; Lewis et al (2014), pp. 1472-1473.

771. The home care nurse visits a child with scarlet fever who is being treated with penicillin G potassium (Pfizerpen). The mother tells the nurse that the child has only voided a small amount of tea-colored urine since the previous day. The mother also reports that the child's appetite has decreased and that the child's face was swollen this morning. How should the nurse interpret these new symptoms?

1. Nothing to be concerned about
2. Signs/symptoms of acute glomerulonephritis
3. Signs/symptoms of the normal progression of scarlet fever
4. Symptoms of an allergic reaction to penicillin G potassium

Level of Cognitive Ability: Analyzing
Client Needs: Health Promotion and Maintenance
Integrated Process: Nursing Process/Analysis
Content Area: Pharmacology: Immune Medications
Priority Concepts: Elimination; Infection

Answer: 2
Rationale: Scarlet fever is an infectious and communicable disease caused by group A beta-hemolytic streptococci. The symptoms identified in the question indicate acute glomerulonephritis, indicative of nephrotoxicity. These symptoms are not normal and should not be ignored. Although the child is receiving penicillin G potassium, these are not symptoms of an allergic reaction.
Priority Nursing Tip: Scarlet fever is transmitted by direct contact with an infected person or droplet spread or indirectly by contact with contaminated articles or the ingestion of contaminated milk or other foods.
Test-Taking Strategy: Eliminate options 1 and 3 because they are comparable or alike. From the remaining options, recalling the complications of scarlet fever and the symptoms of a medication reaction will direct you to the correct option. Review the complications of scarlet fever and the symptoms of acute glomerulonephritis.
Reference(s): Hodgson, Kizior (2014), pp. 927-928; McKinney et al (2013), pp. 1025, 1128-1129.

772. A client who sustained a thoracic cord injury a year ago returns to the clinic for a follow-up visit, and the nurse notes a small reddened area on the coccyx. The client is not aware of the reddened area. After counseling the client to relieve pressure on the area by adhering to a turning schedule, which action by the nurse is **most appropriate**?

1. Teaching the client to feel for reddened areas
2. Asking a family member to assess the skin daily
3. Teaching the client to use a mirror for skin assessment
4. Scheduling the client to return to the clinic daily for a skin check

Level of Cognitive Ability: Applying
Client Needs: Health Promotion and Maintenance
Integrated Process: Nursing Process/Implementation
Content Area: Adult Health: Neurological
Priority Concepts: Client Education; Tissue Integrity

Answer: 3
Rationale: The client should be encouraged to be as independent as possible. The most effective means of skin self-assessment for this client is with the use of a mirror. The redness cannot be felt. Asking a family member to assess the skin daily does not promote independence. It is unnecessary and unrealistic for the client to return to the clinic daily for a skin check.
Priority Nursing Tip: Autonomic dysreflexia may occur with lesions or injuries above T6 and in cervical lesions.
Test-Taking Strategy: Note the strategic words, *most appropriate*. Recall that independence is vital to the rehabilitation of clients. Options 2 and 4 involve others in performing a task that the client can do independently. Option 1 is an inaccurate assessment technique because redness cannot be felt. Option 3 is the only option that addresses client self-assessment. Review: the home care measures for the client with a spinal cord injury.
Reference(s): Lewis et al (2014), pp. 1479-1480; Swearingen (2012), p. 318.

773. The nurse has given instructions to a client who is returning home after an arthroscopy of the knee. The nurse determines that the client understands the home care instructions if the client states the need to follow which instruction?

1. Resume strenuous exercise the following day.
2. Stay off the leg entirely for the rest of the day.
3. Refrain from eating food for the remainder of the day.
4. Report fever or site inflammation to the health care provider.

Level of Cognitive Ability: Evaluating
Client Needs: Health Promotion and Maintenance
Integrated Process: Nursing Process/Evaluation
Content Area: Adult Health: Musculoskeletal
Priority Concepts: Client Education; Health Promotion

Answer: 4
Rationale: After arthroscopy, signs and symptoms of infection should be reported to the health care provider. The client is instructed to avoid strenuous exercise for at least a few days; however, the client can usually walk carefully on the leg after sensation has returned. The client may resume the usual diet.
Priority Nursing Tip: An arthroscopy allows for an endoscopic examination of various joints and is done to diagnose and treat acute and chronic disorders of the joint.
Test-Taking Strategy: Focus on the subject, a client returning home after arthroscopy. Recalling that the procedure is invasive will direct you to option 4. Additionally, the client is always taught which signs and symptoms of infection to report to the health care provider. Review: the home care instructions for the client after **arthroscopy.**
Reference(s): Ignatavicius, Workman (2013), pp. 1116-1117.

774. Allopurinol (Zyloprim) has been prescribed for a client to treat gouty arthritis. The nurse teaches the client to anticipate which prescription if an acute attack occurs?

1. Doubling the dose of the allopurinol
2. Stopping the allopurinol and taking acetylsalicylic acid (aspirin)
3. Stopping the allopurinol and taking a nonsteroidal anti-inflammatory drug
4. Adding colchicine or a nonsteroidal anti-inflammatory drug to the treatment plan

Level of Cognitive Ability: Applying
Client Needs: Health Promotion and Maintenance
Integrated Process: Teaching and Learning
Content Area: Pharmacology: Musculoskeletal Medications
Priority Concepts: Client Education; Pain

Answer: 4
Rationale: Allopurinol helps prevent an attack of gouty arthritis, but it does not relieve the pain. Therefore, another medication such as colchicine or a nonsteroidal anti-inflammatory drug must be added if an acute attack occurs. Because acute attacks may occur more frequently early during the course of therapy with allopurinol, some health care providers recommend taking the two products concurrently during the first 3 to 6 months.
Priority Nursing Tip: Gout is a systemic disease in which urate crystals deposit in joints and other body tissues. Elevated uric acid levels result that can cause uric acid renal stones.
Test-Taking Strategy: Eliminate options 2 and 3 first because it is unlikely that medication will be stopped. From the remaining options, focus on the subject, gouty arthritis; recalling that an acute attack of gouty arthritis is painful will assist you with selecting option 4 because of the anti-inflammatory action of the nonsteroidal anti-inflammatory drug. Review the interventions for an acute attack of **gouty arthritis.**
Reference(s): Ignatavicius, Workman (2013), p. 350.

775. A nursing instructor asks a nursing student to describe live or attenuated vaccines. What should the student tell the instructor about these types of vaccines?
1. Live or attenuated vaccines contain bacterial toxins that have been made inactive by either chemicals or heat.
2. Live or attenuated vaccines contain pathogens made inactive by either chemicals or heat.
3. Live or attenuated vaccines have their virulence (potency) diminished so as to not produce a full-blown clinical illness.
4. Live or attenuated vaccines have been obtained from the pooled blood of many people and provide antibodies to a variety of diseases.

Level of Cognitive Ability: Understanding
Client Needs: Health Promotion and Maintenance
Integrated Process: Teaching and Learning
Content Area: Child Health: Infectious and Communicable Diseases
Priority Concepts: Health Promotion; Immunity

Answer: 3
Rationale: Live or attenuated vaccines have their virulence (potency) diminished so as to not produce a full-blown clinical illness. In response to vaccination, the body produces antibodies and causes immunity to be established. Option 1 identifies toxoids. Option 2 identifies killed or inactivated vaccines. Option 4 identifies human immune globulin.
Priority Nursing Tip: An immunocompromised individual should not receive a vaccine without first consulting with the health care provider.
Test-Taking Strategy: Focus on the subject, live or attenuated vaccines. Noting the word *live* in the question will assist you in eliminating options 1, 2, and 4. Review the different types of vaccines.
Reference(s): McKinney et al (2013), p. 83.

776. A client has received a prescription for lisinopril (Prinivil, Zestril). The nurse teaches the client that which frequent side effect may occur?
1. Cough
2. Polyuria
3. Hypothermia
4. Hypertension

Level of Cognitive Ability: Applying
Client Needs: Health Promotion and Maintenance
Integrated Process: Teaching and Learning
Content Area: Pharmacology: Cardiovascular Medications
Priority Concepts: Client Education; Safety

Answer: 1
Rationale: Cough is a frequent side effect of therapy with any of the angiotensin-converting enzyme (ACE) inhibitors. Fever is an occasional side effect. Proteinuria is another common side effect, but polyuria is not. Hypertension is the reason to administer the medication rather than a side effect.
Priority Nursing Tip: Hypoglycemic reactions can occur in the client with diabetes mellitus who is taking an angiotensin-converting enzyme (ACE) inhibitor.
Test-Taking Strategy: Focus on the subject, lisinopril (Prinivil, Zestril). Recalling that most ACE inhibitor medication names end in "-pril" and that ACE inhibitors are used to treat hypertension will assist you in eliminating option 4. From the remaining options, it is necessary to know that cough is a frequent side effect of these medications. Review: the side effects of lisinopril (Prinivil, Zestril).
Reference(s): Lehne (2013), p. 512.

777. The nurse has provided home-care instructions to a client who is taking lithium carbonate (Lithobid). Which client statement indicates that the client understands the prescribed regimen?
1. "I will restrict my water intake."
2. "I will make sure that my diet contains salt."
3. "I will keep my medication in the refrigerator."
4. "I will be careful to avoid eating foods high in potassium."

Level of Cognitive Ability: Evaluating
Client Needs: Health Promotion and Maintenance
Integrated Process: Nursing Process/Evaluation
Content Area: Pharmacology: Psychiatric Medications
Priority Concepts: Client Education; Safety

Answer: 2
Rationale: Lithium is a mood stabilizer used to treat bipolar disorder. It replaces sodium ions in the cells and induces the excretion of sodium and potassium from the body. Client teaching includes the maintenance of sodium intake in the daily diet and increased fluid intake (at least 1 to 1½ L per day) during maintenance therapy. Lithium is stored at room temperature and protected from light and moisture.
Priority Nursing Tip: Blood samples to check serum lithium levels should be drawn in the morning, 12 hours after the last dose was taken.
Test-Taking Strategy: Focus on the subject, lithium carbonate (Lithobid). Recalling that lithium is a salt that replaces sodium ions and that induces the excretion of sodium and potassium will direct you to the correct option. Review: lithium carbonate (Lithobid).
Reference(s): Lehne (2013), p. 388.

778. An older client is given a prescription for an antipsychotic. The nurse instructs the client and family to report any signs/symptoms of pseudoparkinsonism and tells the family to monitor for what effects indicative of this medication complication?
1. Tremors and hyperpyrexia
2. Motor restlessness and aphasia
3. Stooped posture and a shuffling gait
4. Muscle weakness and decreased salivation

Level of Cognitive Ability: Applying
Client Needs: Health Promotion and Maintenance
Integrated Process: Teaching and Learning
Content Area: Pharmacology: Psychiatric Medications
Priority Concepts: Client Education; Safety

Answer: 3
Rationale: Pseudoparkinsonism is a common extrapyramidal side effect of antipsychotic medications. This condition is characterized by a stooped posture, a shuffling gait, a masklike facial appearance, drooling, tremors, and pill-rolling motions of the fingers. Hyperpyrexia is characteristic of the extrapyramidal side effect of neuroleptic malignant syndrome. Motor restlessness, aphasia, muscle weakness, and decreased salivation are not characteristic of pseudoparkinsonism.
Priority Nursing Tip: Antipsychotic medications improve the thought processes and the behavior of the client with psychotic symptoms, especially clients with schizophrenia.
Test-Taking Strategy: Focus on the subject, signs/symptoms of pseudoparkinsonism. Recalling the characteristics of Parkinson's disease will direct you to the correct option. Review: the characteristics and side/adverse effects of **antipsychotic medications** and **pseudoparkinsonism.**
Reference(s): Lehne (2013), pp. 349-351.

779. A client who is taking tranylcypromine sulfate (Parnate) requests information about foods that are acceptable to eat while taking the medication. Which foods are safe to consume while taking this medication?
1. Yogurt
2. Raisins
3. Oranges
4. Smoked fish

Level of Cognitive Ability: Applying
Client Needs: Health Promotion and Maintenance
Integrated Process: Teaching and Learning
Content Area: Pharmacology: Psychiatric Medications
Priority Concepts: Client Education; Safety

Answer: 3
Rationale: Tranylcypromine sulfate is classified as a monoamine oxidase inhibitor (MAOI); as such, tyramine-containing food should be avoided. Oranges are permissible. Types of food to be avoided include—but are not limited to—those items identified in options 1, 2, and 4. Additionally, beer, wine, caffeinated beverages, pickled meats, yeast preparations, avocados, bananas, and plums are to be avoided.
Priority Nursing Tip: Instruct the client taking an antipsychotic medication to report signs/symptoms of agranulocytosis, including sore throat, fever, and malaise.
Test-Taking Strategy: The food items in options 1, 2, and 4 are comparable or alike. These are food items that are either processed or that contain some type of additive. The only natural food is option 3. Remember that, although bananas, avocados, and plums are natural foods, they are not permitted while taking an MAOI. Review: **tranylcypromine sulfate (Parnate)** and foods that are high in **tyramine.**
Reference(s): Lehne (2013), pp. 370, 378-379.

780. The nurse is performing an assessment on a 3-year-old child with chickenpox. The child's mother tells the nurse that the child keeps scratching at night, and the nurse teaches the mother about measures that will prevent an alteration in skin integrity. Which statement by the mother indicates that teaching was **effective?**
1. "I need to place white gloves on my child's hands at night."
2. "I will apply generous amounts of a cortisone cream to prevent itching."
3. "I will give my child a glass of warm milk at bedtime to help my child sleep."
4. "I need to keep my child in a warm room at night so that the covers will not cause my child to scratch."

Level of Cognitive Ability: Evaluating
Client Needs: Health Promotion and Maintenance
Integrated Process: Nursing Process/Evaluation
Content Area: Child Health: Infectious and Communicable Diseases
Priority Concepts: Client Education; Tissue Integrity

Answer: 1
Rationale: Gloves will keep the child from causing an alteration in skin integrity from scratching. Generous amounts of any topical cream can lead to medication toxicity. Warm milk will have no effect on itching. A warm room will increase the child's skin temperature and make the itching worse.
Priority Nursing Tip: Isolate high-risk children, such as children who have immunosuppressive disorders, from a child with a communicable disease.
Test-Taking Strategy: Note the strategic word, *effective.* Note the subject preventing an alteration in skin integrity in a 3-year-old child with chickenpox. Eliminate option 4 first because this action will promote itching. Option 3 is eliminated next because it is unrelated to skin integrity. From the remaining options, the words *generous amounts* in option 2 should provide you with a clue that this option is incorrect. Review the measures related to the child with **chickenpox**.
Reference(s): Hockenberry, Wilson (2013), p. 424.

781. The nurse is providing instructions to a client with peptic ulcer disease about symptom management. Which statement by the client indicates they are learning about the disease?
1. "I should eat a snack at bedtime."
2. "I can take aspirin to relieve gastric pain."
3. "It is important that I eat slowly and chew my food thoroughly."
4. "I should take my antacid and famotidine (Pepcid) at the same time."

Level of Cognitive Ability: Evaluating
Client Needs: Health Promotion and Maintenance
Integrated Process: Nursing Process/Evaluation
Content Area: Adult Health: Gastrointestinal
Priority Concepts: Client Education; Health Promotion

Answer: 3
Rationale: Eating slowly and chewing thoroughly helps prevent overdistention and reflux. Bedtime snacks are avoided because they can promote nighttime acid secretion. Acetaminophen (Tylenol) is administered for routine pain relief during treatment. All nonsteroidal anti-inflammatory drugs and aspirin are avoided. Antacids will interfere with the absorption of the famotidine (Pepcid), a histamine-2 (H$_2$) receptor antagonist, so they should not be taken at the same time.
Priority Nursing Tip: Famotidine (Pepcid) is a histamine-2 (H$_2$) receptor antagonist that suppresses the secretion of gastric acid, alleviates the symptoms of heartburn, and assists in preventing the complications associated with peptic ulcer disease.
Test-Taking Strategy: Focus on the subject, peptic ulcer disease and client teaching about the disorder. Use the concepts related to digestion to direct you to option 3. Review the teaching points related to the client with **peptic ulcer disease**.
Reference(s): Ignatavicius, Workman (2013), p. 1230; Nix (2013), pp. 359-361.

782. A client with a hiatal hernia asks the nurse about fluids that are safe to drink and that will not irritate the gastric mucosa. What fluid should the nurse tell the client to drink?
1. Apple juice
2. Orange juice
3. Tomato juice
4. Grapefruit juice

Level of Cognitive Ability: Applying
Client Needs: Health Promotion and Maintenance
Integrated Process: Nursing Process/Implementation
Content Area: Adult Health: Gastrointestinal
Priority Concepts: Nutrition; Tissue Integrity

Answer: 1
Rationale: Substances that are irritating to the client with hiatal hernia include tomato products and citrus fruits, which should be avoided. Because caffeine stimulates gastric acid secretion, beverages that contain caffeine, such as coffee, tea, cola, and cocoa, are also eliminated from the diet.
Priority Nursing Tip: With hiatal hernia, a portion of the stomach herniates through the diaphragm and into the thorax.
Test-Taking Strategy: Eliminate options 2, 3, and 4 because they are comparable or alike and are all citrus products. Additionally, option 1 is the least irritating to the stomach. Review: the dietary measures for the client with **hiatal hernia**.
Reference(s): Nix (2013), pp. 356-357.

783. The nurse determines that the client with gastroesophageal reflux disease (GERD) **needs further teaching** regarding diet if which statement is made?

1. "I must avoid coffee, tea, and chocolate."
2. "I should eat four to six small meals a day."
3. "It is important that I drink extra fluids during meals."
4. "I need to avoid snacking for 2 to 3 hours before bedtime."

Level of Cognitive Ability: Evaluating
Client Needs: Health Promotion and Maintenance
Integrated Process: Teaching and Learning
Content Area: Adult Health: Gastrointestinal
Priority Concepts: Client Education; Health Promotion

Answer: 3
Rationale: Gastroesophageal reflux disease (GERD) is the backflow of gastric and duodenal contents into the esophagus. Fluids must be taken between meals rather than with meals to prevent the over distention that leads to reflux. Coffee, tea, cola, and chocolate are eliminated from the diet because they decrease lower esophageal sphincter pressure and can potentiate reflux. Four to six smaller meals per day will help to prevent gastric over distention. One of the primary factors in GERD is an incompetent lower esophageal sphincter. Adequate time needs to pass after snacking and before bedtime to decrease the risk for the reflux of gastric contents.
Priority Nursing Tip: Manifestations of gastroesophageal reflux disease (GERD) include heartburn, epigastric pain, dyspepsia, regurgitation, pain and difficulty with swallowing, and hypersalivation.
Test-Taking Strategy: Focus on the strategic words, *needs further teaching*. These words indicate a negative event query and the need to select the incorrect client statement. Think about the pathophysiology associated with this disorder to answer correctly. Eliminate options 1, 2, and 4 because they indicate that the client has a proper understanding of the dietary management of GERD. Review: the dietary measures for the client with **gastroesophageal reflux disease (GERD).**
Reference(s): Ignatavicius, Workman (2013), p. 1206.

784. When preparing the client with a spinal cord injury who is experiencing bladder spasms and reflex incontinence for discharge to home, the nurse should provide which instruction to prevent the problem?

1. "Avoid caffeine in your diet."
2. "Take your temperature every day."
3. "Limit your fluid intake to 1000 mL per 24 hours."
4. "Catheterize yourself every 2 hours as needed to prevent spasm."

Level of Cognitive Ability: Applying
Client Needs: Health Promotion and Maintenance
Integrated Process: Teaching and Learning
Content Area: Adult Health: Neurological
Priority Concepts: Client Education; Elimination

Answer: 1
Rationale: Caffeine in the diet can contribute to bladder spasms and reflex incontinence; thus, it should be eliminated in the diet of the client with a spinal cord injury. The self-monitoring of the temperature would be useful to detect infection, but it does nothing to alleviate bladder spasms. Limiting fluid intake does not prevent spasm, and it could place the client at further risk for urinary tract infection. Self-catheterization every 2 hours is too frequent and serves no useful purpose.
Priority Nursing Tip: For the client with a spinal cord injury, it is important for the nurse to institute measures to prevent urinary retention. Initiating a bladder control program and ensuring that the client maintains a fluid intake of 2000 mL per day are important measures.
Test-Taking Strategy: Focus on the subject, preventive measures for bladder spasms and reflex incontinence. Eliminate options 3 and 4 first because they place the client at increased risk for urinary tract infection and are therefore not appropriate. From the remaining options, eliminate option 2 because this action would detect infection but does not deal with spasms and incontinence. Review: the measures to prevent **bladder spasms and reflex incontinence.**
Reference(s): Ignatavicius, Workman (2013), p. 1501.

❖ **785.** A client is diagnosed with organic erectile dysfunction and the nurse is collecting subjective data from the client. After the assessment, the nurse explains to the client that which are causes of this disorder? **Select all that apply.**
- ❏ **1.** Stress
- ❏ **2.** Depression
- ❏ **3.** Hypertension
- ❏ **4.** Vascular disease
- ❏ **5.** Diabetes mellitus
- ❏ **6.** Alcohol consumption

Level of Cognitive Ability: Applying
Client Needs: Health Promotion and Maintenance
Integrated Process: Teaching and Learning
Content Area: Developmental Stages: Health Assessment/Physical Exam
Priority Concepts: Client Education; Sexuality

Answer: 3, 4, 5, 6
Rationale: Erectile dysfunction is the inability to achieve or maintain an erection for sexual intercourse. Organic erectile dysfunction is a gradual deterioration of function; the man first notices diminishing firmness and a decrease in frequency of erections. Causes include inflammation of the prostate, urethra, or seminal vesicles; surgical procedures such as prostatectomy; pelvic fractures or lumbosacral injuries; vascular diseases, including hypertension; chronic neurological conditions such as Parkinson's disease or multiple sclerosis; endocrine disorders such as diabetes mellitus or thyroid disorders; smoking and alcohol consumption; drugs; and poor overall health. Functional (not organic) erectile dysfunction usually has a psychological cause.
Priority Nursing Tip: Some factors that cause erectile dysfunction are modifiable, such as smoking and alcohol consumption. It is important for the nurse to inform the client of these modifiable factors and provide assistance in seeking necessary support services.
Test-Taking Strategy: Focus on the subject, organic erectile dysfunction. Noting the word *organic* and recalling that these types of disorders have a physiological cause will direct you to the correct options. Review the causes of **organic erectile dysfunction.**
Reference(s): Ignatavicius, Workman (2013), p. 1642.

786. The nurse determines that the client with atherosclerosis understands dietary modifications to lower the risk of heart disease if which food selection is made?
1. Roast beef
2. Fresh cantaloupe
3. Broiled cheeseburger
4. Mashed potato with gravy

Level of Cognitive Ability: Evaluating
Client Needs: Health Promotion and Maintenance
Integrated Process: Nursing Process/Evaluation
Content Area: Adult Health: Cardiovascular
Priority Concepts: Health Promotion; Nutrition

Answer: 2
Rationale: To lower the risk of heart disease, the diet should be low in saturated fat with the appropriate number of total calories. The diet should include less red meat and more white meat with the skin removed. Dairy products used should be low in fat, and foods with high amounts of empty calories should be avoided.
Priority Nursing Tip: The nurse needs to stress to the client with coronary artery disease that the necessary dietary changes to prevent complications are not temporary and need to be maintained for life.
Test-Taking Strategy: Focus on the subject, lowering the risk of heart disease. Use the fat content of the foods in the options as a guide to answering this question. Eliminate options 1 and 3 first because of the fat content of the described meats. From the remaining options, eliminate option 4 because fresh fruits and vegetables (option 2) are naturally low in fat. Review: the dietary measures that will lower the risk of **heart disease.**
Reference(s): Ignatavicius, Workman (2013), pp. 774-775; Nix (2013), p. 384.

787. A client being discharged to home after angioplasty via the right femoral groin has received the catheter insertion site discharge instructions from the nurse. Which client statement indicates the client understands the instructions?
1. "Coolness or discoloration of the right foot is expected."
2. "I should expect a large area of bruising at the right groin."
3. "Mild discomfort in the right groin may occur, and Tylenol should relieve the pain."
4. "Temperature as high as 101° F is not unusual a few days after the procedure."

Level of Cognitive Ability: Evaluating
Client Needs: Health Promotion and Maintenance
Integrated Process: Nursing Process/Evaluation
Content Area: Adult Health: Cardiovascular
Priority Concepts: Client Education; Perfusion

Answer: 3
Rationale: The client may feel some mild discomfort at the catheter insertion site after angioplasty. This is usually relieved by analgesics such as acetaminophen (Tylenol). The client is taught to report to the health care provider any neurovascular changes to the affected leg; bleeding or bruising at the insertion site; and signs/symptoms of local infection, such as drainage at the site or increased temperature.
Priority Nursing Tip: Following angioplasty, the nurse needs to keep the client on bed rest and maintain the affected extremity in a straight position for 6 to 8 hours (or as prescribed).
Test-Taking Strategy: Focus on the subject, client instructions following angioplasty. Knowing that bleeding and infection are complications of the procedure guides you in eliminating options 2 and 4. From the remaining options, eliminate option 1 knowing that neurovascular status should not be impaired by the procedure or by knowing that the area may be mildly uncomfortable. Review: the complications associated with **angioplasty.**
Reference(s): Ignatavicius, Workman (2013), pp. 704-705; Pagana, Pagana (2013), p. 123.

788. The nurse is teaching dietary modifications to the client with hypertension. The nurse should instruct the client to eat which snack foods?
1. Raw carrots
2. Frozen pizza
3. Cheese and crackers
4. Canned tomato soup

Level of Cognitive Ability: Applying
Client Needs: Health Promotion and Maintenance
Integrated Process: Teaching and Learning
Content Area: Adult Health: Cardiovascular
Priority Concepts: Client Education; Nutrition

Answer: 1
Rationale: Sodium should be avoided by the client with hypertension. Fresh fruits and vegetables are naturally low in sodium. Hypertensive clients are also advised to keep fat intake to less than 30% of their total calories as part of prudent heart living. Each of the incorrect options contains high amounts of sodium, and options 2 and 3 are also likely to be higher in fat.
Priority Nursing Tip: A goal of treatment for the client with hypertension is to lower the blood pressure and prevent or lessen the extent of any organ damage.
Test-Taking Strategy: Focus on the subject, the dietary modifications needed with hypertension. Eliminate options 2, 3, and 4 because they are comparable or alike and because they are all processed food items. Review: the dietary measures for the client with **hypertension**.
Reference(s): Ignatavicius, Workman (2013), pp. 778, 780; Nix (2013), p. 389.

789. The nurse teaches a client with hypertension to recognize the signs and symptoms that may occur during periods of elevated blood pressure. The nurse determines that the client **needs additional teaching** if the client states that which sign/symptom is associated with this condition?
1. Epistaxis
2. Dizziness
3. Blurred vision
4. A feeling of fullness in the head

Level of Cognitive Ability: Evaluating
Client Needs: Health Promotion and Maintenance
Integrated Process: Teaching and Learning
Content Area: Adult Health: Cardiovascular
Priority Concepts: Client Education; Perfusion

Answer: 4
Rationale: A feeling of fullness in the head is more likely associated with a sinus condition. Cerebrovascular symptoms of hypertension include early morning headaches, occipital headaches, blurred vision, lightheadedness, vertigo, dizziness, and epistaxis. The client should be aware of these symptoms and report them if they occur. The client should also be taught to self-monitor the blood pressure.
Priority Nursing Tip: There is no known cause for primary (essential) hypertension. Secondary hypertension occurs as a result of other diseases or conditions.
Test-Taking Strategy: Note the strategic words, *needs additional teaching*. These words indicate a negative event query and ask you to select an option that is an incorrect sign or symptom. Focus on the subject, signs/symptoms of an elevated blood pressure. Option 4 is the vague option, whereas options 1, 2, and 3 are specific and related to hypertension. Review: the signs and symptoms of **hypertension**.
Reference(s): Ignatavicius, Workman (2013), p. 778.

790. Which instruction should the nurse include in the teaching plan for a client taking iron supplements to correct iron deficiency anemia?
1. Eat a low-fiber diet.
2. Limit the intake of fluids.
3. Limit the intake of meat, fish, and poultry.
4. Avoid taking the iron supplements with milk or antacids.

Level of Cognitive Ability: Applying
Client Needs: Health Promotion and Maintenance
Integrated Process: Teaching and Learning
Content Area: Pharmacology: Hematological Medications
Priority Concepts: Client Education; Nutrition

Answer: 4
Rationale: The client should avoid taking the iron supplements with milk or antacids because these items decrease the absorption of iron. The client should also avoid taking the iron with food, if possible. Finally, the client should take in sufficient fiber and fluids to prevent constipation as a side effect of iron therapy. The client should increase the intake of natural sources of iron, such as meats, fish, and poultry.
Priority Nursing Tip: Liquid iron preparations can stain the teeth. The client taking iron in the liquid form needs to be instructed to use a straw to take the medication and perform mouth care after taking the medication.
Test-Taking Strategy: Focus on the subject, iron supplements. Eliminate options 1 and 2 because constipation is a common side effect of iron therapy. Recalling that meat products contain iron helps you eliminate option 3 next. Remember that several medications have impaired absorption with milk products or antacids. Review: the home care measures for the client with **iron deficiency anemia**.
Reference(s): Kee, Hayes, McCuistion (2012), p. 227; Skidmore-Roth (2014), pp. 536-537.

791. A client with a colostomy complains to the nurse of appliance odor. The nurse recommends that the client take in which deodorizing foods?
1. Eggs
2. Yogurt
3. Cucumbers
4. Mushrooms

Level of Cognitive Ability: Applying
Client Needs: Health Promotion and Maintenance
Integrated Process: Teaching and Learning
Content Area: Adult Health: Gastrointestinal
Priority Concepts: Client Education; Elimination

Answer: 2
Rationale: Foods that help eliminate odor with a colostomy include yogurt, buttermilk, cranberry juice, and parsley. Foods that cause odor are many and include alcohol, beans, turnips, radishes, asparagus, onions, cucumbers, mushrooms, cabbage, eggs, and fish.
Priority Nursing Tip: The normal color for the stoma of a colostomy is pink to bright red and shiny, indicating high vascularity.
Test-Taking Strategy: Focus on the subject, deodorizing foods for a client with a colostomy. Remember that foods that cause gas in the client with normal gastrointestinal function also form gas in the gastrointestinal tract of the client with a colostomy. Use basic nutritional knowledge to eliminate options 1, 3, and 4. Review: the foods that cause gas formation and colostomy.
Reference(s): Ignatavicius, Workman (2013), pp. 1252-1253.

792. The nurse is demonstrating colostomy care to a client with a newly created colostomy. The nurse demonstrates the correct cutting of the appliance by making the circle how much larger than the client's stoma?
1. ⅛ inch
2. ¼ inch
3. ½ inch
4. 1 inch

Level of Cognitive Ability: Applying
Client Needs: Health Promotion and Maintenance
Integrated Process: Teaching and Learning
Content Area: Adult Health: Gastrointestinal
Priority Concepts: Client Education; Elimination

Answer: 1
Rationale: The size of the opening for the appliance is generally cut 1/8 inch larger than the size of the client's stoma. This minimizes the amount of exposed skin but does not put pressure on the stoma. Options 2, 3, and 4 leave too much skin area exposed for irritation by gastrointestinal contents.
Priority Nursing Tip: A pale pink colostomy stoma most likely indicates that the client has a low hemoglobin and hematocrit level.
Test-Taking Strategy: Focus on the subject, colostomy care. Remember that the goal is to prevent stoma and skin irritation. Visualizing each of the appliance sizes in the options will direct you to the correct option. Review: the home care instructions for the client with a colostomy.
Reference(s): Ignatavicius, Workman (2013), p. 1252.

793. The nurse teaches a client with a spinal cord injury about measures to prevent autonomic hyperreflexia. Which statement by the client would indicate the **need for additional teaching?**
1. "It is best if I avoid tight clothing and lumpy bedclothes."
2. "I should watch for headache, congestion, and flushed skin."
3. "Symptoms I should watch for include fever and chest pain."
4. "I need to pay close attention to how frequently my bowels move."

Level of Cognitive Ability: Evaluating
Client Needs: Health Promotion and Maintenance
Integrated Process: Teaching and Learning
Content Area: Adult Health: Neurological
Priority Concepts: Client Education; Intracranial Regulation

Answer: 3
Rationale: Autonomic hyperreflexia generally occurs in a spinal cord injury client after the period of spinal shock resolves. It occurs with injuries above T6 and cervical injuries. Symptoms of autonomic hyperreflexia include headache, congestion, flushed skin above the level of injury and cold skin below it, diaphoresis, nausea, and anxiety. Fever and chest pain are not associated with this condition.
Priority Nursing Tip: Triggers of autonomic hyperreflexia include visceral stimulation from a distended bladder or an impacted rectum.
Test-Taking Strategy: Note the strategic words, *need for additional teaching*. These words indicate a negative event query and ask you to select an option that is an incorrect statement. Recalling the signs, symptoms, and causes of autonomic hyperreflexia will direct you to the correct option. Review the signs and/or symptoms of autonomic hyperreflexia.
Reference(s): Ignatavicius, Workman (2013), p. 973.

794. The nurse is discharging a female client from the hospital who has a diagnosis of a thoracic 11 (T11) fracture with cord transection. The nurse has provided home care instructions to the client. Which action would indicate the **need for further teaching** before discharge?

1. The client jokes about no longer needing to worry about birth control.
2. The client states that she will be careful to not eat as many dairy products.
3. The client verbalizes the need to eat her meals at the same time every day.
4. The client states that she will wash her hands, her perineum, and the catheter with soap and water before performing self-catheterization.

Level of Cognitive Ability: Evaluating
Client Needs: Health Promotion and Maintenance
Integrated Process: Teaching and Learning
Content Area: Adult Health: Neurological
Priority Concepts: Client Education; Intracranial Regulation

Answer: 1
Rationale: Female spinal cord trauma clients remain fertile during their reproductive years, and contraception is necessary for those who are sexually active. However, oral contraceptives may increase the risk for thrombophlebitis. Clients with paralysis should avoid dairy products to control the formation of urinary calculi. Meals should be eaten at the same time every day, and they should include fiber and warm solid and liquid foods to promote and maintain the regular evacuation of the bowel. Clients who lack bladder control are taught to self-catheterize using clean technique.
Priority Nursing Tip: With complete transection of the cord, the spinal cord is severed completely, with total loss of sensation, movement, and reflex activity below the level of injury.
Test-Taking Strategy: Note the strategic words, *need for further teaching*. These words indicate a negative event query and ask you to select an option that is an incorrect statement. Remember that the key aspects of dealing with a spinal cord injury client are nutrition and elimination. Options 2, 3, and 4 address these areas. Review: the teaching points for a client with a spinal cord injury.
Reference(s): Ignatavicius, Workman (2013), pp. 974-975.

795. A client has been started on a monoamine oxidase inhibitor (MAOI). Which should the nurse include when teaching the client about the medication?

1. This medication can cause severe drowsiness.
2. The client must avoid foods that contain tyramine.
3. The medication is associated with a high rate of abuse.
4. The medication will begin to alleviate symptoms of depression almost immediately.

Level of Cognitive Ability: Applying
Client Needs: Health Promotion and Maintenance
Integrated Process: Teaching/Learning
Content Area: Pharmacology: Psychiatric Medications
Priority Concepts: Client Education; Safety

Answer: 2
Rationale: MAOIs are used to treat depression. Although MAOIs usually produce hypotension as a side effect, potentially lethal hypertension can occur if the client eats foods that contain tyramine. Such foods include aged cheeses, hot dogs, and beer, among others. Options 1, 3, and 4 are incorrect statements.
Priority Nursing Tip: Instruct the client taking a monoamine oxidase inhibitor (MAOI) to change positions slowly to prevent orthostatic hypotension.
Test-Taking Strategy: Focus on the subject, a client taking a MAOI. Recalling that MAOIs are associated with a food-medication interaction will direct you to the correct option. Review: these food-medication interactions for a monoamine oxidase inhibitor (MAOI).
Reference(s): Varacrolis (2013), pp. 272-273.

796. The nurse is developing a plan of care for an older client with dementia. The nurse develops which realistic outcome for the client?
1. The client will function at the highest level of independence possible.
2. The client will be admitted to a nursing home to have the needs of activities of daily living met.
3. The nursing staff will attend to all of the client's activities of daily living needs during the hospital stay.
4. The client will complete all activities of daily living independently within a 1- to 1½-hour time frame.

Level of Cognitive Ability: Analyzing
Client Needs: Health Promotion and Maintenance
Integrated Process: Nursing Process/Planning
Content Area: Mental Health
Priority Concepts: Cognition; Health Promotion

Answer: 1
Rationale: All clients, regardless of age, need to be encouraged to perform at the highest level of independence possible. This contributes to the client's sense of control and well-being. Options 2 and 3 are not client-centered goals, and a 1- to 1½-hour time frame may not be realistic for an older client with dementia.
Priority Nursing Tip: Providing a safe environment is the priority for a client with dementia.
Test-Taking Strategy: Focus on the subject, a client with dementia. Note the words *realistic outcome for the client*. Eliminate options 2 and 3 first because they are not client centered. From the remaining options, eliminate option 4 because of the unrealistic time frame. Review: the care of the client with **dementia**.
Reference(s): Potter et al (2013), pp. 1239-1240; Varcarolis (2013), pp. 349-350.

797. Percussion is a physical assessment technique that is used to identify which findings? **Select all that apply.**
❏ 1. Fluid in body cavities
❏ 2. Borders of body organs
❏ 3. Consistency of body organs
❏ 4. Mobility of organs and other structures
❏ 5. Resilience and resistance of tissue and organs
❏ 6. Location, size, and density of an underlying structure

Level of Cognitive Ability: Analyzing
Client Needs: Health Promotion and Maintenance
Integrated Process: Nursing Process/Assessment
Content Area: Developmental Stages: Health Assessment/Physical Exam
Priority Concepts: Clinical Judgment; Health Promotion

Answer: 1, 2, 3, 6
Rationale: Percussion involves tapping the body with the fingertips to evaluate the size, borders, and consistency of body organs and assess for fluid in body cavities. Through percussion, the location, size, and density of an underlying structure can be determined. Through palpation, assessment is done via the sense of touch. Measurements of specific physical signs, including resistance, resilience, roughness, texture, and mobility, can be made through palpation.
Priority Nursing Tip: Physical assessment techniques include inspection, palpation, percussion, and auscultation.
Test-Taking Strategy: Focus on the subject, percussion, and recall that percussion involves tapping the body with the fingertips. Visualize the effect of this assessment technique to determine what it would evaluate. Review: the assessment technique of **percussion**.
Reference(s): Jarvis (2012), p. 116; Potter et al (2013), pp. 494, 834.

798. A client is newly diagnosed with chronic obstructive pulmonary disease (COPD). The client returns home after a short hospitalization. The home care nurse should **most importantly** plan teaching strategies that are designed to do what?

1. Promote membership in support groups.
2. Encourage the client to become a more active person.
3. Identify irritants in the home that interfere with breathing.
4. Improve oxygenation and minimize carbon dioxide retention.

Level of Cognitive Ability: Applying
Client Needs: Health Promotion and Maintenance
Integrated Process: Teaching and Learning
Content Area: Adult Health: Respiratory
Priority Concepts: Gas Exchange; Safety

Answer: 4
Rationale: Chronic obstructive pulmonary disease (COPD) is a disease state characterized by airflow obstruction. Improving oxygenation and minimizing carbon dioxide retention are the primary goals. The other options are interventions that will help with the achievement of this primary goal.
Priority Nursing Tip: In COPD, progressive airflow limitation occurs. This is associated with an abnormal inflammatory response of the lungs that is not completely reversible.
Test-Taking Strategy: Note the strategic words, *most importantly.* Use the ABCs—airway, breathing, and circulation—to direct you to the correct option. Review care of the client with **chronic obstructive pulmonary disease (COPD).**
Reference(s): Ignatavicius, Workman (2013), p. 622; Swearingen (2012), p. 112.

799. A client is being discharged from the hospital after a bronchoscopy that was performed a day earlier. After the discharge teaching, the client makes all of the following statements to the nurse. Which statement should the nurse identify as indicating a **need for further teaching**?

1. "I will stop smoking my cigarettes."
2. "I can expect to cough up bright red blood."
3. "I will get help immediately if I start having trouble breathing."
4. "I will use the throat lozenges as directed by the health care provider until my sore throat goes away."

Level of Cognitive Ability: Evaluating
Client Needs: Health Promotion and Maintenance
Integrated Process: Teaching and Learning
Content Area: Adult Health: Respiratory
Priority Concepts: Client Education; Gas Exchange

Answer: 2
Rationale: After bronchoscopy, expectorated secretions are inspected for hemoptysis, and if the client expectorates bright red blood, the health care provider is to be notified. The client needs to avoid smoking. The client should be observed for signs/symptoms of respiratory distress, including dyspnea, changes in respiratory rate, the use of accessory muscles, and changes in or absent lung sounds. A sore throat is common, and lozenges would be helpful to alleviate it.
Priority Nursing Tip: Following bronchoscopy, the nurse needs to maintain the client on an NPO status until the gag reflex returns.
Test-Taking Strategy: Note the strategic words, *need for further teaching.* These words indicate a negative event query and ask you to select an option that is an incorrect statement. Note the words *bright red* in option 2. Remember that bright red blood indicates active bleeding and that this needs to be reported to the health care provider immediately. Review: the care of the client after **bronchoscopy.**
Reference(s): Pagana, Pagana (2013), p. 196.

800. A client who is taking an antipsychotic is preparing for discharge. To facilitate health promotion for this client, what instruction should the nurse provide?

1. Avoid prolonged exposure to the sun.
2. Adhere to a strict tyramine-restricted diet.
3. Recognize the signs and symptoms of a relapse of depression.
4. Have therapeutic blood levels drawn because the medication has a narrow therapeutic range.

Level of Cognitive Ability: Applying
Client Needs: Health Promotion and Maintenance
Integrated Process: Teaching and Learning
Content Area: Pharmacology: Psychiatric Medications
Priority Concepts: Client Education; Psychosis

Answer: 1
Rationale: Antipsychotic medications improve the thought processes and behaviors of a client with psychotic symptoms, especially a client with schizophrenia. Photosensitivity is a side effect of antipsychotic medications. Options 2, 3, and 4 are unrelated to the administration of antipsychotic medication. Option 2 relates to monoamine oxidase inhibitors (MAOIs). Antipsychotics are not used to treat depression. Lithium (Lithobid) is a mood stabilizer that requires monitoring of medication blood levels.
Priority Nursing Tip: Monitor the client taking an antipsychotic medication for anticholinergic and extrapyramidal side effects.
Test-Taking Strategy: Focus on the subject, an antipsychotic medication to eliminate option 3. Eliminate option 2 because this option relates to medications that are monoamine oxidase inhibitors. There is not a narrow range between therapeutic and toxic levels such as there is with lithium carbonate (Lithobid); therefore, option 4 can be eliminated. Review: **antipsychotic medications.**
Reference(s): Lehne (2013), p. 351.

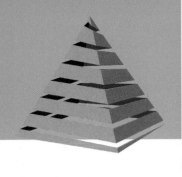
Psychosocial Integrity

❖ **801.** A client with a diagnosis of schizophrenia is experiencing visual hallucinations. The nurse plans care based on the determination that this symptom is related to an alteration in brain function in which lobe of the cerebrum? (**Refer to the figure.**)

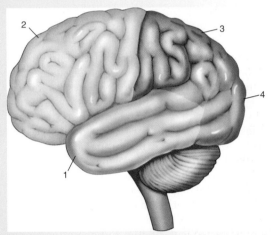

Figure from Patton KT, Thibodeau GA: Anatomy & Physiology, ed 8, St. Louis, 2013, Mosby.

Level of Cognitive Ability: Applying
Client Needs: Psychosocial Integrity
Integrated Process: Nursing Process/Planning
Content Area: Mental Health
Priority Concepts: Clinical Judgment; Psychosis

Answer: 4

Rationale: Visual hallucinations indicate an alteration in brain function in the cerebrum. The occipital lobe is located in the back of the head and is primarily responsible for seeing and receiving information and is responsible for visual hallucinations. The temporal lobe lies beneath the skull on both sides of the brain and is primarily responsible for hearing and receiving information via the ears. Symptoms indicating an alteration of function in the temporal lobe include auditory hallucinations, sensory aphasia, alterations in memory, and altered emotional responses. The frontal lobe is located in the anterior or front area of the brain and is primarily responsible for motor functions, higher thought processes such as decision making, intellectual insight and judgment, and expression of emotion. Symptoms indicating an alteration of function in the frontal lobe include changes in affect, alteration in language production, alteration in motor function, impulsive behavior, and impaired decision making. The parietal lobe lies beneath the skull at the back and top of the head and is primarily responsible for association and sensory perception. Symptoms indicating an alteration of function in the parietal lobe include alterations in sensory perceptions, difficulty with time concepts and calculating numbers, alteration in personal hygiene, and poor attention span.

Priority Nursing Tip: The client experiencing visual hallucinations is seeing things that are not there.

Test-Taking Strategy: Focus on the subject, a client who is experiencing visual hallucinations. Use concepts related to anatomy and physiology of the brain to answer this question. Recalling the location of the occipital lobe and that this lobe is primarily responsible for seeing and receiving information via the eyes will assist in answering correctly. Review: **the lobes of the cerebrum.**

Reference(s): Stuart (2013), pp. 74-75, 78; Varcarolis (2013), pp. 47-48, 272.

802. A client with acute pyelonephritis who is very shy and modest is scheduled for a voiding cystourethrogram. Why should the nurse determine that this client would benefit from increased support and teaching about the procedure?

1. Radioactive material is inserted into the bladder.
2. Radiopaque contrast is injected into the bloodstream.
3. The client must void while the voiding process is filmed.
4. The client must lie on an x-ray table in a cold, barren room.

Level of Cognitive Ability: Analyzing
Client Needs: Psychosocial Integrity
Integrated Process: Nursing Process/Analysis
Content Area: Fundamental Skills: Diagnostic Tests
Priority Concepts: Clinical Judgment; Elimination

Answer: 3
Rationale: Having to void in the presence of others can be very embarrassing for clients, and it may actually interfere with the client's ability to void. The nurse teaches the client about the procedure to try to minimize stress from a lack of preparation and gives the client encouragement and emotional support. Screens may be used in the radiology department to try to provide an element of privacy during this procedure. Options 1, 2, and 4 are incorrect and do not address the subject of support.
Priority Nursing Tip: Pyelonephritis frequently follows untreated urinary tract infections and is associated with increased incidence of anemia, low birth weight, gestational hypertension, preterm labor and delivery, and premature rupture of the membranes.
Test-Taking Strategy: Focus on the subject, a shy and modest client scheduled for a voiding cystourethrogram. Use your knowledge regarding this procedure. Noting the words *shy* and *modest* will direct you to the correct option. Review: the procedure for a voiding cystourethrogram.
Reference(s): Pagana, Pagana (2013), p. 324.

803. A female client who is in a manic state emerges from her room topless while making sexual remarks and lewd gestures toward the staff and her peers. Which intervention should the nurse initiate **first**?

1. Quietly approach the client, escort her to her room, and offer help to get dressed.
2. Confront the client on the inappropriateness of her behavior and offer her a time out.
3. Approach the client in the hallway and insist that she go to her own room immediately.
4. Ask the other clients to ignore her behavior; eventually she will return to her own room.

Level of Cognitive Ability: Applying
Client Needs: Psychosocial Integrity
Integrated Process: Nursing Process/Implementation
Content Area: Mental Health
Priority Concepts: Clinical Judgment; Mood and Affect

Answer: 1
Rationale: A person who is experiencing mania lacks insight and judgment, has poor impulse control, and is highly excitable. The nurse must take control without creating increased stress or anxiety for the client. Insisting that the client go to her room may cause the nurse to be met with a great deal of resistance. Confronting the client and offering her a consequence of time out may be meaningless to her. Asking other clients to ignore her is inappropriate. A quiet but firm approach while distracting the client (walking her to her room and helping her to get dressed) achieves the goal of having the client dressed appropriately and preserving her psychosocial integrity.
Priority Nursing Tip: Bipolar disorder is characterized by episodes of mania and depression with periods of normal mood and activity in between. It is commonly treated with lithium carbonate, which can be toxic and requires regular monitoring of serum lithium levels.
Test-Taking Strategy: Note the strategic word, *first*. Focus on the subject, a client in a manic state. Recalling that the nurse must take control to protect the client will direct you to option 1. Review: the care of the client with mania.
Reference(s): Fortinash, Holoday-Worret (2012), p. 241; Varcarolis (2013), pp. 287, 290.

804. Both the client who had cardiac surgery and the client's family express anxiety regarding how to cope with the recuperative process when they are home alone after discharge. Which available resource should the nurse plan to tell the client and family about?
1. The United Way
2. The local library
3. The American Cancer Society Reach for Recovery
4. The American Heart Association Mended Hearts Club

Level of Cognitive Ability: Applying
Client Needs: Psychosocial Integrity
Integrated Process: Nursing Process/Planning
Content Area: Adult Health: Cardiovascular
Priority Concepts: Anxiety; Perfusion

Answer: 4
Rationale: Most clients and families benefit from knowing that there are available resources to help them cope with the stress of self-care management at home. These can include telephone contact with the surgeon, cardiologist, and nurse; cardiac rehabilitation programs; and community support groups such as the American Heart Association Mended Hearts Club, which is a nationwide program with local chapters. The United Way provides a wide variety of services to people who may not otherwise be able to afford them. The library normally does not provide resources for coping with the recuperative process. The American Cancer Society Reach for Recovery helps women recover after mastectomy.
Priority Nursing Tip: Many hospitals sponsor health fairs, blood pressure screening, and risk factor modification programs. The Internet is a resource that can be used to locate such events.
Test-Taking Strategy: Focus on the subject, the available resource for the client who had cardiac surgery. Note that the options identify three organizations and a library. Eliminate the library first because the client and family need resources to cope, which imply the need for an interactive process. From the remaining options, noting that the client had cardiac surgery will direct you to option 4. Review: the support services for clients who have had cardiac surgery.
Reference(s): Ignatavicius, Workman (2013), p. 853.

805. An older client who has never been hospitalized before is to have a 12-lead electrocardiogram (ECG). Which explanation by the nurse should alleviate the client's anxiety about the test?
1. "It's important to lie still during the procedure."
2. "It should only take about 20 minutes to complete the ECG tracing."
3. "The ECG electrodes are painless and will record the electrical activity of the heart."
4. "The ECG can give the doctor information about what might be wrong with your heart."

Level of Cognitive Ability: Applying
Client Needs: Psychosocial Integrity
Integrated Process: Nursing Process/Implementation
Content Area: Fundamental Skills: Diagnostic Tests
Priority Concepts: Anxiety; Client Education

Answer: 3
Rationale: The ECG uses painless electrodes that are applied to the chest and limbs. The procedure takes less than 5 minutes to complete, and it requires the client to lie still. The ECG measures the heart's electrical activity to determine rate, rhythm, and a variety of abnormalities. Options 1 and 4 are factual statements, but they are not stated to reduce anxiety.
Priority Nursing Tip: An echocardiogram is a noninvasive procedure that evaluates structural and functional changes in the heart. The client must lie still, breathe normally, and refrain from talking during the test.
Test-Taking Strategy: Focus on the subject, alleviating the client's anxiety about a 12-lead electrocardiogram (ECG). Eliminate option 2 because it is inaccurate. Next, eliminate options 1 and 4 because they will not alleviate anxiety. Review: 12-lead electrocardiogram (ECG) and measures to alleviate anxiety.
Reference(s): Pagana, Pagana (2013), p. 367.

806. A spouse of a client who is scheduled for the insertion of an implantable cardioverter-defibrillator (ICD) expresses anxiety about what would happen if the device discharges during physical contact. What information should the nurse provide to the spouse?

1. Physical contact should be avoided whenever possible.
2. The spouse would not feel or be harmed by the countershock.
3. The shock would be felt, but it would not cause the spouse any harm.
4. A warning device sounds before countershock, so there is time to move away.

Level of Cognitive Ability: Applying
Client Needs: Psychosocial Integrity
Integrated Process: Nursing Process/Implementation
Content Area: Adult Health: Cardiovascular
Priority Concepts: Anxiety; Perfusion

Answer: 3
Rationale: Clients and families are often fearful about the activation of the ICD. Their fears are about the device itself and also about the occurrence of life-threatening dysrhythmias that trigger its function. Family members need reassurance that, even if the device activates while they are touching the client, the level of the charge is not high enough to harm the family member, although it will be felt. The ICD emits a warning beep when the client is near magnetic fields, which could possibly deactivate it, but it does not beep before countershock.
Priority Nursing Tip: An ICD monitors cardiac rhythm and detects and terminates episodes of ventricular fibrillation and ventricular tachycardia.
Test-Taking Strategy: Focus on the subject, the client's spouse's anxiety about implantable cardioverter-defibrillator (ICD), and use your knowledge of the function of the ICD to answer this question. This will direct you to the correct option. Remember that the shock would be felt, but it would not cause the spouse any harm. Review: the client teaching points related to the implantable cardioverter-defibrillator (ICD).
Reference(s): Ignatavicius, Workman (2013), p. 742; Lewis et al (2011), p. 834.

807. A client who is scheduled for permanent transvenous pacemaker insertion says to the nurse, "I know I need it, but I'm not sure this surgery is a great idea." Which nursing response will **best** help the nurse assess the client's preoperative concerns?

1. "How does your family feel about the surgery?"
2. "Has anyone taught you about the procedure yet?"
3. "You sound unnecessarily worried. Has anyone told you that the technology is quite advanced now?"
4. "You sound uncertain about the procedure. Can you tell me more about what has you concerned?"

Level of Cognitive Ability: Applying
Client Needs: Psychosocial Integrity
Integrated Process: Communication and Documentation
Content Area: Adult Health: Cardiovascular
Priority Concepts: Anxiety; Communication

Answer: 4
Rationale: Anxiety is common in the client with the need for pacemaker insertion. This can be related to a fear of life-threatening dysrhythmias or of the surgical procedure. Option 4 is the correct choice because it is open-ended and uses clarification as a communication technique to explore the client's concerns. Option 1 is not indicated because it asks about the family and deflects attention away from the client's concerns. Options 2 and 3 are closed ended and are not exploratory.
Priority Nursing Tip: A pacemaker is a temporary or permanent device that provides electrical stimulation and maintains the heart rate when the client's intrinsic pacemaker fails to provide a perfusing rhythm.
Test-Taking Strategy: Note the strategic word, *best*. Use therapeutic communication techniques, focusing on the subject, addressing the client's preoperative concerns. Option 1 can be eliminated first because it addresses the family rather than the client. From the remaining options, the only option that addresses the client's concerns is option 4. Review: therapeutic communication techniques.
Reference(s): Ignatavicius, Workman (2013), p. 741; Potter et al (2013), pp. 320-322.

808. A client with superficial varicose veins says to the nurse, "I hate these things. They're so ugly. I wish I could get them to go away." Which therapeutic response should the nurse make to the client?
1. "You should try sclerotherapy. It's great."
2. "There's not much you can do once you get them."
3. "What have you been told about varicose veins and their management?"
4. "I understand how you feel, but you know, they really don't look too bad."

Level of Cognitive Ability: Applying
Client Needs: Psychosocial Integrity
Integrated Process: Communication and Documentation
Content Area: Adult Health: Cardiovascular
Priority Concepts: Anxiety; Communication

Answer: 3
Rationale: The client expressing distress about physical appearance has a risk for an altered body image. The nurse assesses the client's knowledge and self-management of the condition as a means of empowering the client and helping him or her adapt to the body change. Options 1, 2, and 4 are not therapeutic.
Priority Nursing Tip: Varicose veins occur from the weakening and dilation of vein walls and incompetence of the valves inside the veins. The client may feel pain in the legs with dull aching after standing, a feeling of fullness in the legs, and ankle edema.
Test-Taking Strategy: Use therapeutic communication techniques. With questions that deal with client's feelings, select the option that facilitates the sharing of information and concerns by the client. Options 1, 2, and 4 cut off or limit further comments by the client. Additionally, option 3 addresses assessment, which is the first step of the nursing process. Review: therapeutic communication techniques.
Reference(s): Ignatavicius, Workman (2013), p. 805; Potter et al (2013), pp. 662-663.

809. A client who has been diagnosed with chronic kidney disease (CKD) has been told that hemodialysis will be required. The client becomes angry and states, "I'll never be the same now." What should the nurse identify as a client problem?
1. Anxiety about the hemodialysis
2. Inability to think clearly because of the treatments needed
3. Potential for noncompliance because of concerns about the disease
4. Altered body image because of the physical changes that may occur

Level of Cognitive Ability: Analyzing
Client Needs: Psychosocial Integrity
Integrated Process: Nursing Process/Analysis
Content Area: Adult Health: Renal and Urinary
Priority Concepts: Coping; Mood and Affect

Answer: 4
Rationale: A client with a renal disorder such as CKD may become angry in response to the permanence of the condition. Because of the physical changes and the change in lifestyle that may be required to manage a severe renal condition, the client may experience an altered body image. Anxiety is not appropriate because the client is exhibiting anger at this time. The client is not cognitively impaired, eliminating option 2, and is not stating a refusal to undergo therapy, so therefore eliminate option 3.
Priority Nursing Tip: The client undergoing hemodialysis will either have a subclavian or femoral catheter for short-term or temporary use in acute kidney injury. This will be used until a fistula or graft is created and matures, which typically takes 6 weeks, or the short-term catheter may be required if the permanent fistula has failed because of infection or clotting.
Test-Taking Strategy: Focus on the subject, an angry client who will have hemodialysis and states that he/she will never be the same. Note that the client's statement focuses on the self, which is consistent with altered body image. Review: psychosocial concerns of the client with chronic kidney disease and altered body image.
Reference(s): Ignatavicius, Workman (2013), p. 1552; Potter et al (2013), pp. 662-663.

810. A client with the diagnosis of hyperparathyroidism says to the nurse, "I can't stay on this diet. It is too difficult for me." How should the nurse **best** respond when intervening in this situation?

1. "Why do you think you find this diet plan difficult to adhere to?"
2. "It really isn't difficult to stick to this diet. Just avoid milk products."
3. "You are having a difficult time staying on this plan. Let's discuss this."
4. "It is very important that you stay on this diet to avoid forming renal calculi."

Level of Cognitive Ability: Applying
Client Needs: Psychosocial Integrity
Integrated Process: Nursing Process/Implementation
Content Area: Adult Health: Endocrine
Priority Concepts: Communication; Nutrition

Answer: 3
Rationale: By paraphrasing the client's statement, the nurse can encourage the client to verbalize emotions. The nurse also sends feedback to the client that the message was understood. An open-ended statement or question such as this prompts a thorough response from the client. Option 1 requests information that the client may not be able to express. Option 2 devalues the client's feelings. Option 4 gives advice, which blocks communication.
Priority Nursing Tip: After the nurse determines the cause of a client's difficulty in adhering to a prescribed diet, the nurse can develop a plan of care and refer the client to appropriate community support programs, such as nutritional programs.
Test-Taking Strategy: Note the strategic word, *best.* Use therapeutic communication techniques, and focus on the client's statement. Note that option 3 paraphrases the client's statement. Review: therapeutic communication techniques.
Reference(s): Ignatavicius, Workman (2013), pp. 1406-1407; Potter et al (2013), pp. 320-322.

811. The nurse is caring for a client with newly diagnosed type 1 diabetes mellitus. Which component of a teaching plan is **most important initially**?

1. Knowledge of the diabetic diet
2. Understanding of the diagnosis
3. Monitoring of blood glucose levels
4. Correct technique for administering insulin

Level of Cognitive Ability: Applying
Client Needs: Psychosocial Integrity
Integrated Process: Teaching and Learning
Content Area: Adult Health: Endocrine
Priority Concepts: Client Education; Glucose Regulation

Answer: 2
Rationale: Before educating about a disease process, it is important that the client understands the components of the disease process. Following this teaching, the actual components of diet, blood glucose testing, and insulin injections can be taught.
Priority Nursing Tip: The management of diabetes mellitus is complicated and involves considerable client involvement and education, so it is important for the nurse to ensure the client understands the disease process.
Test-Taking Strategy: Note the strategic words, *most important* and *initially.* All of the options may be appropriate to assess, but note that options 1, 3, and 4 relate to specific components of the teaching. Option 2 is the umbrella option, and considering the principles of teaching and learning, this aspect needs to be assessed before the implementation of teaching. Review: **diabetes mellitus.**
Reference(s): Ignatavicius, Workman (2013), pp. 1458-1460; Potter et al (2013), pp. 329-330.

812. A client with newly diagnosed type 1 diabetes mellitus has been seen for 3 consecutive days in the emergency department with hyperglycemia. During the assessment, the client says to the nurse, "I'm sorry to keep bothering you every day, but I just can't give myself those awful shots." Which therapeutic response should the nurse make?

1. "I couldn't give myself a shot either."
2. "You must learn to give yourself the shots."
3. "Let me see if we can change your medication."
4. "Has someone given you instructions on how to perform them?"

Level of Cognitive Ability: Applying
Client Needs: Psychosocial Integrity
Integrated Process: Communication and Documentation
Content Area: Adult Health: Endocrine
Priority Concepts: Communication; Glucose Regulation

Answer: 4
Rationale: It is important to determine and deal with a client's underlying fear of self-injection. The nurse should determine whether a knowledge deficit exists. Positive reinforcement should occur rather than focusing on negative behaviors. Demanding that the client perform a behavior or skill is inappropriate. The nurse should not offer a change in regimen that cannot be accomplished.
Priority Nursing Tip: Common sites for the injection of insulin include the upper arm, abdomen, thighs, lower back, and buttocks.
Test-Taking Strategy: Use therapeutic communication techniques. Options 1, 2, and 3 are not therapeutic. In addition, option 3 may provide false reassurance regarding a potential change in medications. Review: therapeutic communication techniques and type 1 diabetes mellitus.
Reference(s): Ignatavicius, Workman (2013), p. 1434; Potter et al (2013), pp. 320-322.

813. The nurse requests that a client with diabetes mellitus ask their family members to attend an educational conference about the self-administration of insulin. The client questions why they need to be included. How should the nurse answer this question?

1. "Family members are at risk of developing diabetes."
2. "Family members can take you to your appointments."
3. "Nurses need someone to call and check on a client's progress."
4. "Clients and families often work together to develop strategies for the management of diabetes."

Level of Cognitive Ability: Applying
Client Needs: Psychosocial Integrity
Integrated Process: Communication and Documentation
Content Area: Adult Health: Endocrine
Priority Concepts: Communication; Glucose Regulation

Answer: 4
Rationale: Families and significant others may be included in diabetes education to assist with adjustments of the diabetic regimen. Having positive family members involved will be a support to the client in assuming independent care.
Priority Nursing Tip: Some chronic complications of diabetes mellitus include diabetic retinopathy, diabetic nephropathy, and diabetic neuropathy.
Test-Taking Strategy: Use of therapeutic communication techniques will promote independence in coping with a chronic illness. Options 1, 2, and 3 are not therapeutic. Review: therapeutic communication techniques.
Reference(s): Ignatavicius, Workman (2013), p. 1456; Potter et al (2013), pp. 320-322.

814. A 22-year-old client has recently been diagnosed with polycystic kidney disease. The nurse has a series of discussions with the client that are intended to help the client adjust to the disorder. Which item should the nurse plan to include as part of one of these discussions?
1. Ongoing fluid restriction
2. The need for genetic counseling
3. The risk of hypotensive episodes
4. Depression regarding massive edema

Level of Cognitive Ability: Applying
Client Needs: Psychosocial Integrity
Integrated Process: Nursing Process/Planning
Content Area: Adult Health: Renal and Urinary
Priority Concepts: Client Education; Elimination

Answer: 2
Rationale: Adult polycystic kidney disease is a hereditary disorder that is inherited as an autosomal-dominant trait. Because of this, the client and the extended family should have genetic counseling. Ongoing fluid restriction is unnecessary. The client is likely to have hypertension rather than hypotension. Massive edema is not part of the clinical picture of this disorder.
Priority Nursing Tip: In polycystic kidney disease, a cystic formation and hypertrophy of the kidneys leads to cystic rupture, infection, formation of scar tissue, and damaged nephrons. There is no specific treatment to arrest the progress of the destructive cysts.
Test-Taking Strategy: Focus on the subject of polycystic kidney disease. Use knowledge about the characteristics of this disease. This disease is a hereditary disease that does not have a need for fluid restriction or conditions related to blood pressure. Review: polycystic kidney disease.
Reference(s): Ignatavicius, Workman (2013), pp. 1521-1522; Lewis et al (2011), p. 1143.

815. The nurse is admitting a client to the hospital that is to undergo ureterolithotomy for urinary calculi removal. Which are necessary to assess in order to determine if the client is ready for surgery? **Select all that apply.**
☐ 1. The need for a visit from a support group
☐ 2. The knowledge of postoperative activities
☐ 3. An understanding of the surgical procedure
☐ 4. Expected outcomes of the surgical procedure
☐ 5. Feelings or anxieties about the surgical procedure

Level of Cognitive Ability: Analyzing
Client Needs: Psychosocial Integrity
Integrated Process: Nursing Process/Assessment
Content Area: Adult Health: Renal and Urinary
Priority Concepts: Caregiving; Elimination

Answer: 2, 3, 4, 5
Rationale: Ureterolithotomy is the removal of a calculus from the ureter using either a flank or abdominal incision. The client should have an understanding of the same items as are required for any surgery, including knowledge of the procedures, the expected outcome, the postoperative routines, and any expected discomfort. The client should also be assessed for any concerns or anxieties before surgery. Because no urinary diversion is created during this procedure, the client has no need for a visit from a member of a support group.
Priority Nursing Tip: Problems resulting from urinary calculi are pain, obstruction, tissue trauma, secondary hemorrhage, and infection. A stone analysis will be done after passage to determine the type of stone and assist in determining treatment.
Test-Taking Strategy: Focus on the subject, the client's readiness for surgery. This will assist in directing you to the correct options. Review: preoperative assessment and ureterolithotomy.
Reference(s): Ignatavicius, Workman (2013), p. 1506; Lewis et al (2011), p. 1140.

816. The spouse of a dying client says to the nurse, "I don't think I can come anymore and watch her die. It's chewing me up too much!" Which therapeutic response should the nurse make to the spouse?

1. "It's hard to watch someone you love die. You've been here with your wife every day. Are you taking any time for yourself?"
2. "Focus on your wife's pain rather than yours. I know it's hard, but this isn't about what's happening to you, you know."
3. "I know it's hard for you, but she would know if you're not there, and you would feel so very guilty all of the rest of your days."
4. "I think you're making the right decision. Your wife knows you love her. You don't have to come every day. I'll take care of her."

Level of Cognitive Ability: Applying
Client Needs: Psychosocial Integrity
Integrated Process: Communication and Documentation
Content Area: Mental Health
Priority Concepts: Caregiving; Communication

Answer: 1
Rationale: The most therapeutic response is the one that is empathetic and that reflects the nurse's understanding of the client's, in this case, the husband's, stress and emotional pain. In the correct option, the nurse suggests that the client take time for himself. Option 2 is an example of a nontherapeutic and judgmental attitude that places blame. Option 3 makes statements that the nurse cannot know are true (the client's wife may not in fact know if the husband visits), and it predicts feelings of guilt, which is inappropriate. Option 4 fosters dependency and gives advice, which is nontherapeutic.
Priority Nursing Tip: Respite care provides support to the caregiver(s) of the client requiring long-term care. This allows family members and significant others involved in the client's care time to care for themselves.
Test-Taking Strategy: Use therapeutic communication techniques to answer the question. The correct option is the only option that is therapeutic and that addresses the husband's feelings. Review: **therapeutic communication techniques.**
Reference(s): Stuart (2013), pp. 25-29; Varcarolis (2013), pp. 144-145.

817. An older adult client at the retirement center spits her food out and throws it on the floor. She yells, "This turkey is dry and cold! I can't stand the food here!" How should the nurse respond to the client?

1. "Now look what you've done! You're ruining this meal for the whole community. Aren't you ashamed of yourself?"
2. "I think you had better return to your apartment now. I'll make arrangements for a new meal to be served to you there."
3. "Let me get you another serving that is more to your liking. Would you like to see the chef and select your own serving?"
4. "One of the things that was agreed upon was that anyone who did not use appropriate behavior would be asked to leave the dining room. Please leave now."

Level of Cognitive Ability: Applying
Client Needs: Psychosocial Integrity
Integrated Process: Nursing Process/Implementation
Content Area: Mental Health
Priority Concepts: Communication; Professionalism

Answer: 3
Rationale: Asking the client to accompany the nurse to the kitchen respects the client's need for control, removes the angry client from the dining room, and may offer the nurse an opportunity to assess what is happening with the client. Agency procedure should be followed regarding those who are allowed access to the facility kitchen. Option 1 is angry, aggressive, and nontherapeutic. Option 2 could provoke a regressive struggle between the nurse and the client and cause more anger in the client. In option 4, the nurse is authoritative, and it would not be appropriate to ask the client to leave. This action may set up an aggressive struggle between the nurse and the client.
Priority Nursing Tip: The aging client may experience a sense of loss of control, particularly if she has been moved from her home into a care facility. The nurse should allow the client to exercise as much control as possible through decision making and other means.
Test-Taking Strategy: Use therapeutic communication techniques and your knowledge about the care of an angry client. Option 3 is the only option that addresses the client's angry feelings, and it also provides the nurse with an opportunity to further assess the client. Review: **therapeutic communication techniques.**
Reference(s): Stuart (2013), pp. 581-582; Varcarolis (2013), pp. 120-122.

818. A health care provider prescribes a follow-up home care visit for an older adult client with emphysema. When the home care nurse arrives, the client is smoking. Which statement by the nurse would be therapeutic?
1. "Well, I can see you never got to the stop smoking clinic!"
2. "I'm glad I caught you smoking! Now that your secret is out, let's decide what you are going to do."
3. "I notice that you are smoking. Did you explore the stop smoking program at the senior citizens center?"
4. "I wonder if you realize that you are slowly killing yourself. Why prolong the agony? You can just jump off the bridge!"

Level of Cognitive Ability: Applying
Client Needs: Psychosocial Integrity
Integrated Process: Communication and Documentation
Content Area: Adult Health: Respiratory
Priority Concepts: Communication; Gas Exchange

Answer: 3
Rationale: Clients with emphysema must avoid smoking and all airborne irritants. The nurse who observes a maladaptive behavior in a client should not make judgmental comments and should instead explore an adaptive strategy with the client without being overly controlling. This will place the decision making in the client's hands and provide an avenue for the client to share what may be expressions of frustration about an inability to stop what is essentially a physiological addiction. Option 1 is an intrusive use of sarcastic humor that is degrading to the client. Option 2 is a disciplinary remark and places a barrier between the nurse and the client within the therapeutic relationship. In Option 4, the nurse preaches and is judgmental.
Priority Nursing Tip: Emphysema occurs when there is abnormal permanent enlargement of air spaces distal to the terminal bronchioles, with destruction of alveolar walls without obvious fibrosis.
Test-Taking Strategy: Use therapeutic communication techniques. Option 3 recognizes and addresses the client's behavior and explores an avenue for dealing with the behavior. Review therapeutic communication techniques.
Reference(s): Ignatavicius, Workman (2013), p. 621; Potter et al (2013), pp. 320-322.

819. A client is to have arterial blood gases drawn. While the nurse is performing Allen's test, the client says to the nurse, "What are you doing? No one else has done that!" Which therapeutic response should the nurse make to the client?
1. "I assure you that I am doing the correct procedure. I cannot account for what others do."
2. "This step is crucial to safe blood withdrawal. I would not let anyone take my blood until they did this."
3. "Oh? You have questions about this? You should insist that they all do this procedure before drawing up your blood."
4. "This is a routine precautionary step that simply makes certain your circulation is intact before a blood sample is obtained."

Level of Cognitive Ability: Applying
Client Needs: Psychosocial Integrity
Integrated Process: Communication and Documentation
Content Area: Adult Health: Cardiovascular
Priority Concepts: Client Education; Safety

Answer: 4
Rationale: Allen's test is performed to assess collateral circulation in the hand before drawing a radial artery blood specimen. The therapeutic response provides information to the client. Option 1 is defensive and nontherapeutic in that it offers false reassurance. Option 2 identifies client advocacy, but it is overly controlling and aggressive, and undermines treatment. Option 3 is aggressive, controlling, and nontherapeutic in its disapproving stance.
Priority Nursing Tip: Before an arterial blood gas (ABG) is drawn, the client should rest for 30 minutes to ensure accurate measurement of body oxygenation. If the client is wearing oxygen, it should not be turned off unless the ABG sample is prescribed to be drawn with the client breathing room air.
Test-Taking Strategy: Use therapeutic communication techniques. Option 4 addresses the subject, explaining an Allen's test to a questioning client, and provides information to the client in an appropriate manner. Review: therapeutic communication techniques.
Reference(s): Pagana, Pagana (2013), p. 117; Potter et al (2013), pp. 320-322.

820. A client reports having difficulty concentrating and outbursts of anger, as well as feeling "keyed up" all the time. The nurse obtaining the client's history discovers that the symptoms started about 6 months ago. The client reveals that, around that same time, a best friend was killed in a drive-by shooting while they were talking together. The nurse should suspect which stressor before communicating with the client?

1. Social phobia
2. Panic disorder
3. Posttraumatic stress disorder (PTSD)
4. Obsessive-compulsive disorder (OCD)

Level of Cognitive Ability: Analyzing
Client Needs: Psychosocial Integrity
Integrated Process: Nursing Process/Analysis
Content Area: Mental Health
Priority Concepts: Anxiety; Stress

Answer: 3
Rationale: PTSD is a response to an event that would be markedly distressing to almost anyone. Characteristic symptoms include a sustained level of anxiety, difficulty sleeping, irritability, difficulty concentrating, and outbursts of anger. Panic disorders and social phobia are characterized by a specific fear of an object or situation. OCD involves some repetitive thoughts or behaviors.
Priority Nursing Tip: Common stressors that can result in posttraumatic stress disorder (PTSD) include a natural disaster; terrorist attack; combat experiences; accidents; rape; crime or violence; sexual, physical, and emotional abuse; and re-experiencing the event as flashbacks.
Test-Taking Strategy: Focus on the data in the question. Eliminate options 1 and 2 first because they are comparable or alike. From the remaining options, recalling that OCD relates to a repetitive thought or behavior will direct you to the correct option. Review: posttraumatic stress disorder (PTSD).
Reference(s): Fortinash, Holoday-Worret (2012), pp. 192-193; Varcarolis (2013), p. 159.

821. A client says to the nurse, "I can't get any help with my care! I call and call, but the nurses never answer my light. Last night one of them told me she had other clients besides me! I'm very sick, but the nurses don't care!" Which statement from the nurse is therapeutic?

1. "I think you are being very impatient. The nurses come as quickly as they can."
2. "I can hear your anger. That nurse had no right to speak to you that way. I will report her."
3. "You poor thing! I'm so sorry this happened to you. That nurse should be fired immediately."
4. "It's hard to be in bed and to have to ask for help. You feel that the nurses do not seem to care?"

Level of Cognitive Ability: Applying
Client Needs: Psychosocial Integrity
Integrated Process: Communication and Documentation
Content Area: Mental Health
Priority Concepts: Communication; Professionalism

Answer: 4
Rationale: Empathy is a term that describes the nurse's capacity to enter into the life of another person and to perceive how the client is feeling and what meaning this has for the client. In option 4, the nurse displays empathy and shares perceptions. The sharing of perceptions asks the client to validate the nurse's understanding of what the client is feeling and thinking. It opens the door for the client to share concerns, fears, and anxieties. In option 1, the nurse is assertive and also defends the nursing staff. In option 2, the nurse expresses the client's frustration by labeling the client's feelings as angry and disapproving of the nursing staff. This is splitting, and it is nontherapeutic. Option 3 is a social response, and it is demeaning to the client.
Priority Nursing Tip: The nurse should encourage the client to share thoughts and feelings. This will assist to uncover other feelings, anxieties, or fears the client is having.
Test-Taking Strategy: Use therapeutic communication techniques. Focus on the client's statement in the question. Note the relationship between the client's statement and option 4. In addition, in this option, the nurse validates the client's feelings. Review: therapeutic communication techniques.
Reference(s): Stuart (2013), pp. 32-33, 38; Varcarolis (2013), pp. 144-145.

822. An English-speaking Hispanic man with a newly applied long leg cast has a right proximal fractured tibia. During rounds at night, the nurse finds the client restless, withdrawn, and quiet. Which nursing statement would be appropriate?

1. "Are you uncomfortable?"
2. "Tell me what you are feeling."
3. "You'll feel better in the morning."
4. "I'll get your pain medication right away."

Level of Cognitive Ability: Applying
Client Needs: Psychosocial Integrity
Integrated Process: Communication and Documentation
Content Area: Mental Health
Priority Concepts: Communication; Culture

Answer: 2
Rationale: Option 2 is open-ended and makes no assumptions about the client's psychological or emotional state. Option 1 is incorrect because males in traditional standard Hispanic cultures practice "machismo" in which stoicism is valued, so this client may deny any pain when asked. False reassurance is never therapeutic, which makes option 3 incorrect. Option 4 is incorrect because an assessment is necessary before administering medication for pain.
Priority Nursing Tip: The concept of machismo (manliness) may predominate in the Mexican-American culture. The nurse must be aware of these types of culture issues, so that culturally competent care can be provided.
Test-Taking Strategy: Use therapeutic communication techniques. Recalling that the client's feelings are the priority will direct you to the correct option. Review: **therapeutic communication techniques** and **Hispanic cultures.**
Reference(s): Giger (2013), pp. 214-215; Potter et al (2013), pp. 321-322, 969.

823. A client was started on oral anticoagulant therapy while hospitalized. The client is now being discharged to home and is intermittently confused. The nurse identifies which is the **best** support system for successful anticoagulant therapy monitoring?

1. The client has a home health aide coming to the house for 9 weeks
2. The client was going to stay with a daughter in the daughter's home indefinitely
3. The client was going to have blood work drawn in the home by a local laboratory
4. The client has a good friend living next door who would take the client to the doctor

Level of Cognitive Ability: Analyzing
Client Needs: Psychosocial Integrity
Integrated Process: Nursing Process/Assessment
Content Area: Adult Health: Cardiovascular
Priority Concepts: Family Dynamics; Health Promotion

Answer: 2
Rationale: The client taking anticoagulant therapy should be informed about the medication, its purpose, and the necessity of taking the proper dose at the specified times. If the client is unwilling or unable to comply with the medication regimen, the continuance of the regimen should be questioned. Clients may need support systems in place to enhance compliance with therapy. Option 2 provides a direct support system. Option 1 facilitates reminding the client to take the medication, option 3 facilitates blood work only, and option 4 facilitates medical care.
Priority Nursing Tip: Anticoagulants are administered when there is evidence of or likelihood of clot formation. Such situations include myocardial infarction, unstable angina, atrial fibrillation, deep vein thrombosis, pulmonary embolism, and the presence of mechanical heart valves.
Test-Taking Strategy: Note the strategic word, *best.* Note the subject, the best support system for a client on oral anticoagulant therapy. Note that option 2 is the only option that indicates direct support for the client. Review: the concepts surrounding support systems for the client.
Reference(s): Ignatavicius, Workman (2013), p. 864.

824. A client who has undergone successful femoral-popliteal bypass grafting of the leg says to the nurse, "I hope everything goes well after this and that I don't lose my leg. I'm so afraid that I'll have gone through this for nothing." Which therapeutic response should the nurse make to the client?

1. "I can understand what you mean. I'd be nervous too if I were in your shoes."
2. "This surgery is so successful that I wouldn't be concerned at all if I were you."
3. "Complications are possible, but you have a good deal of control if you make the lifestyle adjustments we talked about."
4. "Stress isn't helpful for you. You should probably just try to relax. You shouldn't worry unless something actually happens."

Level of Cognitive Ability: Applying
Client Needs: Psychosocial Integrity
Integrated Process: Communication and Documentation
Content Area: Adult Health: Cardiovascular
Priority Concepts: Communication; Perfusion

Answer: 3
Rationale: Clients frequently fear that they will ultimately lose a limb or become debilitated in some other way. Option 3 acknowledges the client's concerns and empowers the client to improve his or her health, which will ultimately reduce concern about the risk of complications. Option 1 feeds into the client's anxiety and is not therapeutic. Option 2 gives false reassurance. Option 4 is meant to be reassuring, but it offers no suggestions to empower the client.
Priority Nursing Tip: The client undergoing femoral-popliteal bypass grafting who is returning home should progressively return to his or her normal routine. Additionally, the client should limit pushing or pulling objects for 6 weeks; maintain incision care and report signs of redness, swelling, or discharge; avoid crossing the legs; use prescribed medications; and maintain the prescribed therapeutic diet.
Test-Taking Strategy: Use therapeutic communication techniques. Option 3 is the only option that acknowledges the client's concerns and addresses his or her control over the situation. Review: **therapeutic communication techniques**.
Reference(s): Lewis et al (2011), pp. 789-790; Potter et al (2013), pp. 320-322.

825. A client in the coronary care unit is about to have a pericardiocentesis performed for a rapidly accumulating pericardial effusion. What is the **best** plan for the nurse to implement in order to alleviate the client's apprehension?

1. Tell the client to watch television during the procedure as a distraction.
2. Talk to the client from the foot of the bed and be available to get needed supplies.
3. Stay beside the client and give information and encouragement during the procedure.
4. Tell the client that she (the nurse) will take care of another assigned client at this time, so that she will be unavailable until the procedure is complete.

Level of Cognitive Ability: Applying
Client Needs: Psychosocial Integrity
Integrated Process: Caring
Content Area: Adult Health: Cardiovascular
Priority Concepts: Anxiety; Communication

Answer: 3
Rationale: Clients who develop sudden complications are in situational crisis and need therapeutic intervention. Staying with the client and giving information and encouragement is part of building and maintaining trust in the nurse–client relationship. Options 1 and 4 distance the nurse from the client psychosocially. The nurse should ask another caregiver to be available to get extra supplies if they are needed.
Priority Nursing Tip: A pericardiocentesis involves aspiration of fluid from the pericardium. It is generally done with the guidance of ultrasound so as to minimize complications.
Test-Taking Strategy: Note the strategic word, *best*. Use therapeutic communication techniques. Option 3 is the only option that provides direct contact with and assistance to the client. Review: **therapeutic communication techniques**.
Reference(s): Lewis et al (2011), pp. 848-849; Pagana, Pagana (2013), p. 708; Potter et al (2013), pp. 320-322.

826. The nurse has developed a teaching plan about side effects for the client taking spironolactone (Aldactone). On which psychosocial side effect of the medication should the nurse base the teaching plan?
1. Edema
2. Hair loss
3. Alopecia
4. Decreased libido

Level of Cognitive Ability: Analyzing
Client Needs: Psychosocial Integrity
Integrated Process: Nursing Process/Planning
Content Area: Pharmacology: Cardiovascular Medications
Priority Concepts: Client Education; Fluid and Electrolyte Balance

Answer: 4
Rationale: The nurse should be aware of the fact that the client taking spironolactone may experience body image changes that result from a threatened sexual identity. These are related to decreased libido, gynecomastia in males, and hirsutism in females. Edema and hair loss are not specifically associated with the use of this medication.
Priority Nursing Tip: Spironolactone (Aldactone) is a potassium-retaining diuretic. A primary concern with administering potassium-retaining diuretics is hyperkalemia.
Test-Taking Strategy: Recall your knowledge regarding the side effects of spironolactone. Eliminate options 2 and 3 because they are comparable or alike options. From the remaining options, focusing on the word psychosocial in the question will direct you to the correct option. Review: the side effects of **spironolactone (Aldactone)**.
Reference(s): Hodgson, Kizior (2014), p. 1104; Lehne (2013), pp. 483, 487; Potter et al (2013), pp. 662-663.

827. The nurse is caring for a client who is recovering from an episode of autonomic hyperreflexia. Which therapeutic statement should the nurse make to the client?
1. "How could your home care nurse let this happen?"
2. "Now that this problem is taken care of, I'm sure you'll be fine."
3. "I have some time if you would like to talk about what happened to you."
4. "I'm sure you now understand the importance of preventing this from occurring."

Level of Cognitive Ability: Applying
Client Needs: Psychosocial Integrity
Integrated Process: Communication and Documentation
Content Area: Adult Health: Neurological
Priority Concepts: Communication; Mobility

Answer: 3
Rationale: Option 3 encourages the client to discuss his or her feelings. Options 1 and 4 show disapproval, and option 2 provides false reassurance; these are nontherapeutic techniques.
Priority Nursing Tip: Autonomic dysreflexia occurs with spinal cord lesions or injuries above T6. If autonomic dysreflexia occurs, immediately place the client in high Fowler's position.
Test-Taking Strategy: Use therapeutic communication techniques to identify the correct answer. Remembering to always address the client's concerns and feelings first will direct you to the correct option. Review: **therapeutic communication techniques**.
Reference(s): Ignatavicius, Workman (2013), pp. 973-974; Potter et al (2013), pp. 320-322; Swearingen (2012), pp. 308-309.

828. While assisting a client with a spinal cord injury with activities of daily living, the client states, "I can't do this. I wish I were dead." Which therapeutic response should the nurse make to the client?
1. "Why do you say that?"
2. "You wish you were dead?"
3. "Let's wash your back now."
4. "I'm sure you are frustrated, but things will work out just fine for you."

Level of Cognitive Ability: Applying
Client Needs: Psychosocial Integrity
Integrated Process: Communication and Documentation
Content Area: Adult Health: Neurological
Priority Concepts: Communication; Functional Ability

Answer: 2
Rationale: Clarifying is a therapeutic technique that involves restating what was said to obtain additional information. By asking "why" in option 1, the nurse puts the client on the defensive. Option 3 changes the subject. In option 4, false reassurance is offered. Options 1, 3, and 4 are nontherapeutic and block communication.
Priority Nursing Tip: Trauma to the spinal cord causes partial or complete disruption of the nerve tracts and neurons. Loss of motor function, sensation, reflex activity, and bowel and bladder control may result; therefore, the client is likely to feel a sense of loss of control.
Test-Taking Strategy: Use therapeutic communication techniques. Remember to focus on the client's feelings. Option 2 involves clarifying and restating, and it is the only option that will encourage the client to verbalize feelings and concerns. Review: **therapeutic communication techniques**.
Reference(s): Ignatavicius, Workman (2013), pp. 970, 973-974; Potter et al (2013), pp. 320-322.

829. Family members of a client who attempted suicide are tearful. Which statement by the nurse would be therapeutic?
1. "I'll check on when you will be able to see your loved one."
2. "Believe me when I say that everything possible is being done."
3. "Don't worry. You have absolutely nothing to feel guilty about."
4. "I certainly can see that you are terribly worried about your loved one."

Level of Cognitive Ability: Applying
Client Needs: Psychosocial Integrity
Integrated Process: Caring
Content Area: Mental Health
Priority Concepts: Communication; Professionalism

Answer: 4
Rationale: Option 4 addresses the family's feelings and displays empathy. Options 1, 2, and 3 are communication blocks. Option 1 focuses on an important issue at an inappropriate time. Option 2 uses clichés and false reassurance. Option 3 labels the family's behavior without their validation.
Priority Nursing Tip: All suicide behavior is serious regardless of the intent. Suicide ideation requires constant attention, and typically one-on-one observation. The client at risk must be placed on suicide precautions.
Test-Taking Strategy: Use therapeutic communication techniques. Option 4 involves clarifying, and it is the only option that will encourage the family to verbalize feelings and concerns. Review: **therapeutic communication techniques.**
Reference(s): Fortinash, Holoday-Worret (2012), pp. 71-74; Stuart (2013), pp. 204-205; Swearingen (2012), pp. 700-701.

830. The nurse is caring for an 11-year-old child who has been abused. Which therapeutic action should the nurse include in the plan of care?
1. Encourage the child to fear the abuser.
2. Provide a care environment that allows for the development of trust.
3. Teach the child to make wise choices when confronted with an abusive situation.
4. Have the child point out the abuser if he or she should visit while the child is hospitalized.

Level of Cognitive Ability: Applying
Client Needs: Psychosocial Integrity
Integrated Process: Caring
Content Area: Mental Health
Priority Concepts: Caregiving; Interpersonal Violence

Answer: 2
Rationale: The abused child usually requires long-term therapeutic support. The environment provided during the child's healing must include one in which trust and empathy are modeled and provided for the child. Option 2 is therapeutic because it provides the child with a nurturing and supportive environment in which to begin the healing process. Option 1 reinforces fear, which should not be encouraged. Options 3 and 4 ask the child to behave with a maturity beyond that which would be expected of an 11-year-old child.
Priority Nursing Tip: Nurses are legally required to report all cases of suspected child abuse to the appropriate local or state agency. Documentation of information related to the suspected abuse should be done in an objective manner.
Test-Taking Strategy: Use therapeutic communication techniques. Option 2 is the only option that provides support to the child. Review: **child abuse.**
Reference(s): Fortinash, Holoday-Worret (2012), p. 541; Swearingen (2012), pp. 569-570.

831. Which psychosocial factor obtained during an assessment of an older client places the client at risk for abuse?
1. The client resides in an apartment in a low-income neighborhood.
2. The client shows several signs and symptoms of clinical depression.
3. The client is completely dependent on family members for both food and medicine.
4. The client has been diagnosed with and is receiving treatment for several chronic illnesses.

Level of Cognitive Ability: Analyzing
Client Needs: Psychosocial Integrity
Integrated Process: Nursing Process/Assessment
Content Area: Mental Health
Priority Concepts: Development; Interpersonal Violence

Answer: 3
Rationale: Elder abuse is sometimes the result of frustrated adult children who find themselves caring for dependent parents. Increasing demands by parents for care and financial support can cause resentment and a feeling of being burdened. The issues of abuse are not bound to socioeconomic status (option 1). Option 2 relates to depression rather than the risk for abuse. Option 4 relates to a physical factor rather than a psychosocial factor.
Priority Nursing Tip: Factors that contribute to elder abuse and neglect include long-standing family violence, caregiver stress, and the individual's increasing dependence on others. The interaction between the older adult and caregiver can provide important clues about the relationship.
Test-Taking Strategy: Note the words *psychosocial factor*, and focus on the subject, the risk for elder abuse. Noting the words *completely dependent* in option 3 will direct you to this option. Review the risk factors associated with **elder abuse.**
Reference(s): Fortinash, Holoday-Worret (2012), pp. 542-544; Stuart (2013), pp. 745-746.

832. The nurse is caring for a dying client who says, "Will you be the executor of my will?" How should the nurse **best** respond to this client?
1. "I must decline your offer because I am your nurse."
2. "I will carry out your will according to your wishes."
3. "It is an honor to be named the executor of your will."
4. "Tell me more so that I can understand your thinking."

Level of Cognitive Ability: Applying
Client Needs: Psychosocial Integrity
Integrated Process: Nursing Process/Implementation
Content Area: Leadership/Management: Ethical/Legal
Priority Concepts: Ethics; Health Care Law

Answer: 4
Rationale: The client's question reflects his thoughts about the will and how to obtain an executor, but the question does not reveal why the client is asking the nurse to be executor, and it also does not address other important information. In option 4, the nurse seeks clarification while acknowledging the client's statement. Most agencies do not allow the nurse to be the executor of a client's will (option 3). The other options fail to regard the potential consequences, think critically, or explore the client's motivation and needs.
Priority Nursing Tip: A living will is one example of the execution of the Patient's Bill of Rights (Patient Care Partnership), which reflects acknowledgment of a client's right to participate in his or her health care with an emphasis on client autonomy.
Test-Taking Strategy: Note the strategic word, *best*. Use therapeutic communication techniques. Option 4 is the only option that addresses the client's thoughts and feelings. Review: **therapeutic communication techniques and wills.**
Reference(s): Ignatavicius, Workman (2013), p. 108; Potter et al (2013), pp. 320-322.

833. A client who has urticaria (hives) and pruritus is anxious and says to the nurse, "What am I going to do? I'm getting married next week, and I'll probably be covered in this rash and itching like crazy." Which statement made by the nurse is the most therapeutic?
1. "You're troubled that this will extend into your wedding?"
2. "It's probably just due to prewedding jitters. You'll be fine."
3. "The antihistamine will help a great deal, just you wait and see."
4. "I hope your husband-to-be has a sense of humor and can laugh about this."

Level of Cognitive Ability: Applying
Client Needs: Psychosocial Integrity
Integrated Process: Communication and Documentation
Content Area: Mental Health
Priority Concepts: Anxiety; Communication

Answer: 1
Rationale: The therapeutic communication technique that the nurse uses in option 1 is reflection. In option 2, the nurse minimizes the client's anxiety and fears. In option 3, the nurse talks about antihistamines and asks the client to "wait and see." This is nontherapeutic because the nurse is making promises that may not be kept. In addition, the response is closed-ended and shuts off the client's expression of feelings. In option 4, the nurse uses humor inappropriately and without sensitivity.
Priority Nursing Tip: Antihistamines are used to treat the common cold, rhinitis, nausea and vomiting, motion sickness, urticaria, and as a sleep aid. These medications can cause central nervous system depression if taken with alcohol, opioids, hypnotics, and barbiturates.
Test-Taking Strategy: Use therapeutic communication techniques. Options 2, 3, and 4 are nontherapeutic responses. Option 1 addresses the client's feelings. Review: **therapeutic communication techniques.**
Reference(s): Ignatavicius, Workman (2013), p. 472; Potter et al (2013), pp. 320-322.

834. Which statement made by a client with a spinal cord injury warrants follow-up by the nurse?

1. "I'm so angry that this happened to me."
2. "I'm really looking forward to going home."
3. "I know I will have to make major adjustments in my life."
4. "I would like my family members to be here for my teaching sessions."

Level of Cognitive Ability: Analyzing
Client Needs: Psychosocial Integrity
Integrated Process: Nursing Process/Analysis
Content Area: Adult Health: Neurological
Priority Concepts: Coping; Functional Ability

Answer: 1
Rationale: It is important to allow the client with a spinal cord injury to verbalize his or her feelings. If the client indicates a desire to discuss his or her feelings, the nurse should respond therapeutically. No data in the question indicate that the client will not be going home; therefore, this comment does not require further intervention. Options 3 and 4 indicate that the client understands that changes will be occurring and that family involvement is best.
Priority Nursing Tip: Autonomic dysreflexia is a concern for the client with a spinal cord injury. Autonomic dysreflexia occurs with spinal lesions or injury above T6. Severe hypertension occurs in autonomic dysreflexia; therefore, immediately place the client in the high Fowler's position and eliminate the noxious stimuli causing the problem.
Test-Taking Strategy: Focus on the subject, the client statement that *warrants follow-up*. Noting the word *angry* in option 1 will direct you to this option. Review: **spinal cord injury.**
Reference(s): Ignatavicius, Workman (2013), pp. 970, 973-974.

835. The nurse is caring for a client with a mild cerebral bleed as a result of a cerebral aneurysm rupture. The client tells you he is feeling very restless and anxious before visiting hours. Which comment by the client should assist the nurse in identifying the rationale for the feelings?

1. "I really do not like this stiff neck."
2. "At least I am able to talk to my family."
3. "My family is very supportive of my condition."
4. "I told my daughter I would be fully recovered in no time."

Level of Cognitive Ability: Analyzing
Client Needs: Psychosocial Integrity
Integrated Process: Nursing Process/Analysis
Content Area: Adult Health: Neurological
Priority Concepts: Anxiety; Intracranial Regulation

Answer: 4
Rationale: With a mild bleed from a cerebral aneurysm rupture the client usually remains alert but has nuchal rigidity with possible neurological deficits, depending on the area of the bleed. Because these clients remain alert, they are acutely aware of the neurological deficits and frequently have some degree of body image disturbance. Option 4 alludes to the client's daughter not being given correct information. The remaining client statements are unrelated to anxiety and restlessness.
Priority Nursing Tip: For the client with a cerebral aneurysm, bed rest is usually maintained with the head of the bed elevated 30 to 45 degrees to prevent pressure on the aneurysm site that can lead to rupture.
Test-Taking Strategy: Focus on the subject, that the client is feeling restless and anxious, and note the words *before visiting hours*. Using your knowledge of the effects of this disorder and focusing on the client's behavior will direct you to option 4. Review: the effects of a **cerebral aneurysm rupture.**
Reference(s): Ignatavicius, Workman (2013), pp. 792-793; Potter et al (2013), pp. 662-663.

836. When planning the care of the client with thromboangiitis obliterans (Buerger's disease), the nurse incorporates measures to help the client cope with the lifestyle changes that are needed to control the disease process. The nurse can accomplish this by recommending which support service?

1. Consult with a dietician
2. Pain management clinic
3. Smoking cessation program
4. Referral to a medical social worker

Level of Cognitive Ability: Applying
Client Needs: Psychosocial Integrity
Integrated Process: Nursing Process/Implementation
Content Area: Adult Health: Cardiovascular
Priority Concepts: Health Promotion; Perfusion

Answer: 3
Rationale: Smoking is highly detrimental to the client with Buerger's disease, and clients are recommended to stop completely. Because smoking is a form of chemical dependency, referral to a smoking cessation program may be helpful for many clients. For many clients, symptoms are relieved or alleviated when smoking stops. Options 1, 2, and 4 are not directly related to the physiology associated with this condition.
Priority Nursing Tip: Buerger's disease is an occlusive disease of the median and small arteries and veins. The distal upper and lower limbs are affected most commonly.
Test-Taking Strategy: Focus on the subject, Buerger's disease. Recalling that the treatment goals are the same as for peripheral vascular disease will direct you to the correct option. Review: the treatment goals for **Buerger's disease.**
Reference(s): Ignatavicius, Workman (2013), p. 797; Lewis et al (2011), pp. 875, 881.

837. While assessing a 14-year-old child, the nurse notes bruises and cigarette burns on the child's chest and rope burns on the buttocks. The child states, "I'm afraid to go home because my stepfather will be angry with me for telling on him!" The nurse should make which therapeutic response to the child?

1. "You can't go back there with that man. How do you think your mother will react?"
2. "You must know that your presence in the house will only tease your stepfather more."
3. "I am sorry that this has happened to you, but you will be safe here until plans can be made."
4. "Let's keep this between you, me, and the health care provider until we formulate further plans to assist you."

Level of Cognitive Ability: Applying
Client Needs: Psychosocial Integrity
Integrated Process: Caring
Content Area: Mental Health
Priority Concepts: Caring; Interpersonal Violence

Answer: 3
Rationale: A child who has been physically and sexually abused should be admitted to the hospital. This will provide time for a more comprehensive evaluation while protecting the child from further abuse. The correct option also provides an empathic statement that supports the child to appropriately perceive himself or herself as the victim while assuring the child of protection from abuse. In option 1, the nurse does not respond with a calm and reassuring communication style or maintain a professional attitude. Option 2, which holds an innuendo, appears to accuse the victim of teasing the stepfather and is thus incorrect; it is also judgmental, controlling, and demeaning. The nurse's suggestion in option 4 is not only incorrect but also passive in its stance.
Priority Nursing Tip: Ensuring a safe environment is the priority for a child who is a victim of abuse.
Test-Taking Strategy: Use therapeutic communication techniques, and your knowledge of the care of the child who has been physically abused. Recalling that the priority is the safety of the victim will direct you to option 3. Review: **child abuse.**
Reference(s): Fortinash, Holoday-Worret (2012), pp. 71-74, 541; Swearingen (2012), pp. 569-570.

838. The nurse is caring for a 12-year-old client who has been physically and sexually abused by her father. The father angrily approaches the nurse and says, "I'm taking my daughter home. She's told me what you people are up to, and we're out of here!" Which therapeutic response should the nurse make?

1. "Your daughter will remain here until the doctor discharges her. I'll call hospital security and the police if you attempt to take her."
2. "Try to listen to me, please. If you are insistent and do take your daughter from this unit, the police will most certainly order you to bring her back again."
3. "Your daughter is ill and needs to be here. I know you want to help her to recover and that you will work to help everyone straighten out the circumstances that caused this."
4. "You seem very upset. Let's talk at the nurse's station. I know you're very concerned and that you want to help your daughter. It will be best if you agree to let your daughter stay here for now."

Level of Cognitive Ability: Applying
Client Needs: Psychosocial Integrity
Integrated Process: Communication and Documentation
Content Area: Mental Health
Priority Concepts: Interpersonal Violence; Professionalism

Answer: 4
Rationale: When a suspected abused child is admitted to the hospital for further evaluation and protection, the health care provider will usually work with the parents so that they will agree to the admission. If the parents refuse to do this, the hospital can request an immediate court order to retain the child for a specific length of time. In option 1, the nurse is angry and verbally abusive. It is clear that the nurse has decided that the father is guilty of child abuse. In addition, the nurse is aggressive and challenging; this may antagonize the father and cause the nurse to become a victim of violence as well. In option 2, the command to listen is somewhat demanding. Option 3 seems somewhat pompous and lecturing.
Priority Nursing Tip: Nurses are legally required to report all cases of suspected child abuse to the appropriate local or state agency. A safe environment must be provided for the victim.
Test-Taking Strategy: Use therapeutic communication techniques. Note that the client of the question is the child's father. Note that option 4 addresses the father's behavior yet protects the child. Review: the psychosocial issues related to **child abuse.**
Reference(s): Fortinash, Holoday-Worret (2012), pp. 71-74, 541; Swearingen (2012), pp. 569-570.

839. A client with arterial leg ulcers complains of pain and tells the nurse, "I'm so discouraged. I have had this pain for more than a year now. The pain never seems to go away. I can't do anything, and I feel as though I'll never get better." Which is the **priority** client problem?
1. Fatigue
2. Uneasiness
3. Chronic pain
4. An acute illness

Level of Cognitive Ability: Analyzing
Client Needs: Psychosocial Integrity
Integrated Process: Nursing Process/Analysis
Content Area: Adult Health: Cardiovascular
Priority Concepts: Clinical Judgment; Pain

Answer: 3
Rationale: The major focus of the client's complaint is the experience of pain. Pain that has a duration of more than 3 months is defined as chronic pain and does not indicate an acute illness. There are no data in the question that indicate fatigue or uneasiness.
Priority Nursing Tip: The client with nonhealing arterial ulcerations should monitor the site and report signs of infection. These signs include redness, edema, and warmth at the affected area. In addition, an elevated temperature and change in vital signs may be signs of infection and should be reported.
Test-Taking Strategy: Note the strategic word, *priority.* Focusing on the words *pain for more than a year now* will direct you to the correct option. Review: **chronic pain and leg ulcers.**
Reference(s): Ignatavicius, Workman (2013), pp. 788, 872-873; Swearingen (2012), p. 520.

840. A client with valvular heart disease is being considered for mechanical valve replacement. Which item is **essential** to assess before the surgery is performed?
1. The physical demands of the client's lifestyle
2. The ability to comply with anticoagulant therapy for life
3. The ability to participate in a cardiac rehabilitation program
4. The likelihood of the client experiencing body image problems

Level of Cognitive Ability: Analyzing
Client Needs: Psychosocial Integrity
Integrated Process: Nursing Process/Assessment
Content Area: Adult Health: Cardiovascular
Priority Concepts: Adherence; Clotting

Answer: 2
Rationale: Mechanical valves carry the associated risk of thromboemboli, which require long-term anticoagulation with warfarin sodium (Coumadin). No data in the question indicate that physical demands exist in the client's lifestyle. Not all clients who undergo cardiac surgery require cardiac rehabilitation. Body image problems are important but not critical.
Priority Nursing Tip: A priority concern when the client is taking an anticoagulant is bleeding.
Test-Taking Strategy: Focus on the strategic word, *essential.* Recalling that mechanical valves are thrombogenic will direct you to the correct option. Review: care of the client undergoing a **mechanical valve replacement.**
Reference(s): Ignatavicius, Workman (2013), pp. 760-761; Lewis et al (2011), p. 857.

841. A client who has a history of depression has been prescribed nadolol (Corgard) for the management of angina pectoris. Which item is **most important** when the nurse plans to counsel this client about the effects of this medication?
1. Risk of tachycardia
2. Probability of fatigue
3. High incidence of hypoglycemia
4. Possible exacerbation of depression

Level of Cognitive Ability: Analyzing
Client Needs: Psychosocial Integrity
Integrated Process: Nursing Process/Planning
Content Area: Pharmacology: Cardiovascular Medications
Priority Concepts: Clinical Judgment; Safety

Answer: 4
Rationale: Clients with depression or a history of depression have experienced an exacerbation of depression after beginning therapy with beta-adrenergic blocking agents. These clients should be monitored carefully if these agents are prescribed. The medication would cause bradycardia rather than tachycardia. Fatigue is a possible side effect, but it is not the most important item. Hypoglycemia is a sign that is masked with beta blockers.
Priority Nursing Tip: The goal of treatment for angina is to provide relief of the acute attack, correct the imbalance between myocardial oxygen supply and demand, and prevent the progression of the disease and further attacks to reduce the risk of myocardial infarction.
Test-Taking Strategy: Note the strategic words, *most important.* Focus on the subject, the effects of nadolol. Note the word *depression* in the question to direct you to the correct option. Clients with depression or a history of depression have experienced an exacerbation of depression after beginning therapy with beta-adrenergic blocking agents. These clients should be monitored carefully if these agents are prescribed. Review: **nadolol (Corgard).**
Reference(s): Hodgson, Kizior (2014), pp. 808-809.

842. The nurse is caring for a client with terminal cancer of the throat. The family approaches the nurse and tells the nurse that they have spoken to the health care provider regarding taking their loved one home. The nurse plans to coordinate discharge planning. Which service would be **most** supportive to the client and the family?

1. Hospice care
2. The American Cancer Society
3. The American Lung Association
4. Local religious and social organizations

Level of Cognitive Ability: Applying
Client Needs: Psychosocial Integrity
Integrated Process: Caring
Content Area: Adult Health: Oncology
Priority Concepts: Caregiving; Palliation

Answer: 1
Rationale: Hospice care provides an environment that emphasizes caring rather than curing; the emphasis is on palliative care. One of the major goals of hospice care is that clients be free of pain and other symptoms that do not allow them to maintain a quality life. An interdisciplinary approach is used. Options 2, 3, and 4 would be helpful, but they are not the most supportive of the options provided.
Priority Nursing Tip: Hospice care is a concept of care for terminally ill clients that include the idea of intensive caring rather than intensive care. The client and the family are the focus of nursing care, and the goal is to relieve pain and facilitate an optimal quality of life.
Test-Taking Strategy: Note the strategic word, *most*. Knowledge regarding the goals and services provided by hospice care will assist you with answering the question. Think about what each support service presented in the options will provide for meeting this client's needs. This will assist with directing you to the correct option. Review: **hospice care.**
Reference(s): Ignatavicius, Workman (2013), pp. 108, 110; Potter et al (2013), pp. 719-720.

843. The home care nurse is caring for a client with acute cancer pain. What is the **most appropriate** way to assess the client's pain?

1. The client's pain rating
2. The nurse's impression of the client's pain
3. Verbal and nonverbal clues from the client
4. Pain relief after appropriate nursing intervention

Level of Cognitive Ability: Applying
Client Needs: Psychosocial Integrity
Integrated Process: Caring
Content Area: Fundamental Skills: Pain
Priority Concepts: Clinical Judgment; Pain

Answer: 1
Rationale: The client's perception of pain is the hallmark of pain assessment. Usually noted by the client's rating on a scale of 1 to 10, the assessment is documented and followed with appropriate medical and nursing interventions. The nurse's impression and the verbal and nonverbal clues are subjective data. Pain relief after intervention is appropriate but relates to evaluation.
Priority Nursing Tip: The nurse must assess the client's pain; pain is what the client describes or says that it is. The nurse must not undermedicate the cancer client who is in pain.
Test-Taking Strategy: Note the strategic words, *most appropriate*. Using the steps of the nursing process, note that the correct option addresses the client directly. Review: nursing assessment of **pain.**
Reference(s): Ignatavicius, Workman (2013), p. 48; Potter et al (2013), p. 970.

844. A prenatal client has been told during a health care provider office visit that she is positive for human immunodeficiency virus (HIV). The client cried and was significantly distressed regarding this news. Which client problem statement would this assessment data **best** support?

1. Pain
2. Nonadherence
3. Anticipatory grieving
4. High risk for infection

Level of Cognitive Ability: Analyzing
Client Needs: Psychosocial Integrity
Integrated Process: Caring
Content Area: Maternity: Antepartum
Priority Concepts: Coping; Immunity

Answer: 3
Rationale: A life-threatening diagnosis such as HIV will stimulate the anticipatory grief response. Anticipatory grief occurs when the client, family, and loved ones know that the client will die. The prenatal HIV client is forced to make important changes in her life, frequently resulting in grief related to lost future dreams and diminished self-esteem as a result of an inability to achieve life goals. Although options 1, 2, and 4 may be appropriate problem statements at some point, they do not address the information given in the question.
Priority Nursing Tip: During the prenatal period, the health care providers must focus on preventing opportunistic infections in the client with human immunodeficiency virus (HIV). Procedures that increase the risk of perinatal transmission, such as amniocentesis and fetal scalp sampling, should be avoided.
Test-Taking Strategy: Note the strategic word, *best*. Focus on the data in the question. A client who is distressed and crying is supporting data for the problem statement of anticipatory grieving. Review: **human immunodeficiency virus (HIV)** and **anticipatory grieving.**
Reference(s): McKinney et al (2013), pp. 629-630.

845. The nurse is assessing a client's suicide potential. Which **most important** question should the nurse ask the client?

1. "Why do you want to hurt yourself?"
2. "Do you have a plan to commit suicide?"
3. "Has anyone in your family committed suicide?"
4. "Can you describe how you are feeling right now?"

Level of Cognitive Ability: Analyzing
Client Needs: Psychosocial Integrity
Integrated Process: Nursing Process/Assessment
Content Area: Mental Health
Priority Concepts: Mood and Affect; Safety

Answer: 2
Rationale: When assessing for suicide risk, the nurse must evaluate whether the client has a suicide plan. Clients who have a definitive plan pose a greater risk for suicide. Options 3 and 4 may also be questions that the nurse would ask, but they are not the most important. The nurse avoids the use of the word "why" when communicating with a client. The use of this word may place the client on the defensive; additionally, the client may not even know the reason that he or she wants to hurt himself or herself.
Priority Nursing Tip: The client who has a plan to commit suicide must be placed on suicide precautions.
Test-Taking Strategy: Note the strategic words, *most important.* Recalling the importance of assessing for a suicide plan will direct you to the correct option. Review **suicide.**
Reference(s): Fortinash, Holoday-Worret (2012), p. 515; Swearingen (2012), pp. 700-701.

846. The nurse is caring for a client who is receiving electroconvulsive therapy (ECT) for a major depressive disorder. Which assessment finding should the nurse identify as an unexpected side effect of ECT that requires notifying the health care provider?

1. Confusion
2. Memory loss
3. Hypertension
4. Disorientation

Level of Cognitive Ability: Analyzing
Client Needs: Psychosocial Integrity
Integrated Process: Nursing Process/Assessment
Content Area: Mental Health
Priority Concepts: Clinical Judgment; Mood and Affect

Answer: 3
Rationale: The major side effects of ECT are confusion, disorientation, and memory loss. A change in blood pressure would not be an anticipated side effect and would be a cause for concern. If hypertension occurred after ECT, the health care provider should be notified.
Priority Nursing Tip: Electroconvulsive therapy (ECT) may be used to treat depression. It consists of inducing a seizure by passing an electrical current through electrodes attached to the temples. It is not always effective in clients with dysthymic depression, depression and personality disorders, drug dependence, or depression secondary to situational or social difficulties.
Test-Taking Strategy: Focus on the subject, an unexpected side effect of ECT. Recall the side effects of ECT, and note that options 1, 2, and 4 are comparable or alike. Review: the expected side effects of electroconvulsive therapy (ECT).
Reference(s): Fortinash, Holoday-Worret (2012), p. 620; Stuart (2013), p. 599.

847. During the admission assessment of a client admitted to the hospital for ruptured esophageal varices, the client says, "I deserve this. I brought it on myself." Which therapeutic response should the nurse make to the client?

1. "Would you like to talk to the chaplain?"
2. "Is there some reason you feel you deserve this?"
3. "Not all esophageal varices are caused by alcohol."
4. "That is something to think about when you leave the hospital."

Level of Cognitive Ability: Applying
Client Needs: Psychosocial Integrity
Integrated Process: Communication and Documentation
Content Area: Adult Health: Gastrointestinal
Priority Concepts: Caring; Communication

Answer: 2
Rationale: Ruptured esophageal varices are often a complication of cirrhosis of the liver, and the most common type of cirrhosis is caused by chronic alcohol abuse. It is important to obtain an accurate history regarding the client's alcohol intake. If the client is ashamed or embarrassed, he or she may not respond accurately. Option 2 is open-ended and allows the client to discuss his or her feelings about drinking. Option 1 blocks the nurse–client communication process. Options 3 and 4 are somewhat judgmental.
Priority Nursing Tip: Rupture and resultant hemorrhage of the esophageal varices are primary concerns because this is a life-threatening situation.
Test-Taking Strategy: Use therapeutic communication techniques to direct you to the correct option. Remember that the client's feelings should be addressed first. Review: **therapeutic communication techniques.**
Reference(s): Ignatavicius, Workman (2013), p. 1294; Lewis et al (2011), p. 1075; Potter et al (2013), pp. 320-322.

848. The nurse is performing a neurological assessment on a client with dementia and assessing the function of the frontal lobe of the brain. What should the nurse assess to yield the **best** information about this area of functioning?

1. Eye movements
2. Feelings or emotions
3. Level of consciousness
4. Insight, judgment, and planning

Level of Cognitive Ability: Applying
Client Needs: Psychosocial Integrity
Integrated Process: Nursing Process/Assessment
Content Area: Developmental Stages: Health Assessment/Physical Exam
Priority Concepts: Clinical Judgment; Cognition

Answer: 4
Rationale: Insight, judgment, and planning are part of the function of the frontal lobe. Eye movements are under the control of cranial nerves III, IV, and VI. Feelings and emotions are part of the role of the limbic system. The level of consciousness is controlled by the reticular activating system.
Priority Nursing Tip: A common type of dementia is Alzheimer's disease. Dementia results in a self-care deficit. Long-term and short-term memory loss occur, with impairment in judgment, abstract thinking, problem-solving ability, and behavior.
Test-Taking Strategy: Focus on the subject, the frontal lobe of the brain. Note the strategic word, *best*. Recalling the location of the frontal lobe and that this lobe is primarily responsible for insight and reasoning will assist in answering correctly. Review: **frontal lobe of the brain.**
Reference(s): Ignatavicius, Workman (2013), p. 907; Jarvis (2012), p. 622; Lewis et al (2011), pp. 1408-1409.

849. The client who is dying tells his nurse, "I hope I am worthy of heaven." What intervention should the nurse implement **first** after determining this client is experiencing fear?

1. Help the client express fears.
2. Assess the nature of the client's fears.
3. Help the client identify coping mechanisms that were successful in the past.
4. Document verbal and nonverbal expressions of fear and other significant data.

Level of Cognitive Ability: Applying
Client Needs: Psychosocial Integrity
Integrated Process: Nursing Process/Implementation
Content Area: Developmental Stages: End-of-Life Care
Priority Concepts: Anxiety; Palliation

Answer: 2
Rationale: Fear can range from a paralyzing, overwhelming feeling to a mild concern. Therefore, the nurse would first assess the nature of the client's fears to know how best to help the client. Next, the nurse would help the client express his or her fears. The client's fear may not be limited to the fear of dying, and the nurse needs this information to help the client. After the nurse is aware of the client's fears, the methods that the client used to cope with fear in the past are identified. From the interventions listed, the nurse would document verbal and nonverbal expressions of fear and any other significant data as a final intervention.
Priority Nursing Tip: The nurse should avoid repeated, unnecessary assessments on a dying client. Assessment should be limited to obtaining essential data.
Test-Taking Strategy: Note the strategic word, *first*. Use the steps of the nursing process to assist you with determining the order of priority of the nursing interventions. An assessment of the client's fear would be the first intervention. Review: the care of the **dying client and fear.**
Reference(s): Ignatavicius, Workman (2013), p. 114.

850. Fluoxetine hydrochloride (Prozac) is prescribed for a client with depression. The nurse provides instructions to the client regarding the administration of the medication. Which statement by the client indicates an understanding about administration of the medication?

1. "I should take the medication with my evening meal."
2. "I should take the medication at noon with an antacid."
3. "I should take the medication in the morning when I first arise."
4. "I should take the medication right before bedtime with a snack."

Level of Cognitive Ability: Evaluating
Client Needs: Psychosocial Integrity
Integrated Process: Nursing Process/Evaluation
Content Area: Pharmacology: Psychiatric Medications
Priority Concepts: Client Education; Safety

Answer: 3
Rationale: Fluoxetine hydrochloride is an antidepressant and is administered in the early morning without consideration of meals. Options 1, 2, and 4 are incorrect.
Priority Nursing Tip: For the depressed client, the nurse should assess for homicidal and suicidal ideation and provide safety from suicidal actions. Additional interventions should be to assist with activities of daily living, remind the client of times when he or she felt better and was successful, and spend time with the client to communicate the client's value.
Test-Taking Strategy: Eliminate options 1, 2, and 4 because they are comparable or alike and indicate taking the medication with an antacid or food. Review: **fluoxetine hydrochloride (Prozac).**
Reference(s): Hodgson, Kizior (2014), p. 496.

851. A mother comes to the pediatric clinic because her previously continent 6-year-old son has resumed bedwetting. The nurse assesses the home environment and discovers there is a new baby at home. Which explanation by the nurse describes for the mother the defense mechanism the son is using?
1. Regression
2. Repression
3. Identification
4. Rationalization

Level of Cognitive Ability: Applying
Client Needs: Psychosocial Integrity
Integrated Process: Nursing Process/Implementation
Content Area: Mental Health
Priority Concepts: Client Education; Coping

Answer: 1
Rationale: The defense mechanism of regression is characterized by returning to an earlier form of expressing an impulse. Option 2 is characterized by blocking a wish or desire from conscious expression. Option 3 occurs when a person models behavior after someone else. Option 4 occurs when a person unconsciously falsifies an experience by giving a "rational" explanation.
Priority Nursing Tip: A defense mechanism is a coping mechanism used in an effort to protect the individual from feelings of anxiety. As anxiety increases and becomes overwhelming, the individual copes by using defense mechanisms to protect the ego and decrease anxiety.
Test-Taking Strategy: Focus on the subject, the defense mechanism the child is using. Noting the words *resumed bedwetting* will direct you to the correct option. Review: **defense mechanisms.**
Reference(s): Hockenberry, Wilson (2013), p. 390; McKinney et al (2013), pp. 878, 1120-1121.

852. The nurse is obtaining a health history from an adolescent. Which statement by the adolescent indicates a **need for follow-up** assessment and intervention?
1. "When I get stressed out about school, I just like to be alone."
2. "I find myself very moody. I'm happy one minute and crying the next."
3. "I don't eat anything with any fat in it, and I've lost 8 pounds in 2 weeks."
4. "I can't seem to wake up in the morning. I would sleep until noon if I could."

Level of Cognitive Ability: Analyzing
Client Needs: Psychosocial Integrity
Integrated Process: Nursing Process/Analysis
Content Area: Developmental Stages: Infancy to Adolescence
Priority Concepts: Development; Nutrition

Answer: 3
Rationale: During the adolescent period, there is a heightened awareness of body image and peer pressure to go on excessively restrictive diets. The extreme limitation of omitting all fat in the diet and losing weight during a time of growth suggests inadequate nutrition and a possible eating disorder. Options 1, 2, and 4 are common and normal behaviors or feelings that occur during adolescence.
Priority Nursing Tip: The nurse must remember that the adolescent may be preoccupied with body image and should encourage and support independence. Additionally, the nurse should provide privacy during examination and engage in conversation about the adolescent's interests.
Test-Taking Strategy: Note the strategic words, *need for follow-up.* These words indicate a negative event query and ask you to select the option that identifies a statement made by the adolescent that is of concern. Options 1, 2, and 4 are common and normal behaviors or feelings during adolescence. Option 3 indicates a problem or abnormality. Review: the developmental stage of **adolescence.**
Reference(s): Hockenberry, Wilson (2013), pp. 486, 488.

853. The nurse is caring for a client who has bipolar disorder and is in a manic state. The nurse determines that which menu choice would be **best** for this client?
1. Beef stew, fruit salad, tea
2. Cheeseburger, banana, milk
3. Macaroni and cheese, apple, milk
4. Scrambled eggs, orange juice, coffee with cream and sugar

Level of Cognitive Ability: Analyzing
Client Needs: Psychosocial Integrity
Integrated Process: Nursing Process/Planning
Content Area: Mental Health
Priority Concepts: Mood and Affect; Nutrition

Answer: 2
Rationale: The client in a manic state often has inadequate food and fluid intake as a result of physical agitation. Foods that the client can eat "on the run" are best because the client is too active to sit at meals and use utensils. Additionally, clients in a manic state should not have any products that contain caffeine.
Priority Nursing Tip: For the client in a manic state, the nurse should maintain safety for the client, others, and self. The nurse should maintain large personal space, use a nonaggressive posture, a calm approach, and communicate with a calm, clear tone of voice.
Test-Taking Strategy: Note the strategic word, *best.* Focus on the words *manic state.* Note that options 1, 3, and 4 are comparable or alike in that the client needs to sit to eat some of these food items. Remember the concept of "finger foods" with regard to the client with mania. Review: **bipolar disorder** and **mania.**
Reference(s): Fortinash, Holoday-Worret (2012), p. 239; Swearingen (2012), p. 686; Varcarolis (2013), p. 290.

854. The nurse is caring for a child who is a victim of abuse and has determined that the child uses repression to cope with past life experiences. Which activity should the nurse implement as part of the nursing care plan?
1. Encourage the child to use therapeutic play to act out past experiences.
2. Tell the child to let the past go and concentrate on the present and future.
3. Place the child on medications that will help the child forget the incidents.
4. Have the child talk about the abuse in detail during the first therapy session.

Level of Cognitive Ability: Applying
Client Needs: Psychosocial Integrity
Integrated Process: Nursing Process/Implementation
Content Area: Mental Health
Priority Concepts: Coping; Interpersonal Violence

Answer: 1
Rationale: Therapeutic play is used to reduce the trauma of illness and hospitalizations. It is a nonthreatening avenue through which the child can use artwork, dolls, or puppets to act out frightening life experiences. Option 3 would be extremely threatening to the child and nontherapeutic. Options 2 and 4 devalue the child and force the child to further repress harmful past experiences rather than facing them and moving on.
Priority Nursing Tip: Repression is the unconscious process in which the client blocks undesirable and unacceptable thoughts from conscious expression.
Test-Taking Strategy: Use therapeutic communication techniques to eliminate options 2 and 4. From the remaining options, note the relationship of the words *past life experiences* in the question and *past experiences* in the correct option. Review: **child abuse** and **regression**.
Reference(s): Hockenberry, Wilson (2013), p. 452; McKinney et al (2013), pp. 1471-1472.

855. An older client is brought to the emergency department by a family member with whom she lives. The nurse notes that the client has poor hygiene, contractures, and pressure ulcers on the sacrum, the scapula, and the heels. The client is suspected of which form of victimization?
1. Sexual abuse
2. Physical abuse
3. Emotional abuse
4. Psychological abuse

Level of Cognitive Ability: Analyzing
Client Needs: Psychosocial Integrity
Integrated Process: Nursing Process/Analysis
Content Area: Mental Health
Priority Concepts: Clinical Judgment; Interpersonal Violence

Answer: 2
Rationale: Victimization in a family can take many forms. When analyzing a specific client situation, it is important to understand which form of abuse is being considered. Physical abuse can take the form of battering (hitting, slapping, striking), or it can be more subtle, such as neglect (the failure to meet basic needs). Sexual abuse can involve unwanted sexual remarks, sexual advances, and physical sexual acts. Emotional and psychological abuse can involve inflicting verbal statements that cause mental anguish or alienation of the victim.
Priority Nursing Tip: Victims of abuse are often isolated socially by their abusers.
Test-Taking Strategy: Note the subject, the form of victimization. Focus on the words that relate to physical abuse in the question such as the description of the client. Option 2 is the only choice that fits the description in the question. Review: the signs of **physical abuse** in the older client.
Reference(s): Fortinash, Holoday-Worret (2012), p. 544.

856. A client is admitted to the inpatient mental health unit. When asked her name, she responds, "I am Elizabeth, the Queen of England." What should the nurse recognize this client statement as indicating?
1. Visual illusion
2. Loose association
3. Grandiose delusion
4. Auditory hallucination

Level of Cognitive Ability: Analyzing
Client Needs: Psychosocial Integrity
Integrated Process: Nursing Process/Assessment
Content Area: Mental Health
Priority Concepts: Clinical Judgment; Psychosis

Answer: 3
Rationale: A delusion is an important personal belief that is almost certainly not true and that resists modification. An illusion is a misperception or misinterpretation of externally real stimuli. Loose association is thinking that is characterized by speech in which ideas that are unrelated shift from one subject to another. A hallucination is a false perception.
Priority Nursing Tip: In delusions of grandeur, the client attaches special significance to self in relation to others or the universe and has an exaggerated sense of self that has no basis in reality.
Test-Taking Strategy: Note the subject, what the client's statement indicates. Focus on the word *queen* in the question. Making a reference to being a queen is a grandiose assumption. Review: **grandiose delusions**.
Reference(s): Fortinash, Holoday-Worret (2012), p. 275; Varcarolis (2013), p. 306.

857. A client who has been newly admitted to the mental health unit with a diagnosis of bipolar disorder is trying to organize a dance with the other clients on the unit and is planning an on-unit supper. The nurse should encourage which activity to decrease stimulation with the clients?

1. Seek assistance from other staff members.
2. Engage the help of other clients on the unit to accomplish the task.
3. Stop the planning and firmly tell the client that this task is inappropriate.
4. Postpone organizing the dance and supper and engage the client in a writing activity.

Level of Cognitive Ability: Applying
Client Needs: Psychosocial Integrity
Integrated Process: Nursing Process/Implementation
Content Area: Mental Health
Priority Concepts: Clinical Judgment; Psychosis

Answer: 4
Rationale: Because the client with bipolar disorder is easily stimulated by the environment, sedentary activities are the best outlets for energy release. Most bipolar clients enjoy writing, so the writing task is appropriate. An activity such as planning a dance or supper may be appropriate at some point, but not for the newly admitted client who is likely to have impaired judgment and a short attention span. Options 1 and 2 encourage planning the activity and therefore increase client stimulation. Option 3 could result in an angry outburst by the client.
Priority Nursing Tip: Bipolar disorder is commonly treated with lithium carbonate. This medication can result in toxicity and requires regular monitoring of serum lithium levels.
Test-Taking Strategy: Focus on the subject, the activity that will decrease stimulation. Options 1 and 2 encourage activity and should be eliminated. Option 3 tells the client that the activity is inappropriate, and this could result in an angry outburst by the client. Option 4 is the only choice that limits activity. Review: **bipolar disorder**.
Reference(s): Fortinash, Holoday-Worret (2012), pp. 242, 631; Stuart (2013), p. 315.

858. A client with obsessive-compulsive disorder spends many hours during the day and night washing her hands. The nurse should **initially** allow the client to continue this behavior because it has what effect for the client?

1. Relieves the client's anxiety
2. Decreases the chance of infection
3. Gives the client a feeling of self-control
4. Increases the client's sense of self-esteem

Level of Cognitive Ability: Applying
Client Needs: Psychosocial Integrity
Integrated Process: Nursing Process/Implementation
Content Area: Mental Health
Priority Concepts: Anxiety; Clinical Judgment

Answer: 1
Rationale: The compulsive act provides immediate relief from anxiety and is used to cope with stress, conflict, or pain. Options 2 and 3 are also incorrect interpretations of the client's need to perform this behavior. Although the client may feel the need to increase self-esteem, that is not the primary goal of this behavior.
Priority Nursing Tip: For the client with obsessive-compulsive disorder, the nurse should ensure that basic needs are met, such as food, rest, and grooming. Also, the nurse should help the client identify situations that precipitate compulsive behavior and encourage the client to verbalize thoughts and feelings when these situations arise.
Test-Taking Strategy: Focusing on the strategic word, *initially*, and recalling the effect of compulsive acts will direct you to the correct option. Review: **obsessive-compulsive disorder**.
Reference(s): Fortinash, Holoday-Worret (2012), p. 195; Varcarolis (2013), p. 177.

859. An adolescent is preparing to return home after psychiatric hospitalization for a suicide attempt. Which would be the **least effective** for preparing the client to return home?

1. Identify the family's strengths and weaknesses.
2. Ask that the mother's boyfriend move out of the home.
3. Provide and offer the family appropriate options and resources.
4. Encourage communication and the sharing of feelings among the family members.

Level of Cognitive Ability: Analyzing
Client Needs: Psychosocial Integrity
Integrated Process: Nursing Process/Planning
Content Area: Mental Health
Priority Concepts: Mood and Affect; Safety

Answer: 2
Rationale: Option 2 is clearly the least effective option because there is no information in the question that indicates that the boyfriend's involvement has anything to do with the suicide attempt. Options 1, 3, and 4 offer helpful ways to enhance the family processes.
Priority Nursing Tip: High-risk groups for suicide include clients with a history of previous suicide attempts, family history of suicide attempts, adolescents, older adults, disabled or terminally ill clients, clients with personality disorders, clients with organic brain syndrome or dementia, depressed or psychotic clients, and substance abusers.
Test-Taking Strategy: Note the strategic words, *least effective*. These words indicate a negative event query and ask you to select the option that would be the least helpful. Focus on the data in the question, and note that options 1, 3, and 4 are comparable or alike and that they identify positive measures. Review: client with **suicide**.
Reference(s): Fortinash, Holoday-Worret (2012), p. 514; Swearingen (2012), p. 679.

860. An 11-year-old child scheduled for a diagnostic procedure will have an intravenous line inserted and will receive an intramuscular injection. What form of communication should the nurse use in preparing the child for the procedure?

1. Reassuring the child that he or she will not feel any pain
2. Teaching the parents so that they can explain everything to the child
3. Telling the child not to worry because the doctors take care of everything
4. Using pictures, concrete words, and demonstrations to describe what will happen

Level of Cognitive Ability: Applying
Client Needs: Psychosocial Integrity
Integrated Process: Nursing Process/Implementation
Content Area: Developmental Stages: Infancy to Adolescence
Priority Concepts: Communication; Development

Answer: 4
Rationale: The school-age child understands best with visual aids and concrete language. Option 1 is inaccurate information because the injection will cause some discomfort. Option 2 inappropriately delegates the responsibility for teaching to the parents. Option 3 is not therapeutic.
Priority Nursing Tip: For the school-age child, the nurse should provide reassurance to help in alleviating fears and anxieties. In addition to using pictures, concrete words, and demonstrations to describe what will happen, the nurse can use medical play techniques.
Test-Taking Strategy: Use therapeutic communication techniques. Option 1 presents inaccurate information. In option 2, a nursing responsibility is inappropriately delegated to parents, and option 3 is nontherapeutic. Review: **communication** with the **school-age child.**
Reference(s): Hockenberry, Wilson (2013), pp. 638, 642.

861. The nurse observes an anxious client blocking the hallway, walking three steps forward and then two steps backward. Other clients are agitated and trying to get past the client. How should the nurse intervene?

1. Stand alongside the client and say, "You're very anxious today."
2. Attempt to stop the behavior and say, "You're going to get exhausted."
3. Take the client to the lounge and say, "Relax and watch television now."
4. Walk alongside the client and say, "You're not going anywhere very fast doing this."

Level of Cognitive Ability: Applying
Client Needs: Psychosocial Integrity
Integrated Process: Nursing Process/Implementation
Content Area: Mental Health
Priority Concepts: Anxiety; Communication

Answer: 1
Rationale: An important consideration when alleviating anxiety is to assist the client with recognizing the behavior. Options 2 and 3 do not address the increased anxiety and the need to control the underlying behavior, and they may even escalate the behavior. Option 4 does not raise the client to a functioning level.
Priority Nursing Tip: Cognitive therapy is one treatment modality for anxiety. This therapy involves an active, directive, time-limited, structured approach and is based on the principle that how an individual feels and behaves is determined by how he or she thinks about the world and his or her place in it.
Test-Taking Strategy: Focus on the subject, dealing with a client who is anxious. Note the word *anxious* in the question and in the correct option. Remember that it is important to assist the client with recognizing his or her behavior. Review: communication with a **client** with **anxiety.**
Reference(s): Fortinash, Holoday-Worret (2012), pp. 197-198; Swearingen (2012), pp. 678-679.

862. The nurse is assisting with providing a form of psychotherapy in which the client acts out situations that are of emotional significance. Based on this assessment data, which form of therapy should the nurse expect the health care provider to prescribe?

1. Psychodrama
2. Reality therapy
3. Psychoanalytic therapy
4. Short-term dynamic psychotherapy

Level of Cognitive Ability: Applying
Client Needs: Psychosocial Integrity
Integrated Process: Nursing Process/Implementation
Content Area: Mental Health
Priority Concepts: Coping; Psychosis

Answer: 1
Rationale: Psychodrama involves the enactment of emotionally charged situations. Reality therapy is used for individuals with cognitive impairment. Both short-term dynamic psychotherapy and psychoanalytic therapy depend on techniques that are drawn from psychoanalysis.
Priority Nursing Tip: Psychotherapy consists of three levels: supportive therapy, re-educative therapy, and reconstructive therapy. These modalities use a therapeutic relationship to modify the client's feelings, attitudes, and behaviors.
Test-Taking Strategy: Focus on the subject, the specific form of psychotherapy. Note the words *the client acts out situations*. These words will assist you by providing you with the definition of psychodrama. Review: **psychodrama.**
Reference(s): Fortinash, Holoday-Worret (2012), p. 619; Stuart (2013), p. 626.

863. A manic client is placed in a seclusion room after an outburst of violent behavior that involved a physical assault on another client. Which intervention should the nurse include in her plan of care before seclusion?
1. Ask the client if she understands why the seclusion is necessary.
2. Remain silent because verbal interaction would be too stimulating.
3. Tell the client that she will be allowed to come out when she can behave.
4. Inform the client that she is being secluded to help her regain her self-control.

Level of Cognitive Ability: Applying
Client Needs: Psychosocial Integrity
Integrated Process: Nursing Process/Implementation
Content Area: Mental Health
Priority Concepts: Mood and Affect; Safety

Answer: 4
Rationale: Seclusion is a process in which a client is placed alone in a specially designed room for protection and close supervision. This client is removed to a nonstimulating environment as a result of her behavior. Options 1, 2, and 3 are nontherapeutic actions. Additionally, option 2 implies punishment. It is best to directly inform the client of the purpose of the seclusion.
Priority Nursing Tip: While in seclusion, the client is monitored continuously and must be protected from all sources of harm.
Test-Taking Strategy: Focus on the subject, care to the client in seclusion. Also, use therapeutic communication techniques. Select the option that presents reality most clearly to the client. Option 4 is the only option that provides a clear and direct purpose of the seclusion. Review: **mania and seclusion.**
Reference(s): Varcarolis (2013), p. 457.

864. A client with angina pectoris is extremely anxious after being hospitalized. What should the nurse do to minimize the client's anxiety?
1. Provide care choices to the client.
2. Keep the door open and the hallway lights on at night.
3. Encourage the client to limit visitors to as few as possible.
4. Admit the client to a room as far as possible from the nursing station.

Level of Cognitive Ability: Applying
Client Needs: Psychosocial Integrity
Integrated Process: Nursing Process/Implementation
Content Area: Adult Health: Cardiovascular
Priority Concepts: Anxiety; Caregiving

Answer: 1
Rationale: General interventions to minimize anxiety in the hospitalized client include providing information, social support, and control over choices related to care, as well as acknowledging the client's feelings. Leaving the door open with the hallway lights on may keep the client oriented, but these actions may interfere with sleep and increase anxiety. Limiting visitors reduces social support. Being far from the nursing station is unlikely to reduce anxiety for this client.
Priority Nursing Tip: Angina pectoris is chest pain resulting from myocardial ischemia caused by inadequate myocardial blood and oxygen supply. In addition to anxiety, the client with angina may experience dyspnea, pallor, sweating, palpitations and tachycardia, dizziness and faintness, hypertension, or digestive disturbances.
Test-Taking Strategy: Focus on the subject, minimizing anxiety. Thinking about each option and how it may either increase or minimize anxiety will direct you to the correct option. Review: the interventions used to minimize **anxiety** in the hospitalized client.
Reference(s): Ignatavicius, Workman (2013), p. 835.

865. A client diagnosed with catatonic posturing demonstrates severe withdrawal by lying on the bed with his body pulled into a fetal position. Which intervention should the nurse take to increase interpersonal communication?
1. Ask the client direct questions to encourage talking.
2. Leave the client alone and intermittently check on him.
3. Sit beside the client in silence and occasionally ask open-ended questions.
4. Take the client into the dayroom with the other clients, so that they can help watch him.

Level of Cognitive Ability: Applying
Client Needs: Psychosocial Integrity
Integrated Process: Nursing Process/Implementation
Content Area: Mental Health
Priority Concepts: Caregiving; Psychosis

Answer: 3
Rationale: Clients who are withdrawn may be immobile and mute, and they require consistent, repeated approaches. Intervention includes the establishment of interpersonal contact. The nurse facilitates communication with the client by sitting in silence, asking open-ended questions, and pausing to provide opportunities for the client to respond. Asking this client direct questions is not therapeutic. The client is not to be left alone.
Priority Nursing Tip: Catatonic posturing occurs when the client holds bizarre positions for long periods of time.
Test-Taking Strategy: Focus on the subject, increasing interpersonal communication. Eliminate option 2 because the nurse would not leave the client alone. Option 4 relies on other clients to care for this client; this is inappropriate and it should be eliminated next. From the remaining options, recall that asking direct questions to this client would not be therapeutic. Review: the care of the client with **catatonic posturing.**
Reference(s): Fortinash, Holoday-Worret (2012), pp. 271-272; Varcarolis (2013), p. 310.

866. The nurse is interviewing a client being admitted to the mental health inpatient unit who was involved in a fire 2 months ago. The client is complaining of insomnia, difficulty concentrating, nervousness, hypervigilance, and frequently thinking about fires. The nurse recognizes these complaints to be indications of which disorder?

1. Phobia
2. Dissociative disorder
3. Obsessive-compulsive disorder
4. Posttraumatic stress disorder (PTSD)

Level of Cognitive Ability: Analyzing
Client Needs: Psychosocial Integrity
Integrated Process: Nursing Process/Assessment
Content Area: Mental Health
Priority Concepts: Clinical Judgment; Psychosis

Answer: 4
Rationale: PTSD is precipitated by events that are overwhelming, unpredictable, and sometimes life threatening. Typical symptoms of PTSD include difficulty concentrating, sleep disturbances, intrusive recollections of the traumatic event, hypervigilance, and anxiety. These symptoms are not characteristic of the disorders noted in options 1, 2, and 3.
Priority Nursing Tip: Assist the client with posttraumatic stress disorder to develop adaptive coping mechanisms and to use relaxation techniques.
Test-Taking Strategy: Note the subject, the disorder that the client is experiencing. Focus on the words *fire* and *disorder* in the question regarding the client's complaints. Recalling that having flashbacks of traumatic events is a common symptom of PTSD will direct you to the correct option. Review **posttraumatic stress disorder (PTSD)**.
Reference(s): Stuart (2013), p. 228.

867. A 16-year-old client is hospitalized. Which statement by the client would alert the nurse to a potential developmental problem?

1. "I'd like my hair washed before my friends get here."
2. "Is it okay if I have a couple of friends in to visit me this evening?"
3. "Please tell my friends not to visit, since I'll see them back at school next week."
4. "When my friends get here, I would like to play some computer games with them."

Level of Cognitive Ability: Analyzing
Client Needs: Psychosocial Integrity
Integrated Process: Nursing Process/Assessment
Content Area: Developmental Stages: Infancy to Adolescence
Priority Concepts: Clinical Judgment; Development

Answer: 3
Rationale: Adolescents who withdraw from peers into isolation struggle with developing identity, so option 3 should cause the nurse to be concerned. It is appropriate for the client to ask for hygiene measures to be attended to before the peer group arrives. Option 2 indicates that the client is eager for companionship. Adolescents often develop special interests within their groups that may help them maximize certain skills, such as with computers.
Priority Nursing Tip: For the hospitalized adolescent, separation from friends is a source of anxiety. Additionally, adolescents are not sure whether they want their parents with them when they are hospitalized.
Test-Taking Strategy: Options 1, 2, and 4 are comparable or like and indicate that the client is anticipating the arrival of a peer group, which is appropriate. Option 3 indicates that the client may be withdrawing from appropriate relationships. Review: peer group relationships of **adolescents**.
Reference(s): McKinney et al (2013), p. 884.

868. The nurse obtains an electrocardiogram (ECG) rhythm strip for an adult client who is anxious about the result. The ECG shows that the heart rate is 90 beats per minute. What should the nurse tell the client to relieve anxiety?

1. The rate is normal.
2. There is no need to worry.
3. A slower heart rate is preferred.
4. Medication specific to the problem will be prescribed.

Level of Cognitive Ability: Applying
Client Needs: Psychosocial Integrity
Integrated Process: Nursing Process/Implementation
Content Area: Adult Health: Cardiovascular
Priority Concepts: Clinical Judgment; Perfusion

Answer: 1
Rationale: A normal adult resting pulse rate ranges between 60 and 100 beats per minute; therefore, the rate is normal. The nurse would not tell a client not to worry. Options 3 and 4 indicate that the ECG is abnormal.
Priority Nursing Tip: Obtaining a baseline measurement of the client's vital signs will allow the nurse to determine any changes. The nurse can also measure the client's pulse rate and blood pressure in sitting, standing, and lying positions and compare the readings.
Test-Taking Strategy: Recall knowledge of the basic range of pulse rates for an adult. Option 2 is not therapeutic because telling the client not to worry is an inappropriate action. Eliminate options 3 and 4 because they are comparable or alike and indicate that a problem exists. Review: the **normal adult vital signs**.
References(s): Chernecky, Berger (2013), pp. 462-463; Pagana, Pagana (2013), pp. 367-368.

869. Which is a sign of depression that a client would exhibit when recovering from a myocardial infarction?
1. Reports insomnia at night
2. Consumes 25% of meals and shows little interest when doing client teaching
3. Ignores activity restrictions and does not report the experience of chest pain with activity
4. Expresses apprehension about leaving the hospital and requests that someone stay in the room at night

Level of Cognitive Ability: Analyzing
Client Needs: Psychosocial Integrity
Integrated Process: Nursing Process/Analysis
Content Area: Adult Health: Cardiovascular
Priority Concepts: Clinical Judgment; Mood and Affect

Answer: 2
Rationale: Signs of depression include withdrawal, lack of interest, crying, anorexia, and apathy. Insomnia may be a sign of anxiety or fear. Ignoring symptoms and activity restrictions are signs of denial. Apprehension is a sign of anxiety.
Priority Nursing Tip: The nurse should monitor a depressed client closely for signs of suicidal ideation. If the client presents with increased energy, monitor closely because it could mean the client now has the energy to perform the suicide act.
Test-Taking Strategy: Focus on the subject, sign of depression. Recalling that anorexia and a lack of interest are associated with depression will direct you to the correct option. Review: the signs of depression.
Reference(s): Ignatavicius, Workman (2013), p. 835.

870. A client who recently had a gastrostomy feeding tube inserted refuses to participate in the plan of care, will not make eye contact, and does not speak to family or visitors. Which type of coping mechanism should the nurse assess that the client is using?
1. Distancing
2. Self-control
3. Problem solving
4. Accepting responsibility

Level of Cognitive Ability: Analyzing
Client Needs: Psychosocial Integrity
Integrated Process: Nursing Process/Assessment
Content Area: Mental Health
Priority Concepts: Anxiety; Coping

Answer: 1
Rationale: Distancing is an unwillingness or inability to discuss events. Self-control is demonstrated by stoicism and hiding feelings. Problem solving involves making plans and verbalizing what will be done. Accepting responsibility places the responsibility for a situation on oneself.
Priority Nursing Tip: Coping mechanisms are methods used to decrease anxiety. The use of a coping mechanism can be conscious, unconscious, constructive, destructive, task oriented in relation to direct problem solving, or defense oriented and regulating in response to protect oneself.
Test-Taking Strategy: Note the subject, the type of coping mechanism that the client is using. Focus on the words *will not make eye contact*, and *does not speak to family or visitors* in the question. Noting the client's behavior will direct you to the correct option. Review: coping mechanisms.
Reference(s): Ignatavicius, Workman (2013), p. 1184; Stuart (2013), p. 226.

871. The nurse reviews the preoperative teaching plan for a client scheduled for a radical neck dissection. Which part of the nursing care plan should the nurse **initially** focus on?
1. The financial status of the client
2. Postoperative communication techniques
3. Information given to the client by the surgeon
4. The client's support systems and coping behaviors

Level of Cognitive Ability: Applying
Client Needs: Psychosocial Integrity
Integrated Process: Nursing Process/Planning
Content Area: Fundamental Skills: Perioperative Care
Priority Concepts: Client Education; Clinical Judgment

Answer: 3
Rationale: The first step in client teaching is establishing what the client already knows. This allows the nurse not only to correct any misinformation, but also to determine the starting point for teaching and to implement the education at the client's level. Although options 1, 2, and 4 may be components of the plan, they are not the initial focus.
Priority Nursing Tip: Because of the potential for edema formation, airway patency is always a priority concern for any client who underwent surgery in the neck area.
Test-Taking Strategy: Note the strategic word, *initially*. Remember that determining what the client already knows provides a starting point for teaching. Review: the teaching and learning process.
Reference(s): Ignatavicius, Workman (2013), p. 591.

872. The community health nurse is conducting an awareness workshop on adolescent suicide. What should the nurse discuss as risk factors? **Select all that apply.**

❑ 1. Family violence
❑ 2. Use of alcohol or drugs
❑ 3. Strong peer relationships
❑ 4. Family history of depression
❑ 5. Adequate school performance

Level of Cognitive Ability: Analyzing
Client Needs: Psychosocial Integrity
Integrated Process: Nursing Process/Assessment
Content Area: Mental Health
Priority Concepts: Development; Mood and Affect

Answer: 1, 2, 4
Rationale: Risk factors for suicide among adolescents are depression; a family history of mental health disorders, especially depression and suicide; previous attempts at suicide; family violence or abuse; substance abuse; poor school performance; feelings of worthlessness or hopelessness; and homosexuality.
Priority Nursing Tip: The client who is a suicide risk and is taking an antidepressant must be monitored closely, especially during the period in which the medication begins to take effect, which is in about 4 to 6 weeks. The client experiences an unusual burst of energy once the medication begins to take effect, which may further motivate him or her to carry out the suicide plan.
Test-Taking Strategy: Focus on the subject, the risk factors for suicide. Noting the words *strong* in option 3 and *adequate* in option 5 will assist in eliminating these options as risk factors. Review: risk factors for **suicide** in an adolescent.
Reference(s): Fortinash, Holoday-Worret (2012), pp. 403-404; Varcarolis (2013), pp. 438, 440.

873. A preschool child is placed in traction for the treatment of a femur fracture. The child has started bedwetting, even though he has been toilet trained for a year. The mother is very upset about the situation. The nurse explains to the mother that this behavior should be recognized as which psychosocial adaptation?

1. A body image disturbance
2. Attention-seeking behavior
3. Regressing to earlier developmental behavior
4. A result of an undiagnosed urinary tract infection

Level of Cognitive Ability: Applying
Client Needs: Psychosocial Integrity
Integrated Process: Nursing Process/Implementation
Content Area: Developmental Stages: Infancy to Adolescence
Priority Concepts: Coping; Development

Answer: 3
Rationale: The monotony of immobilization can lead to sluggish intellectual and psychomotor responses. Regressive behaviors are not uncommon in immobilized children, and they usually do not require professional intervention. Body image may or may not be affected by long-term immobilization, but it does not relate to the information presented in the question.
Priority Nursing Tip: The nurse needs to plan care for the hospitalized preschooler recalling that the hospitalized preschooler may be quietly withdrawn and uninterested in the environment and may become uncooperative, refusing to eat or take medication, and repeatedly asking when the parents will be visiting.
Test-Taking Strategy: Focus on the subject, the behavior and psychosocial adaptation of the preschooler. This will eliminate option 1. From the remaining options, recalling that regression is a normal psychological response to immobilization will direct you to option 3. Review: **psychosocial adaptations.**
Reference(s): Hockenberry, Wilson (2013), pp. 390, 1053.

874. The nurse is assessing a client to determine the client's adjustment to presbycusis. Which indicates successful adaptation to this problem?

1. Proper use of a hearing aid
2. Denial of a hearing impairment
3. Withdrawal from social activities
4. Reluctance to answer the telephone

Level of Cognitive Ability: Evaluating
Client Needs: Psychosocial Integrity
Integrated Process: Nursing Process/Evaluation
Content Area: Adult Health: Ear
Priority Concepts: Clinical Judgment; Sensory Perception

Answer: 1
Rationale: Presbycusis occurs as part of the aging process; it is a progressive sensorineural hearing loss. Clients show adequate adaptation by obtaining and regularly using a hearing aid. Some clients may not adapt well to the impairment, denying its presence. Others withdraw from social interactions and contact with others, embarrassed by the problem and the need to wear a hearing aid.
Priority Nursing Tip: Presbycusis is a gradual nerve degeneration associated with aging; it leads to degeneration or atrophy of the ganglion cells in the cochlea and a loss of elasticity of the basilar membranes.
Test-Taking Strategy: Focus on the subject, successful adaptation to the problem. A review of each of the options shows that the only option with positive wording is option 1. The incorrect options indicate a need for further adaptation. Review: **presbycusis.**
Reference(s): Ignatavicius, Workman (2013), pp. 1100-1101.

❖ **875.** The nurse prepares to implement suicide precautions for an acutely suicidal client. What nursing interventions are included with regard to these precautions? **Select all that apply.**
- ❏ 1. Maintain arm's length distance with the client at all times.
- ❏ 2. Ensure that meal trays contain no glass or metal silverware.
- ❏ 3. Carefully watch the client swallow each dose of medication.
- ❏ 4. Conduct one-on-one nursing observation and interaction 24 hours a day.
- ❏ 5. Document client's mood, verbatim statements, and behaviors every 15 to 30 minutes per protocol.
- ❏ 6. Allow the client to totally cover self with the bedcovers during sleep at night as long as the nurse is present.

Level of Cognitive Ability: Applying
Client Needs: Psychosocial Integrity
Integrated Process: Nursing Process/Implementation
Content Area: Mental Health
Priority Concepts: Mood and Affect; Safety

Answer: 1, 2, 3, 4, 5
Rationale: Suicide precautions involve constant observation of the client by the nursing staff. This intense attention from the nurse provides for safety and also allows for constant reassessment of risk. Suicide precautions include maintaining arm's length distance with the client at all times; ensuring that meal trays contain no glass or metal silverware; carefully watching the client swallow each dose of medication; conducting one-on-one nursing observation and interaction 24 hours a day and explaining to the client the procedures involved with suicide precautions; and documenting client's mood, verbatim statements, and behaviors every 15 to 30 minutes per protocol. During observation when the client is sleeping, the client's hands should always be in view and not under the bedcovers.
Priority Nursing Tip: If a client is known to be a risk for suicide, the client must be monitored closely. A staff member must be within arm's length of this client, and any potentially dangerous objects must be removed from the client's environment and living space.
Test-Taking Strategy: Focus on the subject, suicide precautions, and note the words *an acutely suicidal client.* Read each option carefully, keeping safety in mind. The only option that presents a risk is option 6, allowing the client to totally cover self with the bedcovers during sleep at night. Remember that the client's hands should always be in view. Review: nursing interventions related to **suicide precautions.**
References(s): Varcarolis (2013), p. 442.

❖ **876.** A client with a severe ulcer of the right foot is told that a right leg amputation may be necessary. Which signs or client behaviors indicative of anticipatory grief should the nurse monitor the client for? **Select all that apply.**
- ❏ 1. Stating a fear of the future and unknown
- ❏ 2. Engaging in periods of weeping or raging
- ❏ 3. Expressing anger at the medical professionals
- ❏ 4. Expressing a feeling of unreality and disbelief
- ❏ 5. Expressing a desire to run away from the situation
- ❏ 6. Stating that he knows all he needs to know about his condition

Level of Cognitive Ability: Analyzing
Client Needs: Psychosocial Integrity
Integrated Process: Nursing Process/Assessment
Content Area: Mental Health
Priority Concepts: Clinical Judgment; Coping

Answer: 1, 2, 3, 4, 5
Rationale: Anticipatory grief refers to the intellectual and emotional responses and behaviors by which individuals, families, or communities work through the process of modifying self-concept based on the perception of potential loss. Signs of anticipatory grief include fears of the future and the unknown, periods of weeping or raging, anger at medical professionals, a feeling of unreality and disbelief, a desire to run away from the situation, feelings of emptiness or of being lost, a sense of being numb and fatigued, a need to oversee every detail of care, pronounced clinging to or dependency on other family members, and fear of going crazy. A statement by the client that he knows all he needs to know about his condition is not a sign of anticipatory grieving; it may indicate another client problem such as avoidance or fear.
Priority Nursing Tip: The stages of the grief process include denial, bargaining, anger, depression, and acceptance. These stages can be experienced in any order and at any time during the grieving process.
Test-Taking Strategy: Focus on the subject, the signs/client behaviors of anticipatory grief. Recall that anticipatory grief involves the intellectual and emotional responses and behaviors by which an individual works through the process of modifying self-concept based on the perception of potential loss. Read each option, keeping the subject of the question and the definition of anticipatory grief in mind to assist in answering correctly. Review: **anticipatory grief.**
Reference(s): Fortinash, Holoday-Worret (2012), p. 646; Stuart (2013), p. 769.

877. The nurse manager is discussing seclusion procedures with the nursing staff for clients with a mental health disorder. Under which circumstances is seclusion contraindicated? **Select all that apply.**
- ❑ 1. The client has severe dementia.
- ❑ 2. The client requests to be secluded.
- ❑ 3. The client experienced a severe drug overdose.
- ❑ 4. The client presents a clear and present danger to self or others.
- ❑ 5. The client has been legally detained for involuntary treatment and is thought to pose an escape risk.
- ❑ 6. The client has an unstable mental health disorder and nursing staff needs to attend a monthly staff meeting.

Level of Cognitive Ability: Analyzing
Client Needs: Psychosocial Integrity
Integrated Process: Nursing Process/Implementation
Content Area: Mental Health
Priority Concepts: Health Care Law; Safety

Answer: 1, 3, 6
Rationale: Seclusion is the confinement of a client to a room in which the client is prevented from leaving. General contraindications to seclusion include extremely unstable medical or mental health conditions, delirium or dementia leading to inability to tolerate decreased stimulation; severe suicidal tendencies; severe drug reactions or overdoses or the need for close monitoring of drug doses; and desire for punishment of the client or convenience of the staff. Seclusion may be used for the following circumstances: the client presents a clear and present danger to self or others, the client has been legally detained for involuntary treatment and is thought to pose an escape risk, and the client requests to be secluded.
Priority Nursing Tip: Seclusion is used most commonly when a client presents a risk to self or other people in the area. The client must be monitored continuously while in seclusion to ensure his or her safety. A liability issue is present if a client is secluded without reasonable grounds for seclusion.
Test-Taking Strategy: Focus on the subject, contraindications to seclusion. Noting the word *severe* in options 1 and 3 will assist in selecting these options. Noting that option 6 indicates that seclusion is needed for the convenience of the nursing staff will assist in selecting this option. Review: **seclusion.**
Reference(s): Varcarolis (2013), p. 86.

878. During an office visit, a prenatal client with mitral stenosis states that she has been under a lot of stress lately. During the examination, the client questions the nurse about the assessment and behaves anxiously. What is the appropriate nursing action at this time?
1. Tell the client not to worry.
2. Refer the client to a counselor.
3. Ignore the client's unfounded concerns and continue with the assessment.
4. Explain the purpose of the nurse's actions and answer all of the client's questions.

Level of Cognitive Ability: Applying
Client Needs: Psychosocial Integrity
Integrated Process: Nursing Process/Implementation
Content Area: Maternity: Antepartum
Priority Concepts: Clinical Judgment; Communication

Answer: 4
Rationale: In the prenatal cardiac client, stress should be reduced as much as possible. The client should be provided with honest and informed answers to questions to help alleviate unnecessary fears and emotional stress. Explaining the purpose of nursing actions will assist with decreasing the stress level of the client. Options 1, 2, and 3 are nontherapeutic methods of communication at this time.
Priority Nursing Tip: In mitral stenosis, valvular tissue thickens and narrows the valve opening, preventing blood flow through the heart. If the client requires a valve replacement, the nurse should inform the client that thromboembolism is a problem after valve replacement with a mechanical prosthetic valve, and lifetime anticoagulant therapy is required.
Test-Taking Strategy: Use therapeutic communication techniques to answer the question. The client's concerns and feelings should always be addressed, and option 4 is the only choice that does this. Review: **therapeutic communication techniques.**
Reference(s): McKinney et al (2013), pp. 620-621.

879. A postpartum client with gestational diabetes is scheduled for discharge. During the discharge teaching, the client asks the nurse, "Do I have to worry about this diabetes anymore?" Which is the appropriate response by the nurse?

1. "Your blood glucose level is within normal limits now, so you will be all right."
2. "You will only have to worry about the diabetes if you become pregnant again."
3. "You will be at risk for developing gestational diabetes with your next pregnancy and also for developing diabetes mellitus."
4. "When you have gestational diabetes, you have diabetes forever, and you must be treated with medication for the rest of your life."

Level of Cognitive Ability: Applying
Client Needs: Psychosocial Integrity
Integrated Process: Nursing Process/Implementation
Content Area: Maternity: Postpartum
Priority Concepts: Glucose Regulation; Reproduction

Answer: 3
Rationale: The client is at risk for developing gestational diabetes with each pregnancy. The client also has an increased risk for developing diabetes mellitus and needs to comply with follow-up assessments. She also needs to be taught techniques to lower her risk for developing diabetes mellitus, such as weight control. The diagnosis of gestational diabetes mellitus indicates that this client has an increased risk for developing diabetes mellitus, however, with proper care, it may not develop.
Priority Nursing Tip: Pregnant women should be screened for gestational diabetes between 24 and 28 weeks of pregnancy. Insulin rather than oral hypoglycemic agents are prescribed for use during pregnancy.
Test-Taking Strategy: Note the subject, the long-term effect of gestational diabetes. In addition, use therapeutic communication techniques to answer the question and direct you to the correct option. Review: **gestational diabetes.**
Reference(s): Lowdermilk, Perry, Cashion, Alden (2012), p. 704.

880. The nurse is performing an assessment on a 16-year-old client who has been diagnosed with anorexia nervosa. Which statement by the client should the nurse identify as a **priority** requiring a **need for further assessment?**

1. "I check my weight every day without fail."
2. "I exercise 3 to 4 hours every day to keep my slim figure."
3. "I've been told that I am 10% below my ideal body weight."
4. "My best friend was in the hospital with this disorder a year ago."

Level of Cognitive Ability: Analyzing
Client Needs: Psychosocial Integrity
Integrated Process: Nursing Process/Analysis
Content Area: Mental Health
Priority Concepts: Clinical Judgment; Nutrition

Answer: 2
Rationale: Exercising 3 to 4 hours every day is excessive physical activity and unrealistic for a 16-year-old girl. The nurse needs to further assess this statement immediately to find out why the client feels the need to exercise this much to maintain her figure. It is not considered abnormal to check the weight every day; many clients with anorexia nervosa check their weight close to 20 times a day. A weight that exceeds 15% below the ideal weight is significant for clients with anorexia nervosa. Although it is unfortunate that the client's best friend had this disorder, this is not considered a major threat to this client's physical well-being.
Priority Nursing Tip: The onset of anorexia nervosa is often associated with a stressful life event. The client intensely fears obesity, body image is distorted, and the client has a disturbed self-concept.
Test-Taking Strategy: Note the strategic words, *priority* and *need for further assessment.* The words *need for further assessment* indicate a negative event query and ask you to select the option that identifies a concern. Eliminate options 3 and 4 first because these client statements are not significant or abnormal. From the remaining options, knowledge regarding the manifestations associated with anorexia nervosa will direct you to option 2. Review: **anorexia nervosa.**
Reference(s): Fortinash, Holoday-Worret (2012), p. 423; Stuart (2013), p. 490.

881. A client who has confusion as a result of bed rest and a prolonged length of hospital stay receives a prescription for progressive ambulation as tolerated. Which is the **best** nursing intervention to use to implement the prescription?

1. Ambulate to the client's bathroom three times a day.
2. Ambulate in the room for short distances frequently.
3. Ambulate in the hall progressively three times a day.
4. Assist with range-of-motion exercises three times a day.

Level of Cognitive Ability: Analyzing
Client Needs: Psychosocial Integrity
Integrated Process: Nursing Process/Planning
Content Area: Adult Health: Musculoskeletal
Priority Concepts: Clinical Judgment; Sensory Perception

Answer: 3
Rationale: The cause of the client's confusion is bed rest and decreased sensory stimulation from a prolonged length of stay; therefore, the best intervention is to ambulate the client in the hall to increase sensory stimulation. Hopefully the stimulation can help decrease the confusion. Options 1 and 2 do not address the client's need for sensory stimulation. The nurse performs option 4 in preparation for ambulation while the client is on bed rest.
Priority Nursing Tip: Special senses changes that may occur as a result of decreased sensory stimulation and aging include: decreased visual acuity, decreased accommodation in the eyes, decreased peripheral vision and increased sensitivity to glare, presbyopia and cataract formation, possible loss of hearing ability, inability to discern taste of food, decreased sense of smell, changes in touch sensation, and decreased pain awareness.
Test-Taking Strategy: Note the strategic word, *best*. Focus on the subject, client confusion as a result of bed rest and a prolonged length of hospital stay. Eliminate option 4 first because this action should have been performed in preparation for ambulation. Next eliminate options 1 and 2 because they are comparable or alike in that they both address ambulating the client in the hospital room. Review: sensory stimulation.
Reference(s): Perry, Potter, Elkin (2012), pp. 387-388; Potter et al (2013), pp. 757, 759.

882. The nurse is caring for an older client who has been placed in Buck's extension traction after a hip fracture. During the assessment of the client, the nurse notes that the client is disoriented. What is the appropriate nursing intervention for this client?

1. Apply restraints to the client.
2. Ask the family to stay with the client.
3. Ask the laboratory to perform electrolyte studies.
4. Reorient the client frequently and place a clock and a calendar in the client's room.

Level of Cognitive Ability: Applying
Client Needs: Psychosocial Integrity
Integrated Process: Nursing Process/Implementation
Content Area: Adult Health: Musculoskeletal
Priority Concepts: Clinical Judgment; Cognition

Answer: 4
Rationale: An inactive older person may become disoriented as a result of a lack of sensory stimulation. The appropriate nursing intervention would be to frequently reorient the client and place objects such as a clock and a calendar in the client's room to maintain orientation. Restraints may cause further disorientation and should not be applied unless specifically prescribed. Agency policies and procedures should be followed before the application of restraints. The family can assist with the orientation of the client, but it is not appropriate to ask the family to stay with the client. It is not within the scope of nursing practice to prescribe laboratory studies.
Priority Nursing Tip: The nurse should ask the family of a client who is disoriented to bring items from home, such as family photographs for placement at the client's bedside.
Test-Taking Strategy: Focus on the subject, the appropriate intervention for the client who is disoriented. Eliminate option 3 first because it is not within the realm of nursing practice to prescribe laboratory studies. Next eliminate option 1 because restraints may add to the disorientation that the client is experiencing. It is not appropriate to place the responsibility of the client on the family, so option 2 should be eliminated. In addition, note the relationship between the words *disoriented* in the question and *reorient* in option 4. Review: disoriented client.
Reference(s): Ignatavicius, Workman (2013), pp. 950-951, 1157; Lewis et al (2011), pp. 1528-1529.

883. An 8-year-old boy is admitted to the hospital. He was sexually abused by an adult family member, and he is withdrawn and appears frightened. Which describes the **best** plan for the **initial** nursing encounter to convey concern and support?

1. Introduce self and explain to the child that he is safe now that he is in the hospital.
2. Introduce self and tell the child that you would like to sit with him for a little while.
3. Introduce self and then ask the child to express how he feels about the events leading up to this hospital admission.
4. Introduce self, explain your role, and ask the child to act out the sexual encounter with the abuser with the use of art therapy.

Level of Cognitive Ability: Applying
Client Needs: Psychosocial Integrity
Integrated Process: Caring
Content Area: Mental Health
Priority Concepts: Caregiving; Interpersonal Violence

Answer: 2
Rationale: Victims of sexual abuse may exhibit fear and anxiety regarding what has just occurred. In addition, they may fear that the abuse could be repeated. When initiating contact with a child victim of sexual abuse who demonstrates a fear of others, it is best to convey a willingness to spend time and move slowly to initiate activities that may be perceived as threatening. After a rapport is established, the nurse may explore the child's feelings or use various therapeutic modalities to encourage the recounting of the sexual encounter. Option 2 conveys a plan for an initial encounter that establishes trust by sitting with the child in a nonthreatening atmosphere. Option 1 does not convey concern and support by the nurse. Options 3 and 4 may be implemented after trust and rapport are established.
Priority Nursing Tip: Sexual abuse can involve incest, molestation, exhibitionism, use of pornography, prostitution, or pedophilia; the findings associated with sexual abuse may not be easily apparent in the child.
Test-Taking Strategy: Note the strategic words, *best* and *initial*. Use therapeutic communication techniques. Recalling that rapport needs to be established first will direct you to the correct option. Review: **child sexual abuse.**
Reference(s): Hockenberry, Wilson (2013), p. 448.

884. A female victim of a sexual assault is being seen in the crisis center for a third visit. She states that although the rape occurred nearly 2 months ago, she still feels "as though the rape just happened yesterday." How should the nurse respond?

1. "In reality, the rape did not just occur. It has been over 2 months now."
2. "What can you do to alleviate some of your fears about being assaulted again?"
3. "In time, our goal will be to help you move on from these strong feelings about your rape."
4. "Tell me more about those aspects of the rape that cause you to feel like the rape just occurred."

Level of Cognitive Ability: Applying
Client Needs: Psychosocial Integrity
Integrated Process: Communication and Documentation
Content Area: Mental Health
Priority Concepts: Communication; Interpersonal Violence

Answer: 4
Rationale: Option 4 allows for the client to express her ideas and feelings more fully and portrays a unhurried, nonjudgmental, supportive attitude. Clients need to be reassured that their feelings are normal and that they may freely express their concerns in a safe care environment. Although option 1 is true, it immediately blocks communication. Option 2 places the problem solving totally on the client. Option 3 places the client's feelings on hold.
Priority Nursing Tip: For the client who is a victim of rape, rape trauma syndrome may occur. The client may experience sleep disturbances; nightmares; loss of appetite; fears; anxiety; phobias; suspicion; a decrease in activities and motivation; disruptions in relationships with the partner, family, or friends; self-blame, guilt, and shame; lowered self-esteem; feelings of worthlessness; and somatic complaints.
Test-Taking Strategy: Use therapeutic communication techniques. Option 4 specifically addresses the client's feelings and concerns. Remember to always address the client's feelings first. Review: therapeutic communication techniques and sexual assault.
Reference(s): Fortinash, Holoday-Worret (2012), pp. 71-74, 549; Stuart (2013), pp. 747-748.

885. What should the nurse instruct the staff to do when formulating the plan of care for a client with paranoia?
1. Have the client sign a release of information form.
2. Avoid laughing or whispering in front of the client.
3. Increase the socialization of the client with unit peers.
4. Begin educating the client about available social supports.

Level of Cognitive Ability: Applying
Client Needs: Psychosocial Integrity
Integrated Process: Nursing Process/Implementation
Content Area: Mental Health
Priority Concepts: Caregiving; Psychosis

Answer: 2
Rationale: A client experiencing paranoia is distrustful and suspicious of others. The health care team needs to establish rapport and trust with the client. Laughing or whispering in front of the client would increase the client's paranoia. Options 1, 3, and 4 ask the client to trust on a multitude of levels. These options are too intrusive for a client who is paranoid.
Priority Nursing Tip: The client with a paranoid disorder has a concrete, pervasive delusional system characterized by persecutory and grandiose beliefs. The client is often viewed by others as hostile, stubborn, and defensive, and the client commonly exhibits suspiciousness and mistrust of others.
Test-Taking Strategy: Focus on the subject, the plan of care for a client with paranoia. Recalling that the client with paranoia is distrustful and suspicious of others will direct you to the correct option. Review: **paranoia**.
Reference(s): Fortinash, Holoday-Worret (2012), p. 306; Varcarolis (2013), pp. 315-316.

886. The nurse is assessing a client who was just admitted to the psychiatric unit. The client says, "You won't have to worry about me much longer." How should the nurse interpret this statement?
1. An intention of suicide
2. An expression of depression
3. An intention of self-mutilation
4. An expression of hopelessness

Level of Cognitive Ability: Analyzing
Client Needs: Psychosocial Integrity
Integrated Process: Nursing Process/Analysis
Content Area: Mental Health
Priority Concepts: Clinical Judgment; Safety

Answer: 1
Rationale: A client who is at risk for suicide who says, "You won't have to worry about me much longer," is making an expression of a suicidal intent. Although depression, self-mutilation and hopelessness may relate to violence to oneself, the statement that he or she will not be around is a direct comment about the act of suicide.
Priority Nursing Tip: All suicide behavior is extremely serious regardless of the intent. Suicide ideation requires constant attention, and typically, one-on-one observation. The client with a suicide plan must be placed on suicide precautions.
Test-Taking Strategy: Focus on the subject, interpreting the client's statement. Noting the words, *You won't have to worry about me much longer,* will direct you to the correct option. Review: **suicide**.
Reference(s): Fortinash, Holoday-Worret (2012), pp. 309-311; Stuart (2013), p. 337.

887. The nurse notes that an assigned client is lying tense in bed and staring at the cardiac monitor. The client states, "There sure are a lot of wires around there. I sure hope we don't get hit by lightning." Which is the appropriate nursing response?
1. "Your family can stay tonight if they wish."
2. "Would you like a mild sedative to help you relax?"
3. "Oh, don't worry, the weather is supposed to be sunny and clear today."
4. "Yes, all of those wires must be a little scary. Did someone explain to you what the cardiac monitor is for?"

Level of Cognitive Ability: Applying
Client Needs: Psychosocial Integrity
Integrated Process: Nursing Process/Implementation
Content Area: Adult Health: Cardiovascular
Priority Concepts: Anxiety; Communication

Answer: 4
Rationale: The nurse should initially validate the client's concern and then assess the client's knowledge regarding the cardiac monitor. This gives the nurse an opportunity to provide client education if necessary. Options 1, 2, and 3 do not address the client's concern. In addition, pharmacological interventions should be considered only if necessary.
Priority Nursing Tip: The client should be oriented to the room upon admission to the hospital. Any medical equipment should be explained, and explanations should be repeated for the client if necessary. Decreasing sensory stimulation will allow the client to rest, which is important for the process of recovery.
Test-Taking Strategy: Use therapeutic communication techniques. Remember to address the client's feelings first. Option 4 is the only option that addresses the client's feelings. Review: **therapeutic communication techniques**.
Reference(s): Ignatavicius, Workman (2013), p. 288; Potter et al (2013), pp. 320-322.

888. A young adult client with a spinal cord injury tells the nurse, "It's so depressing that I'll never get to have sex again." What is the realistic reply for the nurse to make to the client?

1. "It must feel horrible to know you can never have sex again."
2. "It's still possible to have a sexual relationship, but it will be different."
3. "You're young, so you'll adapt to this more easily than if you were older."
4. "Because of body reflexes, sexual functioning will be no different than before."

Level of Cognitive Ability: Applying
Client Needs: Psychosocial Integrity
Integrated Process: Communication and Documentation
Content Area: Adult Health: Neurological
Priority Concepts: Functional Ability; Sexuality

Answer: 2
Rationale: It is possible to have a sexual relationship after a spinal cord injury, but it is different than what the client will have experienced before the injury. Males may experience reflex erections, although they may not ejaculate. Females can have adductor spasm. Sexual counseling may help the client adapt to changes in sexuality after a spinal cord injury.
Priority Nursing Tip: The complications associated with a spinal cord injury depend on the level of the injury. One complication is autonomic dysreflexia. Autonomic dysreflexia occurs with spinal lesions above the level of T6.
Test-Taking Strategy: Use knowledge regarding the effects of a spinal cord injury and therapeutic communication techniques in chronic conditions to answer correctly. Option 2 addresses the subject of sexual relationships after spinal cord injury; it is accurate; and is a therapeutic response. Review: the effects of a spinal cord injury.
References(s): Ignatavicius, Workman (2013), pp. 974-975; Potter et al (2013), pp. 320-322.

889. A family member of a client with a brain tumor states that he is feeling distraught and guilty for not encouraging the client to seek medical evaluation earlier. What should the nurse incorporate when formulating a response to the family member's statement?

1. There are no symptoms of a brain tumor.
2. It is true that brain tumors are easily recognizable.
3. Brain tumors are never detected until very late in their course.
4. The symptoms of a brain tumor may be easily attributed to another cause.

Level of Cognitive Ability: Applying
Client Needs: Psychosocial Integrity
Integrated Process: Caring
Content Area: Adult Health: Neurological
Priority Concepts: Cellular Regulation; Communication

Answer: 4
Rationale: Signs and symptoms of a brain tumor vary depending on location, and they may easily be attributed to another cause. Symptoms include headache, vomiting, visual disturbances, and changes in intellectual abilities or personality. Seizures occur in some clients. These symptoms can be easily attributed to other causes. The family requires support to assist them during the normal grieving process. Options 1, 2, and 3 are inaccurate.
Priority Nursing Tip: The brain is a common site of metastasis for cancers that originate in the lungs and the breast. Tumors that originate in the brain primarily affect the central nervous system and its associated functions.
Test-Taking Strategy: Eliminate options 1 and 3 first because they contain the closed-ended words "no" and "never," respectively. From the remaining options, recall that the symptoms of a brain tumor may be easily attributed to another cause. Also note the word *may* in the correct option. Review: brain tumor.
Reference(s): Ignatavicius, Workman (2013), p. 1032; Lewis et al (2011), pp. 1445, 1448.

890. A client has a hip fracture repair with a prosthetic implant placed. On the day after the implant, the nurse finds the client surrounded by papers from his briefcase and planning a phone meeting. The nurse plans to discuss activities with the client and should base the discussion on which item?

1. Rest is an essential component of bone healing.
2. Setting limits on a client's behavior is a mandated nursing role.
3. Not keeping up with his job will increase the client's stress level.
4. Immediate involvement in his job will keep the client from becoming bored while on bed rest.

Level of Cognitive Ability: Applying
Client Needs: Psychosocial Integrity
Integrated Process: Nursing Process/Planning
Content Area: Adult Health: Musculoskeletal
Priority Concepts: Clinical Judgment; Mobility

Answer: 1
Rationale: Rest is an essential component of bone healing. Nurses can help clients understand the importance of rest and find ways to balance work demands to promote healing. Stress should be kept to a minimum to promote bone healing. Nurses cannot demand these changes, but they need to encourage clients to choose them. Setting limits on a client's behavior is not a mandated nursing role. It may relieve stress to do work; however, during the immediate period after the cast is applied, it may not be therapeutic.
Priority Nursing Tip: Although rare, a fat embolism can occur as a result of a bone fracture. A fat embolism originates in the bone marrow and occurs when a fat globule is released into the bloodstream. If the nurse suspects this, the nurse must notify the health care provider immediately.
Test-Taking Strategy: Eliminate options 3 and 4 because they are comparable or alike. From the remaining options, note that option 1 is the umbrella option, and it addresses rest after hip fracture repair with a prosthetic implant. Review: the physiological and psychosocial needs of the client hip fracture repair with a prosthetic implant.
References(s): Ignatavicius, Workman (2013), pp. 322, 1145.

891. A charge nurse observes an unlicensed assistive personnel (UAP) talking in an unusually loud voice to a client with delirium. Which action should the charge nurse take?

1. Enter the room and inform the client that everything is all right.
2. Speak to the UAP immediately while in the client's room to solve the problem.
3. Ensure the client's safety, calmly ask the UAP to step outside the room, and inform the UAP that her voice was unusually loud.
4. Explain to the UAP that yelling in the client's room is tolerated only if the client is talking loudly and the UAP needs to get the client's attention.

Level of Cognitive Ability: Applying
Client Needs: Psychosocial Integrity
Integrated Process: Nursing Process/Implementation
Content Area: Leadership/Management: Ethical/Legal
Priority Concepts: Communication; Leadership

Answer: 3
Rationale: The nurse must ascertain that the client is safe and then discuss the matter with the UAP in an area away from the hearing of the client. If the client hears the conversation, the client may become more confused or agitated. Options 1, 2, and 4 are incorrect actions.
Priority Nursing Tip: Methods that can be used to enhance communication include using written words if the client is able to see, read, and write; providing plenty of light in the room; getting the attention of the client before beginning to speak; facing the client when speaking; and talking in a room without distracting noises.
Test-Taking Strategy: Focus on the subject, the action that the charge nurse should take. Use therapeutic communication techniques to answer correctly. Also note that the correct option addresses client safety. Review: therapeutic communication techniques and the care of the client with delirium.
Reference(s): Fortinash, Holoday-Worret (2012), pp. 71-74, 380; Stuart (2013), p. 426.

892. A teenager who has celiac disease arrives at the emergency department complaining of profuse, watery diarrhea after a pizza party the night before. The client states, "I don't want to be different from my friends." What client problem should the nurse focus on when responding to the client?

1. Diarrhea
2. Low self-esteem
3. Deficient fluid volume
4. Increased inflammation

Level of Cognitive Ability: Analyzing
Client Needs: Psychosocial Integrity
Integrated Process: Nursing Process/Analysis
Content Area: Mental Health
Priority Concepts: Communication; Coping

Answer: 2

Rationale: The client expresses concern about being different from friends. Celiac crisis is a medical diagnosis that often involves diarrhea. Although the question states that the client has profuse, watery diarrhea, no data identify an actual deficient fluid volume or increased inflammation.

Priority Nursing Tip: The client with celiac disease has intolerance to gluten, the protein component of wheat, barley, rye, and oats. Consuming products containing these components results in the accumulation of the amino acid glutamine, which is toxic to the intestinal mucosal cells.

Test-Taking Strategy: Focus on the subject of a client feeling different. Focus on the client's statement and note the relationship of the statement and the correct option. Also note that the incorrect options are comparable or alike and identify physiological problems. Review: the defining characteristics of **low self-esteem**.

References(s): Hockenberry, Wilson (2013), pp. 75, 814-815.

---

893. The nurse develops a plan of care for a 1-month-old infant hospitalized for intussusception. Which nursing measure would be **most effective** to provide psychosocial support for the parent–child relationship?

1. Provide educational materials.
2. Encourage the parents to room-in with their infant.
3. Initiate home nutritional support as early as possible.
4. Encourage the parents to go home and get some sleep.

Level of Cognitive Ability: Applying
Client Needs: Psychosocial Integrity
Integrated Process: Caring
Content Area: Child Health: Gastrointestinal
Priority Concepts: Anxiety; Development

Answer: 2

Rationale: Rooming-in is effective for reducing separation anxiety and preserving the parent–child relationship. Educational materials may be beneficial, but they will not provide psychosocial support for the parent–child relationship. Home nutritional support is not usually necessary in the situation described. Parents are under stress when a child is ill and hospitalized, and telling a parent to go home and sleep will not relieve this stress.

Priority Nursing Tip: Intussusception occurs when one portion of the bowel telescopes into another portion of the bowel, and results in obstruction to the passage of intestinal contents. The nurse must monitor for signs and symptoms of obstruction, perforation, and shock, including fever, increased heart rate, changes in level of consciousness or blood pressure, and respiratory distress.

Test-Taking Strategy: Note the strategic words, *most effective.* Focus on the words *parent–child relationship.* The only choice that addresses the parent–child relationship is option 2. Review: **intussusception**.

Reference(s): McKinney et al (2013), p. 879.

---

894. Which comment made by the parents of a male infant who will have a surgical repair of a hernia would **require follow-up** assessment by the nurse?

1. "I understand that surgery will repair the hernia."
2. "I don't know if he will be able to father a child when he grows up."
3. "The day nurse told me to give him sponge baths for a few days after surgery."
4. "I'll need to buy extra diapers because we need to change them more frequently now."

Level of Cognitive Ability: Evaluating
Client Needs: Psychosocial Integrity
Integrated Process: Nursing Process/Assessment
Content Area: Child Health: Gastrointestinal
Priority Concepts: Client Education; Sexuality

Answer: 2

Rationale: The anatomical location of a hernia frequently causes more psychological concern to the parents than does the actual condition or treatment. Options 1, 3, and 4 all indicate accurate understanding. Option 2 is an incorrect comment requiring follow-up.

Priority Nursing Tip: A hernia occurs as a result of a weakened muscle wall. After surgical repair, the client or parents of a child who underwent repair need to be informed about the importance of allowing the site to heal.

Test-Taking Strategy: Focus on the strategic words, *require follow-up.* These words indicate a negative event query and the need to select the incorrect statement. Options 1, 3, and 4 do not require follow-up, whereas option 2 reflects parental fear and identifies a need for further assessment. Review: **hernia repair.**

Reference(s): Hockenberry, Wilson (2013), p. 809.

895. The nurse is leading a crisis intervention group comprised of high school students who have experienced the recent death of a classmate who committed suicide. The students are experiencing disbelief as they review the details of finding the classmate dead in a bathroom. Which should be the **initial** step by the nurse?

1. Ask how the students recovered from a death event in the past.
2. Reinforce the students' ability to work through this death event.
3. Inquire about the students' perception of their classmate's suicide.
4. Reinforce the students' sense of growth through this death experience.

Level of Cognitive Ability: Analyzing
Client Needs: Psychosocial Integrity
Integrated Process: Nursing Process/Implementation
Content Area: Mental Health
Priority Concepts: Communication; Coping

Answer: 3
Rationale: It is essential to determine the students' views. Inquiring about the students' perception of the suicide will specifically identify the appraisal of the suicide and the meaning of the perception. Although option 1 is exploratory, it does not address the "here-and-now" appraisal in terms of the classmate's suicide. Although the nurse is interested in how students have coped in the past, this inquiry should not be the most immediate assessment. Options 2 and 4 are attempts to foster students' self-esteem. Such an approach is premature at this point.
Priority Nursing Tip: The nurse's role in the grief and loss process includes communicating with those involved in the crisis. The nurse must consider the client's culture, religion, family structure, individual life experiences, coping skills, and support systems.
Test-Taking Strategy: Note the strategic word, *initial*. Use the steps of the nursing process to eliminate options 2 and 4. Options 2 and 4 are also comparable or alike in that they are attempts to foster students' self-esteem. From the remaining options, consider the subject of the question, high school students who recently lost a classmate to suicide and select the option that deals with the here and now. The nurse must first determine the students' perception and appraisal of the stressful event. Review: **crisis** and **suicide**.
Reference(s): Fortinash, Holoday-Worret (2012), pp. 492, 647-648; Stuart (2013), pp. 188-189.

896. A hospitalized client has participated in substance abuse therapy group sessions. The nurse is monitoring the client's response to these sessions. Which statement by the client would **best** indicate that the client has assimilated session topics, understood coping response styles, and processed information **effectively** for self-use?

1. "I'll keep all my appointments, and I'll do everything I'm supposed to. I just know nothing will go wrong that way."
2. "I know I'm ready to be discharged. I feel like I'll have no problem saying no and leaving a group of friends if they are drinking."
3. "This group has really helped a lot. I know it will be different when I go home. But I'm sure that my family and friends will all help me, like the people in this group have. They'll all help me, I know they will. They won't let me go back to old ways."
4. "I'm looking forward to leaving here, but I know that I will miss all of you. So, I'm happy, and I'm sad. I'm excited, and I'm scared. I know that I have to work hard to be strong and that everyone isn't going to be as helpful as you all have been. I know it isn't going to be easy, but I'm going to try as hard as I can."

Level of Cognitive Ability: Evaluating
Client Needs: Psychosocial Integrity
Integrated Process: Nursing Process/Evaluation
Content Area: Mental Health
Priority Concepts: Addiction; Coping

Answer: 4
Rationale: With the defense mechanism of denial, the person denies reality. There can be varying degrees of this denial. In option 4 the client is expressing real concern and ambivalence about discharge from the hospital. The client demonstrates an ability to perceive reality in the appraisal regarding the lifestyle changes that will have to be initiated, as well as the fact that the client will have to work hard and develop new friends and meeting places. In option 1 the client is concrete and procedure oriented; again, the client verbalizes denial. Option 2 identifies denial. In option 3 the client is relying heavily on others, and the client's locus of control is external.
Priority Nursing Tip: A defense mechanism is a coping device used in an effort to protect the individual from feelings of anxiety. As anxiety increases and becomes overwhelming, the individual copes by using defense mechanisms to protect the ego and decrease anxiety.
Test-Taking Strategy: Note the strategic words, *best* and *effectively*. Select the option that identifies the most realistic client verbalization. Recalling that a person in denial is unable to face reality will assist you with eliminating options 1, 2, and 3. Review: **denial**.
Reference(s): Fortinash, Holoday-Worret (2012), pp. 184-185; Stuart (2013), pp. 190, 226.

897. A client recovering from a head injury becomes agitated at times. Which action should the nurse incorporate to calm this client?
1. Assign the client a new task to master.
2. Turn on the television to a musical program.
3. Make the client aware that the behavior is undesirable.
4. Talk to the client about the familiar objects, such as family pictures, that are kept in the client's room.

Level of Cognitive Ability: Applying
Client Needs: Psychosocial Integrity
Integrated Process: Caring
Content Area: Adult Health: Neurological
Priority Concepts: Anxiety; Intracranial Regulation

Answer: 4
Rationale: Providing familiar objects will decrease anxiety. Decreasing environmental stimuli also aids in reducing agitation for the head-injured client. Option 1 does not simplify the environment because a new task may be frustrating. Option 2 increases stimuli. In option 3 the nurse uses negative reinforcement to help the client adjust.
Priority Nursing Tip: For the client with a head injury, the nurse should monitor for cerebrospinal fluid (CSF) drainage, such as from the nose. CSF can be distinguished from other fluids by the presence of concentric rings (yellowish stain surrounded by bloody fluid) when the fluid is placed on a white sterile background, such as a gauze pad. CSF also tests positive for glucose when tested using a strip test.
Test-Taking Strategy: Focus on the subject, the measure that will calm a client who is agitated. Identify those options that may increase stimuli, agitation, and frustration. This will assist you with eliminating options 1, 2, and 3. Review: the measures that will relieve agitation.
Reference(s): Ignatavicius, Workman (2013), p. 1026; Lewis et al (2011), p. 1444.

898. A client recovering from a stroke has become irritable and angry regarding limitations. Which is the **best** nursing approach to help the client regain motivation to succeed?
1. Ignore the behavior, knowing that the client is grieving.
2. Allow longer and more frequent visitation by the spouse.
3. Use supportive statements to correct the client's behavior.
4. Tell the client that the nurses are experienced and know how the client feels.

Level of Cognitive Ability: Applying
Client Needs: Psychosocial Integrity
Integrated Process: Caring
Content Area: Adult Health: Neurological
Priority Concepts: Intracranial Regulation; Motivation

Answer: 3
Rationale: Clients who have experienced a stroke have many and varied needs. It is also important to support and praise the client for accomplishments. The client may need his or her behavior pointed out so that correction can take place, and the client's behavior should not be ignored. Spouses of a stroke client are often grieving; therefore, more visitations may not be helpful. Additionally, short visits are often encouraged. Stating that the nurse knows how the client feels is inappropriate.
Priority Nursing Tip: For the client at risk for increased intracranial pressure, the nurse should ensure that the client avoids extreme hip and neck flexion; extreme hip flexion may increase intrathoracic pressure, whereas extreme neck flexion prohibits venous drainage from the brain.
Test-Taking Strategy: Note the strategic word, *best*. Use therapeutic communication techniques to eliminate options 1 and 4. From the remaining choices, option 3 is the only one that addresses the client's behavior described in the question. Review: the psychosocial aspects related to a stroke.
Reference(s): Ignatavicius, Workman (2013), p. 1012.

899. An older client is admitted to the hospital with a fractured hip and is experiencing periods of confusion. The nurse develops a plan of care and should identify which psychosocial outcome?
1. Improved sleep patterns
2. Reduced family fears and anxiety
3. Meeting self-care needs independently
4. Increased ability to concentrate and participate in care

Level of Cognitive Ability: Analyzing
Client Needs: Psychosocial Integrity
Integrated Process: Nursing Process/Planning
Content Area: Adult Health: Musculoskeletal
Priority Concepts: Clinical Judgment; Cognition

Answer: 4
Rationale: The client needs to be able to concentrate and participate in his or her care. When the client is able to do that, the nurse can work with the client to achieve the other outcomes. Options 1 and 3 address physiological needs rather than psychosocial outcomes. Option 2 is a secondary need and does not address the client.
Priority Nursing Tip: For the client who has experienced a hip fracture, the nurse must maintain the leg and hip in proper alignment and prevent internal or external rotation, as well as extreme hip flexion.
Test-Taking Strategy: Focus on the subject, psychosocial outcome, and that the client is confused. Select the option that will have the greatest impact on the client's ability to function psychosocially. Option 2 can be eliminated because it does not address the client. Options 1 and 3 address physiological rather than psychosocial needs. Review: psychosocial outcomes for the client with confusion.
Reference(s): Ignatavicius, Workman (2013), p. 1161.

900. The nurse is caring for a young woman who is dying from breast cancer. Which client behavior is a characteristic of anticipatory grieving?

1. Discusses thoughts and feelings related to loss
2. Has prolonged emotional reactions and outbursts
3. Verbalizes unrealistic goals and plans for the future
4. Ignores untreated medical conditions that require treatment

Level of Cognitive Ability: Analyzing
Client Needs: Psychosocial Integrity
Integrated Process: Nursing Process/Analysis
Content Area: Adult Health: Oncology
Priority Concepts: Clinical Judgment; Coping

Answer: 1
Rationale: The nurse can determine the client's stage of anticipatory grief by observing the client's behavior. Options 2, 3, and 4 are examples of dysfunctional grieving.
Priority Nursing Tip: The nurse's role in the grief and loss process includes communicating with the client, family members, and significant others.
Test-Taking Strategy: Focus on the subject, anticipatory grieving. Note that options 2, 3, and 4 are comparable or alike and indicate dysfunctional grieving. Also noting the words *prolonged*, *unrealistic*, and *ignores* in these options will assist you in eliminating them. Review: anticipatory grieving.
Reference(s): Ignatavicius, Workman (2013), pp. 1598, 1608-1609; Lewis et al (2011), pp. 1323-1324.

901. The nurse determines that a client is beginning to experience shock and hemorrhage as a result of a partial inversion of the uterus. The nurse pages the obstetrician to come immediately and calls for assistance. The client asks in an apprehensive voice, "What is happening to me? I feel so funny, and I know I'm bleeding. Am I dying?" What typical response is the client experiencing during this medical emergency?

1. Panic as a result of shock
2. Anticipatory grieving related to the fear of dying
3. Depression related to postpartum hormonal changes
4. Fear and anxiety related to unexpected and unknown changes

Level of Cognitive Ability: Analyzing
Client Needs: Psychosocial Integrity
Integrated Process: Nursing Process/Assessment
Content Area: Critical Care: Emergency Situations
Priority Concepts: Caregiving; Clinical Judgment

Answer: 4
Rationale: Feelings of loss of control are common causes of anxiety, and the unknown is the most common cause of fear. Apprehension and feelings of impending doom are also associated with shock, but the information in the question does not suggest panic at this point. Anticipatory grieving occurs when there is knowledge of the impending loss, but it is not associated with a sudden situational crisis such as this one. It is far too early for the onset of postpartum depression.
Priority Nursing Tip: For the postpartum client experiencing uterine atony, the nurse should massage the fundus, taking care not to overmassage. If the client is hemorrhaging, the nurse should remain with the client and ask another nurse to contact the health care provider.
Test-Taking Strategy: Note the subject, the response that the client is experiencing. Focus on the words *I feel so funny* in the question and *unexpected and unknown changes* in option 4. Review: fear and anxiety during crisis.
Reference(s): Lowdermilk, Perry, Cashion, Alden (2012), pp. 830-831.

902. A perinatal home care nurse has just assessed the fetal status of a client with a diagnosis of partial placental abruption of 20 weeks' gestation. The client is experiencing new bleeding and reports less fetal movement. The nurse informs the client that the health care provider will be contacted for possible hospital admission. The client begins to cry quietly while holding her abdomen with her hands. She murmurs, "No, no, you can't go, my little man." The nurse should recognize the client's behavior as an indication of which psychosocial reaction?
1. Pain from abdominal tetany
2. Fear of loss and the death of the fetus
3. Grief due to potential loss of the fetus
4. Cognitive confusion as a result of shock

Level of Cognitive Ability: Analyzing
Client Needs: Psychosocial Integrity
Integrated Process: Nursing Process/Analysis
Content Area: Critical Care: Emergency Situations
Priority Concepts: Coping; Reproduction

Answer: 3
Rationale: Grief occurs when a client has knowledge of an impending loss, such as when signs of fetal distress accelerate. The first stages of grieving may be characterized by shock; emotional numbness; disbelief; and strong emotions such as tears, screaming, or anger.
Priority Nursing Tip: In abruption placentae, there is dark red vaginal bleeding, uterine pain or tenderness or both, and uterine rigidity. In placenta previa, there is painless, bright red vaginal bleeding, and the uterus is soft, relaxed, and nontender.
Test-Taking Strategy: Focus on the subject, the client's psychosocial reaction. Options 1 and 4 can be eliminated because there is no indication of pain or confusion. While options 2 and 3 are somewhat similar, one suggests a fetal death and the other a potential loss. There is no indication of fetal death. The client perceives this as a potential loss. With this knowledge, option 3 is the only correct answer. Review: the defining characteristics of grief.
Reference(s): Lowdermilk, Perry, Cashion, Alden (2012), pp. 685, 913.

903. A postoperative client has been vomiting and has absent bowel sounds, and paralytic ileus has been diagnosed. The health care provider prescribes the insertion of a nasogastric tube. The nurse explains the purpose of the tube and the insertion procedure to the client. The client says to the nurse, "I'm not sure I can take any more of this treatment." Which response should the nurse make to the client?
1. "Let's just put the tube down, so that you can get well."
2. "If you don't have this tube put down, you will just continue to vomit."
3. "You are feeling tired and frustrated with your recovery from surgery?"
4. "It is your right to refuse any treatment. I'll notify the health care provider."

Level of Cognitive Ability: Applying
Client Needs: Psychosocial Integrity
Integrated Process: Caring
Content Area: Adult Health: Gastrointestinal
Priority Concepts: Communication; Professionalism

Answer: 3
Rationale: In option 3, the nurse uses empathy. Empathy, comprehending, and sharing a client's frame of reference are important components of the nurse–client relationship. This assists clients with expressing and exploring feelings, which can lead to problem solving. The other options are examples of barriers to effective communication, including option 1, which is stereotyping; option 2, which is defensiveness; and option 4, which is showing disapproval.
Priority Nursing Tip: In the postoperative period, vomiting, abdominal distention, and the absence of bowel sounds may be signs of paralytic ileus.
Test-Taking Strategy: Use therapeutic communication techniques. Option 3 is an open-ended question and a communication tool; it also focuses on the client's feelings. Review: therapeutic communication techniques.
Reference(s): Ignatavicius, Workman (2013), p. 290; Potter et al (2013), pp. 320-322.

Test 4

❖ **904.** The nurse implements de-escalation techniques with a client who is extremely angry and exhibiting increasingly agitated behavior. Which de-escalation techniques should the nurse employ? **Select all that apply.**
   ❑ 1. Avoid verbal struggles.
   ❑ 2. Provide clear options to the client.
   ❑ 3. Place an arm around the client's shoulder.
   ❑ 4. Maintain the client's self-esteem and dignity.
   ❑ 5. Establish what the client considers to be his or her need.
   ❑ 6. Use a firm and aggressive tone of voice when speaking to the client.

Level of Cognitive Ability: Applying
Client Needs: Psychosocial Integrity
Integrated Process: Nursing Process/Implementation
Content Area: Mental Health
Priority Concepts: Anxiety; Safety

Answer: 1, 2, 4, 5
Rationale: When the client is angry and exhibits increasingly agitated behavior, the nurse should employ de-escalation techniques to prevent client violence and assaultive behaviors. These techniques include assessing the situation, using a calm and clear tone of voice when communicating with the client, remaining calm, avoiding verbal struggles, presenting clear options to the client, and maintaining the client's self-esteem and dignity. The nurse should establish what the client considers to be his or her need and maintain a large personal space (touching the client could increase agitation).
Priority Nursing Tip: When using de-escalation techniques, the nurse needs to remain calm and centered. The nurse should encourage the client to use slow breathing, which will help in successful de-escalation.
Test-Taking Strategy: Focus on the subject, de-escalation techniques. In selecting the correct answers, determine if the technique would calm or further agitate the client. Remember the need to maintain a calm approach and a large distance from the client. Review: de-escalation techniques.
Reference(s): Fortinash, Holoday-Worret (2012), pp. 289-290; Stuart (2013), p. 427.

905. A client who is receiving total parenteral nutrition (TPN) tells the nurse, "I'm not sure that I want to receive an infusion of lipids because it could make me obese." What **initial** action should the nurse take?
   1. Inquire how illness affects the client's self-concept.
   2. Ask the provider to discuss the benefits of intralipids.
   3. State that intralipids supply essential fatty acids for life.
   4. Explain how intralipids replace dietary sources of lipids.

Level of Cognitive Ability: Applying
Client Needs: Psychosocial Integrity
Integrated Process: Nursing Process/Implementation
Content Area: Fundamental Skills: Nutrition
Priority Concepts: Caregiving; Nutrition

Answer: 1
Rationale: A client who receives TPN is at risk for developing an essential fatty acid deficiency; however, this client's comment requires more than a simple informational response initially. Thus, the nurse responds with option 1 to assist the client with self-expression and to deal with aspects of illness and treatment. Option 2 delays client self-expression and devalues the client's feelings. Options 3 and 4 provide information only.
Priority Nursing Tip: Total parenteral nutrition is the least desirable form of nutrition and is used when there is no other nutritional alternative. Other forms of administering nutrition such as oral or via a gastrointestinal tube are initiated first.
Test-Taking Strategy: Note the strategic word, *initial*. This should cue you to use therapeutic communication techniques to focus on the client's feelings because the client's feelings must be assessed before the nurse can provide comprehensive information and adapt the information accordingly. Option 1 is the only choice that addresses the client's feelings. Review: therapeutic communication techniques.
Reference(s): Ignatavicius, Workman (2013), pp. 1347-1348; Potter et al (2013), pp. 320-322.

906. A client has terminal cancer and is using opioid analgesics for pain relief. The client is concerned about becoming addicted to the pain medication. Which action by the home care nurse would allay the client's anxiety?

1. Encouraging the client to hold off as long as possible between doses of pain medication
2. Telling the client to take lower doses of medications even though the pain is not well controlled
3. Explaining to the client that the fears are justified but should be of no concern during the final stages of care
4. Explaining to the client that addiction rarely occurs in individuals who are taking medication to relieve pain

Level of Cognitive Ability: Applying
Client Needs: Psychosocial Integrity
Integrated Process: Caring
Content Area: Adult Health: Oncology
Priority Concepts: Caregiving; Pain

Answer: 4
Rationale: Clients who are on opioid analgesics often have well-founded fears about addiction, even in the face of pain. The nurse has the responsibility to provide correct information about the likelihood of addiction while still maintaining adequate pain control. Addiction is rare for individuals who are taking medication to relieve pain. Allowing the client to be in pain, as in options 1 and 2, is not acceptable nursing practice. Option 3 is only partially correct in that it acknowledges the client's fear.
Priority Nursing Tip: The nurse should continually assess the client with terminal cancer for signs of pain. The nurse needs to ensure that measures to reduce and eliminate the pain are effective.
Test-Taking Strategy: Options 1 and 2 are comparable or alike options and should be eliminated. Focusing on the words *allay the client's anxiety* will also assist in selecting the best answer. Review: **pain management**.
Reference(s): Ignatavicius, Workman (2013), pp. 44-45; Lewis et al (2011), p. 147.

907. A client is very anxious about receiving chest physiotherapy (CPT) for the first time at home. When planning for the client's care, which concept about CPT should the home care nurse use to reassure the client?

1. CPT will help the client cough more effectively.
2. There are no risks associated with this procedure.
3. CPT will resolve all of the client's respiratory symptoms.
4. CPT will assist with mobilizing secretions to enhance more effective breathing.

Level of Cognitive Ability: Applying
Client Needs: Psychosocial Integrity
Integrated Process: Teaching and Learning
Content Area: Adult Health: Respiratory
Priority Concepts: Client Education; Gas Exchange

Answer: 4
Rationale: CPT is an intervention to assist with mobilizing and clearing secretions to enhance more effective breathing. CPT will assist the client with coughing if the secretions have been mobilized and the cough stimulus is present. There are risks associated with CPT, including cardiac, gastrointestinal, neurological, and pulmonary effects. It will not resolve all of the client's respiratory symptoms.
Priority Nursing Tip: Contraindications for chest physiotherapy include unstable vital signs, increased intracranial pressure, bronchospasm, history of pathological fractures, rib fractures, and chest incisions.
Test-Taking Strategy: Eliminate options 2 and 3 because they contain the closed-ended words "no" and "all." Option 4 is the umbrella option and contains most of the purposes of CPT. Review: the purpose of **chest physiotherapy (CPT)**.
Reference(s): Lewis et al (2011), p. 1753; Potter et al (2013), pp. 842-843, 1148.

908. A client with cardiomyopathy stops eating, takes long naps, and turns away from the nurse when the nurse talks to the client. The nurse should make which interpretation about this behavior?

1. The client is depressed.
2. The client is noncompliant.
3. The client has intractable pain.
4. The client is unable to tolerate activity.

Level of Cognitive Ability: Analyzing
Client Needs: Psychosocial Integrity
Integrated Process: Nursing Process/Analysis
Content Area: Adult Health: Cardiovascular
Priority Concepts: Clinical Judgment; Mood and Affect

Answer: 1
Rationale: Depression is a common problem related to clients who have long-term and debilitating illnesses. Options 2, 3, and 4 are not related to the symptoms present in the question and therefore are not appropriate interpretations.
Priority Nursing Tip: Cardiomyopathy is a subacute or chronic disorder of the heart muscle. Treatment is palliative, not curative, and the client needs assistance with numerous required lifestyle changes and has a shortened life span.
Test-Taking Strategy: Note the subject, interpretation of the client's behavior. Focus on the words *stops eating, takes long naps, and turns away from the nurse* in the question. On the basis of the data presented, the only appropriate interpretation is depression. Review: the characteristics of **depression**.
Reference(s): Ignatavicius, Workman (2013), pp. 767, 841.

909. The nurse is caring for a pregnant client who has been hospitalized for the stabilization of diabetes mellitus. The client tells the nurse that her husband is caring for their 2-year-old daughter. Which short-term psychosocial outcome should the nurse develop for the client?

1. Be alert to the risks of early labor and birth.
2. Protect the client from injuries that can result from seizures.
3. Teach the client and family about diabetes and its implications.
4. Provide emotional support and education about interrupted family processes related to the pregnant woman's hospitalization.

Level of Cognitive Ability: Analyzing
Client Needs: Psychosocial Integrity
Integrated Process: Nursing Process/Planning
Content Area: Maternity: Antepartum
Priority Concepts: Glucose Regulation; Health Promotion

Answer: 4
Rationale: The short-term psychosocial well-being of the family is at risk as a result of the hospitalization of the client. Options 1 and 2 are unrelated to diabetes mellitus and are more related to gestational hypertension. Teaching about diabetes mellitus is a long-term goal related to diabetes.
Priority Nursing Tip: The pregnant client will need to use insulin to control the blood glucose levels.
Test-Taking Strategy: Eliminate options 1 and 2 because they are unrelated to diabetes mellitus. Next, note the words *short-term psychosocial outcome*, and focus on the data in the question to direct you to option 4. In addition, the incorrect options are comparable or alike in that they are all physiological outcomes. Review: the outcomes for **interrupted family processes**.
Reference(s): Lowdermilk, Perry, Cashion, Alden (2012), p. 694; McKinney et al (2013), p. 616.

910. A new mother is trying to decide whether to have her baby boy circumcised. The nurse should make which statement to assist the mother with making the decision?

1. "I had my son circumcised, and I am so glad."
2. "Circumcision is a difficult decision, but your health care provider is the best, and you know it's better to get it done now than later."
3. "You know they say it prevents cancer and sexually transmitted infections, so I would definitely have my son circumcised."
4. "Circumcision is a difficult decision. There are various controversies surrounding circumcision. Here, read this pamphlet that discusses the pros and cons, and we will talk about any questions that you have after you read it."

Level of Cognitive Ability: Applying
Client Needs: Psychosocial Integrity
Integrated Process: Communication and Documentation
Content Area: Maternity: Newborn
Priority Concepts: Client Education; Communication

Answer: 4
Rationale: Informed decision making is the strategic point when answering this question. The nurse should provide educational materials and answer questions pertaining to the education of the mother. Providing written information to the mother will give her the information she needs to make an educated and informed decision. The nurse's personal thoughts and feelings should not be part of the educational process.
Priority Nursing Tip: The nurse should instruct the mother of a newborn who has been circumcised to monitor urine output and for signs of urinary retention.
Test-Taking Strategy: Use therapeutic communication techniques. Options 1, 2, and 3 are communication blocks because the nurse is providing a personal opinion to the client. Review: **therapeutic communication techniques**.
Reference(s): McKinney et al (2013), pp. 30-31, 518.

911. The nurse is planning care for a client who is experiencing anxiety after a myocardial infarction. Which **priority** nursing intervention should be included in the plan of care?
1. Answer questions with factual information.
2. Provide detailed explanations of all procedures.
3. Limit family involvement during the acute phase.
4. Administer an antianxiety medication to promote relaxation.

Level of Cognitive Ability: Applying
Client Needs: Psychosocial Integrity
Integrated Process: Nursing Process/Implementation
Content Area: Adult Health: Cardiovascular
Priority Concepts: Anxiety; Perfusion

Answer: 1
Rationale: Accurate information reduces fear, strengthens the nurse–client relationship, and assists the client with dealing realistically with the situation. Providing detailed information may increase the client's anxiety. Information should be provided simply and clearly. Limiting family involvement may or may not be helpful. The client's family may be a source of support for the client. Medication should not be used unless necessary.
Priority Nursing Tip: Myocardial infarction causes ischemia to the heart muscle. Ischemia can lead to necrosis of the myocardial tissue if blood flow is not restored.
Test-Taking Strategy: Note the strategic word, *priority*, and the word *anxiety* in the question. Eliminate option 2 first because of the word *detailed*. Eliminate option 4 next because medication should not be the first intervention to alleviate anxiety; however, it may be necessary if other strategies are not effective. From the remaining options, eliminate option 3 because limiting family involvement does not reduce anxiety in all situations. Review: the measures to reduce **anxiety**.
Reference(s): Ignatavicius, Workman (2013), pp. 835, 846.

912. A client recovering from an acute myocardial infarction will be discharged in 1 day. Which client action on the evening before discharge suggests that the client is in the denial phase?
1. Requests a sedative for sleep at 10:00 PM
2. Expresses a hesitancy to leave the hospital
3. Consumes 25% of foods and fluids given for supper
4. Walks up and down three flights of stairs unsupervised

Level of Cognitive Ability: Evaluating
Client Needs: Psychosocial Integrity
Integrated Process: Nursing Process/Evaluating
Content Area: Adult Health: Cardiovascular
Priority Concepts: Clinical Judgment; Coping

Answer: 4
Rationale: Ignoring activity limitations and avoiding lifestyle changes are signs of the denial stage. Walking three flights of stairs should be a supervised activity during this phase of the recovery process. Option 1 is an appropriate client action on the evening before discharge. Option 2 may be a manifestation of anxiety or fear rather than denial. Option 3 is a manifestation of depression rather than denial.
Priority Nursing Tip: Pain relief increases oxygen supply to the myocardium; the nurse should administer morphine sulfate as prescribed as a priority in managing pain in the client having a myocardial infarction.
Test-Taking Strategy: Focus on the subject, the client action that indicates denial. Option 4 is the only option that identifies denial. Option 1 is an appropriate client request. Option 2 identifies anxiety or fear. Option 3 identifies depression. Review: the manifestations associated with **denial**.
Reference(s): Ignatavicius, Workman (2013), pp. 835, 840-841.

913. The nurse is caring for a client with Hodgkin's disease who will be receiving radiation and chemotherapy. Which statement by the client indicates a positive coping mechanism to be used during these treatments?
1. "I won't leave the house bald."
2. "Losing my hair won't bother me."
3. "I will be one of the few who doesn't lose my hair."
4. "I have selected a wig, even though I will miss my own hair."

Level of Cognitive Ability: Evaluating
Client Needs: Psychosocial Integrity
Integrated Process: Nursing Process/Evaluation
Content Area: Adult Health: Oncology
Priority Concepts: Cellular Regulation; Coping

Answer: 4
Rationale: A combination of radiation and chemotherapy often causes alopecia. To make use of positive coping mechanisms, the client must identify personal feelings and positive interventions to deal with side effects. Options 1, 2, and 3 are not positive coping mechanisms.
Priority Nursing Tip: A coping mechanism involves any effort to decrease anxiety.
Test-Taking Strategy: Focus on the subject, a positive coping mechanism. Options 1, 2, and 3 involve avoidance and denial. Option 4 is the only choice that addresses a positive coping mechanism. Review: **coping mechanisms**.
Reference(s): Ignatavicius, Workman (2013), pp. 422-424; Lewis et al (2011), p. 281.

914. A male client is admitted to the hospital with diabetic ketoacidosis (DKA). The client's daughter says to the nurse, "My mother died last month, and now this. I've been trying to follow all of the instructions from the doctor, but what have I done wrong?" Which response should the nurse make to the client's daughter?

1. "Tell me what you think you did wrong."
2. "Maybe we can keep your father in the hospital for a while longer to give you a rest."
3. "You should talk to the social worker about getting you someone at home who is more capable with managing a diabetic's care."
4. "An emotional stress such as your mother's death can trigger DKA in a diabetic client, even though the prescribed regimen is being followed."

Level of Cognitive Ability: Applying
Client Needs: Psychosocial Integrity
Integrated Process: Nursing Process/Implementation
Content Area: Adult Health: Endocrine
Priority Concepts: Communication; Glucose Regulation

Answer: 4
Rationale: Environment, infection, or an emotional stressor can initiate the physiological mechanism of DKA. Options 1 and 3 substantiate the daughter's feelings of guilt and incompetence. Option 2 is not a cost-effective intervention.
Priority Nursing Tip: Diabetic ketoacidosis (DKA) is a life-threatening complication of diabetes mellitus that develops when a severe insulin deficiency occurs. Hyperglycemia progresses to ketoacidosis over a period of several hours to days. DKA occurs in clients with type 1 diabetes mellitus, persons with undiagnosed diabetes, and persons who stop prescribed treatment for diabetes.
Test-Taking Strategy: Identify the option that focuses on therapeutic communication techniques. Eliminate option 2 first because this option is not cost effective. Options 1 and 3 devalue the client (the daughter) and block therapeutic communication, so they are eliminated next. Review: **therapeutic communication techniques** and **diabetic ketoacidosis (DKA).**
Reference(s): Ignatavicius, Workman (2013), p. 1455; Potter et al (2013), pp. 320-322.

915. The nurse has been working with a victim of rape in an outpatient setting for the past 4 weeks. The nurse should identify that which client objective is an unrealistic short-term goal?

1. The client will verbalize feelings about the rape event.
2. The client will resolve feelings of fear and anxiety related to the rape trauma.
3. The client will experience physical healing of the wounds that were incurred during the rape.
4. The client will participate in the treatment plan by following through with treatment options.

Level of Cognitive Ability: Analyzing
Client Needs: Psychosocial Integrity
Integrated Process: Nursing Process/Analysis
Content Area: Mental Health
Priority Concepts: Coping; Interpersonal Violence

Answer: 2
Rationale: Short-term goals include the beginning stages of dealing with the rape trauma. Clients will initially be expected to keep appointments, participate in care, start to explore feelings, and begin to heal the physical wounds that were inflicted at the time of the rape. The resolution of feelings of anxiety and fear is a long-term goal.
Priority Nursing Tip: For the client who is a victim of rape, rape trauma syndrome may occur. The client may experience sleep disturbances; nightmares; loss of appetite; fears; anxiety; phobias; suspicion; a decrease in activities and motivation; disruptions in relationships with partner, family, or friends; self-blame; guilt and shame; lowered self-esteem; feelings of worthlessness; and somatic complaints.
Test-Taking Strategy: Focus on the subject, an unrealistic short-term goal for a rape victim. Consider each option and the reality of it being achieved in the short term. Note the word *resolve* in option 2. This word should provide you with the clue that this option is a long-term goal. Review: the appropriate goals for the client who is a victim of **rape.**
Reference(s): Fortinash, Holoday-Worret (2012), p. 549; Stuart (2013), p. 748.

916. A client is admitted to a surgical unit with a diagnosis of cancer. The client is scheduled for surgery in the morning. When the nurse enters the room and begins the surgical preparation, the client states, "I'm not having surgery. You must have the wrong person! My test results were negative. I'll be going home tomorrow." The nurse recognizes the client's statement as indicative of which ego defense mechanism?

1. Denial
2. Psychosis
3. Delusions
4. Displacement

Level of Cognitive Ability: Analyzing
Client Needs: Psychosocial Integrity
Integrated Process: Nursing Process/Analysis
Content Area: Adult Health: Oncology
Priority Concepts: Cellular Regulation; Coping

Answer: 1
Rationale: By definition, ego defense mechanisms are operations outside of a person's awareness that the ego calls into play to protect against anxiety. Denial is the defense mechanism that blocks out painful or anxiety-inducing events or feelings. In this case, the client cannot deal with the upcoming surgery for cancer and therefore denies the illness. Psychosis and delusions are not defense mechanisms. Displacement is the discharging of pent-up feelings on people who are less dangerous than those who initially aroused the feelings.
Priority Nursing Tip: For the client using defense mechanisms, the nurse should assist the client to identify the source of anxiety and explore methods to reduce anxiety.
Test-Taking Strategy: Focus on the subject, ego defense mechanism. Options 2 and 3 are eliminated first because these are not ego defense mechanisms. From the remaining options, focus on the client's statement to direct you to option 1. Review: ego defense mechanisms.
Reference(s): Ignatavicius, Workman (2013), p. 419; Potter et al (2013), pp. 333, 734.

917. A community health nurse working in an industrial setting has received a memo indicating that a large number of employees will be laid off during the next 2 weeks. An analysis of previous layoffs suggested that workers experienced role crises, indecision, and depression. Using this information, how should the nurse begin to assist employees?

1. Help the workers acquire unemployment benefits to avoid a gap in income.
2. Reduce the staff in the occupational health department of the industrial setting.
3. Notify insurance carriers of the upcoming event to assist with potential health care alterations.
4. Identify referral, counseling, and vocational rehabilitative services for the employees being laid off.

Level of Cognitive Ability: Analyzing
Client Needs: Psychosocial Integrity
Integrated Process: Nursing Process/Planning
Content Area: Mental Health
Priority Concepts: Coping; Stress

Answer: 4
Rationale: In preparation for this crisis, the nurse should identify the services that are available to the employees. These resources will provide immediate avenues for assistance when the layoff occurs. Additional information about the industrial setting is needed to determine whether options 1, 2, and 3 are necessary or possible.
Priority Nursing Tip: One role of the community health nurse is to perform a needs assessment for the individuals with whom he or she is working. The needs assessment is important to identify the potential underlying factors that may play a role in the client's ability to function normally.
Test-Taking Strategy: Use the steps of the nursing process to direct you to option 4. This option refers to the assessment of resources and services for employees. Review: crisis interventions.
Reference(s): Fortinash, Holoday-Worret (2012), pp. 483-484; Stuart (2013), p. 188.

918. A primigravida client comes to the clinic and has been diagnosed with a urinary tract infection. She repeatedly verbalizes concern regarding the safety of the fetus. What should the nurse address **first**?
1. Client's fear
2. Prescribing a sedative
3. Instructions regarding improved hygiene
4. Instructions regarding medication compliance

Level of Cognitive Ability: Analyzing
Client Needs: Psychosocial Integrity
Integrated Process: Nursing Process/Implementation
Content Area: Maternity: Antepartum
Priority Concepts: Anxiety; Infection

Answer: 1
Rationale: The primary concern of this client is the safety of her fetus rather than herself. The priority for the nurse to address at this time is fear. Option 2 is outside the scope of nursing practice. Instructions on medication compliance should come at a later time. Poor hygiene is a contributing factor in urinary tract infections, but there are no data to support that this is the case with this client.
Priority Nursing Tip: Some of the predisposing conditions for urinary tract infection in a pregnant client include a history of urinary tract infections, sickle cell trait, poor hygiene, anemia, and diabetes mellitus.
Test-Taking Strategy: Note the strategic word, *first*. Eliminate option 2 because it is out of the nursing scope of practice. Focusing on the data in the question and noting the words *verbalizes concern* will direct you to the correct option Review: **urinary tract infections** in a pregnant woman and **fear**.
Reference(s): Lowdermilk, Perry, Cashion, Alden (2012), pp. 344-345.

919. The nurse is planning interventions for counseling a maternal client who has been newly diagnosed with sickle cell anemia. Which would be the **most important** psychosocial intervention at this time?
1. Provide emotional support.
2. Avoid discussing the disease.
3. Allow the client to be alone if she is crying.
4. Provide the client with all of the information regarding the disease.

Level of Cognitive Ability: Applying
Client Needs: Psychosocial Integrity
Integrated Process: Caring
Content Area: Maternity: Antepartum
Priority Concepts: Caregiving; Coping

Answer: 1
Rationale: One of the most important nursing roles is providing emotional support to the client and family during the counseling process. Option 2, like option 4, is nontherapeutic. Option 3 is only appropriate if the client requests to be alone; if this is not requested, the nurse is abandoning the client in a time of need. Option 4 overwhelms the client with information while she is trying to cope with the news of the disease.
Priority Nursing Tip: Situations that precipitate sickling in sickle cell anemia include fever, dehydration, and emotional or physical stress. Any condition that increases the need for oxygen or alters the transport of oxygen can result in sickle cell crisis.
Test-Taking Strategy: Note the strategic words, *most important*. Eliminate options 2 and 4 because of the closed-ended words "avoid" and "all." Additionally, these actions are nontherapeutic. From the remaining options, remember that the client's feelings are the priority, and an extremely important role of the nurse is to provide emotional support. Review: the interventions related to providing **emotional support**.
Reference(s): McKinney et al (2013), pp. 622-623.

920. A neonatal intensive care nurse is caring for a newborn immediately after delivery. The newborn has a suspected diagnosis of erythroblastosis fetalis. Which statement should the nurse make to the parents at this time?

1. "Your infant is very sick. The next 24 hours are the most crucial."
2. "This is a common neonatal problem, so you shouldn't be concerned."
3. "There is no need to worry. We have the most updated equipment in this hospital."
4. "You must have many concerns. Please ask me any questions that you have so that I can explain your infant's care."

Level of Cognitive Ability: Applying
Client Needs: Psychosocial Integrity
Integrated Process: Caring
Content Area: Maternity: Newborn
Priority Concepts: Communication; Family Dynamics

Answer: 4
Rationale: Parental anxiety is expected in relation to the care of the infant with erythroblastosis fetalis. This anxiety is caused by a lack of knowledge regarding the disease process, treatments, and expected outcomes. Parents need to be encouraged to verbalize concerns and participate in the care as appropriate. The nurse would not tell the parents to be or to not be concerned. Option 1 will produce anxiety in the parents.
Priority Nursing Tip: Erythroblastosis fetalis is the destruction of red blood cells that results from an antigen–antibody reaction. The nurse should administer Rho(D) immune globulin (RhoGAM) to the mother during the first 72 hours after delivery if the Rh-negative mother delivers an Rh-positive fetus but remains unsensitized.
Test-Taking Strategy: Use therapeutic communication techniques. Eliminate options 2 and 3 because they are comparable or alike and are blocks to communication. Eliminate option 1 because it will produce anxiety in the parents. Remember to address the clients' feelings and concerns. Option 4 is the only choice that encourages communication. Review: **therapeutic communication techniques.**
Reference(s): McKinney et al (2013), pp. 30-31, 721.

❖ **921.** The nurse is preparing a plan of care for a client diagnosed with mania. Which interventions should be included in the plan of care? **Select all that apply.**

❑ 1. Place the client in seclusion.
❑ 2. Ignore any client complaints.
❑ 3. Use a firm and calm approach.
❑ 4. Use short and concise explanations and statements.
❑ 5. Remain neutral and avoid power struggles and value judgments.
❑ 6. Firmly redirect energy into more appropriate and constructive channels.

Level of Cognitive Ability: Analyzing
Client Needs: Psychosocial Integrity
Integrated Process: Nursing Process/Planning
Content Area: Mental Health
Priority Concepts: Mood and Affect; Psychosis

Answer: 3, 4, 5, 6
Rationale: A client with mania will be extremely restless, disorganized, and chaotic. Grandiose plans are extremely out of touch with reality, and judgment is poor. Interventions for the client in acute mania include using a firm and calm approach to provide structure and control, using short and concise explanations or statements because of the client's short attention span, remaining neutral and avoiding power struggles and value judgments, being consistent in approach and expectations and having frequent staff meetings to plan consistent approaches and to set agreed-on limits to avoid manipulation by the client, hearing and acting on legitimate client complaints, and redirecting energy into more appropriate and constructive channels.
Priority Nursing Tip: Clients experiencing mania may also experience a disruption in their sleep pattern. When deciding which clients to place together in a room, special considerations should be made for the client experiencing mania. Ideally they should be in a private room so as not to disturb other clients and to decrease sensory stimulation.
Test-Taking Strategy: Focus on the subject, a client with mania. Read each option and think about the manifestations that occur in the client with mania and how the intervention may or may not assist the client. Eliminate option 1 because of the word *seclusion* and option 2 because of the word *ignore*. Review: the therapeutic interventions for the client with **mania.**
Reference(s): Fortinash, Holoday-Worret (2012), p. 237; Varcarolis (2013), p. 287.

922. The nurse is planning care for a client with an intrauterine fetal demise. Which is an inappropriate goal for this client?
1. The woman and her family will discuss plans for going home without the infant.
2. The woman and her family will express their grief about the loss of their desired infant.
3. The woman will recognize that thoughts of worthlessness and suicide are normal after a loss.
4. The woman and her family will contact their pastor or grief counselor for support after discharge.

Level of Cognitive Ability: Analyzing
Client Needs: Psychosocial Integrity
Integrated Process: Caring
Content Area: Maternity: Postpartum
Priority Concepts: Caregiving; Coping

Answer: 3
Rationale: It is important for the nurse to assess whether the client is undergoing the normal grieving process. Signs that are a cause for concern and that are not part of the normal grieving process include thoughts of worthlessness and suicide. Options 1, 2, and 4 are appropriate goals.
Priority Nursing Tip: For the client with intrauterine fetal demise, there is a risk for disseminated intravascular coagulation (DIC).
Test-Taking Strategy: Focus on the subject, an inappropriate goal. These words should direct you to option 3 because thoughts of worthlessness and suicide are causes for concern. Review: the psychosocial care of the client who has experienced **intrauterine fetal demise**.
Reference(s): Lowdermilk, Perry, Cashion, Alden (2012), pp. 932-934.

923. A client with severe preeclampsia is admitted to the hospital. The client is a student at a local college and insists on continuing her studies while in the hospital, despite being instructed to rest. The client studies approximately 10 hours a day and has numerous visits from fellow students, family, and friends. Which intervention should the nurse use to assist the client with promoting rest?
1. Ask her why she is not complying with the prescription for bed rest.
2. Develop a routine with the client to balance her studies and her rest needs.
3. Include a significant other in helping the client understand the need for bed rest.
4. Instruct the client that the health of the baby is more important than her studies at this time.

Level of Cognitive Ability: Applying
Client Needs: Psychosocial Integrity
Integrated Process: Nursing Process/Implementation
Content Area: Maternity: Antepartum
Priority Concepts: Caregiving; Reproduction

Answer: 2
Rationale: Option 2 involves the client in the decision-making process. In options 1 and 4 the nurse is judging the client's choices and asking probing questions; this will cause a breakdown in communication. Option 3 persuades the client's significant other to disagree with the client's actions. This could cause problems with the relationship between the client and the significant other, and it could also cause conflict in the client's communication with the health care workers.
Priority Nursing Tip: Signs of preeclampsia are hypertension, generalized edema, and proteinuria.
Test-Taking Strategy: Focus on the subject, assisting the client with promoting rest. Options 1, 3, and 4 are blocks to both communication and a therapeutic nurse–client relationship. Option 2 is the most thorough nursing action because it addresses both rest and studies, and involves the client in the decision-making process. Review: the psychosocial care of the client with **preeclampsia**.
Reference(s): Lowdermilk, Perry, Cashion, Alden (2012), pp. 660, 662-663; McKinney et al (2013), p. 593.

924. A pregnant client is newly diagnosed with gestational diabetes. The client cries when receiving this information and keeps repeating, "What have I done to cause this? If only I could live my life over." Considering this statement, which problem should the nurse identify for the client?
1. Injury to the fetus because of maternal distress
2. Low self-esteem because of pregnancy complications
3. Lack of understanding about diabetic self-care during pregnancy
4. Poorly perceived body image caused by complications of pregnancy

Level of Cognitive Ability: Analyzing
Client Needs: Psychosocial Integrity
Integrated Process: Nursing Process/Analysis
Content Area: Maternity: Antepartum
Priority Concepts: Coping; Reproduction

Answer: 2
Rationale: The client is putting the blame for the diabetes on herself, thus lowering her self-esteem. She is expressing fear and grief. There are no data in the question to support the problems in options 1 and 4. Client lack of understanding is important to consider, but not at this time because the client will not be able to comprehend information in her current state.
Priority Nursing Tip: Gestational diabetes occurs in pregnancy in clients not previously diagnosed as diabetic and occurs when the pancreas cannot respond to the demand for more insulin.
Test-Taking Strategy: Focus on the subject, the appropriate problem for the client situation described in the question. Note the words *what have I done*. Options 1, 3, and 4 do not address the concerns the client is having. Review: **low self-esteem.**
Reference(s): Lowdermilk, Perry, Cashion, Alden (2012), p. 703.

925. A client says to the nurse, "I'm going to die, and I wish my family would stop hoping for a cure! I get so angry when they carry on like this! After all, I'm the one who's dying." Which therapeutic response should the nurse make to the client?
1. "Have you shared your feelings with your family?"
2. "I think we should talk more about your anger at your family."
3. "You're feeling angry that your family continues to hope for you to be cured?"
4. "Well, it sounds like you're being pretty pessimistic. After all, years ago people died of pneumonia."

Level of Cognitive Ability: Applying
Client Needs: Psychosocial Integrity
Integrated Process: Caring
Content Area: Mental Health
Priority Concepts: Communication; Coping

Answer: 3
Rationale: Reflection is the therapeutic communication technique that redirects the client's feelings back at the client to validate what the client is saying. Option 3 uses the therapeutic technique of reflection. In option 1, the nurse is attempting to assess the client's ability to openly discuss feelings with family members. In option 2, the nurse attempts to use focusing, but the attempt to discuss central issues seems premature. In option 4, the nurse makes a judgment, and this is not therapeutic in the one-to-one relationship. Although this is an appropriate assessment for this client, the timing is somewhat premature, and it closes off the facilitation of the client's feelings.
Priority Nursing Tip: Successful communication includes appropriateness, efficiency, flexibility, and feedback. Communication also needs to be goal-directed within a professional framework.
Test-Taking Strategy: Use therapeutic communication techniques to answer the question. Option 3 is the only choice that uses a therapeutic technique. Also, note the word *angry* in the question and the correct option. Review: the technique of **reflection.**
Reference(s): Fortinash, Holoday-Worret (2012), pp. 71-74; Varcarolis (2013), pp. 121-123.

926. The nurse is caring for a client who says, "I don't want to talk with you because you're only the nurse. I'll wait for my doctor." What should the nurse say in response to the client?

1. "I'm angry with the way you dismissed me."
2. "I understand. So should I call your health care provider?"
3. "Your health care provider directs me in your nursing care."
4. "So then, you would prefer to speak with your health care provider?"

Level of Cognitive Ability: Applying
Client Needs: Psychosocial Integrity
Integrated Process: Communication and Documentation
Content Area: Mental Health
Priority Concepts: Communication; Professionalism

Answer: 2
Rationale: The nurse uses techniques of therapeutic communication to reflect the client's statement (option 2), redirect feelings back to the client for validation, and focus on the client's desire to talk with the doctor. Options 1 and 3 are nontherapeutic responses and are defensive responses. Option 4 reinforces the client's behavior and does not encourage client expression of feelings.
Priority Nursing Tip: Communication includes both verbal and nonverbal expression. Anxiety in the nurse or client may impede communication.
Test-Taking Strategy: Use therapeutic communication techniques. Option 2 is the only therapeutic response. This response focuses on the client's concern and reflects back the statement made by the client. Review: **therapeutic communication techniques.**
Reference(s): Fortinash, Holoday-Worret (2012), pp. 71-74; Stuart (2013), pp. 27-28.

927. A client is awaiting surgery for the removal of a pancreatic mass, and she tells the nurse that she is scared that she will not wake up after receiving the anesthesia. Which therapeutic response should the nurse make to the client?

1. "This is a very common concern."
2. "Tell me what makes you feel concerned about the anesthesia."
3. "I had surgery a year ago and was afraid of the same thing. I did just fine."
4. "You have the best anesthesiologist in this hospital. There is no need to be scared."

Level of Cognitive Ability: Applying
Client Needs: Psychosocial Integrity
Integrated Process: Communication and Documentation
Content Area: Fundamental Skills: Perioperative Care
Priority Concepts: Anxiety; Communication

Answer: 2
Rationale: This client is concerned about surgery and is expressing fear about the anesthesia. The therapeutic response to the client is the one that encourages the client to express her concerns. Option 1 is a stereotypical response. Option 3 avoids the client's concern and focuses on the nurse's personal experience. Option 4 also avoids the client's concern.
Priority Nursing Tip: The nurse must keep the client undergoing surgery who has received preoperative medications in bed. The call bell should be placed next to the client, and the client should be instructed not to get out of bed and to call for assistance if needed.
Test-Taking Strategy: Use therapeutic communication techniques, and focus on the client's feelings. The only response that addresses the client's feelings is option 2. Review: **therapeutic communication techniques.**
Reference(s): Ignatavicius, Workman (2013), p. 1333; Potter et al (2013), pp. 320-322.

928. A community health nurse visits a recently widowed retired military man. When the nurse visits, the ordinarily immaculate house is in chaos, the client is disheveled and has an alcohol type of odor on his breath. Which therapeutic statement should the nurse make to the client?

1. "I can see this isn't a good time to visit."
2. "You seem to be having a very troubling time."
3. "Do you think your wife would want you to behave like this?"
4. "What are you doing? How much are you drinking and for how long?"

Level of Cognitive Ability: Applying
Client Needs: Psychosocial Integrity
Integrated Process: Communication and Documentation
Content Area: Mental Health
Priority Concepts: Communication; Coping

Answer: 2
Rationale: The therapeutic statement is the one that helps the client explore his situation and express his feelings. Reflection, by telling the client that the nurse feels that he is experiencing a troubled or difficult time, is empathic, and it will assist the client with beginning to ventilate his feelings. Option 1 uses humor to avoid therapeutic intimacy and effective problem solving. Option 3 uses admonishment and tries to shame the client, which is not therapeutic or professional. This social communication belittles the client, will likely cause anger, and may evoke "acting out" by the client. Option 4 uses social communication.
Priority Nursing Tip: Therapeutic communication techniques should always be used when communicating with the client, family, or significant other.
Test-Taking Strategy: Use therapeutic communication techniques. Remember to focus on the client's behavior and feelings. This will direct you to the correct option. Review: **therapeutic communication techniques.**
Reference(s): Stuart (2013), pp. 27-28.

929. A client says to the nurse, "I don't do anything right. I'm such a loser." Which therapeutic statement should the nurse make to the client?

1. "Everything will get better."
2. "You don't do anything right?"
3. "You do things right all the time."
4. "You are not a loser, you are sick."

Level of Cognitive Ability: Applying
Client Needs: Psychosocial Integrity
Integrated Process: Communication and Documentation
Content Area: Mental Health
Priority Concepts: Communication; Coping

Answer: 2
Rationale: Option 2 provides the client with the opportunity to verbalize. With this statement, the nurse can learn more about what the client really means by the statement. Options 1, 3, and 4 are closed statements and do not encourage the client to explore further.
Priority Nursing Tip: Nontherapeutic communication techniques block the communication process and should never be used by the nurse in the communication process.
Test-Taking Strategy: Use therapeutic communication techniques. Option 2 repeats the client's statement and encourages further communication. Review: **therapeutic communication techniques.**
Reference(s): Stuart (2013), pp. 21-22; Varcarolis (2013), p. 118.

930. A client who is experiencing suicidal thoughts greets the nurse with the following statement, "It just doesn't seem worth it anymore. Why not just end it all?" Which response should the nurse make to further assess the client?

1. "Did you sleep at all last night?"
2. "Tell me what you mean by that."
3. "I know you have had a stressful night."
4. "I'm sure that your family is worried about you."

Level of Cognitive Ability: Applying
Client Needs: Psychosocial Integrity
Integrated Process: Communication and Documentation
Content Area: Mental Health
Priority Concepts: Communication; Safety

Answer: 2
Rationale: Option 2 allows the client the opportunity to tell the nurse more about what his or her current thoughts are. Option 1 changes the subject and may block communication. Although option 3 offers empathy to the client, it does not further assess the client. Option 4 is false reassurance and may block communication.
Priority Nursing Tip: The nurse should develop a contract with the suicide client that is written, dated, and signed, and that indicates alternative behavior at times of suicidal thoughts.
Test-Taking Strategy: Note the words *further assess.* Use the steps of the nursing process and therapeutic communication techniques to select the correct option. Options 3 and 4 can be eliminated first because they do not reflect assessment. Both options 1 and 2 relate to assessment, but option 2 is directly related to the subject of the question, suicide, and is the most therapeutic. Review: **therapeutic communication techniques.**
Reference(s): Fortinash, Holoday-Worret (2012), pp. 71-74, 512; Varcarolis (2013), pp. 436, 440-441.

931. A mother says to the nurse, "I am afraid that my child might have another febrile seizure." Which therapeutic communication statement is **best** for the nurse to make to the mother?

1. "Tell me what frightens you the most about seizures."
2. "Tylenol can prevent another seizure from occurring."
3. "Most children will never experience a second seizure."
4. "Why worry about something that you cannot control?"

Level of Cognitive Ability: Applying
Client Needs: Psychosocial Integrity
Integrated Process: Communication and Documentation
Content Area: Child Health: Neurological
Priority Concepts: Communication; Intracranial Regulation

Answer: 1
Rationale: Option 1 is the only response that is an open-ended statement and that provides the mother with an opportunity to express her feelings. Options 2 and 3 are incorrect because the nurse is giving false reassurance that a seizure will not recur or that it can be prevented in this child. Option 4 is incorrect because it blocks communication by giving a flippant response to an expressed fear.
Priority Nursing Tip: For the client experiencing a seizure, the nurse should ensure airway patency, have suction equipment and oxygen available, time the seizure episode, place a pillow or folded blanket under the client's head, loosen restrictive clothing, remove eyeglasses if present, and clear the area of any hazardous objects.
Test-Taking Strategy: Note the strategic word, *best*, and use therapeutic communication techniques to identify the correct answer. Options 2, 3, and 4 violate the principles of therapeutic communication and actually block communication. Review: **therapeutic communication techniques.**
Reference(s): McKinney et al (2013), pp. 30-31, 1433.

932. A client has just given birth to a newborn who has a cleft lip and palate. When planning to talk to the client, the nurse recognizes that the client needs to **first** work through which emotion before maternal bonding can occur?

1. Guilt
2. Grief
3. Anger
4. Depression

Level of Cognitive Ability: Analyzing
Client Needs: Psychosocial Integrity
Integrated Process: Nursing Process/Planning
Content Area: Maternity: Postpartum
Priority Concepts: Caregiving; Coping

Answer: 2
Rationale: The nurse should recognize that a mother will go through the grief process after giving birth to a child with a birth defect. Following the grief process, the mother can begin to focus on bonding with the infant. Options 1, 3, and 4 are incorrect because they are each only one component of the grief process.
Priority Nursing Tip: The nurse's role in the grief and loss process includes communicating with the client and family members. The nurse must consider the client's culture, religion, family structure, individual life experiences, coping skills, and support systems.
Test-Taking Strategy: Note the strategic word, *first*. Options 1, 3, and 4 are incorrect because they are each only one component of the grief process. Review: the **grief process.**
Reference(s): McKinney et al (2013), pp. 1072-1074.

933. An infant who has been diagnosed with acute chalasia is admitted to the hospital. During the nursing history, the mother tells the nurse, "I am concerned that I am somehow causing my infant to vomit after feeding her." Considering this statement, which problem should the nurse identify for the mother?

1. An unrealistic expectation of self
2. Denial that chalasia is a physiological defect
3. Lack of understanding about feeding an infant with chalasia
4. Anxiety about the need for hospitalization of the infant for chalasia

Level of Cognitive Ability: Analyzing
Client Needs: Psychosocial Integrity
Integrated Process: Nursing Process/Analysis
Content Area: Child Health: Gastrointestinal
Priority Concepts: Family Dynamics; Professionalism

Answer: 1
Rationale: The infant is vomiting because of a physiological problem that is not caused by the mother. The misconception that the mother is responsible for the problem is an unrealistic expectation of self and may result in the mother having a decreased perception of her ability to adequately parent the child. The nurse should assist the mother with understanding that she is not responsible for the child's condition. There are no data in the question to support that the mother is experiencing denial that chalasia is a physiological defect. There are insufficient data to support that the mother lacks understanding on feeding techniques for a child with chalasia. The mother's statement does not reflect symptoms of anxiety regarding the child's hospitalization. The mother states a concern regarding her own behavior.
Priority Nursing Tip: Chalasia occurs when there is an abnormal relaxation of a body orifice, such as the cardiac sphincter. This disorder is commonly associated with gastroesophageal reflux disease (GERD).
Test-Taking Strategy: Focus on the subject, that the mother is blaming herself for the child's health problem. The only option that relates to this subject is option 1. Review: psychosocial **parental reactions** to a child's illness.
Reference(s): Hockenberry, Wilson (2013), pp. 617, 781-782.

934. A client who experienced a myocardial infarction (MI) 4 days ago refuses to dangle at the bedside, saying, "If my doctor tells me to do it, I will. Otherwise, I won't." What behavior should the nurse determine that the client is likely displaying?

1. Anger
2. Denial
3. Depression
4. Dependency

Level of Cognitive Ability: Analyzing
Client Needs: Psychosocial Integrity
Integrated Process: Nursing Process/Assessment
Content Area: Adult Health: Cardiovascular
Priority Concepts: Coping; Perfusion

Answer: 4
Rationale: Clients may experience numerous emotional and behavioral responses after an MI. Dependency is one response that may be manifested by the client's refusal to perform any tasks or activities unless specifically approved by the health care provider. Although the client's statement may express anger to some degree, it most specifically addresses dependency. There are no data in the question to support denial or depression.
Priority Nursing Tip: Dependency is evident when the client who sustained a myocardial infarction is totally reliant on staff or others, prefers to be monitored by electrocardiogram (ECG) at all times, and is hesitant to leave the cardiac nursing unit or the hospital.
Test-Taking Strategy: Focus on the subject of a client who refuses to perform tasks after an MI. Begin by eliminating options 2 and 3 because the client is not exhibiting signs of denial or depression. From the remaining options, focus on the client's statement to direct you to option 4. Review: psychosocial reactions after **myocardial infarction** and **dependency**.
Reference(s): Lewis et al (2011), p. 789.

935. The nurse is assessing a 45-year-old client who was admitted to the hospital for urinary calculi. The client received 4 mg of morphine sulfate approximately 2 hours previously. The client states to the nurse, "I'm scared to death that it'll come back. That was the worst pain I ever had. Like a knife going from my right side to my groin." Based on these statements, which problem should the nurse identify for this client at this time?

1. Pain from the calculus in right ureter
2. Lack of understanding about the disease process
3. Anxiety about the anticipation of recurrent severe pain
4. Retention of urine from the obstruction of the urinary tract by calculi

Level of Cognitive Ability: Analyzing
Client Needs: Psychosocial Integrity
Integrated Process: Nursing Process/Analysis
Content Area: Adult Health: Renal and Urinary
Priority Concepts: Anxiety; Clinical Judgment

Answer: 3
Rationale: The client stated, "I'm scared to death that it'll come back." The anticipation of the recurring pain produces anxiety and threatens the client's psychological integrity. There is no evidence that the client has a calculus in the right ureter. There is also no evidence that the client has lack of knowledge or urinary retention.
Priority Nursing Tip: Problems resulting from urinary calculi are pain, obstruction, tissue trauma, secondary hemorrhage, and infection.
Test-Taking Strategy: Focus on the subject, the appropriate client problem based on the client's statement. Note the words *I'm scared to death that it'll come back*, and note the relationship of these words to option 3. Review: the characteristics of **urinary calculi** and **anxiety**.
Reference(s): Ignatavicius, Workman (2013), pp. 49, 1506.

936. The nurse is observing the parents at the bedside of their small-for-gestational-age (SGA) infant, who was born at 27 weeks' gestation. The infant's mother states, "She is so tiny and fragile. I'll never be able to hold her with all those tubes." Considering this statement, which problem should the nurse identify for the mother?

1. Impaired adjustment
2. Trouble with family coping
3. Potential for compromised parenting
4. Difficulty monitoring signs of respiratory difficulty

Level of Cognitive Ability: Analyzing
Client Needs: Psychosocial Integrity
Integrated Process: Nursing Process/Analysis
Content Area: Maternity: Postpartum
Priority Concepts: Coping; Family Dynamics

Answer: 3
Rationale: Parents of a high-risk neonate, such as a preterm SGA infant, are at risk for compromised parenting. Parent–infant bonding is affected if the infant does not exhibit normal newborn characteristics. Option 1 involves the nonacceptance of a health status change or an inability to solve a problem or set a goal. Option 2 involves the identification of trouble with family coping. Option 4 addresses the nurse's role in caring for the infant.
Priority Nursing Tip: For the infant who is small for gestational age, the nurse must maintain airway patency and cardiopulmonary function and maintain the infant's body temperature.
Test-Taking Strategy: Focus on the subject, the appropriate client problem based on the client's statement. Eliminate option 4 first because this is not a role of the parent and is a nursing function. Note the words *"I'll never be able to hold her."* This should assist with directing you to compromised parenting. Review: the psychosocial parental concerns for a **small-for-gestational-age infant.**
Reference(s): McKinney et al (2013), pp. 704, 711-712.

937. A client has just delivered a large-for-gestational-age (LGA) infant by the vaginal route. The client verbalizes concern regarding the infant's facial bruising and causing pain to the site if touched. Which therapeutic statement should the nurse make to alleviate the client's concerns?

1. "I can show you how to gently stroke the face and not cause pain."
2. "It is a normal finding in large babies and nothing to be concerned about."
3. "The bruising is caused by polycythemia, which usually leads to jaundice."
4. "Because the bruising is painful, it is advisable that you not touch the baby's face."

Level of Cognitive Ability: Applying
Client Needs: Psychosocial Integrity
Integrated Process: Nursing Process/Implementation
Content Area: Maternity: Postpartum
Priority Concepts: Communication; Pain

Answer: 1
Rationale: The mother of an LGA infant with facial bruising may be reluctant to interact with the infant because of concern about causing additional pain to the infant. The bruising is temporary. Option 2 does not address the mother's verbalized concerns. The LGA infant may have polycythemia, which can contribute to bruising, but the bruising is not actually caused by the polycythemia. Option 4 advises the mother not to touch the baby's face because the bruising is painful, but touch is an important component of the attachment process. Touching the infant gently with the fingertips should be encouraged.
Priority Nursing Tip: For the infant that is large for gestational age, the nurse should monitor vital signs, monitor blood glucose levels and for signs of hypoglycemia, and initiate early feedings.
Test-Taking Strategy: Note the subject, causing pain to infant's facial bruising if touched and alleviating the client's concern. Eliminate options 2 and 3 first because they do not specifically address the subject of touch. From the remaining options, note the relationship of the word *touch* in the question and the word *stroke* in the correct option. Review: **mother–infant bonding.**
Reference(s): Lowdermilk, Perry, Cashion, Alden (2012), p. 508; McKinney et al (2013), pp. 704, 712.

938. A client with myasthenia gravis is ready to return home. The client confides that she is concerned that her husband will no longer find her physically attractive. What should the nurse include in the plan of care?

1. Encourage the client to start a support group.
2. Tell the client to stop dwelling on the negative.
3. Insist that the client reach out and face this fear.
4. Encourage the client to share her feelings with her husband.

Level of Cognitive Ability: Applying
Client Needs: Psychosocial Integrity
Integrated Process: Caring
Content Area: Adult Health: Neurological
Priority Concepts: Communication; Sexuality

Answer: 4
Rationale: Talking to the client about sharing her feelings with her husband directly addresses the subject of the question. Encouraging the client to start a support group will not address the client's immediate and individual concerns. Options 2 and 3 are blocks to communication and avoid the client's concern.
Priority Nursing Tip: Myasthenia gravis is a neuromuscular disease characterized by considerable weakness and abnormal fatigue of the voluntary muscles. A defect in the transmission of nerve impulses at the myoneural junction occurs.
Test-Taking Strategy: Focus on the subject, the concerns of a client with myasthenia gravis, and use therapeutic communication techniques. Option 4 is the only option that addresses the client's immediate concern. Remember to address the client's feelings and concerns first. Review: **therapeutic communication techniques.**
Reference(s): Ignatavicius, Workman (2013), p. 996; Potter et al (2013), pp. 320-322.

939. A 9-year-old child is hospitalized for 2 months after a car accident. Which intervention should the nurse plan to use to **best** promote psychosocial development?

1. Providing a portable media player (MP3)
2. Tutoring to keep the child up with schoolwork
3. Providing a phone for calling family and friends
4. Placing computer games, a television, and videos at the bedside

Level of Cognitive Ability: Applying
Client Needs: Psychosocial Integrity
Integrated Process: Nursing Process/Planning
Content Area: Developmental Stages: Infancy to Adolescence
Priority Concepts: Development; Health Promotion

Answer: 2
Rationale: The developmental task of the school-age child is industry versus inferiority. The child achieves success by mastering skills and knowledge. Maintaining schoolwork provides for accomplishment and prevents feelings of inferiority that may be caused by lagging behind the rest of the class. The other options provide diversion and are of lesser importance for a child of this age.
Priority Nursing Tip: For the school-age child, the nurse should use photographs, books, dolls, and videos to explain medical procedures.
Test-Taking Strategy: Note the strategic word, *best*. Note the words *psychosocial development* in the query of the question. Note the age of the child, and determine the developmental task for this child. Options 1, 3, and 4 address social and diversional issues, whereas option 2 specifically addresses psychosocial development. Review: psychosocial development of the **school-age child.**
Reference(s): McKinney et al (2013), p. 884.

940. A client who is in halo traction says to the visiting nurse, "I can't get used to this contraption. I can't see properly on the side, and I keep misjudging where everything is." Which therapeutic response should the nurse make to the client?

1. "If I were you, I would have had the surgery rather than suffer like this."
2. "No one ever gets used to that thing! It's horrible. Many of our sports people who are in it complain vigorously."
3. "Halo traction involves many difficult adjustments. Practice scanning with your eyes after standing up and before you move around."
4. "Why do you feel like this when you could have died from a broken neck? This is the way it is for several months. You need to be more accepting, don't you think?"

Level of Cognitive Ability: Applying
Client Needs: Psychosocial Integrity
Integrated Process: Nursing Process/Implementation
Content Area: Adult Health: Neurological
Priority Concepts: Communication; Mobility

Answer: 3

Rationale: In option 3, the nurse employs empathy and reflection. The nurse then offers a strategy for problem solving, which helps increase the peripheral vision of the client in halo traction. In option 1, the nurse undermines the client's faith in the medical treatment being employed by giving advice that is insensitive and unprofessional. In option 2, the nurse provides a social response that contains emotionally charged language that could increase the client's anxiety. In option 4, the nurse uses excessive questioning and gives advice, which is nontherapeutic.

Priority Nursing Tip: Halo traction involves the insertion of pins or screws into the client's skull and application of a circular fixation device and halo jacket or cast; it is used to immobilize the cervical spine. The nurse should instruct the client to notify the health care provider if the halo vest or ring bolts loosen.

Test-Taking Strategy: Seek the option that represents a therapeutic communication technique. Focus on the client's statement, and note that option 3 is the only statement that addresses the client's concern. Review: **therapeutic communication techniques.**

Reference(s): Ignatavicius, Workman (2013), pp. 971, 975; Potter et al (2013), pp. 320-322.

941. An older client has been admitted to the hospital with a hip fracture. The nurse prepares a plan of care for the client and identifies desired outcomes related to surgery and impaired physical mobility. Which statement by the client supports a positive adjustment to the surgery and impairment in mobility?

1. "Hurry up and go away. I want to be alone."
2. "What took you so long? I called for you 30 minutes ago."
3. "I wish you nurses would leave me alone! You are all telling me what to do!"
4. "I find it difficult to concentrate since the surgeon talked with me about the surgery tomorrow."

Level of Cognitive Ability: Evaluating
Client Needs: Psychosocial Integrity
Integrated Process: Nursing Process/Evaluation
Content Area: Adult Health: Musculoskeletal
Priority Concepts: Coping; Mobility

Answer: 4

Rationale: Option 4 reflects an individual with moderate anxiety caused by a difficulty to concentrate. It most appropriately supports a positive adjustment. Option 1 demonstrates withdrawal behavior. Option 2 is a demanding response. Option 3 demonstrates acting out by the client. Demanding, acting out, and withdrawn clients have not coped with or adjusted to the injury or disease.

Priority Nursing Tip: Common fears before surgery include fear of death, fear of pain and discomfort, fear of mutilation or alteration in body image, fear of anesthesia, and fear of disruption of life functioning or patterns.

Test-Taking Strategy: Focus on the subject, positive adjustment to surgery and impairment in mobility. You should easily be able to eliminate options 1, 2, and 3. Remember that age and impaired mobility in combination with medications often contribute to anxiety and difficulty concentrating. Review: **hip fracture** surgery.

Reference(s): Ignatavicius, Workman (2013), p. 321.

942. A client who is quadriplegic frequently makes lewd sexual suggestions and uses profanity. The nurse interprets that the client is inappropriately using displacement. Which problem should the nurse identify as being appropriate for this client?
1. Disuse syndrome
2. Lack of coping skills
3. Negative body image
4. Lack of awareness of surroundings

Level of Cognitive Ability: Analyzing
Client Needs: Psychosocial Integrity
Integrated Process: Nursing Process/Analysis
Content Area: Mental Health
Priority Concepts: Clinical Judgment; Coping

Answer: 2
Rationale: Lack of coping skills is evident when the client demonstrates an impaired ability to adapt to meeting life's demands and roles. This client is displacing feelings onto the environment instead of using them in a constructive fashion. Option 3 may be appropriate, but it has nothing to do with the displacement that the client is currently using. Options 1 and 4 have no relation to this situation.
Priority Nursing Tip: When using displacement as a defense mechanism, the person's feelings toward one person are directed to another who is less threatening to satisfy an impulse with a substitute object.
Test-Taking Strategy: Note that the question addresses the subject of the defense mechanism of displacement. Focus on the information in the subject and remember that the use of displacement indicates lack of coping skills. This will direct you to the correct option. Review: displacement and defense **mechanisms.**
Reference(s): Fortinash, Holoday-Worret (2012), p. 185; Stuart (2013), p. 228.

943. The nurse in the newborn nursery is caring for a preterm infant. Which is the **best** method the nurse can use to assist the parents with developing attachment behaviors?
1. Place family pictures within the infant's view.
2. Encourage the parents to touch and speak to their infant.
3. Report only positive qualities and progress to the parents.
4. Provide information regarding infant development and stimulation.

Level of Cognitive Ability: Applying
Client Needs: Psychosocial Integrity
Integrated Process: Nursing Process/Implementation
Content Area: Maternity: Newborn
Priority Concepts: Caregiving; Family Dynamics

Answer: 2
Rationale: Parents' involvement through touch and voice establishes and initiates the bonding process in the parent–infant relationship. Their active participation builds their confidence and supports the parenting role. Family pictures are ineffective for an infant. Providing information and emphasizing only positives are not incorrect actions, but they do not relate to the attachment process.
Priority Nursing Tip: The primary concern for preterm infants is immaturity of all body systems.
Test-Taking Strategy: Note the strategic word, *best*. Focus on the subject, attachment behaviors. The only option that addresses attachment behaviors is option 2. Review: the measures that promote parent–infant bonding.
Reference(s): McKinney et al (2013), pp. 460-461.

944. A 16-year-old child is admitted to the hospital with hyperglycemia as a result of a failure to follow the diet, insulin, and glucose monitoring regimen. The child states, "I'm fed up with having my life ruled by doctors' prescriptions and machines!" Which is the **priority** client problem?
1. A chronic illness
2. A personal crisis
3. Feelings of loss of control
4. Lack of understanding about nutrition

Level of Cognitive Ability: Analyzing
Client Needs: Psychosocial Integrity
Integrated Process: Nursing Process/Analysis
Content Area: Developmental Stages: Infancy to Adolescence
Priority Concepts: Adherence; Development

Answer: 3
Rationale: Adolescents strive for identity and independence, and the situation describes a common fear of loss of control. Therefore, the priority problem relates to these feelings of loss of control. Although the child has a chronic illness and may be experiencing a personal crisis, the child's statement focuses on loss of control. There is no information in the question that indicates a lack of knowledge.
Priority Nursing Tip: The adolescent may be preoccupied with body image, and the nurse should encourage and support independence.
Test-Taking Strategy: Note the strategic word, *priority*. Focus on the information in the question and the child's statement to direct you to the correct option. Review: The developmental characteristics of the adolescent.
Reference(s): Hockenberry, Wilson (2013), p. 1614; McKinney et al (2013), p. 1401.

945. The client angrily tells the nurse that the health care provider (HCP) purposefully provided incorrect information. Which response to the client would hinder therapeutic communication?

1. "I'm certain that the HCP would not lie to you."
2. "I'm not sure what information you are referring to."
3. "Can you describe the information that you are referring to?"
4. "Do you think it would be helpful to talk to your doctor about this?"

Level of Cognitive Ability: Applying
Client Needs: Psychosocial Integrity
Integrated Process: Communication and Documentation
Content Area: Mental Health
Priority Concepts: Communication; Professionalism

Answer: 1
Rationale: Option 1 hinders communication by disagreeing with the client. This technique could make the client defensive and block further communication. Options 2 and 3 attempt to clarify the information to which the client is referring. Option 4 attempts to explore whether the client is comfortable talking to the HCP about this issue and encourages direct confrontation.
Priority Nursing Tip: Agreeing or disagreeing with the client is a nontherapeutic communication technique.
Test-Taking Strategy: Focus on the subject, the response that would hinder communication. Disagreeing with or challenging a client's response will hinder or block therapeutic communication. Review: **therapeutic communication techniques.**
References: Fortinash, Holoday-Worret (2012), pp. 71-74, 77, 80; Stuart (2013), p. 24.

946. A client with a diagnosis of depression says to the nurse, "I should have died. I've always been a failure." Which therapeutic response should the nurse make to the client?

1. "I see a lot of positive things in you."
2. "You still have a great deal to live for."
3. "Feeling like a failure is part of your illness."
4. "You've been feeling like a failure for some time now?"

Level of Cognitive Ability: Applying
Client Needs: Psychosocial Integrity
Integrated Process: Communication and Documentation
Content Area: Mental Health
Priority Concepts: Communication; Mood and Affect

Answer: 4
Rationale: Responding to the feelings expressed by a client is an effective therapeutic communication technique. The correct option is an example of the use of restating. Options 1, 2, and 3 block communication because they minimize the client's experience and do not facilitate the exploration of the client's expressed feelings.
Priority Nursing Tip: Any client with depression needs to be carefully assessed for a risk for suicide.
Test-Taking Strategy: Use therapeutic communication techniques to answer this question. Remember to address the client's feelings and concerns. Option 4 is the only option that is stated in the form of a question and that is open-ended, thus encouraging the verbalization of feelings. Review: **therapeutic communication techniques.**
Reference(s): Fortinash, Holoday-Worret (2012), pp. 71-74, 504; Varcarolis (2013), p. 253.

947. Two months after a right mastectomy for breast cancer, a client comes to the office for a follow-up appointment. After being diagnosed with cancer in the right breast, the client was told that the risk for cancer in the left breast existed. When asked about her breast self-examination (BSE) practices since the surgery, the client replied, "I don't need to do that anymore." The nurse interprets this response as which coping mechanism?

1. Denial
2. Grief and mourning
3. Change in body image
4. Change in role pattern

Level of Cognitive Ability: Analyzing
Client Needs: Psychosocial Integrity
Integrated Process: Nursing Process/Analysis
Content Area: Adult Health: Oncology
Priority Concepts: Cellular Regulation; Coping

Answer: 1
Rationale: The coping strategy of denying or minimizing a health problem can produce health situations that may be life threatening. Denial can lead to an avoidance of self-care measures, such as taking medications or performing a BSE. Options 2, 3, and 4 are unrelated to the client's statement.
Priority Nursing Tip: Denial is the disowning of consciously intolerable thoughts and impulses.
Test-Taking Strategy: Focus on the subject, the coping mechanism that the client is using. Note the words "*I don't need to do that anymore.*" Eliminate options 2, 3, and 4 because they are not directly related to the client's statement. Review: the indicators of **denial.**
Reference(s): Ignatavicius, Workman (2013), pp. 1598-1599; Potter et al (2013), p. 333.

948. When planning for the care of the client who is dying of cancer, one of the goals is that the client verbalizes his or her acceptance of impending death. Which client statement indicates to the nurse that this goal has been reached?

1. "I just want to live until my 100th birthday."
2. "I would like to have my family here when I die."
3. "I'll be ready to die when my children finish school."
4. "I want to go to my daughter's wedding. Then I'll be ready to die."

Level of Cognitive Ability: Evaluating
Client Needs: Psychosocial Integrity
Integrated Process: Nursing Process/Evaluation
Content Area: Developmental Stages: End-of-Life Care
Priority Concepts: Caregiving; Coping

Answer: 2

Rationale: Acceptance is often characterized by plans for death. Often the client wants loved ones nearby. Options 1, 3, and 4 all reflect the bargaining stage of coping during which the client tries to negotiate with his or her higher power or fate.

Priority Nursing Tip: Outcomes related to care during illness and the dying experience should be based on the client's wishes.

Test-Taking Strategy: Note that options 1, 3, and 4 are comparable or alike. These options all demonstrate negotiating for something else to happen before death occurs. Option 2 is different, and it is the option that reflects acceptance. Review: the stages of death and dying.

Reference(s): Potter et al (2013), pp. 720-722.

949. The nurse is caring for a client with cancer who has a problem with negative body perception related to alopecia. What should the nurse plan to focus on with the client?

1. The importance of rinsing the mouth after eating
2. The use of cosmetics to hide drug-induced rashes
3. The use of wigs, which are often covered by insurance
4. Proper dental hygiene with the use of a foam toothbrush

Level of Cognitive Ability: Applying
Client Needs: Psychosocial Integrity
Integrated Process: Nursing Process/Implementation
Content Area: Adult Health: Oncology
Priority Concepts: Cellular Regulation; Coping

Answer: 3

Rationale: The temporary or permanent thinning or loss of hair, known as alopecia, is common among clients with cancer who are receiving chemotherapy. This often causes a body image disturbance that can be easily addressed with the use of wigs, hats, or scarves. Options 1, 2, and 4 are all unrelated to alopecia.

Priority Nursing Tip: The nurse should provide the client with alopecia from chemotherapy with information on purchasing a wig. The nurse should also inform the client that the hair will grow back, but may be a different color and texture.

Test-Taking Strategy: Focus on the subject of alopecia. Recalling that alopecia refers to hair loss will direct you to the correct option. Review: the interventions used to treat alopecia.

Reference(s): Ignatavicius, Workman (2013), pp. 422-424.

950. A client with hyperaldosteronism has developed kidney failure and says to the nurse, "This means that I will die very soon." What is the appropriate response for the nurse to make to the client?

1. "You will do just fine."
2. "What are you thinking about?"
3. "You sound discouraged today."
4. "I read that death is a beautiful experience."

Level of Cognitive Ability: Applying
Client Needs: Psychosocial Integrity
Integrated Process: Communication and Documentation
Content Area: Adult Health: Endocrine
Priority Concepts: Communication; Coping

Answer: 3

Rationale: Option 3 uses the therapeutic communication technique of reflection, and it both clarifies and encourages the further expression of the client's feelings. Options 1 and 4 deny the client's concerns and provide false reassurance. Option 2 requests an explanation and does not encourage the expression of feelings.

Priority Nursing Tip: The signs and symptoms of acute kidney injury are primarily caused by the retention of nitrogenous wastes, the retention of fluids, and the inability of the kidneys to regulate electrolytes. Kidney failure affects all major body systems and may require dialysis to maintain life.

Test-Taking Strategy: Use therapeutic communication techniques. Note that option 3 facilitates the client's expression of feelings. Remember to focus on the client's feelings. Review: therapeutic communication techniques.

Reference(s): Ignatavicius, Workman (2013), p. 1390; Potter et al (2013), pp. 320-322.

951. A client with diabetes mellitus has expressed frustration with learning the diabetic regimen and insulin administration. Which should be the **initial** action by the home care nurse?
1. Attempt to identify the cause of the frustration.
2. Call the health care provider to discuss the termination of home care services.
3. Offer to administer the insulin on a daily basis until the client is ready to learn.
4. Continue with diabetic teaching, knowing that the client will overcome any frustrations.

Level of Cognitive Ability: Applying
Client Needs: Psychosocial Integrity
Integrated Process: Teaching and Learning
Content Area: Adult Health: Endocrine
Priority Concepts: Client Education; Glucose Regulation

Answer: 1
Rationale: The home care nurse must determine what is causing the client's frustration. Terminating the client from home care services achieves nothing and is considered abandonment unless other follow-up care is arranged. Administering the insulin provides only a short-term solution. Continuing to teach may only further block the learning process.
Priority Nursing Tip: The nurse should assist the client in making the necessary lifestyle adjustments to manage diabetes mellitus.
Test-Taking Strategy: Note the strategic word, *initial* as you select your answer. Use the steps of the nursing process. Assessment is the first step. Of the options presented, options 2, 3, and 4 represent implementation phases of the nursing process. The only assessment option is option 1. Review: **teaching and learning principles** and **diabetes mellitus**.
Reference(s): Ignatavicius, Workman (2013), pp. 1436-1437, 1453; Potter et al (2013), pp. 329-330, 333.

952. A client with cancer is placed on permanent total parenteral nutrition as a means of providing nutrition. Why should the nurse include psychosocial support when planning care for this client?
1. Death is imminent.
2. The client will need to adjust to the idea of living without eating by the usual route.
3. Total parenteral nutrition requires disfiguring surgery for permanent port implantation.
4. Nausea and vomiting occur regularly with this type of treatment and will prevent the client from participating in social activity.

Level of Cognitive Ability: Applying
Client Needs: Psychosocial Integrity
Integrated Process: Nursing Process/Planning
Content Area: Adult Health: Oncology
Priority Concepts: Coping; Nutrition

Answer: 2
Rationale: Permanent total parenteral nutrition is indicated for clients who can no longer absorb nutrients via the enteral route. These clients will no longer take nutrition orally. Options 1, 3, and 4 are inaccurate. There is no indication in the question that death is imminent. Permanent port implantation is not disfiguring. Total parenteral nutrition does not cause nausea and vomiting.
Priority Nursing Tip: Total parenteral nutrition is the administration of a nutritionally complete formula through a central or peripheral intravenous catheter.
Test-Taking Strategy: Focus on the subject, psychosocial support for the client receiving total parenteral nutrition. Note the words *permanent* and *as a means of providing nutrition* in the question, and note the relationship between these words and option 2. Option 2 states *living without eating by the usual route*. Also, knowledge regarding total parenteral nutrition therapy will assist you with eliminating options 1, 3, and 4. Review: **total parenteral nutrition**.
Reference(s): Ignatavicius, Workman (2013), pp. 1348-1349; Potter et al (2013), p. 904.

953. A client who is to be discharged to home with a temporary colostomy says to the nurse, "I know I've changed this thing once, but I just don't know how I'll do it by myself when I'm home alone. Can't I stay here until the surgeon puts it back?" Which therapeutic response should the nurse make to the client?

1. "This is only temporary, but you need to hire a nurse companion until your surgery."
2. "So you're saying that, although you've practiced changing your colostomy bag once, you don't feel comfortable on your own yet?"
3. "Well, your insurance will not pay for a longer stay just to practice changing your colostomy, so you'll have to fight it out with them."
4. "Going home to care for yourself still feels pretty overwhelming? I will schedule you for home visits until you're feeling more comfortable."

Level of Cognitive Ability: Applying
Client Needs: Psychosocial Integrity
Integrated Process: Nursing Process/Implementation
Content Area: Adult Health: Gastrointestinal
Priority Concepts: Anxiety; Communication

Answer: 4
Rationale: The client is expressing feelings of fear and helplessness. Option 4 assists with meeting this client's needs. Option 1 provides information that the client already knows and then problem solves by using a client-centered action, which would probably overwhelm the client. Option 2 is restating, but this response could cause the client to feel more helpless because the client's fears are reflected back to the client. Option 3 provides what is probably accurate information, but the words "just to practice" can be interpreted by the client as belittling.
Priority Nursing Tip: For the client with a colostomy, the nurse should monitor stoma color. A dark blue, purple, or black stoma indicates compromised circulation, requiring health care provider notification.
Test-Taking Strategy: Use therapeutic communication techniques, and focus on the subject of the question, fear of being discharged home without help. This will eliminate options 1 and 3. From the remaining options, remember the subject of the question, and address the client's feelings and concerns. Option 2 is restating, but this intervention could cause the client to feel more helpless. Option 4 addresses the client's fear and dependency (helplessness) needs. Review: therapeutic communication techniques.
Reference(s): Ignatavicius, Workman (2013), p. 1253; Potter et al (2013), pp. 320-322.

954. The parents of a newborn infant with congenital hypothyroidism and Down syndrome tell the nurse how despondent they are that their child was born with these problems. They had many plans for a normal child, and now these will need to be adjusted. On the basis of these statements, the nurse identifies which problem for the parents?

1. Inability to cope with change
2. Anger about lost opportunities
3. Trouble adjusting to a child born with medical issues
4. Depression associated with the birth of a child with defects

Level of Cognitive Ability: Analyzing
Client Needs: Psychosocial Integrity
Integrated Process: Nursing Process/Analysis
Content Area: Maternity: Newborn
Priority Concepts: Coping; Mood and Affect

Answer: 4
Rationale: Depression is a normal part of the grieving process. It is a reaction to practical implications related to loss. The grief process includes intellectual and emotional responses and behaviors by which individuals and families work through the process of modifying their self-concepts on the basis of the perception of potential loss. Characteristics include expressions of sorrow and distress at the potential loss. While the parents may have trouble adjusting and have anger, the best answer is to address their depression and sadness.
Priority Nursing Tip: Down syndrome is a congenital condition that results in moderate to severe retardation and has been linked to an extra G chromosome, chromosome 21 (trisomy 21).
Test-Taking Strategy: Focus on the subject, the appropriate problem based on the parent's statement. Noting the words *how despondent they are* should lead you to the answer regarding depression. Review: depression.
Reference(s): Hockenberry, Wilson (2013), pp. 338-340; Lowdermilk, Perry, Cashion, Alden (2012), pp. 913, 927.

955. The nurse is caring for a client who has been diagnosed with schizophrenia. The client is unable to speak, although there is no known pathological dysfunction. What type of dysfunctional communication is the client experiencing?
1. Mutism
2. Verbigeration
3. Pressured speech
4. Poverty of speech

Level of Cognitive Ability: Analyzing
Client Needs: Psychosocial Integrity
Integrated Process: Communication and Documentation
Content Area: Mental Health
Priority Concepts: Communication; Psychosis

Answer: 1
Rationale: Mutism is the absence of verbal speech. The client does not communicate verbally despite an intact physical and structural ability to speak. Verbigeration is the purposeless repetition of words or phrases. Pressured speech refers to a rapidity of speech that reflects the client's racing thoughts. Poverty of speech involves diminished amounts of speech or monotonic replies.
Priority Nursing Tip: Clients with schizophrenia may experience hallucinations. For a client with hallucinations, safety is the first priority; the nurse should ensure that the client does not have an auditory command telling him or her to harm self or others.
Test-Taking Strategy: Focus on the subject, an inability to speak. This should assist you with eliminating options 2 and 3. From the remaining options, recalling that poverty of speech indicates a diminished amount of speech will assist you with eliminating option 4. Review: **schizophrenia** and **altered speech patterns.**
Reference(s): Stuart (2013), p. 362; Varcarolis (2013), p. 305.

956. A client tells the nurse, "I am a spy for the FBI. I am an eye, an eye in the sky." Which abnormal thought process is the client exhibiting?
1. Echolalia
2. Word salad
3. Clang associations
4. Loosened associations

Level of Cognitive Ability: Analyzing
Client Needs: Psychosocial Integrity
Integrated Process: Nursing Process/Analysis
Content Area: Mental Health
Priority Concepts: Communication; Psychosis

Answer: 3
Rationale: The repetition of words or phrases that are similar in sound and in no other way (rhyming) is one altered thought and language pattern seen in clients with schizophrenia. Clang associations often take the form of rhyming. Echolalia is the involuntary parrot-like repetition of words spoken by others. Word salad is the use of words with no apparent meaning attached to them or to their relationship to one another. Loosened associations occur when the individual speaks with frequent changes of subject and when the content is only obliquely related.
Priority Nursing Tip: Abnormal thought processes displayed by the mentally ill client occur as a result of the psychiatric disorder.
Test-Taking Strategy: Focus on the subject, the abnormal thought process that the client is experiencing. Also, note the client's statement. Recalling that clang associations often take the form of rhyming will direct you to option 3. Review: **schizophrenia, altered thought,** and **language patterns.**
Reference(s): Varcarolis (2013), p. 307.

957. The nurse is planning the hospital discharge of a young client who has been newly diagnosed with type 1 diabetes mellitus. The client tells the nurse that she is concerned about self-administering insulin while in school with other students around. Which statement by the nurse **best** supports the client's need at this time?
1. "Oh, don't worry about that! You'll do fine!"
2. "You could leave school early and take your insulin at home."
3. "You shouldn't be embarrassed by your diabetes. Lots of people have this disease."
4. "You could contact the school nurse, who could provide a private area for you to administer your insulin."

Level of Cognitive Ability: Applying
Client Needs: Psychosocial Integrity
Integrated Process: Nursing Process/Implementation
Content Area: Child Health: Metabolic/Endocrine
Priority Concepts: Coping; Glucose Regulation

Answer: 4
Rationale: When planning this client's role transition, the nurse functions in the role of a problem solver by assisting the client with adapting to his or her illness. In option 4, the nurse offers information that addresses the client's need and that promotes or assists the client with reaching a decision that optimizes a sense of well-being. Options 1 and 3 are inappropriate statements and blocks to communication. Option 2 requires a change in lifestyle.
Priority Nursing Tip: Schools vary with regard to the availability of nursing services. The parents of a child with diabetes mellitus should work with school administration to determine appropriate staff and resources to ensure proper administration of insulin for their child as needed.
Test-Taking Strategy: Note the strategic word, *best.* Use therapeutic communication techniques, and focus on the subject, a concern about self-administering insulin while in school. Options 1 and 3 are comparable or alike because they are nontherapeutic, so eliminate those options first. From the remaining options, select option 4 because it promotes the client's ability to continue the present lifestyle, whereas option 2 requires a change in lifestyle. Review: **developmental stages** and **type 1 diabetes mellitus.**
Reference(s): Hockenberry, Wilson (2013), p. 1006; McKinney et al (2013), pp. 30-31.

958. The nurse prepares a client for a parathyroidectomy when the client states, "I guess I'll have to wear a scarf after this surgery." Considering this statement which problem is appropriate for this client?
1. Denial that the surgery is necessary
2. Trouble coping with the need for surgery
3. Issues with potential changes to body image
4. Anxiety about the scar the surgery will cause

Level of Cognitive Ability: Analyzing
Client Needs: Psychosocial Integrity
Integrated Process: Nursing Process/Analysis
Content Area: Fundamental Skills: Perioperative Care
Priority Concepts: Clinical Judgment; Coping

Answer: 3
Rationale: The client's statement reflects a psychosocial concern regarding his or her appearance after surgery, so option 3 is the correct option. The remaining options identify unsuitable problems that are not supported by the provided client data.
Priority Nursing Tip: The appearance of the incision following parathyroidectomy may be distressing to the client. The nurse should reassure the client that the scar will fade in color and decrease in size over time.
Test-Taking Strategy: Note the subject that the client is expressing a concern about a possible scar. With this in mind, eliminate option 4 because the client is not demonstrating anxious behavior. Next, option 1 can be eliminated because denial is a way of avoiding concerns. Eliminate option 2 because the client expresses a realistic method of coping with a surgical scar. Review: the psychosocial concerns after **parathyroidectomy**.
Reference(s): Ignatavicius, Workman (2013), pp. 1404, 1407; Potter et al (2013), pp. 75-76.

959. The husband of a client with Graves' disease expresses concern regarding his wife's health, because during the past 3 months, she has been experiencing bursts of temper, nervousness, and an inability to concentrate on even trivial tasks. On the basis of this information, the nurse should identify which problem for the client?
1. Grief
2. Socialization issues
3. Issues related to sensory perception
4. Trouble with coping with her disease

Level of Cognitive Ability: Analyzing
Client Needs: Psychosocial Integrity
Integrated Process: Nursing Process/Analysis
Content Area: Adult Health: Endocrine
Priority Concepts: Clinical Judgment; Coping

Answer: 4
Rationale: A client with Graves' disease may become irritable, nervous, or depressed. The signs and symptoms in the question support option 4. The information in the question does not support options 1, 2, and 3.
Priority Nursing Tip: Graves' disease causes an enlarged thyroid gland, also known as goiter. The client may experience palpitations, cardiac dysrhythmias, protruding eyeballs, hypertension, heat intolerance, diaphoresis, weight loss, and diarrhea. Smooth, soft skin and hair; nervousness and fine tremors; and personality changes may also be noted in the client with Graves' disease.
Test-Taking Strategy: Focus on the subject, the appropriate client problem based on the client's behavior. Note the behaviors of bursts of temper, nervousness, and an inability to concentrate on even trivial tasks in the question. This will direct you to option 4. Review: **coping skills.**
Reference(s): Ignatavicius, Workman (2013), pp. 1395-1396.

960. A client who was admitted to the hospital for the treatment of thyroid storm (hyperthyroidism) is preparing for discharge. The client is anxious about his illness and is, at times, emotionally labile. Which intervention should the nurse take at this time in caring for this client?
1. Avoid teaching the client anything about the disease until he is emotionally stable.
2. Assist the client with identifying coping skills, support systems, and potential stressors.
3. Reassure the client that everything will be fine after he returns to his home environment.
4. Confront the client and explain that he must control his behavior if he wants to go home.

Level of Cognitive Ability: Applying
Client Needs: Psychosocial Integrity
Integrated Process: Nursing Process/Implementation
Content Area: Adult Health: Endocrine
Priority Concepts: Anxiety; Caregiving

Answer: 2
Rationale: It is normal for clients who experience thyroid storm (hyperthyroidism) to continue to be anxious and emotionally labile at the time of discharge. The best intervention is to help the client cope with these changes in behavior and to anticipate potential stressors so that symptoms will not be as severe. Options 1 and 3 block communication by either avoiding the issue or providing false reassurance. The confrontation described in option 4 will only heighten his anxiety.
Priority Nursing Tip: Thyroid storm occurs in a client with uncontrollable hyperthyroidism. It can be caused by manipulation of the thyroid gland during surgery and the release of thyroid hormone into the bloodstream; it also can occur from severe infection and stress.
Test-Taking Strategy: Use therapeutic communication techniques. Eliminate options 1 and 3 because they are blocks to communication. From the remaining options, note the words *anxious about his illness*. Eliminate option 4 because it will heighten the client's anxiety. Review: therapeutic communication techniques.
Reference(s): Ignatavicius, Workman (2013), pp. 1395-1396; Potter et al (2013), pp. 320-322.

961. The nurse cares for a client who has been admitted to the hospital for the insertion of a subclavian central venous catheter (CVC). The client is concerned because she is in a professional job where she works with the public. With this assessment data, what client problem would be the **priority**?
1. Poor self-care
2. Body image insecurity
3. Neck range of motion restrictions
4. Uncontrolled pain related to the CVC

Level of Cognitive Ability: Analyzing
Client Needs: Psychosocial Integrity
Integrated Process: Nursing Process/Assessment
Content Area: Mental Health
Priority Concepts: Coping; Functional Ability

Answer: 2
Rationale: Psychosocial assessment includes client data related to psychological and social issues. The CVC can create socially awkward situations and impair the client's security in their body image. The client data presented do not support assessing the client for poor self-care. Although pain and neck range of motion are valid issues for this client, options 3 and 4 are physiological issues and do not relate to the concerns of the client.
Priority Nursing Tip: For central line insertion, tubing change, and line removal, place the client in Trendelenburg or in the supine position if not contraindicated. Instruct the client to perform the Valsalva maneuver to increase pressure in the central veins when the intravenous system is open, such as during tubing changes.
Test-Taking Strategy: Note the strategic word, *priority* and the subject of subclavian CVC. The client data presented do not support poor self-care. Pain and restricted neck movements are physical concerns. Also, note that the client is concerned because she is in a professional job where she works with the public to assist in answering correctly. Review: insertion of a **subclavian central venous catheter (CVC)** and **body image insecurity**.
Reference(s): Ignatavicius, Workman (2013), pp. 223, 891; Potter et al (2013), p. 75.

962. A 12-year-old child is seen in the health care clinic. During the assessment, which finding would suggest to the nurse that the child is experiencing a disruption in the development of self-concept?
1. The child has many friends.
2. The child has a part-time babysitting job.
3. The child has an intimate relationship with a significant other.
4. The child enjoys playing chess and mastering new skills with this game.

Level of Cognitive Ability: Analyzing
Client Needs: Psychosocial Integrity
Integrated Process: Nursing Process/Assessment
Content Area: Developmental Stages: Infancy to Adolescence
Priority Concepts: Development: Health Promotion

Answer: 3
Rationale: The formation of an intimate relationship would not be expected until young adulthood. Friends are important and appropriate for members of this age group. A sense of industry is appropriate for this age group, and it may be exhibited by the child having a part-time job. The increase in self-esteem associated with skill mastery is an important part of development for the school-age child.
Priority Nursing Tip: The school age child is usually highly social, independent, and involved with activities.
Test-Taking Strategy: Note the subject, that the child is experiencing disruption in the development of self-concept. Focus on normal growth and development. Noting the age of the child in the question will assist you with eliminating options 1, 2, and 4. Review: **normal growth and development**.
Reference(s): Hockenberry, Wilson (2013), p. 72; McKinney et al (2013), p. 149.

963. A client who has been newly diagnosed with tuberculosis (TB) is hospitalized and will be on respiratory isolation for at least 2 weeks. Which intervention is appropriate to prevent psychosocial distress in the client?

1. Noting whether the client has visitors
2. Instructing all staff members to not touch the client
3. Giving the client a roommate with TB who persistently tries to talk
4. Removing the calendar and clock in the room so that the client will not obsess about time

Level of Cognitive Ability: Applying
Client Needs: Psychosocial Integrity
Integrated Process: Nursing Process/Implementation
Content Area: Adult Health: Respiratory
Priority Concepts: Coping; Infection

Answer: 1
Rationale: The nurse should note whether the client has visitors and social contacts because the presence of others can offer positive stimulation. Touch may be important to help the client feel socially acceptable. A roommate who insists on talking could create sensory overload. In addition the client on respiratory isolation should be in a private room. The calendar and clock are needed to promote orientation to time.
Priority Nursing Tip: An individual who has received a bacillus Calmette-Guérin vaccine (TheraCys BCG) will have a positive tuberculin skin test result and should be evaluated for tuberculosis with a chest x-ray.
Test-Taking Strategy: Focus on the subject, the intervention to prevent psychosocial distress in the client with tuberculosis. Eliminate option 3 first because the client should be in a private room. From the remaining options, noting that the client will be on respiratory isolation for at least 2 weeks and recalling the basic principles related to sensory overload will direct you to option 1. Review: the psychosocial concerns related to isolation and tuberculosis (TB).
Reference(s): Ignatavicius, Workman (2013), pp. 446-447.

964. The nurse is interviewing a client with chronic obstructive pulmonary disease (COPD) who has a respiratory rate of 35 breaths per minute and who is experiencing extreme dyspnea. On the basis of the nurse's observations, which is the appropriate client problem?

1. Lack of knowledge about COPD
2. Difficulty coping related with a situational crisis
3. Negative self-image because of neurological deficit
4. Restricted verbal communication because of a physical barrier

Level of Cognitive Ability: Analyzing
Client Needs: Psychosocial Integrity
Integrated Process: Nursing Process/Analysis
Content Area: Adult Health: Respiratory
Priority Concepts: Communication; Gas Exchange

Answer: 4
Rationale: A client with COPD may suffer physical or psychological alterations that impair communication. To speak spontaneously and clearly, a person must have an intact respiratory system. Extreme dyspnea is a physical alteration that affects speech. There are no data in the question that support options 1, 2, and 3.
Priority Nursing Tip: For the client with obstructive pulmonary disease (COPD), the nurse should not increase the oxygen flow rate above 2 L/min. Low concentration of oxygen should be administered as prescribed because the stimulus to breathe is a low arterial Po_2 instead of an increased Pco_2.
Test-Taking Strategy: Focus on the subject, that the client is experiencing extreme dyspnea during an interview. Based on this, option 4 is the only option that addresses this subject. Review: communication in a client with a chronic obstructive pulmonary disease (COPD).
Reference(s): Ignatavicius, Workman (2013), pp. 615-616, 623.

965. While inebriated, a client received a severe full-thickness burn to his left leg. Following an unsuccessful response to treatment, an amputation is required. After signing of the informed consent form, the nurse observes that the client appears withdrawn. Which action should the nurse take at this time?

1. Let the client have some time alone to grieve about the future loss of the limb.
2. Teach the client that the injury was a result of alcohol abuse, and suggest counseling.
3. Inform the health care provider of the client's behavior, and request medication to assist with coping.
4. Communicate with the client in a manner that reflects back to the client that he appears to be upset.

Level of Cognitive Ability: Applying
Client Needs: Psychosocial Integrity
Integrated Process: Nursing Process/Implementation
Content Area: Mental Health
Priority Concepts: Communication; Coping

Answer: 4
Rationale: Reflection statements tend to elicit a deeper awareness of feelings. A well-timed reflection can reveal an emotion that has escaped the client's notice. Additionally, option 4 validates the perception that the client is upset. Options 1 and 3 address interventions before assessing the situation. Option 2 is inappropriate and a block to communication.
Priority Nursing Tip: For the client undergoing amputation, the nurse should encourage verbalization regarding loss of the body part and assist the client to identify coping mechanisms to deal with the loss.
Test-Taking Strategy: Use therapeutic communication techniques. Focus on the client's feelings, and select the option that encourages the client to express his feelings and to talk more. This will direct you to option 4. Review: **therapeutic communication techniques.**
Reference(s): Fortinash, Holoday-Worret (2012), pp. 71-74; Potter et al (2013), p. 202; Stuart (2013), pp. 27-28, 30.

966. The nurse is caring for a client with left-sided Bell's palsy. Which statement by the client **requires follow-up** by the nurse?

1. "My left eye is tearing a lot."
2. "I have trouble closing my left eyelid."
3. "I can't taste anything on the left side."
4. "I don't know how I'll live with this stroke."

Level of Cognitive Ability: Evaluating
Client Needs: Psychosocial Integrity
Integrated Process: Nursing Process/Evaluating
Content Area: Adult Health: Neurological
Priority Concepts: Client Education; Inflammation

Answer: 4
Rationale: Bell's palsy is an inflammatory condition that involves the facial nerve (cranial nerve VII). Although it results in facial paralysis, it is not the same as a stroke. Many clients fear that they have had a stroke when the symptoms of Bell's palsy appear, and they commonly believe that the paralysis is permanent. Symptoms resolve, although it may take several weeks. Options 1, 2, and 3 are expected assessment findings of the client with Bell's palsy.
Priority Nursing Tip: Bell's palsy is characterized by the inability to raise the eyebrows, frown, smile, close the eyelids, or puff out the cheeks.
Test-Taking Strategy: Note the strategic words, *requires follow-up*. These words indicate a negative event query and ask you to select an option that is an incorrect client statement. Recalling that this disorder is a temporary condition will direct you to option 4, which identifies an inaccurate understanding of the disorder and thus requires further exploration. Review: **Bell's palsy.**
Reference(s): Ignatavicius, Workman (2013), pp. 1001-1002; Lewis et al (2011), p. 1542.

967. A client has a scheduled office visit due to a new diagnosis of diabetes mellitus. The client tells the nurse that he has trouble maintaining proper health due to anxiety regarding the self-administration of insulin. Which teaching/learning strategy should the nurse **initially** plan to implement?

1. Teach a family member to give the client the insulin.
2. Leave a list of instructions at the bedside for practicing the insulin injections.
3. Insert the needle, and have the client push in the plunger and remove the needle.
4. Give the injection until the client feels confident enough to do so by himself or herself.

Level of Cognitive Ability: Applying
Client Needs: Psychosocial Integrity
Integrated Process: Teaching and Learning
Content Area: Adult Health: Endocrine
Priority Concepts: Anxiety; Client Education

Answer: **3**
Rationale: Some clients find it difficult to insert a needle into their own skin. For these clients, the nurse might assist by selecting the site and inserting the needle. Then, as a first step in self-injection, the client can push in the plunger and remove the needle. Options 1, 2, and 4 place the client in a dependent role.
Priority Nursing Tip: Insulin injected into the abdomen may absorb more evenly and rapidly than at other sites.
Test-Taking Strategy: Note the strategic word, *initially*. Focus on the subject, anxiety regarding the self-administration of insulin. The correct option allows the client to participate in this activity. Eliminate options 1, 2, and 4 because they place the client in a dependent position. Also note that option 3 addresses the subject of self-administration. Review: **anxious client** and **diabetes mellitus**.
Reference(s): Ignatavicius, Workman (2013), p. 1435.

968. A client who is in labor has human immunodeficiency virus (HIV) and says to the nurse, "I know I will have a sick-looking baby." Which appropriate response should the nurse make?

1. "You are very sick, but your baby may not be."
2. "All babies are beautiful. I am sure your baby will be, too."
3. "You have concerns about how HIV will affect your baby?"
4. "There is no reason to worry. Our neonatal unit offers the latest treatments available."

Level of Cognitive Ability: Applying
Client Needs: Psychosocial Integrity
Integrated Process: Communication and Documentation
Content Area: Maternity: Intrapartum
Priority Concepts: Communication; Infection

Answer: **3**
Rationale: Option 3 is the most therapeutic response, and it will elicit the best information. It addresses the therapeutic communication technique of paraphrasing. Option 3 also is an open-ended response that will provide an opportunity for the client to verbalize her concerns. Parents need to know that their baby will not look sick from HIV at birth and that there may be a period of uncertainty before it is known whether the baby has acquired the infection. Options 1 and 2 provide false reassurances. The client should not be told that there is no reason to worry.
Priority Nursing Tip: Infants at risk for human immunodeficiency virus (HIV) infection need to receive all recommended immunizations at the regular schedule; however, no live vaccines should be administered.
Test-Taking Strategy: Use therapeutic communication techniques. Remember to address the client's feelings and concerns. This will direct you to option 3. Review: **therapeutic communication techniques** and **human immunodeficiency virus (HIV)**.
Reference(s): Lowdermilk, Perry, Cashion, Alden (2012), pp. 850-851; McKinney et al (2013), pp. 30-31, 629.

969. A client who is scheduled for an abdominal peritoneoscopy tells the home care nurse, "The surgeon told me to restrict food and liquids for at least 8 hours before this procedure and to use a Fleet enema 4 hours before entering the hospital. Do people ever get into trouble after this procedure?" Which appropriate response should the nurse make to the client?

1. "Any invasive procedure brings risk with it. You need to report any shoulder pain immediately."
2. "You seem to understand the preparation very well. Are you having any concerns about the procedure?"
3. "Trouble? There is never any trouble with this procedure. That's why the surgeon will use local anesthesia."
4. "There are relatively few problems, especially if you are having local anesthesia, but vaginal bleeding should be reported immediately."

Level of Cognitive Ability: Applying
Client Needs: Psychosocial Integrity
Integrated Process: Communication and Documentation
Content Area: Fundamental Skills: Perioperative Care
Priority Concepts: Clinical Judgment; Communication

Answer: 2
Rationale: Abdominal peritoneoscopy is performed to directly visualize the liver, gallbladder, spleen, and stomach after the insufflation of nitrous oxide. During the procedure, a rigid laparoscope is inserted through a small incision in the abdomen. A microscope in the endoscope allows for the visualization of the organs and provides a way to collect a specimen for biopsy or remove small tumors. The appropriate response is the one that facilitates the expression of the client's feelings. Option 1 may increase the client's anxiety. In option 3, the nurse states that no problems are associated with this procedure; this is close-ended and is incorrect. Although option 4 contains accurate information, the word "immediately" can increase the client's anxiety.
Priority Nursing Tip: Following endoscopic procedures in which the throat is sprayed with an anesthetic, the nurse should monitor for the return of a gag reflex before giving the client any oral substance. If the gag reflex has not returned and food or fluids are administered, the client could aspirate.
Test-Taking Strategy: Use therapeutic communication techniques to identify the client's feelings and concerns. Option 2 is the appropriate response because it provides an opportunity for the client to verbalize concerns. Review: **therapeutic communication techniques.**
Reference(s): Chernecky, Berger (2013), pp. 705-706; Potter et al (2013), pp. 320-322.

970. The nurse is caring for a client during a precipitous labor. The nurse should anticipate that the client will require care for which emotional need?

1. Support in maintaining a sense of control
2. Less pain and anxiety than with a normal labor
3. A sense of satisfaction regarding her quick labor
4. Fewer fears regarding the effect of labor on the newborn infant

Level of Cognitive Ability: Analyzing
Client Needs: Psychosocial Integrity
Integrated Process: Nursing Process/Assessment
Content Area: Maternity: Intrapartum
Priority Concepts: Clinical Judgment; Reproduction

Answer: 1
Rationale: The client experiencing a precipitous labor may have more difficulty maintaining control because of the abrupt onset and quick progression of the labor. This may be very different from previous labor experiences; therefore, the client needs support from the nurse to understand and adapt to the rapid progression. The contractions often increase in intensity very quickly, which adds to the client's pain, anxiety, and lack of control. The client may also have an increased amount of concern about the effect of the labor on the newborn infant. A lack of control over the situation in combination with increased pain and anxiety can result in a decreased level of satisfaction with the labor and delivery experience.
Priority Nursing Tip: A precipitous labor is a labor lasting less than 3 hours.
Test-Taking Strategy: Focus on the subject of precipitous labor and the client's reaction to this type of labor in selecting the correct option. Thinking about the definition and characteristics of a precipitous labor will direct you to the correct option. Review: the care of the client with a **precipitous labor.**
Reference(s): McKinney et al (2013), p. 644.

971. The nurse is planning care for a client who presents in active labor with a history of a previous cesarean delivery. The client complains of a "tearing" sensation in the lower abdomen. She is upset, and she expresses concern for the safety of her baby. Which response to the client should the nurse make?

1. "Don't worry, you are in good hands."
2. "You'll have to talk to your doctor about that."
3. "I don't have time to answer questions now. We'll talk later."
4. "I can understand that you are fearful. We are doing everything possible for your baby."

Level of Cognitive Ability: Applying
Client Needs: Psychosocial Integrity
Integrated Process: Nursing Process/Implementation
Content Area: Maternity: Intrapartum
Priority Concepts: Communication; Reproduction

Answer: 4
Rationale: Clients have a concern for the safety of their baby during labor and delivery, especially when a problem arises. Empathy and a calm attitude with realistic reassurances are important aspects of client care. Dismissing or ignoring the client's concerns can lead to increased fear and a lack of cooperation. Option 1 uses a cliché and provides false reassurance. Options 2 and 3 place the client's feelings on hold.
Priority Nursing Tip: Breathing techniques can be used to enhance relaxation for the pregnant client. They also provide a focus for the client during contractions and can interfere with pain sensory transmission.
Test-Taking Strategy: Use therapeutic communication techniques. Eliminate options 2 and 3 because they place the client's feelings on hold. Next eliminate option 1 because the client should not be told to not worry. Review: **therapeutic communication techniques.**
Reference(s): McKinney et al (2013), pp. 30-31, 424-425.

972. A newborn male infant is diagnosed with an undescended testicle (cryptorchidism), and these findings are shared with the parents. The parents ask questions about the condition. The nurse should tell the parents that which condition can occur and have a psychosocial impact if the undescended testicle is not corrected?

1. Atrophy
2. Infertility
3. Malignancy
4. Feminization

Level of Cognitive Ability: Analyzing
Client Needs: Psychosocial Integrity
Integrated Process: Nursing Process/Implementation
Content Area: Maternity: Newborn
Priority Concepts: Client Education; Reproduction

Answer: 2
Rationale: Infertility can occur in males with this condition because proper function of the testes in producing fertile sperm depends on a temperature of less than 98.6° F. The psychological effects of an "empty scrotum" could affect the client's perception of self and the ability to reproduce. Options 1 and 3 are possible physical consequences of a failure to treat cryptorchidism rather than psychosocial consequences. Because all of the hormones that are responsible for secondary sex characteristics continue to be secreted directly into the bloodstream, option 4 is not correct.
Priority Nursing Tip: Cryptorchidism is a condition in which one or both testes fail to descend through the inguinal canal into the scrotal sac.
Test-Taking Strategy: Focusing on the subject of the psychosocial impact of an undescended testicle (cryptorchidism) will assist you with eliminating options 1 and 3. From the remaining options, it is necessary to know that infertility can occur if the condition is not corrected. Review: **undescended testicle (cryptorchidism).**
Reference(s): Hockenberry, Wilson (2013), p. 452; McKinney et al (2013), pp. 497, 1127.

973. The mother of a newborn with hydrocephalus is concerned about the complication of mental retardation. The mother states to the nurse, "I'm not sure if I can care for my baby at home." Which therapeutic response should the nurse make to the mother?

1. "All babies have individual needs."
2. "Mothers instinctively know what is best for their babies."
3. "You have concerns about your baby's condition and care?"
4. "There is no reason to worry. You have a good pediatrician."

Level of Cognitive Ability: Applying
Client Needs: Psychosocial Integrity
Integrated Process: Communication and Documentation
Content Area: Maternity: Newborn
Priority Concepts: Communication; Coping

Answer: 3
Rationale: Paraphrasing is restating the mother's message in the nurse's own words. Option 3 demonstrates the therapeutic technique of paraphrasing. In option 1, the nurse is minimizing the social needs involved with the baby's diagnosis, which is harmful for the nurse–parent relationship. In options 2 and 4, the nurse is offering false reassurance, and these types of responses will block communication.
Priority Nursing Tip: Hydrocephalus results in head enlargement and increased intracranial pressure.
Test-Taking Strategy: Use therapeutic communication techniques to answer the question. Option 3 is the only therapeutic response, and it demonstrates paraphrasing. This is the only option that will provide the client with an opportunity to verbalize her concerns. Review: **therapeutic communication techniques.**
Reference(s): Hockenberry, Wilson (2013), pp. 969-970; McKinney et al (2013), pp. 30-31, 969-970.

974. A preschooler has just been diagnosed with impetigo. The child's mother tells the nurse, "But my children take baths every day." Which therapeutic response should the nurse make to the mother?

1. "You are concerned about how your child got impetigo?"
2. "There is no need to worry. We will not tell your day care provider why your child is absent."
3. "Not only do you have to do a better job of keeping your children clean, you must also wash your hands more frequently."
4. "You should have seen the doctor before the wound became infected, and then you would not have had to worry about the child having impetigo."

Level of Cognitive Ability: Applying
Client Needs: Psychosocial Integrity
Integrated Process: Nursing Process/Implementation
Content Area: Child Health: Infectious and Communicable Diseases
Priority Concepts: Communication; Tissue Integrity

Answer: 1
Rationale: By paraphrasing what the parent tells the nurse, the nurse is addressing the parent's thoughts. Option 1 demonstrates the therapeutic technique of paraphrasing. Options 2, 3, and 4 are blocks to communication because they make the parent feel guilty for the child's illness.
Priority Nursing Tip: A child with an integumentary disorder needs to be monitored for signs of a skin infection or a systemic infection.
Test-Taking Strategy: Use therapeutic communication techniques to answer the question. Option 1 is the only therapeutic technique, and it demonstrates paraphrasing. This is the only option that will provide the client with an opportunity to verbalize her concerns. Options 2, 3, and 4 are blocks to communication. Review: **therapeutic communication techniques and impetigo.**
Reference(s): Hockenberry, Wilson (2013), p. 1018; McKinney et al (2013), pp. 30-31, 1305.

975. The nurse is preparing to care for a child from a culture that is different from the nurse's. What is the **best** way to address the cultural needs of the child and family when the child is admitted to the health care facility?

1. Address only those issues that directly affect the nurse's care of the child.
2. Ask questions, and explain to the family why the questions are being asked.
3. Explain that cultural practices need to be discontinued during hospitalization.
4. Ignore cultural needs because they are not important to health care professionals.

Level of Cognitive Ability: Applying
Client Needs: Psychosocial Integrity
Integrated Process: Caring
Content Area: Fundamental Skills: Cultural Awareness
Priority Concepts: Culture; Professionalism

Answer: 2
Rationale: When caring for individuals from a different culture, it is important to ask questions about their specific cultural needs and means of treatment. An understanding of the family's beliefs and health practices is essential to successful interventions for that particular family. Options 1, 3, and 4 ignore the cultural beliefs and values of the client.
Priority Nursing Tip: When caring for a client from a different culture, the nurse needs to treat the client with respect and appreciate the differences and diversity of beliefs about health, illness, and treatment modalities.
Test-Taking Strategy: Note the strategic word, best. Focus on the subject, cultural needs. Options 1, 3, and 4 are judgmental. In addition, these options are comparable or alike in that they ignore the cultural practices and values of the client. Review: the nursing interventions related to **cultural awareness.**
Reference(s): Hockenberry, Wilson (2013), pp. 56-57.

976. A client with a T1 spinal cord injury has just learned that the cord was completely severed. The client says, "I'm no good to anyone. I might as well be dead." Which response should the nurse make to the client?

1. "You're not a useless person at all."
2. "I'll ask the psychologist to see you about this."
3. "You are feeling pretty bad about things right now."
4. "It makes me uncomfortable when you talk this way."

Level of Cognitive Ability: Applying
Client Needs: Psychosocial Integrity
Integrated Process: Communication and Documentation
Content Area: Adult Health: Neurological
Priority Concepts: Communication; Professionalism

Answer: 3
Rationale: Restating and reflecting keep the lines of communication open and encourage the client to expand on current feelings of unworthiness and loss that require exploration. The nurse can block communication by showing discomfort and disapproval or postponing the discussion of issues. Grief is a common reaction to a loss of function. The nurse facilitates grieving through open communication.
Priority Nursing Tip: Trauma to the spinal cord causes partial or complete disruption of the nerve tracts and neurons.
Test-Taking Strategy: Use therapeutic communication techniques. Options 1, 2, and 4 block communication. Option 3 identifies the therapeutic communication technique of restating and reflecting. Review: **therapeutic communication techniques.**
Reference(s): Ignatavicius, Workman (2013), p. 970; Potter et al (2013), pp. 320-322.

977. The nurse enters the room of a client who has had a myocardial infarction (MI) and finds the client quietly crying. After determining that there is no physiological reason for the client's distress, how should the nurse **best** respond?

1. "Do you want me to call your daughter?"
2. "Can you tell me a little about what has you so upset?"
3. "Try not to be so upset. Psychological stress is bad for your heart."
4. "I understand how you feel. I'd cry, too, if I had a major heart attack."

Level of Cognitive Ability: Analyzing
Client Needs: Psychosocial Integrity
Integrated Process: Communication and Documentation
Content Area: Adult Health: Cardiovascular
Priority Concepts: Anxiety; Communication

Answer: 2
Rationale: Clients with MI often have anxiety or fear. The nurse allows the client to express concerns by showing genuine interest and concern and facilitating communication using therapeutic communication techniques. Option 2 provides the client with an opportunity to express concerns. Options 1, 3, and 4 do not address the client's feelings or promote client verbalization.
Priority Nursing Tip: Cardiac rehabilitation is the process of actively assisting the client with cardiac disease to achieve and maintain a vital and productive life within the limitations of the heart disease.
Test-Taking Strategy: Note the strategic word, *best*. Use therapeutic communication techniques that have an exploratory approach because the question does not identify why the client is upset. This technique helps you eliminate each of the incorrect options. Review: therapeutic communication techniques.
Reference(s): Ignatavicius, Workman (2013), pp. 835, 841; Potter et al (2013), pp. 320-322.

978. A client with a recent complete T4 spinal cord transection tells the nurse that he will walk again as soon as the spinal shock resolves. Which statement provides the **most** accurate basis for planning a response to the client?

1. The client is projecting by insisting that walking is the rehabilitation goal.
2. To speed acceptance, the client needs reinforcement that he will not walk again.
3. Denial can be protective while the client deals with the anxiety created by the new disability.
4. The client needs to move through the grieving process rapidly to benefit from rehabilitation.

Level of Cognitive Ability: Analyzing
Client Needs: Psychosocial Integrity
Integrated Process: Nursing Process/Planning
Content Area: Adult Health: Neurological
Priority Concepts: Coping; Mobility

Answer: 3
Rationale: During the adjustment period that occurs the first few weeks after a spinal cord injury, clients may use denial as a defense mechanism. Denial may decrease anxiety temporarily, and it is a normal part of grieving. After the spinal shock resolves, the prolonged or excessive use of denial may impair rehabilitation. However, rehabilitation programs include psychological counseling to deal with denial and grief.
Priority Nursing Tip: In spinal shock, a sudden depression of reflex activity in the spinal cord occurs below the level of injury (areflexia).
Test-Taking Strategy: Note the strategic word, *most*. Focus on the subject, the physiological effects of a T4 spinal cord injury. The words *walking is the rehabilitation goal*, *speed acceptance*, and *move through the grieving process rapidly*, should be indicators that these are incorrect options. Also, focus on the client's statement, which is an indication of denial, to direct you to option 3. Review: the defining characteristics of denial.
Reference(s): Ignatavicius, Workman (2013), p. 970; Potter et al (2013), pp. 333, 734.

979. The nurse is developing a plan of care for a client scheduled for an above-the-knee leg amputation. Which action should the nurse include in the plan of care when addressing the psychosocial needs of the client?

1. Explain to the client that open grieving is abnormal.
2. Encourage the client to express feelings about body changes.
3. Advise the client to seek psychological treatment after surgery.
4. Discourage sharing with others who have had similar experiences.

Level of Cognitive Ability: Applying
Client Needs: Psychosocial Integrity
Integrated Process: Caring
Content Area: Mental Health
Priority Concepts: Caregiving; Coping

Answer: **2**
Rationale: Surgical incisions or the loss of a body part can alter a client's body image. The onset of problems coping with these changes may occur during the immediate or extended postoperative stage. Nursing interventions primarily involve providing psychological support. The nurse should encourage the client to express how he or she feels about these postoperative changes that will affect his or her life. Option 1 is an incorrect statement because open grieving is normal. Option 3 indicates disapproval, and in option 4, the nurse is giving advice.
Priority Nursing Tip: After amputation, avoid elevating the residual limb on a pillow to prevent hip flexion contractures.
Test-Taking Strategy: Focus on the subject, the psychosocial needs of the client undergoing amputation. Also, use therapeutic communication techniques. Remember to always focus on the client's feelings first. This will direct you to option 2. Review: **therapeutic communication techniques.**
Reference(s): Ignatavicius, Workman (2013), p. 1165; Potter et al (2013), pp. 320-322.

980. A client with pulmonary edema exhibits severe anxiety. The nurse is preparing to carry out the medical prescriptions. Which intervention should the nurse use to meet the needs of the client in a holistic manner?

1. Ask a family member to stay with the client.
2. Give the client the call bell, and encourage its use if the client feels worse.
3. Leave the client alone while gathering required equipment and medications.
4. Stay with the client, and ask another nurse to gather needed equipment and supplies.

Level of Cognitive Ability: Applying
Client Needs: Psychosocial Integrity
Integrated Process: Nursing Process/Implementation
Content Area: Adult Health: Respiratory
Priority Concepts: Anxiety; Gas Exchange

Answer: **4**
Rationale: Pulmonary edema is accompanied by extreme fear and anxiety. Because the client typically experiences a sense of impending doom, the nurse should remain with the client as much as possible. Family members can emotionally support the client, but they are not able to respond to physiological needs and symptoms. In fact, they are typically in psychological distress themselves. Options 2 and 3 do not provide for the psychological needs of the client in distress.
Priority Nursing Tip: If pulmonary edema occurs, the nurse should place the client in a high Fowler's position; administer oxygen; assess the client quickly, including lung sounds; ensure an intravenous access device is in place; prepare for the administration of a diuretic and morphine sulfate and insertion of a Foley catheter; prepare for intubation and ventilator support, if required; and document the event, actions taken, and the client's response.
Test-Taking Strategy: Focus on the subject, a client with pulmonary edema who exhibits severe anxiety. Identify the word *holistic.* This word guides you to consider both the physical and emotional well-being of the client. Option 4 is the only choice that addresses both needs. Review: the psychosocial aspects of care for the client with **pulmonary edema.**
Reference(s): Ignatavicius, Workman (2013), p. 665.

981. The family of a client with a myocardial infarction complicated by cardiogenic shock is visibly anxious and upset about the client's condition. What should the nurse plan to do to provide support to the family?

1. Offer them coffee and other beverages on a regular basis.
2. Insist that they go home to sleep at night to keep up their own strength.
3. Ask the hospital chaplain to sit with them until the client's condition stabilizes.
4. Provide flexibility with visiting times according to the client's condition and family needs.

Level of Cognitive Ability: Applying
Client Needs: Psychosocial Integrity
Integrated Process: Caring
Content Area: Adult Health: Cardiovascular
Priority Concepts: Anxiety; Coping

Answer: 4
Rationale: The use of flexible visiting hours meets the needs of both the client and family for reducing the anxiety levels of both. Offering the family beverages does not provide support. Insisting that the family go home is nontherapeutic. Although the chaplain may provide support, it is unrealistic for the chaplain to stay until the client stabilizes.
Priority Nursing Tip: Cardiogenic shock is failure of the heart to pump adequately, thereby reducing cardiac output and compromising tissue perfusion.
Test-Taking Strategy: Note the subject, the method of providing support to a client's anxious family. Options 2 and 3 may or may not be helpful, depending on the client and family situation. Coffee and beverages, although probably helpful to many, do not provide support. Review: **anxiety** and **myocardial infarction** complicated by **cardiogenic shock**.
Reference(s): Ignatavicius, Workman (2013), p. 841; Potter et al (2013), p. 741.

982. A client with premature ventricular contractions says to the nurse, "I'm so afraid that something bad will happen." Which action by the nurse provides the **most immediate** help to the client?

1. Telephoning the client's family
2. Using a television to distract the client
3. Having a staff member stay with the client
4. Giving reassurance that nothing will happen to the client

Level of Cognitive Ability: Applying
Client Needs: Psychosocial Integrity
Integrated Process: Caring
Content Area: Adult Health: Cardiovascular
Priority Concepts: Anxiety; Caregiving

Answer: 3
Rationale: When a client experiences fear, the nurse can provide a calm, safe environment by offering appropriate reassurance, using therapeutic touch, and having someone remain with the client as much as possible. Options 1 and 2 do not address the client's fear, and option 4 provides false reassurance.
Priority Nursing Tip: For the client experiencing premature ventricular contractions (PVCs), notify the health care provider if the client complains of chest pain or if the PVCs increase in frequency, are multifocal, occur on the T wave (R on T), or occur in runs of ventricular tachycardia.
Test-Taking Strategy: Note the strategic words, *most immediate* in selecting the correct option. Options 1 and 2 are comparable or alike options because they do not address the immediate concern of fear. Next, focusing on the strategic words will direct you to the correct option. Review: measures to reduce a client's **fear**.
Reference(s): Ignatavicius, Workman (2013), pp. 668, 728.

983. A client with Raynaud's disease tells the nurse that he has a stressful job and does not handle stressful situations well. Which life change should the nurse teach the client to consider to help alleviate his stress?

1. Change jobs.
2. Seek help from a psychologist.
3. Consider a stress management program.
4. Use earplugs to minimize environmental noise.

Level of Cognitive Ability: Applying
Client Needs: Psychosocial Integrity
Integrated Process: Nursing Process/Implementation
Content Area: Adult Health: Cardiovascular
Priority Concepts: Perfusion; Stress

Answer: 3
Rationale: Stress can trigger the vasospasm that occurs with Raynaud's disease, so referral to a stress management program or the use of biofeedback training may be helpful. Option 1 is unrealistic. Option 2 is not necessarily required at this time. Option 4 does not specifically address the subject.
Priority Nursing Tip: Raynaud's disease is vasospasm of the arterioles of the upper and lower extremities, which cause constriction of the cutaneous vessels.
Test-Taking Strategy: Focus on the subject, an intervention to alleviate stress. Note the relationship between this subject and option 3. Review: the measures that reduce **stress** and **Raynaud's disease**.
Reference(s): Ignatavicius, Workman (2013), pp. 343, 798; Potter et al (2013), p. 741.

984. A client with a history of pulmonary emboli is scheduled for the insertion of an inferior vena cava filter. The nurse checks on the client 1 hour after the health care provider has explained the procedure and obtained informed consent from the client. The client is lying in bed, wringing his hands, and says to the nurse, "I'm not sure about this. What if it doesn't work and I'm just as bad off as before?" Which problem for the client should the nurse identify at this time?

1. Anxiety
2. Inability to handle the treatment regimen
3. Lack of knowledge about the surgical procedure
4. Fear about the potential risks and outcomes of surgery

Level of Cognitive Ability: Analyzing
Client Needs: Psychosocial Integrity
Integrated Process: Nursing Process/Analysis
Content Area: Adult Health: Respiratory
Priority Concepts: Anxiety; Clinical Judgment

Answer: 4
Rationale: This client has indicated the surgical procedure and its outcome as the object of fear. Anxiety is present when the client cannot identify the source of the uneasy feelings. A client's inability to handle a treatment regimen would be when the client is not making needed adaptations to deal with daily life. Lack of knowledge would be when there is a lack of appropriate information.
Priority Nursing Tip: If a pulmonary embolism is suspected, the nurse should notify the rapid response team; reassure the client and elevate the head of the bed; prepare to administer oxygen; obtain vital signs and check lung sounds; prepare to obtain an arterial blood gas; prepare for the administration of heparin therapy or other therapies; and document the event, the actions taken, and the client's response.
Test-Taking Strategy: Note the subject, the client's concern about the outcome of the surgery. The client is also stating the concerns related to the procedure. Identify the option that addresses surgery, as well as fear. Also note the relationship of the client's statement and option 4. Review: the characteristics of **fear**.
Reference(s): Ignatavicius, Workman (2013), pp. 667, 802; Potter et al (2013), p. 1265.

985. A client has an oral endotracheal tube attached to a mechanical ventilator and is about to begin the weaning process. The nurse determines that which item, that was previously used to minimize the client's anxiety, should now be limited?

1. Radio
2. Television
3. Family visitors
4. Antianxiety medications

Level of Cognitive Ability: Analyzing
Client Needs: Psychosocial Integrity
Integrated Process: Nursing Process/Analysis
Content Area: Adult Health: Respiratory
Priority Concepts: Anxiety; Gas Exchange

Answer: 4
Rationale: Antianxiety medications and opioid analgesics are used cautiously in the client who is being weaned from a mechanical ventilator. These medications may interfere with the weaning process by suppressing the respiratory drive. The client may exhibit anxiety during the weaning process for a variety of reasons; therefore, distractions such as radio, television, and visitors are still very useful.
Priority Nursing Tip: For the client receiving mechanical ventilation, always assess the client first, and then assess the ventilator. Additionally, never set ventilator alarms to the off position.
Test-Taking Strategy: Focus on the subject, the item that should be limited during weaning from a ventilator. Think about the items that could interfere with the client's strength, endurance, and respiratory drive to maintain independent ventilation. Using this as the guideline, the only possible choice is option 4. The side effects of these medications could include sedation, which could interfere with optimal respiratory function. Review: the care of the client who is being weaned from a **mechanical ventilator**.
Reference(s): Ignatavicius, Workman (2013), pp. 681-682, 1711.

986. A client scheduled for pulmonary angiography is fearful about the procedure and asks the nurse if the procedure involves significant pain and radiation exposure. What response should the nurse make to the client to provide reassurance?

1. "The procedure is somewhat painful, but there is minimal exposure to radiation."
2. "Discomfort may occur with needle insertion, and there is minimal exposure to radiation."
3. "There is very mild pain throughout the procedure, and the exposure to radiation is negligible."
4. "There is absolutely no pain, although a moderate amount of radiation must be used to get accurate results."

Level of Cognitive Ability: Applying
Client Needs: Psychosocial Integrity
Integrated Process: Nursing Process/Implementation
Content Area: Adult Health: Respiratory
Priority Concepts: Client Education; Gas Exchange

Answer: 2
Rationale: Pulmonary angiography involves minimal exposure to radiation. The procedure is painless, although the client may feel discomfort with insertion of the needle for the catheter that is used for dye injection. Options 1, 3, and 4 are incorrect.
Priority Nursing Tip: A pulmonary angiography is an invasive procedure that involves inserting a catheter through the antecubital or femoral vein into the pulmonary artery or one of its branches. It also involves an injection of iodine or radiopaque contrast material; therefore, the nurse should assess for an allergy to these substances.
Test-Taking Strategy: Focus on the subject of pulmonary angiography. Eliminate option 4 because of the closed-ended words "absolutely no." From the remaining options, recalling that discomfort occurs with needle insertion will direct you to option 2. Review: **pulmonary angiography.**
Reference(s): Pagana, Pagana (2013), pp. 773-774.

987. The nurse is caring for an anxious client who has an open pneumothorax and a sucking chest wound. An occlusive dressing has been applied to the site. Which intervention by the nurse would **best** relieve the client's anxiety?

1. Staying with the client
2. Distracting the client with television
3. Interpreting the arterial blood gas report
4. Encouraging the client to cough and breathe deeply

Level of Cognitive Ability: Applying
Client Needs: Psychosocial Integrity
Integrated Process: Nursing Process/Implementation
Content Area: Adult Health: Respiratory
Priority Concepts: Anxiety; Gas Exchange

Answer: 1
Rationale: Staying with the client has a twofold benefit. First, it relieves the anxiety of the dyspneic client. In addition, the nurse must stay with the client to observe respiratory status after the application of the occlusive dressing. It is possible that the dressing could convert the open pneumothorax to a closed (tension) pneumothorax, which would result in a sudden decline in respiratory status and a mediastinal shift. If this occurs, the nurse is present and able to remove the dressing immediately. Option 2 is nontherapeutic. Interpreting the arterial blood gas report and promoting coughing and deep breathing have no immediate benefits for the client who is in distress.
Priority Nursing Tip: An open pneumothorax occurs when an opening through the chest wall allows the entrance of positive atmospheric air pressure into the pleural space.
Test-Taking Strategy: Note the strategic word, *best*. Focus on the subject, relieving the anxiety of a client who has an open pneumothorax. Eliminate option 2 first because the client is in distress. From the remaining options, use therapeutic nursing measures to direct you to option 1. Review: the measures used to relieve **anxiety** and **open pneumothorax.**
Reference(s): Ignatavicius, Workman (2013), p. 668.

988. A client with acquired immunodeficiency syndrome (AIDS) shares with the nurse feelings of social isolation since the diagnosis was made. Which strategy should the nurse suggest as the **most** useful way to decrease the client's stated loneliness?
1. Reinstituting contact with the client's family, who live in a distant city
2. Contacting a support group for clients with AIDS that is available in the local region
3. Using the Internet or the computer to facilitate communication while maintaining isolation
4. Using the television and newspapers to maintain a feeling of being "in touch" with the world

Level of Cognitive Ability: Applying
Client Needs: Psychosocial Integrity
Integrated Process: Nursing Process/Implementation
Content Area: Adult Health: Immune
Priority Concepts: Coping; Immunity

Answer: 2
Rationale: The nurse encourages the client to maintain social contact and support and assists the client with reducing barriers to social contact. This can include educating the client's family about the disease and its transmission, as well as suggesting the use of community resources and support groups. Option 1, although feasible, is less likely to address the client's current feelings of loneliness. Options 3 and 4 will not decrease the client's loneliness.
Priority Nursing Tip: Some of the tests that are used to monitor the progression of human immunodeficiency virus (HIV), which is the virus that leads to AIDS, include complete blood cell count, lymphocyte screen, quantitative immunoglobulin, chemistry panel, anergy panel, hepatitis B surface antigen testing, blood cultures, and chest radiography.
Test-Taking Strategy: Note the strategic word, *most.* Eliminate options 3 and 4 first because they are comparable or alike. From the remaining options, note that the wording of option 1 implies that contact has been lost over time, which is not stated in the question. Review: the strategies related to reducing social isolation and acquired immunodeficiency syndrome (AIDS).
Reference(s): Ignatavicius, Workman (2013), pp. 379-380.

989. A client was just told by the primary care health care provider that she will have an exercise stress test to evaluate the client's status after recent episodes of severe chest pain. As the nurse enters the examining room, the client states, "Maybe I shouldn't bother going. I wonder if I should just take more medication instead." Which therapeutic response should the nurse make to the client?
1. "Can you tell me more about how you're feeling?"
2. "Don't you really want to control your heart disease?"
3. "Most people tolerate the procedure well without any complications."
4. "Don't worry. Emergency equipment is available if it should be needed."

Level of Cognitive Ability: Applying
Client Needs: Psychosocial Integrity
Integrated Process: Communication and Documentation
Content Area: Adult Health: Cardiovascular
Priority Concepts: Anxiety; Communication

Answer: 1
Rationale: Anxiety and fear are often present before stress testing. The nurse should explore a client's feelings if concerns are expressed. Option 1 is open ended and is the only choice that is phrased to engender trust and the sharing of concerns by the client. Options 2, 3, and 4 are inappropriate statements and limit communication.
Priority Nursing Tip: A stress test is a noninvasive procedure that studies the heart during activity and detects and evaluates coronary artery disease. Treadmill testing is the most commonly used mode of stress testing.
Test-Taking Strategy: Use therapeutic communication techniques. Remember to focus on the client's feelings. This will direct you to option 1. Review: **therapeutic communication techniques.**
Reference(s): Pagana, Pagana (2013), pp. 227-229; Potter et al (2013), pp. 320-322.

990. The nurse is giving a client with heart failure home care instructions for use after hospital discharge. The client interrupts, saying, "What's the use? I'll never remember all of this, and I'll probably die anyway!" The nurse determines that the client's statement is **most likely** due to which psychosocial concern?
1. Anger about the new medical regimen
2. The teaching strategies used by the nurse
3. Insufficient financial resources to pay for the medications
4. Anxiety about the ability to manage the disease process at home

Level of Cognitive Ability: Analyzing
Client Needs: Psychosocial Integrity
Integrated Process: Nursing Process/Analysis
Content Area: Adult Health: Cardiovascular
Priority Concepts: Anxiety; Perfusion

Answer: 4
Rationale: Anxiety and fear often develop after heart failure, and they can further tax the failing heart. The client's statement is made in the middle of receiving self-care instructions. There is no evidence in the question to support options 1, 2, or 3.
Priority Nursing Tip: Heart failure results in inadequate cardiac output. The diminished cardiac output results in inadequate peripheral tissue perfusion.
Test-Taking Strategy: Note the strategic words, *most likely*. Focus on the subject of a client with heart failure being discharged. Because the client is being prepared for home care, the implication with the question is self-management. Review: the psychosocial concerns of a client with **heart failure**.
Reference(s): Ignatavicius, Workman (2013), pp. 756-757.

991. Before inserting a peripheral intravenous (IV) catheter into a preoperative client, the nurse notes that the client's muscles are tense and she is fidgeting with the bedsheet, stating she does not understand why she has to have the IV. Which statement should the nurse **first** verbalize to the client?
1. "This will be finished before you know it."
2. "Inserting the IV does not hurt very much."
3. "The IV adds fluid into your bloodstream."
4. "The IV catheter is an 18-gauge angiocatheter."

Level of Cognitive Ability: Applying
Client Needs: Psychosocial Integrity
Integrated Process: Communication and Documentation
Content Area: Fundamental Skills: Perioperative Care
Priority Concepts: Anxiety; Communication

Answer: 3
Rationale: In option 3 the nurse uses simple terms to clearly inform the client about the IV's purpose. Option 1 is an unethical statement for the nurse to make because the information is incorrect. Avoiding the client's feelings in option 2, blocks client communication regarding justifiable fears and feelings related to the IV insertion. Option 4 is an unsuitable statement because the client potentially would not understand the word "angiocatheter."
Priority Nursing Tip: Administration of an intravenous solution or medication provides immediate access to the vascular system. This is a benefit of administering solutions or medications via this route, but it can also present a risk. Therefore, it is critical to ensure that the health care provider's prescriptions are checked carefully and the correct solution or medication is administered as prescribed. Always follow the six rights for medication administration.
Test-Taking Strategy: Note the strategic word, *first*. Use therapeutic communication techniques when responding to the client. Nonverbal signals that indicate anxiety should also be noted and addressed using therapeutic communication techniques. Review: **intravenous insertion procedures** and **therapeutic communication techniques**.
Reference(s): Ignatavicius, Workman (2013), pp. 213-214; Potter et al (2013), pp. 320-322.

992. A client who received an implanted port for intermittent chemotherapy says, "I'm not sure if I can handle having a tube coming out of me. What will my friends think?" What should the nurse do **first**?
1. Ask the client if his friends are close to him.
2. Show the client various central line catheters
3. Notify the health care provider of the client's concerns.
4. Explain that implanted ports are subcutaneous and not visible.

Level of Cognitive Ability: Analyzing
Client Needs: Psychosocial Integrity
Integrated Process: Nursing Process/Implementation
Content Area: Pharmacology: Oncology Medications
Priority Concepts: Client Education; Coping

Answer: 4
Rationale: An implanted port is subcutaneous; it is not visible, and it has no external tubing. Tubing is used when an intravenous line is connected, and the port is accessed for therapy. The remaining options do not correct the client's confusion about the implanted port. Notifying the provider is not indicated. Inquiring about the client's friends is a reasonable response, but it can also provide false hope that the friends will be accepting. In addition, the nurse is likely to cause more anxiety and concern by providing information about the catheter's subcutaneous location. Showing various central line catheters is unlikely to be beneficial because the client will not be using them; in addition, this can heighten client anxiety and concerns.
Priority Nursing Tip: Antineoplastic medication causes the rapid destruction of cells, resulting in the release of uric acid. Allopurinol (Zyloprim) may be prescribed to lower the serum uric acid level.
Test-Taking Strategy: Note the strategic word, *first*. Also note the subject, a client who received an implanted port for intermittent chemotherapy and that the client is concerned. Noting the words *not visible* in option 4 will direct you to this option. Review: the concepts related to **implanted catheters** and the **teaching and learning process.**
Reference(s): Ignatavicius, Workman (2013), pp. 218-220; Potter et al (2013), pp. 329-330.

993. A postoperative client displays signs of anxiety when the nurse explains that the intravenous (IV) line will need to be discontinued as a result of an infiltration. Which appropriate statement should the nurse make to the client?
1. "This will be a totally painless experience. It is nothing to worry about."
2. "I'm sure it will be a real relief for you just as soon as I discontinue this IV for good."
3. "Just relax and take a deep breath. This procedure will not take long, and it will be over soon."
4. "I can see that you're anxious. Removal of the IV shouldn't be painful, but the IV will need to be restarted in another location."

Level of Cognitive Ability: Applying
Client Needs: Psychosocial Integrity
Integrated Process: Communication and Documentation
Content Area: Fundamental Skills: Perioperative Care
Priority Concepts: Anxiety; Communication

Answer: 4
Rationale: Option 4 addresses the client's anxiety and honestly informs the client that the IV may need to be restarted. This option uses the therapeutic technique of giving information, and it also acknowledges the client's feelings. Although discontinuing an IV is a painless experience, it is not therapeutic to tell a client not to worry. Option 2 does not acknowledge the client's feelings, and it does not tell the client that an infiltrated IV may need to be restarted. Option 3 does not address the client's feelings.
Priority Nursing Tip: The nurse should avoid venipuncture and placing an intravenous line over an area of flexion to prevent infiltration.
Test-Taking Strategy: Use therapeutic communication techniques, and recall that an infiltrated IV may need to be restarted. This will direct you to option 4. In addition, note that the correct option acknowledges the client's feelings. Review: **therapeutic communication techniques.**
Reference(s): Ignatavicius, Workman (2013), p. 228; Potter et al (2013), pp. 320-322.

994. A client has an initial positive result of an enzyme-linked immunosorbent assay (ELISA) test for human immunodeficiency virus (HIV). The client begins to cry and asks the nurse what this means. What knowledge should the nurse use to provide support to the client?

1. The client is HIV positive, but the client's CD4 cell count is high.
2. The client is HIV positive, but the disease has been detected early.
3. There are occasional false-positive readings with this test, which can be cleared up by repeating it one more time.
4. False-positive results can occur, and more testing is needed before diagnosing the client as being HIV positive.

Level of Cognitive Ability: Applying
Client Needs: Psychosocial Integrity
Integrated Process: Nursing Process/Implementation
Content Area: Adult Health: Immune
Priority Concepts: Client Education; Infection

Answer: 4
Rationale: If the client tests positive for HIV with the ELISA test, the test is repeated because of the potential for a false-positive result (for example, from a recent influenza or hepatitis B vaccine) or a false-negative result if drawn too early after infection. If the test is positive a second time, the Western blot (a more specific test) is done to confirm the finding. The client is not diagnosed as HIV positive unless the Western blot is positive. Some laboratories also run the Western blot a second time with a new specimen before making a final determination.
Priority Nursing Tip: Acquired immunodeficiency syndrome (AIDS) is a viral disease caused by the human immunodeficiency virus.
Test-Taking Strategy: Focus on the subject, the procedure for HIV testing and an affirmative diagnosis. Use knowledge about these procedures and recall that if the client tests positive for HIV with the ELISA test, the test is repeated because of the potential for a false-positive result. Review: **human immunodeficiency virus (HIV) and enzyme-linked immunosorbent assay (ELISA).**
Reference(s): Ignatavicius, Workman (2013), pp. 363-364, 369.

995. When performing an assessment on a client who is suicidal, which question is the **most appropriate** for the nurse to ask?

1. "Do you have a death wish?"
2. "Do you wish your life was over?"
3. "Do you ever think about ending it all?"
4. "Do you have any thoughts of killing yourself?"

Level of Cognitive Ability: Analyzing
Client Needs: Psychosocial Integrity
Integrated Process: Nursing Process/Assessment
Content Area: Mental Health
Priority Concepts: Mood and Affect; Safety

Answer: 4
Rationale: A lethality assessment requires direct communication between the client and the nurse concerning the client's intent. It is important to provide a question that is directly related to lethality. Euphemisms should be avoided.
Priority Nursing Tip: All suicide behavior is serious regardless of the intent. Suicide ideation requires constant attention, and typically one-on-one observation. The client with a plan must be placed on suicide precautions.
Test-Taking Strategy: Note the strategic words, *most appropriate.* Note the relationship between the word *suicidal* in the question and *killing* in the correct option. Although options 1, 2, and 3 infer suicidal intent, option 4 is the most direct. Review: **suicide risk.**
Reference(s): Fortinash, Holoday-Worret (2012), pp. 510, 512, 515; Stuart (2013), p. 328.

996. A client diagnosed with cancer of the bladder is fearful of the potential outcomes of an upcoming cystectomy and urinary diversion. Which statement indicates the client's fear?

1. "I wish I'd never gone to the doctor at all."
2. "I'm so afraid that I won't live through all this."
3. "I'll never feel like myself if I can't go to the bathroom normally."
4. "What if I have no help at home after going through this awful surgery?"

Level of Cognitive Ability: Analyzing
Client Needs: Psychosocial Integrity
Integrated Process: Nursing Process/Analysis
Content Area: Adult Health: Renal and Urinary
Priority Concepts: Anxiety; Clinical Judgment

Answer: 2
Rationale: For fear to be an actual problem, the client must be able to identify the object of fear. In this question, the client is expressing a fear of an uncertain outcome related to cancer and possibly a fear of death. Option 1 is vague and nonspecific. Option 3 reflects a negative self-image. The statement in option 4 reflects potential trouble at home after surgery.
Priority Nursing Tip: The nurse should monitor urinary output closely after bladder surgery. The health care provider's prescriptions and agency policy regarding bladder irrigation should be followed.
Test-Taking Strategy: Note the subject of client fear related to upcoming cystectomy and urinary diversion surgery. Option 1 is a general statement and should be eliminated first. Options 3 and 4 focus on the client after surgery, but they do not contain statements about an uncertain outcome. In option 2, the client expresses a fear of dying after enduring the ordeal of surgery. Review: **characteristics of fear.**
Reference(s): Ignatavicius, Workman (2013), pp. 1512-1513.

997. A client with nephrotic syndrome asks the nurse, "Why should I even bother trying to control my diet and the edema? It doesn't really matter what I do if I can never get rid of this kidney problem, anyway!" What should the nurse select as the **most appropriate** problem for this client?

1. Anxiety
2. Powerlessness
3. Difficulty coping
4. Negative self-image

Level of Cognitive Ability: Analyzing
Client Needs: Psychosocial Integrity
Integrated Process: Nursing Process/Analysis
Content Area: Adult Health: Renal and Urinary
Priority Concepts: Anxiety; Clinical Judgment

Answer: 2
Rationale: Powerlessness is present when the client believes that personal actions will not affect an outcome in any significant way. Because nephrotic syndrome is progressive, the client may feel that personal actions may not affect the disease process. Anxiety is appropriate when the client has a feeling of unease with a vague or undefined source. Difficulty coping occurs when the client has impaired adaptive abilities or behaviors with regard to meeting expected demands or roles. Negative self-image is when there is an alteration in the way that the client perceives his or her body image.
Priority Nursing Tip: The classic manifestations of nephrotic syndrome are massive proteinuria, hypoalbuminemia, and edema.
Test-Taking Strategy: Note the strategic words, *most appropriate*. Focus on the subject, nephrotic syndrome and the client's statement of "It doesn't really matter what I do." This implies that the client feels a lack of control over the situation, and it will direct you to option 2. Review: **powerlessness.**
Reference(s): Ignatavicius, Workman (2013), pp. 1529-1530; Lewis et al (2011), pp. 161, 1134.

998. A client with renal cell carcinoma of the left kidney is scheduled for nephrectomy. The right kidney appears to be normal at this time. The client is anxious about whether dialysis will ultimately be a necessity. Which pieces of information should the nurse provide to the client?

1. It is very likely that the client will need dialysis within 5 to 10 years.
2. One kidney is adequate to meet the needs of the body, as long as it has normal function.
3. There is absolutely no chance of the client needing dialysis because of the nature of the surgery.
4. Dialysis could become likely, but it depends on how well the client complies with fluid restriction after surgery.

Level of Cognitive Ability: Applying
Client Needs: Psychosocial Integrity
Integrated Process: Nursing Process/Implementation
Content Area: Adult Health: Renal and Urinary
Priority Concepts: Client Education; Elimination

Answer: 2
Rationale: Fears about having only one functioning kidney are common among clients who must undergo nephrectomy for renal cancer. These clients need emotional support and reassurance that the remaining kidney should be able to fully meet the body's metabolic needs as long as it has normal function. Options 1, 3, and 4 are inaccurate.
Priority Nursing Tip: For the client who has undergone a nephrectomy, the nurse should monitor specifically for abdominal distention, decreases in urinary output, and alterations in level of consciousness as signs of bleeding; the nurse should also check the bed linens under the client for bleeding.
Test-Taking Strategy: Focus on the subject, a client who is anxious about an upcoming nephrectomy. Eliminate option 3 because of the words *absolutely no chance*. Knowing that there is no need for fluid restriction with a functioning kidney guides you to eliminate option 4 next. From the remaining options, recalling that an individual can donate a kidney without adverse consequences or the need for dialysis will direct you to option 2. Review: the psychosocial aspects related to **nephrectomy.**
Reference(s): Ignatavicius, Workman (2013), p. 1476.

999. A charge nurse is supervising a nursing student who is providing care to a client with end-stage heart failure. The client is withdrawn and reluctant to talk, and she shows little interest in participating in hygienic care or activities. Which statement, if made by the student to the client, indicates that the student **requires teaching** regarding the use of therapeutic communication techniques?

1. "What are your feelings right now?"
2. "Why don't you feel like getting up for your bath?"
3. "These dreams you mentioned, what are they like?"
4. "Many clients with end-stage heart failure fear death."

Level of Cognitive Ability: Analyzing
Client Needs: Psychosocial Integrity
Integrated Process: Teaching and Learning
Content Area: Adult Health: Cardiovascular
Priority Concepts: Communication; Leadership

Answer: 2
Rationale: When the nurse asks a "why" question of the client, the nurse is requesting an explanation for feelings and behaviors when the client may not know the reason. Requesting an explanation is a nontherapeutic communication technique. In option 1, the nurse is encouraging the verbalization of emotions or feelings, which is a therapeutic communication technique. In option 3, the nurse is using the therapeutic communication technique of exploring, which involves asking the client to describe something in more detail or to discuss it more fully. In option 4, the nurse is using the therapeutic communication technique of giving information. Identifying the common fear of death among clients with end-stage heart failure may encourage the client to voice concerns.
Priority Nursing Tip: Communication includes verbal and nonverbal expression.
Test-Taking Strategy: Note the strategic words, *requires teaching*. These words indicate a negative event query and ask you to select an option that is an incorrect statement made by the student. Select the option that is a block to communication. The word *why* in option 2 should guide you to this option. Review: **therapeutic communication techniques.**
Reference(s): Ignatavicius, Workman (2013), pp. 749, 754-755; Potter et al (2013), pp. 320-322.

1000. The nurse is caring for a client with acute pulmonary edema. Which psychosocial strategy should the nurse plan to incorporate into the care of the client?

1. Reducing anxiety
2. Increasing fluid volume
3. Decreasing cardiac output
4. Promoting a positive body image

Level of Cognitive Ability: Applying
Client Needs: Psychosocial Integrity
Integrated Process: Nursing Process/Planning
Content Area: Adult Health: Cardiovascular
Priority Concepts: Clinical Judgment; Gas Exchange

Answer: 1
Rationale: When cardiac output falls as a result of acute pulmonary edema, the sympathetic nervous system is stimulated. Stimulation of the sympathetic nervous system results in the fight-or-flight reaction, which further impairs cardiac function. The goals of treatment are to increase cardiac output and decrease fluid volume. A disturbed body image is not a common problem among clients with acute pulmonary edema.
Priority Nursing Tip: If pulmonary edema occurs, the initial nursing action is to place the client in a high Fowler's position.
Test-Taking Strategy: Focus on the subject, a psychosocial strategy for the client with acute pulmonary edema. Thinking about the physiological occurrences of this condition will assist you with eliminating options 2, 3, and 4. In addition, recalling that severe dyspnea occurs should assist with directing you to the correct option. Review: the care of the client with **pulmonary edema.**
Reference(s): Ignatavicius, Workman (2013), p. 668.

❖ **1001.** A client with acute kidney injury is having trouble remembering information and instructions as a result of altered laboratory values. Which actions should the nurse take when communicating with this client? **Select all that apply.**
   ❑ 1. Give simple, clear directions.
   ❑ 2. Include the family in discussions related to care.
   ❑ 3. Explain treatments using understandable language.
   ❑ 4. Explain the possibility of hemodialysis in simple terms.
   ❑ 5. Give thorough and complete explanations of treatment options.

Level of Cognitive Ability: Applying
Client Needs: Psychosocial Integrity
Integrated Process: Nursing Process/Implementation
Content Area: Adult Health: Renal and Urinary
Priority Concepts: Cognition; Communication

Answer: 1, 2, 3, 4
Rationale: The client with acute kidney injury may have difficulty remembering information and instructions because of anxiety and altered laboratory values. Communications should be clear, simple, and understandable. The family is included whenever possible. Information about treatment should be explained using understandable language. Thorough and complete explanations may be confusing and will not be understandable for the client.
Priority Nursing Tip: The signs and symptoms of acute kidney injury are primarily caused by the retention of nitrogenous wastes, the retention of fluids, and the inability of the kidneys to regulate electrolytes.
Test-Taking Strategy: Focus on the subject, communicating with the client with acute kidney injury who is experiencing an alteration in cognitive function. Recalling the basic principles of effective communication would lead you to recognize that options 1, 2, 3, and 4 are helpful for maintaining effective communication. Review: **effective communication techniques.**
Reference(s): Ignatavicius, Workman (2013), p. 1572; Potter et al (2013), pp. 320-322.

1002. The rehabilitation nurse witnessed a postoperative client who had a coronary artery bypass graft and his spouse arguing after a rehabilitation session. What would be an appropriate statement for the nurse to make to identify the feelings of the client?
   1. "You seem upset."
   2. "Oh, don't let this get you down."
   3. "It will seem better tomorrow. Now smile."
   4. "You shouldn't get upset. It'll affect your heart."

Level of Cognitive Ability: Applying
Client Needs: Psychosocial Integrity
Integrated Process: Communication and Documentation
Content Area: Adult Health: Cardiovascular
Priority Concepts: Communication; Professionalism

Answer: 1
Rationale: Acknowledging the client's feelings without inserting your own values or judgments is a method of therapeutic communication. Therapeutic communication techniques assist with the flow of communication, and they always focus on the client. Option 1 is an open-ended statement that allows the client to verbalize, which gives the nurse a direction or clarification of the client's true feelings. Options 2, 3, and 4 do not encourage verbalization by the client.
Priority Nursing Tip: After arterial revascularization, the nurse should monitor for a sharp increase in pain because pain is frequently the first indicator of postoperative graft occlusion. If signs of graft occlusion occur, notify the health care provider immediately.
Test-Taking Strategy: Use therapeutic communication techniques. Focusing on the subject of identifying the feelings of the client will direct you to option 1. Review: **therapeutic communication techniques.**
Reference(s): Ignatavicius, Workman (2013), pp. 850-851; Potter et al (2013), pp. 320-322.

1003. The nurse is monitoring the neurological status on a client with dementia and assessing the limbic system. Which items should the nurse assess to yield the **best** information about this area of functioning?
   1. Judgment
   2. Emotions
   3. Consciousness
   4. Eye movements

Level of Cognitive Ability: Applying
Client Needs: Psychosocial Integrity
Integrated Process: Nursing Process/Assessment
Content Area: Adult Health: Neurological
Priority Concepts: Intracranial Regulation; Mood and Affect

Answer: 2
Rationale: Feelings and emotions are part of the role of the limbic system. Eye movements are under the control of cranial nerves III, IV, and VI. The level of consciousness is controlled by the reticular activating system. Insight, judgment, and planning are part of the function of the frontal lobe.
Priority Nursing Tip: Clients with dementia are typically dependent on others. Individuals most at risk for abuse include those who are dependent because of their immobility or altered mental status.
Test-Taking Strategy: Note the strategic word, *best*. Also focus on the subject, assessment of the limbic system. Use knowledge of anatomy and physiology concepts related to the neurological system to answer correctly. Remember, feelings and emotions are part of the role of the limbic system. Review: the function of the **limbic system.**
Reference(s): Ignatavicius, Workman (2013), p. 907.

1004. A client is admitted to the mental health unit with a diagnosis of panic disorder. The nurse should check the health care provider's prescription sheet anticipating that which medication, a benzodiazepine, will be prescribed?
1. Doxepin (Silenor)
2. Alprazolam (Xanax)
3. Imipramine (Tofranil)
4. Bupropion (Wellbutrin)

Level of Cognitive Ability: Analyzing
Client Needs: Psychosocial Integrity
Integrated Process: Nursing Process/Analysis
Content Area: Pharmacology: Psychiatric Medications
Priority Concepts: Anxiety; Safety

Answer: 2
Rationale: Alprazolam (Xanax), which is a benzodiazepine antianxiety agent, depresses the central nervous system (CNS) and induces relaxation in clients with panic disorders. Options 1, 3, and 4 are classified as antidepressants, and they act by stimulating the CNS to elevate mood.
Priority Nursing Tip: The immediate nursing action for a client with anxiety is to decrease stimuli in the environment and provide a calm and quiet environment.
Test-Taking Strategy: Focus on the subject, a benzodiazepine, and use knowledge regarding panic disorders and the classification of the medications identified in the options to answer this question. Eliminate options 1, 3, and 4 because they are comparable or alike and all are antidepressants. Review: **Alprazolam (Xanax).**
Reference(s): Hodgson, Kizior (2014), p. 38.

1005. A client with empyema is to undergo decortication to remove inflamed tissue, pus, and debris. On the basis of what understanding about this procedure should the nurse offer emotional support to the client?
1. This problem may decrease the client's life expectancy.
2. The client is likely to be in excruciating pain after surgery.
3. The client will probably have chronic dyspnea after the surgery.
4. Chest tubes will be in place after surgery for some time, and the healing process is slow.

Level of Cognitive Ability: Analyzing
Client Needs: Psychosocial Integrity
Integrated Process: Caring
Content Area: Adult Health: Respiratory
Priority Concepts: Clinical Judgment; Gas Exchange

Answer: 4
Rationale: The client undergoing decortication to treat empyema needs ongoing support from the nurse. This is especially true because the client will have chest tubes in place after surgery, and these must remain until the former pus-filled space is completely obliterated. This may take some time, and it may be discouraging to the client. Progress is monitored by chest x-ray. Options 1, 2, and 3 are not accurate.
Priority Nursing Tip: If the chest tube is pulled out of the chest accidentally, pinch the skin opening together, apply an occlusive sterile dressing, cover the dressing with overlapping pieces of 2-inch tape, and call the health care provider immediately.
Test-Taking Strategy: Focus on the subject, of a client with empyema who will undergo decortication and the need for emotional support. Recalling that chest tubes are a requirement after this surgery will assist in the selection of the correct option. Review: **decortication.**
Reference(s): Ignatavicius, Workman (2013), pp. 659-660.

1006. A client who has never been hospitalized before, who is in a hospital room with a roommate, is having trouble initiating the stream of urine. Knowing that there is no pathological reason for this difficulty, what nursing interventions should be included when assisting the client? **Select all that apply**.

☐ 1. Catheterizing the client
☐ 2. Running tap water in the sink
☐ 3. Assisting the client to a commode behind a closed curtain
☐ 4. Instructing the client to pour warm water over the perineum
☐ 5. Closing the bathroom door and instructing the client to pull the call bell when done

Level of Cognitive Ability: Analyzing
Client Needs: Psychosocial Integrity
Integrated Process: Nursing Process/Implementation
Content Area: Fundamental Skills: Elimination
Priority Concepts: Clinical Judgment; Elimination

Answer: 2, 4, 5
Rationale: A lack of privacy is a key issue that may inhibit the ability of the client to void in the absence of known pathology. Using a commode behind a curtain may inhibit voiding for some individuals, especially with a roommate present. The use of a bathroom is preferable, and this may be supplemented with the use of running water or pouring water over the perineum, as needed. Catheterization is not a nursing intervention and presents a risk of infection. If noninvasive techniques do not work, then the health care provider may prescribe that the client be catheterized.
Priority Nursing Tip: To aid in initiating the stream of urination, the client should be taught to increase ambulation, increase fluid intake unless contraindicated, pour warm water over the perineum, or allow the client to hear running water to promote voiding.
Test-Taking Strategy: Focus on the subject, nursing interventions for a client who is having difficulty voiding. Also, think about the issue related to decreased privacy and its effects on elimination. Review: measures used to assist with promoting urinary elimination.
Reference(s): Potter et al (2013), pp. 1045-1046, 1048.

1007. The client tells the nurse, "I'm scheduled for outpatient surgery, but I live alone and my only child lives 300 miles away. I'm afraid. What happens if something goes wrong after I go home?" Which statement by the nurse is therapeutic?

1. "Don't worry about the details. This procedure is done all the time and generally without any problems. You'll be fine!"
2. "They say managed care is no care! Get an alarm system so that, if you fall, it will alert someone. If necessary, I'll come."
3. "Your concern is well voiced. I advise you to call your son and insist that he come home immediately! You can't be too careful."
4. "You seem very concerned about going home without help. Have you discussed your concerns with both your surgeon and your family?"

Level of Cognitive Ability: Applying
Client Needs: Psychosocial Integrity
Integrated Process: Communication and Documentation
Content Area: Mental Health
Priority Concepts: Communication; Professionalism

Answer: 4
Rationale: The client has verbalized concerns. In option 4, the nurse uses reflection to direct the client's feelings and concerns. In option 1 the nurse provides false reassurance and then minimizes the client's concerns. In option 2 the nurse is ventilating the nurse's own anger, frustration, and powerlessness. In addition the nurse is trying to problem solve for the client but is overly controlling and takes the decision making out of the client's hands. In option 3, the nurse is projecting the client's own fears, and the problem solving suggested by the nurse will increase fear and anxiety in the client.
Priority Nursing Tip: Communication with the client needs to be goal directed and based on the client's concerns.
Test-Taking Strategy: Use therapeutic communication techniques. Remember that the priority is to address the client's feelings, and option 4 is the only option that does this. Review: therapeutic communication techniques.
Reference(s): Fortinash, Holoday-Worret (2012), pp. 71-74; Stuart (2013), pp. 30-31.

1008. During the nursing assessment, the client says, "My surgeon just told me that my cancer has spread, and I have less than 6 months to live." Which nursing response would be therapeutic?

1. "I am sorry. Would you like to discuss this with me some more?"
2. "I am sorry. There are no easy answers in times like this, are there?"
3. "I hope you'll focus on the fact that your doctor says you have 6 months to live and that you'll think of how you'd like to live."
4. "I know it seems desperate, but there have been a lot of breakthroughs. Something might come along in a month or so to change your status drastically."

Level of Cognitive Ability: Applying
Client Needs: Psychosocial Integrity
Integrated Process: Communication and Documentation
Content Area: Adult Health: Oncology
Priority Concepts: Communication; Coping

Answer: 1
Rationale: The client has received very distressing news and is most likely still experiencing shock and denial. In option 1, the nurse invites the client to ventilate feelings. Option 2 is social and expresses the nurse's feelings rather than the client's feelings. Option 3 is patronizing and stereotypical. Option 4 provides social communication and false hope.
Priority Nursing Tip: The nurse should monitor the client's progression through the stages of grieving. Not all clients will progress in the same manner and may progress from one stage to another in no logical order.
Test-Taking Strategy: Use therapeutic communication techniques. Note that option 1 provides the opportunity for the client to express feelings. Remember to focus on the client's feelings. Review: **therapeutic communication techniques.**
Reference(s): Ignatavicius, Workman (2013), p. 419, Potter et al (2013), pp. 320-322.

1009. A client with an endotracheal tube gets easily frustrated when trying to communicate personal needs to the nurse. Which method for communication should the nurse determine may be the **best** for the client?

1. Use a picture or word board.
2. Have the family interpret needs.
3. Devise a system of hand signals.
4. Use a pad of paper and a pencil.

Level of Cognitive Ability: Analyzing
Client Needs: Psychosocial Integrity
Integrated Process: Communication and Documentation
Content Area: Adult Health: Respiratory
Priority Concepts: Clinical Judgment; Communication

Answer: 1
Rationale: The client with an endotracheal tube in place cannot speak, so the nurse devises an alternative communication system with the client. The use of a picture or word board is the simplest method of communication because it requires only pointing at the word or object. The family does not need to bear the burden of communicating the client's needs, and they may not understand them either. The use of hand signals may not be a reliable method because it may not meet all needs, and it is subject to misinterpretation. A pad of paper and a pencil is an acceptable alternative, but it requires more client effort and time.
Priority Nursing Tip: A resuscitation (Ambu) bag must be kept at the bedside of a client with an endotracheal tube or a tracheostomy tube at all times.
Test-Taking Strategy: Note the strategic word, *best*. Options 3 and 4 are not the *best*, and they are therefore eliminated first. Because the family may not necessarily know what the client is trying to communicate, option 2 could cause added frustration for the client. Review: **alternative methods of communication** and a client with an **endotracheal tube.**
Reference(s): Ignatavicius, Workman (2013), p. 679.

1010. The home care nurse visits a client who is receiving total parenteral nutrition, and the client states, "I really miss eating dinner with my family." How should the nurse respond in order to reply to the client therapeutically?
1. "What you are feeling is very common."
2. "Tell me more about your family dinners."
3. "In a few weeks, you may be allowed to eat."
4. "You can sit down to dinner even if you do not eat."

Level of Cognitive Ability: Applying
Client Needs: Psychosocial Integrity
Integrated Process: Communication and Documentation
Content Area: Fundamental Skills: Nutrition
Priority Concepts: Communication; Nutrition

Answer: 2
Rationale: The nurse assists the client with expressing feelings and dealing with the aspects of illness and treatment by clarifying and helping the client to focus on and explore concerns. In option 1, the nurse characterizes and classifies the feelings on the basis of an assumption. Option 3 provides false hope and option 4 blocks communication by giving advice.
Priority Nursing Tip: The delivery of hypertonic solutions into peripheral veins can cause sclerosis, phlebitis, or swelling, and the nurse should monitor for these complications.
Test-Taking Strategy: Use therapeutic communication techniques. It is important that the nurse validate that the client has concerns and allow them to be discussed. The other options do not allow for the communication exchange about concerns. This will direct you to option 2. Review: **therapeutic communication techniques** and **total parenteral nutrition**.
Reference(s): Ignatavicius, Workman (2013), pp. 1348-1349; Potter et al (2013), pp. 320-322.

1011. A client has been receiving imipramine (Tofranil). The nurse notifies the health care provider if which adverse effect to the medication is noted?
1. Increased appetite
2. Increased drowsiness
3. Reported decrease in anxiety
4. Increased sense of well-being

Level of Cognitive Ability: Analyzing
Client Needs: Psychosocial Integrity
Integrated Process: Nursing Process/Implementation
Content Area: Fundamental Skills: Safety
Priority Concepts: Collaboration; Safety

Answer: 2
Rationale: Imipramine is a tricyclic antidepressant that is used to treat various forms of depression and anxiety. The client is also often in psychotherapy while taking this medication. Adverse effects to report to the health care provider include drowsiness, lethargy, and fatigue. Expected effects of the medication include an increased appetite and time spent sleeping, a reduced sense of anxiety, and an improved sense of well-being.
Priority Nursing Tip: The nurse should monitor a depressed client closely for signs of suicidal ideation. If the client presents with increased energy, the nurse should monitor him or her closely because it could mean that the client now has the energy to perform the suicidal act.
Test-Taking Strategy: Focus on the subject, an adverse effect to imipramine (Tofranil). Recall that this medication is an antidepressant. It would seem reasonable to expect options 1, 3, and 4 to occur as positive responses to this medication. Review: **imipramine (Tofranil)**.
Reference(s): Hodgson, Kizior (2014), p. 600; Lehne (2013), pp. 377-378.

1012. A client who is to undergo thoracentesis is afraid of not being able to tolerate the procedure. The nurse interprets that the client needs honest support and reassurance, which can **best** be accomplished by which statement?
1. "I'll be right by your side, but the procedure will be totally painless as long as you don't move."
2. "The procedure only takes 1 to 2 minutes, so you might try to get through it by mentally counting up to 120."
3. "The needle hurts when it goes in, and you must remain still. I'll stay with you throughout the entire procedure and help you hold your position."
4. "The needle is a little uncomfortable going in, but this is controlled by rhythmically breathing in and out. I'll be with you to coach your breathing."

Level of Cognitive Ability: Applying
Client Needs: Psychosocial Integrity
Integrated Process: Communication and Documentation
Content Area: Fundamental Skills: Diagnostic Tests
Priority Concepts: Communication; Gas Exchange

Answer: 3
Rationale: The needle insertion for thoracentesis is painful for the client. The nurse tells the client how important it is to remain still during the procedure so that the needle does not injure visceral pleura or lung tissue. The nurse reassures the client during the procedure and helps the client hold the proper position. Options 1, 2, and 4 are inaccurate statements.
Priority Nursing Tip: The client undergoing thoracentesis should be positioned sitting upright with the arms and shoulders supported by a table or lying in bed toward the affected side with the head of the bed elevated.
Test-Taking Strategy: Note the strategic word, *best* and focus on the subject of thoracentesis. Recalling that the client must remain still during the procedure helps you eliminate option 4 first. Knowing that the procedure may be painful for the client and that it takes longer than 1 to 2 minutes helps you eliminate options 1 and 2. Review: thoracentesis.
Reference(s): Ignatavicius, Workman (2013), pp. 559-560; Pagana, Pagana (2013), pp. 888-890; Potter et al (2013), pp. 320-322.

1013. A client with chronic respiratory failure is dyspneic. The client becomes anxious, which worsens the feelings of dyspnea. The nurse teaches the client which method to **best** interrupt the dyspnea–anxiety–dyspnea cycle?
1. Guided imagery and limiting fluids
2. Relaxation and breathing techniques
3. Biofeedback and coughing techniques
4. Distraction and increased dietary carbohydrates

Level of Cognitive Ability: Applying
Client Needs: Psychosocial Integrity
Integrated Process: Teaching and Learning
Content Area: Adult Health: Respiratory
Priority Concepts: Client Education; Gas Exchange

Answer: 2
Rationale: The anxious client with dyspnea should be taught interventions to decrease anxiety, which include relaxation, biofeedback, guided imagery, and distraction. This will stop the escalation of feelings of anxiety and dyspnea. The dyspnea can be further controlled by teaching the client breathing techniques, which include pursed lip and diaphragmatic breathing. Coughing techniques are useful, but breathing techniques are more effective. Limiting fluids will thicken secretions, and increased dietary carbohydrates will increase the production of carbon dioxide by the body.
Priority Nursing Tip: Clients with a respiratory disorder should be positioned with the head of the bed elevated.
Test-Taking Strategy: Focus on the subject of relieving anxiety and dyspnea, and note the strategic word, *best*. Limiting fluids and increasing carbohydrates are contraindicated and therefore eliminated. From the remaining options, recall that breathing techniques are more effective than coughing techniques. This will direct you to option 2. Review: the measures used to relieve anxiety and dyspnea in the client with respiratory failure.
Reference(s): Ignatavicius, Workman (2013), p. 671; Potter et al (2013), pp. 644, 646-647, 978.

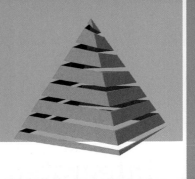

UNIT III

Integrated Processes

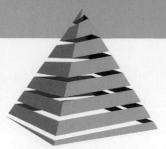

CHAPTER 7

Integrated Processes and the NCLEX-RN® Test Plan

Integrated Processes

In the new test plan implemented in April 2013, the National Council of State Boards of Nursing (NCSBN) identified a test plan framework based on Client Needs. This framework was selected on the basis of the analysis of the findings in a practice analysis study of newly licensed registered nurses in the United States. This study identified the nursing activities performed by entry-level nurses across all settings for all clients. The NCSBN identified four major categories of Client Needs. These categories—Safe and Effective Care Environment, Health Promotion and Maintenance, Psychosocial Integrity, and Physiological Integrity—are described in Chapter 6.

The 2013 NCLEX-RN test plan also identifies four processes, titled Integrated Processes, that are fundamental to the practice of nursing. These processes are integrated throughout the four major categories of Client Needs and include Caring, Communication and Documentation, Teaching and Learning, and Nursing Process (Box 7-1).

Caring

Caring is the essence of nursing, and it is basic to any helping relationship. Caring is central to every encounter that the nurse may have with a client. Through caring, the nurse humanizes the client. Treating the client with respect and dignity is a true expression of caring. In the technological environment of health care, emphasizing the client's individuality counteracts any potential process of depersonalization. Caring is an Integrated Process of the test plan for NCLEX-RN, and the NCSBN describes caring in part as a role of the nurse in providing encouragement, hope, support, and compassion. The process of caring is integral to all Client Needs components of the test plan.

For the NCLEX-RN, the process of caring is primary. It is very easy to become involved with looking at a question

from a technological viewpoint. However, the process of caring must be addressed when reading a test question and when selecting an option. Always address the client's feelings and provide support. Remember that this examination is all about nursing, and nursing is caring (Box 7-2)!

Communication and Documentation

The process of communication occurs as the nurse interacts either verbally or nonverbally with a client. Therapeutic communication techniques are essential to an effective nurse–client relationship. Communication-type test questions are integrated throughout the NCLEX-RN test plan, and they may address a client situation in any health care setting. The NCSBN

BOX 7-1   Integrated Processes

Caring
Communication and Documentation
Teaching and Learning
Nursing Process

BOX 7-2   Caring

A client who has end-stage cancer is admitted to a hospice care facility from her home. Which intervention should the nurse implement to address the client's psychosocial needs?
1. Administer total care for the client.
2. Engage the client in social activities.
3. Allow the client to verbalize feelings.
4. Provide pain medication every 4 hours.

Answer: 3
Focus on the subject, meeting psychosocial needs. The client is experiencing loss from two life-changing experiences: her poor prognosis and the loss of control over the environment, independence, and privacy that accompanies admission to a hospice care facility. To meet the client's psychosocial needs, the nurse should promote a therapeutic relationship and allow the client to verbalize her feelings. Options 1 and 4 manage physical needs. Although total care may be necessary, it does not address psychosocial needs. Providing pain medication is indicated as part of effective pain management; however, this can interfere with therapeutic communication if the client is too sedated. Engaging the client in social activities is unlikely to effectively meet the client's psychosocial needs relating to loss; it is more likely to help diminish loneliness and isolation. Review: interventions to meet the psychosocial needs of a client who is **dying.**

describes communication as the verbal and nonverbal interactions that occur in the health care environment.

When answering a question on the NCLEX-RN, the use of therapeutic communication techniques indicates a correct option, and the use of nontherapeutic communication techniques indicates an incorrect option. In addition, some communication-type questions may focus on psychosocial issues or issues related to client anxiety, fears, or concerns. For communication-type questions, always focus on the client's feelings first. If an option reflects the client's feelings, anxiety, or concerns, select that choice.

Documentation is a critical component of the nurse's responsibilities. The process of documentation serves many purposes; it provides a comprehensive representation of the client's health status and the care given by all members of the interprofessional team. There are many methods of documentation, but the responsibilities surrounding this practice remain the same. The NCSBN describes documentation as the activities associated with the client's medical record that reflect standards of practice and accountability.

When answering a question on the NCLEX-RN related to documentation, consider the ethical and legal responsibilities related to documentation and the specific guidelines related to both narrative and computerized documentation systems (Box 7-3).

Teaching and Learning

Client and family education is a primary nursing responsibility. The NCSBN describes this process as facilitating the acquisition of knowledge, skills, and attitudes that lead to a change in behavior.

The principles related to the teaching and learning process are used when the nurse functions as a teacher. The nurse must remember that the assessment of the client's readiness and motivation to learn is the initial step in the teaching and learning process.

When answering a question on the NCLEX-RN related to the teaching and learning process, use the principles related to teaching and learning theory. If a test question addresses client education, remember that client motivation and readiness to learn are the first priorities (Box 7-4).

BOX 7-4 **Teaching and Learning**

The nurse is preparing a plan regarding home care instructions for the parents of a child with generalized tonic-clonic seizures who is being treated with oral phenytoin (Dilantin). Which instruction should the nurse include in the plan?
1. Monitor the child's intake and output daily.
2. Provide oral hygiene, especially care of the gums.
3. Administer the medication 1 hour before food intake.
4. Check the child's blood pressure before the administration of the medication.

Answer: 2

Focus on the subject, instructions regarding phenytoin. Phenytoin is an anticonvulsant medication and causes gum bleeding and hyperplasia; therefore, a soft toothbrush and gum massage should be instituted to diminish this complication and prevent trauma. Intake, output, and blood pressure are not affected by this medication. Directions for administration of this medication include administering it with food to minimize gastrointestinal upset. Review: client instructions for **phenytoin (Dilantin)**.

BOX 7-3 **Communication and Documentation**

Communication

A client with myasthenia gravis is having difficulty with the motor aspects of speech. The client has difficulty forming words, and the voice has a nasal tone. The nurse should plan to use which communication strategy when working with this client?
1. Encourage the client to speak quickly.
2. Nod continuously while the client is speaking.
3. Repeat what the client has said to verify the message.
4. Engage the client in lengthy discussions to strengthen the voice.

Answer: 3

Focus on the subject, an appropriate communication strategy. The client has speech that is nasal in tone because of cranial nerve involvement in the muscles that govern speech. The nurse should listen attentively and verbally verify what the client has said. Other helpful techniques involve asking questions that require a "yes" or "no" response and developing alternative communication methods (e.g., letter board, picture board, pen and paper, flash cards). Encouraging the client to speak quickly is inappropriate and counterproductive. Continuous nodding may be distracting and is unnecessary. Lengthy discussions will tire the client rather than

strengthen the voice. Review: **communication** strategies for a client with **myasthenia gravis**.

Documentation

The nurse finds a client lying on the floor. The nurse performs an assessment, assists the client back to bed, and completes an incident report. Which should the nurse document on the incident report?
1. The client fell onto the floor.
2. The client climbed over the side rails.
3. The client was found lying on the floor.
4. The nurse was the only responder to the event.

Answer: 3

Focus on the subject, documenting on an incident report. The incident report should contain the client's name, age, and diagnosis and a factual description of the incident, any injuries experienced by those involved, and the outcome of the situation. Option 3 is the only choice that describes the facts as observed by the nurse. The nurse did not witness the events that led up to finding the client on the floor; thus, he or she cannot comment on how the client got to the floor (options 1 and 2). Option 4 is unsuitable documentation on an incident report because it implies that other staff members failed to respond to the event. Review **documentation guidelines** for an **incident report**.

Nursing Process

The steps of the nursing process provide a systematic and organized method of problem solving and providing care to clients. As noted by the NCSBN, the nursing process is a scientific and clinical reasoning approach to client care and includes the steps of assessment, analysis, planning, implementation, and evaluation.

Assessment

Assessment is the first step of the nursing process. It involves a systematic method of collecting data about a client to identify existing or potential (at-risk) client health problems and establish a database. The database provides the foundation for the remaining steps of the nursing process; therefore, a thorough and adequate database is essential. Data collection begins with the first contact with the client. During all successive contacts, the nurse continues to collect information that is significant and relevant to the needs of that client.

During the assessment process, the nurse collects data about the client from a variety of sources. The client is the primary source of data. Family members and significant others are secondary sources of assessment data, and these sources may supplement or verify the information provided by the client. Data may also be obtained from the client's record through the medical history, laboratory results, and diagnostic reports. Medical records from previous admissions may provide additional information about the client. The nurse may also obtain information through consultation with other interprofessional team members who have had contact with the client.

A thorough database is obtained with the use of a health history and a physical assessment. The information collected by the nurse includes both subjective and objective data. Subjective data include the information that the client states. Objective data are the observable, measurable pieces of information about the client, including measurements such as vital signs, laboratory findings, and results of diagnostic tests, as well as information obtained by observing the client. Objective data also include clinical manifestations, such as the signs and symptoms of an illness or disease.

The process of assessment additionally consists of confirming and verifying client data, communicating information obtained through the assessment process, and documenting assessment findings in a thorough and accurate manner.

On the NCLEX-RN, remember that assessment is the first step of the nursing process. When answering these types of questions, focus on the data in the question, and select the option that addresses an assessment action. The only exception to selecting an option that addresses an assessment action is if the question presents an emergency situation. In an emergency situation, an intervention may be the priority. In addition, use the skills of prioritizing and the ABCs—airway, breathing, and circulation—to answer the question. However, if the question asks about the procedure for administering cardiopulmonary resuscitation, then follow the CAB (circulation, airway, breathing) guidelines (Box 7-5).

Analysis

Analysis is the second step of the nursing process. During this step, the nurse focuses on the data gathered during the assessment process and identifies existing or potential health care needs, problems, or both. During this process, the nurse

---

> ### BOX 7-5   Nursing Process: Assessment
>
> The clinic nurse in a well-baby clinic is collecting data regarding the motor development of a 15-month-old child. Which is the highest level of development that the nurse would expect to observe in this child?
> 1. The child turns a doorknob.
> 2. The child unzips a large zipper.
> 3. The child builds a tower of two blocks.
> 4. The child puts on simple clothes independently.
>
> **Answer: 3**
> Focus on the subject, the highest level of development for a 15-month-old child. At the age of 15 months, the nurse would expect that the child could build a tower of 2 blocks. A 24-month-old child would be able to turn a doorknob and unzip a large zipper. At the age of 30 months, the child would be able to put on simple clothes independently. Review: motor development for a **15-month-old child.**

summarizes and interprets the assessment data, organizes and validates the data, and determines the need for additional data. Client assessment data are compared with the normal expected findings and behaviors for the client's age, education, and cultural background. The nurse then draws conclusions regarding the client's unique needs and health care problems or risks.

Client health problems are categorized as potential or at-risk problems that require prevention or as existing problems that are being managed or require interventions. The nurse reports the results of the analysis to the appropriate members of the interprofessional team and documents the client's unique health care problems, needs, or both.

On the NCLEX-RN, questions that address the process of analysis are difficult, because they require an understanding of the principles of physiological responses and an interpretation of the data on the basis of assessment findings or other presented data. Analysis questions require critical thinking and determining the rationale for therapeutic interventions that may be addressed in the case event. These questions may address identification of an existing or potential client problem and the communication and documentation of the results of the process of analysis (Box 7-6).

Planning

Planning is the third step of the nursing process. This step involves the functions of setting priorities, determining goals of care, planning actions, collaborating with other interprofessional team members, establishing evaluative criteria, and communicating the plan of care.

Setting priorities assists the nurse with organizing and planning care that solves the most urgent problems. Priorities may change as the client's level of wellness changes. Both existing and at-risk problems should be considered when establishing priorities. Existing problems are usually more important than at-risk problems. However, at-risk problems may at times take precedence over existing problems.

After priorities are established, the client and the nurse mutually decide on the expected goals. The expected goals serve as a guide for selecting nursing interventions and determining the criteria for evaluation. Before nursing actions are implemented, mechanisms to determine goal achievement and the

Nursing Process: Analysis

A client is admitted to the cardiac unit and placed on telemetry. The nurse reviews the client's laboratory values and notes that the potassium level is 6.3 mEq/L. When analyzing the cardiac rhythm, the nurse would expect to note which electrocardiogram (ECG) finding?
  1. A sinus tachycardia with an extra U wave
  2. A sinus rhythm with a tall, peaked T wave
  3. A sinus rhythm with a depressed ST segment
  4. A sinus tachycardia with a prolonged QT interval

Answer: 2

Focus on the subject, hyperkalemia and the associated ECG finding. A potassium level of more than 5.0 mEq/L indicates hyperkalemia, which can be detected on the ECG by the presence of a tall, peaked T wave. A U wave and a depressed ST segment occur with hypokalemia. A prolonged QT interval indicates hypocalcemia. Review: the manifestations associated with **hyperkalemia.**

phase that involves counseling, teaching, organizing and managing client care, providing care to achieve established goals, supervising and coordinating the delivery of client care, and communicating and documenting the nursing interventions and client responses.

During implementation, the nurse uses intellectual (critical thinking), interpersonal, and technical skills. Intellectual skills involve critical thinking, problem solving, and making judgments. Interpersonal skills involve the ability to communicate, listen, and convey compassion. Technical skills relate to the performance of treatments and procedures and the use of necessary equipment when providing care to the client.

The nurse independently implements actions that include activities that do not require a health care provider's (HCPs) prescription. The nurse also implements actions collaboratively on the basis of the HCP's prescriptions. Sound nursing judgment and working with other interprofessional team members is incorporated into the process of implementation. The implementation step concludes when the nurse's actions are completed and when these actions, including their effects and the client's response, are communicated and documented.

The NCLEX-RN is an examination about nursing, so focus on the nursing action rather than the medical action, unless the question is asking what prescribed medical action is anticipated (Box 7-8).

effectiveness of nursing interventions are established. Unless criteria have been predetermined, it is difficult to know whether the goal has been achieved or the problem has been resolved.

It is important for the nurse to both identify health or social resources available to the client and collaborate with other interprofessional team members when planning the delivery of care. The nurse needs to communicate the plan of care, review the plan of care with the client, and document the plan of care thoroughly and accurately.

When answering questions on the NCLEX-RN, remember that this is a nursing examination. In addition, remember that existing problems are usually more important than at-risk problems, and physiological needs are usually the priority (Box 7-7).

Implementation

Implementation is the fourth step of the nursing process. It includes initiating and completing nursing actions that are required to accomplish defined goals. This step is the action

Evaluation

Evaluation is the fifth and final step of the nursing process. The process of evaluation identifies the degree to which the plans for care and interventions have been successful.

Although evaluation is the final step of the nursing process, it is an ongoing and integral component of each step. The process of data collection and assessment is reviewed to determine if sufficient information was obtained and the information obtained was specific and appropriate. The client's identified

Nursing Process: Planning

The nurse is planning care for a child with an infectious and communicable disease. The nurse should identify which as the **primary** goal?
  1. The child will experience mild discomfort.
  2. The public health department will be notified.
  3. The child will not spread the infection to others.
  4. The child will experience only minor complications.

Answer: 3

Note the strategic word, *primary.* The primary goal for a child with an infectious and communicable disease is to prevent the spread of the infection to others. It is also important for the nurse to prevent discomfort as much as possible, but this is not the primary goal based on the options provided. Although the health department may need to be notified at some point, it is not the primary goal. The child should experience no complications. Review: goals of care for a child with an **infectious and communicable disease.**

Nursing Process: Implementation

The nurse in the postpartum unit checks the temperature of a client who delivered a healthy newborn 4 hours ago. The mother's temperature is 100.8° F. The nurse provides oral hydration to the mother and encourages fluid intake. Four hours later, the nurse rechecks the temperature and notes that it is still 100.8° F. Which appropriate nursing action should the nurse take at this time?
  1. Document the temperature.
  2. Increase the intravenous fluids.
  3. Notify the health care provider.
  4. Continue hydration and recheck the temperature in 4 hours.

Answer: 3

Focus on the subject, a temperature of 100.8° F in a postpartum client. In the postpartum client, a temperature of more than 100.4° F at two consecutive readings is considered febrile, and the health care provider should be notified. Options 1, 2, and 4 are inappropriate actions at this time. Although the nurse should document the temperature, this action delays necessary intervention. A health care provider's prescription is needed to increase intravenous fluids. Continuing hydration and rechecking the temperature in 4 hours also delays necessary intervention. Review: normal **postpartum** assessment findings.

existing and potential problems are evaluated for accuracy and completeness on the basis of the client's specific needs. The plan and expected outcomes are examined to determine whether they are realistic, achievable, measurable, and effective. Interventions are examined to determine their effectiveness for achieving the expected outcomes.

Because evaluation is an ongoing process, it is vital to all steps of the nursing process. It is the continuous process of comparing actual outcomes with the expected outcomes of care, and it provides the means for determining the need to modify the plan of care. Inherent in this step of the nursing process are the communication of evaluation findings and the process of documenting the client's response to treatment, care, and teaching.

Evaluation-type questions on the NCLEX-RN may be written to address a client's response to treatment measures or determine a client's understanding of the prescribed treatment measures (Box 7-9).

BOX 7-9   Nursing Process: Evaluation

A client has been given a prescription for a course of azithromycin (Zithromax). The nurse determines that the medication is having the intended effect if which is noted?
1. The pain is relieved.
2. The blood pressure is lowered.
3. The joint discomfort is reduced.
4. The signs and symptoms of infection are relieved.

Answer: 4

Focus on the subject, the intended effect of azithromycin. Azithromycin is a macrolide antibiotic that is used to treat infection. It is not prescribed for the treatment of pain, high blood pressure, or joint discomfort. Review: **azithromycin (Zithromax).**

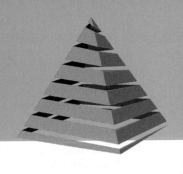

Integrated Processes

Caring

1014. Family members of a Cuban-American client who is terminally ill are visibly upset and crying loudly in the hallways. Which intervention should the nurse implement?
1. Direct the family members to the chapel.
2. Close the doors of the other clients' rooms.
3. Provide a private room for the family and client.
4. Ask the family to quiet down when in the hallways.

Level of Cognitive Ability: Applying
Client Needs: Psychosocial Integrity
Integrated Process: Caring
Content Area: Fundamental Skills: Cultural Awareness
Priority Concepts: Caregiving; Culture

Answer: 3
Rationale: In the Cuban-American culture, loud crying and other physical manifestations of grief are acceptable. The nurse provides culturally sensitive care and a caring approach to the client and family by providing a private room for the family to use to engage in grieving while still fulfilling the duty owed to the other clients. The nurse can direct the family to the chapel upon their request. Closing the doors to other clients' rooms can increase the risk of client injury and annoyance. Asking the grieving family to be considerate and to quiet down can be misinterpreted as being disrespectful.
Priority Nursing Tip: Many Hispanic/Latino clients live in close-knit communities and are often involved in the end-of-life stage of family and friends. The support of their cultural expression to the dying process should be supported by nursing.
Test-Taking Strategy: Focus on the subject, the client and the family who are Cuban Americans and going through the process of grief. Recall the characteristics of this culture, the importance of cultural sensitivity, and the duty owed to all clients. Also recall the grief process and the needs that those involve will experience. This will direct you to the correct option. Review: **cultural awareness.**
Reference(s): Giger (2013), p. 652.

1015. A client comes into the emergency depart-ment in a severe state of anxiety. What is the **priority** nursing intervention at this time?
1. Remaining with the client.
2. Placing the client in a quiet room.
3. Teaching the client deep-breathing exercises.
4. Encouraging the expression of feelings and concerns.

Level of Cognitive Ability: Analyzing
Client Needs: Psychosocial Integrity
Integrated Process: Caring
Content Area: Mental Health
Priority Concepts: Anxiety; Caregiving

Answer: 1
Rationale: If the client is left alone with severe anxiety, he or she may feel abandoned and become overwhelmed. Placing the client in a quiet room is also indicated, but the nurse must stay with the cli-ent. It is not possible to teach the client deep-breathing or relaxation exercises until the anxiety decreases. Encouraging the client to discuss her concerns and feelings would not take place until the anxiety has decreased.
Priority Nursing Tip: Anxiety occurs as a result of a threat that may be misperceived or misinterpreted or of a threat to identity or self-esteem.
Test-Taking Strategy: Because the anxiety state is severe, eliminate options 3 and 4. From the remaining choices, consider the **strate-gic word**, *priority* in the question. Focus on the **subject,** a client in a severe state of anxiety. This should direct you to the correct option. Review: the care of the client with **severe anxiety.**
Reference(s): Varcarolis (2013), p. 169.

1016. A client who is diagnosed with diabe-tes mellitus and requires the immediate amputation of a leg is very upset and states, "This is the doctor's fault! I did everything that I was told to do!" How should the nurse respond to the client's statement?
1. Notify the agency's risk management department
2. Help the client consider alternatives to treatment
3. Allow the client to use anger as a coping mechanism
4. Ask the client to list all previous health care providers

Level of Cognitive Ability: Applying
Client Needs: Psychosocial Integrity
Integrated Process: Caring
Content Area: Mental Health
Priority Concepts: Caregiving; Coping

Answer: 3
Rationale: Anger is a stage in the grieving process and an expected response to impending loss. Usually a client directs the anger toward himself or herself, God or another spiritual being, or the caregivers; thus far the client's behavior demonstrates effective coping. Notifying the risk management department is premature, especially because the client has said nothing about legal action. Analyzing alternative treat-ment options and previous health care providers is likely to interfere with effective coping, and it can delay life-saving treatment.
Priority Nursing Tip: A coping mechanism is a method used to decrease anxiety.
Test-Taking Strategy: Focus on the **subject,** a very upset client. Noting that the client is blaming the doctor and knowledge of the stages of grief associated with loss will direct you to the correct option. Review: the **stages of grief** and expected client expressions.
Reference(s): Ignatavicius, Workman (2013), p. 1165; Stuart (2013), pp. 574-575; Varcarolis (2013), p. 455.

1017. The nurse has an established relationship with the family of a client whose death is imminent. Which intervention should the nurse focus on in order to help the family **most effectively** cope with this experience?
1. Limiting time in the client's room to promote privacy
2. Providing education regarding coping mechanisms to use
3. Identifying spiritual measures that work best for dying clients
4. Answering questions clearly and providing resources as requested

Level of Cognitive Ability: Applying
Client Needs: Psychosocial Integrity
Integrated Process: Caring
Content Area: Developmental Stages: End-of-Life Care
Priority Concepts: Caregiving; Palliation

Answer: 4
Rationale: Maintaining effective and open communication among family members affected by death and grief is important to facilitate decision making and effective coping. The nurse maintains and enhances communication and preserves the family's sense of self-direction and control effectively by answering questions clearly and providing information and resources for decision making as requested by the family. Isolating the family from the client by limiting time in the client's room is inappropriate. The nurse should not provide education about coping mechanisms for family members to use because coping mechanisms directed by the nurse are unlikely to be as effective as the methods that the individuals choose for themselves. Identifying spiritual measures that work best for the dying client generalizes and does not reflect individualized care.
Priority Nursing Tip: People dealing with crisis usually feel helpless and are unable to control the circumstances; therefore, the nurse must facilitate open communication to determine and then meet the persons' needs.
Test-Taking Strategy: Note the strategic words, *most effectively*. Focus on therapeutic communication techniques and the role of the nurse in grieving, loss, and crisis, and then choose the most effective intervention. Also note that the correct option uses the words *as requested*. Review: the therapeutic communication techniques for individuals in crisis.
Reference(s): Ignatavicius, Workman (2013), pp. 115-116; Potter et al (2013), p. 714.

1018. When a client is dead on arrival (DOA) to the emergency department, the family states that they do not want an autopsy performed. Which statement should the nurse make in response to the family?
1. "Autopsies are mandatory for clients who are DOA."
2. "Federal law requires autopsies for clients who are DOA."
3. "The medical examiner makes the decision about autopsies."
4. "I will make sure the medical examiner is aware of your request."

Level of Cognitive Ability: Applying
Client Needs: Safe and Effective Care Environment
Integrated Process: Caring
Content Area: Developmental Stages: End-of-Life Care
Priority Concepts: Health Care Law; Professionalism

Answer: 4
Rationale: The nurse should notify the medical examiner or the coroner when a family wishes to avoid having an autopsy on a deceased family member. Normally the medical examiner will honor the family request unless there is a state law requiring the autopsy. Depending on the state, it is not mandatory for every client who is DOA to have an autopsy. However, many states require an autopsy in specific circumstances, including sudden death, a suspicious death, and death within 24 hours of admission to the hospital. Autopsy is not a requirement under federal law.
Priority Nursing Tip: Special consents are required for performing an autopsy, the use of restraints, receiving blood transfusions, photographing the client, disposal of body parts during surgery, and donating organs after death. It is often times within the client/family's right to deny such a request.
Test-Taking Strategy: Focus on the subject, the laws and issues surrounding autopsy and use therapeutic communication techniques to answer the question. Eliminate options 1 and 2 because these statements are not accurate. From the remaining choices, option 4 is the most therapeutic and caring response to the family. Review: autopsy.
Reference(s): Potter et al (2013), pp. 301, 724.

1019. An older client states, "This is confusing. How am I going to take care of myself?" Which intervention should the nurse implement before discharge?
1. Notify a family member that the client needs assistance.
2. Advise social services to provide follow-up communication.
3. Ask the health care provider to delay discharge for additional teaching.
4. Request a home health care referral from the health care provider (HCP).

Level of Cognitive Ability: Applying
Client Needs: Safe and Effective Care Environment
Integrated Process: Caring
Content Area: Developmental Stages: Early Adulthood to Later Adulthood
Priority Concepts: Caregiving; Safety

Answer: 4
Rationale: With managed care demanding earlier hospital discharges, clients return home with more serious health problems. To make a successful transition to self-care at home for effective health maintenance, clients potentially require support from a home health agency until they can function independently. Engaging a family member in the client's transition to home does not guarantee effective health maintenance for the client; in addition, there may not be a family member available. The HCP may not be able to delay the discharge for client teaching when those services can be provided in the home. Social services cannot assist with postdischarge surveillance of the client's health care because that is not their area of expertise or responsibility.
Priority Nursing Tip: Physiological changes in the older client increase the risk of accidents.
Test-Taking Strategy: Focus on the subject of effective health maintenance of an older client, and remember the client's concern. Note that option 4 is the only action that will ensure that the client receives the necessary assistance until independence is achieved. Review: **home care support services.**
Reference(s): Ignatavicius, Workman (2013), p. 300; Potter et al (2013), pp. 20, 175.

1020. The nurse is interacting with the family of a client who is unconscious as a result of a head injury. Which approach should the nurse use to help the family cope with this situation?
1. Explain equipment and procedures on an ongoing basis.
2. Discourage displays of grief so the client isn't saddened.
3. Encourage the use of limited touch to allow the client to rest.
4. Explain that the client must rest so they must adhere to regular visiting hours.

Level of Cognitive Ability: Applying
Client Needs: Psychosocial Integrity
Integrated Process: Caring
Content Area: Mental Health
Priority Concepts: Coping; Family Dynamics

Answer: 1
Rationale: Families often need assistance to cope with the sudden severe illness of a loved one. The nurse should explain all equipment, treatments, and procedures, and he or she should supplement or reinforce the information given by the health care provider. Displaying grief is a normal process and should not be discouraged. The family should be encouraged to touch and speak to the client and become involved in the client's care in some way if they are comfortable with doing so. The nurse should allow the family to stay with the client whenever possible. This is important for both the client and the family.
Priority Nursing Tip: Families of clients who are acutely ill may experience anticipatory grief. Anticipatory grief occurs before the loss and is associated with an acute, chronic, or terminal illness.
Test-Taking Strategy: Use therapeutic communication techniques to answer this question. The correct option provides the family with information that will help them cope with the situation. Each of the incorrect options puts distance between the family and the client. Review: **grieving and coping.**
Reference(s): Ignatavicius, Workman (2013), p. 94; Potter et al (2013), p. 119.

1021. The nurse admits a client who has right-sided weakness, aphasia, and urinary incontinence. The woman's daughter states, "If this is a stroke, it's the kiss of death." What **initial** response should the nurse make?

1. "Why would you think like that?"
2. "You feel your mother is dying?"
3. "These symptoms are reversible."
4. "A stroke is not the kiss of death."

Level of Cognitive Ability: Applying
Client Needs: Psychosocial Integrity
Integrated Process: Caring
Content Area: Adult Health: Neurological
Priority Concepts: Communication; Coping

Answer: 2
Rationale: Option 2 allows the daughter to verbalize her feelings, begin coping, and adapt to what is happening. By restating, the nurse seeks clarification of the daughter's feelings and offers information that potentially helps ease some of the fears and concerns related to the client's condition and prognosis. Option 1 is a disapproving comment that is likely to interfere with communication. Option 3 is potentially misleading and offers false hope. The nurse could reflect back the statement in option 4 to the daughter to promote communication. However, as it stands, option 4 is a barrier to communication that contradicts the daughter's feelings.
Priority Nursing Tip: A critical factor in the early intervention and treatment of stroke is the accurate identification of stroke manifestations and establishing the onset of manifestations.
Test-Taking Strategy: Note the strategic word, *initial*. Use the principles of therapeutic communication to arrive at the option that allows for clarification of the daughter's feelings. Review: **therapeutic communication techniques.**
Reference(s): Ignatavicius, Workman (2013), p. 1011; Potter et al (2013), pp. 320-322.

1022. A client and her infant have undergone testing for human immunodeficiency virus (HIV), and both clients were found to be positive. The mother is crying. The nurse determines that which intervention will meet the client's **initial** needs at this time?

1. Examining with the mother how she got HIV
2. Listening quietly while the mother talks and cries
3. Describing the progressive stages and treatments of HIV
4. Calling an HIV counselor to make an appointment for the mother and infant

Level of Cognitive Ability: Analyzing
Client Needs: Psychosocial Integrity
Integrated Process: Caring
Content Area: Mental Health
Priority Concepts: Caregiving; Coping

Answer: 2
Rationale: This client has just received devastating news and needs to have someone present with her as she begins to cope with this issue. The nurse needs to sit and actively listen while the mother talks and cries. Examining the mother and describing the progression and treatment of HIV is not appropriate for this stage of coping. Calling an HIV counselor may be helpful, but it is not what the client needs initially.
Priority Nursing Tip: The nurse must maintain issues of confidentiality surrounding human immunodeficiency virus and acquired immunodeficiency syndrome testing while addressing the client's feelings.
Test-Taking Strategy: Note the strategic word, *initial*. Use therapeutic communication techniques, and remember to focus on the client's feelings. This will direct you to the correct option. Review: **therapeutic communication techniques.**
Reference(s): McKinney et al (2013), pp. 30-31, 629-630; Stuart (2013), pp. 25-29.

1023. The nurse cared for a client who died a few minutes ago. Which statement supports the nurse's belief that the client died with dignity?

1. The family thanks the nurse for facilitating such a peaceful death.
2. The nurse states that it is difficult to give that kind of care to a dying client.
3. The health care provider is aware that all of the prescriptions were carried out.
4. The nurse gave increasing doses of pain medication to keep the client well sedated.

Level of Cognitive Ability: Evaluating
Client Needs: Psychosocial Integrity
Integrated Process: Caring
Content Area: Developmental Stages: End-of-Life Care
Priority Concepts: Caregiving; Palliation

Answer: 1
Rationale: The family response is an external perception, and it is extremely important. Families derive a great deal of comfort from knowing that their loved one received the best care possible. Option 1 provides external validation that the client received comprehensive, quality care. Option 2 focuses on the feelings of the nurse, who may be expressing his or her own anxiety. Option 3 focuses on the provider's prescriptions rather than client care. Option 4 reflects on only one aspect of the care of a dying client.
Priority Nursing Tip: Outcomes related to care during illness and the dying experience should be based on the client's wishes. Pain must be controlled; the dying client should be as pain free and comfortable as possible.
Test-Taking Strategy: Focus on the subject of whether the client died with dignity. The only choice that addresses this subject is option 1. Review: the concepts related to **death and dying**.
Reference(s): Ignatavicius, Workman (2013), p. 116; Potter et al (2013), p. 723.

1024. The family of a client diagnosed with Parkinson's disease tells the nurse that the client is having difficulty adjusting to the disorder, and they do not know what to do to help. Which intervention should the nurse suggest to cope with effects of the disease?

1. Plan only a few activities for the client during the day.
2. Assist the client with activities of daily living as much as possible.
3. Cluster activities at the end of the day, when the client is restless and bored.
4. Encourage and reinforce client efforts to exercise and perform activities of daily living.

Level of Cognitive Ability: Applying
Client Needs: Psychosocial Integrity
Integrated Process: Caring
Content Area: Adult Health: Neurological
Priority Concepts: Coping; Functional Ability

Answer: 4
Rationale: The client with Parkinson's disease has a tendency to become withdrawn and depressed, which can be limited by encouraging the client to be an active participant in his or her own care. The family should plan activities intermittently throughout the day to inhibit daytime sleeping and boredom. The family should also give the client encouragement and praise for his or her perseverance in these efforts and help only when necessary.
Priority Nursing Tip: The client with Parkinson's disease should exercise in the morning when energy levels are highest.
Test-Taking Strategy: Focus on the subject of supporting the client in coping with the effects of Parkinson's disease. Recalling that the client should be an active participant in his or her own care will direct you to the correct option. Review: **Parkinson's disease**.
Reference(s): Ignatavicius, Workman (2013), pp. 945-946.

1025. A community health nurse is caring for a group of homeless people. What is the **most immediate** concern when planning for the potential needs of this group?

1. Finding affordable housing for the group
2. Setting up a 24-hour crisis center and hotline
3. Providing peer support through structured support groups
4. Ensuring that adequate food, shelter, and clothing are available

Level of Cognitive Ability: Analyzing
Client Needs: Physiological Integrity
Integrated Process: Caring
Content Area: Leadership/Management: Prioritizing
Priority Concepts: Caregiving; Health Promotion

Answer: 4
Rationale: The question asks about the situation's most immediate concern. The initial community health concern is always attending to people's basic physiological needs of food, shelter, and clothing. Finding affordable housing and providing crisis intervention and peer support are meaningful interventions that may be completed at a later time.
Priority Nursing Tip: Nursing's primary concern is always initially focused on meeting a client's physiological needs.
Test-Taking Strategy: Note the strategic words, *most immediate*. Use Maslow's Hierarchy of Needs theory to answer the question. Option 4 addresses basic physiological needs. Although options 1, 2, and 3 are also appropriate actions, option 4 is the most immediate concern. Review: the needs of the **homeless population**.
Reference(s): Ignatavicius, Workman (2013), p. 33; Potter et al (2013), pp. 118, 123.

1026. A stillborn baby was delivered a few hours ago. After the birth, the family has remained together, holding and touching the baby. Which statement by the nurse should further assist the family with their grieving?
1. "How can I assist you with ways to remember your baby?"
2. "You seem upset. Do you think a tranquilizer would help?"
3. "I feel so bad. I don't understand why this happened either."
4. "I can allow another 15 minutes together for you to grieve."

Level of Cognitive Ability: Applying
Client Needs: Psychosocial Integrity
Integrated Process: Caring
Content Area: Developmental Stages: End-of-Life Care
Priority Concepts: Caregiving; Communication

Answer: 1
Rationale: Nurses should be able to explore measures that assist the family with creating memories of the infant so that the existence of the child is confirmed, and the parents can complete the grieving process. Option 1 identifies this measure and also demonstrates a caring and empathetic client-focused response while providing the family with the option to express their needs. Option 2 devalues the parents' feelings and is inappropriate. Option 3 is inappropriate and reflects a lack of knowledge on the nurse's part. Option 4 appears that the nurse is uncaring.
Priority Nursing Tip: Loss and grief may occur with the birth of a preterm infant, an infant with complications of birth, or an infant with congenital anomalies; it may also occur in a client who is giving up a child for adoption. Beliefs and needs vary widely across individuals, cultures, and religions.
Test-Taking Strategy: Note the words *further assist the family with their grieving*. Use therapeutic communication techniques to choose the option that demonstrates a caring and empathetic response by the nurse and that meets the psychosocial needs of the grieving client and family. Review: therapeutic communication techniques and the grief process.
Reference(s): Hockenberry, Wilson (2013), p. 566; Lowdermilk, Perry, Cashion, Alden (2012), p. 938; McKinney et al (2013), pp. 30-31.

1027. While counseling a prenatal client about her dietary and alcohol consumption habits, the nurse observes that the client has difficulty concentrating and appears agitated. Which should the nurse use as a guideline to proceed with the assessment?
1. Discussion of all the possible consequences of drinking alcohol should be avoided.
2. Women are generally negative to the need to stop drinking during their pregnancy.
3. Evoke maternal guilt to promote motivation to want to work on exiting problems.
4. A nonjudgmental approach may help the nurse gain maternal trust and cooperation.

Level of Cognitive Ability: Applying
Client Needs: Psychosocial Integrity
Integrated Process: Caring
Content Area: Maternity: Antepartum
Priority Concepts: Caregiving; Communication

Answer: 4
Rationale: The potential effects of alcohol abuse during pregnancy for both the mother and fetus have been well documented. The nurse who expresses genuine concern with suspected abusers may motivate positive behavioral changes during the prenatal period. The maternal behaviors of lack of concentration and agitation are frequently seen among childbearing women who are abusing alcohol. Avoiding important topics, making assumptions about the woman's motivations, and evoking guilt are inappropriate guidelines for the nurse to follow in this situation, and they do not address a caring approach.
Priority Nursing Tip: Consumption of alcohol during pregnancy may lead to fetal alcohol syndrome and can cause jitteriness, physical abnormalities, congenital anomalies, and growth deficits in the newborn.
Test-Taking Strategy: Use therapeutic communication techniques, and note the words *difficulty concentrating and appears agitated*. Remembering that it is important to display a caring and nonjudgmental attitude will direct you to the correct option. Review: therapeutic communication techniques and alcohol use during pregnancy.
Reference(s): Lowdermilk, Perry, Cashion, Alden (2012), p. 765; McKinney et al (2013), pp. 30-31, 293.

1028. The nurse is caring for a depressed, withdrawn client who was responsible for an automobile accident that recently resulted in the death of a child. What is the nurse's **initial** action?

1. Allow the client have some time alone to grieve over the loss.
2. Reinforce for the client that the child's death was a result of an accident.
3. Inform the health care provider of the client's possible need for medication to cope.
4. Communicate in a manner that acknowledges and respects the client's depressed state.

Level of Cognitive Ability: Applying
Client Needs: Psychosocial Integrity
Integrated Process: Caring
Content Area: Mental Health
Priority Concepts: Communication; Mood and Affect

Answer: 4

Rationale: The nurse's initial intervention is to encourage the client to express feelings, which is facilitated by establishing a nurse–client relationship that is based upon respect. Option 4 validates the perception that the client is upset. A well-timed reflection can reveal an emotion that has escaped the client's notice. Both options 1 and 3 address interventions before assessing the situation and identifying the client's actual needs. Option 2 is inappropriate and is a block to communication.

Priority Nursing Tip: For any client experiencing depression following a traumatic event, the nurse should be nonjudgmental and supportive. Encourage the client to express their feelings.

Test-Taking Strategy: Note the strategic word, *initial*, while using therapeutic communication techniques. Select the option that encourages the client to express feelings and maintains communication. Remember to always address the client's feelings. Review: **therapeutic communication techniques and depression.**

Reference(s): Fortinash, Holoday-Worret (2012), pp. 71-74; Varcarolis, Halter (2013), pp. 121-123.

1029. The nurse is bathing a client when the client begins to cry. Which action by the nurse is therapeutic at this time?

1. Continue bathing the client and say nothing.
2. Stop the bath, cover the client, and sit with the client.
3. Call the health care provider to report the signs of depression.
4. Stop the bath, cover the client, and allow the client private time.

Level of Cognitive Ability: Applying
Client Needs: Psychosocial Integrity
Integrated Process: Caring
Content Area: Mental Health
Priority Concepts: Caregiving; Communication

Answer: 2

Rationale: If a client begins to cry, the nurse should stay with the client and let the client know that it is all right to cry. The nurse should ask the client what they are thinking or feeling at the time. By continuing the bath or by leaving the client, the nurse appears to be ignoring the client's feelings. Crying alone is not necessarily an indication of depression, and calling the health care provider is a premature action.

Priority Nursing Tip: Used appropriately, silence and listening are therapeutic communication techniques.

Test-Taking Strategy: Focus on the subject, a client who begins to cry. The nurse needs to acknowledge the client's crying and provide emotional support. Option 2 is the only one that provides the appropriate care for an emotional client. Review: **therapeutic communication techniques** and how to support an **emotional client.**

Reference(s): Fortinash, Holoday-Worret (2012), pp. 71-74; Stuart (2013), p. 17.

1030. Older residents are emotionally despondent when their homes are severely damaged by flooding. When planning for the rescue and relocation of these older residents, what is the **initial** item that the community nurse needs to consider?

1. Contacting their families
2. Attending to their emotional needs
3. Arranging for the repair of their homes
4. Attending to their basic physiological needs

Level of Cognitive Ability: Applying
Client Needs: Physiological Integrity
Integrated Process: Caring
Content Area: Leadership/Management: Prioritizing
Priority Concepts: Clinical Judgment; Caregiving

Answer: 4

Rationale: The question asks about the first thing that the nurse needs to consider when planning for the rescue and relocation of these older residents. The initial concerns of community health are always attending to people's basic needs of food, shelter, and clothing. Contacting family, addressing emotional needs, and arranging for home repairs are needs that may be addressed as needed after physiology needs are met.

Priority Nursing Tip: For any client, the nurse should address physiological needs first; then the nurse should assess safety and psychosocial needs.

Test-Taking Strategy: Use Maslow's Hierarchy of Needs theory to answer the question. Option 4 addresses basic physiological needs. Although options 1, 2, and 3 may be appropriate actions at a later time, option 4 is the immediate concern. Review: the care of clients experiencing crisis.

Reference(s): Ignatavicius, Workman (2013), p. 163; Potter et al (2013), pp. 741-743.

1031. The nurse is planning the care of a client who is suicidal who has been newly admitted to the mental health unit. To provide a caring, therapeutic environment, which intervention should be included in the nursing care plan?
1. Placing the client in a private room to ensure privacy and confidentiality
2. Establishing a therapeutic relationship by conveying unconditional positive regard
3. Maintaining a distance of 10 inches in order to ensure the client that personal control will be provided
4. Placing the client in charge of a meaningful unit activity, such as the morning chess tournament

Level of Cognitive Ability: Applying
Client Needs: Psychosocial Integrity
Integrated Process: Caring
Content Area: Mental Health
Priority Concepts: Mood and Affect; Safety

Answer: 2
Rationale: The establishment of a therapeutic relationship with the suicidal client increases feelings of acceptance. Although the suicidal behavior and the client's thinking are unacceptable, the use of unconditional positive regard acknowledges the client in a human-to-human context and increases the client's sense of self-worth. The client would not be placed in a private room because this is an unsafe action that may intensify the client's feelings of worthlessness. Distances of 18 inches or less between two individuals constitutes intimate space. The invasion of this space may be misinterpreted by the client and increase the client's tension and feelings of helplessness. Placing the client in charge of the morning chess tournament is a premature intervention that can overwhelm the client and cause him or her to fail; this can reinforce the client's feelings of worthlessness.
Priority Nursing Tip: Monitor a depressed client closely for signs of suicidal ideation. If the client presents with increased energy, monitor him or her closely because it could mean that the client now has the energy to perform the suicide act.
Test-Taking Strategy: Focus on the subject, providing a therapeutic environment for a client who is suicidal. Option 2 is the only choice that addresses a caring and therapeutic environment. Review: suicide and principles of therapeutic relationship building.
Reference(s): Fortinash, Holoday-Worret (2012), pp. 517-518; Varcarolis (2013), pp. 442-443.

1032. Shortly after a client dies, the nurse asks the family about funeral arrangements. When the family refuses to discuss the issue, which intervention by the nurse is appropriate for their stage of grief?
1. Displaying acceptance of the family's issues.
2. Providing information about funerals in general.
3. Probing for information about funeral arrangements.
4. Asking the family if they would like time alone with the client.

Level of Cognitive Ability: Applying
Client Needs: Psychosocial Integrity
Integrated Process: Caring
Content Area: Developmental Stages: End-of-Life Care
Priority Concepts: Coping; Palliation

Answer: 4
Rationale: The family is exhibiting the first stage of grief: denial. By asking the family if they would like time alone with the client, the nurse supports the family's feelings and allows the family to process the death. Option 1 is a suitable intervention for the acceptance or reorganization and restitution stage of grief. Options 2 and 3 are not appropriate at this time because the family has indicated their desire not to discuss funeral arrangements.
Priority Nursing Tip: Grief usually involves moving through a series of stages or tasks to help resolve the grief. Feelings associated with grief include anger, frustration, loneliness, sadness, guilt, regret, and peace.
Test-Taking Strategy: Focus on the subject of a grieving family. Note the words *at this time* and the stage of grief that the family is demonstrating. This will help you recognize that the family is in denial and direct you to choose the correct option. Review: the grieving process.
Reference(s): Ignatavicius, Workman (2013), p. 116; Potter et al (2013), pp. 722-723.

1033. A client diagnosed with incurable cancer has a life expectancy of a few weeks. Which response indicates that the client's partner is reacting with an expected coping response?

1. Refusing to visit the client
2. Expresses anger with his God
3. Not allowing his partner to die at home
4. Sending the children to live with relatives

Level of Cognitive Ability: Applying
Client Needs: Psychosocial Integrity
Integrated Process: Caring
Content Area: Developmental Stages: End-of-Life Care
Priority Concepts: Coping; Palliation

Answer: 2
Rationale: The expression of anger is a normal response to impending loss, and often the anger is directed internally or at the dying person, God or another spiritual being, or the caregivers. In option 1, the partner is denying the client's situation and needs by refusing to visit. Options 3 and 4 indicate hasty, unilateral decisions made by the partner without considering anyone else's feelings.
Priority Nursing Tip: A coping mechanism is a method used to decrease anxiety. The use of a coping mechanism can be conscious, unconscious, constructive, destructive, task-oriented in relation to direct problem solving, or defense-oriented and regulating in response to protect oneself.
Test-Taking Strategy: Focus on the subject, *an expected coping response.* Recalling the stages of grief associated with loss will direct you to the correct option. Review: **effective coping mechanisms** and the **grief response.**
Reference(s): Ignatavicius, Workman (2013), p. 419; Potter et al (2013), p. 333.

Communication and Documentation

1034. The nurse working on the mental health unit is in the orientation (introductory) phase of the therapeutic nurse–client relationship. Which intervention is representative of this phase of the relationship?

1. The nurse and client determine the contract for time.
2. The client is encouraged to make use of all services depending on need.
3. The client begins to identify with the nurse, and trust and rapport are maintained.
4. The nurse focuses on facilitating the safe expression of feelings on the part of the client.

Level of Cognitive Ability: Applying
Client Needs: Psychosocial Integrity
Integrated Process: Communication and Documentation
Content Area: Mental Health
Priority Concepts: Communication; Professionalism

Answer: 1
Rationale: In the orientation (introductory phase) of the therapeutic nurse–client relationship, the client and nurse meet and determine the contract for time, such as how often to meet, the length of the meetings, and when termination is anticipated to occur. Utilizing services, identification with the nurse, and expression of feelings are appropriate for the working phase of the therapeutic nurse–client relationship.
Priority Nursing Tip: Acceptance, trust, and boundaries are established in the orientation (introductory) phase of the therapeutic nurse–client relationship.
Test-Taking Strategy: Focus on the subject, the orientation (introductory) phase of the therapeutic nurse–client relationship. Recognizing that option 1 contains the only "orienting" actions will assist you in selecting it as the correct option. Review: the phases of the **therapeutic nurse–client relationship.**
Reference(s): Stuart (2013), p. 19.

1035. The partner of a client who has an esophageal tube tells the nurse, "I thought having this tube down her nose the first time would convince her to quit drinking." Which response to the statement should the nurse make?

1. "I think you are a good person to stay with her."
2. "Alcoholism is a disease that affects the whole family."
3. "Have you discussed this subject at the Al-Anon meetings?"
4. "You sound frustrated with dealing with her drinking problem."

Level of Cognitive Ability: Applying
Client Needs: Psychosocial Integrity
Integrated Process: Communication and Documentation
Content Area: Mental Health
Priority Concepts: Addiction; Communication

Answer: 4
Rationale: In option 4, the nurse uses the therapeutic communication techniques of clarifying and focusing to assist the client's partner with expressing feelings about the client's chronic illness. Showing approval (option 1), stereotyping (option 2), and changing the subject (option 3) are nontherapeutic techniques that block communication.
Priority Nursing Tip: Alcohol abuse is an addiction and a relapse in behavior can occur. This can be very frustrating for families to understand and accept.
Test-Taking Strategy: Use therapeutic communication techniques. Remembering to always address the client's feelings will direct you to the correct option. Review: **therapeutic communication techniques.**
Reference(s): Perry, Potter, Ostendorf (2014), p. 639; Potter et al (2013), pp. 320-322.

1036. The nurse has a prescription to institute aneurysm precautions for a client with a cerebral aneurysm. Which item should the nurse document on the plan of care for this client?

1. Limit out-of-bed activities to twice daily.
2. Allow the client to read and watch television.
3. Encourage the client to take his or her own daily bath.
4. Instruct the client to not strain with bowel movements.

Level of Cognitive Ability: Applying
Client Needs: Physiological Integrity
Integrated Process: Communication and Documentation
Content Area: Adult Health: Neurological
Priority Concepts: Clinical Judgment; Intracranial Regulation

Answer: 4
Rationale: Any activity that increases the blood pressure (BP) or impedes venous flow from the brain is prohibited, such as pushing, pulling, sneezing, coughing, or straining. The nurse documents that the client is instructed to avoid straining with bowel movements. Aneurysm precautions usually include placing the client on bed rest in a quiet setting. Lights are kept dim to minimize environmental stimulation. The nurse provides all physical care to minimize increases in the BP. For the same reason, visitors, radio, television, and reading materials are prohibited or limited. Stimulants such as caffeine and nicotine are also prohibited.
Priority Nursing Tip: For a cerebral aneurysm, bed rest is maintained with the head of the bed elevated 30 to 45 degrees (semi-Fowler's to Fowler's position) to prevent pressure on the aneurysm site.
Test-Taking Strategy: Focus on the subject, components of aneurysm precautions, and note these precautions are to limit the amount of stimulation (in any form) that the client receives and to prevent increased intracranial pressure (ICP). With this in mind, options 1, 2, and 3 are not appropriate. Recognizing that straining can increase ICP, will help you identify option 4 as being correct. Review: the components of **aneurysm precautions.**
Reference(s): Ignatavicius, Workman (2013), pp. 1014-1015.

1037. A client diagnosed with type 2 diabetes mellitus was recently hospitalized for hyperglycemic hyperosmolar syndrome (HHS). Upon discharge from the hospital, the client expresses anxiety and concerns about the recurrence of HHS. How should the nurse respond to promote communication with the client?

1. "Do you think you might need to go to the nursing home?"
2. "You have concerns about the treatment of your condition?"
3. "If you take the correct medications, I doubt this will happen again."
4. "Don't worry. I'm sure your family will provide all the help you need."

Level of Cognitive Ability: Applying
Client Needs: Psychosocial Integrity
Integrated Process: Communication and Documentation
Content Area: Mental Health
Priority Concepts: Anxiety; Communication

Answer: 2
Rationale: The nurse should provide time and listen to the client's concerns while attempting to clarify the client's feelings as in option 2. Option 1 is not an appropriate nursing response because it is making suggestions regarding care options without appropriately identifying the client's true concerns. Options 3 and 4 provide inappropriate false hope and disregard the client's concerns.
Priority Nursing Tip: It is inappropriate to tell a client to "not worry" because it is a barrier to effective communication between the client and the nurse.
Test-Taking Strategy: Use therapeutic communication techniques to always address the client's feelings, especially anxiety, to direct you to the correct option. Review: **therapeutic communication techniques**.
Reference(s): Ignatavicius, Workman (2013), pp. 1458-1459; Potter et al (2013), pp. 320-322.

1038. The nurse assesses the client's peripheral intravenous (IV) site and notes that it is cool, pale, swollen, and not infusing. Which condition should the nurse document?

1. Phlebitis
2. Infection
3. Infiltration
4. Thrombosis

Level of Cognitive Ability: Applying
Client Needs: Physiological Integrity
Integrated Process: Communication and Documentation
Content Area: Critical Care: Medications and Intravenous Therapy
Priority Concepts: Clinical Judgment; Tissue Integrity

Answer: 3
Rationale: The infusion stops when the pressure in the tissue exceeds the pressure in the tubing. The pallor, coolness, and swelling of the IV site are the result of IV fluid infusing into the subcutaneous tissue. An IV site is infiltrated when it becomes dislodged from the vein and is lying in subcutaneous tissue, so the nurse concludes that the IV is infiltrated. The nurse needs to remove the infiltrated catheter and insert a new IV. All the remaining options are likely to be accompanied by warmth at the site. Options 1 and 2 also involve the site appearance as reddened.
Priority Nursing Tip: Insert an infusion catheter at a distal site to provide the option of proceeding up the extremity if the vein is ruptured or infiltration occurs; for example, if infiltration occurs from the antecubital vein, the lower veins in the same arm usually cannot be used for further puncture sites.
Test-Taking Strategy: Focus on the subject, an IV site that is cool, pale, swollen, and not infusing. Use your knowledge regarding the clinical indicators of the complications associated with IV therapy to direct you to option 3. Also note that options 1, 2, and 4 are comparable or alike and are characteristic of warmth at the site. Review: the signs of **IV infiltration**.
Reference(s): Ignatavicius, Workman (2013), p. 228.

❖ **1039.** What instruction should the nurse give to the unlicensed assistive personnel (UAP) in preparation for communicating with a hearing impaired client? **Select all that apply.**
  ❏ 1. Speak using a normal tone of voice.
  ❏ 2. Speak clearly when communicating with the client.
  ❏ 3. Speak slowly and directly into the client's impaired ear.
  ❏ 4. Face the client directly when carrying on a conversation.
  ❏ 5. Be aware of signs that the client does not understand the conversation.

Level of Cognitive Ability: Applying
Client Needs: Safe and Effective Care Environment
Integrated Process: Communication and Documentation
Content Area: Adult Health: Ear
Priority Concepts: Communication; Sensory Perception

Answer: 1, 2, 4, 5
Rationale: When communicating with a hearing-impaired client, the caregiver should speak in a normal tone to the client and should not shout. One should talk directly to the client while facing the client and speak clearly. If the client does not seem to understand what is being said, the caregiver should express the statement differently. Moving closer to the client and toward the better ear may facilitate communication, but one must avoid talking directly into the impaired ear.
Priority Nursing Tip: Hearing impairment occurs with aging; usually high-frequency tones are less perceptible.
Test-Taking Strategy: Focus on the subject, communication techniques for a hearing-impaired client. Knowledge regarding effective therapeutic communication techniques will direct you to the correct options. Review: therapeutic communication techniques and the hearing impaired.
Reference(s): Ignatavicius, Workman (2013), p. 1103.

1040. When the nurse is providing care for a client who is not fluent in the English language, what is the **initial** nursing action?
  1. Determine the client's primary language.
  2. Obtain a translation dictionary for the client.
  3. Establish a means of communication using gestures and hand movements.
  4. Obtain a pad and paper so that the client can write and draw to express needs.

Level of Cognitive Ability: Applying
Client Needs: Psychosocial Integrity
Integrated Process: Communication and Documentation
Content Area: Fundamental Skills: Cultural Awareness
Priority Concepts: Communication; Culture

Answer: 1
Rationale: Language is the largest barrier for people who do not speak English or cannot communicate in English effectively. The nurse needs to assess the client's ability to communicate. If the client is not fluent in English, the nurse should first determine his or her primary language. Then a trained medical interpreter designated by the health care facility should be contacted for communication with the client to prevent errors in communication that could lead to client harm. The client should not be expected to use a translation dictionary or use gestures and hand movements because this could cause confusion and errors in communication. Writing or drawing needs on a pad of paper could also cause confusion and lead to error.
Priority Nursing Tip: The nurse should always seek an agency-designated interpreter if a client does not speak or understand the English language. Having a family member or other person interpret for the client can be a breach of confidentiality; additionally, it could lead to misinterpretation of information and resultant errors.
Test-Taking Strategy: Note the strategic word, *initial*. Use the steps of the nursing process to answer correctly. Option 1 is the only option that reflects the first step of the nursing process, assessment. Review: the nursing considerations for caring for a client who is experiencing language-related barriers to communication.
Reference(s): Ignatavicius, Workman (2013), p. 33.

1041. The nurse develops a plan of care to facilitate effective communication for a client who will require a walker for ambulation. Which intervention has **highest priority**?
1. Directing the discussions so that teaching needs are met
2. Focusing directly on the client's message regarding needs
3. Reflecting only facts related to the client's expressed concerns
4. Reacting to the client's responses in a matter of fact, professional manner

Level of Cognitive Ability: Applying
Client Needs: Psychosocial Integrity
Integrated Process: Communication and Documentation
Content Area: Adult Health: Musculoskeletal
Priority Concepts: Caregiving; Communication

Answer: 2
Rationale: For effective communication, the nurse uses active listening and assesses for verbal and nonverbal communication to receive the client's intended message, thus creating an environment in which the client feels comfortable expressing his or her feelings. An authoritarian approach is directive and not permissive, and it is unlikely to create an environment for the free exchange of thoughts and ideas. Reflecting facts only is a barrier to effective communication because subjective information can also provide a stimulus for effective communication. Reacting enthusiastically can be an ineffective strategy for facilitating communication.
Priority Nursing Tip: The nurse should use both verbal and nonverbal communication cues to interpret what the client is trying to express.
Test-Taking Strategy: Note the strategic words, *highest priority.* Eliminate option 3 because of the closed-ended word "only." Next, use therapeutic communication techniques. This will direct you to the correct option. Review: **therapeutic communication techniques.**
Reference(s): Ignatavicius, Workman (2013), pp. 98, 1157; Potter et al (2013), pp. 320-322.

1042. The nurse made an error when documenting vital signs on a client's paper-based medical record. Which procedure should the nurse use when correcting a written narrative error?
1. Document the correction as a late entry.
2. Draw a line through the error to identify it.
3. Cover the error completely using a permanent marker.
4. Conceal the error with correction fluid approved by the facility.

Level of Cognitive Ability: Applying
Client Needs: Safe and Effective Care Environment
Integrated Process: Communication and Documentation
Content Area: Leadership/Management: Ethical/Legal
Priority Concepts: Communication; Health Care Law

Answer: 2
Rationale: If the nurse makes a narrative documentation error in the client's record, the agency's policy should be followed to correct the error. Agency policy usually includes drawing one line through the error, initialing and dating the line, and then providing the correct information. The nurse uses a late entry to document additional information that was not documented at the time that it occurred. The nurse avoids concealing the error with a marker or correction fluid because these actions raise the suspicion of wrongdoing.
Priority Nursing Tip: Principles of documentation must be followed and data recorded accurately, concisely, completely, legibly, and objectively without bias or opinions. Always follow agency protocol for documentation.
Test-Taking Strategy: Focus on the subject, the principles related to a documentation error. Option 2 is the only option that represents application of documentation principles because the remaining options either alter the record in some fashion or incorrectly identify the documentation. Review: the principles related to **documentation.**
Reference(s): Potter et al (2013), p. 351.

1043. When responding to the call bell, the nurse finds the client lying on the floor. After a thorough assessment and appropriate care, the nurse completes an incident report. What information should be included?
1. The client fell out of bed.
2. The client climbed over the side rails.
3. The client was found lying on the floor.
4. The client was restless and got out of bed.

Level of Cognitive Ability: Applying
Client Needs: Safe and Effective Care Environment
Integrated Process: Communication and Documentation
Content Area: Leadership/Management: Ethical/Legal
Priority Concepts: Communication; Health Care Law

Answer: 3
Rationale: The incident report should contain the client's name, age, and diagnosis. It should contain a factual description of the incident, any injuries experienced by those involved, and the outcome of the situation. Option 3 is the only option that describes the facts as observed by the nurse. Options 1, 2, and 4 are interpretations of the situation and are not factual data as observed by the nurse.
Priority Nursing Tip: The incident report is used as a means of identifying risk situations and improving client care. The report form should not be copied or placed in the client's record.
Test-Taking Strategy: Focus on the subject of an incident report and use general documentation guidelines and principles to answer the question. Remembering to focus on factual information when documenting and avoiding the inclusion of interpretations will direct you to option 3. Review: the **documentation principles** related to incident reports.
Reference(s): Huber (2014), pp. 318-319; Potter et al (2013), pp. 305, 358.

1044. A client diagnosed with angina pectoris appears to be very anxious and states, "So, I had a heart attack, right?" Which response should the nurse make to the client?
1. "No. That is not why you are hospitalized."
2. "No, but there could be some minimal damage to your heart."
3. "No, and we will see to it that you do not have a heart attack."
4. "No, but your health care provider wants to monitor and control or eliminate your pain."

Level of Cognitive Ability: Applying
Client Needs: Psychosocial Integrity
Integrated Process: Communication and Documentation
Content Area: Adult Health: Cardiovascular
Priority Concepts: Communication; Perfusion

Answer: 4
Rationale: Angina pectoris occurs as a result of an inadequate blood supply to the myocardium causing pain; managing the condition will help address the client's pain. The nurse will want to correct the client's misconception regarding a heart attack while addressing the client's concerns. Option 1 does not address the client's concerns. Option 2 is not correct because angina involves interrupted blood supply but does not result in cardiac tissue damage. Neither the nurse nor the health care provider can guarantee that a heart attack will not occur as option 3 appears to do.
Priority Nursing Tip: By clarifying the client's condition with the client, the nurse will help minimize stress, which is a contributing factor of angina attacks.
Test-Taking Strategy: Use therapeutic communication techniques and focus on the subject, the difference between the pathology of a heart attack and angina. Option 4 is the only option that demonstrates correct communication techniques and provides accurate information on the client's condition. Review: the pathophysiology associated with angina pectoris and therapeutic communication techniques.
Reference(s): Ignatavicius, Workman (2013), pp. 835, 841; Potter et al (2013), pp. 320-322.

1045. The nurse is caring for a client diagnosed with depression who appears anxious and withdrawn. Which statement is appropriate for the nurse to make when **initially** initiating conversation?
1. "Do you feel like talking today?"
2. "You are wearing your new shoes."
3. "It appears that talking makes you anxious."
4. "Can you tell me how you are feeling today?"

Level of Cognitive Ability: Applying
Client Needs: Psychosocial Integrity
Integrated Process: Communication and Documentation
Content Area: Mental Health
Priority Concepts: Communication; Mood and Affect

Answer: 2
Rationale: When a depressed client is mute or silent, the nurse should use the communication technique of making observations. A statement such as, "You are wearing your new shoes" is an appropriate statement to make to the client because it is open ended and nonthreatening. When the client is not ready to talk, direct questions or statements such as options 1, 3, and 4 can often raise the client's anxiety level.
Priority Nursing Tip: Depression may be mild, moderate, or severe. Treatment may include counseling, antidepressant medication, or electroconvulsive therapy.
Test-Taking Strategy: Note the strategic word, *initially.* Use your understanding of therapeutic communication techniques to eliminate options 1, 3, and 4 because they are comparable or alike and are likely to increase the client's anxiety. Also, note that option 2 is both open ended and nonthreatening. Review: therapeutic communication techniques for the depressed client.
Reference(s): Fortinash, Holoday-Worret (2012), pp. 35, 71-74; Stuart (2013), p. 22.

1046. The nurse is caring for a client diagnosed with delirium who states, "Look at the spiders on the wall." How should the nurse respond?
1. "Would you like me to kill the spiders for you?"
2. "While there may be spiders on the wall, they are not going to hurt you."
3. "I know that you are frightened, but I do not see any spiders on the wall."
4. "You are having a hallucination; I'm sure there are no spiders in this room."

Level of Cognitive Ability: Applying
Client Needs: Psychosocial Integrity
Integrated Process: Communication and Documentation
Content Area: Mental Health
Priority Concepts: Communication; Psychosis

Answer: 3
Rationale: When hallucinations are present, the nurse should reinforce reality with the client while acknowledging their feelings as option 3 does. Options 1 and 2 do not reinforce reality but rather support the legitimacy of the hallucination. Option 4 reinforces reality but does not address the client's feelings.
Priority Nursing Tip: If the client is hallucinating, ask the client to describe the hallucinations. Avoid reacting to the hallucination as if it were real.
Test-Taking Strategy: Use therapeutic communication techniques and focus on the subject, therapeutically responding to a client who is hallucinating. Option 3 is the only option that both supports reality and addresses the client's feelings. Review: therapeutic communication techniques for the client experiencing hallucinations.
Reference(s): Fortinash, Holoday-Worret (2012), pp. 71-74, 275; Varcarolis (2013), p. 315.

1047. While in the hospital, a client was diagnosed with coronary artery disease (CAD). Which question by the nurse is likely to elicit the **most** useful client response for determining the client's degree of adjustment to the new diagnosis?
1. "Is there anyone to help with housework and shopping?"
2. "How do you feel about making changes to your lifestyle?"
3. "Do you understand the schedule for your new medications?"
4. "Did you make a follow-up appointment with your provider?"

Level of Cognitive Ability: Applying
Client Needs: Health Promotion and Maintenance
Integrated Process: Communication and Documentation
Content Area: Adult Health: Cardiovascular
Priority Concepts: Communication; Coping

Answer: 2
Rationale: Exploring feelings assists the nurse with determining the individualized plan of care for the client who is adjusting to a new diagnosis. Option 2 is the best question to ask the client because it is likely to elicit the most revealing information about the client's feelings about CAD and the requisite lifestyle changes that can help maintain health and wellness. The remaining choices are aspects of post–hospital care, but they are unlikely to uncover as much information about the client's adjustment to CAD because they are closed-ended questions.
Priority Nursing Tip: Increased cholesterol levels, low-density lipoproteins (LDL) levels, and triglyceride levels place the client at risk for coronary artery disease.
Test-Taking Strategy: Note the strategic word, *most*. Use therapeutic communication techniques. Open-ended questions are needed to explore the client's reactions to or feelings about an identified situation. Closed-ended responses generally elicit a "yes" or "no" response exclusively. All of the incorrect options are closed-ended responses. Review: therapeutic communication techniques.
Reference(s): Ignatavicius, Workman (2013), p. 834; Potter et al (2013), pp. 320-322.

1048. A client with a long leg cast who has been using crutches to ambulate for 1 week reports pain, fatigue, and frustration with crutch walking. How should the nurse respond when the client states, "I feel like I will always be crippled"?

1. "Tell me what makes this so bothersome for you."
2. "I know how you feel. I had to use crutches before, too."
3. "Why don't you take a couple of days off of work and rest?"
4. "Just remember, you'll be done with the crutches in another month."

Level of Cognitive Ability: Applying
Client Needs: Psychosocial Integrity
Integrated Process: Communication and Documentation
Content Area: Adult Health: Musculoskeletal
Priority Concepts: Communication; Coping

Answer: 1
Rationale: Option 1 demonstrates the therapeutic communication technique of clarification and validation and indicates that the nurse is dealing with the client's problem from the client's perspective. Option 2 devalues the client's feelings and thus blocks communication. Option 3 gives advice and is a communication block. Option 4 provides false reassurances because the client may not be done with the crutches in another month. Additionally, it does not focus on the present problem.
Priority Nursing Tip: The nurse should monitor for compartment syndrome in a client who has a cast. This is a condition in which pressure increases in a confined anatomical space, leading to decreased blood flow, ischemia, and dysfunction of the tissues.
Test-Taking Strategy: Use therapeutic communication techniques. Option 1 is the only response that encourages communication. The remaining options are comparable or alike because they are blocks to communication. Review: therapeutic communication techniques.
Reference(s): Ignatavicius, Workman (2013), pp. 1157-1158; Potter et al (2013), pp. 320-322.

1049. A teenaged client is discharged from the hospital after surgery with instructions to use a cane for the next 6 months. What question **best** demonstrates the nurse's ability to use therapeutic communication techniques to **effectively** assess the teenager's feelings about using a cane?

1. "How do you feel about needing a cane to walk?"
2. "Do you have questions about ambulating with a cane?"
3. "Are you worried about what your friends will think about your cane?"
4. "What types of problems do you think you'll have ambulating with a cane?"

Level of Cognitive Ability: Applying
Client Needs: Psychosocial Integrity
Integrated Process: Communication and Documentation
Content Area: Developmental Stages: Infancy to Adolescence
Priority Concepts: Communication; Coping

Answer: 1
Rationale: The nurse effectively uses therapeutic communication techniques when posing an open-ended question to elicit assessment data about how the teenager feels about using a cane. The remaining options are closed-ended questions. Option 3 makes assumptions about how the teenager feels while options 2 and 4 focus on the physical aspects of using the cane.
Priority Nursing Tip: The nurse should instruct the client using a cane to inspect the rubber tip on the cane regularly for worn places. A worn tip will need to be replaced.
Test-Taking Strategy: Note the strategic words, *best* and *effectively* in the question. Focus on the subject, the teenager's feelings about the use of the cane. Note the relationship of the subject and option 1. Also use therapeutic communication techniques and avoid responses that include communication blocks. Review: **therapeutic communication techniques.**
Reference(s): Ignatavicius, Workman (2013), pp. 98, 1157-1158; Potter et al (2013), pp. 320-322.

1050. After the surgical repair of a fractured hip, an older adult client has consistently refused to engage in ambulation as prescribed. Which statement by the nurse will **best** encourage the client's need to ambulate?

1. "What is it about getting out of bed that concerns you?"
2. "If you are afraid of the pain, I can give you medication to help."
3. "If you don't get up and start walking, your recovery will take much longer."
4. "Being dependent on others must be a depressing for an active person like yourself."

Level of Cognitive Ability: Applying
Client Needs: Psychological Integrity
Integrated Process: Communication and Documentation
Content Area: Developmental Stages: Early adulthood to later adulthood
Priority Concepts: Adherence; Communication

Answer: 1
Rationale: Early ambulation during the postoperative period is very important to a client's health and recovery, but many different factors may be contributing to the client's refusal to ambulate as prescribed. Asking an open-ended question that encourages a discussion about getting out of bed is the best option available to allow the nurse to facilitate the client's plan of care. Pain may be a concern for the client, but again, the nurse is making an unfounded assumption. While it is true that the recovery might be prolonged by not ambulating and the client may be depressed, these statements make assumptions about the reason the client is refusing to comply with the plan of care.
Priority Nursing Tip: Effective communication with the client is a necessary factor in determining the underlying reasons for noncompliance with the plan of care.
Test-Taking Strategy: Note the strategic word, *best*. Use the principles of therapeutic communication techniques, and your understanding that non-compliance may have many and varied reasons will help direct you to the correct option. Review: **therapeutic communication techniques** and the factors that contribute to **noncompliance**.
Reference(s): Ignatavicius, Workman (2013), p. 99; Potter et al (2013), pp. 320-322.

1051. A client has developed thrombophlebitis in the left leg. Which intervention should the nurse document in the client's plan of care while the client is on bed rest?

1. Elevating the left leg
2. Keeping the left leg flat
3. Engaging in activity as tolerated
4. Maintaining bathroom privileges

Level of Cognitive Ability: Applying
Client Needs: Physiological Integrity
Integrated Process: Communication and Documentation
Content Area: Adult Health: Cardiovascular
Priority Concepts: Clinical Judgment; Clotting

Answer: 1
Rationale: The nurse plans to elevate the affected extremity because this facilitates venous return by using gravity to improve blood return to the heart, decreases venous pressure, and helps relieve edema and pain. Option 2 does not facilitate venous return and thus is not indicated for a client with thrombophlebitis. Options 3 and 4 are unsuitable activities for a client on bed rest.
Priority Nursing Tip: Thrombophlebitis is an inflammation of a vein, often accompanied by clot formation that can present serious circulatory problems.
Test-Taking Strategy: Focus on the subject, thrombophlebitis, and think about the pathophysiology associated with this condition and how gravity affects venous blood flow and edema. This will direct you to option 1. Review: the nursing care for a client with **thrombophlebitis**.
Reference(s): Ignatavicius, Workman (2013), p. 800.

1052. A client who is experiencing paranoid thinking involving his food being poisoned is admitted to the mental health unit. Which communication technique should the nurse use to encourage the client to communicate his fears?

1. Open-ended questions and silence
2. Offering personal opinions about the need to eat
3. Verbalizing reasons why the client may choose not to eat
4. Focusing on self-disclosure of the nurse's own food preferences

Level of Cognitive Ability: Applying
Client Needs: Physiological Integrity
Integrated Process: Communication and Documentation
Content Area: Mental Health
Priority Concepts: Communication; Psychosis

Answer: 1
Rationale: Open-ended questions and silence are strategies that are used to encourage clients to discuss their feelings in a descriptive manner. Options 2 and 3 are not helpful to the client because they do not encourage the expression of personal feelings. Option 4 is not a client-centered intervention.
Priority Nursing Tip: Avoid whispering in the presence of a client who is paranoid because this will intensify his or her feelings of paranoia.
Test-Taking Strategy: Use your knowledge of therapeutic communication techniques to identify the usefulness of the techniques suggested in option 1. The communication techniques identified in options 2, 3, and 4 are nontherapeutic and are blocks to communication. Review: **therapeutic communication techniques and paranoid behavior.**
Reference(s): Fortinash, Holoday-Worret (2012), pp. 71-74; Varcarolis (2013), pp. 120-123.

1053. The nurse is preparing a client for electroconvulsive therapy (ECT). After the client signs the informed consent form for the procedure, a family member states, "I don't think that this ECT will be helpful, especially since it makes people's memory worse." What form of communication should the nurse implement to address the family member's concern?

1. Ask other family members and the client if they think that ECT makes people worse.
2. Immediately reassure the client and family that ECT will help and that the memory loss is only temporary.
3. Involve the family member in a dialogue to ascertain how the family member arrived at this conclusion.
4. Reinforce with the client and the family member that depression causes more memory impairment than ECT.

Level of Cognitive Ability: Applying
Client Needs: Psychosocial Integrity
Integrated Process: Communication and Documentation
Content Area: Mental Health
Priority Concepts: Communication; Mood and Affect

Answer: 3
Rationale: In option 3, the nurse is looking for data to assist with clarifying information about the procedure with the family which is necessary in order to deal effectively with their concerns. Option 1 may place family members on the defensive and promote conflict among them. Option 2 does not acknowledge the family member's statement and concerns. Option 4 addresses content clarification but not the assessment process, and it is not the most therapeutic action.
Priority Nursing Tip: Electroconvulsive therapy (ECT) may be prescribed to treat depression. It consists of inducing a seizure by passing an electrical current through the brain via electrodes attached to the temples. ECT is not a permanent cure. It is true that some clients experience temporary memory loss, but it usually centers on the time period around the treatment itself.
Test-Taking Strategy: Use therapeutic communication techniques and the steps of the nursing process. Remember that assessment is the first step in the nursing process. In option 3, the nurse gathers more data via the assessment process and addresses the family member's thoughts and feelings. Review: **therapeutic communication techniques and electroconvulsive therapy (ECT).**
Reference(s): Fortinash, Holoday-Worret (2012), pp. 71-74, 286; Stuart (2013), pp. 596-597, 600.

Teaching and Learning

1054. A client diagnosed with tuberculosis (TB) is provided instructions concerning home care in preparation for discharge. Which client statement indicates a **need for further teaching**?

1. "I need to place used tissues in a plastic bag when I am home."
2. "I need to eat foods that are high in iron, protein, and vitamin C."
3. "It is not necessary to maintain respiratory isolation when I am at home."
4. "If I miss a dose of medication, I should then resume my regular schedule."

Level of Cognitive Ability: Evaluating
Client Needs: Physiological Integrity
Integrated Process: Teaching and Learning
Content Area: Adult Health: Respiratory
Priority Concepts: Adherence; Client Education

Answer: **4**
Rationale: Because of the resistant strains of TB, the nurse must emphasize that noncompliance regarding medication could lead to an infection that is difficult to treat and that may cause total drug resistance. Medication doses should not be skipped. If a TB medication dose is missed it needs to be taken as soon as remembered. Options 1, 2, and 3 are correct in their description of appropriated self-management of the infection.
Priority Nursing Tip: For the hospitalized client, private negative airflow pressure rooms and personal respiratory protection devices are required with airborne diseases such as tuberculosis. A mask must be worn by the client when he or she leaves the room.
Test-Taking Strategy: Note the strategic words, *need for further teaching*. These words indicate a negative event query and ask you to select an option that is an incorrect statement. General principles related to medication administration will direct you to option 4. Review: **tuberculosis (TB)**.
Reference(s): Ignatavicius, Workman (2013), pp. 657-658; Lehne (2013), pp. 1129-1130.

❖ **1055.** The nurse is planning discharge teaching for a client diagnosed and treated for tuberculosis (TB). Which instruction should be included in order to minimize the spread of TB? **Select all that apply.**

❑ 1. All used dishes should be sterilized.
❑ 2. Close contacts should be tested for TB.
❑ 3. Soiled tissues should be disposed of properly.
❑ 4. House isolation is required for at least 8 months.
❑ 5. The mouth should always be covered when coughing.

Level of Cognitive Ability: Applying
Client Needs: Safe and Effective Care Environment
Integrated Process: Teaching and Learning
Content Area: Fundamental Skills: Infection Control
Priority Concepts: Client Education; Infection

Answer: **2, 3, 5**
Rationale: Tuberculosis is a communicable disease, and the nurse must teach the client measures to prevent its spread. Any close contacts with the client must be tested and treated if the results of the screening test are positive. Because it is an airborne disease, the client must properly dispose of used tissues and needs to cover the mouth when coughing. There is no evidence to suggest that sterilizing dishes would break the chain of infection with pulmonary TB. It is not necessary for the client to isolate herself or himself to the house. Once the client is treated and results of three sputum cultures are negative, she or he will not spread the infection.
Priority Nursing Tip: Multidrug resistant strains of tuberculosis can result from improper compliance, noncompliance with treatment programs, or development of mutations in tubercle bacillus; the nurse must include the importance of medication compliance when teaching the client with tuberculosis (TB).
Test-Taking Strategy: Focus on the subject, minimizing the spread of tuberculosis. Also focusing on the pathophysiology of TB and the associated communicability factors and risks will assist you in answering correctly. Review: the home care principles related to **tuberculosis (TB)** and **airborne disease transmission precautions**.
Reference(s): Ignatavicius, Workman (2013), p. 657.

1056. A client is receiving intravenous (IV) antibiotic therapy at home via an intermittent IV catheter. In order to facilitate the early detection of IV therapy complications, which intervention should be included in the client's education?
1. Protect the IV site continually.
2. Keep the IV site clean and dry.
3. Report local pain, drainage, or edema.
4. Apply pressure to the IV site if it dislodges.

Level of Cognitive Ability: Applying
Client Needs: Safe and Effective Care Environment
Integrated Process: Teaching and Learning
Content Area: Fundamental Skills: Safety
Priority Concepts: Client Education, Safety

Answer: 3
Rationale: The nurse instructs the client to report clinical indicators of an IV site infection, including pain, drainage, and edema because the early detection of infection decreases the risk of septicemia, tissue loss, and devastating complications. The remaining options are reasonable aspects of client teaching for IV therapy at home, but they are not surveillance methods.
Priority Nursing Tip: Any solution administered by the intravenous route directly enters the client's circulatory system. Strict aseptic technique is necessary to prevent infection.
Test-Taking Strategy: Focus on the subject, early detection of IV therapy complications. Eliminate options 1, 2, and 4 because these choices describe aspects of IV care to help prevent complications, but they do not contribute to early detection. Review: the principles of IV site care.
Reference(s): Potter et al (2013), p. 925.

1057. The home care nurse provides instructions about the management of pruritus to a client diagnosed with jaundice. Which statement made by the client suggests to the nurse that the client **needs further teaching**?
1. "I need to wear loose cotton clothing."
2. "A tepid water bath should help stop the itching."
3. "Keeping the house warmer is likely to lessen the itching"
4. "I need to take the prescribed antihistamines as I'm supposed to."

Level of Cognitive Ability: Evaluating
Client Needs: Physiological Integrity
Integrated Process: Teaching and Learning
Content Area: Adult Health: Gastrointestinal
Priority Concepts: Client Education; Tissue Integrity

Answer: 3
Rationale: Pruritus is caused by the accumulation of bile salts in the skin and results from obstructed biliary excretion. The client would be instructed to keep the house temperature cool in order to minimize the itching. The client should avoid the use of alkaline soap, and he or she should wear loose, soft, cotton clothing. Antihistamines may relieve the itching, as will tepid water and emollient baths.
Priority Nursing Tip: Jaundice results when the liver is unable to metabolize bilirubin or when edema, fibrosis, and scarring of the hepatic bile ducts interfere with normal bile and bilirubin secretion.
Test-Taking Strategy: Note the strategic words, *needs further teaching*. These words indicate a negative event query and ask you to select an option that is an incorrect statement. Recalling that heat causes vasodilation will assist with directing you to the correct option. Review: the measures that assist with alleviating **pruritus**.
Reference(s): Ignatavicius, Workman (2013), p. 471; Lewis et al (2011), pp. 466, 1081.

1058. The nurse has provided home care instructions to a client who has been hospitalized for a transurethral resection of the prostate (TURP). Which statement by the client indicates the **need for further teaching**?

1. "Prune juice needs to be included in my diet."
2. "I need to avoid strenuous activity for 4 to 6 weeks."
3. "My intake of water needs to be at least 6 to 8 glasses daily."
4. "I can't lift or push objects that weigh more than 30 pounds."

Level of Cognitive Ability: Evaluating
Client Needs: Physiological Integrity
Integrated Process: Teaching and Learning
Content Area: Adult Health: Renal and Urinary
Priority Concepts: Client Education; Safety

Answer: 4

Rationale: The client needs to be advised to avoid strenuous activity for 4 to 6 weeks and avoid lifting items that weigh more than 20 pounds. Straining during defecation is avoided to prevent bleeding. Prune juice is a satisfactory bowel stimulant. The client needs to consume a daily intake of at least 6 to 8 glasses of nonalcoholic fluids to minimize clot formation.

Priority Nursing Tip: Following transurethral resection of the prostate (TURP), monitor for hemorrhage. Postoperative continuous bladder irrigation (CBI) may be prescribed, which prevents catheter obstruction from clots.

Test-Taking Strategy: Note the strategic words, *need for further teaching*. These words indicate a negative event query and ask you to select an option that is an incorrect statement. Options 2 and 3 can be eliminated first because they are general postoperative teaching points. Considering the anatomical location of the surgical procedure, it is reasonable to think that constipation needs to be avoided; therefore, eliminate option 1. Also note that lifting items that weigh 30 pounds is excessive. Review: **transurethral resection of the prostate (TURP)** discharge teaching points.

Reference(s): Ignatavicius, Workman (2013), pp. 1636, 1641.

1059. The nurse is providing home care instructions to a client who will be receiving intravenous (IV) therapy. What is the **most important** measure the nurse should stress in order to prevent an infection at the IV site?

1. Keep a dressing over the insertion site.
2. Assess the IV site for redness and edema.
3. Change the IV tubing every 48 to 72 hours.
4. Wash the hands well before handling the IV site.

Level of Cognitive Ability: Analyzing
Client Needs: Safe and Effective Care Environment
Integrated Process: Teaching and Learning
Content Area: Fundamental Skills: Infection Control
Priority Concepts: Client Education; Infection

Answer: 4

Rationale: Option 4 emphasizes the need to perform thorough hand washing before handling the IV site or equipment to reduce the risk of introducing potential pathogens that are likely to cause an infection, and it is the most important measure. Option 1 helps maintain the IV catheter securely and prevents a mode of entry for potential pathogens. Option 2 helps with the early detection of infection. Changing the IV fluid and tubing (option 3) helps reduce the risk of overgrowth of microorganisms from within the system.

Priority Nursing Tip: Signs of infection at the site of an intravenous line include redness, swelling, and drainage.

Test-Taking Strategy: Note the strategic words, *most important*, which indicates that all options may be correct and you need to select the most important measure. Focus on the subject, preventing infection at an IV site. Remember that the top priority for infection prevention always includes proper hand-washing technique. Review: **standard precautions** and their role in preventing **infection**.

Reference(s): Ignatavicius, Workman (2013), pp. 223, 440-441.

1060. A client is being treated for an atrial dysrhythmia with quinidine gluconate. Which statement by the client indicates to the nurse that the medication instructions about what to do if a dose is missed have been understood?
1. "I should call my health care provider."
2. "I should take the next prescribed dose as usual."
3. "I should take the dose as soon as I realize I've missed it."
4. "I take two doses of the medication at the next scheduled time."

Level of Cognitive Ability: Evaluating
Client Needs: Physiological Integrity
Integrated Process: Teaching and Learning
Content Area: Pharmacology: Cardiovascular Medications
Priority Concepts: Client Education; Safety

Answer: 2
Rationale: Quinidine gluconate needs to be taken exactly as prescribed. Because of the action and effects of this medication, the client should be instructed to take the medication if remembered within 2 hours of the missed dose, or omit the dose and then resume the normal schedule. There is no need to call the doctor. It is not safe to take the dose whenever it is remembered or to take an extra dose.
Priority Nursing Tip: Quinidine gluconate is an antidysrhythmic medication. The client must be instructed to take the medication exactly as prescribed.
Test-Taking Strategy: Focus on the subject, the principles related to quinidine gluconate administration. Think about the action and effect of the medication. Only option 2 expresses the appropriate measures to take when this medication dose is forgotten. Review: the basic principles associated with medication administration and quinidine gluconate.
Reference(s): Kee, Hayes, McCuistion (2012), p. 635.

1061. Which is the **best** recommendation for the nurse to provide to a client to save lives and prevent burn injuries in the event of a fire in the home?
1. Place escape ladders in the bedrooms.
2. Install a whole-house sprinkler system.
3. Keep fresh batteries in smoke detectors.
4. Mount fire extinguishers in several areas.

Level of Cognitive Ability: Applying
Client Needs: Safe and Effective Care Environment
Integrated Process: Teaching and Learning
Content Area: Fundamental Skills: Safety
Priority Concepts: Client Education; Safety

Answer: 3
Rationale: The early detection of smoke using a smoke detector and immediate evacuation from the house have significant and positive effects on mortality rates. This is because the smoke alarm activates before the appearance of open flames, which gives people in the house a chance to evacuate without burn injuries. Option 1 helps people in the house escape from second-story rooms safely, but it does not alert the people to the fire before flames are evident, thus exposing them to the risk of burn injury. Installing a sprinkler system is very expensive (option 2), and this is usually not done in private residences. Fire extinguishers are a good idea to have in the kitchen and other areas for small fires, but they are not designed to extinguish large fires.
Priority Nursing Tip: In the hospital, remember the mnemonic RACE (Rescue the client, Activate the fire alarm, Confine the fire, and Extinguish the fire) to set priorities in the event of a fire.
Test-Taking Strategy: Note the strategic word, *best*. Focus of the subject, measure to save lives and prevent burn injuries in the event of a fire in the home. This will direct you to the correct option. Review: the principles of fire safety.
Reference(s): Potter et al (2013), pp. 367, 386.

1062. A client has had same-day surgery to insert a ventilating tube into the tympanic membrane. Which statement assures the nurse that the client understands the discharge instructions?

1. "I will use a shower cap when taking a shower."
2. "I was told to try and avoid taking medications for pain."
3. "Swimming is allowed only if I keep my head above water."
4. "I need to wash my hair quickly; taking 2 minutes or less."

Level of Cognitive Ability: Evaluating
Client Needs: Physiological Integrity
Integrated Process: Teaching and Learning
Content Area: Adult Health: Ear
Priority Concepts: Client Education; Sensory Perception

Answer: 1
Rationale: After the insertion of tubes into the tympanic membrane, it is important to avoid getting water in the ears. A shower cap or earplug may be used when showering, if allowed by the health care provider. Swimming, showering without a shower cap or ear plugs, and washing the hair are avoided after surgery until the time frame designated for each is identified by the surgeon The client should take medication as advised for postoperative discomfort.
Priority Nursing Tip: Ventilating tubes inserted into the tympanic membranes are tiny, white, spool-shaped tubes. If the tubes fall out, it is not an emergency, but the health care provider should be notified.
Test-Taking Strategy: Note the words *understands the discharge instructions.* Eliminate option 3 because of the closed-ended word "only," and eliminate option 4 because of the word *quickly.* From the remaining choices, focusing on the anatomical location of the surgery will direct you to option 1. Review: client instructions after the insertion of ventilating tubes into the **tympanic membrane.**
Reference(s): Ignatavicius, Workman (2013), p. 1094.

1063. The nurse has completed diet teaching for a client on a low-sodium diet for the treatment of hypertension. Which statement by the client should indicate to the nurse that there is a **need for further teaching?**

1. "Frozen foods are usually lowest in sodium."
2. "This diet will help lower my blood pressure."
3. "This diet is not a replacement for my antihypertensive medications."
4. "The reason I need to lower my salt intake is to reduce fluid retention."

Level of Cognitive Ability: Evaluating
Client Needs: Physiological Integrity
Integrated Process: Teaching and Learning
Content Area: Adult Health: Cardiovascular
Priority Concepts: Client Education; Nutrition

Answer: 1
Rationale: A low-sodium diet is used as an adjunct to antihypertensive medications for the treatment of hypertension. Sodium retains fluid, which leads to hypertension as a result of increased fluid volume. Frozen foods use salt as a preservative, which increases their sodium content. Canned foods are extremely high in sodium. Fresh foods are best.
Priority Nursing Tip: Emphasize to the client with hypertension that dietary changes are not temporary and must be maintained for life.
Test-Taking Strategy: Note the strategic words, *need for further teaching.* These words indicate a negative event query and ask you to select an option that is an incorrect statement. Eliminate options 2, 3, and 4 because these are accurate statements related to hypertension. Also, recall that "fresh is best"; fresh foods are lowest in sodium. Review: the treatment of **hypertension** and foods high in **sodium.**
Reference(s): Nix (2013), p. 389.

1064. The nurse is giving dietary instructions to a client who has been prescribed cyclosporine (Sandimmune). Which food item should the nurse instruct the client to avoid?

1. Red meats
2. Orange juice
3. Grapefruit juice
4. Green leafy vegetables

Level of Cognitive Ability: Applying
Client Needs: Physiological Integrity
Integrated Process: Teaching and Learning
Content Area: Pharmacology: Immune Medications
Priority Concepts: Client Education; Safety

Answer: 3
Rationale: A compound in grapefruit juice inhibits the metabolism of cyclosporine. Thus, drinking grapefruit juice can raise cyclosporine levels by 50% to 100%, greatly increasing the risk of toxicity. The foods in options 1, 2, and 4 are acceptable to consume.
Priority Nursing Tip: Cyclosporine (Sandimmune) is an immunosuppressant medication that can be toxic and cause kidney damage.
Test-Taking Strategy: Focus on the subject, the food item to avoid. This creates a negative event query and requires you to select something the client should avoid ingesting. Use general medication guidelines to assist in answering the question, and remember that grapefruit juice should not be administered with medications. Review: the nursing considerations related to cyclosporine (Sandimmune).
Reference(s): Hodgson, Kizior (2014), p. 293.

1065. The nurse performs an initial assessment on a pregnant client and determines that the client is at risk for toxoplasmosis. What should the nurse teach the client to prevent exposure to this disease?
1. Eat raw meats.
2. Wash your hands only before meals.
3. Avoid exposure to litter boxes used by cats.
4. Use topical corticosteroid treatments prophylactically.

Level of Cognitive Ability: Applying
Client Needs: Safe and Effective Care Environment
Integrated Process: Teaching and Learning
Content Area: Maternity: Antepartum
Priority Concepts: Client Education; Infection

Answer: 3
Rationale: Infected house cats transmit toxoplasmosis through the feces. Handling litter boxes can transmit the disease to the pregnant client. Meats that are undercooked can harbor microorganisms that can cause infection. Hands should be washed frequently throughout the day. The use of topical corticosteroids will not prevent exposure to the disease.
Priority Nursing Tip: Toxoplasmosis is an infection that can be transmitted to the fetus across the placenta. This infection can cause spontaneous abortion in the first trimester.
Test-Taking Strategy: Eliminate option 2 because of the closed-ended word "only." Option 1 represents an extreme statement and can also be eliminated. From the remaining choices, focusing on the words *prevent exposure* in the question will direct you to option 3. Review: the causes of **toxoplasmosis.**
Reference(s): McKinney et al (2013), p. 630.

1066. A home care nurse is instructing a mother of a child diagnosed with cystic fibrosis (CF) about the appropriate dietary measures. Which diet should the nurse tell the mother that the child needs to consume?
1. Low-calorie, low-fat diet
2. High-calorie, restricted fat
3. Low-calorie, low-protein diet
4. High-calorie, high-protein diet

Level of Cognitive Ability: Applying
Client Needs: Physiological Integrity
Integrated Process: Teaching and Learning
Content Area: Child Health: Throat/Respiratory
Priority Concepts: Client Education; Nutrition

Answer: 4
Rationale: Children with CF are managed with a high-calorie, high-protein diet. Pancreatic enzyme replacement therapy and fat-soluble vitamin supplements are administered. Fat restriction is not necessary.
Priority Nursing Tip: Cystic fibrosis is a progressive and incurable disorder, and respiratory failure is a common cause of death; organ transplantations may be an option to increase survival rates.
Test-Taking Strategy: Eliminate options 1 and 2 first because they are comparable or alike, and both restrict fat. From the remaining choices, focus on the subject of nutritional needs of a child with cystic fibrosis (CF) and the pathophysiology related to CF; this will direct you to option 4. Review: the diet plan for the child with **cystic fibrosis (CF).**
Reference(s): Hockenberry, Wilson (2013), p. 751; McKinney et al (2013), p. 1190.

1067. When should the nurse schedule crutch walking instructions for a client who is to be scheduled for knee replacement surgery?
1. Before surgery
2. On the first postoperative day
3. On the second postoperative day
4. At the time of discharge after surgery

Level of Cognitive Ability: Applying
Client Needs: Physiological Integrity
Integrated Process: Teaching and Learning
Content Area: Adult Health: Musculoskeletal
Priority Concepts: Client Education; Mobility

Answer: 1
Rationale: It is best to assess crutch-walking ability and instruct the client with regard to the use of the crutches before surgery because this task can be difficult to learn when the client is in pain and not used to the imbalance that may occur after surgery. Options 2, 3, and 4 are not the appropriate times to teach a client about crutch walking.
Priority Nursing Tip: For the client undergoing knee replacement surgery, the nurse should plan to begin continuous passive motion 24 to 48 hours postoperatively as prescribed to exercise the knee and provide moderate flexion and extension.
Test-Taking Strategy: Focus on the subject, the time to schedule crutch walking instructions. Note that options 2, 3, and 4 are comparable or alike in that they address the postoperative period. Review: knee replacement surgery.
Reference(s): Ignatavicius, Workman (2013), p. 329.

1068. A client with a short leg plaster cast reports intense itching under the cast. The nurse provides instructions to the client regarding relief measures for the itching. Which statement by the client indicates an understanding of the measures used to relieve the itching?

1. "I can use the blunt part of a ruler to scratch the area."
2. "I can trickle small amounts of water down inside the cast."
3. "I need to obtain assistance when placing an object into the cast for the itching."
4. "I can use a hair dryer on the low setting and allow the air to blow into the cast."

Level of Cognitive Ability: Evaluating
Client Needs: Physiological Integrity
Integrated Process: Teaching and Learning
Content Area: Adult Health: Musculoskeletal
Priority Concepts: Client Education; Mobility

Answer: 4
Rationale: Itching is a common complaint of clients with casts. Objects should not be put inside a cast because of the risk of scratching the skin and providing a point of entry for bacteria. A plaster cast can break down when wet. Therefore, the best way to relieve itching is with the forceful injection of air inside the cast.
Priority Nursing Tip: The health care provider is notified immediately if circulatory impairment occurs in the extremity with a cast.
Test-Taking Strategy: Eliminate options 1 and 3 first because they are comparable or alike and indicate putting objects inside the cast. Next, focus on the subject, proper cast care, to direct you to option 4. Review: client teaching regarding cast care.
Reference(s): Ignatavicius, Workman (2013), p. 1151; Lewis et al (2011), p. 1601.

1069. Disulfiram (Antabuse) has been prescribed for a client, and the nurse provides instructions to the client about the medication. Which statement by the client indicates the **need for further teaching?**

1. "I must be careful taking cold medicines."
2. "I will have to check my aftershave lotion."
3. "I'll be fine as long as I don't drink alcohol."
4. "I need to be careful with ingredients when I cook."

Level of Cognitive Ability: Evaluating
Client Needs: Physiological Integrity
Integrated Process: Teaching and Learning
Content Area: Pharmacology: Psychiatric Medications
Priority Concepts: Client Education; Safety

Answer: 3
Rationale: Clients who are taking disulfiram must be taught that substances that contain alcohol can trigger an adverse reaction. Sources of hidden alcohol include foods (soups, sauces, and vinegars), medicine (cold medicine), mouthwashes, and skin preparations (alcohol rubs and aftershave lotions).
Priority Nursing Tip: Disulfiram is an alcohol deterrent that may be prescribed for alcoholic dependence. The medication sensitizes the client to alcohol, so a disulfiram-alcohol reaction occurs if alcohol is ingested.
Test-Taking Strategy: Note the strategic words, *need for further teaching*. These words indicate a negative event query and ask you to select an option that is an incorrect statement. Remember that disulfiram is used for clients who have alcoholism, and any form of alcohol must be avoided with this medication. Review: disulfiram (Antabuse).
Reference(s): Lehne (2013), p. 449.

1070. The nurse has provided instructions to a client who is receiving external radiation therapy. Which statement by the client indicates a **need for further teaching** regarding self-care related to the radiation therapy?

1. "I need to eat a high-protein diet."
2. "I need to avoid exposure to sunlight."
3. "I need to wash my skin with a mild soap and pat it dry."
4. "I need to apply pressure on the irritated area to prevent bleeding."

Level of Cognitive Ability: Evaluating
Client Needs: Physiological Integrity
Integrated Process: Teaching and Learning
Content Area: Adult Health: Oncology
Priority Concepts: Client Education; Tissue Integrity

Answer: 4
Rationale: The client receiving external radiation therapy should avoid pressure on the irritated area and wear loose-fitting clothing. Specific health care provider instructions would be necessary to obtain if an alteration in skin integrity occurred as a result of the radiation therapy. Options 1, 2, and 3 are accurate measures regarding radiation therapy.
Priority Nursing Tip: The client undergoing external radiation therapy does not emit radiation and does not pose a hazard to anyone else.
Test-Taking Strategy: Note the strategic words, *need for further teaching*. These words indicate a negative event query and ask you to select an option that is an incorrect statement. The word *pressure* in option 4 is an indication that this is an inappropriate measure. Review: the client teaching points related to skin care and radiation therapy.
Reference(s): Ignatavicius, Workman (2013), p. 413.

1071. The nurse has provided instructions to a client regarding the testicular self-examination (TSE). Which statement by the client indicates that the client **needs further teaching** regarding TSE?
1. "I know to report any small lumps."
2. "I should examine myself every 2 months."
3. "I should examine myself after I take a warm shower."
4. "I know it's normal to feel something that is cord-like in the back."

Level of Cognitive Ability: Evaluating
Client Needs: Health Promotion and Maintenance
Integrated Process: Teaching and Learning
Content Area: Adult Health: Oncology
Priority Concepts: Client Education; Health Promotion

Answer: 2
Rationale: TSE should be performed every month. Small lumps or abnormalities should be reported. The spermatic cord finding is normal. After a warm bath or shower, the scrotum is relaxed, which makes it easier to perform TSE.
Priority Nursing Tip: Teach the client how to perform TSE; a day of the month is selected and the exam is performed on the same day each month after a shower or bath when the hands are warm and soapy and the scrotum is warm.
Test-Taking Strategy: Note the strategic words, *needs further teaching*. These words indicate a negative event query and the need to select the incorrect client statement. Remembering that breast self-examination needs to be performed monthly may assist you with recalling that TSE is also performed monthly. Review: the procedure for testicular self-examination (TSE).
Reference(s): Ignatavicius, Workman (2013), p. 1643; Potter et al (2013), p. 549.

1072. A client diagnosed with acquired immuno-deficiency syndrome (AIDS) is reporting fatigue. Which strategy should the nurse teach the client to conserve energy after discharge from the hospital?
1. Bathe before eating breakfast.
2. Sit for as many activities as possible.
3. Stand in the shower instead of taking a bath.
4. Group all tasks to be performed early in the morning.

Level of Cognitive Ability: Applying
Client Needs: Physiological Integrity
Integrated Process: Teaching and Learning
Content Area: Adult Health: Immune
Priority Concepts: Client Education; Functional Ability

Answer: 2
Rationale: The client is taught to conserve energy by sitting for as many activities as possible, including dressing, shaving, preparing food, ironing, and so on. The client should also sit in a shower chair instead of standing while showering. The client needs to prioritize activities such as eating breakfast before bathing, and he or she should intersperse each major activity with a period of rest.
Priority Nursing Tip: Acquired immunodeficiency syndrome (AIDS) is a disorder caused by the human immunodeficiency virus (HIV) and characterized by generalized dysfunction of the immune system.
Test-Taking Strategy: Focus on the subject of conserving energy. Think about the amount of exertion required by the client to perform each of the activities described in the options. Options 3 and 4 are obviously taxing for the client and are thus eliminated first. From the remaining choices, recall that bathing may take away energy that could be used for eating and so is not helpful. Review: the measures that conserve energy.
Reference(s): Ignatavicius, Workman (2013), pp. 371, 375-376.

❖ **1073.** The nurse is providing home care instructions to the partner of a client who is confused and will be cared for at home. Which instructions should the nurse provide to help minimize the client's confusion? **Select all that apply.**
- ❑ 1. Turn the lights off at dusk.
- ❑ 2. Maintain a predictable routine.
- ❑ 3. Use simple, clear communication.
- ❑ 4. Limit the number of choices given to the client.
- ❑ 5. Encourage frequent visits from family and friends.
- ❑ 6. Display a calendar and a clock in the client's room.

Level of Cognitive Ability: Applying
Client Needs: Psychosocial Integrity
Integrated Process: Teaching and Learning
Content Area: Mental Health
Priority Concepts: Client Education; Cognition

Answer: 2, 3, 4, 6
Rationale: The caregiver of a confused client is taught measures and techniques that will keep the client oriented and calm. Sensory overload or tasks and activities that are overwhelming for the client will cause disorientation and additional confusion. Therefore, any measures or activities that will increase sensory overload are avoided. Some helpful techniques include turning the lights on at dusk to avoid the sundown syndrome of increased confusion and combative behavior; maintaining a predictable routine; using simple, clear communication; limiting the number of choices given to the client; limiting the number of visitors who come to see the client; and displaying a calendar and a clock around the house and in the client's room.
Priority Nursing Tip: The nurse should encourage the family of a confused client to help him or her maintain independence. Constant encouragement with a simple step-by-step approach with the client is most helpful.
Test-Taking Strategy: Focus on the subject, measures that will minimize confusion. Think about each listed intervention, and remember that measures or activities that will increase sensory overload or are overwhelming for the client are to be avoided. This principle will assist you with selecting the correct measures. Review: the care of the client with **confusion**.
Reference(s): Fortinash, Holoday-Worret (2012), pp. 380-381; Stuart (2013), p. 429.

1074. A 10-year-old child has been diagnosed with type 1 diabetes mellitus. What instruction should the nurse provide concerning the need to monitor the child's insulin needs?
1. The child should be taught to self-monitor insulin needs.
2. The parents will need to be available to monitor the child's insulin needs.
3. The child's school teacher will assume responsibility of insulin need monitoring.
4. Close friends and family will need to be involved with monitoring the child's insulin needs.

Level of Cognitive Ability: Applying
Client Needs: Physiological Integrity
Integrated Process: Teaching and Learning
Content Area: Developmental Stages: Infancy to Adolescence
Priority Concepts: Client Education; Development

Answer: 1
Rationale: Most children 9 years old or older can understand the principles of monitoring their own insulin requirements. They are usually responsible enough to determine the appropriate intervention needed to maintain their health. Parents, friends, and family cannot always be available. The school teacher should not be expected to take responsibility for health care interventions.
Priority Nursing Tip: The abdomen is the preferred site for infusion set sites and injections. It is easy to see and reach, and offers the quickest absorption.
Test-Taking Strategy: Focus on the subject, a 10-year-old child with type 1 diabetes mellitus. Noting the age of the child will indicate that the child is able to take control and responsibility regarding his health care situation. Eliminate options 2, 3, and 4 because they are comparable or alike and rely on other individuals to care for the child. Review: the **growth and development** of a 10-year-old child.
Reference(s): Hockenberry, Wilson (2013), pp. 459, 1005.

1075. The nurse instructs a client diagnosed with oral candidiasis (thrush) about caring for the disorder. Which statement by the client indicates a **need for additional teaching?**
1. "I can eat foods that are liquid or pureed."
2. "I should eliminate spicy foods from my diet."
3. "It's best if I don't drink citrus juices or hot liquids."
4. "I need to rinse my mouth four times daily with mouthwash."

Level of Cognitive Ability: Evaluating
Client Needs: Physiological Integrity
Integrated Process: Teaching and Learning
Content Area: Adult Health: Immune
Priority Concepts: Client Education; Infection

Answer: 4
Rationale: Clients with thrush cannot tolerate commercial mouthwashes because the high alcohol concentration in these products can cause pain and discomfort of the lesions. A solution of warm water or mouthwash formulas without alcohol are better tolerated and may promote healing. A change in diet to liquid or pureed food often eases the discomfort of eating. The client should avoid spicy foods, citrus juices, and hot liquids.
Priority Nursing Tip: Candidiasis can be oral or vaginal. Antifungal medications are used to treat this infection. The nurse should encourage increased fluid intake and monitor the client's temperature when the client has an infection and is taking antifungal medication.
Test-Taking Strategy: Note the strategic words, *need for additional teaching*. These words indicate a negative event query and ask you to select an option that is an incorrect statement. In addition, noting the words *commercial mouthwash* in option 4 will direct you to this option. Review: the client teaching points related to **candidiasis (thrush).**
Reference(s): Ignatavicius, Workman (2013), p. 1193.

1076. The nurse has given instructions about site care to a hemodialysis client who had an implantation of an arteriovenous (AV) fistula in the right arm. Which statement by the client indicates a **need for further teaching?**
1. "I will need to sleep on my right side."
2. "It's important that I don't carry heavy objects with the right arm."
3. "I will perform range-of-motion exercises routinely on my right arm."
4. "It's important that I report any right arm redness or drainage at the site."

Level of Cognitive Ability: Evaluating
Client Needs: Physiological Integrity
Integrated Process: Teaching and Learning
Content Area: Adult Health: Renal and Urinary
Priority Concepts: Perfusion; Safety

Answer: 1
Rationale: Routine instructions to the client with an AV fistula, graft, or shunt include avoiding sleeping with the body weight on the extremity with the access site, avoiding carrying heavy objects or compressing the extremity that has the access site, performing routine range-of-motion exercises of the affected extremity, and reporting signs and symptoms of infection.
Priority Nursing Tip: Arterial steal syndrome can occur as a result of the presence of an arteriovenous (AV) fistula. This is a syndrome that can develop after the insertion of an arteriovenous fistula when too much blood is diverted to the vein and arterial perfusion to the hand is compromised.
Test-Taking Strategy: Note the strategic words, *need for further teaching*. These words indicate a negative event query and ask you to select an option that is an incorrect statement. Recalling the importance of maintaining the patency of the AV fistula will direct you to the correct option. Review: the home care instructions for a client with an AV fistula.
Reference(s): Ignatavicius, Workman (2013), p. 1562.

1077. The nurse provides instructions to a client about applying a nitroglycerin patch (Transderm-Nitro). What statement indicates that the client is using correct technique?
1. "A second patch will be applied if chest pain occurs."
2. "I will apply the patch to a nonhairy area of the body."
3. "I will remove the patch when bathing and reapply it after the bath."
4. "I will remove the patch after gently rubbing the area to activate the medication."

Level of Cognitive Ability: Evaluating
Client Needs: Physiological Integrity
Integrated Process: Teaching and Learning
Content Area: Pharmacology: Cardiovascular Medications
Priority Concepts: Client Education; Safety

Answer: 2
Rationale: Topical nitroglycerin is applied to a nonhairy part of the body. It is used on a scheduled basis and is not prescribed specifically for the occurrence of chest pain. The ointment is not rubbed into the skin; it is reapplied only as directed.
Priority Nursing Tip: Nitroglycerin is a vasodilator and will lower the blood pressure. The nurse needs to wear gloves when applying the topical preparation to a client.
Test-Taking Strategy: Focus on the subject, understanding the instructions for applying a nitroglycerin patch. Noting the word *nonhairy* in option 2 will direct you to this choice. Review: the client teaching points for using topical **nitroglycerin.**
Reference(s): Ignatavicius, Workman (2013), p. 838.

1078. The nurse is giving medication instructions to a client who is receiving furosemide (Lasix). Which client statement indicates a **need for further teaching**?
  1. "I need to change positions slowly."
  2. "I need to be careful to not get overheated in warm weather."
  3. "I need to talk to my health care provider about the use of alcohol."
  4. "I need to avoid the use of salt substitutes because they contain potassium."

Level of Cognitive Ability: Evaluating
Client Needs: Physiological Integrity
Integrated Process: Teaching and Learning
Content Area: Pharmacology: Cardiovascular Medications
Priority Concepts: Client Education; Safety

Answer: 4
Rationale: Furosemide is a potassium-losing diuretic, so there is no need to avoid high-potassium products, such as a salt substitute. Orthostatic hypotension is a risk, and the client must use caution when changing positions and with exposure to warm weather. The client needs to discuss the use of alcohol with the health care provider.
Priority Nursing Tip: The nurse should monitor the electrolyte values, specifically the potassium value, when the client is receiving a potassium-losing diuretic.
Test-Taking Strategy: Note the strategic words, *need for further teaching*. These words indicate a negative event query and ask you to select an option that is an incorrect statement. Focus on the subject of a client who is receiving furosemide (Lasix). Recalling that furosemide is a potassium-losing diuretic and that diuretic therapy can induce orthostatic hypotension will direct you to the correct option. Review: furosemide (Lasix).
Reference(s): Hodgson, Kizior (2014), pp. 524-525; Ignatavicius, Workman (2013), p. 179.

1079. A client has been prescribed a clonidine patch (Catapres-TTS), and the nurse has instructed the client regarding the use of the patch. Which client statement indicates a **need for further teaching**?
  1. "I intend to change the patch every 7 days."
  2. "I need to trim the patch if an edge becomes loose."
  3. "It's important to put the patch on a hairless site on my torso."
  4. "It's alright to leave the patch in place during bathing or showering."

Level of Cognitive Ability: Evaluating
Client Needs: Physiological Integrity
Integrated Process: Teaching and Learning
Content Area: Pharmacology: Cardiovascular Medications
Priority Concepts: Client Education; Safety

Answer: 2
Rationale: The clonidine patch should not be trimmed because it will alter the medication dose. If it becomes slightly loose, it should be covered with an adhesive overlay from the medication package. If it becomes very loose or falls off, it should be replaced. It is changed every 7 days, and is left in place when bathing or showering. The clonidine patch should be applied to a hairless site on the torso or the upper arm. The patch is discarded by folding it in half with the adhesive sides together.
Priority Nursing Tip: Clonidine (Catapres-TTS) is a centrally acting sympatholytic that is used to treat hypertension. The client is instructed not to discontinue the medication because abrupt withdrawal can cause severe rebound hypertension.
Test-Taking Strategy: Note the strategic words, *need for further teaching*. These words indicate a negative event query and ask you to select an option that is an incorrect statement. Noting the words *trim the patch* will direct you to option 2 because this client's action would alter the medication dose. Review: the clonidine patch (Catapres-TTS).
Reference(s): Hodgson, Kizior (2014), p. 267.

1080. Cholestyramine (Questran) is prescribed, and the nurse provides instructions to the client about the medication. Which client statement indicates a **need for further teaching**?
  1. "I should take this medication with meals."
  2. "I need to mix the medication with juice or applesauce."
  3. "I should increase my fluid intake while taking this medication."
  4. "I should call my health care provider immediately if it causes constipation."

Level of Cognitive Ability: Evaluating
Client Needs: Physiological Integrity
Integrated Process: Teaching and Learning
Content Area: Pharmacology: Cardiovascular Medications
Priority Concepts: Client Education; Safety

Answer: 4
Rationale: Common side effects of cholestyramine (Questran) include constipation, nausea, indigestion, and flatulence. Therefore, it is not necessary to contact the health care provider immediately if constipation occurs. Questran must be administered with food to be effective. This medication should not be taken dry, and it can be mixed in water, juice, carbonated beverages, applesauce, or soup. Increasing fluids will minimize the constipating effects of the medication.
Priority Nursing Tip: Cholestyramine (Questran) is a bile acid sequestrant used to lower the cholesterol level, and client compliance is a problem because of its taste and palatability. Mixing the medication with flavored products or fruit juices can improve the taste.
Test-Taking Strategy: Note the strategic words, *need for further teaching*. These words indicate a negative event query and ask you to select an option that is an incorrect statement. Select option 4 because of the word *immediately* and because normally measures can be taken to prevent constipation rather than immediately calling the health care provider. Review: the side effects of cholestyramine (Questran).
Reference(s): Hodgson, Kizior (2014), pp. 234-236.

1081. The nurse is preparing written medication instructions for a client who is prescribed colestipol hydrochloride (Colestid). What should the nurse instruct the client to take to counteract unintended medication effects?
1. Vitamin C
2. Vitamin B$_{12}$
3. B-complex vitamins
4. Fat-soluble vitamins

Level of Cognitive Ability: Applying
Client Needs: Physiological Integrity
Integrated Process: Teaching and Learning
Content Area: Pharmacology: Cardiovascular Medications
Priority Concepts: Client Education; Safety

Answer: 4
Rationale: Colestipol, which is a bile-sequestering agent, is used to lower blood cholesterol levels. However, the bile salts (which are rich in cholesterol) interfere with the absorption of the fat-soluble vitamins A, D, E, and K, as well as folic acid. With ongoing therapy, the client is at risk for the deficiency of these vitamins and is counseled to take them as supplements.
Priority Nursing Tip: Bile acid sequestrants bind with acids in the intestines, which prevents reabsorption of cholesterol.
Test-Taking Strategy: Focus on the subject, considerations for administration of colestipol hydrochloride (Colestid) and counteracting unintended medication effects. This will help you recall that bile-sequestering agents interfere with the absorption of fat-soluble vitamins and will assist you with eliminating options 1, 2, and 3. Also, select option 4 because it is the umbrella option. Review: client teaching points regarding colestipol hydrochloride (Colestid).
Reference(s): Lehne (2013), p. 616.

Nursing Process

Assessment

1082. Which data should the nurse expect to obtain during the admission assessment of a child with the diagnosis of irritable bowel syndrome?
1. Reports of frequent incidents of frothy diarrhea
2. Reports of frequent foul-smelling ribbon stools
3. Reports of profuse, watery diarrhea and vomiting daily
4. Reports of diffuse abdominal pain unrelated to meals or activity

Level of Cognitive Ability: Analyzing
Client Needs: Physiological Integrity
Integrated Process: Nursing Process/Assessment
Content Area: Child Health: Gastrointestinal
Priority Concepts: Clinical Judgment; Elimination

Answer: 4
Rationale: Irritable bowel syndrome causes diffuse abdominal pain unrelated to meals or activity. Alternating constipation and diarrhea with the presence of undigested food and mucus in the stools may also be noted. Option 1 is a clinical manifestation of lactose intolerance. Option 2 is a clinical manifestation of Hirschsprung's disease. Option 3 is a clinical manifestation of celiac disease.
Priority Nursing Tip: Stress and emotional factors may contribute to the occurrence of irritable bowel syndrome.
Test-Taking Strategy: Focus on the subject, manifestations of irritable bowel syndrome. Noting the name of the syndrome will direct you to option 4 because you would expect abdominal pain to occur in clients with this disorder. Review: the clinical manifestations associated with irritable bowel syndrome.
Reference(s): McKinney et al (2013), p. 1084.

1083. A child diagnosed with hemophilia is brought into the emergency department after being hit on the neck with a baseball. What is the focus of the nurse's **immediate** assessment?
1. Airway obstruction
2. Factor VIII deficiency
3. Spontaneous hematuria
4. Headache and slurred speech

Level of Cognitive Ability: Analyzing
Client Needs: Physiological Integrity
Integrated Process: Nursing Process/Assessment
Content Area: Child Health: Hematological
Priority Concepts: Clinical Judgment; Clotting

Answer: 1
Rationale: Trauma to the neck may cause bleeding into the tissues of the neck, which may compromise the airway. Factor VIII deficiency is not a symptom of hemophilia, but rather a common form of the disease. Although hematuria is a symptom of hemophilia, it is not associated with neck injury. Headache and slurred speech are associated with head trauma.
Priority Nursing Tip: Hemophilia is transmitted as an X-linked recessive disorder. (It may also occur as a result of a gene mutation.) Bleeding is the primary concern.
Test-Taking Strategy: Note the strategic word, *immediate*. Focus on the location of the injury. Use the ABCs—airway, breathing, and circulation—to answer this question. Remember that airway assessment is always assessed immediately. This will direct you to option 1. Review: the care of the child with hemophilia.
Reference(s): Hockenberry, Wilson (2013), p. 758; McKinney et al (2013), p. 1253.

1084. The nurse caring for a child diagnosed with rubeola (measles) notes that the health care provider has documented the presence of Koplik's spots. On the basis of this documentation, which observation is expected?
1. Pinpoint petechiae noted on both legs
2. Whitish vesicles located across the chest
3. Petechiae spots that are reddish and pinpoint on the soft palate
4. Small, blue-white spots with a red base found on the buccal mucosa

Level of Cognitive Ability: Analyzing
Client Needs: Physiological Integrity
Integrated Process: Nursing Process/Assessment
Content Area: Child Health: Infectious and Communicable Diseases
Priority Concepts: Clinical Judgment; Infection

Answer: 4
Rationale: In rubeola (measles), Koplik's spots appear approximately 2 days before the appearance of the rash. These are small, blue-white spots with a red base that are found on the buccal mucosa. The spots last approximately 3 days, after which time they slough off. Options 1, 2, and 3 are incorrect.
Priority Nursing Tip: Rubeola (measles) is transmitted via airborne particles, direct contact with infectious droplets, or transplacental contact. The nurse must implement airborne precautions when caring for the hospitalized client with rubeola.
Test-Taking Strategy: Eliminate options 1 and 3 first because they are comparable or alike and address petechiae spots. Focusing on the subject of Koplik's spots will direct you to the correct option. Review: the presentation of Koplik's spots and rubeola (measles).
Reference(s): McKinney et al (2013), pp. 1009, 1013.

1085. Which assessment finding should the nurse expect to note in the child hospitalized with a diagnosis of nephrotic syndrome?
1. Weight loss
2. Constipation
3. Hypotension
4. Abdominal pain

Level of Cognitive Ability: Analyzing
Client Needs: Physiological Integrity
Integrated Process: Nursing Process/Assessment
Content Area: Child Health: Renal and Urinary
Priority Concepts: Clinical Judgment; Fluid and Electrolyte Balance

Answer: 4
Rationale: Clinical manifestations associated with nephrotic syndrome include edema, anorexia, fatigue, and abdominal pain from the presence of extra fluid in the peritoneal cavity. Diarrhea caused by the edema of the bowel occurs and may cause decreased absorption of nutrients. Increased weight and a normal blood pressure are noted.
Priority Nursing Tip: The primary objectives of therapeutic management for nephrotic syndrome are to reduce the excretion of urinary protein, maintain protein-free urine, reduce edema, prevent infection, and minimize complications.
Test-Taking Strategy: Focus on the subject, the physiology and manifestations associated with nephrotic syndrome. Recalling that edema is a clinical manifestation will direct you to option 4. Review: the clinical manifestations of nephrotic syndrome.
Reference(s): McKinney et al (2013), p. 1132.

1086. A child is admitted to the hospital with a suspected diagnosis of von Willebrand's disease. On assessment of the child, which symptom would **most likely** be noted?
1. Hematuria
2. Presence of hematomas
3. Presence of hemarthrosis
4. Bleeding from the mucous membranes

Level of Cognitive Ability: Analyzing
Client Needs: Physiological Integrity
Integrated Process: Nursing Process/Assessment
Content Area: Child Health: Hematological
Priority Concepts: Clinical Judgment; Clotting

Answer: 4
Rationale: The primary clinical manifestations of von Willebrand's disease are bruising and mucous membrane bleeding from the nose, mouth, and gastrointestinal tract. Prolonged bleeding after trauma and surgery, including tooth extraction, may be the first evidence of abnormal hemostasis in those with mild disease. In females, menorrhagia and profuse postpartum bleeding may occur. Bleeding associated with von Willebrand's disease may be severe and lead to anemia and shock, but unlike what is seen in clients with hemophilia, deep bleeding into joints and muscles is rare. Options 1, 2, and 3 are characteristic of those signs found in clients with hemophilia.
Priority Nursing Tip: von Willebrand's disease is a disorder that causes platelets to adhere to damaged endothelium and is characterized by an increased tendency to bleed from mucous membranes.
Test-Taking Strategy: Note the strategic words, *most likely*. Think about the pathophysiology of this disorder and recall that options 1, 2, and 3 are characteristic of hemophilia to assist you with eliminating these options and direct you to option 4. Review: the clinical manifestations of von Willebrand's disease.
Reference(s): McKinney et al (2013), p. 1252.

1087. A client prescribed dextroamphetamine (Adderall XR) reports to the nurse difficulty falling asleep at night. In order to minimize sleep disorders, when should the nurse instruct the client to take the medication?
1. Before a bedtime snack
2. Upon awaking in the morning
3. Two hours before going to bed
4. At least 6 hours before bedtime

Level of Cognitive Ability: Applying
Client Needs: Physiological Integrity
Integrated Process: Nursing Process/Assessment
Content Area: Pharmacology: Neurological Medications
Priority Concepts: Client Education; Safety

Answer: 4
Rationale: Dextroamphetamine is a central nervous system (CNS) stimulant that acts by releasing norepinephrine from the nerve endings. The client should take the medication at least 6 hours before going to bed at night to prevent disturbances with sleep. Therefore, options 1, 2, and 3 are incorrect.
Priority Nursing Tip: The client taking a central nervous system (CNS) stimulant needs to be instructed to avoid foods containing caffeine to prevent additional stimulation.
Test-Taking Strategy: Focus on the subject, dextroamphetamine (Adderall XL) and difficulty sleeping. Think about the action and purpose of this medication. Evaluate each of the options in terms of how far removed the scheduled dose is from the client's bedtime. This will direct you to option 4. Review: the effects of **dextroamphetamine (Adderall)**.
Reference(s): Kee, Hayes, McCuistion (2012), p. 288; Lehne (2013), p. 428.

1088. The nurse is assessing the level of consciousness of a child with a head injury and documents that the child is obtunded. On the basis of this documentation, which observation did the nurse note?
1. The child is unable to think clearly and rapidly.
2. The child is unable to recognize place or person.
3. The child always requires considerable stimulation for arousal.
4. The child has limited interaction with the environment unless aroused.

Level of Cognitive Ability: Analyzing
Client Needs: Physiological Integrity
Integrated Process: Nursing Process/Assessment
Content Area: Child Health: Neurological
Priority Concepts: Cognition; Intracranial Regulation

Answer: 4
Rationale: If the child is obtunded, the child sleeps unless aroused and, when aroused, has limited interaction with the environment. Option 1 describes confusion. Option 2 describes disorientation. Option 3 describes stupor.
Priority Nursing Tip: Do not place a client with a head injury in a flat or Trendelenburg's position because of the risk of increased intracranial pressure.
Test-Taking Strategy: Focus on the subject, that the child is obtunded. Knowledge regarding the standard terms used to identify level of consciousness will direct you to option 4. Review: the assessment of the **levels of consciousness**.
Reference(s): McKinney et al (2013), p. 1419.

1089. The home health nurse is performing an assessment of the psychosocial adjustment of a client in a body cast. What need has **priority**?
1. The amount of home care support available
2. The amount of sensory stimulation provided
3. The ability to perform activities of daily living
4. The type of transportation available for follow-up care

Level of Cognitive Ability: Analyzing
Client Needs: Psychosocial Integrity
Integrated Process: Nursing Process/Assessment
Content Area: Adult Health: Musculoskeletal
Priority Concepts: Coping; Mobility

Answer: 2
Rationale: A psychosocial assessment of the client who is immobilized would most appropriately include the need for sensory stimulation as a priority. This assessment should also include such factors as body image, past and present coping skills, and the coping methods used during the period of immobilization. Although home care support, the ability to perform activities of daily living, and transportation are components of an assessment, they are not specifically related to psychosocial adjustment.
Priority Nursing Tip: Assess the client in a body cast for respiratory impairment and paralytic ileus, which are possible complications of the body cast.
Test-Taking Strategy: Focus on the subject, the assessment of the psychosocial adjustment of a client in a body cast. Note the strategic word, *priority*. Option 3 can be eliminated first because it relates to physiological integrity rather than psychosocial integrity. Eliminate options 1 and 4 next because they are most closely related to the physical support of, rather than the psychosocial needs of, the client. Review: the components of a **psychosocial assessment** of a client in a **body cast.**
Reference(s): Ignatavicius, Workman (2013), pp. 104, 1158.

1090. The nurse is caring for a client diagnosed with acquired immunodeficiency syndrome (AIDS). Which sign/symptom indicates the presence of an opportunistic respiratory infection?

1. Nausea and vomiting
2. Fever and exertional dyspnea
3. An arterial blood gas pH of 7.40
4. A respiratory rate of 20 breaths per minute

Level of Cognitive Ability: Analyzing
Client Needs: Physiological Integrity
Integrated Process: Nursing Process/Assessment
Content Area: Adult Health: Immune
Priority Concepts: Immunity; Infection

Answer: 2
Rationale: Fever and exertional dyspnea are signs of *Pneumocystis jiroveci* pneumonia, which is a common, life-threatening opportunistic infection that afflicts those with AIDS. Option 1 is not associated with respiratory infection. Options 3 and 4 are normal findings.
Priority Nursing Tip: A client with human immunodeficiency virus (HIV) or acquired immunodeficiency syndrome (AIDS) is at risk for developing a life-threatening opportunistic infection. Monitor the client closely for signs/symptoms of infection and report these signs immediately if they occur.
Test-Taking Strategy: Focus on the subject, opportunistic respiratory infection in a client with AIDS. Eliminate options 3 and 4 first because they are comparable or alike and are normal findings. For the remaining options, focusing on the subject, a respiratory infection, will direct you to option 2. Review: the signs of *Pneumocystis jiroveci* pneumonia.
Reference(s): Ignatavicius, Workman (2013), pp. 366, 375.

1091. An adult client seeks treatment in an ambulatory care clinic for reports of a left earache, nausea, and a full feeling in the left ear. The client has an elevated temperature. Which assessment question should the nurse ask **first?**

1. "Do you have a history of a recent brain abscess?"
2. "Do you have a chronic hearing problem in the left ear?"
3. "Do you obtain pain relief with acetaminophen (Tylenol)?"
4. "Do you have a history of a recent upper respiratory infection (URI)?"

Level of Cognitive Ability: Analyzing
Client Needs: Physiological Integrity
Integrated Process: Nursing Process/Assessment
Content Area: Adult Health: Ear
Priority Concepts: Clinical Judgment; Sensory Perception

Answer: 4
Rationale: Otitis media in the adult is typically one-sided and presents as an acute process with earache; nausea; and possible vomiting, fever, and fullness in the ear. The client may complain of diminished hearing in that ear during the acute process. The nurse takes a client history first, assessing whether the client has had a recent URI. It is unnecessary to question the client about a brain abscess. The nurse may ask the client if anything relieves the pain, but ear infection pain is usually not relieved until antibiotic therapy is initiated.
Priority Nursing Tip: Infants and children have eustachian tubes that are shorter, wider, and straighter, which makes them more prone to otitis media.
Test-Taking Strategy: Focus on the subject, the relationship between an upper respiratory infection and otitis media. Noting the strategic word, *first* will direct you to option 4. Review: the causes of **otitis** media.
Reference(s): Ignatavicius, Workman (2013), p. 1092.

1092. The home care nurse visits an older client experiencing limited range of motion who is upset about urinary incontinence. Which should the nurse determine is a potential environmental contributor to the client's problem?
1. Nightlights in the hallways
2. Large, unmovable furniture
3. A bathroom at each end of the house
4. The commode seat being at a 15-inch height

Level of Cognitive Ability: Analyzing
Client Needs: Physiological Integrity
Integrated Process: Nursing Process/Assessment
Content Area: Adult Health: Renal and Urinary
Priority Concepts: Elimination; Safety

Answer: 4
Rationale: A bathroom with a low commode seat is a potential barrier to voiding for an older adult. The low seat is likely to increase the time that it takes for the client to lower the body down onto the seat. This increases the risk of incontinence because reaching a low level can be very difficult for a client with limited range of motion who is at risk for falls or needs an assistive device for ambulation. The nurse helps resolve the client's problem with incontinence by recommending a raised toilet seat that can be attached to a standard commode or toilet. Nightlights, a fixed floor plan as a result of heavy furniture, and conveniently located bathrooms should facilitate voiding.
Priority Nursing Tip: Urinary incontinence places the client at a higher risk for skin breakdown because of the increased skin moisture. Therefore, the nurse should implement practices to keep the skin clean and dry and teach the client these practices.
Test-Taking Strategy: Focus on the subject of an environmental barrier to normal voiding. Eliminate option 1, 2, and 3 because they contribute to the client safely reaching the bathroom for voiding. Also, noting the words *15-inch height* will direct you to option 4. Review: the measures that promote **normal voiding**.
Reference(s): Ignatavicius, Workman (2013), p. 1506; Potter et al (2013), p. 1047.

1093. The nurse prepares to administer a continuous intravenous (IV) infusion through a peripheral IV to a dehydrated client. Which **priority** assessment should the nurse obtain before initiating the IV infusion?
1. Daily body weight
2. Serum electrolytes
3. Intake and output records
4. Status of the client's dominant side

Level of Cognitive Ability: Analyzing
Client Needs: Physiological Integrity
Integrated Process: Nursing Process/Assessment
Content Area: Fundamental Skills: Fluids and Electrolytes
Priority Concepts: Clinical Judgment; Fluid and Electrolyte Balance

Answer: 1
Rationale: The nurse obtains the client's baseline body weight as a priority before beginning the IV infusion because body weight is a sensitive and specific indicator of fluid volume status when body weights are compared on a daily basis. This means that as a client receives or accumulates fluid, body weight quickly and proportionately increases and vice versa. The remaining options may also be reasonable assessments to complete before initiating an IV infusion. However, intake, output, and serum electrolytes are potentially affected by more confounding factors; thus, they are less specific and sensitive to fluctuations in body fluid. Determining the client's dominant side assists in deciding a site for inserting the initial IV catheter, but it provides no information about fluid volume status.
Priority Nursing Tip: Clients with respiratory, cardiac, renal, or liver disease, older clients, and very young children are at risk for circulatory overload and may not be able to tolerate an excessive body fluid volume.
Test-Taking Strategy: Focus on the subject, continuous intravenous (IV) infusion through a peripheral IV to a dehydrated client. Note the strategic word, *priority*. Review the options to determine the best method for the nurse to use to evaluate fluid status. Body weight is the best option because it is the most sensitive and specific measurement listed. Review: the care of the client with **dehydration**.
Reference(s): Ignatavicius, Workman (2013), p. 175.

1094. A client is scheduled for an arteriogram using a radiopaque dye. Which **most important** item should the nurse assesses before the procedure?
1. Vital signs
2. Intake and output
3. Height and weight
4. Allergy to iodine or shellfish

Level of Cognitive Ability: Analyzing
Client Needs: Physiological Integrity
Integrated Process: Nursing Process/Assessment
Content Area: Fundamental Skills: Diagnostic Tests
Priority Concepts: Clinical Judgment; Safety

Answer: 4
Rationale: Allergy to iodine or seafood is associated with allergy to the radiopaque dye that is used for medical imaging examinations. Informed consent is necessary because an arteriogram requires the injection of a radiopaque dye into the blood vessel. Although options 1, 2, and 3 are components of the preprocedure assessment, the risks of allergic reaction and possible anaphylaxis are the most critical.
Priority Nursing Tip: If anaphylaxis occurs after the injection of a radiopaque dye, the nurse immediately assesses the client's respiratory status and provides respiratory support and asks another nursing staff member to contact the health care provider.
Test-Taking Strategy: Note the strategic words, *most important*. Focusing on the subject of arteriogram using a radiopaque dye will help you recall the risk of anaphylaxis related to the dye; this will direct you to option 4. Review: the preprocedure care for **angiography**.
Reference(s): Chernecky, Berger (2013), pp. 165-166; Pagana, Pagana (2013), p. 121.

1095. The nurse is performing a cardiovascular assessment on a client. Which item should the nurse assess to obtain the **best** information about the client's left-sided heart function?
1. The status of breath sounds
2. The presence of peripheral edema
3. The presence of hepatojugular reflux
4. The presence of jugular vein distention

Level of Cognitive Ability: Analyzing
Client Needs: Physiological Integrity
Integrated Process: Nursing Process/Assessment
Content Area: Adult Health: Cardiovascular
Priority Concepts: Gas Exchange; Perfusion

Answer: 1
Rationale: The client with heart failure may present different symptoms depending on whether the right or the left side of the heart is failing. The assessment of breath sounds provides information about left-sided heart function. Peripheral edema, hepatojugular reflux, and jugular vein distention are all signs of right-sided heart function.
Priority Nursing Tip: Signs of left ventricular failure are evident in the pulmonary system. Signs of right ventricular failure are evident in the systemic circulation.
Test-Taking Strategy: Focus on the subject, the status of left-sided heart function and the strategic word, *best*. Remember "left" and "lungs." Options 2, 3, and 4 reflect right-sided heart failure. Review: the signs of right- and left-sided **heart failure**.
Reference(s): Ignatavicius, Workman (2013), pp. 748-749.

1096. The nurse is obtaining a history from a client who was admitted to the hospital with a thrombotic stroke. The nurse assesses the client, knowing that the client **most likely** experienced which sign/symptom before the stroke occurred?
1. No symptoms at all
2. Throbbing headaches
3. Transient hemiplegia and loss of speech
4. Unexplained episodes of loss of consciousness

Level of Cognitive Ability: Analyzing
Client Needs: Physiological Integrity
Integrated Process: Nursing Process/Assessment
Content Area: Adult Health: Neurological
Priority Concepts: Clinical Judgment; Intracranial Regulation

Answer: 3
Rationale: Cerebral thrombosis does not occur suddenly. During the few hours or days before a thrombotic stroke, the client may experience a transient loss of speech, hemiplegia, or paresthesias on one side of the body. Other signs and symptoms of thrombotic stroke vary, but they may include dizziness, cognitive changes, or seizures. Headache is rare, and a loss of consciousness is not likely to occur.
Priority Nursing Tip: A stroke is a syndrome in which the cerebral circulation is interrupted, causing neurological deficits. Cerebral anoxia lasting longer than 10 minutes causes cerebral infarction with irreversible change.
Test-Taking Strategy: Focus on the subject, symptoms of a stroke and the strategic words, *most likely*. Option 1 is eliminated first because the client experiencing a stroke will likely experience symptoms. From the remaining choices, focus on the type of stroke addressed in the question to direct you to option 3. Review: the signs and symptoms of a **thrombotic stroke**.
Reference(s): Ignatavicius, Workman (2013), pp. 1005-1006.

1097. A client in a long-term care facility has had a series of gastrointestinal (GI) diagnostic tests, including an upper and lower GI series and endoscopies. Upon return to the long-term care facility, which **priority** assessment should the nurse focus on?
1. The comfort level
2. Activity tolerance
3. The level of consciousness
4. The hydration and nutrition status

Level of Cognitive Ability: Applying
Client Needs: Physiological Integrity
Integrated Process: Nursing Process/Assessment
Content Area: Fundamental Skills: Diagnostic Tests
Priority Concepts: Fluid and Electrolyte Balance; Safety

Answer: 4
Rationale: Many of the diagnostic studies to identify GI disorders require that the GI tract be cleaned (usually with laxatives and enemas) before testing. In addition, the client most often takes nothing by mouth before and during the testing period. Because the studies may be done over a period that exceeds 24 hours, the client may become dehydrated and/or malnourished. Although options 1, 2, and 3 may be components of the assessment, option 4 is the priority.
Priority Nursing Tip: After endoscopic procedures that involve the use of a local throat anesthetic, monitor for the return of a gag reflex before giving the client any oral substance. If the gag reflex has not returned, the client could aspirate.
Test-Taking Strategy: Note the strategic word, *priority*. Use Maslow's Hierarchy of Needs theory to direct you to option 4. Hydration and nutrition are the priorities. Review: the care of the client after **diagnostic GI tests.**
Reference(s): Chernecky, Berger (2013), pp. 1138-1140.

1098. Which aspect(s) of the client should the nurse focus on when assessing a client for the vegetative signs of depression?
1. Level of self-esteem
2. Level of suicidal ideation
3. Ability to think, concentrate, and make rational decisions
4. Appetite, weight, sleep patterns, and psychomotor activity

Level of Cognitive Ability: Analyzing
Client Needs: Physiological Integrity
Integrated Process: Nursing Process/Assessment
Content Area: Mental Health
Priority Concepts: Cognition; Mood and Affect

Answer: 4
Rationale: The vegetative signs of depression are changes in physiological functioning that occur during depression. These include changes in appetite, weight, sleep patterns, and psychomotor activity. Options 1, 2, and 3 represent psychological assessment categories.
Priority Nursing Tip: An inappropriate appearance and indications of poor hygiene practices may be signs of depression, manic disorder, dementia, organic brain disease, or another disorder.
Test-Taking Strategy: Focus on the subject, the vegetative signs of depression. Recalling that these are physiological changes and use of Maslow's Hierarchy of Needs theory will direct you to the correct option. Review: the assessment of **depression.**
Reference(s): Swearingen (2012), pp. 702-703; Varcarolis, Halter (2013), pp. 255-256, 260.

1099. A client diagnosed with cirrhosis of the liver is receiving oral triamterene (Dyrenium) daily. Which would indicate to the nurse that the client is experiencing an adverse effect of the medication?
1. Dry skin
2. Excitability
3. Constipation
4. Hyperkalemia

Level of Cognitive Ability: Analyzing
Client Needs: Physiological Integrity
Integrated Process: Nursing Process/Assessment
Content Area: Pharmacology: Cardiovascular Medications
Priority Concepts: Clinical Judgment; Safety

Answer: 4
Rationale: Triamterene is a potassium-retaining diuretic. Adverse effects include hyperkalemia, dehydration, hyponatremia, and lethargy. Although the concern with most diuretics is hypokalemia, this is a potassium-retaining medication, which means that the concern with the administration of this medication is hyperkalemia. Other effects include nausea, vomiting, cramping, diarrhea, headache, ataxia, drowsiness, confusion, and fever.
Priority Nursing Tip: The client with cirrhosis needs to consume foods high in thiamine. Thiamine is present in a variety of foods of plant and animal origin. Pork products are especially rich in this vitamin.
Test-Taking Strategy: Focus on the subject, oral triamterene (Dyrenium) and think about the classification of the medication. Recalling that this is a potassium-retaining medication will direct you to the correct option. Review: oral **triamterene (Dyrenium).**
Reference(s): Hodgson, Kizior (2014), pp. 1210-1211.

1100. The nurse is preparing a woman in labor for an amniotomy. Which **priority** data should the nurse assess before the procedure?
1. Fetal heart rate
2. Maternal heart rate
3. Fetal scalp sampling
4. Maternal blood pressure

Level of Cognitive Ability: Analyzing
Client Needs: Physiological Integrity
Integrated Process: Nursing Process/Assessment
Content Area: Maternity: Antepartum
Priority Concepts: Reproduction; Safety

Answer: 1
Rationale: Fetal well-being must be confirmed before and after amniotomy. Fetal heart rate should be checked by Doppler or with the application of the external fetal monitor. Although maternal vital signs may be assessed, fetal heart rate is the priority. A fetal scalp sampling cannot be done when the membranes are intact.
Priority Nursing Tip: Amniotomy (artificial rupture of the membranes) can be used to induce labor when the condition of the cervix is favorable (ripe), or to augment labor if the progress begins to slow.
Test-Taking Strategy: Note the strategic word, *priority*. Eliminate option 3 first, knowing that a fetal scalp sampling cannot be done before an amniotomy. Eliminate options 2 and 4 next, noting that they are comparable or alike and address maternal vital signs. Option 1 addresses fetal well-being. Review: preprocedure care for **amniotomy**.
Reference(s): McKinney et al (2013), pp. 344, 412.

1101. The nurse is monitoring a client who is receiving an oxytocin (Pitocin) infusion for the induction of labor. The nurse should suspect water intoxication if which sign or symptom is noted?
1. Fatigue
2. Lethargy
3. Sleepiness
4. Tachycardia

Level of Cognitive Ability: Analyzing
Client Needs: Physiological Integrity
Integrated Process: Nursing Process/Assessment
Content Area: Pharmacology: Reproductive/Maternity/Newborn Medications
Priority Concepts: Fluid and Electrolyte Balance; Safety

Answer: 4
Rationale: During an oxytocin infusion, the woman is monitored closely for signs of water intoxication, including tachycardia, cardiac dysrhythmias, shortness of breath, nausea, and vomiting. The remaining options are not associated with water intoxication.
Priority Nursing Tip: An oxytocin (Pitocin) infusion is discontinued if uterine contraction frequency is less than 2 minutes, the duration is longer than 90 seconds, or fetal distress is noted.
Test-Taking Strategy: Focus on the subject of water intoxication. Think about the physiological response that occurs when fluid overload exists to direct you to option 4. In addition, note that options 1, 2, and 3 are comparable or alike, so eliminate these options. Review: the signs of **water intoxication**.
Reference(s): McKinney et al (2013), p. 418.

1102. The nurse reviews the record of a client who is receiving external radiation therapy and notes documentation of a skin finding as moist desquamation. Which finding on assessment of the client should the nurse expect to observe?
1. A rash
2. Dermatitis
3. Reddened skin
4. Weeping of the skin

Level of Cognitive Ability: Analyzing
Client Needs: Physiological Integrity
Integrated Process: Nursing Process/Assessment
Content Area: Adult Health: Oncology
Priority Concepts: Clinical Judgment; Tissue Integrity

Answer: 4
Rationale: Moist desquamation occurs when the basal cells of the skin are destroyed. The dermal level is exposed, which results in the leakage of serum. A rash, dermatitis, and reddened skin may occur with external radiation, but these conditions are not described as moist desquamation.
Priority Nursing Tip: The nurse should teach the client receiving radiation therapy to wash the irradiated area gently each day with warm water alone or mild soap and water. The client should use the hand rather than a washcloth to wash the area.
Test-Taking Strategy: Options 1, 2, and 3 are eliminated because they are comparable or alike, and they describe a dry rather than a moist skin alteration. In addition, note the relationship between the word *moist* in the question and *weeping* in the correct option. Review: the signs associated with **moist desquamation**.
Reference(s): Ignatavicius, Workman (2013), p. 413; Lewis et al (2011), pp. 284-286.

1103. The nurse is performing an assessment on a pregnant client with a history of cardiac disease. Which body area is venous congestion **most** commonly noted in?
1. Vulva
2. Around the eyes
3. Fingers of the hands
4. Around the abdomen

Level of Cognitive Ability: Analyzing
Client Needs: Physiological Integrity
Integrated Process: Nursing Process/Assessment
Content Area: Maternity: Antepartum
Priority Concepts: Clinical Judgment; Reproduction

Answer: **1**
Rationale: Assessment of the cardiovascular system includes observation for venous congestion that can develop into varicosities. Venous congestion is most commonly noted in the legs, the vulva, or the rectum. Although edema may be noted in the fingers and around the eyes, edema in these areas would not be directly associated with venous congestion. It would be difficult to assess for edema in the abdominal area of a client who is pregnant.
Priority Nursing Tip: Varicose veins can occur in the second and the third trimesters of pregnancy. They result from weakening walls of the veins or valves and venous congestion.
Test-Taking Strategy: Focus on the strategic word, *most*, and note the subject, venous congestion. From the options provided, the only body area in which venous congestion would be noted is the vulva. Review: **venous congestion in a pregnancy.**
Reference(s): McKinney et al (2013), p. 248.

1104. A client who has been receiving long-term diuretic therapy is admitted to the hospital with a diagnosis of dehydration. The nurse should assess for which sign that correlates with this fluid imbalance?
1. Decreased pulse
2. Bibasilar crackles
3. Increased blood pressure
4. Increased urinary specific gravity

Level of Cognitive Ability: Applying
Client Needs: Physiological Integrity
Integrated Process: Nursing Process/Assessment
Content Area: Fundamental Skills: Fluids and Electrolytes
Priority Concepts: Clinical Judgment; Fluid and Electrolyte Balance

Answer: **4**
Rationale: Assessment findings with fluid volume deficit are increased pulse and respirations, weight loss, poor skin turgor, dry mucous membranes, decreased urine output, concentrated urine with increased specific gravity, increased hematocrit, and altered level of consciousness. The assessment findings in options 1, 2, and 3 are not associated findings in dehydration.
Priority Nursing Tip: The nurse needs to monitor for signs of dehydration and electrolyte imbalances in a client receiving diuretic therapy.
Test-Taking Strategy: Focus on the subject, a client with dehydration. Think about the pathophysiology associated with dehydration to direct you to the correct option. Review: the manifestations of dehydration.
Reference(s): Lewis et al (2011), p. 309.

1105. A client who is at 35 weeks of gestation calls the nurse at the clinic and reports a sudden discharge of fluid from the vagina. Based on the data provided, which condition should the nurse suspect?
1. Miscarriage
2. Preterm labor
3. Intrauterine fetal demise
4. Premature rupture of the membranes

Level of Cognitive Ability: Analyzing
Client Needs: Physiological Integrity
Integrated Process: Nursing Process/Assessment
Content Area: Maternity: Intrapartum
Priority Concepts: Clinical Judgment; Reproduction

Answer: **4**
Rationale: Premature rupture of the membranes is usually manifested by a sudden discharge of fluid from the vagina before 37 weeks of gestation. Miscarriage is typically manifested by vaginal bleeding and abdominal pain. Preterm labor is typically manifested by uterine contractions, cramping, and pressure before 37 weeks of gestation. Intrauterine fetal demise is usually manifested by an absence of fetal movements and heartbeat.
Priority Nursing Tip: Infection can cause premature rupture of the membranes, premature labor, and postpartum endometritis.
Test-Taking Strategy: Focus on the subject of a client who is at 35 weeks of gestation and reports a sudden discharge of fluid from the vagina. Note that all of the conditions noted in the options may occur during this time; therefore, the answer needs to be determined by looking at the clinical manifestations. Recall that amniotic fluid, rather than blood, would be expelled in premature rupture of the membranes; this will assist in eliminating option 1. From the remaining options, it is necessary to know which signs and symptoms are associated with each disorder in order to answer correctly. Review: **premature rupture of the membranes.**
Reference(s): McKinney et al (2013), pp. 644-646.

1106. The clinic nurse reviews the chart of a client diagnosed with stage III Lyme disease. On assessment of the client, which clinical manifestation should the nurse expect to note?
1. Palpitations
2. A cardiac dysrhythmia
3. A generalized skin rash
4. Enlarged and inflamed joints

Level of Cognitive Ability: Analyzing
Client Needs: Physiological Integrity
Integrated Process: Nursing Process/Assessment
Content Area: Adult Health: Integumentary
Priority Concepts: Immunity; Inflammation

Answer: 4
Rationale: Stage III Lyme disease develops within a month to several months after initial infection. It is characterized by arthritic symptoms such as arthralgia and enlarged or inflamed joints, which can persist for several years after the initial infection. A rash occurs during stage I, and cardiac and neurological dysfunction occur during stage II.
Priority Nursing Tip: The typical ring-shaped rash of Lyme disease does not occur in all clients. Many clients never develop a rash. Additionally, if a rash does occur, it can arise anywhere on the body, not only at the site of the bite.
Test-Taking Strategy: Eliminate options 1 and 2 first because they are comparable or alike cardiac symptoms. Focusing on the subject of signs and symptoms of stage III Lyme disease will direct you to option 4. Review: the clinical manifestations associated with Lyme disease.
Reference(s): Ignatavicius, Workman (2013), pp. 352-353; Lewis et al (2011), pp. 1661-1662.

1107. The nurse assigned to care for a child with a basilar skull fracture reviews the child's record and notes that the health care provider has documented the presence of Battle's sign. Which should the nurse expect to observe in the child?
1. Bruising behind the ear
2. The presence of epistaxis
3. A bruised periorbital area
4. An edematous periorbital area

Level of Cognitive Ability: Analyzing
Client Needs: Physiological Integrity
Integrated Process: Nursing Process/Assessment
Content Area: Child Health: Neurological
Priority Concepts: Clinical Judgment; Intracranial Regulation

Answer: 1
Rationale: The most serious type of skull fracture is a basilar skull fracture. Two classic findings associated with this type of skull fracture are Battle's sign and raccoon eyes. Battle's sign is the presence of bruising or ecchymosis behind the ear caused by a leaking of blood into the mastoid sinuses. Raccoon eyes occur as a result of blood leaking into the frontal sinus and causing an edematous and bruised periorbital area.
Priority Nursing Tip: Leakage of cerebrospinal fluid (CSF) from the ears or nose may accompany basilar skull fracture. CSF can be distinguished from other body fluids because the drainage will separate into bloody and yellow concentric rings on dressing material, called a halo sign. The CSF fluid also tests positive for glucose.
Test-Taking Strategy: Eliminate options 3 and 4 first because they are comparable or alike. Focusing on the subject of the description of Battle's sign will direct you to option 1. Review: Battle's sign.
Reference(s): McKinney et al (2013), p. 1428.

1108. Which finding would indicate the presence of Kernig's sign?
1. Calf pain when the foot is dorsiflexed
2. Pain when the chin is pulled down to the chest
3. The inability of the child to extend the legs fully when lying supine
4. The flexion of the hips when the neck is flexed from a lying position

Level of Cognitive Ability: Analyzing
Client Needs: Physiological Integrity
Integrated Process: Nursing Process/Assessment
Content Area: Child Health: Neurological
Priority Concepts: Inflammation; Intracranial Regulation

Answer: 3
Rationale: Kernig's sign is the inability of the child to extend the legs fully when lying supine. Brudzinski's sign is flexion of the hips when the neck is flexed from a supine position. Both of these signs are frequently present in clients with bacterial meningitis. Nuchal rigidity is also present with bacterial meningitis, and it occurs when pain prevents the child from touching the chin to the chest. Homans' sign is elicited when pain occurs in the calf region when the foot is dorsiflexed.
Priority Nursing Tip: Meningitis is transmitted by droplet infection. Precautions for this disease include placing the client in a private room or with a cohort client and use of a standard precaution mask.
Test-Taking Strategy: Focus on the subject, characteristics of Kernig's sign. It is necessary to know that Kernig's sign is the inability of the child to extend the legs fully when lying supine. Review: the assessment findings associated with Kernig's sign.
Reference(s): McKinney et al (2013), pp. 1438-1439.

1109. A home care nurse assesses an older client's functional status and ability to perform activities of daily living (ADLs). What is the focus area of the nurse's assessment?
1. Everyday routines
2. Self-care activities
3. Household management
4. Endurance and flexibility

Level of Cognitive Ability: Applying
Client Needs: Health Promotion and Maintenance
Integrated Process: Nursing Process/Assessment
Content Area: Adult Health: Musculoskeletal
Priority Concepts: Functional Ability; Health Promotion

Answer: 2
Rationale: To evaluate the client's functional status, the nurse assesses the client's ability to perform self-care or ADLs, including bathing, toileting, ambulating, dressing, and feeding. Everyday routines, household management, and physical condition are not components of functional status.
Priority Nursing Tip: For the client having a problem with performing activities of daily living (ADLs), an occupational therapist should be consulted. An occupational therapist develops adaptive devices that can help the client perform ADLs.
Test-Taking Strategy: Focus on the subject of the ability to perform ADLs. Recalling that ADLs refer to self-care needs will direct you to option 2. Review: the concepts of **activities of daily living (ADLs)**.
Reference(s): Potter et al (2013), pp. 259-260.

1110. The nurse is assessing a client with Addison's disease for signs of hyperkalemia. Which sign/symptom should the nurse observe with this electrolyte imbalance?
1. Polyuria
2. Cardiac dysrhythmias
3. Dry mucous membranes
4. Prolonged bleeding time

Level of Cognitive Ability: Analyzing
Client Needs: Physiological Integrity
Integrated Process: Nursing Process/Assessment
Content Area: Adult Health: Endocrine
Priority Concepts: Clinical Judgment; Fluid and Electrolyte Balance

Answer: 2
Rationale: The inadequate production of aldosterone in clients with Addison's disease causes the inadequate excretion of potassium and results in hyperkalemia. The clinical manifestations of hyperkalemia are the result of altered nerve transmission. The most harmful consequence of hyperkalemia is its effect on cardiac function. Options 1, 3, and 4 are not manifestations that are associated with Addison's disease or hyperkalemia.
Priority Nursing Tip: A low-potassium diet is usually indicated for hyperkalemia, which may be caused by disorders such as impaired renal function, Addison's disease, and potassium-retaining diuretics.
Test-Taking Strategy: Focus on the subject of Addison's disease and hyperkalemia. Think about the effects of potassium on the body and remember that hyperkalemia has a direct effect on cardiac function. This will direct you to option 2. Review: the pathophysiology associated with **Addison's disease** and the effects of **hyperkalemia**.
Reference(s): Ignatavicius, Workman (2013), p. 1382.

1111. When a client experiences respiratory distress, blood for an arterial blood gas (ABG) assessment is drawn from the radial artery. The nurse performs an Allen's test before the blood is drawn to determine the circulatory adequacy of which vessel?
1. Ulnar
2. Carotid
3. Brachial
4. Femoral

Level of Cognitive Ability: Applying
Client Needs: Physiological Integrity
Integrated Process: Nursing Process/Assessment
Content Area: Fundamental Skills: Acid-Base
Priority Concepts: Acid-Base Balance; Clotting

Answer: 1
Rationale: Before radial puncture for obtaining an arterial specimen for ABGs, Allen's test is performed to determine adequate ulnar circulation. Failure to assess collateral circulation could result in severe ischemic injury to the hand if damage to the radial artery occurs with arterial puncture. Allen's test does not determine the adequacy of carotid, brachial, or femoral circulation.
Priority Nursing Tip: After obtaining an arterial blood gas specimen, the nurse should ensure that pressure is placed over the area of the puncture for at least 5 or 10 minutes and longer if the client is taking an anticoagulant.
Test-Taking Strategy: Note the words *radial artery* in the question. Focus on the subject, arterial blood gas (ABG) assessment drawn from the radial artery and think about the anatomy of the blood vessels. This will eliminate options 2, 3, and 4. Review the purpose and procedure of **Allen's test**.
Reference(s): Chernecky, Berger (2013), p. 212.

1112. A pregnant client with diabetes mellitus arrives at the health care clinic for a follow-up visit. What **priority** assessment should the nurse perform?
1. Urine for specific gravity
2. For the presence of edema
3. Urine for glucose and ketones
4. Blood pressure, pulse, and respirations

Level of Cognitive Ability: Analyzing
Client Needs: Physiological Integrity
Integrated Process: Nursing Process/Assessment
Content Area: Maternity: Antepartum
Priority Concepts: Glucose Regulation; Reproduction

Answer: 3
Rationale: The nurse assesses the pregnant client with diabetes mellitus for glucose and ketones in the urine at each prenatal visit because the physiological changes of pregnancy can drastically alter insulin requirements. The assessment of urine for specific gravity; the presence of edema; and blood pressure, pulse, and respirations are more related to the client with gestational hypertension.
Priority Nursing Tip: Most oral hypoglycemic agents are not prescribed for use during pregnancy because of their teratogenic effects.
Test-Taking Strategy: Focus on the subject of a pregnant client with diabetes mellitus and the strategic word, *priority*. The only option that specifically addresses diabetes mellitus is option 3. Review: the **prenatal care** of the client with **diabetes mellitus.**
Reference(s): Lowdermilk, Perry, Cashion, Alden (2012), p. 694; McKinney et al (2013), p. 607.

Analysis

1113. A client had arterial blood gases drawn. The results are a pH of 7.34, a partial pressure of carbon dioxide of 37 mm Hg, a partial pressure of oxygen of 79 mm Hg, and a bicarbonate level of 19 mEq/L. Which disorder should the nurse interpret that the client is experiencing?
1. Metabolic acidosis
2. Metabolic alkalosis
3. Respiratory acidosis
4. Respiratory alkalosis

Level of Cognitive Ability: Analyzing
Client Needs: Physiological Integrity
Integrated Process: Nursing Process/Analysis
Content Area: Fundamental Skills: Acid-Base
Priority Concepts: Acid-Base Balance; Perfusion

Answer: 1
Rationale: Metabolic acidosis occurs when the pH falls to less than 7.35 and the bicarbonate level falls to less than 22 mEq/L. With metabolic alkalosis, the pH rises to more than 7.45 and the bicarbonate level rises to more than 27 mEq/L. With respiratory acidosis, the pH drops to less than 7.35 and the carbon dioxide level rises to more than 45 mm Hg. With respiratory alkalosis, the pH rises to more than 7.45 and the carbon dioxide level falls to less than 35 mm Hg.
Priority Nursing Tip: Causes of metabolic acidosis include diabetes mellitus or diabetic ketoacidosis, excessive ingestion of acetylsalicylic acid (aspirin), a high-fat diet, insufficient metabolism of carbohydrates, malnutrition, renal insufficiency or renal failure, and severe diarrhea.
Test-Taking Strategy: Knowing that a pH of 7.34 is acidotic assists you with eliminating options 2 and 4 first since they are comparable or alike. From the remaining choices, focus on the subject that involves a metabolic condition that exists when the bicarbonate follows the same up or down pattern as the pH; this will help you to choose option 1 over option 3. Review: the analysis of **arterial blood gas results** and **metabolic acidosis.**
Reference(s): Chernecky, Berger (2013), pp. 208-210; Ignatavicius, Workman (2013), pp. 202-203, 205.

1114. A client diagnosed with advanced cirrhosis of the liver is not tolerating protein well, as evidenced by abnormal laboratory values. The nurse should anticipate that which medication will be prescribed for the client?
1. Folic acid (Folvite)
2. Lactulose (Enulose)
3. Thiamine (vitamin B_1)
4. Ethacrynic acid (Edecrin)

Level of Cognitive Ability: Analyzing
Client Needs: Physiological Integrity
Integrated Process: Nursing Process/Analysis
Content Area: Pharmacology: Gastrointestinal Medications
Priority Concepts: Clinical Judgment; Safety

Answer: 2
Rationale: Ammonia levels are usually elevated in the client with cirrhosis. The administration of lactulose aids in the clearance of ammonia via the gastrointestinal tract. Folic acid and thiamine are vitamins, which may be used as supplemental therapy to treat clients with liver disease. Ethacrynic acid is a diuretic.
Priority Nursing Tip: The client with cirrhosis often has low total protein levels as a result of inadequate nutrition and decreased synthesis by the liver. However, excess protein is not helpful because a function of the liver is to metabolize protein. A diseased liver may not metabolize protein well.
Test-Taking Strategy: To answer this question correctly, focus on the subject of advanced liver disease and its associated pathophysiology. Recall that lactulose is a standard form of medication therapy for this condition. Review: advanced **cirrhosis of the liver** and the purpose of **lactulose.**
Reference(s): Hodgson, Kizior (2014), p. 657; Ignatavicius, Workman (2013), pp. 1294, 1303.

1115. The nurse is caring for a child with kidney disease and is analyzing the child's laboratory results. The nurse notes a sodium level of 148 mEq/L. On the basis of this finding, which clinical manifestation should the nurse expect to note in the child?
1. Lethargy
2. Diaphoresis
3. Cold, wet skin
4. Dry, sticky mucous membranes

Level of Cognitive Ability: Analyzing
Client Needs: Physiological Integrity
Integrated Process: Nursing Process/Analysis
Content Area: Child Health: Metabolic/Endocrine
Priority Concepts: Clinical Judgment; Fluid and Electrolyte Balance

Answer: 4
Rationale: Hypernatremia occurs when the sodium level is more than 145 mEq/L. Clinical manifestations include intense thirst, oliguria, agitation, restlessness, flushed skin, peripheral and pulmonary edema, dry and sticky mucous membranes, nausea, and vomiting. Options 1, 2, and 3 are not associated with the clinical manifestations of hypernatremia.
Priority Nursing Tip: Altered cerebral function is a common manifestation of hypernatremia.
Test-Taking Strategy: Focus on the subject of a child with kidney disease. Note the data in the question and determine that the sodium level is elevated and that the child is experiencing hypernatremia. Eliminate options 2 and 3 because they are comparable or alike. From the remaining choices, recalling that agitation and restlessness (not lethargy) are associated with hypernatremia will direct you to the correct option. Review: the normal sodium level and the clinical manifestations associated with hypernatremia.
Reference(s): McKinney et al (2013), p. 991.

1116. The nurse is caring for an infant who is admitted to the hospital with a diagnosis of hemolytic disease. Which finding should the nurse expect to note in this infant when reviewing the laboratory results?
1. Decreased bilirubin count
2. Elevated blood glucose level
3. Decreased red blood cell count
4. Decreased white blood cell count

Level of Cognitive Ability: Analyzing
Client Needs: Physiological Integrity
Integrated Process: Nursing Process/Analysis
Content Area: Child Health: Hematological
Priority Concepts: Cellular Regulation; Clinical Judgment

Answer: 3
Rationale: The two primary pathophysiologic alterations associated with hemolytic disease are anemia and hyperbilirubinemia. The red blood cell count is decreased because red blood cell production cannot keep pace with red blood cell destruction. Hyperbilirubinemia results from the red blood cell destruction that accompanies this disorder and from the normally decreased ability of the neonate's liver to conjugate and excrete bilirubin efficiently from the body. Hypoglycemia is associated with hypertrophy of the pancreatic islet cells and increased levels of insulin. The white blood cell count is not related to this disorder.
Priority Nursing Tip: Iron is found predominantly in hemoglobin and acts as a carrier of oxygen from the lungs to the tissues and indirectly aids in the return of carbon dioxide to the lungs.
Test-Taking Strategy: Focus on the subject of an infant with hemolytic disease. Noting the word *hemolytic* in the diagnosis will direct you to the correct option. Review: the clinical manifestations associated with hemolytic disease.
Reference(s): Hockenberry, Wilson (2013), pp. 263-265.

1117. The nurse is performing an assessment of a child who is to receive a measles, mumps, and rubella (MMR) vaccine. The nurse notes that the child is allergic to eggs. Which intervention has **priority**?
1. Eliminating this vaccine from the immunization schedule
2. Administering epinephrine (Adrenalin) before the administration of the MMR
3. Administering diphenhydramine (Benadryl) and acetaminophen (Tylenol) before administering the MMR vaccine
4. Taking a careful history about the allergy and reporting this to the health care provider before administering the MMR vaccine

Level of Cognitive Ability: Analyzing
Client Needs: Health Promotion and Maintenance
Integrated Process: Nursing Process/Analysis
Content Area: Child Health: Infectious and Communicable Diseases
Priority Concepts: Health Promotion; Immunity

Answer: 4
Rationale: Live measles vaccine is produced by chick embryo cell culture, so the possibility of an anaphylactic hypersensitivity in children with egg allergies should be considered. The nurse should take a thorough history of the allergy to a previous MMR and report this to the health care provider. If this is the first MMR, the health care provider should be aware of the egg sensitivity before administering the vaccine or any pre-injection medication.
Priority Nursing Tip: Contraindications of the measles, mumps, and rubella (MMR) vaccine include severe allergic reaction to a previous dose or vaccine component (gelatin, neomycin, eggs), pregnancy, or known immunodeficiency.
Test-Taking Strategy: Use the steps of the nursing process and the strategic word, *priority*, to direct you to option 4. Option 1 can be eliminated first because a vaccine would not be eliminated from the immunization schedule. Options 2 and 3 can be eliminated next, knowing that the use of medications before a vaccine is not normal procedure. Review: the procedures related to the administration of vaccines and the measles, mumps, and rubella (MMR) vaccine.
Reference(s): McKinney et al (2013), p. 85.

1118. Intravenous immune globulin (IVIG) therapy is prescribed for a child with idiopathic thrombocytopenic purpura (ITP). What is the expected result of this medication?
1. Urine positive for glucose and negative for protein
2. Urine specific gravity of 1.020 and negative for red blood cells
3. Blood urea nitrogen (BUN) 22 mg/dL and creatinine levels of 2.1 mg/dL
4. White blood cell count 18,000 cells/mm³ and platelets 355,000 cells/mm³

Level of Cognitive Ability: Analyzing
Client Needs: Physiological Integrity
Integrated Process: Nursing Process/Analysis
Content Area: Child Health: Hematological
Priority Concepts: Cellular Regulation; Clinical Judgment

Answer: 4
Rationale: IVIG is usually effective to rapidly increase the platelet count. It is thought to act by interfering with the attachment of antibody-coded platelets to receptors on the macrophage cells of the reticuloendothelial system. Corticosteroids may be prescribed to enhance vascular stability and decrease the production of antiplatelet antibodies. Options 1, 2, and 3 are unrelated to the administration of this medication.
Priority Nursing Tip: Manifestations of idiopathic thrombocytopenic purpura (ITP) are first noted in the skin and mucous membranes. Large ecchymotic areas or a petechial rash on the arms, legs, upper chest, and neck may be noted.
Test-Taking Strategy: Focus on the subject of IVIG therapy for a child with idiopathic thrombocytopenic purpura (ITP). Note the relationship between the name of the diagnosis *thrombocytopenic purpura* and the word *platelets* in the correct option. This relationship may assist with directing you to the correct option. Review: idiopathic thrombocytopenic purpura (ITP) and the purpose of intravenous immune globulin (IVIG).
Reference(s): McKinney et al (2013), p. 1242.

1119. A child was diagnosed with acute post-streptococcal glomerulonephritis and renal insufficiency. Which laboratory result should the nurse expect to note in the child?
1. Urine positive for glucose and negative for protein
2. Urine specific gravity of 1.020 and negative for red blood cells
3. Blood urea nitrogen (BUN) 22 mg/dL and creatinine levels of 2.1 mg/dL
4. White blood cells (WBC) 18,000 cells/mm³ and platelets 355,000 cells/mm³

Level of Cognitive Ability: Analyzing
Client Needs: Physiological Integrity
Integrated Process: Nursing Process/Analysis
Content Area: Child Health: Renal and Urinary
Priority Concepts: Clinical Judgment; Elimination

Answer: 3
Rationale: With poststreptococcal glomerulonephritis, a urinalysis will reveal hematuria with red cell casts. Proteinuria is also present. If renal insufficiency is severe, the BUN and creatinine levels will be elevated. The WBC is usually within normal limits, and mild anemia is common. Platelets would be lower, whereas glucose is not related.
Priority Nursing Tip: In glomerulonephritis, inflammation of the glomeruli results from an antigen–antibody reaction produced by an infection elsewhere in the body. Loss of kidney function develops.
Test-Taking Strategy: Focus on the subject of a child with acute poststreptococcal glomerulonephritis and renal insufficiency. Recalling that the BUN and creatinine levels are laboratory studies that relate to the renal system will direct you to option 3. Review the clinical manifestations associated with **acute poststreptococcal glomerulonephritis**.
Reference(s): McKinney et al (2013), p. 1129.

1120. A child is admitted to the hospital with a suspected diagnosis of bacterial endocarditis. The child has been experiencing fever, malaise, anorexia, and a headache, and diagnostic studies are performed on the child. Which studies will **primarily** confirm the diagnosis?
1. A blood culture
2. A sedimentation rate
3. A white blood cell count
4. An electrocardiogram (ECG)

Level of Cognitive Ability: Analyzing
Client Needs: Physiological Integrity
Integrated Process: Nursing Process/Analysis
Content Area: Child Health: Cardiovascular
Priority Concepts: Clinical Judgment; Infection

Answer: 1
Rationale: The diagnosis of bacterial endocarditis is primarily established on the basis of a positive blood culture of the organisms and the visualization of vegetation on echocardiographic studies. Other laboratory tests that may help confirm the diagnosis are an elevated sedimentation rate and the C-reactive protein level. An ECG is not usually helpful for the diagnosis of bacterial endocarditis.
Priority Nursing Tip: Instruct the parents of a child who had bacterial endocarditis of the need to inform the dentist and any other health care providers about the condition. Prophylactic antibiotics may be prescribed before dental procedures or any other invasive disorders to prevent the recurrence of endocarditis.
Test-Taking Strategy: Note the strategic word, *primarily*. Focus on the subject of bacterial endocarditis and its causes. The only test that will confirm the presence of an organism is the blood culture. Review: the diagnostic studies associated with **bacterial endocarditis**.
Reference(s): McKinney et al (2013), p. 1225.

1121. The nurse is caring for a client with an intracranial aneurysm. The nurse interprets that which observation is related to the dysfunction of cranial nerve III (oculomotor nerve)?
1. Mild drowsiness
2. Ptosis of the left eyelid
3. Diminished mental acuity
4. Less frequent spontaneous speech

Level of Cognitive Ability: Analyzing
Client Needs: Physiological Integrity
Integrated Process: Nursing Process/Analysis
Content Area: Adult Health: Neurological
Priority Concepts: Intracranial Regulation; Sensory Perception

Answer: 2
Rationale: Ptosis of the eyelid is caused by pressure on and the dysfunction of cranial nerve III, the oculomotor nerve. Options 1, 3, and 4 identify early signs of a deteriorating level of consciousness.
Priority Nursing Tip: Cranial nerve III, the oculomotor nerve, controls pupillary constriction, upper eyelid elevation, and most eye movement.
Test-Taking Strategy: Focus on the subject of cranial nerve III dysfunction. Recalling the function of this nerve and that it is the oculomotor nerve will direct you to option 2. Review: the function of **cranial nerve III (oculomotor nerve)**.
Reference(s): Ignatavicius, Workman (2013), pp. 912, 1046.

1122. A client with thrombotic stroke experiences periods of emotional lability. The client alternately laughs and cries and intermittently becomes irritable and demanding. What should the nurse interpret this behavior as indicating?
1. That the client is not adapting well to the disability
2. That the problem is likely to get worse before it gets better
3. That the client is experiencing the usual sequelae of a stroke
4. That the client is experiencing the side effects of prescribed anticoagulants

Level of Cognitive Ability: Analyzing
Client Needs: Psychosocial Integrity
Integrated Process: Nursing Process/Analysis
Content Area: Adult Health: Neurological
Priority Concepts: Intracranial Regulation; Mood and Affect

Answer: 3
Rationale: After a thrombotic stroke, the client often experiences periods of emotional lability, which are characterized by sudden bouts of laughing or crying or by irritability, depression, confusion, or being demanding. This is a normal part of the clinical picture of the client with this health problem, although it may be difficult for health care personnel and family members to deal with it. The other options are incorrect.
Priority Nursing Tip: A critical factor in the early intervention and treatment of stroke is the accurate identification of stroke manifestations and establishing the onset of the manifestations. Stroke screening scales may be used to quickly identify stroke manifestations.
Test-Taking Strategy: Focus on the subject of emotional liability after thrombotic stroke. Eliminate option 4 first because anticoagulants do not cause emotional lability. From the remaining choices, recalling the emotional changes that accompany a thrombotic stroke will direct you to option 3. Review: the effects of a thrombotic stroke.
Reference(s): Ignatavicius, Workman (2013), p. 1012.

1123. A nonstress test is performed on a client, and the results are documented as "two or more fetal heart rate (FHR) accelerations of 15 beats/min lasting 15 seconds in association with fetal movement." How does the nurse interpret these findings?
1. Unsatisfactory
2. A reactive nonstress test
3. A nonreactive nonstress test
4. Unclear for accurate interpretation

Level of Cognitive Ability: Analyzing
Client Needs: Physiological Integrity
Integrated Process: Nursing Process/Analysis
Content Area: Maternity: Antepartum
Priority Concepts: Clinical Judgment; Reproduction

Answer: 2
Rationale: A reactive nonstress test (normal/negative) indicates a healthy fetus. It is described as two or more FHR accelerations of at least 15 beats/min and lasting at least 15 seconds from the beginning of the acceleration to the end in association with fetal movement during a 20-minute period. An unsatisfactory test cannot be interpreted because of the poor quality of the FHR. A nonreactive nonstress test (abnormal) is described as no accelerations or accelerations of less than 15 beats/min or lasting less than 15 seconds in duration throughout any fetal movement during the testing period.
Priority Nursing Tip: Fetal heart rate accelerations are transient increases in the fetal heart rate that often accompany contractions or are caused by fetal movement. Episodic accelerations are thought to be a sign of fetal well-being and adequate oxygen reserve.
Test-Taking Strategy: Focus on the subject, results of a nonstress test. Eliminate options 1 and 4 first because they are comparable or alike. From the remaining choices, remembering that a reactive nonstress test is a normal or negative test will assist with directing you to option 2. Review: the nonstress test.
Reference(s): McKinney et al (2013), pp. 309-310.

1124. The nurse is developing a plan of care for a client in Buck's (extension) traction. The nurse should determine that which is a **priority** client problem?
1. Immobility
2. Trouble bathing
3. Infection at pin sites
4. Need for sensory stimulation

Level of Cognitive Ability: Analyzing
Client Needs: Physiological Integrity
Integrated Process: Nursing Process/Analysis
Content Area: Adult Health: Musculoskeletal
Priority Concepts: Clinical Judgment; Mobility

Answer: 1
Rationale: The priority client problem in Buck's traction is immobility. Options 2 and 4 may also be appropriate for the client in traction, but immobility presents the greatest risk for the development of complications. Buck's traction is a skin traction, and there are no pin sites.
Priority Nursing Tip: Buck's (extension) skin traction is used to alleviate muscle spasms and immobilize a lower limb by maintaining a straight pull on the limb with the use of weights. It is often used in the preoperative period for a client who sustained a hip fracture.
Test-Taking Strategy: Focus on the subject, Buck's traction and its possible complications. Eliminate option 3 first because there are no pin sites with Buck's traction. From the remaining choices, focus on the strategic word, *priority*, recalling that the client experiences immobility when in traction. This will direct you to option 1. Review: the care of the client in Buck's traction.
Reference(s): Ignatavicius, Workman (2013), pp. 1153, 1160-1161.

1125. A pregnant client diagnosed with mitral valve prolapse is prescribed anticoagulant therapy during pregnancy. The nurse reviews the client's medical record, expecting to note that which medication is prescribed?
1. Oral intake of warfarin (Coumadin) daily
2. Intravenous infusion of heparin sodium daily
3. Subcutaneous administration of terbutaline daily
4. Subcutaneous administration of heparin sodium daily

Level of Cognitive Ability: Analyzing
Client Needs: Physiological Integrity
Integrated Process: Nursing Process/Analysis
Content Area: Maternity: Antepartum
Priority Concepts: Clinical Judgment; Safety

Answer: 4
Rationale: Pregnant women with mitral valve prolapse are frequently given anticoagulant therapy during pregnancy because they are at greater risk for thromboembolic disease during the antenatal, intrapartal, and postpartum periods. Heparin, which does not pass the placental barrier, is a safe anticoagulant therapy during pregnancy, and it would be administered by the subcutaneous route. Warfarin (Coumadin) is contraindicated during pregnancy because it passes the placental barrier and causes potential fetal malformations and hemorrhagic disorders. Terbutaline is a medication that is indicated for preterm labor management.
Priority Nursing Tip: Bleeding is the primary concern for a client taking an anticoagulant, thrombolytic, or antiplatelet medication.
Test-Taking Strategy: Focus on the subject, mitral valve prolapse, anticoagulant therapy, and medication safety during pregnancy. Eliminate options 1 and 3 first because warfarin is contraindicated in pregnancy, and terbutaline may be indicated; however, it is for preterm labor management. From the remaining choices, select option 4 because of the word *subcutaneous*. Review: the treatment measures for the pregnant client with **mitral valve prolapse**.
Reference(s): McKinney et al (2013), pp. 618-620.

1126. The nurse continues to assess a client who is in the late first stage of labor for progress and fetal well-being. At the last vaginal exam, the client was fully effaced, 8 cm dilated, vertex presentation, and station −1. Which observation would indicate that the fetus was in fetal distress?
1. The fetal heart rate slowly drops to 110 beats/min during strong contractions, recovering to 138 beats/min immediately afterward.
2. Fresh meconium is found on the examiner's gloved fingers after a vaginal exam, and the fetal monitor pattern remains essentially unchanged.
3. Fresh, thick meconium is passed with a small gush of liquid, and the fetal monitor shows late decelerations with a variable descending baseline.
4. The vaginal exam continues to reveal some old meconium staining, and the fetal monitor demonstrates a U-shaped pattern of deceleration during contractions, recovering to a baseline of 140 beats/min.

Level of Cognitive Ability: Analyzing
Client Needs: Physiological Integrity
Integrated Process: Nursing Process/Analysis
Content Area: Maternity: Intrapartum
Priority Concepts: Perfusion; Reproduction

Answer: 3
Rationale: Meconium staining alone is not a sign of fetal distress. Meconium passage is a normal physiological function that is frequently noted with a fetus of more than 38 weeks' gestation. Fresh meconium in combination with late decelerations and a variable descending baseline is an ominous signal of fetal distress caused by fetal hypoxia. It is not unusual for the fetal heart rate to drop to less than the 140 to 160 beats/min range in late labor during contractions, and, in a healthy fetus, the fetal heart rate will recover between contractions. Old meconium staining may be the result of a prenatal trauma that is resolved.
Priority Nursing Tip: In the event of fetal distress, prepare the client for emergency cesarean delivery.
Test-Taking Strategy: Note the subject, fetal distress. Eliminate options 1 and 4 first because they both indicate a recovering fetal heart rate. From the remaining choices, eliminate option 2 because of the words *fetal monitor pattern remains essentially unchanged*. Review: signs of fetal distress.
Reference(s): Lowdermilk, Perry, Cashion, Alden (2012), p. 448.

1127. The nurse is caring for a child with seizures who is being treated with carbamazepine (Tegretol). The nurse reviews the laboratory report for the results of the drug plasma level and determines that the plasma level is in a therapeutic range if which is noted?
1. 1 mcg/mL
2. 10 mcg/mL
3. 18 mcg/mL
4. 20 mcg/mL

Level of Cognitive Ability: Applying
Client Needs: Physiological Integrity
Integrated Process: Nursing Process/Analysis
Content Area: Pharmacology: Neurological Medications
Priority Concepts: Clinical Judgment; Safety

Answer: 2
Rationale: When carbamazepine is administered, plasma levels of the medication need to be monitored periodically to check for the child's absorption of the medication. The amount of the medication prescribed is based on the results of this laboratory test. The therapeutic plasma level of carbamazepine is 3 to 14 mcg/mL. Option 1 indicates a low level that possibly necessitates an increased medication dose. Options 3 and 4 identify elevated levels that indicate the need to decrease the medication dose.
Priority Nursing Tip: Adverse effects of carbamazepine (Tegretol) appear as blood dyscrasias, including aplastic anemia, agranulocytosis, thrombocytopenia, and leukopenia; cardiovascular disturbances; thrombophlebitis; dysrhythmias; and dermatological effects.
Test-Taking Strategy: Focus on the subject, therapeutic plasma level of carbamazepine, to answer the question. Recalling that the therapeutic plasma level is 3 to 14 mcg/mL will direct you to option 2. Review: the therapeutic plasma level of **carbamazepine (Tegretol).**
Reference(s): Hodgson, Kizior (2014), p. 182.

1128. The nurse performs an assessment on a client with a history of heart failure. The client has been taking diuretics on a long-term basis. The nurse reviews the medication record, knowing that which medication, if prescribed for this client, would place the client at risk for hypokalemia?
1. Bumetanide
2. Triamterene (Dyrenium)
3. Spironolactone (Aldactone)
4. Amiloride and hydrochlorothiazide (Midamor)

Level of Cognitive Ability: Analyzing
Client Needs: Physiological Integrity
Integrated Process: Nursing Process/Analysis
Content Area: Pharmacology: Cardiovascular Medications
Priority Concepts: Clinical Judgment; Fluid and Electrolyte Balance

Answer: 1
Rationale: Bumetanide is a loop diuretic. The client on this medication would be at risk for hypokalemia. Triamterene (Dyrenium), Spironolactone (Aldactone) and Amiloride and hydrochlorothiazide (Midamor) are potassium-retaining diuretics.
Priority Nursing Tip: Natriuretic peptides are neuroendocrine peptides that are used to identify the client with heart failure (HF). The brain natriuretic peptide (BNP) is synthesized in the cardiac ventricle muscle. The higher the BNP level, the more severe the HF. If the BNP is elevated, the dyspnea is caused by HF; if it is normal, the dyspnea is caused by a pulmonary problem.
Test-Taking Strategy: Focus on the subject of the identification of potassium-losing diuretic. Recalling that bumetanide is a loop diuretic will direct you to option 1. Also note that options 2, 3, and 4 are comparable or alike and are potassium-retaining diuretics. Review: **loop diuretics.**
Reference(s): Hodgson, Kizior (2014), pp. 154-155.

1129. The home care nurse is preparing to visit a client with a diagnosis of Ménière's disease. The nurse reviews the health care provider prescriptions and expects to educate the client on which dietary measure?
1. A low-fiber diet with decreased fluids
2. A low-sodium diet and fluid restriction
3. A low-fat diet with a restriction of citrus fruits
4. A low-carbohydrate diet and the elimination of red meats

Level of Cognitive Ability: Analyzing
Client Needs: Physiological Integrity
Integrated Process: Nursing Process/Analysis
Content Area: Adult Health: Ear
Priority Concepts: Client Education; Sensory Perception

Answer: 2
Rationale: Dietary changes such as salt and fluid restrictions that reduce the amount of endolymphatic fluid are sometimes prescribed for clients with Ménière's disease. Options 1, 3, and 4 are not prescribed for this disorder.
Priority Nursing Tip: A priority nursing intervention in the care of a client with Ménière's syndrome is instituting safety measures because severe vertigo can occur.
Test-Taking Strategy: Focus on the subject, a client with Ménière's disease. Recalling that salt and fluid restrictions are sometimes necessary to reduce the amount of endolymphatic fluid will assist with directing you to the correct option. Review: the pathophysiology and treatment of **Ménière's disease.**
Reference(s): Ignatavicius, Workman (2013), p. 1096.

1130. The nurse is caring for a client who has been diagnosed with tuberculosis. The client is receiving 600 mg of oral rifampin (Rifadin) daily. Which laboratory finding would indicate to the nurse that the client is experiencing an adverse effect?

1. A total bilirubin level of 0.5 mg/dL
2. A sedimentation rate of 15 mm/hour
3. Alanine aminotransferase (ALT) of 80 units/L
4. A white blood cell count of 6000 cells/mm³

Level of Cognitive Ability: Analyzing
Client Needs: Physiological Integrity
Integrated Process: Nursing Process/Analysis
Content Area: Pharmacology: Respiratory Medications
Priority Concepts: Clinical Judgment; Safety

Answer: 3
Rationale: Adverse or toxic effects of rifampin include hepatotoxicity, hepatitis, jaundice, blood dyscrasias, Stevens-Johnson syndrome, and antibiotic-related colitis. The nurse monitors for increased liver function, bilirubin, blood urea nitrogen, and uric acid levels because elevations indicate an adverse effect. The normal ALT level is 10 to 40 units/L. The normal total bilirubin level is less than 1.5 mg/dL. The normal sedimentation rate is 0 to 30 mm/hour. A normal white blood cell count is 4500 to 11,000 cells/mm³.
Priority Nursing Tip: A side effect of rifampin (Rifadin), an antituberculosis medication, is red-orange colored body secretions.
Test-Taking Strategy: Focus on the subject, rifampin (Rifadin) and diagnostic results that would indicate a possible adverse effect. Recalling that the medication is metabolized in the liver will assist you with eliminating options 2 and 4 because these laboratory studies are not directly related to assessing liver function. From the remaining choices, knowledge of normal laboratory values will direct you to option 3. Review: oral **rifampin (Rifadin)** and these normal **laboratory values.**
Reference(s): Chernecky, Berger (2013), pp. 117-118; Hodgson, Kizior (2014), pp. 1036-1038; Kee, Hayes, McCuistion (2012), pp. 451, 456.

1131. A home care nurse is assessing a client who is taking prazosin (Minipress). Which statement by the client would support the **need for further teaching** regarding medication compliance?

1. "If I feel dizzy, I'll skip my dose for a few days."
2. "I can't see the numbers on the label to know how much salt is in the food."
3. "I understand why I have to keep taking the pills even when my blood pressure is normal."
4. "If I have a cold, I shouldn't take any over-the-counter remedies without consulting my doctor."

Level of Cognitive Ability: Analyzing
Client Needs: Physiological Integrity
Integrated Process: Nursing Process/Analysis
Content Area: Pharmacology: Cardiovascular Medications
Priority Concepts: Clinical Judgment; Safety

Answer: 1
Rationale: Prazosin (Minipress) is used to treat hypertension. The side effects of prazosin are dizziness and impotence. The client needs to be instructed to call the health care provider if these side effects occur. Holding (skipping) medication will cause an abrupt rise in blood pressure. Option 2 indicates difficulty taking care of oneself. Options 3 and 4 indicate client understanding regarding the medication.
Priority Nursing Tip: Instruct the client taking prazosin (Minipress) to change positions slowly to prevent orthostatic hypotension.
Test-Taking Strategy: Focus on the subject, prazosin (Minipress) and guidelines for addressing medication compliance. Note the strategic words, *need for further teaching.* These words indicate a negative event query and ask you to select an option that is an incorrect statement. Noting the words, "I'll skip my dose," will direct you to option 1. Review: medication administration guidelines and **prazosin (Minipress).**
Reference(s): Hodgson, Kizior (2014), pp. 973-974.

1132. A client manages peptic ulcer disease (PUD) with excessive amounts of oral antacids. Signs/symptoms of which acid-base imbalance should the nurse assess for?
1. Metabolic acidosis
2. Metabolic alkalosis
3. Respiratory acidosis
4. Respiratory alkalosis

Level of Cognitive Ability: Analyzing
Client Needs: Physiological Integrity
Integrated Process: Nursing Process/Analysis
Content Area: Fundamental Skills: Acid-Base
Priority Concepts: Acid-Base Balance; Clinical Judgment

Answer: 2
Rationale: Oral antacids can be effective treatment for PUD when administered properly, but when they are taken in excess they can lead to metabolic alkalosis (a pH of more than 7.45 and a bicarbonate ion [HCO_3] level of more than 27 mEq/L). As effective therapy for PUD, antacids bind with the hydrochloric acid (HCl^-) of gastric secretions and halt the corrosive action of the HCl^-. However, antacids are alkaline substances, and excessive administration can exceed the kidney's ability to clear the excess HCO_3, which leads to the accumulation of HCO_3, an increased pH, and metabolic alkalosis. Metabolic acidosis occurs when the pH is low and the HCO_3 is low; respiratory acidosis occurs when the pH is low and the partial pressure of carbon dioxide (Pco_2) is high; and respiratory alkalosis occurs when the pH is high and the Pco_2 is low.
Priority Nursing Tip: To prevent interactions with other medications and the interference with the action of other medications, allow 1 hour between antacid administration and the administration of other medications.
Test-Taking Strategy: Focus on the subject, the use of antacids, and the possible outcome of that behavior. With this in mind, eliminate options 3 and 4 first because they are comparable and alike because both involve respiratory components. Knowing that the word *antacids* means *working against acids* will help you choose the correct option. Review: the causes of **metabolic alkalosis**.
Reference(s): Ignatavicius, Workman (2013), p. 207.

1133. The nurse is assessing a 39-year-old Caucasian client with a blood pressure (BP) of 152/92 mm Hg at rest, a total cholesterol level of 180 mg/dL, and a fasting blood glucose level of 90 mg/dL. On which risk factor for coronary artery disease should the nurse place **priority**?
1. Age
2. Hypertension
3. Hyperlipidemia
4. Glucose intolerance

Level of Cognitive Ability: Analyzing
Client Needs: Health Promotion and Maintenance
Integrated Process: Nursing Process/Analysis
Content Area: Adult Health: Cardiovascular
Priority Concepts: Health Promotion; Perfusion

Answer: 2
Rationale: Hypertension, cigarette smoking, and hyperlipidemia are major risk modifiable factors for coronary artery disease. Glucose intolerance, obesity, and response to stress are also contributing factors. An age of more than 40 years is a nonmodifiable risk factor. A cholesterol level of 180 mg/dL and a blood glucose level of 90 mg/dL are within the normal range. The nurse places priority on major risk factors that need modification.
Priority Nursing Tip: The goal of treatment for the client with coronary artery disease is to alter the atherosclerotic progression.
Test-Taking Strategy: Focus on the subject of risk factors for coronary artery disease, and note the strategic word, *priority*. Note that the only abnormal value is the BP. Review: the risk factors associated with coronary artery disease.
Reference(s): Ignatavicius, Workman (2013), p. 832.

1134. The nurse is caring for a client who has just returned to the nursing unit after an intravenous pyelogram (IVP). What is the nurse's **priority** for the postprocedure care of this client?
  1. Maintaining the client on bed rest
  2. Ambulating the client in the hallway
  3. Encouraging the increased intake of oral fluids
  4. Encouraging the client to try to void frequently

Level of Cognitive Ability: Analyzing
Client Needs: Physiological Integrity
Integrated Process: Nursing Process/Analysis
Content Area: Fundamental Skills: Diagnostic Tests
Priority Concepts: Clinical Judgment; Elimination

Answer: 3
Rationale: After IVP, the client should take in increased fluids to aid in the clearance of the dye used for the procedure. The client is usually allowed activity as tolerated, without any specific activity guidelines. It is unnecessary to void frequently after the procedure.
Priority Nursing Tip: An informed consent is required for a diagnostic procedure that is invasive.
Test-Taking Strategy: Note the strategic word, *priority*. Option 4 has no useful purpose and is eliminated first. From the remaining choices, recall that there are no activity guidelines after this procedure. Recalling that fluids are necessary to promote the clearance of the dye from the client's system will direct you to option 3. Review: **intravenous pyelogram (IVP).**
Reference(s): Pagana, Pagana (2013), pp. 783-785.

1135. The nurse is caring for a client with myasthenia gravis who is vomiting and complaining of abdominal cramps and diarrhea. The nurse notes that the client is hypotensive and experiencing facial muscle twitching. Which possible situation does this assessment data support?
  1. Myasthenic crisis
  2. Cholinergic crisis
  3. Systemic infection
  4. A reaction to plasmapheresis

Level of Cognitive Ability: Analyzing
Client Needs: Physiological Integrity
Integrated Process: Nursing Process/Analysis
Content Area: Adult Health: Neurological
Priority Concepts: Clinical Judgment; Mobility

Answer: 2
Rationale: Signs and symptoms of cholinergic crisis include nausea, vomiting, abdominal cramping, diarrhea, blurred vision, pallor, facial muscle twitching, pupillary miosis, and hypotension. It is caused by overmedication with cholinergic (anticholinesterase) medications, and it is treated by withholding medications. Myasthenic crisis is an exacerbation of myasthenic symptoms caused by undermedication with anticholinesterase medications. There are no data in the question to support options 1, 3, and 4.
Priority Nursing Tip: In myasthenia gravis, a cholinergic crisis is caused by overmedication with an anticholinesterase medication.
Test-Taking Strategy: Focus on the subject of the client's diagnosis of myasthenia gravis, and the treatment for this disorder. Recalling the effects of cholinergic medications and focusing on the data in the question will direct you to the correct option. Review: the clinical manifestations associated with **cholinergic crisis** and **myasthenia gravis.**
Reference(s): Ignatavicius, Workman (2013), pp. 993-994.

1136. The nurse is assigned to care for a child with juvenile idiopathic arthritis (JIA). What is the child's **priority** problem?
  1. Acute pain
  2. Potential difficulty with everyday tasks
  3. Impaired mobility causing potential injury
  4. Negative view of body because of activity intolerance

Level of Cognitive Ability: Analyzing
Client Needs: Physiological Integrity
Integrated Process: Nursing Process/Analysis
Content Area: Child Health: Neurological
Priority Concepts: Clinical Judgment; Pain

Answer: 1
Rationale: All of the problems identified in the options are appropriate for the child with JIA; however, acute pain must be managed before other problems can be addressed.
Priority Nursing Tip: There are no definitive tests to diagnose juvenile idiopathic arthritis.
Test-Taking Strategy: Note the strategic word, *priority*. Use Maslow's Hierarchy of Needs theory, and remember that physiological needs (option 1) receive the highest priority. Option 2 identifies a potential problem rather than an actual problem. Option 3 addresses safety and security needs. Option 4 addresses body image. Review: the care of a child with **juvenile idiopathic arthritis (JIA).**
Reference(s): McKinney et al (2013), pp. 1370-1371.

1137. A child is admitted to the hospital with a suspected diagnosis of idiopathic thrombocytopenic purpura (ITP) and diagnostic studies are performed. Which diagnostic result is indicative of this disorder?
1. An elevated platelet count
2. Elevated hemoglobin and hematocrit levels
3. A bone marrow examination showing an increased number of megakaryocytes
4. A bone marrow examination indicating an increased number of immature white blood cells

Level of Cognitive Ability: Analyzing
Client Needs: Physiological Integrity
Integrated Process: Nursing Process/Analysis
Content Area: Child Health: Hematological
Priority Concepts: Clinical Judgment; Clotting

Answer: 3
Rationale: The laboratory manifestations of ITP include the presence of a low platelet count of usually less than 20,000 cells/mm³. Thrombocytopenia is the only laboratory abnormality expected with ITP. If there has been significant blood loss, there is evidence of anemia in the blood cell count. If a bone marrow examination is performed, the results with ITP show a normal or increased number of megakaryocytes, which are the precursors of platelets. Option 4 indicates the bone marrow result that would be found in a child with leukemia.
Priority Nursing Tip: For the client with idiopathic thrombocytopenic purpura (ITP), platelet transfusions may be administered when platelet counts are less than 20,000 cells/mm³.
Test-Taking Strategy: Focus on the subject of ITP and associated diagnostic tests. Think about the pathophysiology of this diagnosis. Recalling that megakaryocytes are the precursors of platelets will assist with directing you to the correct option. Review: **idiopathic thrombocytopenic purpura (ITP)**.
Reference(s): Hockenberry, Wilson (2013), pp. 886-887.

1138. The mother explains to the nurse that her infant is vomiting after meals, and it is now becoming more frequent and forceful. During the assessment, the nurse notes visible peristaltic waves moving from left to right across the infant's abdomen. On the basis of these findings, which condition should the nurse suspect?
1. Colic
2. Intussusception
3. Congenital megacolon
4. Hypertrophic pyloric stenosis

Level of Cognitive Ability: Analyzing
Client Needs: Physiological Integrity
Integrated Process: Nursing Process/Analysis
Content Area: Child Health: Gastrointestinal
Priority Concepts: Clinical Judgment; Safety

Answer: 4
Rationale: In pyloric stenosis, the vomitus contains sour, undigested food but no bile, the child is constipated, and visible peristaltic waves move from left to right across the abdomen. A movable, palpable, firm, olive-shaped mass in the right upper quadrant may be noted. Crying during the evening hours, appearing to be in pain, but eating well and gaining weight are clinical manifestations of colic. An infant who suddenly becomes pale, cries out, and draws the legs up to the chest is demonstrating physical signs of intussusception. Ribbon-like stool, bile-stained emesis, the absence of peristalsis, and abdominal distention are symptoms of congenital megacolon (Hirschsprung's disease).
Priority Nursing Tip: In pyloric stenosis, the nurse should monitor for signs of dehydration and electrolyte imbalances.
Test-Taking Strategy: Focus on the subject of an infant who is vomiting after meals, and it is now becoming more frequent and forceful. Note all the child's assessment data and the possible diagnoses. Consider each condition presented in the options, and think about the clinical manifestations of each. Recalling the manifestations associated with pyloric stenosis will direct you to the correct option. Also, recalling that stenosis means "narrowing" will direct you to the correct option. Review: the clinical manifestations of **pyloric stenosis**.
Reference(s): Hockenberry, Wilson (2013), pp. 807-808; McKinney et al (2013), pp. 1095-1096.

1139. The nurse is reviewing the laboratory analysis of cerebrospinal fluid (CSF) obtained during a lumbar puncture from a child who is suspected of having bacterial meningitis. Which result would **most likely** confirm this diagnosis?

1. Clear CSF with low protein and low glucose
2. Cloudy CSF with low protein and low glucose
3. Cloudy CSF with high protein and low glucose
4. Decreased pressure and cloudy CSF with high protein

Level of Cognitive Ability: Analyzing
Client Needs: Physiological Integrity
Integrated Process: Nursing Process/Analysis
Content Area: Child Health: Neurological
Priority Concepts: Clinical Judgment; Infection

Answer: **3**
Rationale: A diagnosis of meningitis is made by testing CSF obtained by lumbar puncture. In the case of bacterial meningitis, findings usually include increased pressure and cloudy CSF with high protein and low glucose. Therefore, options 1, 2, and 4 are incorrect.
Priority Nursing Tip: Pneumococcal conjugate vaccine is recommended for all children beginning at age 2 months to protect against meningitis.
Test-Taking Strategy: Focus on the subject of the laboratory analysis results of CSF associated with bacterial meningitis. Note the strategic words, *most likely*. Eliminate options 1 and 4 first because clear CSF and decreased pressure are not likely to be found with an infectious process such as meningitis. From the remaining choices, recalling that high protein indicates a possible diagnosis of meningitis will direct you to option 3. Review: the findings in **bacterial meningitis**.
Reference(s): McKinney et al (2013), pp. 1414, 1438-1439.

1140. A child is admitted to the pediatric unit with a diagnosis of acute gastroenteritis. The nurse monitors the child for signs of hypovolemic shock as a result of fluid and electrolyte losses that have occurred in the child. Which finding would indicate the presence of compensated shock?

1. Bradycardia
2. Hypotension
3. Profuse diarrhea
4. Capillary refill time greater than 2 seconds

Level of Cognitive Ability: Analyzing
Client Needs: Physiological Integrity
Integrated Process: Nursing Process/Analysis
Content Area: Child Health: Gastrointestinal
Priority Concepts: Fluid and Electrolyte Balance; Infection

Answer: **4**
Rationale: Shock may be classified as compensated or decompensated. In compensated shock, the child becomes tachycardic in an effort to increase the cardiac output. The blood pressure remains normal. The capillary refill time may be prolonged and more than 2 seconds, and the child may become irritable as a result of increasing hypoxia. The most prevalent cause of hypovolemic shock is fluid and electrolyte losses associated with gastroenteritis. Diarrhea is not a sign of shock; rather, it is a cause of the fluid and electrolyte imbalance.
Priority Nursing Tip: Rotavirus is a cause of serious gastroenteritis and is a nosocomial (hospital-acquired) pathogen that is most severe in children 3 to 24 months old. Children younger than 3 months have some protection because of maternally acquired antibodies.
Test-Taking Strategy: Focus on the subject of compensated shock. Recalling that hypotension is a late sign of shock in children will assist you with eliminating option 2. Recalling that tachycardia rather than bradycardia occurs in shock will assist you with eliminating option 1. From the remaining choices, focusing on the subject of signs of shock will direct you to option 4. Review: the signs of **compensated shock** in a child.
Reference(s): McKinney et al (2013), pp. 854-855.

1141. The mother tells the nurse that the teacher has reported that the child appears to be daydreaming and staring off into space numerous times throughout the day, yet during the remainder of the day, the child is alert and participates in classroom activities. The nurse should suspect that the child has which problem?

1. School phobia
2. Absence seizures
3. Behavioral problem
4. Attention-deficit/hyperactivity syndrome

Level of Cognitive Ability: Analyzing
Client Needs: Physiological Integrity
Integrated Process: Nursing Process/Analysis
Content Area: Child Health: Neurological
Priority Concepts: Clinical Judgment; Intracranial Regulation

Answer: 2

Rationale: Absence seizures are a type of generalized seizure. They consist of a sudden, brief (usually 5 to 10 seconds) arrest of the child's motor activities accompanied by a blank stare and a loss of awareness. The child's posture is maintained at the end of the seizure, and the child returns to activity that was in process as though nothing has happened. School phobia includes physical symptoms that usually occur at home and that may prevent the child from attending school. Behavior problems would be noted by more overt symptoms than the ones described in this question. A child with attention-deficit/hyperactivity syndrome becomes easily distracted, is fidgety, and has difficulty following directions.

Priority Nursing Tip: Instruct the parents of a child with a seizure disorder to note the time of onset, precipitating events, and behavior before and after the seizure, if one occurs.

Test-Taking Strategy: Focus on the subject, the child appears to be daydreaming and staring off into space numerous times throughout the day, yet during the remainder of the day, the child is alert and participates in classroom activities. Note the possible diagnoses and the relationship of the information and option 2. Review: **absence seizures.**

Reference(s): McKinney et al (2013), p. 1434.

1142. A mother and her 3-week-old infant arrive at the well-baby clinic for a rescreening test for phenylketonuria (PKU). The nurse reviews the results of the serum phenyl-alanine levels and notes that the level is 1.0 mg/dL. What should the nurse interpret this level as?

1. Normal
2. Inconclusive
3. Requiring a repeat study
4. Elevated and indicating PKU

Level of Cognitive Ability: Understanding
Client Needs: Physiological Integrity
Integrated Process: Nursing Process/Analysis
Content Area: Maternity: Newborn
Priority Concepts: Clinical Judgment; Health Promotion

Answer: 1

Rationale: The normal PKU level is less than 2 mg/dL. With early postpartum discharge, screening is often performed when the infant is less than 2 days old because of the concern that the infant will be lost to follow-up. Infants should be rescreened by the time that they are 14 days old if the initial screening was done when the infant was 24 to 48 hours old.

Priority Nursing Tip: All 50 states require routine screening of all newborns for phenylketonuria.

Test-Taking Strategy: Focus on the subject regarding the normal phenylalanine level. Recalling that the normal level is less than 2 mg/dL will direct you to option 1. Also note that options 2, 3, and 4 are comparable or alike and indicate an other-than-normal finding. Review: the PKU screening test.

Reference(s): McKinney et al (2013), p. 1380.

Planning

1143. The nurse is caring for a client who is receiving total parenteral nutrition through a central venous catheter. Which action should the nurse plan to implement to decrease the risk of infection in this client?
1. Track the client's oral temperature.
2. Administer antibiotics intravenously.
3. Evaluate the differential of the leukocytes.
4. Use sterile technique for dressing changes.

Level of Cognitive Ability: Applying
Client Needs: Safe and Effective Care Environment
Integrated Process: Nursing Process/Planning
Content Area: Fundamental Skills: Infection Control
Priority Concepts: Infection; Nutrition

Answer: 4
Rationale: Sterile technique is vital during dressing changes of a central venous catheter (CVC). CVCs are large-bore catheters that can serve as a direct-entry point for microorganisms into the heart and circulatory system. Using aseptic technique helps avoid catheter-related infections by preventing the introduction of potential pathogens to the site. Options 1, 2, and 3 are reasonable nursing interventions for a client with a CVC; however, none of these actions prevents infection. Options 1 and 3 are assessment methods, and option 2 is implemented after the confirmation of an existing infection.
Priority Nursing Tip: Use sterile technique when caring for a client receiving total parenteral nutrition (TPN). Because the TPN solution has a high concentration of glucose, it is a medium for bacterial growth.
Test-Taking Strategy: Focus on the subject of preventing infection. Note the relationship between "infection" in the question and "sterile" in the correct option. In addition, the only option that will prevent infection is option 4. Review: the care of a client receiving total **parenteral nutrition** and **infection control**.
Reference(s): Ignatavicius, Workman (2013), pp. 1348-1349; Potter et al (2013), pp. 421-422.

1144. The nurse develops a plan of care for a client with a spica cast that covers a lower extremity. Which action should the nurse include in the plan of care to promote bowel elimination?
1. Use a bedside commode.
2. Ambulate to the bathroom.
3. Administer an enema daily.
4. Use a low-profile (fracture) bedpan.

Level of Cognitive Ability: Applying
Client Needs: Physiological Integrity
Integrated Process: Nursing Process/Planning
Content Area: Adult Health: Musculoskeletal
Priority Concepts: Clinical Judgment; Mobility

Answer: 4
Rationale: A client with a spica cast (body cast) that covers a lower extremity cannot bend at the hips to sit up. A low-profile bedpan or fracture pan is designed for use by clients with body or leg casts and for clients who have difficulty raising the hips to use a standard bedpan; therefore, using a commode or the bathroom is contraindicated. Daily enemas are not a part of routine care.
Priority Nursing Tip: Inform the client and family about keeping the cast clean and dry. The material of a cast can crumble if it becomes wet. This presents a risk of altered skin integrity and subsequent infection.
Test-Taking Strategy: Focus on the subject of spica cast care and the words *covers a lower extremity*. Therefore, choose the measure that promotes elimination for a client who cannot flex the hip. Review: the care of the client with a **spica cast**.
Reference(s): Ignatavicius, Workman (2013), p. 1152.

1145. The nurse is caring for a postpartum client with thromboembolytic disease. Which intervention is **most important** to include when planning care to prevent the complication of pulmonary embolism?
1. Enforce bed rest.
2. Monitor the vital signs frequently.
3. Assess the breath sounds frequently.
4. Administer prescribed anticoagulant therapy.

Level of Cognitive Ability: Analyzing
Client Needs: Physiological Integrity
Integrated Process: Nursing Process/Planning
Content Area: Maternity: Postpartum
Priority Concepts: Clotting; Reproduction

Answer: 4
Rationale: The purposes of anticoagulant therapy for the treatment of thromboembolytic disease are to prevent the formation of a clot and to prevent a clot from moving to another area, thus preventing pulmonary embolism. Although options 1, 2, and 3 may be implemented for a client with thromboembolytic disease, option 4 will specifically assist in the prevention of pulmonary embolism.
Priority Nursing Tip: Medications containing aspirin should not be given to clients receiving anticoagulant therapy, because aspirin prolongs the clotting time and increases the risk of bleeding.
Test-Taking Strategy: Note the strategic words, *most important*. Focus on the subject of preventing the complication of pulmonary embolism. Recall that anticoagulant therapy is prescribed to treat thromboembolytic disease. Review: the interventions for the client with **thromboembolytic disease** that will prevent **pulmonary embolism**.
Reference(s): McKinney et al (2013), p. 677.

1146. After reviewing a client's serum electrolyte levels, the provider prescribes an isotonic intravenous (IV) infusion. Which IV solution should the nurse plan to administer?
1. 5% dextrose in water
2. 10% dextrose in water
3. 3% sodium chloride solution
4. 0.45% sodium chloride solution

Level of Cognitive Ability: Understanding
Client Needs: Physiological Integrity
Integrated Process: Nursing Process/Planning
Content Area: Fundamental Skills: Fluids & Electrolytes
Priority Concepts: Clinical Judgment; Fluid and Electrolyte Balance

Answer: 1
Rationale: Five percent dextrose in water is an isotonic solution, which means that the osmolality of this solution matches normal body fluids. Other examples of isotonic fluids include 0.9% sodium chloride solution (normal saline) and lactated Ringer's solution. Ten percent dextrose in water and 3% sodium chloride solution are hypertonic solutions, and 0.45% sodium chloride solution is hypotonic.
Priority Nursing Tip: Isotonic solutions are isotonic to human cells, and thus very little osmosis occurs.
Test-Taking Strategy: To answer this question accurately, focus on the subject of the tonicity of various IV solutions and note the word "isotonic." It is necessary to recall that 5% dextrose in water is an isotonic solution. Review: the tonicity of IV fluids.
Reference(s): Perry, Potter, Ostendorf (2014), p. 694.

1147. The nurse is admitting a client who recently underwent a bilateral adrenalectomy. Which intervention is **essential** for the nurse to include in the client's plan of care?
1. Prevent social isolation.
2. Consider occupational therapy.
3. Discuss changes in body image.
4. Avoid stress-producing situations.

Level of Cognitive Ability: Analyzing
Client Needs: Physiological Integrity
Integrated Process: Nursing Process/Planning
Content Area: Adult Health: Endocrine
Priority Concepts: Clinical Judgment; Stress

Answer: 4
Rationale: Adrenalectomy can lead to adrenal insufficiency. Adrenal hormones are essential to maintaining homeostasis in response to stressors. Options 1, 2, and 3 are not essential interventions specific to this client's problem.
Priority Nursing Tip: Assist a client to identify the source of stress and explore methods to reduce stress.
Test-Taking Strategy: Note the strategic word, *essential*. This indicates the need to prioritize. Remember that, according to Maslow's Hierarchy of Needs theory, physiological needs come first. The stress reaction involves physiological processes. Review: the postoperative effects of an adrenalectomy.
Reference(s): Ignatavicius, Workman (2013), pp. 1387-1388.

1148. A perinatal client is admitted to the obstetric unit during an exacerbation of a heart condition. When planning for the nutritional requirements of the client, about which dietary intervention should the nurse consult with the dietitian?
1. A low-calorie diet to prevent weight gain
2. A diet low in fluids and fiber to decrease blood volume
3. A diet adequate in fluids and fiber to decrease constipation
4. Unlimited sodium intake to increase circulating blood volume

Level of Cognitive Ability: Analyzing
Client Needs: Physiological Integrity
Integrated Process: Nursing Process/Planning
Content Area: Maternity: Antepartum
Priority Concepts: Nutrition; Perfusion

Answer: 3
Rationale: Constipation can cause the client to use Valsalva's maneuver. This maneuver can cause blood to rush to the heart and overload the cardiac system. A low-calorie diet is not recommended during pregnancy. Diets low in fluid and fiber can cause a decrease in blood volume that can deprive the fetus of nutrients; it can also lead to constipation. Therefore, adequate fluid intake and high-fiber foods are important. Sodium should be restricted to some degree as prescribed by the health care provider because this will cause an overload to the circulating blood volume and contribute to cardiac complications.
Priority Nursing Tip: Encourage adequate nutrition for the pregnant client with a cardiac condition to prevent anemia. Anemia could worsen the cardiac status.
Test-Taking Strategy: Focus on the subjects, the physiology of the cardiac system, the maternal and fetal needs, and the factors that increase the workload on the heart to answer the question. Think about what would increase the workload of the heart to direct you to option 3. Review: nursing measures for the pregnant client with cardiac disease.
Reference(s): Lowdermilk, Perry, Cashion, Alden (2012), p. 715.

1149. The nurse is developing a plan of care for a client on bed rest. During the planning, the nurse includes measures to limit the complications of prolonged immobility. Which intervention should the nurse include in the plan?

1. Maintain the client in a supine position.
2. Provide a daily fluid intake of 1000 mL.
3. Limit the intake of milk and milk products.
4. Monitor for signs of a low serum calcium level.

Level of Cognitive Ability: Applying
Client Needs: Physiological Integrity
Integrated Process: Nursing Process/Planning
Content Area: Adult Health: Musculoskeletal
Priority Concepts: Clinical Judgment; Mobility

Answer: **3**
Rationale: The formation of renal and urinary calculi is a complication of immobility. Limiting milk and milk products is the best measure to prevent the formation of calcium stones. A supine position increases urinary stasis; therefore, this position should be limited or avoided. Daily fluid intake should be 2000 mL or more per day. The nurse should monitor for signs and symptoms of hypercalcemia, such as nausea, vomiting, polydipsia, polyuria, and lethargy.
Priority Nursing Tip: The client with calcium oxalate stones may be prescribed to follow a diet decreasing the intake of foods high in calcium and avoiding oxalate food sources. This type of diet will help reduce the urinary oxalate content of urine and stone formation. Oxalate food sources include items such as tea, almonds, cashews, chocolate, cocoa, beans, spinach, and rhubarb.
Test-Taking Strategy: Focus on the subject of the complications of prolonged immobility. Option 1 should be eliminated first because it refers to maintaining an immobile client in one position. Eliminate option 2 next, noting the amount of fluid in this option. From the remaining choices, recalling the effect of the movement of calcium into the blood from the bones will direct you to option 3. Review: the complications of **immobility**.
Reference(s): Ignatavicius, Workman (2013), p. 101; Potter et al (2013), p. 1134.

1150. The nurse determines that a Mantoux tuberculin skin test is positive. Which diagnostic test should the nurse anticipate to be prescribed to accurately diagnose tuberculosis (TB)?

1. Chest x-ray
2. Sputum culture
3. Complete blood cell count
4. Computed tomography scan of the chest

Level of Cognitive Ability: Applying
Client Needs: Physiological Integrity
Integrated Process: Nursing Process/Planning
Content Area: Adult Health: Respiratory
Priority Concepts: Clinical Judgment; Infection

Answer: **2**
Rationale: Although the findings of the chest x-ray examination are important, it is not possible to make a diagnosis of TB solely on the basis of this examination because other diseases can mimic the appearance of TB. The demonstration of tubercle bacilli bacteriologically is essential for establishing a diagnosis. The microscopic examination of sputum for acid-fast bacilli is usually the first bacteriologic evidence of the presence of tubercle bacilli. Options 3 and 4 will not diagnose TB.
Priority Nursing Tip: Tuberculosis (TB) has an insidious onset, and many clients are not aware that the symptoms are associated to TB until the disease is well advanced.
Test-Taking Strategy: Focus on the subject of diagnosing TB. Recalling that the presence of tubercle bacilli indicates TB will direct you to the correct option. Review: the tests used to diagnose **tuberculosis (TB)**.
Reference(s): Ignatavicius, Workman (2013), p. 655.

1151. The home care nurse is preparing a plan of care for a client with Ménière's syndrome who is experiencing severe vertigo. Which nursing intervention should the nurse include in the plan of care to assist the client with controlling the vertigo?

1. Instruct the client to cut down on cigarette smoking.
2. Encourage the client to increase the daily fluid intake.
3. Encourage the client to avoid sudden head movements.
4. Instruct the client to increase the amount of sodium in the diet.

Level of Cognitive Ability: Applying
Client Needs: Physiological Integrity
Integrated Process: Nursing Process/Planning
Content Area: Adult Health: Ear
Priority Concepts: Client Education; Sensory Perception

Answer: 3
Rationale: Ménière's syndrome refers to dilation of the endolymphatic system by overproduction or decreased resorption of endolymphatic fluid. The nurse instructs the client to make slow head movements to prevent worsening of the vertigo. Clients are advised to stop smoking because of its vasoconstrictive effects. Dietary changes such as salt and fluid restrictions that reduce the amount of endolymphatic fluid are sometimes prescribed.
Priority Nursing Tip: Instruct the client experiencing an episode of vertigo to avoid watching television because flickering of lights may exacerbate symptoms.
Test-Taking Strategy: Identify the subject of the question, severe vertigo. Note the relationship between the words *severe vertigo* and the correct option, which recommends the avoidance of sudden head movements. Noting the words *cut down* in option 1 will assist you with eliminating this option. Recalling that salt and fluid restrictions are sometimes prescribed will also assist you with eliminating options 2 and 4. Review: the measures that will reduce **vertigo** in the client with **Ménière's syndrome**.
Reference(s): Ignatavicius, Workman (2013), pp. 1096-1097.

1152. A client is admitted to a mental health unit with a diagnosis of anorexia nervosa. When planning care for this client, which **primary** intervention should health promotion focus on?

1. Providing a supportive environment
2. Examining intrapsychic conflicts and past issues
3. Emphasizing social interaction with clients who are withdrawn
4. Helping the client identify and examine dysfunctional thoughts and beliefs

Level of Cognitive Ability: Applying
Client Needs: Psychosocial Integrity
Integrated Process: Nursing Process/Planning
Content Area: Mental Health
Priority Concepts: Clinical Judgment; Nutrition

Answer: 4
Rationale: Health promotion focuses on helping clients identify and examine dysfunctional thoughts, as well as identifying and examining the values and beliefs that maintain these thoughts. Providing a supportive environment is important, but it is not as primary as option 4 for this client. Examining intrapsychic conflicts and past issues is not directly related to the client's problem. Emphasizing social interaction is not appropriate at this time.
Priority Nursing Tip: Explain treatments and procedures to a client in a quiet and simple manner. Always allow the client the opportunity to express fears.
Test-Taking Strategy: Note the strategic word, *primary*. Focus on the subject of health promotion in a client diagnosed with anorexia nervosa. Option 4 is the only choice that is specifically client centered. This option also focuses on assessment, which is the first step of the nursing process. Review: the care of the client with **anorexia nervosa**.
Reference(s): Fortinash, Holoday-Worret (2012), pp. 427-428; Varcarolis (2013), p. 234.

1153. The nurse is preparing discharge plans for a hospitalized client who attempted suicide. Which intervention should the nurse include in the plan as an **immediate** resource?

1. Scheduling weekly follow-up appointments
2. Establishing contracts with available crisis resources
3. Encouraging family and friends to be with the client at all times
4. Providing phone numbers for the hospital and health care provider

Level of Cognitive Ability: Applying
Client Needs: Psychosocial Integrity
Integrated Process: Nursing Process/Planning
Content Area: Mental Health
Priority Concepts: Mood and Affect; Safety

Answer: 2
Rationale: Crisis times may occur between appointments. Contracts facilitate a client's feeling of responsibility for keeping a promise, which gives him or her control. Providing phone numbers will not ensure available and immediate crisis intervention. Family and friends cannot always be present.
Priority Nursing Tip: Discharge planning and follow-up care are important for the continued well-being of the client with a mental health disorder. Aftercare case managers are used to facilitate the client's adaptation back into the community and provide early referral if the treatment plan is unsuccessful.
Test-Taking Strategy: Focus on the subject, the availability of immediate resources for the client who attempted suicide and the strategic word, *immediate*. Eliminate option 3 first because this is unrealistic. Options 1 and 4 will not necessarily provide immediate resources. Review: the discharge plans for the client who attempted **suicide**.
Reference(s): Fortinash, Holoday-Worret (2012), pp. 513-514; Varcarolis (2013), pp. 442-443.

1154. The nurse is developing a plan of care for a newborn diagnosed with bilateral club feet. Which instruction should the nurse plan to include in the parents education?
1. The regimen of manipulation and casting is effective in all cases of bilateral club feet.
2. Genetic testing is wise for future pregnancies because other children born to this couple may also be affected.
3. If casting is needed, it will begin at birth and continue for 12 weeks, at which time the condition will be reevaluated.
4. Surgery performed immediately after birth has been found to be the most effective for achieving a complete recovery.

Level of Cognitive Ability: Applying
Client Needs: Physiological Integrity
Integrated Process: Nursing Process/Planning
Content Area: Child Health: Musculoskeletal
Priority Concepts: Client Education; Mobility

Answer: 3
Rationale: For the infant with clubfoot, casting should begin at birth and continue for at least 12 weeks or until maximum correction is achieved. At this time, corrective shoes may provide support to maintain alignment, or surgery can be performed. Surgery is usually delayed until the child is 4 to 12 months old. Options 1 and 4 are inaccurate. Option 2 does not specifically address the subject of the question.
Priority Nursing Tip: The nurse needs to monitor the child with a cast or brace for signs of neurovascular impairment. If signs occur, the health care provider is notified immediately.
Test-Taking Strategy: Focus on the subject, parent instructions for the child with bilateral club feet. Eliminate option 2 because it does not specifically address the subject of the question, and it relates to the future. Eliminate option 4 because of the word *immediately.* From the remaining choices, note that option 3 provides accurate information and that option 1 contains the closed-ended word "all." Review: the treatment plan for bilateral club feet.
Reference(s): Hockenberry, Wilson (2013), pp. 1071-1072.

1155. The nurse is planning to assist with obtaining a set of arterial blood gas measurements for a client. Which items should the nurse plan to provide to optimally maintain the integrity of the specimen?
1. A syringe that contains a preservative
2. A heparinized syringe and a bag of ice
3. A heparinized syringe and a preservative
4. A syringe that contains a preservative and a bag of ice

Level of Cognitive Ability: Applying
Client Needs: Physiological Integrity
Integrated Process: Nursing Process/Planning
Content Area: Fundamental Skills: Laboratory Values
Priority Concepts: Clinical Judgment; Acid-Base Balance

Answer: 2
Rationale: The arterial blood gas sample is obtained using a heparinized syringe. The sample of blood is placed on ice and sent to the laboratory immediately. A preservative is not used.
Priority Nursing Tip: Assist with the specimen draw for an arterial blood gas by preparing a heparinized syringe (if one is not already prepackaged); otherwise the blood may clot.
Test-Taking Strategy: Focus on the subject of arterial blood gas measurements; specific knowledge regarding this procedure is needed to answer this question. Remember that an arterial blood gas sample is obtained using a heparinized syringe, is placed on ice, and sent to the laboratory immediately. Review: arterial blood gas measurement.
Reference(s): Pagana, Pagana (2013), p. 117.

1156. A client is experiencing diabetes insipidus as a result of cranial surgery. Which of these anticipated therapies should the nurse who is caring for the client plan to implement?
1. Fluid restriction
2. Administering diuretics
3. Increased sodium intake
4. Intravenous (IV) replacement of fluid losses

Level of Cognitive Ability: Analyzing
Client Needs: Physiological Integrity
Integrated Process: Nursing Process/Planning
Content Area: Adult Health: Neurological
Priority Concepts: Clinical Judgment; Fluid and Electrolyte Balance

Answer: 4
Rationale: The client with diabetes insipidus excretes large amounts of extremely dilute urine. This usually occurs as a result of decreased synthesis or the release of antidiuretic hormone in clients with conditions such as head injury, surgery near the hypothalamus, or increased intracranial pressure. Corrective measures include allowing ample oral fluid intake, administering IV fluid as needed to replace sensible and insensible losses, and administering vasopressin (Pitressin). Diuretics are not administered. Sodium is not administered because the serum sodium level is usually high, as is the serum osmolality.
Priority Nursing Tip: For the client with diabetes insipidus, monitor electrolyte values and monitor for signs of dehydration, and maintain an adequate intake of fluids.
Test-Taking Strategy: Focus on the subject, diabetes insipidus as a result of cranial surgery, and recall that a large fluid loss is the problem in this client. This will assist you with eliminating options 1 and 2. From the remaining choices, recalling that the serum sodium level is already elevated in clients with this disorder or knowing that fluid replacement is the most direct form of therapy for fluid loss will direct you to option 4. Review: the treatment for **diabetes insipidus**.
Reference(s): Ignatavicius, Workman (2013), pp. 1031, 1378-1379.

1157. The nurse is caring for a client diagnosed with dementia who has needs related to nutrition. Which appropriate goal should the nurse plan for with this client?
1. Client will be free of hallucinations.
2. Client will feed self with cueing within 24 hours.
3. Client will be oriented to place by the time of discharge.
4. Client will correctly identify objects in his or her room by the time of discharge.

Level of Cognitive Ability: Applying
Client Needs: Physiological Integrity
Integrated Process: Nursing Process/Planning
Content Area: Mental Health
Priority Concepts: Cognition; Nutrition

Answer: 2
Rationale: Option 2 identifies a goal that is directly related to the client's ability to care for himself or herself. Options 1, 3, and 4 are not related to the client's needs.
Priority Nursing Tip: In dementia, long-term and short-term memory loss occurs, with impairment in judgment, abstract thinking, problem solving, and behavior.
Test-Taking Strategy: Focus on the subject, needs of a client with dementia. Option 2 is the only option that addresses a physiological need. In addition, on the basis of Maslow's Hierarchy of Needs theory, physiological needs take precedence. This will direct you to the correct option. Review: the goals for a client with **nutritional needs** who has **dementia**.
Reference(s): Potter et al (2013), pp. 1239, 1249-1250.

1158. The nurse is preparing to care for an infant diagnosed with pertussis. Which **priority** problem should the nurse address when planning care?
1. Infection
2. Fluid overload
3. Inability to sleep
4. Inability to expectorate secretions

Level of Cognitive Ability: Analyzing
Client Needs: Physiological Integrity
Integrated Process: Nursing Process/Planning
Content Area: Child Health: Throat/Respiratory
Priority Concepts: Clinical Judgment; Gas Exchange

Answer: 4
Rationale: The priority problem for the child with pertussis relates to adequate air exchange. Because of the copious, thick secretions that occur with pertussis and the small airways of an infant, air exchange is critical. Infection is an important consideration, but airway is the priority. A deficient fluid volume is more likely to occur in this infant because of the thick secretions and vomiting. Sleep patterns may be disturbed because of the coughing, but this is not the critical issue.
Priority Nursing Tip: For the client with a respiratory problem, reduce environmental factors that cause coughing spasms, such as dust, smoke, and sudden changes in temperature.
Test-Taking Strategy: Use the ABCs—airway, breathing, and circulation—and note the strategic word, priority. Airway is always the priority. This should direct you to the correct option. Review: the care of the infant with **pertussis**.
Reference(s): McKinney et al (2013), pp. 1024-1025.

1159. The nurse is planning care for an infant who has a diagnosis of hypertrophic pyloric stenosis and is scheduled for surgery. Which intervention should the nurse include into the plan of care to meet the infant's preoperative needs?

1. Administer enemas until returns are clear.
2. Provide the mother privacy to breast-feed every 2 hours.
3. Monitor the intravenous (IV) infusion, intake, output, and weight.
4. Provide small, frequent feedings of glucose, water, and electrolytes.

Level of Cognitive Ability: Analyzing
Client Needs: Physiological Integrity
Integrated Process: Nursing Process/Planning
Content Area: Child Health: Gastrointestinal
Priority Concepts: Clinical Judgment; Safety

Answer: 3
Rationale: Preoperatively, important nursing responsibilities for the child with hypertrophic pyloric stenosis include monitoring the IV infusion, intake, output, and weight and obtaining urine specific gravity measurements. Additionally, weighing the infant's diapers provides information regarding output. Enemas until clear would further compromise the fluid volume status. Preoperatively, the infant receives nothing by mouth unless otherwise prescribed by the health care provider.
Priority Nursing Tip: When preparing the infant with hypertrophic pyloric stenosis for surgery, monitor intake and output, the number and character of stools, and patency of the nasogastric tube used for stomach decompression.
Test-Taking Strategy: Focus on the subject of preoperative care of a child with pyloric stenosis. Eliminate options 2 and 4 because the infant needs to receive nothing by mouth during the preoperative period. Eliminate option 1 because enemas would further compromise the fluid balance status. Review: the preoperative care of the infant with pyloric stenosis.
Reference(s): McKinney et al (2013), pp. 1095-1096.

1160. A client who was a victim of a gunshot incident states, "I feel like I am losing my mind. I keep hearing the gunshots and seeing my friend lying on the ground." Which strategy should the nurse include when **initially** formulating a therapeutic relationship?

1. Teaching the client a variety of relaxation techniques
2. Asking the psychiatrist to prescribe appropriate medication
3. Encouraging the client to talk about the incident and feelings related to it
4. Encouraging the client to think about just how lucky he or she is to still be alive

Level of Cognitive Ability: Analyzing
Client Needs: Psychosocial Integrity
Integrated Process: Nursing Process/Planning
Content Area: Mental Health
Priority Concepts: Clinical Judgment; Communication

Answer: 3
Rationale: When developing a therapeutic relationship, it is important to acknowledge and validate the client's feelings. Although teaching the client relaxation techniques may be helpful at some point, it is not related to the subject of the question. Options 2 and 4 are nontherapeutic techniques, and they do not promote a therapeutic relationship.
Priority Nursing Tip: The nurse should always encourage the client to express thoughts and feelings as they address identified areas of concern.
Test-Taking Strategy: Focus on the subject initiating a therapeutic relationship with a gunshot victim, and note the strategic word, *initially*. Eliminate options 2 and 4 because they do not encourage further discussion about the client's feelings. Teaching the client how to relax may be helpful at some point, but not at the beginning of the therapeutic relationship. Remember to address the client's feelings. Review: therapeutic communication techniques.
Reference(s): Stuart (2013), pp. 25-29.

1161. The nurse is caring for a hospitalized child with a diagnosis of rheumatic fever who has developed carditis. The mother asks the nurse to explain the meaning of carditis. On which description of this complication of rheumatic fever should the nurse base her response?

1. Involuntary movements affecting the legs, arms, and face
2. Inflammation of all parts of the heart, primarily the mitral valve
3. Tender, painful joints, especially in the elbows, knees, ankles, and wrists
4. Red skin lesions that start as flat or slightly raised macules, usually over the trunk, and that spread peripherally

Level of Cognitive Ability: Analyzing
Client Needs: Physiological Integrity
Integrated Process: Nursing Process/Planning
Content Area: Child Health: Cardiovascular
Priority Concepts: Client Education; Inflammation

Answer: 2
Rationale: Carditis is the inflammation of all parts of the heart, primarily the mitral valve, and it is a complication of rheumatic fever. Option 1 describes chorea. Option 3 describes polyarthritis. Option 4 describes erythema marginatum.
Priority Nursing Tip: Initiate seizure precautions if a child with rheumatic fever is experiencing chorea.
Test-Taking Strategy: Focus on the subject of the complications of rheumatic fever–induced carditis. Note the relationship between the word "carditis" in the question and "heart" in the correct option. Review: the characteristics of **rheumatic fever** and **carditis**.
Reference(s): McKinney et al (2013), pp. 1229-1230.

1162. The nurse receives a telephone call from the emergency department and is told that a 7-month-old infant with febrile seizures will be admitted to the pediatric unit. What should the nurse anticipate the need for when planning care for the admission of the infant?

1. Restraints at the bedside
2. A code cart at the bedside
3. Suction equipment and an airway at the bedside
4. A padded tongue blade taped to the head of the bed

Level of Cognitive Ability: Applying
Client Needs: Physiological Integrity
Integrated Process: Nursing Process/Planning
Content Area: Child Health: Neurological
Priority Concepts: Intracranial Regulation: Safety

Answer: 3
Rationale: Suctioning may be required during a seizure to remove secretions that obstruct the airway. An airway should also be readily available. During a seizure, the infant should be placed in a side-lying position, but he or she should not be restrained. It is not necessary to place a code cart at the bedside, but a cart should be readily available on the nursing unit. A padded tongue blade should never be used; in fact, nothing should be placed in the mouth during a seizure.
Priority Nursing Tip: If a child experiences a seizure, lower the child to the floor and protect the child's head from injury.
Test-Taking Strategy: Use the ABCs—airway, breathing, and circulation—to answer the question. Option 3 is the only choice that specifically relates to the airway. Review: nursing interventions for an infant with seizures.
Reference(s): Hockenberry, Wilson (2013), pp. 963-964.

1163. A 10-month-old infant is hospitalized for respiratory syncytial virus (RSV). The nurse develops a plan of care for the infant. On the basis of the developmental stage of the infant, what should the nurse include in the plan of care?
1. Restrain the infant with a total body restraint to prevent any tubes from being dislodged.
2. Follow the home feeding schedule, and allow the infant to be held only when the parents visit.
3. Wash hands, wear a mask when caring for the infant, and keep the infant as quiet as possible.
4. Provide a consistent routine, and touch, rock, and cuddle the infant throughout the hospitalization.

Level of Cognitive Ability: Applying
Client Needs: Physiological Integrity
Integrated Process: Nursing Process/Planning
Content Area: Developmental Stages: Infancy to Adolescence
Priority Concepts: Development; Health Promotion

Answer: 4
Rationale: A 10-month-old infant is in the trust versus mistrust stage of psychosocial development, according to Erik Erikson, and the sensorimotor period of cognitive development, according to Jean Piaget. Hospitalization may have an adverse effect. A consistent routine accompanied by touching, rocking, and cuddling will help the child develop trust and provide sensory stimulation. Total body restraint is unnecessary and an incorrect action. Touching and holding the infant only when the parents visit will not provide adequate stimulation and interpersonal contact for the infant. RSV is not airborne (a mask is not required), and it is usually transmitted by the hands.
Priority Nursing Tip: According to Erikson's theory of psychosocial development, each psychosocial crisis must be resolved for the child or adult to progress emotionally. Unsuccessful resolution can leave the person emotionally disabled.
Test-Taking Strategy: Focus on the subject, a 10-month-old infant who is hospitalized with RSV and appropriate interventions based on the child's developmental state. Note the age and diagnosis of the infant. Eliminate options 1 and 2 because of the closed-ended words "total" and "only," respectively. Review: respiratory syncytial virus (RSV) and the developmental stages.
Reference(s): McKinney et al (2013), p. 1167.

1164. A pediatric nurse is informed that a child with a diagnosis of Reye's syndrome is being admitted to the hospital. The nurse develops a plan of care for the child that includes which **priority** nursing action?
1. Monitoring for hearing loss
2. Monitoring intake and output (I&O)
3. Repositioning the child every 2 hours
4. Providing a quiet environment with dimmed lighting

Level of Cognitive Ability: Analyzing
Client Needs: Physiological Integrity
Integrated Process: Nursing Process/Planning
Content Area: Child Health: Neurological
Priority Concepts: Intracranial Regulation; Safety

Answer: 4
Rationale: Cerebral edema is a progressive part of the disease process of Reye's syndrome. A priority component of care for a child with Reye's syndrome is maintaining effective cerebral perfusion and controlling intracranial pressure. Decreasing stimuli in the environment would decrease the stress on the cerebral tissue, as well as neuron responses. Hearing loss does not occur in clients with this disorder. Although monitoring I&O may be a component of the plan, it is not the priority nursing action. Changing the body position every 2 hours would not affect the cerebral edema and intracranial pressure directly. The child should be in a head-elevated position to decrease the progression of cerebral edema and promote the drainage of cerebrospinal fluid.
Priority Nursing Tip: The nurse needs to assess the neurological status of a child with Reye's syndrome. Signs of neurological deterioration need to be reported immediately.
Test-Taking Strategy: Note the strategic word, priority. Recalling that increased intracranial pressure is a concern for the child with Reye's syndrome will direct you to option 4. Review: the plan of care for the child with Reye's syndrome.
Reference(s): Hockenberry, Wilson (2013), p. 956; McKinney et al (2013), p. 1444.

1165. A nursing student is preparing to conduct a clinical conference regarding cerebral palsy. Which characteristic related to this disorder should the student plan to include in the discussion?

1. Cerebral palsy is an infectious disease of the central nervous system.
2. Cerebral palsy is an inflammation of the brain as a result of a viral illness.
3. Cerebral palsy is a chronic disability characterized by difficulty with muscle control.
4. Cerebral palsy is a congenital condition that results in moderate to severe retardation.

Level of Cognitive Ability: Applying
Client Needs: Physiological Integrity
Integrated Process: Nursing Process/Planning
Content Area: Child Health: Musculoskeletal
Priority Concepts: Functional Ability; Mobility

Answer: 3
Rationale: Cerebral palsy is a chronic disability that is characterized by difficulty with controlling the muscles because of an abnormality in the extrapyramidal or pyramidal motor system. Meningitis is an infectious process of the central nervous system. Encephalitis is an inflammation of the brain that occurs as a result of viral illness or central nervous system infections. Down syndrome is an example of a congenital condition that results in moderate to severe retardation.
Priority Nursing Tip: Provide the parents of a child with cerebral palsy with information about the disorder, treatment plan, and support services, including support groups.
Test-Taking Strategy: Eliminate options 1 and 2 first because they are comparable or alike. From the remaining choices, note the relationship between "palsy" in the question and "muscles" in the correct option. Review: the characteristics associated with cerebral palsy.
Reference(s): Hockenberry, Wilson (2013), pp. 1095-1096.

1166. A nursing student is asked to conduct a clinical conference about autism. Which characteristic associated with autism should the student plan to include?

1. Normal social play that ceases by age 5
2. Lack of social interaction and awareness
3. The consistent imitation of others' actions
4. Normal verbal but abnormal nonverbal communication

Level of Cognitive Ability: Applying
Client Needs: Psychosocial Integrity
Integrated Process: Nursing Process/Planning
Content Area: Child Health: Neurological
Priority Concepts: Functional Ability; Mood and Affect

Answer: 2
Rationale: Autism is a severe developmental disorder that begins in infancy or toddlerhood. A primary characteristic is a lack of social interaction and awareness. Social behaviors in children with autism include a lack of or abnormal imitations of others' actions and a lack of or abnormal social play. Additional characteristics include a lack of or impaired verbal communication and marked abnormal nonverbal communication.
Priority Nursing Tip: For the child with autism, determine the child's routines, habits, and preferences and maintain consistency as much as possible. Provide support to parents.
Test-Taking Strategy: Focus on the subject of characteristics of autism. It is necessary to recall that the primary characteristic is a lack of social interaction and awareness. Review: the characteristics associated with autism.
Reference(s): Hockenberry, Wilson (2013), pp. 590-591.

❖ **1167.** A charge nurse reviews the postoperative plan of care formulated for a child after a tonsillectomy. Which interventions are appropriate for this client? **Select all that apply.**
❑ 1. Offer clear, cool liquids when awake.
❑ 2. Administer pain medication as prescribed
❑ 3. Monitor for bleeding from the surgical site.
❑ 4. Suction every 15 minutes and PRN as necessary.
❑ 5. Initially eliminate milk or milk products from the diet.

Level of Cognitive Ability: Applying
Client Needs: Physiological Integrity
Integrated Process: Nursing Process/Planning
Content Area: Child Health: Throat/Respiratory
Priority Concepts: Clinical Judgment; Safety

Answer: 1, 2, 3, 5
Rationale: After tonsillectomy, clear, cool liquids are encouraged. Options 2 and 3 are important interventions after any type of surgery. Suction equipment should be available, but suctioning is not performed unless there is an airway obstruction. Milk and milk products are avoided initially because they coat the throat; this causes the child to clear the throat, thereby increasing the risk of bleeding.
Priority Nursing Tip: After tonsillectomy, suction equipment should be available, but suctioning is not done unless there is airway obstruction because it will disrupt the integrity of the surgical site and cause bleeding.
Test-Taking Strategy: Focus on the subject of post-tonsillectomy interventions. Think about the location and complications of this procedure to answer correctly. Review: postoperative care for tonsillectomy.
Reference(s): McKinney et al (2013), p. 1157.

1168. The school nurse is preparing to perform health screening for scoliosis on children ages 9 through 14. Which instruction should the nurse plan to provide to the child?

1. Lie flat and lift the legs straight up.
2. Lie on the right side and then roll to the left side while the arms are held overhead.
3. Walk 10 feet forward and then 10 feet backward with the arms held overhead at both sides.
4. Stand with weight equally on both feet with the legs straight, and the arms hanging loosely at both sides.

Level of Cognitive Ability: Applying
Client Needs: Health Promotion and Maintenance
Integrated Process: Nursing Process/Planning
Content Area: Developmental Stages: Health Assessment/Physical Exam
Priority Concepts: Health Promotion; Mobility

Answer: 4
Rationale: To perform this screening test, the child should be asked to disrobe or wear underpants only so that the chest, back, and hips can be clearly seen. The child is asked to stand with weight equally on both feet with the legs straight and the arms hanging loosely at both sides. The nurse assesses the child's posture, spinal column, shoulder height, and leg lengths. Lying down positions and walking forward and backward are incorrect assessment techniques.
Priority Nursing Tip: A complication after surgical treatment of scoliosis is superior mesenteric artery syndrome. This disorder is caused by mechanical changes in the position of the child's abdominal contents that occurs during surgery.
Test-Taking Strategy: Focus on the subject, plan of care for scoliosis screening procedure. Recall the anatomical location of this disorder and then visualize the screening procedure and the preparation required to adequately assess for this disorder. Review: screening procedure for scoliosis.
Reference(s): Hockenberry, Wilson (2013), p. 1077.

1169. The nurse is preparing a plan of care for a child diagnosed with leukemia who is scheduled to receive chemotherapy. Which intervention should the nurse include in the plan of care?

1. Monitor rectal temperatures every 4 hours.
2. Monitor the mouth and anus each shift for signs of breakdown.
3. Encourage the child to consume fresh fruits and vegetables to maintain nutritional status.
4. Provide meticulous mouth care several times daily using an alcohol-based mouthwash and a toothbrush.

Level of Cognitive Ability: Analyzing
Client Needs: Physiological Integrity
Integrated Process: Nursing Process/Planning
Content Area: Child Health: Oncological
Priority Concepts: Cellular Regulation; Infection

Answer: 2
Rationale: When the child is receiving chemotherapy, the nurse should assess the mouth and anus each shift for ulcers, erythema, or breakdown. The nurse should avoid taking rectal temperatures. Oral temperatures are also avoided if mouth ulcers are present. Axillary or temporal temperatures should be taken to prevent alterations in skin integrity. Bland, nonirritating foods and liquids should be provided to the child. Fresh fruits and vegetables need to be avoided because they can harbor organisms. Chemotherapy can cause neutropenia, and the child should be maintained on a low-bacteria diet if the white blood cell count is low. Meticulous mouth care should be performed, but the nurse should avoid alcohol-based mouthwashes and should use a soft-bristled toothbrush.
Priority Nursing Tip: Chemotherapy can cause life-threatening neutropenia and thrombocytopenia.
Test-Taking Strategy: Focus on the subject, interventions for the child receiving chemotherapy. Think about the adverse effects that can occur with chemotherapy to assist in answering correctly. Remember that life-threatening neutropenia and thrombocytopenia can occur. Review: the care of the child receiving chemotherapy.
Reference(s): McKinney et al (2013), p. 1279.

1170. The nurse is preparing to admit a client from the postanesthesia care unit who has had microvascular decompression of the trigeminal nerve. Which equipment should the nurse ask the unlicensed assistive personnel to make sure is at the bedside when the client arrives?

1. Flashlight and pulse oximeter
2. Cardiac monitor and suction equipment
3. Padded bed rails and suction equipment
4. Blood pressure cuff and cardiac monitor

Level of Cognitive Ability: Applying
Client Needs: Physiological Integrity
Integrated Process: Nursing Process/Planning
Content Area: Adult Health: Neurological
Priority Concepts: Clinical Judgment; Intracranial Regulation

Answer: 1
Rationale: The postoperative care of the client having microvascular decompression of the trigeminal nerve is the same as for the client undergoing craniotomy. This client requires hourly neurological assessment as well as monitoring of the cardiovascular and respiratory statuses. Therefore, a flashlight and pulse oximetry are necessary items. Cardiac monitoring and padded bed rails are not indicated unless there is a special need based on a client history of cardiac disease or seizures, respectively. Suctioning is performed cautiously and only when necessary after craniotomy to avoid increasing the intracranial pressure.
Priority Nursing Tip: After surgery for microvascular decompression of the trigeminal nerve, the client's pain is compared with the preoperative pain level.
Test-Taking Strategy: Focus on the subject of required assessments and the necessary equipment for a client who just had microvascular decompression of the trigeminal nerve. The client is not necessarily at risk for seizures postoperatively, so option 3 is eliminated first. Eliminate options 2 and 4 next because no data in the question indicate that the client had a history of a cardiac problem. In addition, knowing that the procedure is performed via craniotomy enables you to recall that suctioning is done cautiously and only when necessary and also that neurological assessment is needed, so a flashlight would be required to perform a neurological assessment. Review: the care of the client after **microvascular decompression of the trigeminal nerve.**
Reference(s): Ignatavicius, Workman (2013), p. 1001; Potter et al (2013), pp. 476, 478-479, 555.

1171. The nurse is receiving a client from the emergency department who has a diagnosis of Guillain-Barré syndrome. The client's chief complaint is an ascending paralysis that has reached the level of the waist. Which items should the nurse plan to have available for emergency use?

1. Nebulizer and pulse oximeter
2. Blood pressure cuff and flashlight
3. Flashlight and incentive spirometer
4. Cardiac monitor and intubation tray

Level of Cognitive Ability: Applying
Client Needs: Physiological Integrity
Integrated Process: Nursing Process/Planning
Content Area: Adult Health: Neurological
Priority Concepts: Gas Exchange; Mobility

Answer: 4
Rationale: The client with Guillain-Barré syndrome is at risk for respiratory failure as a result of ascending paralysis. An intubation tray should be available for emergency use. Another complication of this syndrome is cardiac dysrhythmias, which necessitates the need for cardiac monitoring. Although some of the items in options 1, 2, and 3 may be kept at the bedside (e.g., pulse oximeter, blood pressure cuff, flashlight), they are not necessarily needed for emergency use in this situation.
Priority Nursing Tip: Monitor respiratory and cardiac status closely and prepare to initiate respiratory support for the client with Guillain-Barré syndrome.
Test-Taking Strategy: Focus on the subject, equipment needed for possible emergency use in a client with Guillain-Barré syndrome that is experiencing ascending paralysis. These words tell you that the correct answer will be an option that contains equipment that is not routinely used to provide care. With this in mind, eliminate options 2 and 3 first because a flashlight is needed for routine neurological assessment. From the remaining choices, recalling the complications of this syndrome will direct you to the correct option. Review: the nursing care measures for the client with **Guillain-Barré syndrome.**
Reference(s): Ignatavicius, Workman (2013), pp. 989-990.

1172. The nurse in the newborn nursery is informed that a newborn infant whose mother is Rh negative will be admitted to the nursery. When planning care for the infant's arrival, which action should the nurse take?

1. Obtain the newborn infant's blood type and direct Coombs' results from the laboratory.
2. Obtain the necessary equipment from the blood bank needed for an exchange transfusion.
3. Call the maintenance department and ask for a phototherapy unit to be brought to the nursery.
4. Obtain a vial of vitamin K from the pharmacy and prepare to administer an injection to prevent isoimmunization.

Level of Cognitive Ability: Applying
Client Needs: Physiological Integrity
Integrated Process: Nursing Process/Planning
Content Area: Maternity: Newborn
Priority Concepts: Clinical Judgment; Perfusion

Answer: 1
Rationale: To further plan for the newborn infant's care, the infant's blood type and direct Coombs' results must be known. Umbilical cord blood is taken at the time of delivery to determine blood type, Rh factor, and antibody titer (direct Coombs' test) of the newborn infant. The nurse should obtain these results from the laboratory. Options 2 and 3 are inappropriate at this time, and additional data are needed to determine whether these actions are needed. Option 4 is incorrect because vitamin K is given to prevent hemorrhagic disease of the newborn infant.
Priority Nursing Tip: For the infant with erythroblastosis fetalis, the newborn's blood is replaced with Rh-negative blood to stop the destruction of the newborn's red blood cells; the Rh-negative blood is replaced with the newborn's own blood gradually.
Test-Taking Strategy: Focus on the subject, the mother being Rh negative. Note the relationship between the subject of the question and option 1. In addition, note that option 1 is the only option that addresses assessment. Review: **Rh incompatibilities.**
Reference(s): Hockenberry, Wilson (2013), pp. 869-870.

1173. The nurse is preparing to assist to administer a chemotherapeutic agent via intraperitoneal (IP) therapy. In which position should the nurse plan to place the client before administering this therapy?

1. Supine
2. Semi-Fowler's
3. Trendelenburg's
4. Dorsal recumbent

Level of Cognitive Ability: Applying
Client Needs: Physiological Integrity
Integrated Process: Nursing Process/Planning
Content Area: Adult Health: Oncological Medications
Priority Concepts: Clinical Judgment; Safety

Answer: 2
Rationale: IP therapy is the administration of chemotherapeutic agents into the peritoneal cavity. This therapy is used for intraabdominal malignancies such as ovarian and gastrointestinal tumors that have moved into the peritoneum after surgery. The client should be placed in a semi-Fowler's position for this infusion because the client may experience nausea and vomiting caused by increasing pressure on the internal organs. Additionally, this treatment may also place pressure on the diaphragm. The positions indicated in options 1, 3, and 4 would increase pressure in the peritoneal cavity.
Priority Nursing Tip: Malignancies of the abdomen may be treated with the instillation of chemotherapeutic agents into the peritoneal cavity or with external radiation.
Test-Taking Strategy: Focus on the subject, care of the client receiving IP therapy. Recalling that this therapy can increase intraabdominal pressure and cause nausea and vomiting will assist you in eliminating options 1, 3, and 4. Review: care of the client receiving **chemotherapy.**
Reference(s): Ignatavicius, Workman (2013), p. 236; Potter et al (2013), pp. 572, 794.

1174. A client who initially denied abusing alcohol is being discharged from the mental health unit. The client now states that he will "get some help" to live a healthier lifestyle. For which support group should the nurse provide the client with information?

1. Al-Anon
2. Fresh Start
3. Families Anonymous
4. Alcoholics Anonymous

Level of Cognitive Ability: Understanding
Client Needs: Safe and Effective Care Environment
Integrated Process: Nursing Process/Planning
Content Area: Mental Health
Priority Concepts: Addiction; Health Promotion

Answer: 4
Rationale: Alcoholics Anonymous is a major self-help organization for the treatment of alcoholism. Option 1 is a group for families of alcoholics. Option 2 is for nicotine addicts. Option 3 is for the parents of children who abuse substances.
Priority Nursing Tip: As part of the assessment of a client who abuses alcohol, the nurse should ask about the type of alcohol used, how much is consumed, and for how many years.
Test-Taking Strategy: Focus on the subject, resources for a client who is personally dealing with alcohol abuse. Note the relationship of this subject and option 4. Review: Alcoholics Anonymous.
Reference(s): Fortinash, Holoday-Worret (2012), pp. 354-355; Varcarolis (2013), p. 379.

1175. A client with a stroke is prepared for discharge from the hospital. The health care provider has prescribed range-of-motion (ROM) exercises for the client's right side. Which intervention should the home care nurse's plan include when planning for the client's care?

1. Implements ROM exercises to the point of pain for the client
2. Considers the use of active, passive, or active-assisted exercises in the home
3. Encourages the client to be dependent on the home care nurse to complete the exercise program
4. Develops a schedule that involves ROM exercises every 2 hours while awake, even if the client is fatigued

Level of Cognitive Ability: Applying
Client Needs: Physiological Integrity
Integrated Process: Nursing Process/Planning
Content Area: Adult Health: Neurological
Priority Concepts: Clinical Judgment; Mobility

Answer: 2
Rationale: The home care nurse must consider all forms of ROM for the client. Even if the client has right hemiplegia, the client can assist with some of his or her own rehabilitative care. In addition, the goal of home care nursing is for the client to assume as much self-care and independence as possible. The nurse needs to teach so that the client becomes self-reliant. Options 1 and 4 are incorrect from a physiological standpoint.
Priority Nursing Tip: The nurse should assist the client who had a stroke establish a balanced exercise and rest program.
Test-Taking Strategy: Focus on the subject, appropriate implementation of ROM exercise. Options 1 and 4 can be eliminated first because these actions may be harmful to the client. From the remaining choices, recall that dependency is not in the best interest of a client's sense of health promotion, which will help you eliminate option 3. In addition, note that option 2 is the umbrella option. Review: basic knowledge related to range-of-motion (ROM).
Reference(s): Ignatavicius, Workman (2013), pp. 1111-1112; Potter et al (2013), pp. 1149, 1158.

Implementation

1176. A client diagnosed with heart failure is receiving furosemide (Lasix) and digoxin (Lanoxin) daily. When the nurse enters the room to administer the morning doses, the client complains of anorexia, nausea, and yellow vision. Which intervention should the nurse take **first**?
1. Administer the medications.
2. Contact the health care provider.
3. Check the morning serum digoxin level.
4. Check the morning serum potassium level.

Level of Cognitive Ability: Applying
Client Needs: Physiological Integrity
Integrated Process: Nursing Process/Implementation
Content Area: Pharmacology: Cardiovascular Medications
Priority Concepts: Clinical Judgment; Safety

Answer: 3
Rationale: The nurse should check the result of the digoxin level that was drawn because the client's symptoms are compatible with digoxin toxicity. A low potassium level may contribute to digoxin toxicity, so checking the serum potassium level may give useful additional information, but the digoxin level should be checked first. The medications should be withheld until both levels are known. If the digoxin level is elevated or the potassium level is not within the normal range, then the health care provider should be notified. If the morning digoxin level is within the therapeutic range, then the client's complaints are unrelated to the digoxin.
Priority Nursing Tip: The nurse must count the apical heart rate for 1 full minute in a client who is receiving digoxin (Lanoxin). If the rate is less than 60 beats per minute, the medication is withheld and further investigation is done, because this finding could indicate digoxin toxicity.
Test-Taking Strategy: Note the strategic word, *first*. This will assist you with determining that the nurse's action is to further investigate the cause of the client's complaints. Recalling the manifestations of digoxin toxicity and noting the relationship of the name of the medication and option 3 will direct you to the correct option. Review: the nursing interventions if **digoxin (Lanoxin)** toxicity is suspected.
Reference(s): Hodgson, Kizior (2014), p. 353.

1177. The nurse is checking the fundus of a postpartum woman and notes that the uterus is soft and spongy. Which nursing action is appropriate **initially**?
1. Notify the health care provider.
2. Encourage the mother to ambulate.
3. Massage the fundus gently until it is firm.
4. Document fundal position, consistency, and height.

Level of Cognitive Ability: Applying
Client Needs: Physiological Integrity
Integrated Process: Nursing Process/Implementation
Content Area: Maternity: Postpartum
Priority Concepts: Clinical Judgment; Reproduction

Answer: 3
Rationale: If the fundus is boggy (soft), it should be massaged gently until it is firm and the client is observed for increased bleeding or clots. Option 2 is an inappropriate action at this time. The nurse should document the fundal position, consistency, and height; the need to perform fundal massage; and the client's response to the intervention. The health care provider will need to be notified if uterine massage is not helpful.
Priority Nursing Tip: The nurse needs to gently massage the fundus of a client experiencing uterine atony and take care not to overmassage.
Test-Taking Strategy: Note the strategic word, *initially*. Note the relationship of the data in the question (soft and spongy) and the data in the correct option (massage the fundus gently until it is firm). Review: the nursing interventions related to **uterine atony.**
Reference(s): McKinney et al (2013), p. 668.

1178. A primipara is being evaluated in the clinic during her second trimester of pregnancy. The nurse checks the fetal heart rate (FHR) and notes that it is 190 beats/min. What is the appropriate **initial** nursing action?
1. Document the finding.
2. Tell the client that the FHR is fast.
3. Consult with the health care provider.
4. Recheck the FHR with the client in the standing position.

Level of Cognitive Ability: Applying
Client Needs: Physiological Integrity
Integrated Process: Nursing Process/Implementation
Content Area: Maternity: Antepartum
Priority Concepts: Clinical Judgment; Perfusion

Answer: 3
Rationale: The FHR should be between 120 and 160 beats/min. In this situation, the FHR is elevated from the normal range, and the nurse should consult with the health care provider. The FHR would be documented, but option 3 is the appropriate action. The nurse would not tell the client that the FHR is fast at this point in time. Option 4 is an inappropriate action.
Priority Nursing Tip: The normal fetal heart rate is 160 to 170 beats/min in the first trimester, but slows with fetal growth to 120 to 160 beats/min near or at term. The health care provider must be notified if the fetal heart rate is outside these parameters.
Test-Taking Strategy: Focus on the subject, a fetal heart rate (FHR) of 190 beats/min as well the strategic word, *initial*. Recalling that the normal FHR is between 120 and 160 beats/min will direct you to option 3. Review: the **normal FHR.**
Reference(s): McKinney et al (2013), p. 251.

1179. A client tells the clinic nurse that her skin is very dry and irritated. Which product should the nurse suggest that the client apply to the dry skin?
1. Myoflex
2. Aspercreme
3. Topical emollient
4. Acetic acid solution

Level of Cognitive Ability: Applying
Client Needs: Health Promotion and Maintenance
Integrated Process: Nursing Process/Implementation
Content Area: Adult Health: Integumentary
Priority Concepts: Client Education; Tissue Integrity

Answer: 3
Rationale: A topical emollient is used for dry, cracked, and irritated skin. Aspercreme and Myoflex are used to treat muscular aches. Acetic acid solution is used for irrigating, cleansing, and packing wounds infected with *Pseudomonas aeruginosa*.
Priority Nursing Tip: To sustain the hydrating effect, it is best to apply cream or ointment emollients (moisturizers) after bathing.
Test-Taking Strategy: Focus on the subject, treatment for dry and irritated skin. Note the relationship of the subject and the word *emollient* in option 3. Review: treatment for **dry and irritated skin.**
Reference(s): Perry, Potter, Ostendorf (2014), pp. 505, 509.

1180. A client with a history of hypertension has been prescribed triamterene (Dyrenium). The nurse provides information to the client about the medication and tells the client to avoid consuming which fruit?
1. Pears
2. Apples
3. Bananas
4. Cranberries

Level of Cognitive Ability: Applying
Client Needs: Health Promotion and Maintenance
Integrated Process: Nursing Process/Implementation
Content Area: Adult Health: Cardiovascular Medications
Priority Concepts: Client Education; Nutrition

Answer: 3
Rationale: Triamterene is a potassium-retaining diuretic, and the client should avoid foods that are high in potassium. Fruits that are naturally higher in potassium include avocados, bananas, oranges, mangoes, cantaloupe, strawberries, nectarines, papayas, and dried prunes.
Priority Nursing Tip: Normal potassium levels range from 3.5 to 5.0 mEq/L. A potassium level outside of these parameters needs to be reported.
Test-Taking Strategy: Focus on the subject, the fruit that the client needs to avoid. Note that this is a negative event query asking you to choose the fruit the client should not eat. Recall that triamterene (Dyrenium) is a potassium-retaining diuretic and dietary concerns related to the medication. Review: **triamterene and food items that are high in potassium.**
Reference(s): Hodgson, Kizior (2014), pp. 1210-1211; Kee, Hayes, McCuistion (2012), p. 650.

1181. A client in the late, active, first stage of labor has just reported a gush of vaginal fluid. The nurse observes a fetal monitor pattern of variable decelerations during contractions followed by a brief acceleration. After that, there is a return to baseline until the next contraction, when the pattern is repeated. On the basis of these data, what is the nurse's **initial** intervention?
1. Take the client's vital signs.
2. Perform a Leopold's maneuver.
3. Perform a manual sterile vaginal exam.
4. Test the vaginal fluid with a Nitrazine strip.

Level of Cognitive Ability: Applying
Client Needs: Physiological Integrity
Integrated Process: Nursing Process/Implementation
Content Area: Maternity: Intrapartum
Priority Concepts: Perfusion; Reproduction

Answer: 3
Rationale: Variable deceleration with brief acceleration after a gush of amniotic fluid is a common clinical manifestation of cord compression caused by occult or frank prolapse of the umbilical cord. A manual vaginal exam can detect the presence of the cord in the vagina, which confirms the problem. On the basis of the data in the question, options 1, 2, and 4 are not initial actions.
Priority Nursing Tip: Compression of the cord between the fetal head and the forceps used during delivery can cause a drop in the fetal heart rate (FHR). The FHR and pattern are checked, reported, and recorded before and after forceps are applied.
Test-Taking Strategy: Note the strategic word, *initial.* Focusing on the data in the question and determining the significance of the data will direct you to option 3. Review: the signs of **cord compression.**
Reference(s): Hockenberry, Wilson (2013), p. 459; McKinney et al (2013), p. 659.

1182. The nurse prepares to administer an enteral feeding to a client through a nasogastric tube (NGT). Which is the **priority** intervention for the nurse to complete before administering the feeding?

1. Determining tube placement
2. Auscultating the bowel sounds
3. Measuring the intake and output
4. Establishing the client's baseline weight

Level of Cognitive Ability: Applying
Client Needs: Physiological Integrity
Integrated Process: Nursing Process/Implementation
Content Area: Fundamental Skills: Safety
Priority Concepts: Clinical Judgment; Safety

Answer: 1
Rationale: The nurse avoids injecting any substance into a client's NGT before verifying tube placement because NGTs can migrate out of the stomach. If the NGT is not in the correct location, subsequent injections or feedings through the tube can lead to serious complications such as aspiration. Options 2, 3, and 4 are not priorities before administering an enteral feeding.
Priority Nursing Tip: Following insertion of a nasogastric tube, an abdominal x-ray study should be done to confirm placement of the tube. If the tube is incorrectly placed, the client is at risk for aspiration.
Test-Taking Strategy: Note the strategic word, *priority*. Use the ABCs—airway, breathing, and circulation—and the steps of the nursing process to answer the question. Option 1 relates to assessment and the risk of aspiration. Review: the nursing interventions when initiating a **nasogastric tube (NG) tube feeding**.
Reference(s): Ignatavicius, Workman (2013), p. 1345.

❖ **1183.** The nurse is asked to assist another health care team member with providing care for a client. On entering the client's room, the nurse notes that the client is placed in this position (refer to figure). After maintaining the client position, what should the nurse interpret that this client is **most likely** being treated for?

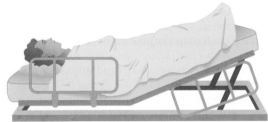

Figure from Black J, Hawks J: *Medical-surgical nursing: clinical management for positive outcomes*, ed 8, Philadelphia, 2009, Saunders.

1. Shock
2. A head injury
3. Respiratory insufficiency
4. Increased intracranial pressure

Level of Cognitive Ability: Analyzing
Client Needs: Physiological Integrity
Integrated Process: Nursing Process/Implementation
Content Area: Adult Health: Cardiovascular
Priority Concepts: Clinical Judgment; Perfusion

Answer: 1
Rationale: A client in shock is placed in a modified Trendelenburg's position that includes elevating the legs, leaving the trunk flat, and elevating the head and shoulders slightly. This position promotes increased venous return from the lower extremities without compressing the abdominal organs against the diaphragm. The Trendelenburg position is no longer recommended for hypotensive clients because the client is predisposed to aspiration and worsens gas exchange. Options 2, 3, and 4 identify conditions in which the head of the client's bed would be elevated.
Priority Nursing Tip: Shock results from the loss of circulatory fluid volume, which is usually caused by hemorrhage. Shock can also be caused by sepsis or hypovolemia (dehydration).
Test-Taking Strategy: Note the strategic words, *most likely*. Focus on the subject of the position identified in the figure. Eliminate options 2 and 4 first because they are comparable or alike, and they both relate to a neurological condition. From the remaining choices, eliminate option 3, recalling that the head of the bed is elevated for respiratory conditions. Review: the care of the client with **shock**.
Reference(s): Ignatavicius, Workman (2013), p. 818.

1184. The nurse needs to administer 7.5 mg of a medication intramuscularly. The medication label reads "10 mg/mL." How much medication should the nurse prepare to administer? **Fill in the blank.**

_____ mL

Level of Cognitive Ability: Analyzing
Client Needs: Physiological Integrity
Integrated Process: Nursing Process/Implementation
Content Area: Fundamental Skills: Medication/IV Calculations
Priority Concepts: Clinical Judgment; Safety

Answer: 0.75 mL
Rationale: Use the following formula to calculate the medication dose:

Formula:

$$\frac{\text{Desired}}{\text{Available}} \times \text{Volume} = \text{mL per dose}$$

$$\frac{7.5 \text{ mg}}{10 \text{ mg}} \times 1 \text{ mL} = 0.75 \text{ mL}$$

Priority Nursing Tip: After performing a medication calculation problem, make sure that the answer or the amount of medication to be administered makes sense and is not an excessive or extremely small dose.
Test-Taking Strategy: Focus on the subject, mL of medication per dose. Use the formula to determine the correct dosage, and use a calculator to verify your answer. Review: the formula for **calculating a medication dose.**
Reference(s): Potter et al (2013), pp. 574-577.

1185. A client diagnosed with obsessive-compulsive rituals often misses the unit's morning activities because of a bed-making ritual. What nursing action would be therapeutic?

1. Verbalize tactful, mild disapproval of the behavior.
2. Discuss the social implications of the behavior with the client.
3. Help the client to make the bed so that the task can be finished quicker.
4. Offer reflective feedback, such as, "I see that you have made your bed several times."

Level of Cognitive Ability: Applying
Client Needs: Psychosocial Integrity
Integrated Process: Nursing Process/Implementation
Content Area: Mental Health
Priority Concepts: Clinical Judgment; Anxiety

Answer: 4
Rationale: Reflective feedback acknowledges the client's behavior. Verbalizing disapproval would increase the client's anxiety and reinforce the need to perform the ritual. The client is usually aware of the implications of the behavior. Helping with the ritual is nontherapeutic and also reinforces the behavior.
Priority Nursing Tip: If a client is experiencing anxiety, assist the client to perform relaxation techniques.
Test-Taking Strategy: Focus on the subject, a client with obsessive-compulsive rituals. Recalling that the purpose of the ritual is to relieve anxiety would assist you with eliminating options 1 and 2 because these actions would increase the client's anxiety. Eliminate option 3 because there is no therapeutic value in participating in the ritual. Review: the appropriate interventions for the client with **obsessive-compulsive behavior.**
Reference(s): Fortinash, Holoday-Worret (2012), pp. 195-196; Varcarolis (2013), p. 181.

1186. A client who has undergone internal fixation after fracturing a left hip has developed a reddened left heel. What should the nurse obtain to manage this problem?

1. Trapeze
2. Bed cradle
3. Draw sheet
4. Alternating pressure mattress

Level of Cognitive Ability: Applying
Client Needs: Physiological Integrity
Integrated Process: Nursing Process/Implementation
Content Area: Adult Health: Musculoskeletal
Priority Concepts: Clinical Judgment; Tissue Integrity

Answer: 4
Rationale: The reddened heel results from the pressure of the foot against the mattress. An alternating pressure mattress is effective at minimizing pressure points. The bed cradle will keep the linens off of the client's lower extremities but will not assist with the management of a reddened heel. A draw sheet and trapeze are of general use for this client, but they are not specific for dealing with the reddened heel.
Priority Nursing Tip: The nurse should perform frequent skin assessments on the immobile client.
Test-Taking Strategy: Note the subject, a reddened left heel after internal fixation surgery. Eliminate option 2 first because it is unnecessary and not helpful. Eliminate options 1 and 3 next because, although they are generally helpful for the client's mobility, they are not related to the subject of the question. Option 4 addresses the problem stated in the question. Review: the measures that prevent **skin breakdown in the immobile client.**
Reference(s): Ignatavicius, Workman (2013), pp. 100-101.

1187. The nurse is caring for an infant after pyloromyotomy performed to treat hypertrophic pyloric stenosis. In which position should the nurse place the infant after surgery?
1. Flat on the operative side
2. Flat on the unoperative side
3. Prone with the head of the bed elevated
4. Supine with the head of the bed elevated

Level of Cognitive Ability: Applying
Client Needs: Physiological Integrity
Integrated Process: Nursing Process/Implementation
Content Area: Child Health: Gastrointestinal
Priority Concepts: Clinical Judgment; Safety

Answer: 3
Rationale: After pyloromyotomy, the head of the bed is elevated, and the infant is placed prone to reduce the risk of aspiration. Options 1, 2, and 4 are incorrect positions after this type of surgery. The surgeon's prescriptions for positioning should always be followed.
Priority Nursing Tip: Following pyloromyotomy to treat hypertrophic pyloric stenosis, small frequent feedings are introduced as prescribed. This is followed by a gradual increase in the amount and interval between feedings until a full feeding schedule had been reinstated.
Test-Taking Strategy: Focus on the subject, proper positioning after pyloromyotomy. Consider the anatomical location of the surgical procedure and the risks associated with the procedure to answer the question. Visualize each of the positions identified in the options. Keeping in mind that aspiration is a major concern will direct you to option 3. Review: the nursing care measures after **pyloromyotomy**.
Reference(s): McKinney et al (2013), pp. 1096-1097.

1188. A mother of a child with mumps calls the health care clinic to tell the nurse that the child has been lethargic and vomiting. What instruction should the nurse give to the mother?
1. To continue to monitor the child
2. That lethargy and vomiting are normal manifestations of mumps
3. To bring the child to the clinic to be seen by the health care provider
4. That, as long as there is no fever, there is nothing to be concerned about

Level of Cognitive Ability: Applying
Client Needs: Physiological Integrity
Integrated Process: Nursing Process/Implementation
Content Area: Child Health: Infectious and Communicable Diseases
Priority Concepts: Clinical Judgment; Infection

Answer: 3
Rationale: Mumps generally affects the salivary glands, but it can also affect multiple organs. The most common complication is septic meningitis, with the virus being identified in the cerebrospinal fluid. Common signs include nuchal rigidity, lethargy, and vomiting. The child should be seen by the health care provider.
Priority Nursing Tip: Inform the parents of a child with mumps that bed rest should be encouraged until the parotid swelling subsides.
Test-Taking Strategy: Focus on the subject, a child with mumps who has been lethargic and vomiting. Recalling that meningitis is a complication of mumps will direct you to option 3. Review: the complications of **mumps** and the associated clinical manifestations.
Reference(s): McKinney et al (2013), p. 1021.

1189. The nurse is reviewing the health care provider's prescriptions for a child who was admitted to the hospital with vaso-occlusive pain crisis from sickle cell anemia. Which health care provider prescription should the nurse question?
1. Bed rest
2. Intravenous fluids
3. Supplemental oxygen
4. Meperidine hydrochloride (Demerol)

Level of Cognitive Ability: Applying
Client Needs: Safe and Effective Care Environment
Integrated Process: Nursing Process/Implementation
Content Area: Child Health: Hematological
Priority Concepts: Collaboration; Safety

Answer: 4
Rationale: Meperidine hydrochloride is contraindicated for ongoing pain management because of the increased risk of seizures associated with the use of the medication. The management of vaso-occlusive pain generally includes the use of strong opioid analgesics such as morphine sulfate or hydromorphone (Dilaudid). These medications are usually most effective when given as a continuous infusion or at regular intervals around the clock. Options 1, 2, and 3 are appropriate prescriptions for treating vaso-occlusive pain crisis.
Priority Nursing Tip: The priority of care for a child with vaso-occlusive pain crisis from sickle cell anemia is to provide hydration and relieve pain.
Test-Taking Strategy: Focus on the subject, the prescription to question for treatment of vaso-occlusive pain crisis. Remember that meperidine hydrochloride is associated with an increased risk of seizures. Review: the care of the child with **sickle cell crisis**.
Reference(s): McKinney et al (2013), p. 1248.

1190. The nurse is caring for an infant with laryngomalacia (congenital laryngeal stridor). In which position should the nurse place the infant to decrease the incidence of stridor?
1. Prone
2. Supine
3. Supine with the neck flexed
4. Prone with the neck hyperextended

Level of Cognitive Ability: Applying
Client Needs: Physiological Integrity
Integrated Process: Nursing Process/Implementation
Content Area: Child Health: Throat/Respiratory
Priority Concepts: Gas Exchange; Safety

Answer: 4
Rationale: The prone position with the neck hyperextended improves the child's breathing. Options 1, 2, and 3 are not appropriate positions.
Priority Nursing Tip: A child experiencing respiratory difficulty is never left unattended.
Test-Taking Strategy: Focus on the subject, positioning a child diagnosed with laryngomalacia in order to minimize stridor. Visualize each of the positions identified in the options and how they may or may not improve breathing to assist with directing you to option 4. Review: the care of the infant with **laryngomalacia**.
Reference(s): McKinney et al (2013), p. 1158.

1191. The nurse in the newborn nursery prepares to admit a newborn with spina bifida, myelomeningocele. Which nursing action is **most important** for the care for this infant?
1. Monitoring the temperature
2. Monitoring the blood pressure
3. Inspecting the anterior fontanel for bulging
4. Monitoring the specific gravity of the urine

Level of Cognitive Ability: Applying
Client Needs: Physiological Integrity
Integrated Process: Nursing Process/Implementation
Content Area: Maternity: Newborn
Priority Concepts: Intracranial Regulation; Tissue Integrity

Answer: 3
Rationale: Intracranial pressure is a complication that is associated with spina bifida. A sign of intracranial pressure in the newborn infant with spina bifida is a bulging anterior fontanel. The newborn infant is at risk for infection before the surgical procedure and the closure of the gibbus, and monitoring the temperature is an important intervention; however, assessing the anterior fontanel for bulging is most important. A normal saline dressing is placed over the affected site to maintain the moisture of the sac and its contents. This prevents tearing or breakdown of skin integrity at the site. Blood pressure is difficult to assess during the newborn period, and it is not the best indicator of infection or a potential complication. Urine concentration is not well developed during the newborn stage of development.
Priority Nursing Tip: In myelomeningocele, the sac (defect) is covered by a thin membrane and is prone to leakage or rupture.
Test-Taking Strategy: Focus on the strategic words, *most important*. Eliminate options 2 and 4 first because blood pressure and specific gravity are common assessments, but they are not as reliable indications of changes in the status of a newborn as they would be for an older child. From the remaining choices, focusing on the strategic words will direct you to option 3. Review: the care of the infant with spina bifida.
Reference(s): McKinney et al (2013), p. 1423.

1192. During the assessment of a child, the nurse notes that the child's genitals are swollen. The nurse suspects that the child is being sexually abused. Which action by the nurse is of **primary** importance?
1. Document the child's physical findings.
2. Report the case because abuse is suspected.
3. Refer the family to appropriate support groups.
4. Assist the family with identifying resources and support systems.

Level of Cognitive Ability: Applying
Client Needs: Psychosocial Integrity
Integrated Process: Nursing Process/Implementation
Content Area: Leadership/Management: Ethical/Legal
Priority Concepts: Health Care Law; Interpersonal Violence

Answer: 2
Rationale: The primary legal responsibility of the nurse when child abuse is suspected is to report the case. All 50 states require health care professionals to report all cases of suspected abuse. Although documenting the assessment findings, assisting the family, and referring the family to appropriate resources and support groups is important, the primary legal responsibility is to report the case. While the remaining options are appropriate, reporting the findings has priority.
Priority Nursing Tip: The nurse needs to document information related to suspected child abuse in an objective manner.
Test-Taking Strategy: Focus on the subject, the possible sexual abuse of a child. Recall that abuse is a crime. Keeping this in mind will direct you to the correct option. Review: the responsibilities of the nurse when **child abuse** is suspected.
Reference(s): McKinney et al (2013), pp. 860-861, 1471-1472.

1193. The nurse is planning care for an infant with a diagnosis of an encephalocele located in the occipital area. Which item should the nurse use to assist with positioning the child to avoid pressure on the encephalocele?
1. Sandbags
2. Sheepskin
3. Feather pillows
4. Foam half donut

Level of Cognitive Ability: Applying
Client Needs: Physiological Integrity
Integrated Process: Nursing Process/Implementation
Content Area: Child Health: Integumentary
Priority Concepts: Safety; Tissue Integrity

Answer: 4
Rationale: The infant is positioned to avoid pressure on the lesion. If the encephalocele is in the occipital area, a foam half donut may be useful for positioning to prevent this pressure. A sandbag, sheepskin, or feather pillow will not protect the encephalocele from pressure.
Priority Nursing Tip: The nurse needs to monitor the infant with encephalocele closely for signs of neurological deterioration.
Test-Taking Strategy: Note that options 1, 2, and 3 are comparable or alike in that they would require the head to remain flat and therefore would not protect the lesion. Review: the nursing care associated with a child with an **encephalocele**.
Reference(s): Hockenberry, Wilson (2013), p. 1103.

1194. The nurse is caring for a child with a head injury. The nurse notes that the health care provider has documented decorticate posturing. During the assessment of the child, the nurse notes the extension of the upper extremities and the internal rotation of the upper arms and wrists. The nurse also notes that the lower extremities are extended, with some internal rotation noted at the knees and feet. On the basis of these findings, what is the **initial** nursing action?
   1. Document the findings.
   2. Notify the health care provider.
   3. Attempt to flex the child's lower extremities.
   4. Continue to monitor the child for any posturing.

Level of Cognitive Ability: Applying
Client Needs: Physiological Integrity
Integrated Process: Nursing Process/Implementation
Content Area: Critical Care: Emergency Situations
Priority Concepts: Clinical Judgment; Intracranial Regulation

Answer: 2
Rationale: Decorticate (flexion) posturing refers to the flexion of the upper extremities and the extension of the lower extremities. Plantar flexion of the feet may also be observed. Decerebrate (extension) posturing involves the extension of the upper extremities with the internal rotation of the upper arms and wrists. The lower extremities will extend with some internal rotation noted at the knees and feet. The progression from decorticate to decerebrate posturing usually indicates deteriorating neurological function and warrants health care provider notification. While documentation is appropriate, it is not the initial action in this situation. The other options are not appropriate.
Priority Nursing Tip: Decorticate (flexion) posturing is seen with severe dysfunction of the cerebral cortex. Decerebrate (extension) posturing is a sign of dysfunction at the level of the midbrain.
Test-Taking Strategy: Focus on the subject, decerebrate and decorticate positioning. Also note the strategic word *initial*. Recalling that progression from decorticate to decerebrate posturing usually indicates deteriorating neurological function will direct you to option 2. Review: **decerebrate and decorticate posturing.**
Reference(s): McKinney et al (2013), pp. 1419-1420.

1195. A child with a diagnosis of hepatitis B is being cared for at home. The mother of the child calls the health care clinic and tells the nurse that the jaundice seems to be worsening. Which response should the nurse make to the mother?
   1. "The hepatitis may be spreading."
   2. "It is necessary to isolate the child from the others."
   3. "The jaundice may appear to get worse before it resolves."
   4. "You need to bring the child to the health care clinic to see the health care provider."

Level of Cognitive Ability: Applying
Client Needs: Physiological Integrity
Integrated Process: Nursing Process/Implementation
Content Area: Child Health: Gastrointestinal
Priority Concepts: Clinical Judgment; Infection

Answer: 3
Rationale: The parents should be instructed that jaundice may appear to get worse before it resolves. The parents of a child with hepatitis should also be taught the danger signs that could indicate a worsening of the child's condition, specifically changes in neurological status, bleeding, and fluid retention. The statements in options 1, 2, and 4 are incorrect.
Priority Nursing Tip: Proper handwashing and standard precautions can help prevent the spread of viral hepatitis.
Test-Taking Strategy: Focus on the subject, the physiology associated with hepatitis to answer this question. Remember that jaundice worsens before it resolves. This will direct you to the correct option. Review: the instructions for the parents of a child with **hepatitis B.**
Reference(s): McKinney et al (2013), p. 1109.

1196. The nurse is preparing to suction a trache-otomy on an infant. The nurse prepares the equipment for the procedure and should turn the suction to which setting?
1. 60 mm Hg
2. 90 mm Hg
3. 110 mm Hg
4. 120 mm Hg

Level of Cognitive Ability: Applying
Client Needs: Physiological Integrity
Integrated Process: Nursing Process/Implementation
Content Area: Fundamental Skills: Safety
Priority Concepts: Gas Exchange; Safety

Answer: 2
Rationale: The suctioning procedure for pediatric clients varies from that used for adults. Suctioning in infants and children requires the use of a smaller suction catheter and lower suction settings as compared with those used for adults. Suction settings for a neonate are usually 60 to 80 mm Hg; for an infant, 80 to 100 mm Hg; and, for larger children, 100 to 120 mm Hg. The health care provider prescription and agency procedures are always followed.
Priority Nursing Tip: The nurse should always hyperoxygenate the infant before performing respiratory suctioning.
Test-Taking Strategy: Focus on the subject of the suctioning of an infant's tracheotomy. Recalling the procedure that is used for an adult will assist with directing you to option 2. Review: the suctioning procedure of a **tracheotomy** on an infant.
Reference(s): Hockenberry, Wilson (2013), p. 691; McKinney et al (2013), p. 941.

1197. The nurse is caring for a client who begins to experience seizure activity while in bed. Which action should the nurse implement to prevent aspiration?
1. Raise the head of the bed
2. Loosen restrictive clothing
3. Remove the pillow and raise the padded side rails
4. Position the client on the side if possible, with the head flexed forward

Level of Cognitive Ability: Applying
Client Needs: Physiological Integrity
Integrated Process: Nursing Process/Implementation
Content Area: Adult Health: Neurological
Priority Concepts: Intracranial Regulation; Safety

Answer: 4
Rationale: Positioning the client on one side with the head flexed forward allows the tongue to fall forward and facilitates the drainage of secretions, which could help prevent aspiration. The nurse would not raise the head of the client's bed. The nurse would remove restrictive clothing and the pillow and raise the padded side rails, if present, but these actions would not decrease the risk of aspiration. Rather, they are general safety measures to use during seizure activity.
Priority Nursing Tip: Never place anything into the mouth of a client experiencing a seizure.
Test-Taking Strategy: Focus on the subject of preventing aspiration. Eliminate option 2 first because it is unrelated to the subject of the question. Focus on the ABCs—airway, breathing, and circulation—and then visualize the effect that each of the remaining options would have on airway and aspiration to direct you to the correct option. Review: the care of the client with **seizures** to prevent **aspiration**.
Reference(s): Ignatavicius, Workman (2013), p. 935.

1198. A client who has experienced a stroke has episodes of coughing while swallowing liquids. The client has developed a temperature of 101° F, an oxygen saturation of 91% (down from 98% previously), is slightly confused, and has noticeable dyspnea. Which action should the nurse take?
1. Notify the health care provider.
2. Encourage the client to cough and deep breathe.
3. Administer an acetaminophen (Tylenol) suppository.
4. Administer a bronchodilator prescribed on an as-needed basis.

Level of Cognitive Ability: Applying
Client Needs: Physiological Integrity
Integrated Process: Nursing Process/Implementation
Content Area: Adult Health: Neurological
Priority Concepts: Clinical Judgment; Gas Exchange

Answer: 1
Rationale: The client is exhibiting clinical signs and symptoms of aspiration, which include fever, dyspnea, decreased arterial oxygen levels, and confusion. Other symptoms that occur with this complication are difficulty with managing saliva or coughing or choking while eating. Because the client has developed a complication that requires medical intervention, the most appropriate action is to contact the health care provider. The remaining options are not related to the management of aspiration.
Priority Nursing Tip: During the acute phase of a stroke, monitor the client for signs of increased intracranial pressure because the client is most at risk during the first 72 hours after the stroke.
Test-Taking Strategy: Focus on the subject, a client who has experienced a stroke and episodes of coughing while swallowing liquids, as well as the client's specific sign/symptoms. This will indicate that aspiration has most likely occurred. Eliminate options 2, 3, and 4 because these actions will not assist with alleviating this life-threatening condition. Review: the appropriate nursing interventions for managing **aspiration**.
Reference(s): Ignatavicius, Workman (2013), p. 1017.

1199. The nurse is providing care to a client after a bone biopsy. Which action should the nurse take as part of aftercare for this procedure?
1. Monitor the vital signs once per day.
2. Keep the area in a dependent position.
3. Administer intramuscular opioid analgesics.
4. Monitor the site for swelling, bleeding, or hematoma formation.

Level of Cognitive Ability: Applying
Client Needs: Physiological Integrity
Integrated Process: Nursing Process/Implementation
Content Area: Adult Health: Musculoskeletal
Priority Concepts: Clinical Judgment; Safety

Answer: 4
Rationale: Nursing care after bone biopsy includes monitoring the site for swelling, bleeding, or hematoma formation. The vital signs are monitored every 4 hours for 24 hours. The biopsy site is elevated for 24 hours to reduce edema. A dependent position will increase the risk for bleeding. The client usually requires mild analgesics; more severe pain usually indicates that complications are arising.
Priority Nursing Tip: Inform the client that mild to moderate discomfort is normal after a bone biopsy.
Test-Taking Strategy: Focus on the subject, care of the client following bone biopsy. Begin to answer this question by recalling that after this procedure the client must have periodic assessments. With this in mind, eliminate option 1 because the time frame is too infrequent. Knowing that the procedure is done under local anesthesia helps you eliminate option 3 next. From the remaining choices, recall the principles related to circulation and positioning to direct you to option 4. Review: the care of a client after bone biopsy.
Reference(s): Chernecky, Berger (2013), p. 244.

1200. The nurse is caring for a client who is going to have an arthrogram involving the use of a contrast medium. Which action by the nurse is the **priority**?
1. Determining the presence of client allergies
2. Asking if the client has any last-minute questions
3. Telling the client to try to void before leaving the unit
4. Emphasizing to the client the importance of remaining still during the procedure

Level of Cognitive Ability: Applying
Client Needs: Physiological Integrity
Integrated Process: Nursing Process/Implementation
Content Area: Adult Health: Musculoskeletal
Priority Concepts: Clinical Judgment; Safety

Answer: 1
Rationale: Because of the risk of allergy to contrast medium, the nurse places the highest priority on assessing whether the client has an allergy to iodine or shellfish. The nurse also reinforces information about the test and reminds the client about the need to remain still during the procedure. It is helpful to have the client void before the procedure for comfort.
Priority Nursing Tip: The priority nursing action before any procedure involving the injection of a contrast medium is to assess the client for any allergies.
Test-Taking Strategy: Note the strategic word, *priority*. Recalling the risk associated with the administration of contrast medium will direct you to option 1. Review: the preprocedure care for an **arthrogram**.
Reference(s): Chernecky, Berger (2013), pp. 166-167.

1201. The nurse responds to a call bell and finds a client lying on the floor after a fall. The nurse suspects that the client's arm may be broken. Which **immediate** action should the nurse take?
1. Immobilize the arm
2. Take a set of vital signs
3. Call the radiology department
4. Tell the client that there is no permanent damage

Level of Cognitive Ability: Applying
Client Needs: Physiological Integrity
Integrated Process: Nursing Process/Implementation
Content Area: Adult Health: Musculoskeletal
Priority Concepts: Clinical Judgment; Mobility

Answer: 1
Rationale: When a fracture is suspected, it is imperative that the area be splinted before the client is moved. Emergency help should be called for if the client is external to a hospital, and a health care provider is called if the client is hospitalized. Vital signs would be taken, but this is not the immediate action. The health care provider rather than the nurse prescribes an x-ray examination. The nurse should remain with the client and provide realistic reassurance. The client would not be told that there is no permanent damage.
Priority Nursing Tip: If a fracture is suspected, immobilize the extremity by splinting, including the joints above and below the fracture site. Monitor circulatory status closely after splinting the extremity.
Test-Taking Strategy: Note the strategic word, *immediate*. Eliminate option 3 because the health care provider will prescribe radiology films. Option 4 is eliminated next because the nurse does not make statements to the client that could provide false reassurance. From the remaining choices, noting that a fracture is suspected will direct you to the correct option. Review: the care of the client with a suspected extremity fracture.
Reference(s): Ignatavicius, Workman (2013), p. 1150.

1202. The nurse is caring for a 14-year-old child who is hospitalized and placed in Crutchfield traction. The child is having difficulty adjusting to the length of the hospital confinement. Which nursing action would be appropriate to meet the child's needs?
  1. Allow the child to play loud music in the hospital room.
  2. Let the child wear his or her own clothing when friends visit.
  3. Allow the child to have his or her hair dyed if the parent agrees.
  4. Allow the child to keep the shades closed and the room darkened at all times.

Level of Cognitive Ability: Applying
Client Needs: Psychosocial Integrity
Integrated Process: Nursing Process/Implementation
Content Area: Developmental Stages: Infancy to Adolescence
Priority Concepts: Clinical Judgment; Development

Answer: 2
Rationale: An adolescent needs to identify with peers and has a strong need to belong to a group. The child should be allowed to wear his or her own clothes to feel a sense of belonging to the group. The adolescent likes to dress like the group and to wear similar hairstyles. Loud music may disturb others in the hospital. Because Crutchfield traction involves the use of skeletal pins, hair dye is not appropriate. The child's request for a darkened room is indicative of a possible problem with depression that may require further evaluation and intervention.
Priority Nursing Tip: Hospitalized adolescents become upset if friends go on with their lives, excluding them. For the hospitalized adolescent, separation from friends is a source of anxiety.
Test-Taking Strategy: Focus on the subject, a 14-year-old child having difficulty adjusting to the length of the hospital confinement. Specific knowledge of Crutchfield traction and its limitations, as well as of growth and development concepts, will direct you to option 2. Review: growth and development and the care of the child in Crutchfield traction and developmental stages.
Reference(s): McKinney et al (2013), p. 884.

1203. The nurse receives a telephone call from the emergency department and is told that a client in leg traction will be admitted to the nursing unit. The nurse prepares for the arrival of the client and asks the unlicensed assistive personnel to obtain which item that will be **essential** for helping the client move in bed while in leg traction?
  1. A foot board
  2. Extra pillows
  3. A bed trapeze
  4. An electric bed

Level of Cognitive Ability: Applying
Client Needs: Physiological Integrity
Integrated Process: Nursing Process/Implementation
Content Area: Adult Health: Musculoskeletal
Priority Concepts: Clinical Judgment; Mobility

Answer: 3
Rationale: A trapeze is essential to allow the client to lift straight up while being moved so that the amount of pull exerted on the limb in traction is not altered. A foot board and extra pillows do not facilitate moving. Either an electric bed or a manual bed can be used for traction, but this does not specifically assist the client with moving in bed.
Priority Nursing Tip: For the client in traction, ensure that pulleys in the traction device are not obstructed and ropes in the pulleys move freely.
Test-Taking Strategy: Note the strategic word, *essential*. Attempt to visualize the items identified in the options, and focus on the subject of helping the client in leg traction to move in bed. This will direct you to the correct option. Review: the care of the client in leg traction.
Reference(s): Ignatavicius, Workman (2013), pp. 1153-1154; Potter et al (2013), p. 1153.

1204. A pregnant client is receiving rehabilitative services for alcohol abuse. How should the nurse provide supportive care?

1. Minimize communication with supportive family members.
2. Encourage the client to stop counseling after the infant is born.
3. Avoid the discussion of the alcohol problem and recovery with the client.
4. Encourage the client to participate in care and identify supportive strategies that are helpful.

Level of Cognitive Ability: Applying
Client Needs: Health Promotion and Maintenance
Integrated Process: Nursing Process/Implementation
Content Area: Maternity: Antepartum
Priority Concepts: Addiction; Reproduction

Answer: 4
Rationale: The nurse provides supportive care by encouraging the client to participate in care. Communication with family members is important and the nurse should not avoid discussing the client's problem with the client. Counseling needs to continue after the infant is born.
Priority Nursing Tip: Fetal alcohol syndrome is caused by maternal alcohol use during pregnancy.
Test-Taking Strategy: Focus on the subject, supportive care to a pregnant client for alcohol abuse. Option 4 provides the client with an active role in care. Options 1, 2, and 3 create barriers for long-term success in dealing with the problem. Review **alcohol abuse in pregnancy.**
Reference(s): Hockenberry, Wilson (2013), pp. 92, 351-352; McKinney et al (2013), pp. 293, 559.

1205. A client in the second trimester of pregnancy is being assessed at the health care clinic. The nurse performing the assessment notes that the fetal heart rate is 100 beats/min. Which nursing action would be appropriate **initially**?

1. Document the findings as normal.
2. Notify the health care provider of the finding.
3. Inform the mother that the assessment is normal and everything is fine.
4. Instruct the mother to return to the clinic in 1 week for the reevaluation of the fetal heart rate.

Level of Cognitive Ability: Applying
Client Needs: Physiological Integrity
Integrated Process: Nursing Process/Implementation
Content Area: Maternity: Antepartum
Priority Concepts: Perfusion; Reproduction

Answer: 2
Rationale: The fetal heart rate should be between 120 and 160 beats/min during pregnancy. A fetal heart rate of 100 beats/min would require that the health care provider be notified and the client be further evaluated. Although the nurse would document the findings, the most appropriate nursing action is to notify the health care provider. Options 3 and 4 are inaccurate nursing actions.
Priority Nursing Tip: The fetal heart rate is usually about twice the maternal heart rate. However, a fetal heart rate outside the parameters of 120 and 160 beats/min during pregnancy warrants health care provider notification.
Test-Taking Strategy: Note the strategic word, *initially*. Options 3 and 4 are comparable or alike and inaccurate, so they can be eliminated first. From the remaining choices, focus on the subject of fetal heart rate recalling that the normal range for the fetal heart rate is between 120 and 160 beats/min; this will direct you to option 2. Review: normal **fetal heart rate.**
Reference(s): Hockenberry, Wilson (2013), p. 416.

1206. A client is admitted to the hospital with a diagnosis of a leaking cerebral aneurysm and is scheduled for surgery. Which intervention should the nurse implement during the preoperative period?

1. Place the client on bed rest.
2. Allow the client to ambulate to the bathroom.
3. Obtain a bedside commode for the client's use.
4. Encourage the client to be up at least twice per day.

Level of Cognitive Ability: Applying
Client Needs: Physiological Integrity
Integrated Process: Nursing Process/Implementation
Content Area: Adult Health: Neurological
Priority Concepts: Clinical Judgment; Intracranial Regulation

Answer: 1
Rationale: The client is placed on aneurysm precautions, and the client's activity is kept to a minimum to prevent Valsalva's maneuver. Clients often hold their breath and strain while pulling up to get out of bed. This exertion may cause a rise in blood pressure, which increases bleeding. Clients who have bleeding aneurysms in any vessel will have activity curtailed. Therefore, options 2, 3, and 4 are incorrect actions.
Priority Nursing Tip: The primary concern for a client with a cerebral aneurysm is rupture.
Test-Taking Strategy: Focus on the subject, the client's diagnosis of a leaking cerebral aneurysm and the words *preoperative period*. Eliminate options 2, 3, and 4 because they are comparable or alike in that they all involve out-of-bed activity and are incorrect. Review: **aneurysm** precautions.
Reference(s): Ignatavicius, Workman (2013), pp. 1014-1015.

1207. A health care provider calls the nurse to obtain the daily laboratory results of a client who is receiving total parenteral nutrition. Which is the **most important** laboratory result for the nurse to present to the health care provider?
1. White blood cell count
2. Serum electrolyte levels
3. Arterial blood gas levels
4. Hemoglobin and hematocrit levels

Level of Cognitive Ability: Analyzing
Client Needs: Physiological Integrity
Integrated Process: Nursing Process/Implementation
Content Area: Critical Care: Parenteral Nutrition
Priority Concepts: Clinical Judgment; Nutrition

Answer: 2
Rationale: Total parenteral nutrition solutions contain amino acids and dextrose in solution with electrolytes, trace elements, and other agents added. The provider uses the electrolyte values (including sodium, potassium, and chloride) and the glucose level to determine the effectiveness of the solution, make changes to the solution as necessary, and decrease the client's risk of a fluid and electrolyte imbalance. It is important to monitor the serum glucose because parenteral nutrition is usually composed of 10% or more dextrose in water. Options 1, 3, and 4 can be suitable tests for a client who is receiving total parenteral nutrition, but these results cover a narrower range of information than serum electrolytes.
Priority Nursing Tip: Assess the client who is to receive total parenteral nutrition for a history of glucose intolerance. If the client receives the solution too rapidly, does not receive enough insulin, or contracts an infection, hyperglycemia can occur.
Test-Taking Strategy: Note the strategic words, *most important* to choose the laboratory test that provides better information than the other options. Eliminate options 1, 3, and 4 because the results of these tests provide less information than serum electrolytes. Review: the composition of **total parenteral nutrition.**
Reference(s): Ignatavicius, Workman (2013), p. 1348.

Evaluation

1208. The nurse is evaluating the effects of care for the client with nephrotic syndrome. Which diagnostic result demonstrates the **least** amount of improvement over 2 days of care?
1. Serum albumin 1.9 g/dL, up to 2.0 g/dL
2. Initial weight 208 pounds, down to 203 pounds
3. Blood pressure 160/90 mm Hg, down to 130/78 mm Hg
4. Daily intake and output record of 2100 mL intake and 1900 mL output and 2000 mL intake and 2900 mL output

Level of Cognitive Ability: Evaluating
Client Needs: Physiological Integrity
Integrated Process: Nursing Process/Evaluation
Content Area: Adult Health: Renal and Urinary
Priority Concepts: Clinical Judgment; Safety

Answer: 1
Rationale: The goal of therapy in nephrotic syndrome is to heal the leaking glomerular membrane. This would then control edema by stopping the loss of protein in the urine. Fluid balance and albumin levels are monitored to determine the effectiveness of therapy. The least amount of improvement is in the serum albumin level because the normal albumin level is 3.5 to 5.0 g/dL. Option 2 represents a loss of fluid that slightly exceeds 2 L and represents a significant improvement. Option 3 shows improvement because both systolic and diastolic blood pressures are lower. Option 4 represents an increased fluid loss, which indicates improvement.
Priority Nursing Tip: For the client with nephrotic syndrome, bed rest is important if severe edema is present.
Test-Taking Strategy: Note the strategic word, *least.* Option 2 illustrates the greatest improvement and is eliminated first. Option 4 is also a significant improvement and is eliminated next. From the remaining choices, noting that the blood pressure has decreased significantly will direct you to option 1. Review: the care of the client with **nephrotic syndrome.**
Reference(s): Ignatavicius, Workman (2013), pp. 1529-1530.

1209. A client is being discharged to home after the application of a plaster leg cast. The nurse determines that the client understands the proper care of the cast when the client states the need to engage in which action?
1. Avoid getting the cast wet.
2. Cover the casted leg with warm blankets.
3. Use the fingertips to lift and move the leg.
4. Use a padded coat hanger end to scratch under the cast.

Level of Cognitive Ability: Evaluating
Client Needs: Physiological Integrity
Integrated Process: Nursing Process/Evaluation
Content Area: Adult Health: Musculoskeletal
Priority Concepts: Client Education; Mobility

Answer: 1
Rationale: A plaster cast must remain dry to keep its strength. Air should circulate freely around the cast to help it dry. Additionally, the cast also gives off heat as it dries. The cast should be handled using the palms of the hands rather than the fingertips until it is fully dry. The client should never scratch under the cast. A cool hair dryer may be used to relieve an itch.
Priority Nursing Tip: The client with a plaster cast needs to be taught to keep the cast clean and dry.
Test-Taking Strategy: Focus on the subject, cast care. Option 4 is dangerous to skin integrity and is eliminated first. Recalling that the cast needs to dry eliminates option 2. Knowing that a wet cast can be dented with the fingertips causing pressure underneath helps you eliminate option 3. Remember that plaster casts, when they have dried after application, should not become wet. Review: the home care instructions for a client with a **plaster cast**.
Reference(s): Ignatavicius, Workman (2013), p. 1151.

1210. A client is being discharged to home while recovering from acute kidney injury. The client demonstrates an understanding of the therapeutic dietary regimen when indicating a need to limit which dietary factor?
1. Fats
2. Vitamins
3. Potassium
4. Carbohydrates

Level of Cognitive Ability: Evaluating
Client Needs: Physiological Integrity
Integrated Process: Nursing Process/Evaluation
Content Area: Adult Health: Renal and Urinary
Priority Concepts: Client Education; Nutrition

Answer: 3
Rationale: Most of the excretion of potassium and the control of potassium balance are normal functions of the kidneys. In the client with renal failure, potassium intake must be restricted as much as possible (30 to 50 mEq/day). The primary mechanism of potassium removal with acute kidney injury is dialysis. Options 1, 2, and 4 are not normally restricted in the client with acute kidney injury unless a secondary health problem warrants the need to do so.
Priority Nursing Tip: Foods that are low in potassium include green beans, applesauce, cabbage, lettuce, peppers, grapes, blueberries, cooked summer squash or turnip greens, pineapple, or raspberries.
Test-Taking Strategy: Focusing on the subject, a client recovering from acute kidney injury, will assist you with answering this question. Recalling that potassium balance and excretion are controlled by the kidney will direct you to option 3. Review: **acute kidney injury**.
Reference(s): Ignatavicius, Workman (2013), pp. 1543, 1545.

1211. The nurse teaches the client with a history of anxiety and command hallucinations to harm self or others appropriate management techniques. Which client statement indicates that the client understands these techniques?
1. "I can go to group and talk about my feelings to hurt myself or others."
2. "If I take my prescribed medication as I'm supposed too, I won't be as anxious."
3. "I can call my counselor so that I can talk about my feelings and not hurt anyone."
4. "If I get enough sleep and eat well, I won't be as likely to get anxious and hear things."

Level of Cognitive Ability: Evaluating
Client Needs: Psychosocial Integrity
Integrated Process: Nursing Process/Evaluation
Content Area: Mental Health
Priority Concepts: Anxiety; Psychosis

Answer: 3
Rationale: There may be an increased risk for impulsive or aggressive behavior if a client is receiving command hallucinations to harm self or others. The client should be asked if he or she has intentions to hurt himself or herself or others. Talking about auditory hallucinations can interfere with the subvocal muscular activity that is associated with a hallucination. Options 1, 2, and 4 are general interventions, but they are not specific to anxiety and hallucinations.
Priority Nursing Tip: Monitor the client experiencing command hallucinations for signs of increasing fear, anxiety, or agitation.
Test-Taking Strategy: Focus on the subject, anxiety and hallucinations. Options 1, 2, and 4 are all interventions that a client can do to aid wellness. Option 3 is specific to the subject and indicates self-responsible commitment and control over the client's own behavior. Review: the interventions for **anxiety** and **hallucinations**.
Reference(s): Fortinash, Holoday-Worret (2012), p. 274; Varcarolis (2013), pp. 315-316.

1212. A perinatal client has been instructed about the prevention of genital tract infections. Which statement by the client indicates an understanding of these preventive measures?
1. "I can douche anytime I want."
2. "I can wear my tight-fitting jeans."
3. "I should avoid the use of condoms."
4. "I should wear underwear with a cotton panel liner."

Level of Cognitive Ability: Evaluating
Client Needs: Health Promotion and Maintenance
Integrated Process: Nursing Process/Evaluation
Content Area: Maternity: Antepartum
Priority Concepts: Infection; Sexuality

Answer: 4
Rationale: Wearing items with a cotton panel liner allows for air movement in and around the genital area. Douching is to be avoided. Wearing tight clothes irritates the genital area and does not allow for air circulation. Condoms should be used to minimize the spread of genital tract infections.
Priority Nursing Tip: Instruct the client with a genital tract infection to avoid the use of perfumed toilet paper, sanitary napkins, and feminine hygiene sprays. These items will irritate the genital area.
Test-Taking Strategy: Focus on the subject, the client's understanding of infection control. Options 1, 2, and 3 are all incorrect statements regarding prevention of infections. Review: the prevention measures associated with genital tract infections.
Reference(s): Lowdermilk, Perry, Cashion, Alden (2012), p. 161.

1213. The nurse has given the client information about the use of sublingual nitroglycerin tablets. The client has a prescription for as-needed use if chest pain occurs. Which client statement helps assure the nurse that the client understands how to self-administer the medication?
1. "I will keep the nitroglycerin in a shirt pocket close to my body."
2. "I will avoid using the medication until the chest pain actually begins and intensifies."
3. "If I get a headache when I first start taking the nitroglycerin, then I will take an aspirin"
4. "I will discard unused nitroglycerin tablets 3 to 6 months after the bottle is opened, and obtain a new prescription."

Level of Cognitive Ability: Evaluating
Client Needs: Physiological Integrity
Integrated Process: Nursing Process/Evaluation
Content Area: Pharmacology: Cardiovascular Medications
Priority Concepts: Client Education; Safety

Answer: 4
Rationale: Nitroglycerin may be self-administered sublingually 5 to 10 minutes before an activity that triggers chest pain. Tablets should be discarded 3 to 6 months after opening the bottle (per expiration date), and a new bottle of pills should be obtained from the pharmacy. Nitroglycerin is unstable and is affected by heat and cold, so it should not be kept close to the body (warmth) in a shirt pocket; rather, it should be kept in a jacket pocket or a purse. Headache often occurs with early use and diminishes in time. Acetaminophen (Tylenol) may be used to treat headache.
Priority Nursing Tip: The nurse needs to teach a client taking nitroglycerin to store the medication in a dark, tightly closed bottle. Additionally, the client needs to be informed that tablets will not relieve chest pain if they have expired.
Test-Taking Strategy: Focus on the subject, self-administration of nitroglycerin. Recalling that nitroglycerin loses its potency in 3 to 6 months will direct you to option 4. Review: the client teaching points related to nitroglycerin.
Reference(s): Ignatavicius, Workman (2013), p. 838.

1214. A client has had a laryngectomy for throat cancer and has started oral intake. The nurse determines that the client has tolerated the first stage of dietary advancement if the client takes which type of diet without aspirating or choking?

1. Bland
2. Full liquids
3. Clear liquids
4. Semisolid foods

Level of Cognitive Ability: Evaluating
Client Needs: Physiological Integrity
Integrated Process: Nursing Process/Evaluation
Content Area: Adult Health: Oncology
Priority Concepts: Nutrition; Safety

Answer: 4
Rationale: Oral intake after laryngectomy is started with semisolid foods. When the client can manage this type of food, liquids may be introduced. A bland diet is not appropriate. The client may not be able to tolerate the texture of some of the solid foods that would be included in a bland diet. Thin liquids are not given until the risk of aspiration is negligible.
Priority Nursing Tip: Following laryngectomy (radical neck dissection) place the client in a semi-Fowler's to Fowler's position to maintain a patent airway and minimize edema.
Test-Taking Strategy: Focus on the subject, swallowing and aspiration concerns related to a postoperative laryngectomy. Eliminate options 2 and 3 first, and recall that a client with swallowing difficulty will not be able to manage liquids. From the remaining choices, recall that a bland diet provides no control over the consistency or texture of the food. Review: the dietary measures for a client after laryngectomy.
Reference(s): Ignatavicius, Workman (2013), p. 593; Potter et al (2013), p. 1017.

1215. An older client who is a victim of elder abuse and his family have been attending counseling sessions for the past month. Which statement, if made by the abusive family member, would indicate that he or she has learned more positive coping skills?

1. "I will be more careful to make sure that my father's needs are 100% met."
2. "I am so sorry and embarrassed that the abusive event occurred. It won't happen again."
3. "I feel better equipped to care for my father now that I know where to turn if I need assistance."
4. "Now that my father is going to move into my home with me, I will have to stop drinking alcohol."

Level of Cognitive Ability: Evaluating
Client Needs: Psychosocial Integrity
Integrated Process: Nursing Process/Evaluation
Content Area: Mental Health
Priority Concepts: Coping; Interpersonal Violence

Answer: 3
Rationale: Elder abuse is sometimes caused by family members who are being expected to care for their aging parents. This care can cause the family to become overextended, frustrated, or financially depleted. Knowing where to turn in the community for assistance with caring for an aging family member can bring much-needed relief. Using these alternatives is a positive coping skill for many families. Options 1, 2, and 4 are statements of good faith or promises, which may or may not be kept in the future.
Priority Nursing Tip: When working with caregivers, assess the need for respite care or the need for other support systems.
Test-Taking Strategy: Focus on the subject, positive coping skills. Option 3 is the only choice that identifies a means of coping with the issues and that outlines a definitive plan for how to handle the pressure associated with the father's care. Review: the concepts related to elder abuse.
Reference(s): Fortinash, Holoday-Worret (2012), p. 546; Stuart (2013), p. 746.

1216. The nurse is caring for a term infant who is 24 hours old who had a confirmed episode of hypoglycemia when 1 hour old. Which observation by the nurse would indicate the **need for follow-up?**

1. Weight loss of 4 ounces and dry, peeling skin
2. Blood glucose level of 40 mg/dL before the last feeding
3. Breast-feeding for 20 minutes or more, with strong sucking
4. High-pitched cry, drinking 10 to 15 mL of formula per feeding

Level of Cognitive Ability: Evaluating
Client Needs: Physiological Integrity
Integrated Process: Nursing Process/Evaluation
Content Area: Maternity: Newborn
Priority Concepts: Clinical Judgment; Glucose Regulation

Answer: 4
Rationale: Hypoglycemia causes central nervous system symptoms (high-pitched cry), and it is also exhibited by a lack of strength for eating enough for growth. At 24 hours old, a term infant should be able to consume at least 1 ounce of formula per feeding. A high-pitched cry is indicative of neurological involvement. Weight loss over the first few days of life and dry, peeling skin are normal findings for term infants. Blood glucose levels are acceptable at 40 mg/dL during the first few days of life. Breast-feeding for 20 minutes with a strong suck is an excellent finding.
Priority Nursing Tip: In the newborn, a low blood glucose level is prevented through early feedings.
Test-Taking Strategy: Note the strategic words, *need for follow up.* These words indicate a negative event query and ask you to select an option that is an abnormal finding. Focus on the subject, signs/symptoms of hypoglycemia. Eliminate options 1, 2, and 3 because these are comparable or alike and are normal findings. The words *high-pitched cry* should direct you to option 4. Review: normal newborn findings and the indications of hypoglycemia.
Reference(s): Hockenberry, Wilson (2013), p. 267.

1217. A home care nurse visits a child with a diagnosis of celiac disease. Which finding **best** indicates that a gluten-free diet is being maintained and has been **effective?**

1. The child is free of diarrhea.
2. The child is free of bloody stools.
3. The child tolerates dietary wheat and rye.
4. A balanced fluid and electrolyte status is noted on the laboratory results.

Level of Cognitive Ability: Evaluating
Client Needs: Physiological Integrity
Integrated Process: Nursing Process/Evaluation
Content Area: Child Health: Gastrointestinal
Priority Concepts: Clinical Judgment; Elimination

Answer: 1
Rationale: Watery diarrhea is a frequent clinical manifestation of celiac disease. The absence of diarrhea indicates effective treatment. Bloody stools are not associated with this disease. The grains of wheat and rye contain gluten and are not allowed. A balance of fluids and electrolytes does not necessarily demonstrate the improved status of celiac disease.
Priority Nursing Tip: The nurse needs to instruct the parents of a child with celiac disease about lifelong elimination of gluten sources.
Test-Taking Strategy: Note the strategic words, *best* and *effective.* Focus on the subject, a child with celiac disease. Recalling that watery diarrhea is a manifestation of celiac disease will direct you to option 1. Review: the manifestations of celiac disease.
Reference(s): McKinney et al (2013), pp. 1104-1105.

1218. The nurse is assisting with caring for a woman in labor who is receiving oxytocin (Pitocin) by intravenous infusion. The nurse monitors the client, knowing that which finding indicates an adequate contraction pattern?

1. One contraction per minute, with resultant cervical dilation
2. Four contractions every 5 minutes, with resultant cervical dilation
3. One contraction every 10 minutes, without resultant cervical dilation
4. Three to 5 contractions in a 10-minute period, with resultant cervical dilation

Level of Cognitive Ability: Evaluating
Client Needs: Physiological Integrity
Integrated Process: Nursing Process/Evaluation
Content Area: Maternity: Intrapartum
Priority Concepts: Clinical Judgment; Reproduction

Answer: 4
Rationale: The preferred oxytocin dosage is the minimal amount necessary to maintain an adequate contraction pattern characterized by 3 to 5 contractions in a 10-minute period, with resultant cervical dilation. If contractions are more frequent than every 2 minutes, contraction quality may be decreased.
Priority Nursing Tip: A woman in labor who is receiving oxytocin (Pitocin) should not be left unattended.
Test-Taking Strategy: Focus on the subject of an adequate contraction pattern in a client receiving oxytocin (Pitocin); this will assist you with eliminating option 3. Eliminate options 1 and 2 next because they are comparable or alike. Review: the expected effects of oxytocin (Pitocin).
Reference(s): McKinney et al (2013), p. 417.

1219. A home care nurse is assigned to visit a preschooler who has a diagnosis of scarlet fever and is on bed rest. What data obtained by the nurse would indicate that the child is coping with the illness and bed rest?

1. The child insists that his mother stay in the room.
2. The child is coloring and drawing pictures in a notebook.
3. The mother keeps providing new activities for the child to do.
4. The child sucks his thumb whenever he does not get what he asked for.

Level of Cognitive Ability: Evaluating
Client Needs: Health Promotion and Maintenance
Integrated Process: Nursing Process/Evaluation
Content Area: Developmental Stages: Infancy to Adolescence
Priority Concepts: Coping; Development

Answer: 2
Rationale: According to Jean Piaget, for the preschooler, play is the best way for children to understand and adjust to life's experiences. They are able to use pencils and crayons, and they can draw stick figures and other rudimentary things. A child with scarlet fever needs quiet play, and drawing will provide that. Options 1, 3, and 4 do not address positive coping mechanisms.
Priority Nursing Tip: Scarlet fever is transmitted via direct contact with an infected person or droplet spread; or indirectly by contact with infected articles, ingestion of contaminated milk, or other foods.
Test-Taking Strategy: Note the subject of the coping behavior of a preschooler with scarlet fever. Think about the developmental level of a preschooler. Look at the analysis of data by the nurse to determine if the child is coping with the disease and bed rest. Option 2 is a positive coping mechanism for preschoolers. Options 1, 3, and 4 do not address positive coping mechanisms. Review: the expected developmental level of a **preschooler** and the effects of bed rest on a child.
Reference(s): McKinney et al (2013), pp. 74, 126, 1026.

1220. A client has just taken a dose of trimethobenzamide (Tigan). When the client states relief of which sign/symptom, can the nurse determine that the medication has been **effective**?

1. Nausea
2. Heartburn
3. Constipation
4. Abdominal pain

Level of Cognitive Ability: Evaluating
Client Needs: Physiological Integrity
Integrated Process: Nursing Process/Evaluation
Content Area: Pharmacology: Gastrointestinal Medications
Priority Concepts: Clinical Judgment; Safety

Answer: 1
Rationale: Trimethobenzamide (Tigan) is an antiemetic agent that is used for the treatment of nausea and vomiting. The medication is not used to treat heartburn, constipation, or abdominal pain.
Priority Nursing Tip: Antinausea medications cause drowsiness; therefore, safety is a concern when they are administered.
Test-Taking Strategy: Note the strategic word, *effective*. Focus on the subject, the intended effect of trimethobenzamide. Recalling that trimethobenzamide is an antiemetic will direct you to option 1. Review: the action of **trimethobenzamide (Tigan)**.
Reference(s): Skidmore-Roth (2014), pp. 1211-1212.

1221. The nurse is providing instructions to the mother of a child with a diagnosis of strabismus of the left eye, and the nurse reviews the procedure for patching the child. Which statement by the mother indicates that the mother understands the procedure?

1. "I will place the patch on both eyes."
2. "I will place the patch on the left eye."
3. "I will place the patch on the right eye."
4. "I will alternate the patch from the right eye to the left eye every hour."

Level of Cognitive Ability: Evaluating
Client Needs: Physiological Integrity
Integrated Process: Nursing Process/Evaluation
Content Area: Child Health: Eye/Ear
Priority Concepts: Client Education; Sensory Perception

Answer: 3
Rationale: Patching may be used for the treatment of strabismus to strengthen the weak eye. With this treatment, the good eye is patched; this encourages the child to use the weaker eye. The treatment is most successful when it is performed during the preschool years. The schedule for patching is individualized and prescribed by the ophthalmologist.
Priority Nursing Tip: Strabismus is also known as "squint" or "lazy eye."
Test-Taking Strategy: Focus of the subject, patching the eye related to the treatment of strabismus. Remembering that this condition involves a lazy eye will direct you to the correct option. It makes sense to patch the unaffected eye to strengthen the muscles in the affected eye. Review: the procedure for **eye patching** and **strabismus**.
Reference(s): McKinney et al (2013), p. 1505.

1222. The nurse is assessing a client with gestational hypertension who was admitted to the hospital 48 hours ago. Which current assessment data would indicate that the condition has not yet resolved?
1. Urinary output is increased
2. Presence of trace urinary protein
3. Client complaints of blurred vision
4. Blood pressure reading at prenatal baseline

Level of Cognitive Ability: Evaluating
Client Needs: Physiological Integrity
Integrated Process: Nursing Process/Evaluation
Content Area: Maternity: Antepartum
Priority Concepts: Perfusion; Reproduction

Answer: 3
Rationale: Client complaints of headache or blurred vision indicate a worsening of the condition and warrant immediate further evaluation. Options 1, 2, and 4 are all signs that the gestational hypertension is being resolved.
Priority Nursing Tip: Signs of preeclampsia are hypertension and proteinuria.
Test-Taking Strategy: Note the words, *not yet resolved*. This indicates a negative event query and asks you to select an option that in an abnormal finding. Focus on the subject, to identify a symptom of gestational hypertension that still exists. Options 1 and 4 can be eliminated first because they are normal findings. From the remaining choices, note that option 2 contains the word "trace" and is the most normal finding of options 2 and 3. Review: the clinical manifestations associated with **gestational hypertension**.
Reference(s): McKinney et al (2013), p. 593.

1223. A client has begun medication therapy with betaxolol (Kerlone). The nurse determines that the client is experiencing the intended effect of therapy if which observation is noted?
1. Edema present at 3+
2. Weight loss of 5 pounds within 2 days
3. Pulse rate increased from 58 to 74 beats/min
4. Blood pressure decreased from 142/94 mm Hg to 128/82 mm Hg

Level of Cognitive Ability: Evaluating
Client Needs: Physiological Integrity
Integrated Process: Nursing Process/Evaluation
Content Area: Pharmacology: Cardiovascular Medications
Priority Concepts: Clinical Judgment; Perfusion

Answer: 4
Rationale: Betaxolol is a beta-adrenergic blocking agent used to lower blood pressure, relieve angina, or eliminate dysrhythmias. Side/adverse effects include bradycardia and symptoms of heart failure, such as weight gain and increased edema.
Priority Nursing Tip: Beta-adrenergic blocking agents are used with caution in clients with diabetes mellitus because they may mask the symptoms of hypoglycemia.
Test-Taking Strategy: Focus on the subject, the intended effect of the betaxolol. Remember that beta-adrenergic blocking agent medication names end with the suffix -*lol*. Recalling the action of the medication will direct you to option 4. Review: the intended effects of **betaxolol (Kerlone)**.
Reference(s): Lehne (2013), pp. 175-176; Potter et al (2013), p. 459.

1224. The nurse has taught a client who is prescribed a xanthine bronchodilator about beverages to avoid. The nurse determines that the client understands the information if the client chooses which beverage from the dietary menu?
1. Cola
2. Coffee
3. Chocolate milk
4. Cranberry juice

Level of Cognitive Ability: Evaluating
Client Needs: Physiological Integrity
Integrated Process: Nursing Process/Evaluation
Content Area: Pharmacology: Respiratory Medications
Priority Concepts: Client Education; Safety

Answer: 4
Rationale: Cola, coffee, and chocolate contain xanthine and should be avoided by the client who is taking a xanthine bronchodilator. This could lead to an increased incidence of cardiovascular and central nervous system side effects that can occur with the use of these types of bronchodilators.
Priority Nursing Tip: Theophylline, a bronchodilator, increases the risk of digoxin toxicity and decreases the effects of lithium and phenytoin (Dilantin).
Test-Taking Strategy: Note that options 1, 2, and 3 are comparable or alike in that they all contain some form of stimulant. Review: the dietary measures for the client taking a **xanthine bronchodilator**.
Reference(s): Lehne (2013), pp. 967, 976.

1225. A client is prescribed glipizide (Glucotrol) once daily. What intended effect of this medication should the nurse observe for?
1. Weight loss
2. Resolution of infection
3. Decreased blood glucose
4. Decreased blood pressure

Level of Cognitive Ability: Evaluating
Client Needs: Physiological Integrity
Integrated Process: Nursing Process/Evaluation
Content Area: Pharmacology: Endocrine Medications
Priority Concepts: Clinical Judgment; Glucose Regulation

Answer: 3
Rationale: Glipizide is an oral hypoglycemic agent that is taken in the morning. It is not used to enhance weight loss, treat infection, or decrease blood pressure.
Priority Nursing Tip: Clients prescribed hypoglycemic agents require education regarding the possible side and adverse effects, including signs of hypoglycemia.
Test-Taking Strategy: Focus on the subject, the intended effect of glipizide. Recalling that this medication is an oral hypoglycemic will direct you to option 3. Review: the action of **glipizide (Glucotrol)**.
Reference(s): Hodgson, Kizior (2014), p. 542.

1226. A client regularly takes both nonsteroidal anti-inflammatory drugs (NSAIDs) and misoprostol (Cytotec). The nurse should monitor the client for the relief of which sign/symptom?
1. Diarrhea
2. Bleeding
3. Infection
4. Epigastric pain

Level of Cognitive Ability: Evaluating
Client Needs: Physiological Integrity
Integrated Process: Nursing Process/Evaluation
Content Area: Pharmacology: Gastrointestinal Medications
Priority Concepts: Clinical Judgment; Pain

Answer: 4
Rationale: The client who regularly takes NSAIDs is prone to gastric mucosal injury, which gives the client epigastric pain as a symptom. Misoprostol is administered to prevent this occurrence. Diarrhea can be a side effect of the medication, but its relief is not an intended effect. Bleeding and infection are unrelated to the question.
Priority Nursing Tip: Nonsteroidal anti-inflammatory drugs (NSAIDs) are contraindicated in clients with hypersensitivity or liver or renal disease.
Test-Taking Strategy: Focus on the subject, the relief of a sign/symptom in a client taking both NSAIDs and misoprostol (Cytotec). This tells you that the medication is being given to treat or prevent the occurrence of a specific sign/symptom. Recalling that NSAIDs can cause gastric mucosal injury will direct you to option 4. Review: the action and indications for the use of **misoprostol (Cytotec)**.
Reference(s): Hodgson, Kizior (2014), p. 788.

1227. A client has received a dose of an as-needed medication called loperamide (Imodium). The nurse evaluates the client after administration to see if the client has relief of which sign/symptom?
1. Diarrhea
2. Tarry stools
3. Constipation
4. Abdominal pain

Level of Cognitive Ability: Evaluating
Client Needs: Physiological Integrity
Integrated Process: Nursing Process/Evaluation
Content Area: Pharmacology: Gastrointestinal Medications
Priority Concepts: Clinical Judgment; Elimination

Answer: 1
Rationale: Loperamide is an antidiarrheal agent, and it is commonly administered after loose stools. It is used for the management of acute diarrhea and also for chronic diarrhea, such as with inflammatory bowel disease. It can also be used to reduce the volume of drainage from an ileostomy. It is not intended to treat any of the other options.
Priority Nursing Tip: Goals for a client with diarrhea is to identify and treat the underlying cause, treat dehydration, replace fluids and electrolytes, relieve abdominal discomfort and cramping, and reduce the passage of stool.
Test-Taking Strategy: Focus on the subject, the intended effect of loperamide. Recalling that this medication is an antidiarrheal agent will direct you to option 1. Review: the purpose of **loperamide (Imodium)**.
Reference(s): Hodgson, Kizior (2014), p. 705.

1228. The nurse has provided discharge instructions to the parent of a child who has undergone heart surgery. Which statement by the parent would indicate the **need for further instruction**?

1. "My child can return to school for full days 2 weeks after discharge."
2. "I should allow my child to play inside but omit outside play at this time."
3. "I should have my child avoid crowds and people for 2 week after discharge."
4. "I should call the health care provider if my child develops faster or harder breathing than normal."

Level of Cognitive Ability: Evaluating
Client Needs: Safe and Effective Care Environment
Integrated Process: Nursing Process/Evaluation
Content Area: Child Health: Cardiovascular
Priority Concepts: Client Education; Safety

Answer: 1
Rationale: The child may return to school the third week after hospital discharge, but he or she should go to school for half days for the first week. Outside play should be omitted for several weeks, with inside play allowed as tolerated. The child should avoid crowds of people for 2 weeks after discharge, including crowds at day care centers and churches. If any difficulty with breathing occurs, the parent should notify the health care provider.
Priority Nursing Tip: Following cardiac surgery, the parents should be instructed the keep the child away from crowds for 2 weeks after discharge to decrease the risk of contracting an infection.
Test-Taking Strategy: Note the strategic words, *need for further instruction*. This indicates a negative event query and asks you to select an option that is an incorrect statement. Recalling the principles related to the prevention of infection and the complications of surgery will direct you to option 1. Review: the home care instructions for a child after **heart surgery**.
Reference(s): McKinney et al (2013), p. 1224.

1229. A client has been taking nadolol (Corgard) for the past month. Which finding would indicate a therapeutic effect of the medication?

1. The client is afebrile.
2. The client has clear breath sounds.
3. The client reports no episodes of headache.
4. The client has a blood pressure of 118/72 mm Hg.

Level of Cognitive Ability: Evaluating
Client Needs: Physiological Integrity
Integrated Process: Nursing Process/Evaluation
Content Area: Pharmacology: Cardiovascular Medications
Priority Concepts: Clinical Judgment; Perfusion

Answer: 4
Rationale: Nadolol is a beta-adrenergic blocking agent that is used to treat hypertension. Therefore, a blood pressure within the normal range would indicate an effective response to the medication. Options 1, 2, and 3 are unrelated to the action of this medication.
Priority Nursing Tip: Beta blockers may be prescribed to treat angina, dysrhythmias, hypertension, migraine headaches, glaucoma, and prevent myocardial infarction.
Test-Taking Strategy: Focus on the subject, the therapeutic effect of nadolol. Remember that an evaluation-type question addresses a client's response to a treatment measure. In addition, recalling that medication names that end with *-lol* are beta-blocking agents will direct you to option 4. Review: the therapeutic effects of **nadolol (Corgard)**.
Reference(s): Hodgson, Kizior (2014), p. 808.

1230. The nurse is assigned to care for a client diagnosed with acquired immunodeficiency syndrome (AIDS) who is receiving amphotericin B for a fungal respiratory infection. Which would indicate an adverse effect of the medication?

1. Hypokalemia
2. Hyperkalemia
3. Hypocalcemia
4. Hypercalcemia

Level of Cognitive Ability: Evaluating
Client Needs: Physiological Integrity
Integrated Process: Nursing Process/Evaluation
Content Area: Pharmacology: Immune Medications
Priority Concepts: Clinical Judgment; Safety

Answer: 1
Rationale: Clients receiving amphotericin B may develop hypokalemia, which can be severe and lead to extreme muscle weakness and electrocardiogram changes. Distal renal tubular acidosis commonly occurs, and this contributes to the development of hypokalemia. High potassium levels do not occur. The medication does not cause calcium levels to fluctuate.
Priority Nursing Tip: Amphotericin B is nephrotoxic and the nurse should monitor the client closely for signs of nephrotoxicity such as decreased urine output and elevated blood urea nitrogen levels or creatinine levels.
Test-Taking Strategy: Focus on the subject, an adverse effect of amphotericin B and recall that it is an antifungal medication. It is necessary to recall that hypokalemia is an adverse effect of this medication. This will direct you to the correct option. Review: **amphotericin B**.
Reference(s): Hodgson, Kizior (2014), p. 62.

1231. A client is seen in the health care clinic, and a diagnosis of conjunctivitis is made. The nurse provides instructions to the client regarding the care of the disorder while at home. Which statement by the client indicates the **need for further instruction**?

1. "I can use an ophthalmic analgesic ointment at night if I have eye discomfort."
2. "I do not need to be concerned about spreading this infection to others in my family."
3. "I should apply warm compresses before instilling antibiotic drops if purulent discharge is present in my eye."
4. "I should perform saline eye irrigation before instilling the antibiotic drops into my eye if purulent discharge is present."

Level of Cognitive Ability: Evaluating
Client Needs: Safe and Effective Care Environment
Integrated Process: Nursing Process/Evaluation
Content Area: Adult Health: Eye
Priority Concepts: Client Education; Infection

Answer: 2
Rationale: Conjunctivitis is highly contagious. Antibiotic drops are usually administered four times a day. Ophthalmic analgesic ointment or drops may be instilled, especially at bedtime because discomfort becomes more noticeable when the eyelids are closed. When purulent discharge is present, saline eye irrigations or applications of warm compresses to the eye may be necessary before instilling the medication.
Priority Nursing Tip: Instruct the client with conjunctivitis about the importance of infection control measures such as good handwashing and not sharing towels and washcloths.
Test-Taking Strategy: Note the strategic words, *need for further instruction*. This indicates a negative event query and asks you to select an incorrect statement. Knowing that this disorder is considered highly contagious will direct you to option 2. Review: the management of the client with **conjunctivitis**.
Reference(s): Ignatavicius, Workman (2013), p. 1056.

1232. The nurse reviews the nursing care plan of a hospitalized child who is immobilized as a result of skeletal traction. The nurse notes concerns related to the child's development because of immobilization and hospitalization. Which evaluative statement indicates a positive outcome for the child?

1. The fracture heals without complications.
2. The caregivers verbalize safe and effective home care.
3. The child maintains normal joint and muscle integrity.
4. The child displays age-appropriate developmental behaviors.

Level of Cognitive Ability: Evaluating
Client Needs: Health Promotion and Maintenance
Integrated Process: Nursing Process/Evaluation
Content Area: Developmental Stages: Infancy to Adolescence
Priority Concepts: Development; Health Promotion

Answer: 4
Rationale: Regression and inappropriate developmental behaviors may be displayed in response to immobilization and hospitalization. With individualized care planning, a positive outcome of age-appropriate behavior can be achieved. Options 1, 2, and 3 are appropriate evaluative statements for an immobilized child, but they do not directly address the child's development.
Priority Nursing Tip: For the hospitalized child who is immobilized, focus on the child's ability and needs. Accept regression in the child but encourage independence.
Test-Taking Strategy: Focus on the subject, concerns regarding growth and development. Recalling that issues with development involve an individual not performing age-appropriate tasks will direct you to option 4. All choices are evaluative statements, but only option 4 addresses development. Review: **developmental stages**.
Reference(s): McKinney et al (2013), p. 1345.

1233. The nurse has been encouraging the intake of oral fluids for a client in labor to improve hydration. Which indicates a successful outcome of this action?

1. Ketones in the urine
2. A urine specific gravity of 1.020
3. A blood pressure of 150/90 mm Hg
4. The continued leaking of amniotic fluid during labor

Level of Cognitive Ability: Evaluating
Client Needs: Physiological Integrity
Integrated Process: Nursing Process/Evaluation
Content Area: Maternity: Intrapartum
Priority Concepts: Fluid and Electrolyte Balance; Reproduction

Answer: 2
Rationale: Urine specific gravity measures the concentration of the urine. During the first stage of labor, the renal system has a tendency to concentrate urine. Labor and birth require hydration and caloric intake to replenish energy expenditure and promote efficient uterine function. An elevated blood pressure and ketones in the urine are not expected outcomes related to labor and hydration. After the membranes have ruptured, it is expected that amniotic fluid may continue to leak.
Priority Nursing Tip: The woman in labor is at risk for hypovolemia because of the dehydrating effects of labor. However, if the laboring woman is receiving intravenous fluids, the risk of hypervolemia is present.
Test-Taking Strategy: Focus on the subject, a successful outcome related to oral intake. Recalling the relationship of oral intake to urine concentration will direct you to option 2. Review: the importance of hydration for the woman in labor.
Reference(s): Lowdermilk, Perry, Cashion, Alden (2012), pp. 446, 450-451; Pagana, Pagana (2013), p. 950.

1234. A goal for a postpartum client has been developed that states, "The client will remain free of infection during her hospital stay." Which assessment data would support that the goal has been met?

1. Loss of appetite
2. Absence of fever
3. Presence of chills
4. Abdominal tenderness

Level of Cognitive Ability: Evaluating
Client Needs: Physiological Integrity
Integrated Process: Nursing Process/Evaluation
Content Area: Maternity: Postpartum
Priority Concepts: Infection; Reproduction

Answer: 2
Rationale: Fever is the first indication of an infection. Therefore, the absence of a fever indicates that an infection is not present. Loss of appetite, chills, and abdominal tenderness can indicate the presence of an infection.
Priority Nursing Tip: In the postpartum client, a temperature up to 100.4° F is normal due to the dehydrating effects of labor.
Test-Taking Strategy: Focus on the subject, the physical indications of an infection. The question is asking for a means of evaluating the effectiveness of a goal that relates to infection. Options 1, 3, and 4 indicate possible signs of infection and that the goal has not been met. Review: the signs of postpartum infection.
Reference(s): McKinney et al (2013), p. 682.

1235. The nurse is monitoring the nutritional status of a client who is receiving enteral nutrition. Which should the nurse monitor as the **best** clinical indicator of the client's nutritional status?

1. Daily weight
2. Calorie count
3. Skinfold measurement
4. Serum prealbumin level

Level of Cognitive Ability: Evaluating
Client Needs: Physiological Integrity
Integrated Process: Nursing Process/Evaluation
Content Area: Fundamental Skills: Nutrition
Priority Concepts: Clinical Judgment; Nutrition

Answer: 4
Rationale: A serum prealbumin level is the most important parameter for determining the effectiveness of a client's nutritional management and nutritional status. Because prealbumin is a major plasma protein with a short half-life, it is sensitive to changes in protein synthesis and catabolism, and it is thus the best clinical indicator of nutritional status. It is a better nutritional index than a daily weight because body weight can be skewed quickly by changes in total body fluid. It is also a better index than anthropomorphic measurements because nutritional status is not necessarily related to skinfold thickness. The calorie count reports the total calories provided to the client without data regarding the client's use of the calories and nutrients.
Priority Nursing Tip: Enteral nutrition provides liquefied foods into the gastrointestinal tract via a tube.
Test-Taking Strategy: Note the strategic word, *best*. This tells you that the correct option is a better indicator of nutritional status than the remaining options. Remember that the prealbumin is a major plasma protein and is sensitive to changes in protein synthesis and catabolism. Review: the methods of monitoring nutritional status of a client who is receiving enteral nutrition.
Reference(s): Ignatavicius, Workman (2013), p. 1342.

1236. An adult client with hyperkalemia is prescribed sodium polystyrene sulfonate (Kayexalate). Which serum potassium level is a clinical indicator of **effective** therapy?
1. 4.9 mEq/L
2. 5.4 mEq/L
3. 5.8 mEq/L
4. 6.2 mEq/L

Level of Cognitive Ability: Evaluating
Client Needs: Physiological Integrity
Integrated Process: Nursing Process/Evaluation
Content Area: Fundamental Skills: Laboratory Values
Priority Concepts: Clinical Judgment; Fluid and Electrolyte Balance

Answer: 1
Rationale: The normal serum potassium level for an adult is 3.5 to 5.0 mEq/L. Option 1 is the only option that reflects a value within this range. Options 2, 3, and 4 identify hyperkalemic levels.
Priority Nursing Tip: Electrocardiographic changes in hyperkalemia include tall peaked T waves, flat P waves, widened QRS complexes, and prolonged PR intervals.
Test-Taking Strategy: Note the strategic word, *effective*. Without knowing the mechanism of action of sodium polystyrene sulfonate, compare each value with normal serum potassium levels. Note that only one value is within normal limits and that effective therapy is very likely to achieve normal results. Review: the expected effects of this medication and the normal potassium level and sodium polystyrene sulfonate (Kayexalate).
Reference(s): Hodgson, Kizior (2014), pp. 1094-1095; Kee, Hayes, McCuistion (2012), p. 235; Pagana, Pagana (2013), p. 741.

1237. The nurse assesses a client after abdominal surgery who has a nasogastric tube (NG) in place that is connected to suction. Which observation by the nurse indicates **most** reliably that the tube is functioning properly?
1. The suction gauge reads low intermittent suction.
2. The client indicates that pain is a 3 on a scale of 1 to 10.
3. The distal end of the NG tube is pinned to the client's gown.
4. The client denies nausea and has 250 mL of fluid in the suction collection container.

Level of Cognitive Ability: Evaluating
Client Needs: Physiological Integrity
Integrated Process: Nursing Process/Evaluation
Content Area: Adult Health: Gastrointestinal
Priority Concepts: Clinical Judgment; Safety

Answer: 4
Rationale: An NG tube connected to suction is used postoperatively to decompress and rest the bowel. The gastrointestinal tract lacks peristaltic activity as a result of manipulation during surgery. The client should not experience symptoms of ileus (nausea and vomiting) if the tube is functioning properly. Although the nurse makes pertinent observations of the tube to ensure that it is secure and properly connected to suction, the client is assessed for the effect. A pain indicator of 3 is an expected finding in a postoperative client.
Priority Nursing Tip: To determine the true or actual amount of nasogastric drainage during a nursing shift, subtract the amount of irrigating solution used during the shift from the amount of drainage in the collection device.
Test-Taking Strategy: Focus on the subject that the nasogastric tube (NG) is functioning properly. Recalling the purpose of an NG tube in a postoperative client will direct you to option 4. Review: the care of the client with a nasogastric tube (NG).
Reference(s): Ignatavicius, Workman (2013), p. 290; Potter et al (2013), p. 1119.

1238. The nurse is caring for a client who has returned from the postanesthesia care unit after prostatectomy. The client has a three-way Foley catheter with an infusion of continuous bladder irrigation (CBI). Which color description of the urinary drainage should lead the nurse to determine that the flow rate is adequate?

1. Dark cherry
2. Clear as water
3. Pale yellow or slightly pink
4. Concentrated yellow with small clots

Level of Cognitive Ability: Evaluating
Client Needs: Physiological Integrity
Integrated Process: Nursing Process/Evaluation
Content Area: Adult Health: Renal and Urinary
Priority Concepts: Clinical Judgment; Elimination

Answer: 3
Rationale: The infusion of bladder irrigant is not at a preset rate; rather, it is increased or decreased to maintain urine that is a clear, pale yellow color or has just a slight pink tinge. The infusion rate should be increased if the drainage is cherry colored or if clots are seen. Alternatively, the rate can be slowed down slightly if the returns are as clear as water.
Priority Nursing Tip: If the client is receiving an infusion of continuous bladder irrigation (CBI), use only sterile bladder irrigation solution or the prescribed solution to prevent water intoxication.
Test-Taking Strategy: Note the subject, an indication of an adequate flow rate of CBI. With this in mind, eliminate option 4 because clots are not expected. Next, eliminate options 1 and 2 as reflecting inadequate or excessive irrigation flow, respectively. Review: the care of the client with of continuous bladder irrigation (CBI).
Reference(s): Ignatavicius, Workman (2013), pp. 290, 1478.

1239. The nurse who is caring for a client with Graves' disease is concerned about the client's calorie intake because of the resulting hypercatabolic state of the disorder. Which situation indicates a successful outcome for this concern?

1. The client verbalizes the need to avoid snacking between meals.
2. The client discusses the relationship between mealtime and the blood glucose level.
3. The client maintains a normal weight or gradually gains weight if it is below normal.
4. The client demonstrates knowledge regarding the need to consume a diet that is high in fat and low in protein.

Level of Cognitive Ability: Evaluating
Client Needs: Physiological Integrity
Integrated Process: Nursing Process/Evaluation
Content Area: Adult Health: Endocrine
Priority Concepts: Immunity; Nutrition

Answer: 3
Rationale: Graves' disease causes a state of chronic nutritional and caloric deficiency caused by the metabolic effects of excessive T3 and T4. Clinical manifestations are weight loss and increased appetite. Therefore, it is a nutritional goal that the client will not lose additional weight and he or she will gradually return to the ideal body weight, if necessary. To accomplish this, the client must be encouraged to eat frequent high-calorie, high-protein, and high-carbohydrate meals and snacks.
Priority Nursing Tip: Provide a high-calorie diet to a client with Graves' disease because of the increased metabolic effects that is characteristic of the disorder.
Test-Taking Strategy: Focus on the subject, the client's need to manage his/her hypercatabolic state. Options 1 and 4 would not be beneficial for a client in a hypercatabolic state. Option 2 can be eliminated because discussing the fluctuation in the blood glucose level will not be helpful for a client who is hypermetabolic. Review: imbalanced nutrition and Graves' disease.
Reference(s): Ignatavicius, Workman (2013), pp. 1366-1367, 1395.

1240. The nurse is reviewing the results of a client's phenytoin (Dilantin) level that was drawn that morning. What result indicates the client has reached a therapeutic drug level?

1. 3 mcg/mL
2. 8 mcg/mL
3. 15 mcg/mL
4. 24 mcg/mL

Level of Cognitive Ability: Understanding
Client Needs: Physiological Integrity
Integrated Process: Nursing Process/Evaluation
Content Area: Pharmacology: Neurological Medications
Priority Concepts: Clinical Judgment; Safety

Answer: 3
Rationale: The therapeutic range for serum phenytoin levels is 10 to 20 mcg/mL in clients with normal serum albumin levels and renal function. A level below this range indicates that the client is not receiving sufficient medication and is at risk for seizure activity. In this case, the medication dose should be adjusted upward. A level above the therapeutic range indicates that the client is entering the toxic range and is at risk for toxic side effects of the medication. In this case, the dose should be adjusted downward.
Priority Nursing Tip: The client prescribed phenytoin (Dilantin) needs to be informed of the need for monitoring therapeutic serum drug levels to assess for toxicity.
Test-Taking Strategy: Focus on the subject, the therapeutic drug serum level. Recalling that this level for phenytoin is 10 to 20 mcg/mL will direct you to option 3. Review: **phenytoin (Dilantin)**.
Reference(s): Hodgson, Kizior (2014), p. 947.

1241. The nurse instructs a parent regarding the appropriate actions to take when the toddler has a temper tantrum. Which statement by the parent indicates a successful outcome of the teaching?

1. "I will ignore the tantrums as long as there is no physical danger."
2. "I will give frequent reminders that only bad children have tantrums."
3. "I will send my child to a room alone for 10 minutes after every tantrum."
4. "I will reward my child with candy at the end of each day without a tantrum."

Level of Cognitive Ability: Evaluating
Client Needs: Health Promotion and Maintenance
Integrated Process: Nursing Process/Evaluation
Content Area: Developmental Stages: Infancy to Adolescence
Priority Concepts: Client Education; Development

Answer: 1
Rationale: Ignoring a negative attention-seeking behavior is considered the best way to extinguish it, provided that the child is safe from injury. Option 2 is untrue and negative. Option 3 gives attention to the tantrum and also exceeds the recommended time of 1 minute per year of age for a time out. Providing candy for rewards is unhealthy and unlikely to be effective at the end of the day.
Priority Nursing Tip: Anticipate temper tantrums from a toddler. Ensure a safe environment if the toddler displays physical acting-out behaviors.
Test-Taking Strategy: Focus on the subject, toddler tantrum management. Recalling that ignoring a tantrum is the best way to extinguish it will direct you to option 1. Review: the interventions for the child who has **temper tantrums**.
Reference(s): McKinney et al (2013), p. 138.

1242. The nurse is caring for a client who is in seclusion. Which client statement indicates to the nurse that the seclusion is no longer necessary?

1. "I am in control of myself now."
2. "I need to use the restroom right away."
3. "I'd like to go back to my room and be alone for a while."
4. "I can't breathe in here. It feels like the walls are closing in on me."

Level of Cognitive Ability: Evaluating
Client Needs: Psychosocial Integrity
Integrated Process: Nursing Process/Evaluation
Content Area: Mental Health
Priority Concepts: Clinical Judgment; Safety

Answer: 1
Rationale: Option 1 indicates that the client may be safely removed from seclusion. The client in seclusion must be assessed at regular intervals (usually every 15 to 30 minutes) for physical needs, safety, and comfort. Option 2 indicates a physical need that could be met with a urinal, bedpan, or commode; it does not indicate that the client has calmed down enough to leave the seclusion room. Option 3 could be an attempt to manipulate the nurse; it gives no indication that the client will control himself or herself when alone in the room. Option 4 could be handled by supportive communication or an as-needed medication, if indicated; it does not necessitate discontinuing seclusion.
Priority Nursing Tip: Within 1 hour of the initiation of restraints or seclusion of a client with a mental health disorder, the psychiatrist must make a face-to-face assessment and evaluation of the client. Agency and state policies and procedures regarding the use of restraints and seclusion are always followed.
Test-Taking Strategy: Focus on the subject, removing a client from seclusion. Recalling the purpose and the use of seclusion will direct you to option 1. Review: seclusion procedures.
Reference(s): Stuart, G. (2013), p. 588; Varcarolis (2013), pp. 85-86.

1243. The nurse has developed a plan of care to include interventions focused on reassuming self-care for a client who is in traction. The nurse evaluates the plan of care and determines that which observation indicates a successful outcome?

1. The client refuses care.
2. The client allows the family to assist in the care.
3. The client assists in self-care as much as possible.
4. The client allows the nurse to complete the care on a daily basis.

Level of Cognitive Ability: Evaluating
Client Needs: Physiological Integrity
Integrated Process: Nursing Process/Evaluation
Content Area: Adult Health: Musculoskeletal
Priority Concepts: Clinical Judgment; Health Promotion

Answer: 3
Rationale: A successful outcome for reassuming self-care is for the client to do as much of the self-care as possible. The nurse should promote independence in the client and allow the client to perform as much self-care as is optimal considering the client's condition. The nurse would determine that the outcome is unsuccessful if the client refuses care or allows others to perform the care.
Priority Nursing Tip: To maintain self-esteem and client dignity, the nurse should encourage and maintain client independence in the performance of activities of daily living as much as possible.
Test-Taking Strategy: Focus on the subject, reassuming of self-care. Option 1 can be eliminated first because the client is refusing care. Note that options 2 and 4 are comparable or alike in that they indicate relying on others to perform care. Review: successful outcomes related to self-care.
Reference(s): Ignatavicius, Workman (2013), pp. 1157-1158.

❖ **1244.** The nurse is monitoring a male client with a spinal cord injury who is experiencing spinal shock. Which findings indicate that the spinal shock is resolving? **Select all that apply.**
- ❑ 1. Flaccidity
- ❑ 2. Presence of a gag reflex
- ❑ 3. Positive Babinski's reflex
- ❑ 4. Development of hyperreflexia
- ❑ 5. Return of the bulbocavernous reflex
- ❑ 6. Return of reflex emptying of the bladder

Level of Cognitive Ability: Evaluating
Client Needs: Physiological Integrity
Integrated Process: Nursing Process/Evaluation
Content Area: Adult Health: Neurological
Priority Concepts: Intracranial Regulation; Mobility

Answer: 3, 4, 5, 6
Rationale: Spinal shock is associated with acute injury to the spinal cord with temporary suppression of reflexes controlled by segments below the level of injury. It may last for 1 to 6 weeks. Indications that spinal shock is resolving include return of reflexes, development of hyperreflexia rather than flaccidity, and return of reflex emptying of the bladder. The return of the bulbocavernous reflex in male clients is also an early indicator of recovery from spinal shock. Babinski's reflex (dorsiflexion of the great toe with fanning of the other toes when the sole of the foot is stroked) is an early returning reflex. The gag reflex is not lost in spinal shock; therefore, its presence is not an indication of resolving spinal shock.
Priority Nursing Tip: For clients with spinal cord injuries above the level of T6, autonomic dysreflexia may occur as a result of autonomic nervous system overstimulation. The clinical manifestations include severe hypertension, throbbing headaches, diaphoresis, nasal stuffiness, flushing above the level of the injury, and bradycardia.
Test-Taking Strategy: Focus on the subject, indications that spinal shock is resolving. As you read each option, recall that spinal shock is associated with acute injury to the spinal cord with temporary suppression of reflexes controlled by segments below the level of injury. This will assist in eliminating flaccidity and the presence of a gag reflex as signs that spinal shock is resolving. Review: the indications that spinal shock is resolving.
Reference(s): Ignatavicius, Workman (2013), pp. 969-970.

❖ **1245.** The nurse is caring for a client on mechanical ventilation via an oral endotracheal tube. What are the possible causes of the high-pressure alarm sounding? **Select all that apply.**
- ❑ 1. A kink in the tube
- ❑ 2. The client fighting the ventilator
- ❑ 3. Increased secretions in the airway
- ❑ 4. A cuff leak in the endotracheal tube
- ❑ 5. The client biting on the endotracheal tube
- ❑ 6. The ventilator tubing disconnecting from the endotracheal tube

Level of Cognitive Ability: Evaluating
Client Needs: Physiological Integrity
Integrated Process: Nursing Process/Evaluation
Content Area: Adult Health: Respiratory
Priority Concepts: Clinical Judgment; Gas Exchange

Answer: 1, 2, 3, 5
Rationale: The high-pressure alarm sounds when the peak inspiratory pressure reaches the set alarm limit. Causes include obstruction of the endotracheal tube because of the client lying on the tube or water or a kink in the tubing; the client being anxious or fighting the ventilator; an increased amount of secretions in the airways or a mucous plug; the client coughing, gagging, or biting on the oral endotracheal tube; decreased airway size related to wheezing or bronchospasm; pneumothorax; and displacement of the artificial airway and the endotracheal tube slipping into the right main stem bronchus. The low-pressure alarm sounds when there is a leak or disconnection in the ventilator circuit or a leak in the client's artificial airway cuff.
Priority Nursing Tip: The nurse never shuts the alarms on a ventilator to the off position.
Test-Taking Strategy: Focus on the subject, the triggers of the high-pressure alarm. Recalling that the high-pressure alarm sounds when the peak inspiratory pressure reaches the set alarm limit assists in eliminating options 4 and 6. In addition, remember that "L" in "low" can be associated with "L" in "leak" for low-pressure alarms. Review: the causes of ventilator alarms.
Reference(s): Ignatavicius, Workman (2013), p. 680.

Test 5

1246. The clinic nurse is observing a student perform a complete physical assessment on a client. During the respiratory assessment, the clinic nurse determines that the student is using which physical assessment technique? **Refer to figure.**

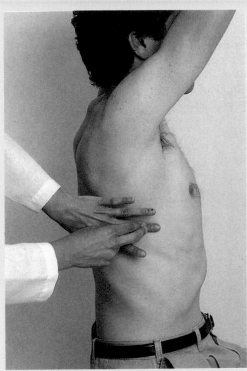

Figure from Wilson SF, Giddens JF: *Health assessment for nursing practice*, ed 5, St. Louis, 2013, Mosby.

1. Palpation
2. Inspection
3. Percussion
4. Auscultation

Level of Cognitive Ability: Evaluating
Client Needs: Health Promotion and Maintenance
Integrated Process: Nursing Process/Evaluating
Content Area: Developmental Stages: Health Assessment/Physical Exam
Priority Concepts: Gas Exchange; Health Promotion

Answer: 3
Rationale: To perform percussion, the nurse places the middle finger of the nondominant hand against the body's surface. The tip of the middle finger of the dominant hand strikes the top of the middle finger of the nondominant hand. Palpation is performed using the sense of touch. Inspection is the process of observation. Auscultation involves listening to the sounds produced by the body.
Priority Nursing Tip: When auscultating breath sounds, instruct the client to breathe through the mouth. Monitor the client for dizziness and provide a rest period if dizziness occurs.
Test-Taking Strategy: Focus on the subject, identifying assessment techniques. Recalling the definition of each technique listed in the options will direct you to option 3. Remember that inspection is observing, palpation uses the sense of touch, and auscultating is listening. Review: **physical assessment techniques and percussion.**
Reference(s): Jarvis (2012), pp. 116, 475.

1247. The nurse is reviewing a plan of care prepared by a nursing student for an infant being admitted to the hospital with a diagnosis of heart failure (HF). Which intervention should the nurse recognize as needing revision?

1. Elevate the head of the bed.
2. Provide oxygen during stressful periods.
3. Limit the time that the infant is allowed to bottle-feed.
4. Wake the infant for feedings to ensure adequate nutrition.

Level of Cognitive Ability: Evaluating
Client Needs: Physiological Integrity
Integrated Process: Nursing Process/Evaluation
Content Area: Child Health: Cardiovascular
Priority Concepts: Development; Perfusion

Answer: 4
Rationale: Awaking the child is not therapeutic in this situation. Measures that will decrease the workload on the heart include limiting the time that the infant is allowed to bottle-feed or breast-feed, elevating the head of the bed, allowing for uninterrupted rest periods, and providing oxygen during stressful periods.
Priority Nursing Tip: An early sign of heart failure in an infant is tachycardia, especially during rest or with slight exertion.
Test-Taking Strategy: Note the words, *needing revision*. This is a negative event query and asks you to select an incorrect option. Review each option carefully, and recall that the goal for an infant with HF is to decrease the workload on the heart. Option 4 is the only option that will not ensure this goal. Review: the measures associated with caring for the **infant with heart failure**.
Reference(s): Hockenberry, Wilson (2013), pp. 837-838.

1248. The nurse has provided self-care activity instructions to a client after the insertion of an internal cardioverter-defibrillator (ICD). The nurse determines that **further instruction is needed** if the client makes which statement?

1. "I need to avoid doing anything where there would be rough contact with the ICD insertion site."
2. "I can perform activities such as swimming, driving, or operating heavy equipment as I need to do them."
3. "I should try to avoid doing strenuous things that would make my heart rate go up to or above the rate cut-off on the ICD."
4. "I should keep away from electromagnetic sources such as transformers, large electrical generators, and metal detectors as well as running motors."

Level of Cognitive Ability: Evaluating
Client Needs: Safe and Effective Care Environment
Integrated Process: Nursing Process/Evaluation
Content Area: Adult Health: Cardiovascular
Priority Concepts: Client Education; Perfusion

Answer: 2
Rationale: Post-discharge instructions typically include avoiding the following: tight clothing or belts over the ICD insertion site; rough contact with the ICD insertion site; electromagnetic fields, such as those surrounding electrical transformers; radio, television, and radar transmitters; metal detectors; and the running motors of cars or boats. Clients must also alert health care providers or dentists to the presence of the device because certain procedures such as diathermy, electrocautery, and magnetic resonance imaging may need to be avoided to prevent device malfunction. Clients should follow the specific advice of a health care provider regarding activities that are potentially hazardous to the self or others, such as swimming, driving, or operating heavy equipment.
Priority Nursing Tip: The nurse who is caring for the client after insertion of an internal cardioverter-defibrillator needs to assess the device settings. Care is similar to that implemented after insertion of a permanent pacemaker.
Test-Taking Strategy: Note the strategic words, *further instruction is needed*, and that this indicates a negative event query. Options 1 and 4 can be eliminated first because they are similar to standard post-pacemaker insertion instructions. From the remaining choices, noting the words *heavy equipment* in option 2 will direct you to this option. Review: the client teaching points for **internal cardioverter-defibrillator (ICD)**.
Reference(s): Ignatavicius, Workman (2013), pp. 741-742.

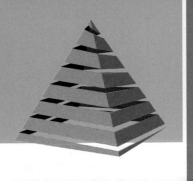

Comprehensive Test

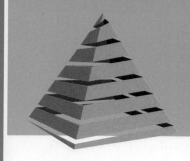
Comprehensive Test

❖ **1249.** The nurse is monitoring a client who is receiving a blood transfusion when the client complains of diaphoresis, warmth, and a backache. The nurse suspects a transfusion reaction and should take which actions? **Select all that apply.**
❑ 1. Remove the IV catheter.
❑ 2. Document the occurrence.
❑ 3. Stop the blood transfusion.
❑ 4. Contact the health care provider.
❑ 5. Hang 0.9% sodium chloride solution.

Level of Cognitive Ability: Applying
Client Needs: Physiological Integrity
Integrated Process: Nursing Process/Implementation
Content Area: Critical Care: Blood Administration
Priority Concepts: Clinical Judgment; Safety

Answer: 2, 3, 4, 5
Rationale: If a client experiences a transfusion reaction, the nurse stops the transfusion and prevents the infusion of any additional blood; then the nurse hangs a bag of 0.9% sodium chloride solution. This maintains IV access and helps maintain the client's intravascular volume. The health care provider is notified, as is the blood bank. The nurse also documents the occurrence, the actions taken, and the client's response. To preserve the IV access, the nurse should not remove the catheter and discontinue the IV site.
Priority Nursing Tip: If the client experiences a transfusion reaction, stay with the client and monitor the vital signs.
Test-Taking Strategy: Note the subject, actions to take if a transfusion reaction occurs. Focus on the physiological occurrence of a transfusion reaction. Read each option carefully and recall that an IV site is needed to administer fluids and emergency medications. Review: interventions when a **transfusion reaction** occurs.
Reference(s): Ignatavicius, Workman (2013), pp. 900-901; Potter et al (2013), pp. 912-913.

1250. The nurse assesses a client admitted to the hospital with rib fractures to identify the risk for potential complications. The nurse notes that the client has a history of emphysema. After the assessment, the nurse ensures that which interventions are documented in the plan of care? **Select all that apply.**

❏ 1. Maintain the client in a position of comfort.
❏ 2. Collect sputum specimens at the hour of sleep.
❏ 3. Offer medication to suppress the cough as needed.
❏ 4. Administer small, frequent meals with plenty of fluids.
❏ 5. Have the client cough and breathe deeply 20 minutes after pain medication is given.
❏ 6. Administer 4 to 6 liters of oxygen when the client's pulse oximetry drops below 90%.

Level of Cognitive Ability: Analyzing
Client Needs: Physiological Integrity
Integrated Process: Nursing Process/Implementation
Content Area: Adult Health: Respiratory
Priority Concepts: Gas Exchange; Pain

Answer: 1, 4, 5
Rationale: Clients with rib fractures need interventions focused on their ability to maintain an effective breathing pattern and support the body in the healing process. Breathing effort is supported when the client is maintained in a comfortable position. Giving the client small frequent meals with plenty of fluids prevents the client from doing too much eating activity at one time and provides hydration to keep sputum liquefied for easier expectoration. Giving the client prescribed pain medication first and then having the client cough and deep breath will encourage the client to complete these actions while limiting the amount of pain from doing them. If sputum specimen collection is prescribed, the specimen should be collected early in the morning upon the client's awakening. Clients with emphysema are not given cough suppressants because expectoration of sputum is essential to airway clearance. Giving the client with emphysema a high flow of oxygen would halt the hypoxic drive and cause apnea.
Priority Nursing Tip: Monitor the client with rib fractures for changes in respiratory rate or depth. Alterations in respiratory patterns can be caused by pain or a complication of the fractures.
Test-Taking Strategy: Note the subject, interventions for the client with emphysema who experienced a rib fracture. Focus on the data in the question and note that the client has emphysema. Recalling the pathophysiology associated with emphysema will assist in determining the correct options. Review: the complications that can occur in the client with **emphysema**.
Reference(s): Ignatavicius, Workman (2013), pp. 618, 621; Lewis et al (2014), p. 588.

1251. A client has been given a prescription to begin using nitroglycerin transdermal medication patches in the management of coronary artery disease. The nurse instructs the client about this medication administration system and provides which information?

1. Apply a new medication patch every 7 days.
2. Wait 1 day to apply a new medication patch if it becomes dislodged.
3. Place the medication patch in the area of a skinfold to promote better adherence.
4. Apply the medication patch in the morning and leave it in place for 12 to 16 hours as directed.

Level of Cognitive Ability: Applying
Client Needs: Physiological Integrity
Integrated Process: Teaching and Learning
Content Area: Pharmacology: Cardiovascular Medications
Priority Concepts: Client Education; Safety

Answer: 4
Rationale: Nitroglycerin is a coronary vasodilator used in the management of coronary artery disease. The client is generally advised to apply a new medication patch each morning and leave it in place for 12 to 16 hours as the health care provider prescribes. The client needs the medication patch applied daily, not every 7 days, to ensure proper dosing is released as prescribed by the health care provider. The client can apply a new medication patch if it becomes dislodged because the dose is released continuously in small amounts through the skin. The client should avoid placing the medication patch in skinfolds or excoriated areas for appropriate absorption.
Priority Nursing Tip: Instruct the client using nitroglycerin transdermal patches to rotate the application sites daily.
Test-Taking Strategy: Focus on the subject, client instructions for using a nitroglycerin patch. Specific information related to this type of medication administration system is needed to answer this question. Reading each option carefully and recalling that tolerance can occur with this medication will direct you to option 4. Review: the procedures related to **transdermal medication patches**.
Reference(s): Lehne (2013), pp. 622, 629.

1252. A 9-year-old child is newly diagnosed with type 1 diabetes mellitus. The nurse is planning for home care with the child and his family and determines that which is an age-appropriate activity for this child for health maintenance?
1. Administering insulin drawn up by an adult
2. Self-administering insulin with adult supervision
3. Making independent decisions with regard to sliding-scale coverage of insulin
4. Having an adult assist in the self-administration of insulin and glucose monitoring

Level of Cognitive Ability: Analyzing
Client Needs: Health Promotion and Maintenance
Integrated Process: Nursing Process/Planning
Content Area: Developmental Stages: Infancy to Adolescence
Priority Concepts: Development; Glucose Regulation

Answer: 2
Rationale: School-age children have the cognitive and motor skills to draw up and administer insulin with adult supervision. Developmentally, they do not yet have the maturity to make independent decisions such as about sliding-scale coverage without adult validation. Options 1 and 4 suppress the maximum level of independence appropriate to the level of this child.
Priority Nursing Tip: The developmental task of the school-age child is developing social, physical, and learning skills. The nurse should encourage the school-age child with diabetes mellitus to become involved with his or her care.
Test-Taking Strategy: Focus on the subject, age-appropriate activities for a 9-year-old child. Focusing on the age of the child will assist in eliminating options 1 and 4. From the remaining choices, recalling that in this age group decision making is a cognitive skill that develops later than motor skills will direct you to option 2. Review: growth and development of the 9-year-old child.
Reference(s): McKinney et al (2013), pp. 1404-1405.

1253. The nurse teaches a pregnant client to perform Kegel exercises. Which statement by the client indicates an understanding of the purpose of these types of exercises?
1. "The exercises will help reduce backache."
2. "The exercises will help prevent ankle edema."
3. "The exercises will help prevent urinary tract infections."
4. "The exercises will help strengthen the pelvic floor in preparation for delivery."

Level of Cognitive Ability: Evaluating
Client Needs: Health Promotion and Maintenance
Integrated Process: Nursing Process/Evaluation
Content Area: Maternity: Antepartum
Priority Concepts: Health Promotion; Reproduction

Answer: 4
Rationale: Kegel exercises assist in strengthening the pelvic floor (pubococcygeal muscle). Pelvic tilt exercises help reduce backaches. Leg elevation assists in preventing ankle edema. Instructing a client to drink 8 ounces of fluids 6 times a day helps prevent urinary tract infections.
Priority Nursing Tip: Kegel exercises strengthen the pelvic floor and will assist in alleviating the urinary urgency and frequency that occur in the first and third trimester of pregnancy.
Test-Taking Strategy: Focus on the subject, Kegel exercises. Thinking about how these exercises are performed will assist in answering correctly. Remember that Kegel exercises will help strengthen the pelvic floor muscles. Review: the purpose of Kegel exercises.
Reference(s): Lowdermilk, Perry, Cashion, Alden (2012), pp. 91, 345; McKinney et al (2013), p. 794.

1254. The care provider prescribes an antibiotic, and 650 mg needs to be administered intravenously every 6 hours. The medication label reads as follows: reconstitute with 4.8 mL of bacteriostatic water to yield 2 g in 5 mL. How many mL should the nurse withdraw from the vial for one dose? **Fill in the blank. Record the answer using one decimal place.**

Answer: _____ mL

Level of Cognitive Ability: Applying
Client Needs: Physiological Integrity
Integrated Process: Nursing Process/Implementation
Content Area: Fundamental Skills: Medications/ IV Calculations
Priority Concepts: Clinical Judgment; Safety

Answer: 1.6 mL
Rationale: Convert 2 g to mg and then use the formula for calculating medication doses. In the metric system, to convert larger to smaller, multiply by 1000 or move the decimal three places to the right. Therefore, 2 g = 2000 mg.

Formula:

$$\frac{\text{Desired}}{\text{Available}} \times mL = mL \text{ per dose}$$

$$\frac{650\,mg}{2000\,mg} \times 5\,mL = 1.625\,mL = 1.6\,mL$$

Priority Nursing Tip: Common equivalent to remember is 1000 mg = 1 g. Always use the dosage strength provided on the medication label when determining accurate dose.
Test-Taking Strategy: Focus on the subject, the amount of medication to be administered for one dose. Identify the components of the question and what the question is asking. In this case, the question asks for the milliliters per dose. Convert grams to milligrams first. Next, use the formula to determine the correct dose, knowing that 2000 mg = 5.0 mL. Finally record the answer using one decimal place. Review: **medication calculations**.
Reference(s): Potter et al (2013), pp. 573-574.

1255. A child with sickle cell disease is admitted to the hospital for treatment of vaso-occlusive pain crisis. The nurse should plan for which interventions in the care of the client? **Select all that apply.**
  ❏ 1. Increase fluid intake.
  ❏ 2. Administer oxygen.
  ❏ 3. Perform frequent pain assessment.
  ❏ 4. Administer intravenous (IV) fluids.
  ❏ 5. Administer meperidine hydrochloride (Demerol).

Level of Cognitive Ability: Analyzing
Client Needs: Safe and Effective Care Environment
Integrated Process: Nursing Process/Implementation
Content Area: Fundamental Skills: Pain
Priority Concepts: Clinical Judgment; Pain

Answer: 1, 2, 3, 4
Rationale: Management of the severe pain that occurs with vaso-occlusive crisis includes frequent pain assessment and the use of strong opioid analgesics, such as morphine sulfate and hydromorphone hydrochloride (Dilaudid). Meperidine hydrochloride is contraindicated because of its side effects and increased risk of seizures. Fluids are necessary to promote hydration, so options 1 and 4 are appropriate. Oxygen is administered to increase tissue perfusion.
Priority Nursing Tip: To prevent the sickling of blood cells in the client with sickle cell disease, it is important to maintain adequate hydration and blood flow through oral and intravenously administered fluids.
Test-Taking Strategy: Focus on the subject, care of the client with vaso-occlusive pain crisis. Use the ABCs—airway, breathing, and circulation—to assist to answer correctly. Also recall that meperidine hydrochloride is contraindicated because of its side effects and increased risk of seizures. Review: care of the client with **sickle cell disease**.
Reference(s): McKinney et al (2013), p. 1248.

1256. A newborn infant receives the first dose of hepatitis B vaccine (Recombivax HB, Engerix-B) within 12 hours of birth. The nurse instructs the mother regarding the immunization schedule for this vaccine and should tell the mother that the second vaccine is administered at which time periods?

1. 3 years of age and then during the adolescent years
2. 8 months of age and then 1 year after the initial dose
3. 6 months of age and then 8 months after the initial dose
4. 1 to 2 months of age and then 6 months after the initial dose

Level of Cognitive Ability: Applying
Client Needs: Health Promotion and Maintenance
Integrated Process: Teaching and Learning
Content Area: Child Health: Infectious and Communicable Diseases
Priority Concepts: Development; Health Promotion

Answer: 4
Rationale: The vaccination schedule for an infant whose mother tests negative for hepatitis B consists of a series of 3 immunizations given at 0 months (birth), 1 to 2 months of age, and then 6 months after the initial dose. An infant whose mother tests positive receives hepatitis B immune globulin (HepaGam B) along with the first dose of the hepatitis vaccine within 12 hours of birth.
Priority Nursing Tip: Immunization schedules must be followed. The nurse needs to document immunization administration on a vaccination card for parents to maintain a record of immunizations administered.
Test-Taking Strategy: Focus on the subject, the hepatitis B vaccine schedule. Knowledge regarding the immunization schedule for hepatitis B vaccine is required to answer this question. Remember that the vaccination schedule consists of a series of three immunizations given at 0 months (birth), 1 to 2 months of age, and then 6 months after the initial dose. Review the hepatitis B vaccine schedule if you are unfamiliar with it.
Reference(s): Hockenberry, Wilson (2013), p. 209; Lowdermilk, Perry, Cashion, Alden (2012), p. 583.

1257. The nurse assesses the client with a diagnosis of thyroid storm. Which manifestations associated with thyroid storm indicate the need for **immediate** nursing intervention?

1. Polyuria, nausea, and severe headaches
2. Hypotension, translucent skin, and obesity
3. Fever, tachycardia, and systolic hypertension
4. Profuse diaphoresis, flushing, and constipation

Level of Cognitive Ability: Analyzing
Client Needs: Physiological Integrity
Integrated Process: Nursing Process/Assessment
Content Area: Adult Health: Endocrine
Priority Concepts: Clinical Judgment; Thermoregulation

Answer: 3
Rationale: The excessive amounts of thyroid hormone cause a rapid increase in the metabolic rate, thereby causing the manifestations of thyroid storm such as fever, tachycardia, and hypertension. When these signs present themselves, the nurse must take quick action to prevent deterioration of the client's health because death can ensue. Priority interventions include maintaining a patent airway and stabilizing the hemodynamic status. Options 1, 2, and 4 do not indicate the need for immediate nursing intervention.
Priority Nursing Tip: Maintaining a patent airway and monitoring vital signs closely are priority interventions for the client with thyroid storm.
Test-Taking Strategy: Note the strategic word, *immediate*. Tachycardia, hypertension, and a fever indicate hemodynamic instability and take precedence over the manifestations identified in options 1, 2, and 4. Additionally option 3 is the only choice that identifies all the manifestations of thyroid storm. Review: thyroid storm.
Reference(s): Ignatavicius, Workman (2013), p. 1399.

1258. A client is hospitalized for ingesting an overdose of acetaminophen (Tylenol). The nurse prepares to administer which specific antidote for this medication overdose?

1. Protamine sulfate
2. Phytonadione (Vitamin K)
3. Acetylcysteine (Acetadote)
4. Naloxone hydrochloride (Narcan)

Level of Cognitive Ability: Analyzing
Client Needs: Physiological Integrity
Integrated Process: Nursing Process/Planning
Content Area: Critical Care: Emergency Situations
Priority Concepts: Clinical Judgment; Safety

Answer: 3
Rationale: Acetylcysteine restores sulfhydryl groups that are depleted by acetaminophen metabolism. Protamine sulfate is the antidote for heparin. Vitamin K is the antidote for warfarin sodium (Coumadin). Naloxone hydrochloride reverses respiratory depression.
Priority Nursing Tip: Acetaminophen (Tylenol) is contraindicated in clients with hepatic or renal disease, alcoholism, and/or hypersensitivity.
Test-Taking Strategy: Focus on the subject, the antidote for acetaminophen overdose. Recalling the specific antidotes for both heparin and warfarin sodium will assist in eliminating options 1 and 2. Next, recalling that naloxone hydrochloride reverses respiratory depression will assist in eliminating option 4. Review: the antidote for acetaminophen (Tylenol) overdose.
Reference(s): Hodgson, Kizior (2014), p. 11.

1259. The nurse is caring for a client at risk for suicide. Which client behavior is **most** indicative that the client may be contemplating suicide?
1. The client shares that he is finally happy.
2. The client sits and cries for long periods of time.
3. The client prefers to spend long periods of time alone.
4. The client reports a variety of sleep pattern disturbances.

Level of Cognitive Ability: Analyzing
Client Needs: Psychosocial Integrity
Integrated Process: Nursing Process/Analysis
Content Area: Mental Health
Priority Concepts: Moods and Affect; Safety

Answer: 1
Rationale: If a client displays a suicidal ideation and is able to share a plan, it should be taken very seriously and suicide precautions should be implemented. Option 1 shows a contentment that is often a sign that a suicide plan has been created. Options 2, 3, and 4 are indicative of depression but are not as definitive as option 1 in regard to suicide.
Priority Nursing Tip: A sudden change in affect and mood with the client at risk for suicide needs to be further explored because it may indicate a suicide plan has been developed.
Test-Taking Strategy: Note the strategic word, *most*, and focus on the subject, suicide. Recalling that signs of suicidal ideation are the formulation of a suicidal plan and a change in behavior will direct you to option 1. Review: assessment of the client at risk for **suicide**.
Reference(s): Stuart (2013), p. 337; Varcarolis (2013), p. 441.

1260. The nurse is reviewing the record of a client who was admitted to the hospital for diagnostic studies after a fainting spell. The nurse notes that the client is receiving olanzapine (Zyprexa). Which disorder or condition should the nurse suspect in the client?
1. History of schizophrenia
2. History of diabetes mellitus
3. History of diabetes insipidus
4. History of coronary artery disease

Level of Cognitive Ability: Analyzing
Client Needs: Physiological Integrity
Integrated Process: Nursing Process/Analysis
Content Area: Mental Health
Priority Concepts: Psychosis; Safety

Answer: 1
Rationale: Olanzapine is an antipsychotic medication used in the management of manifestations associated with psychotic disorders. It is the first-line treatment for schizophrenia, targeting both the positive and the negative symptoms. Options 2, 3, and 4 are not indicated uses for this medication.
Priority Nursing Tip: Instruct the client who is taking olanzapine (Zyprexa) to change positions slowly to avoid orthostatic hypotension.
Test-Taking Strategy: Focus on the subject, olanzapine (Zyprexa). Recalling that this medication is an antipsychotic will direct you to option 1. Review: the antipsychotic medication **olanzapine (Zyprexa)**.
Reference(s): Hodgson, Kizior (2014), pp. 863-864.

1261. A client is admitted to the hospital for a thyroidectomy. While preparing the client for surgery, the nurse assesses the client for psychosocial problems that may cause preoperative anxiety and determines which client fear is a realistic source of anxiety?
1. Sexual dysfunction and infertility
2. Imposed dietary restrictions after discharge
3. Developing gynecomastia and hirsutism postoperatively
4. Changes in body image secondary to the location of the incision

Level of Cognitive Ability: Analyzing
Client Needs: Psychosocial Integrity
Integrated Process: Nursing Process/Assessment
Content Area: Adult Health: Endocrine
Priority Concepts: Anxiety; Coping

Answer: 4
Rationale: Because the incision is in the neck area, the client may be fearful of having a large scar postoperatively. Sexual dysfunction and infertility could possibly occur if the entire thyroid gland is removed, and the client is not placed on thyroid replacement medications. The client will not have specific dietary restrictions after discharge. Having all or part of the thyroid gland removed will not cause gynecomastia or hirsutism.
Priority Nursing Tip: The appearance of a thyroidectomy incision can be distressing to the client. Reassure him or her that the scar will fade in color and that the scar can be easily covered by a scarf or other item.
Test-Taking Strategy: Focus on the subject, possible psychosocial problems related to a thyroidectomy. Recalling the location of the thyroid gland will direct you to the correct option. Review: the psychosocial concerns of the client after **thyroidectomy**.
Reference(s): Ignatavicius, Workman (2013), p. 1402.

1262. A provider prescribes lipids (fat emulsion) intravenously for a client receiving total parenteral nutrition. Which should the nurse assess before beginning the infusion?

1. Allergies
2. Vital signs
3. History of seizures
4. Serum glucose level

Level of Cognitive Ability: Analyzing
Client Needs: Physiological Integrity
Integrated Process: Nursing Process/Assessment
Content Area: Critical Care: Medications and Intravenous Therapy
Priority Concepts: Nutrition; Safety

Answer: 1

Rationale: Before administering any medication, the nurse assesses for allergies to all of the agent's components. Fat emulsions such as intralipids contain an emulsifying agent made from egg yolks, so clients who are hypersensitive to eggs are at risk for developing hypersensitivity reactions. Options 2, 3, and 4 are unrelated to administering lipids.

Priority Nursing Tip: Lipids (fat emulsion) contain egg yolk phospholipids. If the client has an egg allergy, the health care provider is contacted before administration of the solution.

Test-Taking Strategy: Focus on the subject, nursing responsibilities before administering lipids. This will direct you to option 1. Remember that the nurse always assesses for allergies before administering any medication or intravenous solution. Review: the nursing responsibilities related to the administration of **lipids**.

Reference(s): Lewis, et al (2014), p. 901.

1263. A client is admitted to the hospital with a myocardial infarction and is not experiencing chest pain at this time. The nurse reviews the electrocardiogram (ECG) rhythm strip, notes that the PR intervals are 0.16 seconds, and determines that which is the appropriate interpretation?

1. A normal finding
2. An abnormal finding
3. An impending reinfarction
4. First-degree atrioventricular (AV) block

Level of Cognitive Ability: Analyzing
Client Needs: Physiological Integrity
Integrated Process: Nursing Process/Assessment
Content Area: Adult Health: Cardiovascular
Priority Concepts: Clinical Judgment; Perfusion

Answer: 1

Rationale: The PR interval represents the time it takes for the cardiac impulse to spread from the atria to the ventricles. The PR interval range is 0.12 to 0.2 seconds. Therefore, the finding is normal. Options 2, 3, and 4 all indicate an abnormal finding, so they are not appropriate responses.

Priority Nursing Tip: When performing an electrocardiogram (ECG), the nurse should document on the ECG requisition form any cardiac medications the client is taking.

Test-Taking Strategy: Focus on the subject, the PR interval. Eliminate options 2, 3, and 4 because they are comparable or alike and indicate abnormal findings. Review: basic **electrocardiogram (ECG)** findings.

Reference(s): Potter et al (2013), p. 825.

1264. The nurse administers 30 units of NPH insulin at 7:00 AM to a client with a blood glucose level of 200 mg/dL. The nurse monitors the client for a hypoglycemic reaction, knowing that NPH insulin peaks in approximately how many hours following administration?

1. 1 hour
2. 2 to 3 hours
3. 4 to 12 hours
4. 16 to 24 hours

Level of Cognitive Ability: Applying
Client Needs: Physiological Integrity
Integrated Process: Nursing Process/Assessment
Content Area: Pharmacology: Endocrine
Priority Concepts: Clinical Judgment; Glucose Regulation

Answer: 3

Rationale: NPH is an intermediate-acting insulin with a peak time in 4 to 12 hours. Option 1 and 2 do not describe the peak time for an intermediate-acting insulin. Option 4 describes the duration time of NPH insulin.

Priority Nursing Tip: Instruct the client with diabetes mellitus to recognize the signs and symptoms of hypoglycemia and hyperglycemia and the actions to take if these complications occur.

Test-Taking Strategy: Focus on the subject, peak time of NPH insulin. Knowledge of the onset, peak, and duration of NPH insulin is required. Recalling that NPH is an intermediate-acting insulin will direct you to option 3. Review: the various types of **insulin**, specifically **NPH insulin**.

Reference(s): Lehne (2013), p. 712.

1265. A client with a psychotic disorder is being treated with haloperidol (Haldol). Which sign/symptom should the nurse monitor the client for that indicates an adverse effect of this medication?
1. Nausea
2. Hypotension
3. Blurred vision
4. Excessive drooling

Level of Cognitive Ability: Analyzing
Client Needs: Physiological Integrity
Integrated Process: Nursing Process/Assessment
Content Area: Mental Health
Priority Concepts: Psychosis; Safety

Answer: 4
Rationale: Adverse effects of antipsychotic medications include marked drowsiness and lethargy, extrapyramidal symptoms including parkinsonism effects (drooling), dystonias, akathisia, and tardive dyskinesia. Option 4 is a parkinsonism effect of this medication, excessive drooling. Options 1, 2, and 3, or nausea, hypotension, and blurred vision are occasional side effects.
Priority Nursing Tip: Monitor the serum glucose level in a client taking an antipsychotic medication because these medications can elevate the blood glucose level.
Test-Taking Strategy: Focus on the subject, an adverse effect of haloperidol. Noting the word *excessive* in option 4 will direct you to the correct option. Review: the adverse effects of antipsychotics, specifically, haloperidol (Haldol).
Reference(s): Hodgson, Kizior (2014), p. 559.

1266. A home care nurse visits an older client with acute gouty arthritis. Indomethacin (Indocin) has been prescribed for the client. The nurse teaches the client about the medication and determines there is a **need for further teaching** when the client makes which statement?
1. "I'll rest if I am having pain."
2. "I need to call the office if I notice a rash."
3. "I can take a pill whenever I need to for pain."
4. "I'll watch for any swollen feet or fingers or any stomach distress."

Level of Cognitive Ability: Evaluating
Client Needs: Physiological Integrity
Integrated Process: Teaching and Learning
Content Area: Pharmacology: Musculoskeletal Medications
Priority Concepts: Client Education; Safety

Answer: 3
Rationale: Indomethacin may alleviate pain but is administered on a scheduled time frame, not on an as-needed schedule. Option 1 can be effective to relieve gouty arthritis pain. Option 2 could indicate hypersensitivity to the medication. The client should be instructed to monitor for swelling and gastric distress, which can be caused by the medication.
Priority Nursing Tip: Encourage the client with gout to comply with prescribed therapy to prevent elevated uric acid levels, which can trigger a gout attack.
Test-Taking Strategy: Note the strategic words, *need for further teaching*. These words indicate a negative event query and the need to select the incorrect client statement. Recalling the action and purpose of indomethacin and using general medication guidelines will direct you to option 3. Review: client teaching points for indomethacin (Indocin).
Reference(s): Hodgson, Kizior (2014), pp. 610-611; Lehne (2013), p. 899.

1267. The nurse is teaching a community group about violence in the family. Which statement by a group member would indicate a **need for further teaching**?
1. "Abusers use fear and intimidation."
2. "Abusers usually have poor self-esteem."
3. "Abusers are often jealous or self-centered."
4. "Abuse occurs more in low-income families."

Level of Cognitive Ability: Evaluating
Client Needs: Psychosocial Integrity
Integrated Process: Teaching and Learning
Content Area: Mental Health
Priority Concepts: Client Education; Interpersonal Violence

Answer: 4
Rationale: Personal characteristics of abusers include low self-esteem, immaturity, dependence, insecurity, and jealousy. The statement in option 4 that abuse occurs more in low-income families is inaccurate. Options 1, 2, and 3 describe characteristics of abusers who often use fear and intimidation to the point where their victims will do anything just to avoid further abuse.
Priority Nursing Tip: In family violence situations, encourage individual therapy for the abuser that focuses on preventing violent behavior and repairing relationships.
Test-Taking Strategy: Note the strategic words, *need for further teaching*. These words indicate a negative event query and the need to select the incorrect statement. Use knowledge regarding the characteristics related to family violence to direct you to the correct option. Review: the characteristics of an abuser and family violence.
Reference(s): Stuart (2013), pp. 735-736; Varcarolis (2013), pp. 408-409.

1268. Which actions should the nurse implement to prevent ventilator-associated pneumonia (VAP) in the client who is intubated and on mechanical ventilation?
1. Practice meticulous hand hygiene.
2. Maintain the head of the bed elevation at 10 degrees.
3. Perform suctioning of oral cavity secretions every 4 hours.
4. Have the respiratory therapist change the ventilator circuit tubing every 4 hours.

Level of Cognitive Ability: Applying
Client Needs: Safe and Effective Care Environment
Integrated Process: Nursing Process/Implementation
Content Area: Adult Health: Respiratory
Priority Concepts: Health Promotion; Infection

Answer: 1
Rationale: Because normal upper airway defenses are bypassed, clients who are intubated with mechanical ventilation are at risk for VAP. Prevention includes effective handwashing before and after suctioning, when touching ventilator equipment, and when in contact with respiratory secretions. Options 2 and 3 are incorrect because to prevent aspiration of colonized secretions from the oral cavity the client will need more frequent oral cavity suctioning and at least 30 degrees head of the bed elevation. Option 4 is incorrect because the more frequently the circuit is broken, the greater the risk for pathogen entry.
Priority Nursing Tip: Remember when providing nursing care to a client with a respiratory infection that the best methods of preventing the spread of infection are handwashing and the proper disposal of secretions.
Test-Taking Strategy: Focus on the subject, preventing VAP. Option 1 provides evidence-based nursing care. Options 2, 3, and 4 are quantitatively inappropriate. Review: actions to prevent ventilator-associated pneumonia (VAP).
Reference(s): Ignatavicius, Workman (2013), p. 681.

1269. The charge nurse asks a new nurse in orientation about suicide and suicide intentions. The charge nurse determines that the new nurse understands the concepts associated with this topic if the new nurse makes which statement?
1. "Only the psychotic individual commits suicide."
2. "Suicidal attempts are attention-seeking behaviors."
3. "Suicide runs in the family, so there is nothing that health care personnel can do about it."
4. "Many individuals who commit suicide have talked about their suicidal intentions to others."

Level of Cognitive Ability: Evaluating
Client Needs: Psychosocial Integrity
Integrated Process: Nursing Process/Evaluation
Content Area: Mental Health
Priority Concepts: Mood and Affect; Safety

Answer: 4
Rationale: Most people who do commit suicide have given definite clues or warnings about their intentions. The individual who is suicidal is not necessarily psychotic. A suicide attempt is not an attention-seeking behavior, and each act should be taken very seriously. Suicide is not an inherited condition. Options 1, 2, and 3 are considered myths regarding suicide.
Priority Nursing Tip: The client who is at risk for suicide is never allowed to be alone. The nurse must remain with the client at all times.
Test-Taking Strategy: Focus on the subject, suicide and suicide intentions. Eliminate option 1 because of the close-ended word "only." Eliminate option 2 because of the phrase "attention-seeking behaviors." Eliminate option 3 because of the statement, "There is nothing that health care personnel can do about it." Review: concepts related to suicide.
Reference(s): Stuart (2013), p. 326; Varcarolis (2013), p. 440.

1270. A client wanders in and out of other clients' rooms, taking their possessions while singing to herself and then giggling for no apparent reason. The nurse reacts therapeutically by taking which action?

1. Putting arms around the client, saying, "You're okay. You just need a hug."
2. Saying, "I can see you are very anxious today. Let's go and play the piano."
3. Taking the client to the seclusion room until she cooperates with unit rules.
4. Taking the client to the lounge and saying, "Sit here and try to behave yourself."

Level of Cognitive Ability: Analyzing
Client Needs: Psychosocial Integrity
Integrated Process: Nursing Process/Implementation
Content Area: Mental Health
Priority Concepts: Anxiety; Coping

Answer: 2
Rationale: The use of a defense mechanism allows a person to avoid the painful experience of anxiety or transform it into a more tolerable symptom, such as regression. Regression allows the threatened client to move backward developmentally to a stage in which more security is felt. The recognition of regression is a signal that the client feels anxious. Option 2 will help the client feel less anxious. Option 1 does not address the client's anxiety. Options 3 and 4 are restrictive and degrading.
Priority Nursing Tip: Ensure safety for a client using a defense mechanism.
Test-Taking Strategy: Focus on the subject, the client's behaviors expressing a defense mechanism. Recall that because anxiety consumes energy, it should be redirected into a healthier task. This will direct you to the correct option. Review: **defense mechanisms.**
Reference(s): Stuart (2013), pp. 224-225; Varcarolis (2013), p. 172.

1271. The nurse is caring for a human immunodeficiency virus (HIV)–positive pregnant client. Which procedure needs to be avoided to help prevent the transmission of HIV from the woman to her fetus during the intrapartum period?

1. Cesarean birth
2. Epidural anesthesia
3. External fetal heart rate monitoring
4. Direct (internal) fetal heart rate monitoring

Level of Cognitive Ability: Analyzing
Client Needs: Safe and Effective Care Environment
Integrated Process: Nursing Process/Implementation
Content Area: Maternity: Intrapartum
Priority Concepts: Infection; Safety

Answer: 4
Rationale: Health care professionals must use caution during the intrapartal period to reduce the risk of the transmission of HIV to the fetus. Any procedure that exposes blood or body fluids from the mother to the fetus should be avoided. Direct (internal) fetal monitoring is a procedure that may expose the fetus to maternal blood or body fluids and therefore should be avoided. Options 1, 2, and 3 are not invasive measures that place the fetus at risk in the intrapartum period.
Priority Nursing Tip: The transmission of human immunodeficiency virus (HIV) occurs primarily by the exchange of blood or body fluids.
Test-Taking Strategy: Note the subject, the transmission of HIV from the woman to her fetus during the intrapartum period. All of the options address procedures that may take place during the intrapartum period, but only option 4 is invasive with regard to the fetus. Recalling that transmission of HIV occurs primarily by the exchange of body fluids will direct you to the correct option. Review: **HIV transmission,** specifically during the **intrapartum period.**
Reference(s): Lowdermilk, Perry, Cashion, Alden (2012), p. 156.

1272. During electroconvulsive therapy (ECT), the client receives oxygen by mask via positive pressure ventilation. The nurse determines that positive pressure ventilation is necessary for which reason?

1. Seizure activity depresses respirations.
2. Anesthesia is routinely administered during the ECT procedure.
3. Muscle relaxants are given to prevent injury during the seizure.
4. Decreased oxygen to the brain increases confusion and disorientation.

Level of Cognitive Ability: Analyzing
Client Needs: Physiological Integrity
Integrated Process: Nursing Process/Implementation
Content Area: Mental Health
Priority Concepts: Gas Exchange; Safety

Answer: 3
Rationale: A short-acting skeletal muscle relaxant is administered during this procedure to prevent injuries during the seizure. The client receives positive pressure ventilation until the muscle relaxant is metabolized, usually within 2 to 3 minutes. Options 1, 2, and 4 do not address the specific reason for positive pressure ventilation.
Priority Nursing Tip: After electroconvulsive therapy (ECT), assess the gag reflex before giving the client fluids.
Test-Taking Strategy: Focus on the subject, electroconvulsive therapy (ECT) and the need for positive pressure ventilation. Think about how this procedure is performed. Recalling that a muscle relaxant is administered during this procedure will direct you to the correct option. Review: **electroconvulsive therapy (ECT).**
Reference(s): Stuart (2013), p. 598.

1273. A client is in a coma of unknown cause, and the health care provider has written several prescriptions for the client including the need for intubation. Which procedure should the nurse withhold until the client is properly intubated?
1. Gastric feeding
2. Urethral catheterization
3. Finger stick for blood glucose level
4. Venipuncture for complete blood cell (CBC) count

Level of Cognitive Ability: Applying
Client Needs: Physiological Integrity
Integrated Process: Nursing Process/Implementation
Content Area: Adult Health: Neurological
Priority Concepts: Gas Exchange; Safety

Answer: 1
Rationale: Intubation should always precede gastric feeding to prevent pulmonary aspiration. Options 2, 3, and 4 identify procedures that can be initiated before intubation of the client.
Priority Nursing Tip: Airway management is the priority concern for a client in a coma.
Test-Taking Strategy: Focus on the ABCs—airway, breathing, and circulation. Recalling that the comatose client is at risk for aspiration will direct you to the correct option. Review: care of a client in a coma.
Reference(s): Ignatavicius, Workman (2013), pp. 674-675; Potter et al (2013), pp. 1031, 1035.

1274. The nurse is monitoring a client with chronic kidney disease (CKD). Which assessment finding should the nurse report to the health care provider?
1. Pallor
2. Fatigue
3. Lethargy
4. Petechiae

Level of Cognitive Ability: Analyzing
Client Needs: Physiological Integrity
Integrated Process: Nursing Process/Analysis
Content Area: Adult Health: Renal and Urinary
Priority Concepts: Clinical Judgment; Clotting

Answer: 4
Rationale: CKD can cause damage to many body systems. Hematological manifestations that can occur with this disease include anemia and bleeding. Abnormal bleeding (petechiae; purpura; bruising; bleeding from the mucous membranes, nose, or gums; vaginal bleeding; or intestinal bleeding) should be reported to the health care provider because it can be life-threatening. Pallor, fatigue, and lethargy are clinical manifestations associated with anemia.
Priority Nursing Tip: Chronic kidney disease (CKD) affects all major body systems and requires dialysis or kidney transplantation to maintain life.
Test-Taking Strategy: Focus on the subject, the assessment finding that should be reported with CKD. Recalling that the presence of petechiae is a sign of bleeding will direct you to this option. Review: the complications of chronic kidney disease (CKD).
Reference(s): Ignatavicius, Workman (2013), p. 1549.

1275. The nurse is providing instructions to a client regarding quinapril hydrochloride (Accupril). The nurse should give which instruction to the client?
1. Take the medication with food only.
2. Expect a therapeutic effect immediately.
3. Discontinue the medication if nausea occurs.
4. Rise slowly from a lying to a sitting position.

Level of Cognitive Ability: Applying
Client Needs: Physiological Integrity
Integrated Process: Teaching and Learning
Content Area: Pharmacology: Cardiovascular Medications
Priority Concepts: Client Education; Safety

Answer: 4
Rationale: Accupril is an angiotensin-converting enzyme (ACE) inhibitor. It is used in the treatment of hypertension. The client should be instructed to rise slowly from a lying to sitting position and to permit the legs to dangle from the bed momentarily before standing to reduce the hypotensive effect. The medication does not need to be taken with meals. It may be given without regard to food. A full therapeutic effect may be noted in 1 to 2 weeks. If nausea occurs, the client should be instructed to take a non-cola carbonated beverage and salted crackers or dry toast.
Priority Nursing Tip: If the client is receiving an antihypertensive medication, the nurse should instruct the client and family in the technique for monitoring blood pressure.
Test-Taking Strategy: Focus on the subject, client instructions regarding quinapril hydrochloride. Eliminate option 1 because of the closed-ended word "only." Recalling that medication names that end with the letters "-pril" indicate that the medication is an ACE inhibitor and ACE inhibitors are used in the treatment of hypertension will direct you to the correct option. Review: **quinapril hydrochloride (Accupril)**.
Reference(s): Hodgson, Kizior (2014), p. 1011.

1276. The nurse is providing emergency treatment for a client in ventricular tachycardia and is preparing to defibrillate the client. Which nursing action provides for the safest environment during a defibrillation attempt?

1. Ensuring that no lubricant is on the paddles
2. Placing the charged paddles one at a time on the client's chest
3. Holding the client's upper torso stable while the defibrillation is performed
4. Performing a visual and verbal check that all assisting personnel are clear of the client and the client's bed

Level of Cognitive Ability: Applying
Client Needs: Safe and Effective Care Environment
Integrated Process: Nursing Process/Implementation
Content Area: Critical Care: Emergency Situations
Priority Concepts: Perfusion; Safety

Answer: 4
Rationale: Safety during defibrillation is essential for preventing injury to the client and the personnel assisting with the procedure. The person performing the defibrillation ensures that all personnel are standing clear of the bed by a verbal and visual check of "all clear." For the shock to be effective, some type of conductive medium (e.g., lubricant, gel) must be placed between the paddles and the skin. Both paddles are placed on the client's chest.
Priority Nursing Tip: Before defibrillating a client, ensure that the oxygen is shut off to avoid the hazard of fire and be sure that no one is touching the bed or the client.
Test-Taking Strategy: Focus on the subject, safest environment with defibrillation. Option 4 is the umbrella option and involves a verbal and visual check of "all clear" providing for the safety of all involved. Review: the procedure for **defibrillation**.
Reference(s): Ignatavicius, Workman (2013), p. 737.

1277. A client is receiving heparin sodium by continuous intravenous infusion. Which adverse effect of this therapy should the nurse monitor the client?

1. Tinnitus
2. Ecchymoses
3. Increased pulse rate
4. Decreased blood pressure

Level of Cognitive Ability: Analyzing
Client Needs: Physiological Integrity
Integrated Process: Nursing Process/Assessment
Content Area: Pharmacology: Hematological Medications
Priority Concepts: Clotting; Safety

Answer: 2
Rationale: Heparin sodium is an anticoagulant. The client who receives heparin sodium is at risk for bleeding. The nurse monitors for signs of bleeding, which includes bleeding from the gums, ecchymoses on the skin, cloudy or pink-tinged urine, tarry stools, and body fluids that test positive for occult blood. Options 1, 3, and 4 are not related side or adverse effects of this medication.
Priority Nursing Tip: The antidote to heparin sodium is protamine sulfate.
Test-Taking Strategy: Focus on the subject, adverse effects of heparin sodium administration. Recalling that this medication is an anticoagulant will direct you to the correct option. Review: the nursing care related to the administration of **heparin sodium**.
Reference(s): Hodgson, Kizior (2014), p. 561.

1278. A client is admitted to the emergency department with complaints of severe, radiating chest pain. The client is extremely restless, frightened, and dyspneic. Immediate admission prescriptions include oxygen by nasal cannula at 4 liters per minute; troponin, creatinine phosphokinase, and isoenzymes blood levels; a chest x-ray; and a 12-lead ECG. Which action should the nurse take **first**?
1. Obtain the 12-lead ECG.
2. Draw the blood specimens.
3. Apply the oxygen to the client.
4. Call radiology to schedule the chest x-ray study.

Level of Cognitive Ability: Analyzing
Client Needs: Physiological Integrity
Integrated Process: Nursing Process/Implementation
Content Area: Critical Care: Emergency Situations
Priority Concepts: Clinical Judgment; Gas Exchange

Answer: 3
Rationale: The first action would be to apply the oxygen because the client can be experiencing myocardial ischemia. The ECG can provide evidence of cardiac damage and the location of myocardial ischemia. However, oxygen is the priority to prevent further cardiac damage. Drawing the blood specimens would be done after oxygen administration and just before or after the ECG, depending on the situation. Although the chest x-ray can show cardiac enlargement, having the chest x-ray would not influence immediate treatment.
Priority Nursing Tip: Troponin levels elevate as early as 3 hours after myocardial injury.
Test-Taking Strategy: Note the strategic word, *first*. Remember that the immediate goal of therapy is to prevent myocardial ischemia. The only choice that will achieve that goal is option 3. Also, use the ABCs—airway, breathing, and circulation—to direct you to the correct option. Review: care of the client with a **myocardial infarction**.
Reference(s): Ignatavicius, Workman (2013), p. 836.

1279. Chemical cardioversion is prescribed for the client with atrial fibrillation. The nurse who is assisting in preparing the client should expect that which medication specific for chemical cardioversion would be needed?
1. Lidocaine (Xylocaine)
2. Nifedipine (Procardia)
3. Amiodarone (Cordarone)
4. Nitroglycerin (Nitro-Bid, Nitrostat, others)

Level of Cognitive Ability: Analyzing
Client Needs: Physiological Integrity
Integrated Process: Nursing Process/Implementation
Content Area: Critical Care: Emergency Situations
Priority Concepts: Perfusion; Safety

Answer: 3
Rationale: Amiodarone is an antidysrhythmic that is useful in restoring normal sinus rhythm for the client experiencing atrial fibrillation. Lidocaine is used for control of ventricular dysrhythmias. Both nifedipine and nitroglycerin are vasodilators.
Priority Nursing Tip: Provide continuous cardiac monitoring for a client undergoing chemical cardioversion and receiving an antidysrhythmic.
Test-Taking Strategy: Focus on the subject, a specific medication for chemical cardioversion. Recalling the action and classification of these medications and that amiodarone is an antidysrhythmic for both atrial and ventricular dysrhythmias will direct you to the correct option. Review: **amiodarone (Cordarone)** and **chemical cardioversion**.
Reference(s): Hodgson, Kizior (2014), pp. 50, 52.

1280. A registered nurse is observing a new nurse auscultate the breath sounds of a client. Which incorrect action by the new nurse should lead the registered nurse to determine **further teaching is needed?**
1. Uses the bell of the stethoscope
2. Asks the client to sit straight up
3. Places the stethoscope directly on the client's skin
4. Has the client breathe slowly and deeply through the mouth

Level of Cognitive Ability: Analyzing
Client Needs: Physiological Integrity
Integrated Process: Nursing Process/Assessment
Content Area: Developmental Stages: Health Assessment/Physical Exam
Priority Concepts: Gas Exchange; Leadership

Answer: 1
Rationale: The bell of the stethoscope is not used to auscultate breath sounds. The client ideally should sit up and breathe slowly and deeply through the mouth. The diaphragm of the stethoscope, which is warmed before use, is placed directly on the client's skin, not over a gown or clothing.
Priority Nursing Tip: When auscultating breath sounds, the nurse should listen to at least one full respiration in each location (anterior, posterior, and lateral).
Test-Taking Strategy: Focus on the subject, auscultating breath sounds. Note the strategic words, *further teaching is needed* indicating a negative event query and the need to select the incorrect action by the new nurse. Visualizing each action and the procedure for auscultating breath sounds will direct you to the correct option. Review: **auscultation** as a basic physical assessment technique.
Reference(s): Potter et al (2013), pp. 494-495.

1281. The home health nurse cares for an obese adult client. In the client's medical record, the nurse reads, "The client has a sprained right ankle, has not exercised for more than 1 week, and has missed the last two physical therapy appointments." The client says, "I attend therapy for my ankle and I do my exercises three times a day." Which response should the nurse use with the client?

1. "Show me the exercises that you perform in physical therapy."
2. "You will never heal if you skip the physical therapy sessions."
3. "Your progress sounds fine. Is more physical therapy scheduled?"
4. "I see that you missed the last two physical therapy appointments."

Level of Cognitive Ability: Applying
Client Needs: Psychosocial Integrity
Integrated Process: Nursing Process/Implementation
Content Area: Mental Health
Priority Concepts: Adherence; Communication

Answer: 4
Rationale: In option 4, the nurse employs the therapeutic communication technique of confrontation. Because the client is employing avoidance, the nurse presents the facts according to the medical record to assess the client's perspective without accusing, threatening, or humiliating the client about the missed physical therapy. By confronting, the nurse assists the client with problem solving. Option 1 is potentially helpful when the client is complying with therapy. In option 2, the nurse provides an opinion and this statement admonishes the client for the behavior. In option 3, the nurse is nontherapeutic in giving approval and is mirroring the client's avoidance and passivity by not dealing directly with the problem of missed appointments.
Priority Nursing Tip: The nurse needs to employ therapeutic communication techniques to encourage the client to express thoughts and feelings as he or she addresses identified problem areas.
Test-Taking Strategy: Focus on therapeutic communication techniques, specifically confrontation. Option 4 is the only option that promotes problem solving by additional client assessment. Review: therapeutic communication techniques.
Reference(s): Potter et al (2013), pp. 320-322.

1282. A client with unstable ventricular tachycardia (VT) loses consciousness and becomes pulseless after an initial treatment with a dose of lidocaine (Xylocaine) intravenously. Which item should the nurse caring for the client **immediately** obtain?

1. A pacemaker
2. A defibrillator
3. A second dose of lidocaine
4. An electrocardiogram machine

Level of Cognitive Ability: Analyzing
Client Needs: Physiological Integrity
Integrated Process: Nursing Process/Analysis
Content Area: Critical Care: Emergency Situations
Priority Concepts: Clinical Judgment; Perfusion

Answer: 2
Rationale: For the client with VT who becomes pulseless, the health care provider or qualified advanced cardiac life support personnel immediately defibrillate the client. In the absence of this equipment, cardiopulmonary resuscitation is initiated immediately. Options 1, 3, and 4 are not items that are needed immediately in this situation.
Priority Nursing Tip: Ventricular tachycardia (VT) occurs as a result of a repetitive firing of an irritable ventricular ectopic focus at a rate of 140 to 250 beats per minute or more.
Test-Taking Strategy: Note the strategic word, *immediately*, and that the client is in VT. Options 3 and 4 should be eliminated first, because lidocaine was unsuccessful and option 4 is of no use in this situation. From the remaining choices, focusing on the subject, ventricular tachycardia, will direct you to option 2. Review: the immediate measures for **ventricular tachycardia (VT)**.
Reference(s): Gahart, Nazareno (2012), p. 848; Ignatavicius, Workman (2013), p. 723; Lehne (2013), pp. 587-588.

1283. The nurse has done preoperative teaching with a client scheduled for percutaneous insertion of an inferior vena cava (IVC) filter. Which client statement indicates the **need for further teaching** about the procedure?
1. "This is done under general anesthesia."
2. "This procedure is rarely associated with complications."
3. "It may cause congestion when clots get trapped at the filter."
4. "This could possibly eliminate the need for anticoagulant therapy."

Level of Cognitive Ability: Evaluating
Client Needs: Physiological Integrity
Integrated Process: Teaching and Learning
Content Area: Adult Health: Cardiovascular
Priority Concepts: Client Education; Perfusion

Answer: 1
Rationale: The percutaneous approach uses local anesthesia. Complications after insertion of an IVC filter are rare. When they do occur, they include air embolism, improper placement, and filter migration. Venous congestion can occur from accumulation of thrombi on the filter, but the process usually occurs gradually. There is usually no need for anticoagulant therapy after surgery.
Priority Nursing Tip: A vena cava (IVC) filter traps emboli to prevent pulmonary emboli.
Test-Taking Strategy: Note the strategic words, *need for further teaching*. These words indicate a negative event query and the need to select the incorrect client statement. Noting the words *percutaneous insertion* in the question should direct you to the correct option. General anesthesia is not used in this procedure. Review: percutaneous insertion of an **inferior vena cava (IVC) filter.**
Reference(s): Ignatavicius, Workman (2013), pp. 667, 802.

1284. A client with a head injury and a feeding tube continuously tries to remove the tube. The nurse contacts the health care provider who prescribes the use of restraints. After checking the agency's policy and procedure regarding the use of restraints, the nurse uses which method in restraining the client?
1. Belt restraint
2. Waist restraint
3. Wrist restraints
4. Mitten restraints

Level of Cognitive Ability: Applying
Client Needs: Safe and Effective Care Environment
Integrated Process: Nursing Process/Implementation
Content Area: Adult Health: Neurological
Priority Concepts: Intracranial Regulation; Safety

Answer: 4
Rationale: Mitten restraints are useful for this client because the client cannot pull against them, creating resistance that could lead to increased intracranial pressure (ICP). Belt and waist restraints prevent the client from getting up or falling out of bed or off a stretcher but do nothing to limit hand movement. Wrist restraints cause resistance.
Priority Nursing Tip: Always follow agency procedures for the use of a restraint. Monitor the client with a restraint closely. Restrained clients easily become entangled in the restraint device in attempts to get out of the device.
Test-Taking Strategy: Focus on the subject, a restraint that safely limits hand movement for this client. Eliminate options 1 and 2 because they do not address this subject. From the remaining choices, thinking about the concern of ICP in a client with a head injury will direct you to the correct option. Review: care of the client with a **head injury** and **restraints.**
Reference(s): Ignatavicius, Workman (2013), pp. 1021-1022; Potter et al (2013), pp. 390, 392.

1285. The registered nurse has oriented a new nurse to basic procedures for continuous electrocardiogram (ECG) monitoring. Which action by the new nurse while initiating cardiac monitoring on a client should indicate to the registered nurse the **need for further teaching**?
1. Clipped small areas of hair under the area planned for electrode placement
2. Stated the need to change the electrodes and inspect the skin every 24 hours
3. Stated the need to use hypoallergenic electrodes for clients who are sensitive
4. Cleansed the skin with povidone-iodine (Betadine) before applying the electrodes

Level of Cognitive Ability: Evaluating
Client Needs: Safe and Effective Care Environment
Integrated Process: Teaching and Learning
Content Area: Adult Health: Cardiovascular
Priority Concepts: Leadership; Safety

Answer: 4
Rationale: The skin is cleansed with soap and water (not povidone-iodine), denatured with alcohol, and allowed to air dry before electrodes are applied. The other three options are correct measures.
Priority Nursing Tip: Motion artifact noted on the cardiac monitor is caused by client movement.
Test-Taking Strategy: Note the strategic words, *need for further teaching*. These words indicate a negative event query and the need to select the incorrect action. Visualize this procedure and eliminate options 2 and 3 because they are correct procedure. From the remaining choices, remember that povidone-iodine is used to cleanse the skin usually before some type of invasive procedure that breaks the skin barrier. ECG monitoring does not break the skin. Review: the procedure for initiating **electrocardiogram (ECG) monitoring.**
Reference(s): Chernecky, Berger (2013), pp. 462-463.

1286. A client has been defibrillated at 360 joules (monophasic) and the attempts to convert the ventricular fibrillation (VF) were unsuccessful. Based on an evaluation of the situation, the nurse determines that which action would be **best**?
1. Terminating the resuscitation effort
2. Preparing for the administration of sodium bicarbonate intravenously
3. Performing cardiopulmonary resuscitation (CPR) for 5 cycles or about 2 minutes
4. Performing cardiopulmonary resuscitation (CPR) for 5 minutes, then defibrillating three more times at 400 joules

Level of Cognitive Ability: Analyzing
Client Needs: Physiological Integrity
Integrated Process: Nursing Process/Analysis
Content Area: Critical Care: Emergency Situations
Priority Concepts: Clinical Judgment; Perfusion

Answer: 3
Rationale: Defibrillation is an asynchronous countershock used to terminate pulseless ventricular tachycardia (VT) or ventricular fibrillation (VF). The defibrillator is charged to 120 to 200 joules (biphasic) or 300 joules (monophasic) for one countershock from the defibrillator, and then CPR is immediately resumed and continued for 5 cycles or about 2 minutes. The rhythm is reassessed after 2 minutes and if VF or pulseless VT continues, the defibrillator is charged to give a second shock at the same energy level previously used. CPR is resumed after the shock if needed and the life support protocol is continued. There is no information in the question to indicate that life support should be terminated. Sodium bicarbonate may be prescribed but is not the best action. Giving CPR for 5 minutes may not help oxygenation to the brain and myocardium and is not the best action.
Priority Nursing Tip: An automatic external defibrillator (AED) is used by laypersons and emergency medical technicians for prehospital cardiac arrest.
Test-Taking Strategy: Focus on the subject, the treatment for VF. There is no information in the question to indicate that life support should be terminated, so option 1 is eliminated first. From the remaining choices, focusing on the strategic word, *best* and recalling the treatment for VF will direct you to option 3. Review: the treatment for **ventricular fibrillation (VF)**.
Reference(s): Ignatavicius, Workman (2013), p. 737.

1287. The nurse is inserting an oropharyngeal airway into an assigned client. The nurse plans to use which correct insertion procedure?
1. Flex the client's neck.
2. Leave any dentures in place.
3. Suction the client's mouth once per shift.
4. Insert the airway with the tip pointed upward.

Level of Cognitive Ability: Applying
Client Needs: Physiological Integrity
Integrated Process: Nursing Process/Implementation
Content Area: Adult Health: Respiratory
Priority Concepts: Gas Exchange; Safety

Answer: 4
Rationale: The airway is inserted with the tip pointed upward and is then rotated downward once the flange has reached the client's teeth. The client should be positioned supine, with the neck hyperextended if possible. Before insertion of an oropharyngeal airway, any dentures or partial plates should be removed from the client's mouth. An airway should be selected that is an appropriate size. After insertion, the client's mouth is suctioned every hour or as necessary. The airway is removed for inspection of the mouth every 2 to 4 hours.
Priority Nursing Tip: Monitor the client with an oral airway inserted closely for the need of suctioning and for signs of airway obstruction.
Test-Taking Strategy: Focus on the subject, proper insertion of an oral airway. Eliminate option 3 because this is not part of the insertion procedure. Next eliminate option 1 because the neck is hyperextended (unless contraindicated) to open the airway. From the remaining options recall that dentures should be removed because they are a potential source of airway obstruction. Review: the procedure for inserting an **oropharyngeal airway**.
Reference(s): Potter et al (2013), pp. 845-846.

1288. The home care nurse visits a client who started wandering around at 10:00 PM each evening and got out of the house for the first time last night. The family asks for help. Which therapeutic response should the nurse make to the family?

1. "What prevented her from leaving the house in the past?"
2. "You cannot handle this alone because she could get hurt."
3. "I think you need to consider a nursing home immediately."
4. "This is a common problem known as sundowner's syndrome."

Level of Cognitive Ability: Applying
Client Needs: Safe and Effective Care Environment
Integrated Process: Nursing Process/Implementation
Content Area: Fundamental Skills: Safety
Priority Concepts: Cognition; Safety

Answer: 1
Rationale: The nurse responds to the family by assessing the situation and collecting additional data regarding the change in the client's behavior. The best response focuses on the family's problem so the nurse can help develop potential strategies. Option 2 is giving advice. Option 3 is histrionic, invalidates the family's attempt to manage the client's care, and potentially causes resentment. Option 4 provides the nurse's conclusion based on an incomplete assessment; other factors may be causing confusion.
Priority Nursing Tip: Providing a safe environment is the priority for a client with confusion.
Test-Taking Strategy: Use therapeutic communication techniques and the steps of the nursing process because the nurse needs more information before planning care; thus, selecting the option that relates to assessment directs you to the correct option. Review: therapeutic communication techniques and interventions for wandering clients.
Reference(s): Potter et al (2013), pp. 320-322, 380.

1289. The home care nurse is doing an assessment interview with an older adult client who asks the nurse to buy some groceries for her because she is not feeling well today. Which statement should the nurse use in response?

1. "I am not allowed to buy groceries for clients."
2. "Let's discuss how we can solve this problem."
3. "Do you have any support systems for shopping?"
4. "Nurses are professionals and do not run errands."

Level of Cognitive Ability: Applying
Client Needs: Psychosocial Integrity
Integrated Process: Communication and Documentation
Content Area: Mental Health
Priority Concepts: Care Coordination; Communication

Answer: 2
Rationale: The nurse's duty is to help the client; but in helping the client, the nurse's first action is to finish the assessment and then find immediate and long-term solutions to the problem. In option 1 the nurse uses a passive approach and hides behind policies and rules, even though this can be true. In option 3 the nurse asks a closed-ended question, which is unlikely to further nurse–client communication. Option 4 is inappropriate and indicates that the nurse thinks more of status than of helping the client.
Priority Nursing Tip: Identify the local elder care services for the older client and assist the client in making contacts that will help meet his or her needs.
Test-Taking Strategy: Focus on therapeutic communication techniques. Option 2 is the only choice that addresses the client's problem and provides the means to problem solve. Review therapeutic communication techniques.
Reference(s): Potter et al (2013), pp. 320-322.

1290. The nurse is caring for a client who is being treated with an intravenous (IV) bolus of lidocaine hydrochloride (Xylocaine). What should the nurse monitor because of the actions and the effects of this medication?

1. Urinary pH
2. Radial pulse
3. Temperature
4. Blood pressure

Level of Cognitive Ability: Analyzing
Client Needs: Physiological Integrity
Integrated Process: Nursing Process/Implementation
Content Area: Pharmacology: Cardiovascular Medications
Priority Concepts: Perfusion; Safety

Answer: 4
Rationale: Lidocaine hydrochloride is an antidysrhythmic. The nurse is responsible for monitoring the client's respiratory status and blood pressure while he or she is being treated with an IV bolus of this medication. The urinary pH and temperature are not related to this medication. It is best to monitor the apical pulse in this client.
Priority Nursing Tip: Class I antidysrhythmics can cause nausea, vomiting, diarrhea, hypotension, and heart failure and worsen or cause new dysrhythmias.
Test-Taking Strategy: Think about the classification of this medication. Focus on the ABCs—airway, breathing, and circulation—to answer the question. This should direct you to the correct option. Review: nursing responsibilities when a client receives lidocaine hydrochloride (Xylocaine).
Reference(s): Gahart, Nazareno (2012), pp. 848-849; Hodgson, Kizior (2014), p. 690.

1291. A client has a prescription for seizure precautions. Which interventions should be included in the plan of care? **Select all that apply.**
- ❏ 1. Have suction equipment readily available.
- ❏ 2. Keep all the lights on in the room at night.
- ❏ 3. Keep a padded tongue blade at the bedside.
- ❏ 4. Assist the client to ambulate in the hallway.
- ❏ 5. Monitor the client closely while showering.
- ❏ 6. Push the lock-out button on the electric bed to keep the bed in the lowest position.

Level of Cognitive Ability: Analyzing
Client Needs: Safe and Effective Care Environment
Integrated Process: Nursing Process/Implementation
Content Area: Fundamental Skills: Safety
Priority Concepts: Intracranial Regulation; Safety

Answer: 1, 4, 5, 6
Rationale: Suction equipment should be readily available to remove accumulated secretions after the seizure. The client should be accompanied during activities such as bathing and walking, so that assistance is readily available and injury is minimized if a seizure begins. The bed is maintained in a low position for safety. A quiet, restful environment is provided as part of seizure precautions. This includes undisturbed times for sleep, while using a nightlight (not all lights) for safety. A padded tongue blade is not kept at the bedside because nothing is inserted into the client's mouth during the seizure. Agency procedures regarding seizure precautions are always followed.
Priority Nursing Tip: Monitoring airway and maintaining safety are the priorities during a seizure.
Test-Taking Strategy: Focus on the subject, seizure precautions. Noting the word *all* in option 2 will assist in eliminating this option. Next recalling that nothing is inserted into the client's mouth during the seizure will assist in eliminating option 3. Review: care of the client on seizure precautions.
Reference(s): Potter et al (2013), pp. 387, 392-394.

1292. The nurse is monitoring a nursing student who is caring for a child who sustained a head injury from a fall. Which action by the nursing student indicates a **need for further teaching?**
1. Forcing fluids
2. Performing neurological assessments
3. Keeping the child in a sitting-up position
4. Keeping the child awake as much as possible

Level of Cognitive Ability: Evaluating
Client Needs: Physiological Integrity
Integrated Process: Teaching and Learning
Content Area: Child Health: Neurological
Priority Concepts: Clinical Judgment; Intracranial Regulation

Answer: 1
Rationale: A child with a head injury is at risk for increased intracranial pressure (ICP). Forcing fluids may cause fluid overload and increased ICP. Additionally, the nurse should not "force" the client to do something. Neurological assessments must be performed to monitor for increased ICP. Sitting up will decrease fluid retention in cerebral tissue and promote drainage. Keeping the child awake will assist in accurate evaluation of any cerebral edema that is present and will detect early coma.
Priority Nursing Tip: An early sign of increased intracranial pressure (ICP) is a change in level of consciousness.
Test-Taking Strategy: Focus on the subject, neurological assessment to monitor for increased ICP. Note strategic words, *need for further teaching.* This indicates a negative event query and the need to select the incorrect intervention. Use the knowledge regarding increased ICP. Eliminate options 2, 3, and 4 because they are correct in terms of monitoring for and preventing increased ICP. Additionally noting the word *forcing* in option 1 will direct you to this choice. Review: measures to prevent increased **intracranial pressure (ICP).**
Reference(s): Hockenberry, Wilson (2013), p. 942.

1293. The nurse has conducted a stress management seminar for clients in an ambulatory care setting. Which statement by a client would indicate a **need for further teaching**?

1. "I can use those guided imagery techniques I've learned anywhere and anytime."
2. "Biofeedback might be nice, but I don't like the idea of having to use equipment."
3. "Using confrontation with coworkers should solve my problems at work quickly."
4. "The progressive muscle relaxation technique should ease my tension headaches."

Level of Cognitive Ability: Evaluating
Client Needs: Psychosocial Integrity
Integrated Process: Teaching and Learning
Content Area: Mental Health
Priority Concepts: Client Education; Coping

Answer: 3
Rationale: Confrontation is a communication technique, not a stress management technique. It may also exacerbate stress, at least in the short term, rather than alleviate it. Biofeedback, progressive muscle relaxation, meditation, and guided imagery are techniques that the nurse can teach the client to reduce the physical impact of stress on the body and promote a feeling of self-control for the client. Biofeedback entails electronic equipment, whereas the others require no adjuncts, such as tapes, once the technique is learned.
Priority Nursing Tip: Assist the client to identify the source of anxiety and explore methods to reduce anxiety.
Test-Taking Strategy: Note the strategic words, *need for further teaching*. These words indicate a negative event query and the need to select the incorrect statement. Recalling the methods of stress management techniques guides you to option 3, which is a communication technique rather than a stress management technique. Review: **stress management techniques**.
Reference(s): Potter et al (2013), pp. 741, 743; Varcarolis (2013), p. 282.

1294. The nurse is caring for a client with a peptic ulcer. In assessing the client for gastrointestinal perforation, the nurse determines that which should be monitored?

1. Slow, strong pulses
2. Increase in bowel sounds
3. Positive guaiac stool tests
4. Sudden, severe abdominal pain

Level of Cognitive Ability: Analyzing
Client Needs: Physiological Integrity
Integrated Process: Nursing Process/Assessment
Content Area: Adult Health: Gastrointestinal
Priority Concepts: Tissue Integrity; Pain

Answer: 4
Rationale: Sudden, severe abdominal pain is a sign of perforation. When perforation occurs, the pulse will more likely be weak and rapid. The nurse may be unable to hear bowel sounds at all. Positive guaiac stool results indicate the presence of bleeding but are not necessarily indicative of perforation.
Priority Nursing Tip: Gastrointestinal perforation is a life-threatening emergency. If signs of perforation are present, notify the health care provider immediately.
Test-Taking Strategy: Focus on the subject, the signs of perforation. Correlate perforation with sudden, severe abdominal pain. Remember that the nurse may be unable to hear bowel sounds and that the pulse will most likely be weak and rapid. Positive guaiac stool results are not specific to perforation. Review: the signs of **gastrointestinal perforation**.
Reference(s): Ignatavicius, Workman (2013), p. 1227.

1295. Intravenous human albumin is prescribed for a client with burns of the anterior chest and both legs. The nurse reviews the client's medical record to identify the presence of any existing conditions that would be a contraindication in the use of human albumin. The nurse contacts the health care provider before administering the human albumin if which is noted in the client's record?

1. Diabetes mellitus
2. Multiple myeloma
3. Renal insufficiency
4. Lymphocytic leukemia

Level of Cognitive Ability: Analyzing
Client Needs: Physiological Integrity
Integrated Process: Nursing Process/Analysis
Content Area: Critical Care: Blood Administration
Priority Concepts: Collaboration; Safety

Answer: 3
Rationale: Human albumin is classified as a blood derivative and is contraindicated in severe anemia, cardiac failure, history of allergic reaction, renal insufficiency, and when no albumin deficiency is present. It is used with caution in clients with low cardiac reserve, pulmonary disease, or hepatic or renal failure.
Priority Nursing Tip: When any type of blood derivative is prescribed, review the client's chart to determine if the client's belief is Jehovah's Witness. Health care professionals should make every effort to incorporate the client's values and beliefs into the treatment plan.
Test-Taking Strategy: Focus on the subject, a contraindication to infusing human albumin. Eliminate options 2 and 4 first because they are comparable or alike in that they are oncological disorders. From the remaining choices, recalling that albumin restores intravascular volume will assist in directing you to the correct option. Review: **blood derivatives**, specifically **human albumin**.
Reference(s): Gahart, Nazareno (2012), p. 30.

1296. A newborn is in the neonatal intensive care unit for respiratory distress syndrome (RDS) and surfactant replacement therapy has been given. The nurse evaluates the infant 1 hour after the surfactant therapy and determines that the infant's condition has improved somewhat. Which option, if observed by the nurse, indicates improvement?
1. Unequal breath sounds
2. Increased work of breathing
3. Decreased need for supplemental oxygen
4. Increased level of carbon dioxide (CO_2) in the blood gas analysis

Level of Cognitive Ability: Evaluating
Client Needs: Physiological Integrity
Integrated Process: Nursing Process/Evaluation
Content Area: Maternity: Newborn
Priority Concepts: Development; Gas Exchange

Answer: 3
Rationale: A decreased need for supplemental oxygen indicates an improvement in the infant's ability to use oxygen. Unequal breath sounds may indicate atelectasis or blocked airways. The increased work of breathing indicates air hunger and the need for further support. Increased levels of CO_2 would indicate increasing respiratory acidosis and not improvement of the condition.
Priority Nursing Tip: Respiratory distress syndrome (RDS) is a serious lung disorder caused by immaturity and inability to produce surfactant, resulting is hypoxia and acidosis.
Test-Taking Strategy: Focus on the subject, surfactant replacement therapy in a newborn with respiratory distress syndrome (RDS). Noting the word *increased* in options 2 and 4 will assist in eliminating these options. From the remaining choices, recall that "unequal" does not indicate improvement. Review the expected effects of surfactant therapy and respiratory distress syndrome (RDS).
Reference(s): Hockenberry, Wilson (2013), pp. 268-270.

1297. The nurse is evaluating the effectiveness of antimicrobial therapy for a client with infective endocarditis. The nurse determines that which finding documented in the client's health record is the **least** reliable indicator of **effectiveness**?
1. Clear breath sounds
2. Systolic heart murmur
3. Temperature of 98.8° F
4. Negative blood cultures

Level of Cognitive Ability: Evaluating
Client Needs: Physiological Integrity
Integrated Process: Nursing Process/Evaluation
Content Area: Adult Health: Cardiovascular
Priority Concepts: Infection; Perfusion

Answer: 2
Rationale: A systolic heart murmur, once present in the client, will not resolve spontaneously and is therefore the least reliable indicator. Clear breath sounds are a normal finding, and in this instance could mean resolution of heart failure, if that was accompanying the endocarditis. Negative blood cultures and normothermia indicate resolution of infection.
Priority Nursing Tip: Endocarditis is an inflammation of the inner lining of the heart and valves.
Test-Taking Strategy: Focus on the subject, effective indicator of antimicrobial therapy for a client with infective endocarditis. Note the strategic word, *effectiveness* and the word *least*. This creates a negative event query and asks you to look for the finding that will not respond to antimicrobial therapy and is an abnormal finding. The only choice that meets these criteria is option 2, which does not resolve once it has developed. Review: care of the client with infective endocarditis.
Reference(s): Ignatavicius, Workman (2013), pp. 700-701, 764; Lewis et al (2014), p. 812.

1298. The nurse is caring for a client with continuous electrocardiogram (ECG) monitoring. The nurse notes that the ECG complexes are very small and hard to evaluate. Which setting on the ECG monitor console should the nurse check?
1. Power button
2. Low rate alarm
3. High rate alarm
4. Amplitude or "gain"

Level of Cognitive Ability: Applying
Client Needs: Safe and Effective Care Environment
Integrated Process: Nursing Process/Implementation
Content Area: Adult Health: Cardiovascular
Priority Concepts: Perfusion; Safety

Answer: 4
Rationale: The amplitude, commonly called "gain," regulates the size of the complex and can be adjusted up and down to some degree. The power button turns the machine on and off. The low and high alarm settings indicate the heart rate limits beyond which an alarm will sound.
Priority Nursing Tip: An electrocardiogram (ECG) reflects the electrical activity of cardiac cells and records electrical activity at a speed of 25 mm/second.
Test-Taking Strategy: Focus on the subject, ECG complexes that are small and hard to evaluate. Eliminate options 2 and 3 first because they are comparable or alike. From the remaining choices, noting the relation of the subject to the word *amplitude* (meaning size or strength) in option 4 will direct you to this choice. Review: the procedure for the use of an electrocardiogram (ECG) monitor.
Reference(s): Mosby's Dictionary (2013), p. 83.

1299. The nurse is monitoring a client who has received antidysrhythmic therapy for the treatment of premature ventricular contractions (PVCs). Which observation in the PVCs would indicate to the nurse that this therapy is ineffective?

1. Occur in pairs
2. Be unifocal in appearance
3. Be fewer than six per minute
4. Fall after the end of the T wave

Level of Cognitive Ability: Evaluating
Client Needs: Physiological Integrity
Integrated Process: Nursing Process/Evaluation
Content Area: Critical Care: Medications and Intravenous Therapy
Priority Concepts: Clinical Judgment; Perfusion

Answer: 1
Rationale: PVCs are considered dangerous when they are frequent (more than six per minute), occur in pairs or couplets, are multifocal (multiform), or fall on the T wave.
Priority Nursing Tip: The health care provider must be notified when premature ventricular contractions (PVCs) occur.
Test-Taking Strategy: Focus on the subject, antidysrhythmic therapy for PVCs. The word, *ineffective,* indicates a negative event query and the need to select the option that identifies that the therapy is not working. Knowledge regarding the occurrence of PVCs and the situations in which they may be dangerous to the client will direct you to the correct option. Review: the significance of **premature ventricular contractions (PVCs).**
Reference(s): Ignatavicius, Workman (2013), p. 728.

1300. The nurse is reviewing the client's arterial blood gas results. Which finding would indicate that the client has respiratory acidosis?

1. pH 7.5, Pco_2 of 30
2. pH 7.3, Pco_2 of 50
3. pH 7.3, HCO_3 of 19
4. pH 7.5, HCO_3 of 30

Level of Cognitive Ability: Analyzing
Client Needs: Physiological Integrity
Integrated Process: Nursing Process/Analysis
Content Area: Fundamental Skills: Acid-Base
Priority Concepts: Acid-Base Balance; Gas Exchange

Answer: 2
Rationale: In respiratory acidosis, the pH is decreased and an opposite effect is seen in the Pco_2 (pH decreased, Pco_2 elevated). Option 1 indicates respiratory alkalosis; option 3 indicates possible metabolic acidosis; and option 4 indicates possible metabolic alkalosis.
Priority Nursing Tip: If the client has a condition that causes an obstruction of the airway or depresses the respiratory system, monitor for respiratory acidosis.
Test-Taking Strategy: Focus on the subject, respiratory acidosis. Recalling that the pH is decreased in acidosis will assist in eliminating options 1 and 4. Next, remember that in respiratory acidosis, the Pco_2 has an opposite effect from the pH. This will direct you to option 2. Review: the acid-base findings in **respiratory acidosis.**
Reference(s): Ignatavicius, Workman (2013), p. 205.

1301. The nurse is assigned to care for a client with a chest tube attached to closed chest drainage. What should the nurse determine is an indicator the client's lung has completely expanded?

1. Pleuritic chest pain has resolved
2. The oxygen saturation is greater than 92%
3. Fluctuations in the water-seal chamber ceased
4. Suction in the chest drainage system is no longer needed

Level of Cognitive Ability: Evaluating
Client Needs: Physiological Integrity
Integrated Process: Nursing Process/Evaluation
Content Area: Adult Health: Respiratory
Priority Concepts: Clinical Judgment; Gas Exchange

Answer: 3
Rationale: When the lung has completely expanded, there is no longer air in the pleural space causing fluctuations in the water-seal chamber. Thus, an indication that a chest tube is ready for removal is when fluctuations in the water-seal chamber cease. Although air is known to be an irritant to pleural tissue, cessation of pleuritic pain does not indicate that the lung is expanded. The chest tube acts as an irritant and therefore contributes to pain. Adequate oxygen saturation does not imply that the lung has fully reexpanded. Use or nonuse of suction in the chest drainage system is not necessarily governed by the degree of lung expansion. Suction is indicated when gravity is not sufficient to drain air and pleural fluid or if the client has a poor respiratory effort and cough.
Priority Nursing Tip: Fluctuation in the water seal chamber stops if the tube is obstructed, if a dependent loop exists, if the suction is not working properly, or if the lung has reexpanded.
Test-Taking Strategy: Focus on the subject, indicators that a lung has fully reexpanded, specifically in the chest tube drainage system. Eliminate options 1 and 2 because they are not directly related to a chest tube drainage system. From the remaining choices, recalling the functioning of chest tubes will direct you to option 3. Review: **chest tube drainage systems.**
Reference(s): Potter et al (2013), p. 872.

❖ **1302.** The nurse is caring for a child with leukemia and notes that the platelet count is 20,000 cells/mm³. Based on this finding, the nurse should include which interventions in the plan of care? **Select all that apply.**
- ❑ 1. Monitor stools for blood.
- ❑ 2. Clean oral cavity with soft swabs.
- ❑ 3. Provide appropriate play activities.
- ❑ 4. Check the rectal temperature every 4 hours.
- ❑ 5. Administer acetaminophen (Tylenol) suppositories for fever.

Level of Cognitive Ability: Applying
Client Needs: Physiological Integrity
Integrated Process: Nursing Process/Implementation
Content Area: Child Health: Oncological
Priority Concepts: Cellular Regulation; Safety

Answer: 1, 2, 3
Rationale: A platelet count of 20,000/mm³ places the child at risk for bleeding. Options 1, 2, and 3 are accurate interventions. Taking rectal temperatures and the use of suppositories are avoided because of the risk of rectal bleeding.
Priority Nursing Tip: Bleeding precautions are instituted when the platelet count is low. Neutropenic precautions are instituted when the neutrophil count is low.
Test-Taking Strategy: Focus on the subject, bleeding when a child has leukemia. Recalling the interventions related to bleeding precautions will assist in directing you to the correct options. Also note that options 4 and 5 are **comparable or alike** and relate to insertion of an object in the rectum. Review: interventions for the child at risk for bleeding.
Reference(s): McKinney et al (2013), pp. 1276-1277.

1303. The nurse working in the mental health unit is collecting data on a newly admitted client. Which is a **primary** source of data collection?
1. Client
2. Police officer
3. Family member
4. Client's medical record

Level of Cognitive Ability: Applying
Client Needs: Psychosocial Integrity
Integrated Process: Nursing Process/Assessment
Content Area: Mental Health
Priority Concepts: Clinical Judgment; Communication

Answer: 1
Rationale: Assessments are conducted by many professionals, including nurses, psychiatrists, social workers, dietitians, and other therapists. The primary source of data is the client. Secondary sources of data may need to be collected if the client is experiencing psychosis, muteness, or catatonia. These sources of data include family, friends, neighbors, police officers, health care workers, and medical records.
Priority Nursing Tip: As appropriate, the client is always the best source of data when performing an assessment.
Test-Taking Strategy: Note the strategic word, *primary*, and focus on the subject, primary source of data collection. Recognizing that the only primary source of data is the client will assist in eliminating options 2, 3, and 4. Review: **primary and secondary data sources.**
Reference(s): Jarvis (2012), pp. 7-8, 29.

1304. The nurse evaluates the arterial blood gas (ABG) results of a client who is receiving supplemental oxygen. Which finding would indicate that the oxygen level was adequate?
1. A Po₂ of 45 mm Hg
2. A Po₂ of 50 mm Hg
3. A Po₂ of 60 mm Hg
4. A Po₂ of 80 mm Hg

Level of Cognitive Ability: Evaluating
Client Needs: Physiological Integrity
Integrated Process: Nursing Process/Evaluation
Content Area: Fundamental Skills: Acid-Base
Priority Concepts: Clinical Judgment; Gas Exchange

Answer: 4
Rationale: The normal Po₂ level is 80 to 100 mm Hg. Options 1, 2, and 3 are low values and do not indicate adequate oxygen levels.
Priority Nursing Tip: The normal arterial blood gas pH value is 7.35 to 7.45.
Test-Taking Strategy: Focus on the subject, a normal Po₂ level. Select the option that identifies the highest oxygen level. This will direct you to the correct option. Review: interpretation of the results of **arterial blood gas (ABG).**
Reference(s): Chernecky, Berger (2013), p. 208.

1305. A client has been taking lisinopril (Prinivil) for 3 months. The client complains to the nurse of a persistent dry cough that began about 1 month ago. The nurse interprets that which is the **most likely** reason for the client's complaint?

1. Caused by neutropenia as a result of therapy
2. Caused by a concurrent upper respiratory infection
3. An expected, though bothersome, side effect of therapy
4. An indication that the client will show signs of heart failure

Level of Cognitive Ability: Analyzing
Client Needs: Physiological Integrity
Integrated Process: Nursing Process/Analysis
Content Area: Pharmacology: Respiratory Medications
Priority Concepts: Gas Exchange; Safety

Answer: 3
Rationale: A frequent side effect of therapy with any of the angiotensin-converting enzyme (ACE) inhibitors, such as lisinopril, is the appearance of a persistent, dry cough. The cough generally does not improve while the client is taking the medication. Clients are advised to notify the health care provider if the cough becomes very troublesome to them. The other options are incorrect interpretations.
Priority Nursing Tip: Angiotensin-converting enzyme (ACE) inhibitors may be prescribed to treat hypertension. Instruct the client that if dizziness or any other side effect occurs and persists to notify the health care provider.
Test-Taking Strategy: Note the strategic words, *most likely* in the question. Focus on the subject, lisinopril, and specifically side effects of this ACE inhibitor. Eliminate options 1 and 2 first because they are comparable or alike and focus on infection. From the remaining choices, it is necessary to know the frequent side effects of this medication to direct you to the correct option. Review: the side effects of lisinopril (Prinivil).
Reference(s): Hodgson, Kizior (2014), p. 699.

1306. The nurse is developing a plan of care for a client with acquired immunodeficiency syndrome (AIDS). The nurse should document which appropriate goal in the plan of care?

1. The client has no increased platelet aggregation.
2. The client has a urinary output of 50 mL per hour.
3. The client does not experience respiratory distress.
4. The client has no evidence of a dissecting aortic aneurysm.

Level of Cognitive Ability: Analyzing
Client Needs: Physiological Integrity
Integrated Process: Nursing Process/Planning
Content Area: Adult Health: Immune
Priority Concepts: Immunity; Infection

Answer: 3
Rationale: A common, life-threatening opportunistic infection that occurs in clients with AIDS is *Pneumocystis jiroveci* pneumonia. Its symptoms include fever, exertional dyspnea, and nonproductive cough. The absence of respiratory distress is one of the goals that the nurse sets as a priority. Options 1, 2, and 4 are not specifically related to the subject of the question.
Priority Nursing Tip: Acquired immunodeficiency syndrome (AIDS) has a long incubation period, sometimes 10 years or longer. Manifestations may not appear until late in the infection.
Test-Taking Strategy: Focus on the subject, AIDS. Option 3 is the only choice that is directly related to the client's diagnosis. In addition, use the ABCs—airway, breathing, and circulation—to answer the question. Review: care of the client with **acquired immunodeficiency syndrome (AIDS)**.
Reference(s): Ignatavicius, Workman (2013), pp. 366, 375-376.

1307. A client with active tuberculosis (TB) is to be admitted to a medical-surgical unit. Which action should the nurse take when planning a bed assignment?
1. Place the client in a private, well-ventilated room.
2. Plan to transfer the client to the intensive care unit.
3. Assign the client to a double room and places a "strict handwashing" sign outside the door.
4. Assign the client to a double room because intravenous antibiotics will be administered.

Level of Cognitive Ability: Applying
Client Needs: Safe and Effective Care Environment
Integrated Process: Nursing Process/Planning
Content Area: Fundamental Skills: Infection Control
Priority Concepts: Infection; Safety

Answer: 1
Rationale: According to category-specific (respiratory) isolation precautions, a client with TB requires a private room. The room needs to be well ventilated and should have at least 6 to 12 exchanges of fresh air per hour and should be ventilated to the outside if possible. Therefore, option 1 is the only correct choice.
Priority Nursing Tip: The nurse must wear a high-efficiency particulate air (HEPA) mask whenever entering the room of a client with tuberculosis.
Test-Taking Strategy: Focus on the subject, active TB. Eliminate options 3 and 4 because they are comparable or alike in that they involve assignment to a double room. From the remaining choices, recalling the need for respiratory isolation precautions will direct you to the correct option. Review: care of the client with **active tuberculosis (TB)**.
Reference(s): Ignatavicius, Workman (2013), p. 657.

1308. A client develops an irregular heart rate. Which statement by the client indicates to the nurse that the client is ready for learning?
1. "I feel weak with an irregular pulse "
2. "What is it like to have a pacemaker?"
3. "All my medications will be changed now."
4. "How can this heart rate problem affect me?"

Level of Cognitive Ability: Analyzing
Client Needs: Psychosocial Integrity
Integrated Process: Teaching and Learning
Content Area: Adult Health: Cardiovascular
Priority Concepts: Client Education; Health Promotion

Answer: 4
Rationale: Learning depends on two things: physical and emotional readiness to learn. A good time to teach is when the client indicates an interest in learning, is motivated, and is physically capable of concentrating on learning. Option 4 addresses the client's readiness because the client is directly asking about the disorder. Option 1 indicates that the client is potentially physically incapable of learning at this time. The client indicates wanting to learn about pacemakers in option 2; however, the client has formed a hasty conclusion because the need for a pacemaker has not been determined. In option 3, by assuming that the medications will change, the client is emotionally unprepared for learning because the statement is based on incomplete data.
Priority Nursing Tip: The client's readiness to learn is the priority in the teaching and learning process.
Test-Taking Strategy: Focus on the subject, the client's readiness to learn about an irregular heart rate. Note that option 4 directly addresses the client's diagnosis. Also note the words *heart rate* in the question and the correct option. Review: adult **teaching-learning principles**.
Reference(s): Potter et al (2013), pp. 329-330.

1309. A health care provider prescribes lipids (fat emulsion) for a client who is receiving total parenteral nutrition (TPN). The nurse should explain to the client that the fat emulsion is administered for which reason?
1. To provide essential fatty acids
2. As a supplement to fluid intake
3. To decrease the risk of phlebitis
4. During the night in place of TPN

Level of Cognitive Ability: Applying
Client Needs: Physiological Integrity
Integrated Process: Teaching and Learning
Content Area: Fundamental Skills: Nutrition
Priority Concepts: Client Education; Nutrition

Answer: 1
Rationale: Lipids are a brand of intravenous fat emulsion administered to clients who are at risk for developing an essential fatty acid deficiency, such as those receiving TPN. Fat emulsions help meet caloric and nutritional needs that cannot be met by glucose administration alone. Fat emulsions are not administered to increase the amount of body fluids and they do not decrease the incidence of phlebitis. Fat emulsions neither replace TPN nor do they require infusion during the night.
Priority Nursing Tip: Monitor renal function tests in a client receiving lipids (fat emulsion). Abnormal renal function tests may indicate an excess of amino acids.
Test-Taking Strategy: Focus on the subject, intravenous fat emulsion, and use the principles about lipids to choose the correct option. Note the relationship of the words *lipids* in the question and *fatty acids* in the correct option. Remember that fat emulsion is administered to prevent fatty acid deficiency. Review: the purpose of administering **fat emulsion** during **TPN therapy.**
Reference(s): Lewis et al (2014), p. 901.

1310. A client with valvular heart disease is at risk for developing heart failure. What should the nurse assess as the **priority** when monitoring for heart failure?
1. Heart rate
2. Breath sounds
3. Blood pressure
4. Activity tolerance

Level of Cognitive Ability: Analyzing
Client Needs: Physiological Integrity
Integrated Process: Nursing Process/Assessment
Content Area: Adult Health: Cardiovascular
Priority Concepts: Gas Exchange; Perfusion

Answer: 2
Rationale: Breath sounds are the best way to assess for the onset of heart failure. The presence of crackles or an increase in crackles is an indicator of fluid in the lungs caused by heart failure. Options 1, 3, and 4 are components of the assessment but are less reliable indicators of heart failure.
Priority Nursing Tip: Signs of left-sided heart failure are evident by pulmonary manifestations.
Test-Taking Strategy: Note the strategic word, *priority*. Focus on the subject, heart failure resulting from valvular heart disease. Use of the ABCs—airway, breathing, and circulation—will direct you to option 2. Review: assessment of **heart failure.**
Reference(s): Ignatavicius, Workman (2013), p. 748.

1311. The nurse is caring for a client receiving fludrocortisone acetate (Florinef) for the treatment of Addison's disease. The nurse monitors the client for improvement, knowing that which is the anticipated therapeutic effect of this medication?
1. Promote electrolyte balance.
2. Stimulate thyroid production.
3. Stimulate the immune response.
4. Stimulate thyrotropin production.

Level of Cognitive Ability: Evaluating
Client Needs: Physiological Integrity
Integrated Process: Nursing Process/Evaluation
Content Area: Pharmacology: Endocrine Medications
Priority Concepts: Fluid and Electrolyte Balance; Safety

Answer: 1
Rationale: Florinef is a long-acting oral medication with mineralocorticoid and moderate glucocorticoid activity that may be used for long-term management of Addison's disease. Mineralocorticoids act on the renal distal tubules to enhance the reabsorption of sodium and chloride ions and the excretion of potassium and hydrogen ions. The client can rapidly develop hypotension and fluid and electrolyte imbalance if the medication is discontinued abruptly. The medication does not affect the immune response or thyroid or thyrotropin production.
Priority Nursing Tip: Addisonian crisis is a life-threatening disorder caused by acute adrenal insufficiency. It can cause hyponatremia, hyperkalemia, hypoglycemia, and shock.
Test-Taking Strategy: Focus on the subject, Addison's disease. Remember that Addison's disease produces deficiencies of glucocorticoids, mineralocorticoids, and androgens. Eliminate options 2 and 4 first because they are comparable or alike. From the remaining choices, recalling that Addison's disease is not related to the immune system will direct you to the correct option. Review: the action of **fludrocortisone acetate (Florinef).**
Reference(s): Ignatavicius, Workman (2013), pp. 1383-1384; Lilley, Rainforth Collins, Harrington, Snyder (2014b), pp. 537-538.

1312. The nurse is assessing the leg pain of a client who has just undergone right femoral-popliteal artery bypass grafting. Which question would be **most** useful in determining whether the client is experiencing graft occlusion?
1. "Can you describe what the pain feels like?"
2. "Can you rate the pain on a scale of 1 to 10?"
3. "Did you get any relief from the last dose of pain medication?"
4. "Can you compare this pain to the pain you felt before surgery?"

Level of Cognitive Ability: Analyzing
Client Needs: Physiological Integrity
Integrated Process: Nursing Process/Assessment
Content Area: Adult Health: Cardiovascular
Priority Concepts: Pain; Perfusion

Answer: 4
Rationale: The most frequent indication that a graft is occluding is the return of pain that is similar to that experienced preoperatively. Standard pain assessment techniques also include the items described in options 1, 2, and 3, but these will not help differentiate current pain from preoperative pain.
Priority Nursing Tip: Discourage prolonged sitting with leg dependency after femoral-popliteal artery bypass grafting because it may cause pain and edema and increase the risk of venous thrombosis.
Test-Taking Strategy: Focus on the subject, the assessment question that will help differentiate expected postoperative pain from pain that indicates graft occlusion. Note the strategic word, *most*. Eliminate options 1, 2, and 3 because they are comparable or alike and are standard pain assessment questions. Review: care of the client after **right femoral-popliteal artery bypass grafting.**
Reference(s): Ignatavicius, Workman (2013), p. 849; Potter et al (2013), pp. 320-322.

1313. A client has implemented dietary and other lifestyle changes to manage hypertension. The nurse determines that the client has been **most** successful if the client has which follow-up blood pressure reading?
1. 164/90 mm Hg
2. 156/89 mm Hg
3. 140/94 mm Hg
4. 128/84 mm Hg

Level of Cognitive Ability: Evaluating
Client Needs: Physiological Integrity
Integrated Process: Nursing Process/Evaluation
Content Area: Adult Health: Cardiovascular
Priority Concepts: Clinical Judgment; Perfusion

Answer: 4
Rationale: Normal blood pressure readings are less than 120/80 mm Hg. A blood pressure reading between 120/80 mm Hg and 139/89 mm Hg is considered to be a prehypertensive state. From the readings provided in the options, option 4 identifies the most successful outcome, although the reading indicates a prehypertensive state.
Priority Nursing Tip: Evaluate the dietary patterns and sodium intake for a client with hypertension. Sodium promotes fluid retention, elevating the blood pressure.
Test-Taking Strategy: Note the strategic word, *most*. Option 4 identifies a reading that is closest to normal even though it identifies a prehypertensive state. Review: **hypertension.**
Reference(s): Ignatavicius, Workman (2013), pp. 775-777.

1314. A client is scheduled to have surgery. The nurse should place **priority** on determining whether the surgeon wants which medications held in the preoperative period?
1. Furosemide (Lasix)
2. Famotidine (Pepcid)
3. Warfarin (Coumadin)
4. Multivitamin with minerals

Level of Cognitive Ability: Analyzing
Client Needs: Physiological Integrity
Integrated Process: Nursing Process/Analysis
Content Area: Fundamental Skills: Perioperative Care
Priority Concepts: Collaboration; Safety

Answer: 3
Rationale: The nurse is careful to question the surgeon about whether warfarin should be administered in the preoperative period. This medication is often withheld for a period of time preoperatively to minimize the risk of hemorrhage during surgery. The other medications may also be withheld if specifically prescribed, but usually they are discontinued as part of an NPO (nothing by mouth) after midnight prescription.
Priority Nursing Tip: In the preoperative client, the nurse should review the client's medication list and question the health care provider about medications that should be withheld.
Test-Taking Strategy: Note the strategic word, *priority*. Recalling that warfarin is an anticoagulant and that when a client is taking an anticoagulant a risk for bleeding exists will direct you to the correct option. Review: **anticoagulant medication therapy and preoperative nursing care.**
Reference(s): Ignatavicius, Workman (2013), p. 253.

1315. A client's medical record states a history of intermittent claudication. In collecting data about this symptom, the nurse should ask the client about which symptom?
1. Chest pain that is dull and feels like heartburn
2. Leg pain that is sharp and occurs with exercise
3. Chest pain that is sudden and occurs with exertion
4. Leg pain that is achy and gets worse as the day progresses

Level of Cognitive Ability: Applying
Client Needs: Physiological Integrity
Integrated Process: Nursing Process/Assessment
Content Area: Adult Health: Cardiovascular
Priority Concepts: Gas Exchange; Perfusion

Answer: 2
Rationale: Intermittent claudication is a symptom characterized by a sudden onset of leg pain that occurs with exercise and is relieved by rest. It is the classic symptom of peripheral arterial insufficiency. Chest pain can occur for a variety of reasons, including indigestion or angina pectoris. Venous insufficiency is characterized by an achy type of leg pain that intensifies as the day progresses.
Priority Nursing Tip: A client with peripheral arterial disease may achieve some pain relief by dangling the affected leg over the side of the bed or sleeping in a chair with the legs in a dependent position to allow gravity to maximize blood flow.
Test-Taking Strategy: Focus on the subject, intermittent claudication. Recalling that claudication refers to leg pain will assist in eliminating options 1 and 3. The word *intermittent* in the question will direct you to the correct option. Review: **intermittent claudication**.
Reference(s): Ignatavicius, Workman (2013), p. 696; Lewis et al (2014), pp. 834-835.

1316. A client has just been diagnosed with right leg deep vein thrombosis (DVT). Which intervention should the nurse implement?
1. Ice packs to the right leg
2. Elevation of the right leg
3. Hourly calf measurements
4. Vigorous range of motion to the right leg

Level of Cognitive Ability: Applying
Client Needs: Physiological Integrity
Integrated Process: Nursing Process/Implementation
Content Area: Adult Health: Cardiovascular
Priority Concepts: Clotting; Safety

Answer: 2
Rationale: Treatment for DVT may require bed rest, leg elevation, and application of warm moist heat to the affected leg. The client may have calf measurements prescribed once per shift or once per day, but they would not be obtained hourly. Option 1 is incorrect because heat, not cold, may be prescribed. Option 4 is dangerous to the client because vigorous activity after clot formation can cause pulmonary embolus.
Priority Nursing Tip: Intravenous heparin sodium therapy may be prescribed to treat deep vein thrombosis (DVT).
Test-Taking Strategy: Focus on the subject, deep vein thrombosis. Use knowledge of the treatment for DVT as well as concepts related to gravity and the applications of heat and cold to answer the question. Review: the interventions for **deep vein thrombosis (DVT)**.
Reference(s): Ignatavicius, Workman (2013), p. 800.

1317. A client is scheduled to have a serum digoxin (Lanoxin) level obtained. The nurse determines the blood sample should be drawn at which time?
1. Just before a dose is given
2. One hour after a dose is given
3. Just after a dose has been given
4. One-half hour after a dose is given

Level of Cognitive Ability: Applying
Client Needs: Physiological Integrity
Integrated Process: Nursing Process/Planning
Content Area: Pharmacology: Cardiovascular Medications
Priority Concepts: Clinical Judgment; Safety

Answer: 1
Rationale: The purpose of a serum digoxin level is to obtain the serum concentration of the medication to ensure that it is in the therapeutic range. Serum digoxin levels are most often drawn before a dose, although they may be drawn 6 to 8 hours after a dose was administered. Drawing the medication before a dose ensures that the level is not falsely elevated.
Priority Nursing Tip: The therapeutic serum drug level for digoxin is 0.5 to 2.0 ng/dL.
Test-Taking Strategy: Focus on the subject, the best time to draw a blood sample to do a serum digoxin level. Eliminate options 2, 3, and 4 because they are comparable or alike. Each of these options requires the blood sample to be drawn within a relatively short period after the client has been given the medication. Review: The **serum digoxin (Lanoxin) level** blood test.
Reference(s): Hodgson, Kizior (2014), pp. 351-353; Ignatavicius, Workman (2013), p. 726; Lehne (2013), pp. 566-567.

1318. The nurse assesses the environmental safety of a client receiving home oxygen therapy. Which observation by the nurse indicates the client **needs further teaching?**
1. Oxygen used 30 feet from a gas stove
2. Oxygen tank stored in the tank holder
3. "No smoking" sign posted at the front door
4. Oxygen concentrator propped against a wall

Level of Cognitive Ability: Evaluating
Client Needs: Safe and Effective Care Environment
Integrated Process: Teaching and Learning
Content Area: Fundamental Skills: Safety
Priority Concepts: Client Education; Safety

Answer: 4
Rationale: The oxygen concentrator should be free and clear of walls or other enclosed spaces to allow adequate air circulation around the unit; otherwise, the unit can overheat and increase the risk of fire. Clients should avoid using oxygen within 10 feet of open flames because oxygen fuels a fire. Oxygen tanks are secured in a holder to stabilize and protect the tank, and a "no smoking" sign should be in view to alert visitors about the risk.
Priority Nursing Tip: Instruct the client using an oxygen concentrator or any other respiratory device requiring electricity for use to notify the electric company. In case of a power failure, the electric company will know the medical urgency of restoring your power.
Test-Taking Strategy: Focus on the subject, environmental safety when using home oxygen. The strategic words, *needs further teaching* indicate a negative event query and the need to select the incorrect client action. Recalling the principles of safe oxygen use will direct you to the correct option. Review: **oxygen safety principles.**
Reference(s): Perry, Potter, Ostendorf (2014), p. 589.

1319. The nurse has finished suctioning the tracheostomy of a client. Which item should the nurse monitor to determine the **effectiveness** of the procedure?
1. Breath sounds
2. Capillary refill
3. Respiratory rate
4. Oxygen saturation level

Level of Cognitive Ability: Evaluating
Client Needs: Physiological Integrity
Integrated Process: Nursing Process/Evaluation
Content Area: Adult Health: Respiratory
Priority Concepts: Clinical Judgment; Gas Exchange

Answer: 1
Rationale: After suctioning a client either with or without an artificial airway, the breath sounds are auscultated to determine the extent to which the airways have been cleared of respiratory secretions. The other assessment items are not as precise as breath sounds for this purpose.
Priority Nursing Tip: Monitor the client closely during suctioning. Discontinue suctioning if the client's heart rate decreases from baseline by 20 beats per minute, increases from baseline by 40 beats per minute, dysrhythmias occur, or if the pulse oximetry reading decreases to less than 90%.
Test-Taking Strategy: Note the strategic word, *effectiveness.* Focus on the subject, evaluating the effectiveness of suctioning. Recalling that the purpose of suctioning is to clear the airways of secretions will direct you to the correct option. Review: the procedure for **suctioning a tracheostomy.**
Reference(s): Perry, Potter, Ostendorf (2014), pp. 645-646; Potter et al (2013), p. 861.

1320. The nurse has given client directions for proper use of aluminum hydroxide tablets. The client indicates an understanding of the medication if which statement is made?
1. "I should take the tablet at the same time as an antacid."
2. "I should swallow the tablet whole with a full glass of water."
3. "I should take each dose with a laxative to prevent constipation."
4. "I should chew the tablet thoroughly and then drink 4 ounces of water."

Level of Cognitive Ability: Evaluating
Client Needs: Physiological Integrity
Integrated Process: Nursing Process/Evaluation
Content Area: Pharmacology: Gastrointestinal Medications
Priority Concepts: Client Education; Safety

Answer: 4
Rationale: Aluminum hydroxide tablets should be chewed thoroughly before swallowing. This prevents them from entering the small intestine undissolved. They should not be swallowed whole. Antacids should be taken at least 2 hours apart from other medications to prevent interactive effects. Constipation is a side effect of aluminum products, but the client should not take a laxative with each dose. This promotes laxative abuse. The client should first try other means to prevent constipation.
Priority Nursing Tip: If the client is taking an aluminum product such as aluminum hydroxide tablets, the client should be instructed to increase intake of dietary fiber.
Test-Taking Strategy: Focus on the subject, antacids, specifically aluminum hydroxide. Eliminate option 1 using general knowledge of antacid interactive effects. Next, eliminate option 3 because it does not promote healthy bowel function. From the remaining choices, use principles of digestion and medication use to direct you to the correct option. Review: client teaching points related to the use of **aluminum hydroxide.**
Reference(s): Kee, Hayes, McCuistion (2012), p. 720; Lehne (2013), p. 996.

1321. The nurse is checking a client's disposable closed chest drainage system at the beginning of the shift and notes continuous bubbling in the water-seal chamber. What should the nurse determine is the cause?
1. The system is intact.
2. A pneumothorax is resolving.
3. The suction to the system is shut off.
4. There is an air leak somewhere in the system.

Level of Cognitive Ability: Analyzing
Client Needs: Physiological Integrity
Integrated Process: Nursing Process/Analysis
Content Area: Adult Health: Respiratory
Priority Concepts: Clinical Judgment; Gas Exchange

Answer: 4
Rationale: Continuous bubbling in the water-seal chamber through both inspiration and expiration indicates that air is leaking into the system. A resolving pneumothorax would show intermittent bubbling in the water-seal chamber with respiration. Shutting the suction off to the system stops bubbling in the suction control chamber, but does not affect the water-seal chamber.
Priority Nursing Tip: Ensure that all connections are secure in a chest tube drainage system.
Test-Taking Strategy: Focus on the subject, continuous bubbling in the water-seal chamber. The words *continuous bubbling* should provide you with the clue that an air leak is present. Review: the principles associated with a **chest tube drainage system.**
Reference(s): Potter et al (2013), p. 872.

1322. A client is suspected of having pulmonary tuberculosis. Which signs/symptoms of tuberculosis should the nurse assess the client for?
1. High fever and chest pain
2. Increased appetite, dyspnea, and chills
3. Weight gain, insomnia, and night sweats
4. Low-grade fever, fatigue, and productive cough

Level of Cognitive Ability: Analyzing
Client Needs: Physiological Integrity
Integrated Process: Nursing Process/Assessment
Content Area: Adult Health: Respiratory
Priority Concepts: Gas Exchange; Infection

Answer: 4
Rationale: The client with pulmonary tuberculosis generally has a productive or nonproductive cough, anorexia and weight loss, fatigue, low-grade fever, chills and night sweats, dyspnea, hemoptysis, and chest pain. Breath sounds may reveal crackles.
Priority Nursing Tip: If pulmonary tuberculosis is active, caseation and inflammation may be seen on the chest x-ray.
Test-Taking Strategy: Focus on the subject, tuberculosis, specifically its signs and symptoms. Remember that when an option has more than one part, all of the parts of that choice must be correct if the entire option is to be correct. Eliminate options 2 and 3 first because the client will not have an increased appetite or weight gain. From the remaining choices, it is necessary to know that the fever will be low grade. Review: assessment findings related to **pulmonary tuberculosis.**
Reference(s): Ignatavicius, Workman (2013), pp. 654-655.

1323. The nurse is preparing to implement emergency care measures for the client who has just experienced pulmonary embolism. Which health care provider prescription should the nurse implement **first**?
1. Apply oxygen.
2. Administer morphine sulfate.
3. Start an intravenous (IV) line.
4. Obtain an electrocardiogram (ECG).

Level of Cognitive Ability: Analyzing
Client Needs: Physiological Integrity
Integrated Process: Nursing Process/Implementation
Content Area: Critical Care: Emergency Situations
Priority Concepts: Clinical Judgment; Gas Exchange

Answer: 1
Rationale: The client needs oxygen immediately because of hypoxemia, which is most often accompanied by respiratory distress and cyanosis. The client should also have an IV line for the administration of emergency medications such as morphine sulfate. An ECG is useful in determining the presence of possible right ventricular hypertrophy. All of the interventions listed are appropriate, but the client needs the oxygen first.
Priority Nursing Tip: If pulmonary embolism is suspected, notify the rapid response team immediately.
Test-Taking Strategy: Note the strategic word, *first.* Use the ABCs—airway, breathing, and circulation. This will direct you to the correct option. Review: care of the client with **pulmonary embolism.**
Reference(s): Ignatavicius, Workman (2013), p. 665.

❖ **1324.** Which interventions should the nurse include in the plan of care for a client who is scheduled for bronchoscopy? **Select all that apply.**
- ❑ 1. Remove any dentures.
- ❑ 2. Remove contact lenses.
- ❑ 3. Let the client eat or drink.
- ❑ 4. Ensure that the informed consent is signed.
- ❑ 5. Have the client void before transport to endoscopy.

Level of Cognitive Ability: Analyzing
Client Needs: Physiological Integrity
Integrated Process: Nursing Process/Planning
Content Area: Adult Health: Respiratory
Priority Concepts: Gas Exchange; Safety

Answer: 1, 2, 4, 5
Rationale: If the client has any contact lenses, dentures, or other prostheses, they are removed before sedation is administered to him or her. The client must sign an informed consent because the procedure is invasive. For comfort reasons, the client also should be asked about the need to void before transport to the endoscopy department. The client is not allowed to eat or drink usually for 6 to 8 hours (or as specified by the health care provider) before the procedure to prevent the risk of aspiration.
Priority Nursing Tip: After bronchoscopy, avoid giving the client anything orally until the gag reflex returns.
Test-Taking Strategy: Focus on the subject, bronchoscopy, and think about what is involved. Recalling that for many invasive procedures the client must be on nothing by mouth status (NPO) will assist in answering correctly. Review: care of the client undergoing bronchoscopy.
Reference(s): Ignatavicius, Workman (2013), pp. 260, 559; Pagana, Pagana (2013), p. 194.

1325. A client who has no history of immunosuppressive disease and is at low risk for tuberculosis has a Mantoux tuberculin skin test. The results indicate an area of induration that is 8 mm in size. How should the nurse interpret this result?
1. Active tuberculosis
2. A negative response
3. A history of tuberculosis
4. Past exposure to tuberculosis

Level of Cognitive Ability: Analyzing
Client Needs: Physiological Integrity
Integrated Process: Nursing Process/Analyzing
Content Area: Adult Health: Respiratory
Priority Concepts: Gas Exchange; Infection

Answer: 2
Rationale: Induration of 15 mm or more is considered positive for clients in low-risk groups. More than 5 mm of induration is considered a positive result for clients with known or suspected human immunodeficiency virus infection, persons with organ transplants, persons in close contact with a known case of tuberculosis, and those with a chest x-ray study suggestive of previous tuberculosis. More than 10 mm of induration is considered positive in all other high-risk groups, such as intravenous drug users.
Priority Nursing Tip: A positive Mantoux tuberculin skin test reaction does not mean that active disease is present but indicates previous exposure to tuberculosis or the presence of inactive (dormant) disease.
Test-Taking Strategy: Focus on the subject, Mantoux tuberculin skin test results. Note the words, *at low risk.* Noting that the area of induration measures 8 mm will direct you to the correct option. Review: the normal parameters for the **Mantoux tuberculin skin test.**
Reference(s): Chernecky, Berger (2013), pp. 764-765; Pagana, Pagana (2013), pp. 933-934.

1326. A client has a prescription to have a set of arterial blood gases (ABGs) drawn, and the intended site is the radial artery. The nurse ensures that which is positive before the ABGs are drawn?
1. Allen test
2. Turner's sign
3. Babinski reflex
4. Brudzinski's sign

Level of Cognitive Ability: Analyzing
Client Needs: Physiological Integrity
Integrated Process: Nursing Process/Assessment
Content Area: Adult Health: Respiratory
Priority Concepts: Acid-Base Balance; Clinical Judgment

Answer: 1
Rationale: The Allen test is performed before drawing ABGs. Both the radial and ulnar arteries are occluded and then pressure on the ulnar artery is released. Observation is made in the distal circulation. If the results are positive, then the client has adequate circulation and the radial artery may be used. Turner's sign is the bluish discoloration of the flanks and is indicative of pancreatitis. The Babinski reflex is checked by stroking upward on the sole of the foot. Brudzinski's sign tests for nuchal rigidity by bending the head down toward the chest.
Priority Nursing Tip: Arterial blood for blood gas analysis can be obtained through puncture of the radial or femoral artery or through an arterial catheter.
Test-Taking Strategy: Focus on the subject, ABGs drawn from the radial artery pretest. Recalling the purpose of each test listed in the options will direct you to the correct option. Review: Allen test.
Reference(s): Pagana, Pagana (2013), p. 117.

1327. A client has been taking benzonatate (Tessalon) as prescribed. Which action should the nurse tell the client that this medication should do?

1. Increase comfort level
2. Decrease anxiety level
3. Calm the persistent cough
4. Take away nausea and vomiting

Level of Cognitive Ability: Applying
Client Needs: Physiological Integrity
Integrated Process: Teaching and Learning
Content Area: Pharmacology: Respiratory Medications
Priority Concepts: Client Education; Gas Exchange

Answer: **3**
Rationale: Benzonatate is a locally acting antitussive. Its effectiveness is measured by the degree to which it decreases the intensity and frequency of cough, without eliminating the cough reflex. Options 1, 2, and 4 are not intended effects of this medication.
Priority Nursing Tip: Instruct the client taking an antitussive to notify the health care provider if the cough lasts longer than 1 week and a fever or rash occurs.
Test-Taking Strategy: Focus on the subject, benzonatate (Tessalon). Recalling that benzonatate is a locally acting antitussive will direct you to the correct option. Review: **benzonatate (Tessalon).**
Reference(s): Lehne (2013), p. 982.

1328. The nurse is assessing a client with a suspected rib fracture. Which typical signs/symptoms should the nurse observe for?

1. Pain on expiration, deep rapid respirations
2. Pain on inspiration, deep rapid respirations
3. Pain on expiration, shallow guarded respirations
4. Pain on inspiration, shallow guarded respirations

Level of Cognitive Ability: Analyzing
Client Needs: Physiological Integrity
Integrated Process: Nursing Process/Assessment
Content Area: Adult Health: Respiratory
Priority Concepts: Clinical Judgment; Gas Exchange

Answer: **4**
Rationale: The client with fractured ribs typically has pain over the fracture site with inspiration and to palpation. Respirations are shallow, and guarding of the area is often noted. Bruising may or may not be present. Therefore, options 1, 2, and 3 are incorrect.
Priority Nursing Tip: An intercostal nerve block may be prescribed for the client with a rib fracture if the pain is severe.
Test-Taking Strategy: Focus on the subject, suspected rib fracture. Think about the movement of the chest wall on inspiration and expiration. Remember that pain will occur on inspiration, and respirations will be shallow. Review: the signs related to a **rib fracture.**
Reference(s): Ignatavicius, Workman (2013), p. 682; Lewis et al (2014), p. 543.

1329. A client with a flail chest caused by four fractured rib segments is experiencing severe pain when trying to breathe. Which characteristics of a flail chest should the nurse observe the client for?

1. Cyanosis and slow respirations
2. Slight bradypnea with shallow breaths
3. Pallor and paradoxical chest movement
4. Severe dyspnea and paradoxical chest movement

Level of Cognitive Ability: Analyzing
Client Needs: Physiological Integrity
Integrated Process: Nursing Process/Assessment
Content Area: Adult Health: Respiratory
Priority Concepts: Clinical Judgment; Gas Exchange

Answer: **4**
Rationale: The client with flail chest is in obvious respiratory distress. The client has severe dyspnea and cyanosis accompanied by paradoxical chest movement. Respirations are shallow, rapid, and grunting in nature.
Priority Nursing Tip: In flail chest, paradoxical respirations (inward movement of a segment of the thorax during inspiration, with outward movement during expiration) occur.
Test-Taking Strategy: Focus on the subject, flail chest from rib fractures. Remember that for an option to be correct, all parts of that choice must also be correct. With this in mind, eliminate options 2 and 3 because of the words *slight* and *pallor*. Choose between the remaining options, knowing that this client would be tachypneic, rather than having slow respirations. Review: the clinical manifestations associated with **flail chest.**
Reference(s): Ignatavicius, Workman (2013), p. 683; Lewis et al (2014), pp. 543-544.

1330. The nurse is assigned to care for a client with pneumonia. The nurse reviews the nursing progress notes and sees documentation that the client experiences dyspnea when doing activities. Which action should the nurse implement in the client's care?
1. Encourage deep, rapid breathing during activity.
2. Provide stimulation in the environment to maintain client alertness.
3. Observe vital signs and oxygen saturation periodically during activity.
4. Schedule activities before giving respiratory medications or treatments.

Level of Cognitive Ability: Applying
Client Needs: Physiological Integrity
Integrated Process: Nursing Process/Planning
Content Area: Adult Health: Respiratory
Priority Concepts: Clinical Judgment; Gas Exchange

Answer: 3
Rationale: The nurse monitors vital signs, including oxygen saturation, before, during, and after activity to gauge client response. Activities should be planned after giving the client respiratory medications or treatments to increase activity tolerance. The client should use pursed-lip and diaphragmatic breathing to lower oxygen consumption during activity. Finally, the environment should be conducive to rest because the client is easily fatigued.
Priority Nursing Tip: Home care instructions for the client with pneumonia who is discharged from the hospital include notifying the health care provider if chills, fever, dyspnea, hemoptysis, or increased fatigue occurs.
Test-Taking Strategy: Focus on the subject, activity intolerance by the client with pneumonia. Use the ABCs—airway, breathing, and circulation—to direct you to the correct option. Review: the interventions for a client with pneumonia and dyspnea.
Reference(s): Ignatavicius, Workman (2013), pp. 621-622; Lewis et al (2014), p. 527.

1331. The nurse is admitting a newborn infant to the nursery and notes that the health care provider has documented that the newborn has gastroschisis. The nurse plans care, knowing that in this condition, where is the viscera?
1. Inside the abdominal cavity and under the skin
2. Inside the abdominal cavity and under the dermis
3. Outside the abdominal cavity and not covered with a sac
4. Outside the abdominal cavity but inside a translucent sac covered with peritoneum and amniotic membrane

Level of Cognitive Ability: Applying
Client Needs: Physiological Integrity
Integrated Process: Nursing Process/Assessing
Content Area: Maternity: Newborn
Priority Concepts: Development; Elimination

Answer: 3
Rationale: Gastroschisis is an abdominal wall defect in which the viscera are outside the abdominal cavity and not covered with a sac. Embryonal weakness in the abdominal wall causes herniation of the gut on one side of the umbilical cord during early development. Options 1 and 2 describe an umbilical hernia. Option 4 describes an omphalocele.
Priority Nursing Tip: Altered skin integrity and infection are the priority concerns for the infant with gastroschisis.
Test-Taking Strategy: Focus on the subject, gastroschisis. Eliminate options 1 and 2 first because they are comparable or alike. From the remaining choices, recalling the definition of gastroschisis will direct you to the correct option. Review: gastroschisis.
Reference(s): McKinney et al (2013), p. 1078.

1332. The nurse is performing an assessment on a 6-month-old infant suspected of having hydrocephalus. Which finding is associated with this diagnosis?
1. A bulging anterior fontanel
2. An elevated apical heart rate
3. The presence of protein in the urine
4. A drop in blood pressure from baseline

Level of Cognitive Ability: Analyzing
Client Needs: Physiological Integrity
Integrated Process: Nursing Process/Assessment
Content Area: Child Health: Neurological
Priority Concepts: Development; Intracranial Regulation

Answer: 1
Rationale: A bulging anterior fontanel indicates an increase in cerebrospinal fluid collection in the cerebral ventricle, which occurs in hydrocephalus. An elevated apical heart rate, proteinuria, and a drop in blood pressure are not specifically related to increasing cerebrospinal fluid in the brain tissue.
Priority Nursing Tip: In hydrocephalus, there are thin, widely separated bones of the head that produce a cracked-pot sound (known as Macewen's sign) on percussion.
Test-Taking Strategy: Focus on the subject, hydrocephalus. Recall that this relates to excessive fluid buildup in the cranial cavity to answer this question. Remember that fluid accumulation in the cranial cavity will exert pressure on the soft brain tissue. This will cause the anterior fontanel to expand. Additionally correlate the word *hydrocephalus* in the question with *anterior fontanel* in option 1. Review: the findings associated with **hydrocephalus**.
Reference(s): McKinney et al (2013), pp. 1423-1424.

1333. A 10-day postpartum breast-feeding client telephones the postpartum unit complaining of a reddened, painful breast and elevated temperature. Based on assessment of the client's complaints, which action should the nurse tell the client to do?
1. "Breast-feed only with the unaffected breast."
2. "Stop breast-feeding because you probably have an infection."
3. "Notify your health care provider because you may need medication."
4. "Continue breast-feeding because this is a normal response in breast-feeding mothers."

Level of Cognitive Ability: Analyzing
Client Needs: Physiological Integrity
Integrated Process: Nursing Process/Assessment
Content Area: Maternity: Postpartum
Priority Concepts: Infection; Reproduction

Answer: 3
Rationale: Based on the signs and symptoms presented by the client (particularly the elevated temperature), the health care provider needs to be notified because an antibiotic that is tolerated by the infant, as well as the mother, may be prescribed. The mother should continue to nurse on both breasts, but should start the infant on the unaffected breast while the affected breast lets down.
Priority Nursing Tip: Medications, including over-the-counter medications, need to be avoided in the breast-feeding mother unless prescribed, because they may be unsafe when breast-feeding.
Test-Taking Strategy: Focus on the subject, breast-feeding with a reddened, painful breast, and elevated temperature. Option 4 can be eliminated first because the client's complaints are not normal. Eliminate option 2 because it does not encourage the continuation of breast-feeding or notification of the health care provider. Option 1 also does not encourage continuation of normal breast-feeding and could possibly lead to engorgement, creating more discomfort and pain for the mother. Review: **postpartum complications**.
Reference(s): Lowdermilk, Perry, Cashion, Alden (2012), p. 629; McKinney et al (2013), p. 541.

1334. The nurse notes that the health care provider has written a prescription for prednisone for a client. The nurse contacts the health care provider about revision of the client's medication plan if which medication is noted on the client's medication record?
1. Furosemide (Lasix)
2. Oxycodone (OxyContin)
3. Acetaminophen (Tylenol)
4. Acetylsalicylic acid (aspirin)

Level of Cognitive Ability: Analyzing
Client Needs: Physiological Integrity
Integrated Process: Nursing Process/Assessment
Content Area: Pharmacology: Endocrine Medications
Priority Concepts: Collaboration; Safety

Answer: 4
Rationale: Prednisone is irritating to the gastrointestinal (GI) tract, which could be worsened by the use of other products that have the same side effect. Therefore, products such as aspirin and nonsteroidal anti-inflammatory drugs are not used during corticosteroid therapy. The medications identified in the remaining options are not a concern.
Priority Nursing Tip: Monitor the client taking prednisone for hyperglycemia and hypokalemia.
Test-Taking Strategy: Focus on the subject, the adverse effects of prednisone. Think about these adverse effects and recalling that aspirin is irritating to the GI tract will assist in answering the question. Review: the side effects of **prednisone**.
Reference(s): Lehne (2013), pp. 917-918.

❖ **1335.** The nurse talks to students at a high school about sexually transmitted infections (STIs). Which **effective** methods of preventing STIs does the nurse include in the discussion? **Select all that apply.**
   ❑ 1. Some birth control pills prevent STIs.
   ❑ 2. STIs do not transmit through oral sex.
   ❑ 3. Diaphragms are a barrier against STIs.
   ❑ 4. Abstinence prevents transmission of STIs.
   ❑ 5. Proper condom use provides STI protection.
   ❑ 6. Multiple sex partners increase the risk of STIs.

Level of Cognitive Ability: Analyzing
Client Needs: Safe and Effective Care Environment
Integrated Process: Teaching and Learning
Content Area: Fundamental Skills: Infection Control
Priority Concepts: Client Education; Sexuality

Answer: 4, 5, 6
Rationale: Effective measures to avoid STIs include abstinence, using condoms properly, and avoiding multiple partners, and the nurse should provide this factual information to the high school students. The nurse also includes information about ineffective methods of preventing STIs, including birth control pills, oral sex, and diaphragms.
Priority Nursing Tip: All sexual contacts of a client with a sexually transmitted infection also must be treated for the infection.
Test-Taking Strategy: Note the strategic word, *effective*. Focus on the subject, preventing STIs, not pregnancy. This focus will eliminate options 1, 2, and 3. Review: the methods of protection against sexually transmitted infections (STIs).
Reference(s): Lewis et al (2014), p. 1272; Potter et al (2013), pp. 547, 686.

1336. The nurse provides discharge instructions to a client after implantation of a permanent pacemaker. The nurse should tell the client to avoid exposure to which item?
   1. Hair dryers
   2. Electric blankets
   3. Electric toothbrushes
   4. Airport metal detectors

Level of Cognitive Ability: Applying
Client Needs: Safe and Effective Care Environment
Integrated Process: Teaching and Learning
Content Area: Adult Health: Cardiovascular
Priority Concepts: Clinical Judgment; Safety

Answer: 4
Rationale: A pacemaker is shielded from interference from most electrical devices. Devices to be forewarned about include those with a strong electric current or magnetic field, such as antitheft devices in stores, metal detectors used in airports, and radiation therapy (if applicable and which might require relocation of the pacemaker). Radios, televisions, electric blankets, toasters, microwave ovens, heating pads, and hair dryers are considered to be safe.
Priority Nursing Tip: The client with a pacemaker should be instructed to hold a cell phone on the ear on the side of the body opposite the pacemaker.
Test-Taking Strategy: Focus on the subject, the item to avoid after after implantation of a permanent pacemaker. Note that option 4 uses the word *metal*. Review: home care measures for the client with a pacemaker.
Reference(s): Ignatavicius, Workman (2013), p. 741.

1337. A client with low back pain asks the nurse which type of exercise will strengthen the lower back muscles. Which **best** exercise should the nurse tell the client to participate in?
   1. Tennis
   2. Diving
   3. Canoeing
   4. Swimming

Level of Cognitive Ability: Applying
Client Needs: Health Promotion and Maintenance
Integrated Process: Teaching and Learning
Content Area: Fundamental Skills: Pain
Priority Concepts: Client Education; Pain

Answer: 4
Rationale: Walking and swimming are very beneficial in strengthening back muscles for the client with low back pain. The other options involve twisting and pulling of the back muscles, which is not helpful to the client experiencing back pain.
Priority Nursing Tip: The client with chronic low back pain should be encouraged to lose weight and maintain a healthy weight. This will decrease stress on the back muscles.
Test-Taking Strategy: Note the strategic word, *best* in the question. Recalling that low back pain is aggravated by any activity that twists or turns the spine, evaluate each of the options according to this guideline. This will enable you to eliminate options 1, 2, and 3. Review: home care measures for the client with **low back pain.**
Reference(s): Ignatavicius, Workman (2013), p. 962.

1338. The nurse is caring for a child with a diagnosis of Kawasaki disease, and the mother of the child asks the nurse about the disorder. Which description of this disorder should the nurse base the response to the mother on?
1. It is an acquired cell-mediated immunodeficiency disorder.
2. It is a chronic multisystem autoimmune disease characterized by the inflammation of connective tissue.
3. It is also called mucocutaneous lymph node syndrome and is a febrile generalized vasculitis of unknown etiology.
4. It is an inflammatory autoimmune disease that affects the connective tissue of the heart, joints, and subcutaneous tissues.

Level of Cognitive Ability: Applying
Client Needs: Physiological Integrity
Integrated Process: Teaching and Learning
Content Area: Child Health: Cardiovascular
Priority Concepts: Client Education; Inflammation

Answer: 3
Rationale: Kawasaki disease, also called mucocutaneous lymph node syndrome, is a febrile generalized vasculitis of unknown etiology. Option 1 describes human immunodeficiency virus infection. Option 2 describes systemic lupus erythematosus. Option 4 describes rheumatic fever.
Priority Nursing Tip: Cardiac involvement is the most serious complication of Kawasaki disease; aneurysms can develop.
Test-Taking Strategy: Focus on the subject, Kawasaki disease. Knowledge regarding the description of Kawasaki disease is required to answer this question. Remember Kawasaki disease is a febrile generalized vasculitis of unknown etiology. Review: **Kawasaki disease.**
Reference(s): Hockenberry, Wilson (2013), pp. 858-859.

1339. The nurse is preparing to teach the parents of a child with anemia about the dietary sources of iron that are easy for the body to absorb. Which food item should the nurse include in the teaching plan?
1. Fruits
2. Poultry
3. Apricots
4. Vegetables

Level of Cognitive Ability: Applying
Client Needs: Health Promotion and Maintenance
Integrated Process: Teaching and Learning
Content Area: Child Health: Hematological
Priority Concepts: Client Education; Nutrition

Answer: 2
Rationale: Dietary sources of iron that are easy for the body to absorb include meat, poultry, and fish. Vegetables, fruits, cereals, and breads are also dietary sources of iron, but they are harder for the body to absorb.
Priority Nursing Tip: For anemia, instruct the parents and child about the food items that are high in iron such as meats; egg yolk; breads and cereals; and dark green, leafy vegetables.
Test-Taking Strategy: Focus on the subject, food sources that are high in iron and easy to absorb. Options 1 and 3 are comparable or alike and should be eliminated first. From the remaining choices, focusing on the words *easy for the body to absorb* assists in eliminating option 4. Review: **dietary sources of iron.**
Reference(s): McKinney et al (2013), pp. 1242-1243.

1340. The nurse is caring for a child with a patent ductus arteriosus. The nurse reviews the child's assessment data, knowing that which is characteristic of this disorder?
1. It involves an opening between the two atria.
2. It produces abnormalities in the atrial septum.
3. It involves an opening between the two ventricles.
4. It involves an artery that connects the aorta and the pulmonary artery during fetal life.

Level of Cognitive Ability: Applying
Client Needs: Physiological Integrity
Integrated Process: Nursing Process/Assessment
Content Area: Child Health: Cardiovascular
Priority Concepts: Development; Perfusion

Answer: 4
Rationale: Patent ductus arteriosus is described as an artery that connects the aorta and the pulmonary artery during fetal life. It generally closes spontaneously within a few hours to several days after birth. It allows abnormal blood flow from the high-pressure aorta to the low-pressure pulmonary artery, resulting in a left-to-right shunt. Options 1, 2, and 3 are not characteristics of this cardiac defect.
Priority Nursing Tip: In patent ductus arteriosus, a machinery-like murmur is present.
Test-Taking Strategy: Focus on the subject, patent ductus arteriosus. Knowledge regarding the characteristics associated with patent ductus arteriosus is required to answer this question. Remember patent ductus arteriosus is an artery that connects the aorta and the pulmonary artery during fetal life. Review: **patent ductus arteriosus.**
Reference(s): McKinney et al (2013), p. 1214.

❖ **1341.** Which clinical manifestations are consistent with infants who have congenital hypothyroidism? **Select all that apply.**
   ☐ 1. Irritability
   ☐ 2. Hoarse cry
   ☐ 3. Bradycardia
   ☐ 4. Constipation
   ☐ 5. Fused fontanels
   ☐ 6. Excessive sleeping

Level of Cognitive Ability: Analyzing
Client Needs: Physiological Integrity
Integrated Process: Nursing Process/Assessment
Content Area: Child Health: Metabolic/Endocrine
Priority Concepts: Development; Thermoregulation

Answer: 2, 3, 4, 6
Rationale: The infant with congenital hypothyroidism may display the following signs: skin mottling, a large fontanel, a large tongue, hypotonia, slow reflexes, bradycardia, and a distended abdomen. Other signs and symptoms include prolonged jaundice, lethargy, constipation, feeding problems, coldness to touch, umbilical hernia, hoarse cry, and excessive sleeping.
Priority Nursing Tip: Most of the assessment findings that are seen in hypothyroidism reflect slowed or depressed effects, such as lethargy, constipation, and excessive sleeping.
Test-Taking Strategy: Focus on the subject, congenital hypothyroidism. Recall that symptoms of hypothyroidism are clinical manifestations of a slow metabolism or altered neurological or physical development. Irritability would be seen in infants with hyperactive metabolism. Fused fontanels would be present in hyperthyroidism; large fontanels are often seen in hypothyroidism. Review: the manifestations of **hypothyroidism.**
Reference(s): Hockenberry, Wilson (2013), p. 309; McKinney et al (2013), pp. 1383, 1385.

1342. Desmopressin acetate (DDAVP) is prescribed via intranasal route for a child with von Willebrand's disease, and the nurse instructs the parents regarding the administration of this medication. Which statement by the parents indicates a **need for further teaching?**
   1. "We need to refrigerate the DDAVP."
   2. "We need to increase our child's fluid intake."
   3. "Nausea and abdominal cramps can occur as a side effect of the medication."
   4. "Headache and drowsiness may be a sign of water intoxication that can occur with the medication."

Level of Cognitive Ability: Evaluating
Client Needs: Physiological Integrity
Integrated Process: Teaching and Learning
Content Area: Pharmacology: Hematological Medications
Priority Concepts: Fluid and Electrolyte Balance; Safety

Answer: 2
Rationale: Parents should be instructed to reduce fluid intake during initial treatment because the treatment will prevent continued fluid loss and the result will be fluid buildup. The medication should be refrigerated, but freezing should be avoided. Side effects of the medication include facial flushing, nasal congestion, increased blood pressure, nausea, abdominal cramps, decreased urination, and vulval pain. Signs and symptoms of water intoxication include headache, drowsiness and confusion, weight gain, seizures, and coma.
Priority Nursing Tip: Willebrand's disease is a hereditary bleeding disorder and is characterized by a deficiency of or a defect in a protein termed von Willebrand factor.
Test-Taking Strategy: Note the strategic words, *need for further teaching.* These words indicate a negative event query and the need to select the incorrect client statement. Noting the word *increase* in option 2 and thinking about the action of the medication will direct you to this option. Review: the action, use, and side effects of **desmopressin acetate (DDAVP).**
Reference(s): McKinney et al (2013), pp. 1120-1121.

1343. A child is brought to the emergency department after being bitten in the arm by a neighborhood dog. The nurse performs a focused assessment, cleanses the wound as prescribed, and continues to perform a thorough assessment on the child. Which is the **priority** question for the nurse to ask the mother of the child?

1. "How old is the dog?"
2. "Did the dog have rabies?"
3. "Are the child's immunizations up-to-date?"
4. "Did the dog have all of its recommended shots?"

Level of Cognitive Ability: Analyzing
Client Needs: Health Promotion and Maintenance
Integrated Process: Nursing Process/Assessment
Content Area: Child Health: Infectious and Communicable Diseases
Priority Concepts: Immunity; Infection

Answer: 3
Rationale: When a bite occurs, the injury site of the bite should be cleansed carefully and the child should be given tetanus prophylaxis if immunizations are not up-to-date. Option 3 is the priority consideration. Options 1, 2, and 4 identify information that may have to be obtained, but are not the priority questions. Additionally the mother may not have the answers to these questions.
Priority Nursing Tip: Always obtain an immunization history from the parent when the child is brought to the emergency department.
Test-Taking Strategy: Note the strategic word, *priority*. Option 3 is the only option that focuses on the needs of the child. Review: care of a child who receives a **dog bite**.
Reference(s): Hockenberry, Wilson (2013), pp. 715-716.

1344. The nurse is providing instructions to the mother of a child who had a myringotomy with insertion of tympanostomy tubes. Which action should the nurse tell the mother to take if the tubes fall out?

1. "Bring the child to the emergency department immediately."
2. "It is not an emergency, but it is best to call the health care clinic."
3. "It is important to replace them immediately so that the surgical opening does not close."
4. "Clean the tubes with half-strength hydrogen peroxide for 30 minutes and then replace them into the child's ears."

Level of Cognitive Ability: Applying
Client Needs: Physiological Integrity
Integrated Process: Teaching and Learning
Content Area: Child Health: Eye/Ear
Priority Concepts: Client Education; Sensory Perception

Answer: 2
Rationale: The mother should be assured that if the tympanostomy tubes fall out, it is not an emergency, but it is best if the health care provider or health care clinic is notified. The size and appearance of the tympanostomy tubes should be described to the mother following surgery so that she will be familiar with their appearance. Options 1, 3, and 4 are incorrect.
Priority Nursing Tip: After myringotomy with insertion of tympanostomy tubes, instruct the parents to keep the child's ears dry.
Test-Taking Strategy: Focus on the subject, tympanostomy tubes falling out. Option 1 is eliminated first because it will cause concern in the mother and is incorrect. Next, eliminate options 3 and 4 because they are comparable or alike and relate to replacing the tubes. Review: home care instructions after **myringotomy** with insertion of **tympanostomy tubes**.
Reference(s): McKinney et al (2013), p. 1154; Hockenberry, Wilson (2013), pp. 718-719.

1345. The mother of a child calls the health care clinic and tells the nurse that the child has developed a bloody nose. Which action should the nurse instruct the mother to do?
1. Pinch the nostrils for 5 minutes and then recheck for bleeding.
2. Maintain the child in a sitting position with the head tilted backward.
3. Lay the child down with a pillow tucked under the neck and stay with the child to keep the child calm.
4. Have the child sit with the head tilted forward and hold pressure on the soft part of the nose for a period of 10 minutes.

Level of Cognitive Ability: Applying
Client Needs: Physiological Integrity
Integrated Process: Nursing Process/Implementation
Content Area: Child Health: Throat/Respiratory
Priority Concepts: Client Education; Clotting

Answer: 4
Rationale: The child should be positioned erect, sitting with head tilted forward to avoid blood dripping posteriorly to the pharynx. The soft part of the nose should be tightly pinched against the center wall for 10 minutes, and the mother should be instructed that this pinch should be timed by a clock, not estimated. The mother should be told not to release pressure for 10 minutes. The child is encouraged to remain calm and quiet and to breathe through the mouth.
Priority Nursing Tip: For epistaxis, if bleeding cannot be controlled, packing or cauterization of the bleeding vessel may be prescribed.
Test-Taking Strategy: Focus on the subject, controlling a bloody nose. Visualize the positions presented in the options to direct you to option 4. Review: the interventions used when **epistaxis** occurs.
Reference(s): Hockenberry, Wilson (2013), p. 888.

1346. The nurse is assessing a child admitted to the hospital with a diagnosis of rheumatic fever. Which significant question should the nurse ask the child's mother during the assessment?
1. "Has your child had difficulty urinating?"
2. "Has your child been exposed to anyone with chickenpox?"
3. "Has any family member had a sore throat within the past few weeks?"
4. "Has any family member had a gastrointestinal disorder in the past few weeks?"

Level of Cognitive Ability: Analyzing
Client Needs: Physiological Integrity
Integrated Process: Nursing Process/Assessment
Content Area: Child Health: Throat/Respiratory
Priority Concepts: Infection; Inflammation

Answer: 3
Rationale: Rheumatic fever characteristically presents 2 to 6 weeks after an untreated or partially treated group A beta-hemolytic streptococcal infection of the respiratory tract. Initially the nurse determines whether any family member has had a sore throat or unexplained fever within the past few weeks. Options 1, 2, and 4 are unrelated to the assessment findings of rheumatic fever.
Priority Nursing Tip: The parents of a child with a history of rheumatic fever should be informed if anyone in their child's school develops a streptococcal throat infection.
Test-Taking Strategy: Focus on the subject, rheumatic fever. Note the word *significant*. Recalling that rheumatic fever characteristically presents 2 to 6 weeks following a streptococcal infection of the respiratory tract will direct you to the correct option. Review: **rheumatic fever**.
Reference(s): McKinney et al (2013), p. 1229.

1347. The parents of a child with mumps express concern that their child will develop orchitis as a result of having mumps and ask the nurse about the signs of this complication. What should the nurse tell the parents is a sign of this complication?
1. Fever
2. Facial swelling
3. Swollen glands
4. Difficulty urinating

Level of Cognitive Ability: Applying
Client Needs: Physiological Integrity
Integrated Process: Teaching and Learning
Content Area: Child Health: Infectious and Communicable Diseases
Priority Concepts: Client Education; Infection

Answer: 1
Rationale: Unilateral orchitis occurs more frequently than bilateral orchitis. About 1 week after the appearance of parotitis, there is an abrupt onset of testicular pain, tenderness, fever, chills, headache, and vomiting. The affected testicle becomes red, swollen, and tender. Atrophy, resulting in sterility, occurs only in a small number of cases. Facial swelling and swollen glands normally occur in mumps. Difficulty urinating is not a sign of this complication.
Priority Nursing Tip: Warmth and local support with snug, fitting underpants can be used to relieve orchitis.
Test-Taking Strategy: Focus on the subject, orchitis. Eliminate options 2 and 3 first because they are comparable or alike. Recalling that "-itis" indicates inflammation will direct you to option 1. Review: the characteristics of **orchitis**.
Reference(s): McKinney et al (2013), p. 1021.

1348. A maternity nurse is teaching a pregnant client about the physiological effects and hormone changes that occur in pregnancy. The client asks the nurse about the purpose of estrogen. Which information should the nurse provide to the client about estrogen?

1. It maintains the uterine lining for implantation.
2. It stimulates metabolism of glucose and converts the glucose to fat.
3. It prevents the involution of the corpus luteum and maintains the production of progesterone until the placenta is formed.
4. It stimulates uterine development to provide an environment for the fetus and stimulates the breasts to prepare for lactation.

Level of Cognitive Ability: Applying
Client Needs: Physiological Integrity
Integrated Process: Teaching and Learning
Content Area: Maternity: Antepartum
Priority Concepts: Client Education; Reproduction

Answer: 4
Rationale: Estrogen stimulates uterine development to provide an environment for the fetus and stimulates the breasts to prepare for lactation. Progesterone maintains the uterine lining for implantation and relaxes all smooth muscle. Human placental lactogen stimulates the metabolism of glucose and converts the glucose to fat. Human chorionic gonadotropin prevents involution of the corpus luteum and maintains the production of progesterone until the placenta is formed.
Priority Nursing Tip: During the proliferative phase of the menstrual cycle, estrogen stimulates proliferation and growth in the endometrium.
Test-Taking Strategy: Focus on the subject, the purpose of estrogen during pregnancy. Specific knowledge regarding the functions of various hormones related to pregnancy is required to answer this question. Remember that estrogen stimulates uterine development to provide an environment for the fetus and stimulates the breasts to prepare for lactation. Review: purpose of estrogen.
Reference(s): McKinney et al (2013), p. 241.

1349. The nurse has explained the reason that the health care provider has chosen laser surgery to treat a client's cervical cancer. Which statement by the client indicates an understanding of the explanation?

1. "I want to be asleep during my procedure."
2. "I have too much cancer to be removed with surgery."
3. "I am young and the laser prevents cancer tissue from regrowing."
4. "The health care provider is able to see all the edges of my cancer clearly."

Level of Cognitive Ability: Evaluating
Client Needs: Physiological Integrity
Integrated Process: Nursing Process/Evaluation
Content Area: Adult Health: Oncology
Priority Concepts: Client Education; Cellular Regulation

Answer: 4
Rationale: Laser therapy is performed in an outpatient setting and is used when all boundaries of the lesion are visible. Laser surgery is painless, and the client would not receive general anesthesia. Laser therapy does not prevent regrowth.
Priority Nursing Tip: Minimal bleeding is associated with cervical laser surgery.
Test-Taking Strategy: Focus on the subject, laser surgery for cervical cancer. Thinking about the procedure involved in laser surgery will direct you to the correct option. Review: this type of treatment for cervical cancer.
Reference(s): Ignatavicius, Workman (2013), p. 1625.

1350. The nurse is monitoring a client with hypercalcemia. Which assessment finding indicates a **need for follow-up**?
1. Increased peristalsis
2. Decreased capillary refill
3. Increased deep tendon reflexes
4. Decreased abdominal circumference

Level of Cognitive Ability: Analyzing
Client Needs: Physiological Integrity
Integrated Process: Nursing Process/Assessment
Content Area: Fundamental Skills: Fluids & Electrolytes
Priority Concepts: Clotting; Fluid and Electrolyte Balance

Answer: 2
Rationale: The client with hypercalcemia is at risk for formation of blood clots. Clotting is more likely to occur in the lower legs, pelvic region, and areas where blood flow is blocked (causing constriction). The nurse should assess for impaired blood flow by measuring calf circumference with a soft tape measure and assess temperature, color, and capillary refill. Decreased capillary refill may be indicative of a clot. The client with hypercalcemia may also exhibit decreased peristalsis, decreased deep tendon reflexes, altered level of consciousness, hypoactive or absent bowel sounds, or increased abdominal circumference as a result of decreased peristalsis.
Priority Nursing Tip: Hypercalcemia is present when the serum calcium level exceeds 10 mg/dL.
Test-Taking Strategy: Note the strategic words, *need for follow-up*. This phrase indicates a negative event query and the need to select an option that is an abnormal assessment finding. Note that options 1 and 4 are comparable or alike and relate to the gastrointestinal system. From the remaining options, it is necessary to know that hypercalcemia can cause blood clots; this knowledge will direct you to the correct option. Review: the manifestations associated with hypercalcemia.
Reference(s): Ignatavicius, Workman (2013), pp. 190-191.

1351. The nurse is monitoring the function of a client's chest tube. The chest tube is attached to a chest drainage system. The nurse notes that the fluid in the water-seal chamber is below the 2-cm mark. What should the nurse determine based on this finding?
1. There is a leak in the system.
2. Suction should be added to the system.
3. This is caused by client pneumothorax.
4. Water should be added to the chamber.

Level of Cognitive Ability: Analyzing
Client Needs: Physiological Integrity
Integrated Process: Nursing Process/Analysis
Content Area: Adult Health: Respiratory
Priority Concepts: Gas Exchange; Safety

Answer: 4
Rationale: The water-seal chamber should be filled to the 2-cm mark to provide an adequate water seal between the external environment and the client's pleural cavity. The water seal prevents air from reentering the pleural cavity. Because evaporation of water can occur, the nurse should remedy this problem by adding sterile water until the level is again at the 2-cm mark. The other interpretations are incorrect.
Priority Nursing Tip: Excessive bubbling in the water seal chamber of the chest tube drainage system indicates an air leak in the system.
Test-Taking Strategy: Focus on the subject, the water-seal chamber of a chest drainage system is below the 2-cm mark. Recalling that the chamber needs to be filled to the 2-cm mark will direct you to option 4. Review: the principles associated with care of **chest tubes**.
Reference(s): Potter et al (2013), p. 869.

1352. A client has decided to use transcutaneous electrical nerve stimulation (TENS) as prescribed by the health care provider for the relief of chronic pain, and the nurse has provided instructions to the client regarding the TENS unit. Which statement by the client would indicate a **need for further teaching** regarding this pain relief measure?

1. "I understand that this will help relieve the pain."
2. "This unit will eliminate the need for taking so many pain medications."
3. "I am not real happy that I have to stay in the hospital for this treatment."
4. "I am not sure that I am going to like those electrodes attached to my skin."

Level of Cognitive Ability: Evaluating
Client Needs: Physiological Integrity
Integrated Process: Teaching and Learning
Content Area: Fundamental Skills: Pain
Priority Concepts: Client Education; Pain

Answer: 3
Rationale: It is not necessary for the client to remain in the hospital for this treatment. The TENS unit is a portable unit, and the client controls the system for relieving pain and reducing the need for analgesics. It is attached to the skin of the body by electrodes.
Priority Nursing Tip: Usually a physical therapist administers and teaches the client about transcutaneous electrical nerve stimulation (TENS) therapy. The nurse is responsible for ensuring that the client understands how to use this therapy before discharge from the hospital.
Test-Taking Strategy: Note the strategic words, *need for further teaching*. These words indicate a negative event query and the need to select the incorrect client statement. Options 1 and 2 can be eliminated first because they are comparable or alike. From the remaining choices, select option 3, because it would not be a very cost-effective pain management technique if the client required hospitalization. Review: the principles related to **transcutaneous electrical nerve stimulation (TENS).**
Reference(s): Ignatavicius, Workman (2013), pp. 59-60.

1353. A client with chronic kidney disease has a protein restriction in the diet. Which source of incomplete protein should the nurse include in a teaching plan to be chosen in the diet?

1. Fish
2. Eggs
3. Milk
4. Nuts

Level of Cognitive Ability: Applying
Client Needs: Physiological Integrity
Integrated Process: Teaching and Learning
Content Area: Adult Health: Renal and Urinary
Priority Concepts: Client Education; Nutrition

Answer: 4
Rationale: The client whose diet has a protein restriction should be careful to ensure that the proteins eaten are incomplete proteins with the highest biological value. Nuts are the only option that is not a complete protein. Foods such as meat, fish, milk, and eggs are complete proteins, which are not recommended for the client with chronic kidney disease.
Priority Nursing Tip: Proteins build and repair body tissues, regulate fluid balance, maintain acid-base balance, produce antibodies, provide energy, and produce enzymes and hormones.
Test-Taking Strategy: Focus on the subject, protein composition of various foods and a client with chronic kidney disease. Eliminate options 2 and 3 first because they are animal proteins and are dairy products. From the remaining choices, note the words *incomplete protein* to direct you to option 4. Review: foods that are complete and incomplete proteins.
Reference(s): Nix (2013), p. 51.

1354. A newborn infant is diagnosed with imperforate anus. Which is an appropriate description of this disorder to provide to the parents?

1. The presence of fecal incontinence
2. Incomplete development of the anus
3. The infrequent and difficult passage of dry stools
4. Invagination of a section of the intestine into the distal bowel

Level of Cognitive Ability: Applying
Client Needs: Physiological Integrity
Integrated Process: Nursing Process/Planning
Content Area: Maternity: Newborn
Priority Concepts: Development; Elimination

Answer: 2
Rationale: Imperforate anus (anal atresia, anal agenesis) is the incomplete development or absence of the anus in its normal position in the perineum. Option 1 describes encopresis. Encopresis generally affects preschool and school-age children. Option 3 describes constipation. Constipation can affect any child at any time, although it peaks at age 2 to 3 years. Option 4 describes intussusception.
Priority Nursing Tip: Monitor the newborn infant with imperforate anus for the presence of stool in the urine and vagina; this could indicate a fistula.
Test-Taking Strategy: Focus on the subject, imperforate anus. Noting the relationship between the disorder "imperforate anus" and "incomplete development of the anus" in option 2 should direct you to this option. Review: **imperforate anus.**
Reference(s): McKinney et al (2013), p. 1078.

1355. The nurse is providing bottle-feeding instructions to the mother of a newborn infant. The nurse provides instructions regarding the amount of formula to be given, knowing that what is the approximate stomach capacity for a newborn?
1. 5 to 10 mL
2. 10 to 20 mL
3. 30 to 90 mL
4. 75 to 100 mL

Level of Cognitive Ability: Applying
Client Needs: Health Promotion and Maintenance
Integrated Process: Teaching and Learning
Content Area: Maternity: Newborn
Priority Concepts: Development; Nutrition

Answer: 2
Rationale: The stomach capacity of a newborn is approximately 10 to 20 mL. It is 30 to 90 mL for a 1-week-old infant and 75 to 100 mL for a 2- to 3-week-old infant.
Priority Nursing Tip: Instruct the mother not to heat a bottle of formula in a microwave oven.
Test-Taking Strategy: Focus on the subject, the stomach capacity for a newborn. Note the word *newborn*. This should assist in eliminating options 3 and 4. From the remaining choices, visualize the amounts in options 1 and 2. Noting that 5 mL is a very small amount should assist in directing you to option 2. Review: stomach capacities of pediatric ages, specifically the **newborn**.
Reference(s): McKinney et al (2013), p. 1069.

1356. A mother who is breast-feeding her newborn infant is experiencing nipple soreness, and the nurse provides teaching regarding measures to relieve the soreness. Which statement by the mother indicates an understanding of the teaching?
1. "I need to avoid rotating breast-feeding positions so that the nipple will toughen."
2. "I need to stop nursing during the period of nipple soreness to allow the nipples to heal."
3. "I need to nurse less frequently and substitute a bottle feeding until the nipples become less sore."
4. "I need to position my infant with her ear, shoulder, and hip in straight alignment and place her stomach against me."

Level of Cognitive Ability: Evaluating
Client Needs: Health Promotion and Maintenance
Integrated Process: Nursing Process: Evaluation
Content Area: Maternity: Postpartum
Priority Concepts: Client Education; Health Promotion

Answer: 4
Rationale: Comfort measures for nipple soreness include positioning the infant with the ear, shoulder, and hip in straight alignment and with the infant's stomach against the mother's. Additional measures include rotating breast-feeding positions, breaking suction with the little finger, nursing frequently, beginning feeding on the less sore nipple, not allowing the infant to chew on the nipple or to sleep holding the nipple in the mouth, and applying tea bags soaked in warm water to the nipple. Options 1, 2, and 3 are incorrect client statements.
Priority Nursing Tip: The nurse needs to assess the newborn's ability to attach to the mother's breast and suck.
Test-Taking Strategy: Focus on the subject, nipple soreness with breast-feeding. Note the words *indicates an understanding*. Visualize each of the options in terms of how it may or may not lessen the nipple soreness to direct you to option 4. Review: the measures to reduce **nipple soreness** in a mother who is **breast-feeding**.
Reference(s): McKinney et al (2013), pp. 542-543.

1357. A client with acute myocardial infarction receives therapy with alteplase (tissue plasminogen activator, recombinant; t-PA). Which finding indicates to the nurse that the client is experiencing a possible complication?
1. Epistaxis
2. Vomiting
3. ECG changes
4. Absent pedal pulses

Level of Cognitive Ability: Analyzing
Client Needs: Physiological Integrity
Integrated Process: Nursing Process/Analysis
Content Area: Pharmacology: Cardiovascular Medications
Priority Concepts: Clotting; Safety

Answer: 1
Rationale: Bleeding is an adverse effect of t-PA therapy. The bleeding can be superficial or internal and can be spontaneous. Options 2, 3, and 4 are not side or adverse effects of t-PA therapy.
Priority Nursing Tip: Bleeding is the primary concern for a client taking an anticoagulant, thrombolytic, or antiplatelet medication.
Test-Taking Strategy: Focus on the subject, t-PA therapy. Recalling that this medication is a thrombolytic and that epistaxis is a bloody nose will direct you to option 1. Review: the side and adverse effects of **alteplase (tissue plasminogen activator, recombinant; t-PA)**.
Reference(s): Lehne (2013), pp. 655, 660-661.

1358. The nurse is performing an assessment on a mother who just delivered a healthy newborn. When checking the uterine fundus the nurse should expect to note that the fundus is positioned at which location?

1. To the right of the abdomen
2. At the level of the umbilicus
3. Above the level of the umbilicus
4. One fingerbreadth above the symphysis pubis

Level of Cognitive Ability: Analyzing
Client Needs: Physiological Integrity
Integrated Process: Nursing Process/Assessment
Content Area: Maternity: Postpartum
Priority Concepts: Clinical Judgment; Reproduction

Answer: 2
Rationale: Immediately after delivery, the uterine fundus should be at the level of the umbilicus or one to three fingerbreadths below it and in the midline of the abdomen. A fundus that is not located in the midline may indicate a full bladder. If the fundus is above the umbilicus, this may indicate that blood clots in the uterus need to be expelled by fundal massage.
Priority Nursing Tip: The postpartum period starts immediately after delivery and is usually completed by week 6 after delivery.
Test-Taking Strategy: Focus on the subject, position of the uterine fundus postdelivery. Note the words *just delivered*. Use knowledge regarding normal anatomy and visualize each description in the options to direct you to the correct option. Review: **uterine fundus** positions.
Reference(s): McKinney et al (2013), p. 441.

1359. The nurse obtains the vital signs on a mother who delivered a healthy newborn 2 hours ago and notes that the mother's temperature is 102° F. What is the appropriate nursing action at this time?

1. Notify the health care provider.
2. Remove the blanket from the client's bed.
3. Document the finding and recheck the temperature in 4 hours.
4. Administer acetaminophen (Tylenol) and recheck the temperature in 4 hours.

Level of Cognitive Ability: Applying
Client Needs: Physiological Integrity
Integrated Process: Nursing Process/Implementation
Content Area: Maternity: Postpartum
Priority Concepts: Reproduction; Thermoregulation

Answer: 1
Rationale: Vital signs usually return to normal within the first hour postpartum if no complications arise. A slight elevation in the temperature may be noted if the client is experiencing dehydrating effects that can occur from labor. A temperature of 102° F indicates infection, and the health care provider should be notified. Options 2, 3, and 4 are inaccurate nursing interventions for a temperature of 102° F 2 hours after delivery.
Priority Nursing Tip: A temperature of 100.4° F is normal during the first 24 hours postpartum because of dehydration, a temperature of 100.4° F or greater after 24 hours postpartum indicates infection.
Test-Taking Strategy: Focus on the subject, temperature of 102° F 2 hours postdelivery. Note that the mother delivered 2 hours ago. Think about the normal postpartum findings. It is most appropriate in this situation to report the findings because a temperature of 102° F can indicate infection. Review: normal **vital signs after delivery**.
Reference(s): McKinney et al (2013), p. 441.

1360. The nurse in the postpartum unit is caring for a mother after vaginal delivery of a healthy newborn. The client received epidural anesthesia for the delivery. One-half hour after admission to the postpartum unit, the nurse checks the client and suspects the presence of a vaginal hematoma. Which finding would be the **best** indicator of the presence of this type of hematoma?

1. Changes in vital signs
2. Signs of vaginal bruising
3. Client complaints of a tearing sensation
4. Client complaints of intense vaginal pressure

Level of Cognitive Ability: Analyzing
Client Needs: Physiological Integrity
Integrated Process: Nursing Process/Assessment
Content Area: Maternity: Postpartum
Priority Concepts: Perfusion; Reproduction

Answer: 1
Rationale: Changes in vital signs indicate hypovolemia in the anesthetized postpartum woman with a vaginal hematoma. Vaginal bruising may be present, but this may be a result of the delivery process and additionally is not the best indicator of the presence of a hematoma. Because the client received anesthesia, she would not feel pain or pressure.
Priority Nursing Tip: Monitor the postpartum client for abnormal pain or perineal pressure, especially when forceps delivery has occurred.
Test-Taking Strategy: Focus on the subject, vaginal hematoma and signs and symptoms, and note the strategic word, *best*. Noting that the client received an epidural anesthetic will assist in eliminating options 3 and 4. From the remaining choices, recalling the pathophysiology associated with the development of a hematoma and use of the ABCs—airway, breathing, and circulation—will direct you to the correct option. Review: the signs of a **vaginal hematoma**.
Reference(s): McKinney et al (2013), pp. 670-671.

❖ **1361.** A client with acute kidney injury has an elevated blood urea nitrogen (BUN). The client is experiencing difficulty remembering information because of uremia. Which interventions should the nurse use when communicating with this client? **Select all that apply.**

❑ 1. Give simple, clear directions.
❑ 2. Include the family in discussions related to care.
❑ 3. Give thorough, lengthy explanations of procedures.
❑ 4. Explain treatments using understandable language.
❑ 5. Use as many teaching methods as available to provide discharge instructions.

Level of Cognitive Ability: Applying
Client Needs: Psychosocial Integrity
Integrated Process: Communication and Documentation
Content Area: Adult Health: Renal and Urinary
Priority Concepts: Cognition; Communication

Answer: 1, 2, 4
Rationale: The client with acute kidney injury may have difficulty remembering information and instructions because of anxiety and the increased level of the BUN. The nurse should avoid giving lengthy explanations about procedures because this information may not be remembered by the client and could increase client anxiety. Communications should be clear, simple, and understandable. The family should be included whenever possible. Using several methods for teaching can be overwhelming for the client. The nurse should assess the client's learning needs and select a method that will facilitate learning.
Priority Nursing Tip: Provide emotional support to the client who is having memory difficulties and allow the client the opportunity to express concerns and fears.
Test-Taking Strategy: Focus on the subject, communication with a client who is experiencing difficulty remembering information. Use the knowledge of the basic principles of effective communication and teaching and learning principles to eliminate each of the incorrect options. Review: **basic communication techniques** and **teaching and learning principles.**
Reference(s): Ignatavicius, Workman (2013), pp. 1475, 1547; Potter et al (2013), pp. 329-330.

1362. The nurse in the newborn nursery receives a telephone call from the delivery room and is told that a postterm small for gestational age (SGA) newborn will be admitted to the nursery. The nurse develops a plan of care for the newborn and decides which is the **priority** to monitor?

1. Urinary output
2. Blood glucose levels
3. Total bilirubin levels
4. Hemoglobin and hematocrit

Level of Cognitive Ability: Analyzing
Client Needs: Physiological Integrity
Integrated Process: Nursing Process/Planning
Content Area: Maternity: Newborn
Priority Concepts: Clinical Judgment; Development

Answer: 2
Rationale: The most common metabolic complication in the SGA newborn is hypoglycemia, which can produce central nervous system abnormalities and mental retardation if not corrected immediately. Urinary output, although important, is not the highest priority action; however, the postterm SGA newborn is typically dehydrated from placental dysfunction. Hemoglobin and hematocrit levels are monitored because the postterm SGA newborn exhibits polycythemia, although this also does not require immediate attention. The polycythemia contributes to increased bilirubin levels, usually beginning on the second day after delivery.
Priority Nursing Tip: Initiate early feedings in the postterm small for gestational age (SGA) newborn and monitor for signs of aspiration.
Test-Taking Strategy: Note the strategic word, *priority*. Recalling that the most common metabolic complication in the SGA newborn is hypoglycemia will direct you to the correct option. Review: the **small for gestational age (SGA) newborn.**
Reference(s): McKinney et al (2013), pp. 711-712.

1363. The nurse in the postpartum unit reviews a client's record and notes that a new mother was administered methylergonovine maleate intramuscularly after delivery. The nurse understands this medication was administered for which action?

1. Decrease uterine contractions.
2. Prevent postpartum hemorrhage.
3. Maintain a normal blood pressure.
4. Reduce the amount of lochia drainage.

Level of Cognitive Ability: Analyzing
Client's Needs: Physiological Integrity
Integrated Process: Nursing Process/Assessment
Content Area: Pharmacology: Reproductive/ Maternity/Newborn Medications
Priority Concepts: Perfusion; Reproduction

Answer: 2
Rationale: Methylergonovine maleate, an oxytocic, is an agent used to prevent or control postpartum hemorrhage by contracting the uterus. The first dose is usually administered intramuscularly, and then if it needs to be continued, it is given by mouth. It increases the strength and frequency of contractions and may elevate blood pressure. There is no relationship between the action of this medication and lochia drainage.
Priority Nursing Tip: Monitor the blood pressure closely in a client receiving methylergonovine maleate because this medication produces vasoconstriction. If an increase in blood pressure is noted, withhold the medication and notify the health care provider.
Test-Taking Strategy: Focus on the subject, methylergonovine maleate, and note the client is postpartum. Recalling that this medication is an oxytocic agent will direct you to the correct option. Review: **methylergonovine maleate.**
Reference(s): McKinney et al (2013), pp. 668, 673.

1364. The nurse in the newborn nursery receives a telephone call and is informed that a newborn infant with Apgar scores of 1 and 4 will be brought to the nursery. The nurse quickly prepares for the arrival of the newborn and determines that which is the **priority** intervention?
1. Connect the resuscitation bag to oxygen.
2. Turn on the apnea and cardiorespiratory monitor.
3. Prepare for the insertion of an intravenous (IV) line with D$_5$W.
4. Set up the radiant warmer control temperature at 36.5° C (97.6° F).

Level of Cognitive Ability: Analyzing
Client Needs: Physiological Integrity
Integrated Process: Nursing Process/Implementation
Content Area: Critical Care: Emergency Situations
Priority Concepts: Clinical Judgment; Gas Exchange

Answer: 1
Rationale: The top priority action for a newborn infant with low Apgar scores is airway, which would involve preparing respiratory resuscitation equipment. Options 2, 3, and 4 are also important, although they are of lower priority. The newborn infant's cardiopulmonary status would be monitored by a cardiorespiratory monitoring device. Setting up an IV with D$_5$W would provide circulatory support. The radiant warmer will provide an external heat source, which is necessary to prevent further respiratory distress.
Priority Nursing Tip: The newborn's Apgar score is assessed and recorded at 1 minute and at 5 minutes after birth.
Test-Taking Strategy: Note the strategic word, *priority* with the word intervention. This question asks you to prioritize care planning based on information about a newborn's condition. Use the ABCs—airway, breathing, and circulation—to direct you to option 1. Although options 2, 3, and 4 are a component of the plan of care, option 1 is the priority. Review: care of the newborn with a **low Apgar score**.
Reference(s): McKinney et al (2013), p. 360.

1365. The nurse is caring for a client in labor who has butorphanol tartrate (Stadol) prescribed for the relief of labor pain. During the administration of the medication, the nurse should ensure that which **priority** item is readily available?
1. Naloxone (Narcan)
2. Meperidine hydrochloride (Demerol)
3. An intravenous form of an antiemetic
4. An intravenous solution of normal saline

Level of Cognitive Ability: Analyzing
Client Needs: Physiological Integrity
Integrated Process: Nursing Process/Planning
Content Area: Maternity: Intrapartum
Priority Concepts: Gas Exchange; Safety

Answer: 1
Rationale: Butorphanol tartrate is an opioid analgesic that provides systemic pain relief during labor. The nurse should ensure that naloxone and resuscitation equipment are readily available to treat respiratory depression, should it occur. Meperidine hydrochloride is also an opioid analgesic that may be used for pain relief, but it also causes respiratory depression. Although an antiemetic may be prescribed for vomiting, antiemetics may enhance the respiratory depressant effects of the butorphanol tartrate. Although an IV access is desirable, the administration of normal saline is unrelated to the administration of this medication.
Priority Nursing Tip: If the client in labor receives an opioid analgesic, it is imperative to have Naloxone (Narcan), the antidote for respiratory depression, readily available especially if delivery is expected to occur during peak medication absorption time.
Test-Taking Strategy: Focus on the strategic word, *priority*. Recalling that butorphanol tartrate causes respiratory depression will direct you to the correct option. Review: **butorphanol tartrate (Stadol)** and its use during **labor**.
Reference(s): McKinney et al (2013), p. 399.

1366. Methylergonovine maleate is prescribed for a woman who has just delivered a healthy newborn. Which is the **priority** assessment to check before administering the medication?

1. Lochia
2. Uterine tone
3. Blood pressure
4. Deep tendon reflexes

Level of Cognitive Ability: Analyzing
Client Needs: Physiological Integrity
Integrated Process: Nursing Process/Assessment
Content Area: Pharmacology: Reproductive/ Maternity/Newborn Medications
Priority Concepts: Perfusion; Safety

Answer: 3
Rationale: Methylergonovine maleate, an oxytocic, is an agent used to prevent or control postpartum hemorrhage by contracting the uterus. The immediate dose is administered intramuscularly, and then, if still needed, it is administered orally. It causes uterine contractions and may elevate the blood pressure. A priority assessment before administration of methylergonovine maleate is blood pressure. Methylergonovine maleate is to be administered cautiously in the presence of hypertension, and the health care provider should be notified if hypertension is present. Options 1 and 2 are general components of care in the postpartum period. Option 4 is most specifically related to the administration of magnesium sulfate.
Priority Nursing Tip: Methylergonovine maleate is an ergot alkaloid and can produce arterial vasoconstriction and arterial vasospasm of the coronary arteries.
Test-Taking Strategy: Note the strategic word, *priority* and use the ABCs—airway, breathing, and circulation—to direct you to option 3. Options 1 and 2 can be eliminated first because lochia and uterine tone are comparable or alike and are general assessments related to the postpartum period. Blood pressure is a method of assessing circulation. Additionally option 4 can be eliminated because it most specifically relates to the administration of magnesium sulfate. Review: the nursing responsibilities related to the administration of **methylergonovine maleate**.
Reference(s): McKinney et al (2013), p. 668.

1367. The nurse provides instructions to a client who is taking allopurinol (Zyloprim) for the treatment of gout. Which statement by the client indicates an understanding of the medication?

1. "I should put ice on my lips if they swell."
2. "I need to take the medication 2 hours after I eat."
3. "I need to drink at least eight glasses of liquids every day."
4. "I can use an antihistamine lotion if I get a rash that is itchy."

Level of Cognitive Ability: Evaluating
Client Needs: Physiological Integrity
Integrated Process: Nursing Process/Evaluation
Content Area: Pharmacology: Musculoskeletal Medications
Priority Concepts: Client Education; Safety

Answer: 3
Rationale: Clients taking allopurinol are encouraged to drink 3000 mL of fluid a day. If the client develops a rash, irritation of the eyes, or swelling of the lips or mouth, he or she should contact the health care provider because this may indicate hypersensitivity. Allopurinol is to be given with or immediately following meals or milk.
Priority Nursing Tip: Instruct the client taking allopurinol (Zyloprim) for the treatment of gout not to take large doses of vitamin C while taking this medication because kidney stones may occur.
Test-Taking Strategy: Focus on the subject, allopurinol. Note the words *indicates an understanding*. Options 1 and 4 can be eliminated first because they indicate hypersensitivity, which is not a normal expected response. From the remaining choices, recalling that the medication should be taken with food or milk will direct you to the correct option. Review: client instructions related to **allopurinol (Zyloprim)**.
Reference(s): Hodgson, Kizior (2014), pp. 36-37.

1368. A rubella vaccine is administered to a client who delivered a healthy newborn 2 days ago. The nurse provides instructions to the client regarding the potential risks associated with this vaccination. Which statement by the client indicates an understanding of the medication?

1. "I need to stay out of the sunlight for 3 days."
2. "The injection site may itch, but I can scratch it if I need to."
3. "I need to avoid sexual intercourse for 2 to 3 months after the vaccination."
4. "I need to prevent becoming pregnant for 2 to 3 months after the vaccination."

Level of Cognitive Ability: Evaluating
Client Needs: Physiological Integrity
Integrated Process: Nursing Process/Evaluation
Content Area: Maternity: Postpartum
Priority Concepts: Health Promotion; Safety

Answer: 4
Rationale: Rubella vaccine is a live attenuated virus that evokes an antibody response and provides immunity for approximately 15 years. Because rubella is a live vaccine, it will act as the virus and is potentially teratogenic in the organogenesis phase of fetal development. The client needs to be informed about the potential effects this vaccine may have and the need to avoid becoming pregnant for a period of 2 to 3 months afterward. Sunlight has no effect on the person who is vaccinated. The vaccine may cause local or systemic reactions, but all are mild and short-lived. Abstinence from sexual intercourse is not necessary, unless another form of effective contraception is not being used.
Priority Nursing Tip: Individuals who are immunocompromised should not receive the Rubella vaccine.
Test-Taking Strategy: Focus on the subject, a rubella vaccine. Recall the effect of live vaccines on pregnancy and fetal development. Remembering that viruses can cross the placental barrier will direct you to the correct option. Review: the potential risks rubella vaccine.
Reference(s): McKinney et al (2013), pp. 439-440.

1369. The school nurse is planning to give a class on testicular self-examination (TSE) at a local high school. The nurse plans to include which instruction on a written handout to be given to the students?

1. Perform the self-examination every other month.
2. Perform the self-examination after a cold shower.
3. Expect the self-examination to be slightly painful.
4. Roll the testicle between the thumb and forefinger.

Level of Cognitive Ability: Applying
Client Needs: Health Promotion and Maintenance
Integrated Process: Teaching and Learning
Content Area: Developmental Stages: Health Assessment/Physical Exam
Priority Concepts: Client Education; Health Promotion

Answer: 4
Rationale: TSE is a self-screening examination for testicular cancer, which predominantly affects men in their late teens and twenties. The self-examination is performed once a month, as is breast self-examination. As an aid to remember to do it, the examination should be done on the same day each month. The scrotum is held in one hand and the testicle is rolled between the thumb and forefinger of the other hand. The self-examination should not be painful. It is easiest to do either during or after a warm shower (or bath) when the scrotum is relaxed.
Priority Nursing Tip: The nurse should teach the client how to perform testicular self-examination (TSE). The nurse should tell the client to gently lift each testicle, and that each one should feel like an egg, should be firm but not hard, and smooth with no lumps. Also teach the client to notify the health care provider if any changes are noted.
Test-Taking Strategy: Focus on the subject, testicular self-examination, and read each option carefully. Knowledge of physical examination techniques will direct you to the correct option. Review: testicular self-examination (TSE).
Reference(s): Potter et al (2013), p. 549.

1370. A 32-year-old female client has a history of fibrocystic disorder of the breasts. The nurse determines that the client understands the nature of the disorder if the client states that symptoms are **most likely** to occur at which time?
1. After menses
2. Before menses
3. In the spring months
4. In the winter months

Level of Cognitive Ability: Evaluating
Client Needs: Physiological Integrity
Integrated Process: Nursing Process/Evaluation
Content Area: Adult Health: Reproductive
Priority Concepts: Client Education; Sexuality

Answer: 2
Rationale: The client with fibrocystic breast disorder experiences worsening of symptoms (breast lumps, painful breasts, and possible nipple discharge) before the onset of menses. This is associated with cyclical hormone changes. Clients should understand that this is part of the clinical picture of this disorder. Options 1, 3, and 4 are incorrect.
Priority Nursing Tip: Fibrocystic breast changes occur most frequently in women between 35 and 50 years of age but often begin as early as 20 years of age.
Test-Taking Strategy: Note the strategic words, *most likely*. This implies that there is a predictable variation in symptoms. Focus on the disorder and use knowledge of the effects of the various hormonal changes that occur in the body to direct you to the correct option. Review: the cyclical hormonal changes that occur in the female and the characteristics of **fibrocystic disorder of the breasts.**
Reference(s): Ignatavicius, Workman (2013), p. 1589.

1371. A client has received a dose of dimenhydrinate (Dramamine). The nurse determines that the medication is **effective** if the client obtains relief of which problem?
1. Chills
2. Headache
3. Ringing in the ears
4. Nausea and vomiting

Level of Cognitive Ability: Evaluating
Client Needs: Physiological Integrity
Integrated Process: Nursing Process/Evaluation
Content Area: Pharmacology: Gastrointestinal Medications
Priority Concepts: Clinical Judgment; Safety

Answer: 4
Rationale: Dimenhydrinate is used to treat and prevent the symptoms of dizziness, vertigo, and nausea and vomiting that accompany motion sickness. The other options are incorrect.
Priority Nursing Tip: Instruct the client to take dimenhydrinate (Dramamine) with food or milk.
Test-Taking Strategy: Focus on the subject, dimenhydrinate (Dramamine) medication effectiveness. Note the strategic word, *effective*. Recalling that this medication is used to treat motion sickness will direct you to option 4. Review: **dimenhydrinate (Dramamine).**
Reference(s): Hodgson, Kizior (2014), p. 359.

1372. A client is preparing for discharge 10 days after a radical vulvectomy. The nurse determines that the client has the **best** understanding of the measures to prevent complications if the client plans to do which after discharge?
1. Walk
2. Housework
3. Drive a car
4. Sit in a chair all day

Level of Cognitive Ability: Evaluating
Client Needs: Physiological Integrity
Integrated Process: Nursing Process/Evaluation
Content Area: Adult Health: Oncology
Priority Concepts: Client Education; Safety

Answer: 1
Rationale: The client should resume activity slowly, and walking is a beneficial activity. The client should know to rest when fatigue occurs. Activities to be avoided include driving, heavy housework, wearing tight clothing, crossing the legs, and prolonged standing or sitting. Sexual activity is usually prohibited for 4 to 6 weeks after surgery.
Priority Nursing Tip: After radical vulvectomy, monitor the client closely for signs of infection.
Test-Taking Strategy: Note the strategic word, *best*. With this in mind, evaluate each of the options in terms of the stress or harm it could cause to the perineal area. This will direct you to option 1. Review: teaching points for the client after radical **vulvectomy.**
Reference(s): Lewis et al (2014), pp. 1296, 1299.

1373. The nurse is caring for the client with silicosis who has massive pulmonary fibrosis. The nurse monitors the client for emotional reactions related to the chronic respiratory disease. Which emotional reaction, if expressed by the client, indicates a need for **immediate** intervention?

1. Anxiety
2. Depression
3. Suicidal ideation
4. Ineffective coping

Level of Cognitive Ability: Analyzing
Client Needs: Psychosocial Integrity
Integrated Process: Nursing Process/Analysis
Content Area: Mental Health
Priority Concepts: Mood and Affect; Safety

Answer: 3
Rationale: Suicidal ideation is not a normal emotional reaction with this condition. If it is expressed, it warrants immediate intervention. Common emotional reactions to a disease such as massive pulmonary fibrosis may be the same as for chronic airflow limitation and include anxiety, ineffective coping, and depression.
Priority Nursing Tip: Silicosis is a type of occupational lung disease and is caused by exposure to environmental or occupational fumes, dust, vapors, gases, bacterial or fungal antigens, and allergens.
Test-Taking Strategy: Note the strategic word, *immediate*. This will direct you to the correct option. Review: **suicidal ideation.**
Reference(s): Ignatavicius, Workman (2013), pp. 629, 632; Lewis et al (2014), pp. 540-541.

1374. At the beginning of the work shift, the nurse is checking a client who has returned from the postanesthesia care unit after transurethral resection of the prostate (TURP). The client has bladder irrigation running via a three-way Foley catheter. The nurse should notify the health care provider if which color of urine is noted in the urinary drainage bag?

1. Pale pink
2. Bright red
3. Dark pink
4. Tea-colored

Level of Cognitive Ability: Applying
Client Needs: Physiological Integrity
Integrated Process: Nursing Process/Implementation
Content Area: Adult Health: Renal and Urinary
Priority Concepts: Clotting; Elimination

Answer: 2
Rationale: Bright red bleeding should be reported because it could indicate complications related to active bleeding. If the bladder irrigation is infusing at a sufficient rate, the urinary drainage will be pale pink. A dark pink color (sometimes referred to as punch-colored) indicates that the speed of the irrigation should be increased. Tea-colored urine is not seen after TURP but may be noted in the client with renal failure or other renal disorders.
Priority Nursing Tip: After transurethral resection of the prostate (TURP), expect red to light pink urine for 24 hours, turning to amber in 3 days.
Test-Taking Strategy: Focus on the subject, color of urine after a TURP. Recall that hemorrhage is a complication after any surgical procedure. Remember also that the purpose of bladder irrigation is to flush out blood and clots that could otherwise accumulate in the bladder after surgery. With this in mind, select option 2 because bright red drainage indicates a potential complication such as bleeding. Review: care of the client after **transurethral resection of the prostate (TURP).**
Reference(s): Ignatavicius, Workman (2013), p. 1636.

1375. Phenelzine sulfate (Nardil) is being administered to a client with depression. The client suddenly complains of a severe occipital headache radiating frontally, and neck stiffness and soreness, and is vomiting. On further assessment, the client exhibits signs of hypertensive crisis. Which medication should the nurse plan to prepare, which is the antidote for hypertensive crisis?

1. Protamine sulfate
2. Calcium gluconate
3. Phentolamine (OraVerse)
4. Phytonadione (Vitamin K)

Level of Cognitive Ability: Applying
Client Needs: Physiological Integrity
Integrated Process: Nursing Process/Planning
Content Area: Critical Care: Emergency Situations
Priority Concepts: Clinical Judgment; Safety

Answer: 3
Rationale: The manifestations of hypertensive crisis include hypertension, occipital headache radiating frontally, neck stiffness and soreness, nausea, vomiting, sweating, fever and chills, clammy skin, dilated pupils, and palpitations. Tachycardia, bradycardia, and constricting chest pain may also be present. The antidote for hypertensive crisis is phentolamine and a dosage by intravenous injection is administered. Protamine sulfate is the antidote for heparin. Calcium gluconate is used for magnesium overdose. Vitamin K is the antidote for warfarin (Coumadin) overdose.
Priority Nursing Tip: Phenelzine sulfate (Nardil) is a monoamine oxidase inhibitor and the client has to be taught to avoid foods that contain tyramine to prevent hypertensive crisis.
Test-Taking Strategy: Focus on the subject, the antidote for phenelzine sulfate. Knowledge regarding the antidotes for various medications and disorders is required to answer this question. Remember that the antidote for hypertensive crisis is phentolamine. Review: **phentolamine (OraVerse).**
Reference(s): Hodgson, Kizior (2014), p. 938.

1376. The nurse is caring for a 25-year-old client who will undergo bilateral orchiectomy for testicular cancer. The nurse should make it a **priority** to explore which potential psychological concern with this client?
1. Postoperative pain
2. Postoperative swelling
3. Loss of reproductive ability
4. Length of recuperative period

Level of Cognitive Ability: Applying
Client Needs: Psychosocial Integrity
Integrated Process: Caring
Content Area: Adult Health: Oncology
Priority Concepts: Cellular Regulation; Coping

Answer: 3
Rationale: Although the client will need factual information about the postoperative period and recuperation, the nurse should place priority on addressing loss of reproductive ability as a psychological concern. The radical effects of this surgery in the reproductive area make it likely that the client may have some difficulty in adjustment to this consequence of surgery.
Priority Nursing Tip: Infertility is a concern after bilateral orchiectomy. Options such as sperm banking should be discussed with the client in the preoperative period.
Test-Taking Strategy: Focus on the subject, a client undergoing a bilateral orchiectomy for testicular cancer. Note the strategic word, *priority*. Eliminate options 1, 2, and 4 because they are general concerns of any surgical procedure. Option 3 is specific to a bilateral orchiectomy. Review: the psychosocial issues related to an **orchiectomy**.
Reference(s): Ignatavicius, Workman (2013), p. 1646.

1377. The nurse is assisting in participating in a prostate screening clinic for men. Which sign of prostatism should the nurse question each client about?
1. Absence of postvoid dribbling
2. Ability to stop voiding quickly
3. Excessive force in urinary stream
4. Hesitancy when initiating urinary stream

Level of Cognitive Ability: Applying
Client Needs: Health Promotion and Maintenance
Integrated Process: Nursing Process/Assessment
Content Area: Adult Health: Renal and Urinary
Priority Concepts: Elimination; Health Promotion

Answer: 4
Rationale: Signs of prostatism that may be reported to the nurse are reduced force and size of urinary stream, intermittent stream, hesitancy in beginning the flow of urine, inability to stop urinating quickly, a sensation of incomplete bladder emptying after voiding, and an increase in episodes of nocturia. These symptoms are the result of pressure of the enlarging prostate on the client's urethra.
Priority Nursing Tip: The risk of prostatic hypertrophy increases in men with each decade after the age of 50 years.
Test-Taking Strategy: Focus on the subject, prostatism. Eliminate options 1, 2, and 3 because they are comparable or alike and indicate no difficulty with proper emptying of the bladder. Review: the signs of **prostatism**.
Reference(s): Ignatavicius, Workman (2013), p. 1630.

1378. A client being seen in the ambulatory care clinic has a history of being treated for syphilis infection. The nurse interprets that the client has been reinfected if which characteristic is noted in a penile lesion?
1. Papular areas and erythema
2. Cauliflower-like appearance
3. Induration and absence of pain
4. Multiple vesicles, with some that have ruptured

Level of Cognitive Ability: Analyzing
Client Needs: Physiological Integrity
Integrated Process: Nursing Process/Assessment
Content Area: Adult Health: Integumentary
Priority Concepts: Infection; Sexuality

Answer: 3
Rationale: The characteristic lesion of syphilis is painless and indurated. The lesion is referred to as a chancre. Scabies is characterized by erythematous, papular eruptions. Genital warts are characterized by cauliflower-like growths, or growths that are soft and fleshy. Genital herpes is accompanied by the presence of one or more vesicles that then rupture and heal.
Priority Nursing Tip: A diagnosis of syphilis is made by microscopic examination of primary and secondary lesion tissues and serology (Venereal Disease Research Laboratory [VDRL] or rapid plasma reagin [RPR] test).
Test-Taking Strategy: Focus on the subject, penile lesion. To answer this question accurately, it is necessary to be familiar with the characteristics of skin lesions of the various sexually transmitted infections. Remember that the characteristic lesion of syphilis is painless and indurated. Review: the appearance of lesions associated with **syphilis**.
Reference(s): Ignatavicius, Workman (2013), pp. 1654-1656.

1379. An adult client has been admitted to the hospital with a 3-day history of uncontrolled vomiting and diarrhea. Which should the nurse assess for in this client?
1. Excitability
2. Bradycardia
3. Hypertension
4. Tenting of the skin

Level of Cognitive Ability: Analyzing
Client Needs: Physiological Integrity
Integrated Process: Nursing Process/Assessment
Content Area: Fundamental Skills: Fluids & Electrolytes
Priority Concepts: Clinical Judgment; Fluid & Electrolyte Balance

Answer: 4
Rationale: The client described in the question will most likely be dehydrated because of uncontrolled vomiting and diarrhea. The nurse assesses this client for weight loss, lethargy, or headache; sunken eyes; poor skin turgor (such as tenting); flat neck and peripheral veins; tachycardia; and low blood pressure.
Priority Nursing Tip: Dehydration occurs when the fluid intake of the body is not sufficient to meet the fluid needs of the body.
Test-Taking Strategy: Focus on the subject, a 3-day history of uncontrolled vomiting and diarrhea. Recalling that a client who has a 3-day episode of uncontrolled vomiting and diarrhea is at risk for dehydration will direct you to the correct option. Review: the signs of dehydration.
Reference(s): Ignatavicius, Workman (2013), pp. 173-176.

1380. An adult client with renal insufficiency has been placed on a fluid restriction of 1200 mL per day. The nurse discusses the fluid restriction with the dietitian and then plans to allow the client to have how many milliliters of fluid from 7:00 AM to 3:00 PM?
1. 400 mL
2. 600 mL
3. 800 mL
4. 1000 mL

Level of Cognitive Ability: Applying
Client Needs: Physiological Integrity
Integrated Process: Nursing Process/Planning
Content Area: Adult Health: Renal and Urinary
Priority Concepts: Collaboration; Fluid and Electrolyte Balance

Answer: 2
Rationale: When a client is on fluid restriction, the nurse informs the dietary department and discusses the allotment of fluid per shift with the dietitian. When calculating how to distribute a fluid restriction, the nurse usually allows half of the daily allotment (600 mL) during the day shift, when the client eats two meals and takes most medications. Another two-fifths (480 mL) is allotted to the evening shift, with the balance (120 mL) allowed during the nighttime.
Priority Nursing Tip: The prescribed daily fluid allotment should be spaced appropriately throughout the day so the client does not become thirsty.
Test-Taking Strategy: Focus on the subject, a fluid restriction of 1200 mL per day. To answer this question accurately, you must be familiar with fluid restriction and the general principles related to fluid distribution over a 24-hour period. Remember that the nurse usually allows half of the daily allotment (600 mL) during the day shift. Review: these principles and calculation of fluid distribution in the client with renal insufficiency.
Reference(s): Potter et al (2013), p. 900.

1381. A client with chronic kidney disease (CKD) has learned about managing diet and fluid restriction between dialysis treatments. The nurse determines that the client is compliant with the therapeutic regimen if the client gains no more than approximately how much weight between hemodialysis treatments?
1. 2 to 4 kg
2. 5 to 6 kg
3. 0.5 to 0.9 kg
4. 1 to 1.5 kg

Level of Cognitive Ability: Evaluating
Client Needs: Physiological Integrity
Integrated Process: Nursing Process/Evaluation
Content Area: Adult Health: Renal and Urinary
Priority Concepts: Adherence; Fluid and Electrolyte Balance

Answer: 4
Rationale: The health care provider will prescribe the amount of fluid that the client is allowed to gain between dialysis treatments, but usually a limit of 1 to 1.5 kg of weight gain between dialysis treatments helps prevent hypotension that tends to occur during dialysis with the removal of larger fluid loads. The nurse determines that the client is compliant with fluid restriction if this weight gain is not exceeded.
Priority Nursing Tip: The client should be weighed before and after dialysis to determine fluid loss.
Test-Taking Strategy: Focus on the subject, appropriate weight gain between hemodialysis treatments. It may be helpful in answering this question to recall that 1 L of fluid weighs approximately 1 kg. Recalling that there are approximately 6 L of blood circulating in the body will assist in eliminating options 1 and 2 as being amounts that are too large. Correspondingly, option 3 is eliminated because the amount is too small, representing only 500 to 900 mL of fluid. Review: teaching points for the client with chronic kidney disease (CKD).
Reference(s): Ignatavicius, Workman (2013), p. 1553.

1382. A client was admitted to the surgical unit after right total knee replacement performed 2 hours earlier. Which observation by the nurse indicates the need to contact the surgeon?
1. Pale pink and warm right foot
2. Pain relieved by an opioid analgesic
3. Ability to flex and extend the right foot
4. Hemovac wound suction drainage of 175 mL per hour

Level of Cognitive Ability: Analyzing
Client Needs: Physiological Integrity
Integrated Process: Nursing Process/Assessment
Content Area: Adult Health: Musculoskeletal
Priority Concepts: Collaboration; Safety

Answer: 4
Rationale: After total knee replacement, the knee incision may have a wound suction drain in place. Drainage of 175 mL per hour is excessive and should be reported. Output from the drain is generally less than 300 mL per shift. The neurovascular status of the affected leg is assessed, and findings should be within normal limits. The client should have intact capillary refill and adequate color, temperature, sensation, and motion of the limb. Incisional pain should be relieved by opioid analgesic administration.
Priority Nursing Tip: After total knee replacement, the health care provider prescribes physical therapy to exercise the knee and strengthen surrounding muscles.
Test-Taking Strategy: Focus on the subject, postoperative observation. Note the words *need to contact the surgeon*, which indicate that you need to select an abnormal finding. Options 1 and 3 represent normal neurovascular and musculoskeletal status and are eliminated first. Knowing that surgery causes the client pain, which is then relieved by analgesics, will assist in eliminating option 2. This leaves option 4 as the correct option given the wording of this question. Review: expected findings following a **total knee replacement**.
Reference(s): Ignatavicius, Workman (2013), pp. 329-330; Potter et al (2013), pp. 1190-1191.

1383. A client is being discharged from the hospital after removal of chest tubes that were inserted following thoracic surgery. When providing home care instructions to the client, which client statement indicates a **need for further teaching**?
1. "I need to avoid heavy lifting for the first 4 to 6 weeks."
2. "I need to take my temperature to detect a possible infection."
3. "I need to remove the chest tube site dressing as soon as I get home."
4. "I need to report any difficulty with breathing to the health care provider."

Level of Cognitive Ability: Evaluating
Client Needs: Physiological Integrity
Integrated Process: Teaching and Learning
Content Area: Adult Health: Respiratory
Priority Concepts: Client Education; Gas Exchange

Answer: 3
Rationale: Upon removal of a chest tube, a dressing is usually placed over the chest tube site. This is maintained in place until the health care provider says it may be removed. The client should avoid heavy lifting for the first 4 to 6 weeks after discharge to facilitate continued wound healing. The client is taught to monitor and report any respiratory difficulty or increased temperature.
Priority Nursing Tip: Depending on the health care provider's preference when the chest tube is removed, the client may be asked to take a deep breath, exhale, and bear down (Valsalva maneuver).
Test-Taking Strategy: Note the strategic words, *need for further teaching*. These words indicate a negative event query and the need to select the incorrect client statement. Recalling that signs of infection and respiratory difficulty should be monitored and reported helps eliminate options 2 and 4 first. From the remaining choices, recalling that either heavy lifting should be avoided postoperatively or that removal of the chest tube site dressing disturbs the occlusive seal to the site will direct you to option 3. Review: teaching points after removal of a **chest tube**.
Reference(s): Perry, Potter, Ostendorf (2014), pp. 668-670.

1384. The nurse is administering epoetin alfa (Epogen) to a client with chronic kidney disease (CKD). Which adverse effect of this therapy should the nurse monitor the client for?
1. Anemia
2. Hypertension
3. Iron intoxication
4. Bleeding tendencies

Level of Cognitive Ability: Analyzing
Client Needs: Physiological Integrity
Integrated Process: Nursing Process/Assessment
Content Area: Pharmacology: Hematological Medications
Priority Concepts: Cellular Regulation; Safety

Answer: 2
Rationale: The client taking epoetin alfa is at risk of hypertension and seizure activity as the most serious adverse effects of therapy. This medication is used to treat anemia. The medication does not cause iron intoxication. Bleeding tendencies is not an adverse effect of this medication.
Priority Nursing Tip: The initial effects of epoetin alfa (Epogen) can be seen within 1 to 2 weeks, and the hematocrit level reaches normal levels in 2 to 3 months.
Test-Taking Strategy: Focus on the subject, epoetin alfa. Knowledge regarding the adverse effects of this medication is needed to answer this question. Remember that the client taking epoetin alfa is at risk of hypertension and seizure activity as the most serious adverse effects of therapy. Review: **epoetin alfa (Epogen).**
Reference(s): Hodgson, Kizior (2014), p. 424.

1385. A client is taking lansoprazole (Prevacid) for the chronic management of Zollinger-Ellison syndrome. The nurse determines that the client **best** understands this disorder and the medication regimen if the client states to take which product for pain?
1. Naprosyn (Aleve)
2. Ibuprofen (Motrin)
3. Acetaminophen (Tylenol)
4. Acetylsalicylic acid (aspirin)

Level of Cognitive Ability: Evaluating
Client Needs: Physiological Integrity
Integrated Process: Teaching and Learning
Content Area: Pharmacology: Gastrointestinal Medications
Priority Concepts: Client Education; Safety

Answer: 3
Rationale: Zollinger-Ellison syndrome is a hypersecretory condition of the stomach. The client should take acetaminophen for pain relief. The client should not take medications that irritate the stomach lining. Irritants would include aspirin and nonsteroidal anti-inflammatory medications (Naprosyn and ibuprofen).
Priority Nursing Tip: Common side effects of lansoprazole (Prevacid) include headache, diarrhea, abdominal pain, and nausea.
Test-Taking Strategy: Focus on the subject, the purpose and use of lansoprazole. Eliminate options 1 and 2 first because they are both nonsteroidal anti-inflammatory medications. Note the strategic word, *best*. From the remaining choices, select acetaminophen over aspirin because it is least irritating to the stomach. Review: **lansoprazole (Prevacid).**
Reference(s): Lehne (2013), pp. 999-1000.

1386. The client scheduled for a transurethral resection prostatectomy (TURP) has listened to the surgeon's explanation of the surgery. The client later asks the nurse to explain again how the prostate is going to be removed. The nurse should tell the client that the prostate will be removed through which location?
1. The urethra
2. A lower abdominal incision
3. An upper abdominal incision
4. An incision made in the perineal area

Level of Cognitive Ability: Applying
Client Needs: Physiological Integrity
Integrated Process: Teaching and Learning
Content Area: Adult Health: Renal and Urinary
Priority Concepts: Client Education; Elimination

Answer: 1
Rationale: A TURP is done through the urethra. An instrument called a resectoscope is used to remove the tissue using high-frequency current. A lower abdominal incision is used for suprapubic or retropubic prostatectomy. An upper abdominal incision is not used. An incision between the scrotum and anus is made when a perineal prostatectomy is performed.
Priority Nursing Tip: A transurethral resection prostatectomy (TURP) is the procedure most commonly used for benign prostatic hypertrophy (BPH) and there is little risk of impotence.
Test-Taking Strategy: Focus on the subject, prostate removal during a TURP. Note the relationship between the name of the procedure "transurethral" in the question and the word *urethra* in the correct option. Review: **transurethral resection prostatectomy (TURP).**
Reference(s): Ignatavicius, Workman (2013), pp. 1633, 1635-1636.

1387. The nurse should tell a client who is scheduled for a bone marrow biopsy that the specimen can be withdrawn from which site?
1. Ribs
2. Femur
3. Scapula
4. Sternum

Level of Cognitive Ability: Applying
Client Needs: Physiological Integrity
Integrated Process: Teaching and Learning
Content Area: Adult Health: Musculoskeletal
Priority Concepts: Client Education; Safety

Answer: 4
Rationale: The most common sites for bone marrow biopsy in the adult are the iliac crest and the sternum. These areas are rich in bone marrow and are easily accessible for testing. The femur, scapula, and ribs are not sites for bone marrow biopsy.
Priority Nursing Tip: The bone marrow biopsy site should be monitored for bleeding and for signs of infection.
Test-Taking Strategy: Focus on the subject, a bone marrow biopsy. Recalling the anatomy and physiology related to the bones and bone marrow will direct you to the correct option. Review: the procedure for a **bone marrow biopsy.**
Reference(s): Pagana, Pagana (2013), pp. 172-173.

1388. A client is taking amiloride (Midamor) 10 mg orally daily for the treatment of hypertension. Which instruction should the nurse give the client regarding its use?
1. Take the medication in the morning with breakfast.
2. Withhold the medication if the blood pressure is high.
3. Eat foods with extra sodium while taking this medication.
4. Take the medication 2 hours after lunch on an empty stomach.

Level of Cognitive Ability: Applying
Client Needs: Physiological Integrity
Integrated Process: Teaching and Learning
Content Area: Pharmacology: Cardiovascular Medications
Priority Concepts: Client Education; Safety

Answer: 1
Rationale: Amiloride is a potassium-retaining diuretic used to treat edema or hypertension. A daily dose should be taken in the morning to avoid nocturia. Increased blood pressure is not a reason to hold the medication, and it may be an indication for its use. Sodium should be restricted if used as an antihypertensive. The dose should be taken with food to increase bioavailability.
Priority Nursing Tip: Instruct the client taking a potassium-sparing diuretic to avoid foods that are high in potassium.
Test-Taking Strategy: Focus on the subject, client instructions regarding the use of amiloride. Noting the client's diagnosis and recalling that this medication is a potassium-retaining diuretic will direct you to option 1. Review: client teaching points related to this **amiloride (Midamor).**
Reference(s): Kee, Hayes, McCuistion (2012), p. 650.

1389. The nurse is preparing a poster for a booth at a health fair to promote primary prevention of cervical cancer. Which recommendation should the nurse include on the poster?
1. Use a commercial douche on a daily basis.
2. Perform monthly breast self-examination (BSE).
3. Seek treatment promptly if cervical infection is suspected.
4. Use oral contraceptives as a preferred method of birth control.

Level of Cognitive Ability: Applying
Client Needs: Health Promotion and Maintenance
Integrated Process: Teaching and Learning
Content Area: Adult Health: Oncology
Priority Concepts: Client Education; Cellular Regulation

Answer: 3
Rationale: Early treatment of cervical infection can help prevent chronic cervicitis, which can lead to dysplasia of the cervix. Cervical dysplasia is an early cell change that is considered to be premalignant. Douches and oral contraceptives do not decrease the risk for this type of cancer. BSE is useful for early detection of breast cancer, but is unrelated to cervical cancer.
Priority Nursing Tip: Risk factors for cervical cancer include early first intercourse (before age 17), multiple sex partners, or male partners with multiple sex partners.
Test-Taking Strategy: Focus on the subject, primary prevention of cervical cancer. Eliminate option 2 because it is unrelated to cervical cancer. From the remaining choices, recalling the risk factors associated with this type of cancer will direct you to the correct option. Review: the risk factors associated with **cervical cancer.**
Reference(s): Ignatavicius, Workman (2013), pp. 1624-1625.

1390. What is the purpose of the nurse administering diphenhydramine (Benadryl) before a blood transfusion?

1. To prevent urticaria
2. To avoid fever and chills
3. To enhance clotting factors
4. To expand the blood volume

Level of Cognitive Ability: Applying
Client Needs: Physiological Integrity
Integrated Process: Nursing Process/Implementation
Content Area: Pharmacology: Immune Medications
Priority Concepts: Tissue Integrity; Safety

Answer: 1

Rationale: The clinical indicators of urticaria are a rash accompanied by pruritus. Urticaria is a manifestation of a transfusion reaction when it occurs during a blood transfusion and is preventable by premedicating the client with an antihistamine, such as diphenhydramine. Options 2, 3, and 4 are incorrect. Clients can also be premedicated with acetaminophen (Tylenol) to help prevent fever and chills.

Priority Nursing Tip: Diphenhydramine (Benadryl) is an antihistamine and can cause drowsiness.

Test-Taking Strategy: Focus on the subject, the purpose of the diphenhydramine before a blood transfusion. Eliminate options 3 and 4 first because enhancing the blood's clotting factors is undesirable, and the transfusion expands the client's blood volume. Recalling the classification of diphenhydramine will direct you to the correct option. Review: the purpose of **diphenhydramine (Benadryl)**.

Reference(s): Hodgson, Kizior (2014), p. 362.

1391. A client is admitted to the hospital with a diagnosis of infiltrating ductal carcinoma of the breast. Which expected manifestation should the nurse assess the client for?

1. Bilateral palpable masses
2. Pain in the breast and edema
3. A fixed, irregularly shaped mass
4. A round-shaped mass that is moveable

Level of Cognitive Ability: Applying
Client Needs: Physiological Integrity
Integrated Process: Nursing Process/Assessment
Content Area: Adult Health: Oncology
Priority Concepts: Cellular Regulation; Sexuality

Answer: 3

Rationale: Infiltrating ductal carcinoma of the breast usually presents as a fixed, irregularly shaped mass. The mass is usually single and unilateral and is painless, nontender, and hard to the touch.

Priority Nursing Tip: With carcinoma of the breast, the mass is usually felt in the upper outer quadrant, beneath the nipple, or in the axilla.

Test-Taking Strategy: Focus on the subject, infiltrating ductal carcinoma of the breast. Using the principles of anatomy and knowledge regarding the characteristics of a cancerous lesion will assist in eliminating options 1 and 4 first. Choose option 3 over option 2, recalling that pain is generally a late sign of a disorder and that involvement of the ducts makes it more likely that the mass does not move (fixed). Review: the characteristics of **breast cancer**.

Reference(s): Ignatavicius, Workman (2013), p. 1592.

1392. A mother of a 9-year-old child newly diagnosed with diabetes mellitus is very concerned about the child going to school and participating in social events. The nurse develops a plan of care and should formulate which goal?

1. The child's normal growth and development will be maintained.
2. The child will use effective coping mechanisms to manage anxiety.
3. The child and family will discuss all aspects of the illness and its treatments.
4. The child and family will integrate diabetes care into patterns of daily living.

Level of Cognitive Ability: Creating
Client Needs: Psychosocial Integrity
Integrated Process: Nursing Process/Planning
Content Area: Child Health: Metabolic/Endocrine
Priority Concepts: Glucose Regulation; Health Promotion

Answer: 4

Rationale: To effectively manage social events in the child's life, the family and the child need to integrate the care and management of diabetes into their daily living. The other options may be appropriate goals, but they do not deal with social issues.

Priority Nursing Tip: For a child with diabetes mellitus, plan to initiate a consultation with the diabetic specialist to develop an individualized plan of care for the child.

Test-Taking Strategy: Focus on the subject, a child diagnosed with diabetes mellitus and concern about social events. Noting the relationship of this subject and the words *into patterns of daily living* will direct you to the correct option. Review: goals of care for a child with **diabetes mellitus.**

Reference(s): Hockenberry, Wilson (2013), pp. 1005-1006; McKinney et al (2013), pp. 1404-1405, 1408.

❖ **1393.** The nurse performs an assessment on a client with cancer and notes that the client is receiving pain medication via this type of catheter. **(Refer to the figure.)** What should the nurse document that the client has?

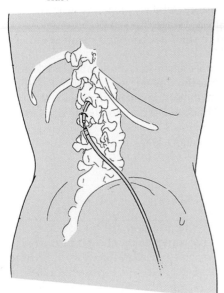

From Lewis S, Dirksen S, Heitkemper M, et al: *Medical-surgical nursing: assessment and management of clinical problems,* ed 8, St. Louis, 2011, Elsevier.

1. Epidural catheter
2. Hickman catheter
3. Central venous catheter (CVC)
4. Patient-controlled analgesia (PCA) pump

Level of Cognitive Ability: Analyzing
Client Needs: Physiological Integrity
Integrated Process: Nursing Process/Implementation
Content Area: Fundamental Skills: Pain
Priority Concepts: Pain; Safety

Answer: 1
Rationale: An epidural catheter is placed in the epidural space. The epidural space lies between the dura mater and the vertebral column. When an opioid is injected into the epidural space, it binds to opiate receptors located on the dorsal horn of the spinal cord and blocks the transmission of pain impulses to the cerebral cortex of the brain. Because the opioid does not cross the blood-brain barrier, pain relief results from drug levels in the spinal cord rather than in the plasma, with little central or systemic distribution of the medication. A Hickman catheter is a vascular access device that is surgically inserted, tunneled through the subcutaneous tissue, and is used to manage long-term intravenous therapy. A CVC is inserted into a large vein (typically the internal or external jugular or the superior vena cava) that leads to the right atrium of the heart. A PCA pump is the device that allows the client to self-administer pain medication.
Priority Nursing Tip: The epidural method of administration of pain medication reduces the amount needed to control pain; therefore, the client experiences fewer side effects.
Test-Taking Strategy: Focus on the subject, the catheter type for pain medication. Recall knowledge of anatomy to answer the question. Noting the location of the catheter site will direct you to the correct option. Review: the placement and use of an **epidural catheter.**
Reference(s): Ignatavicius, Workman (2013), p. 1029; Perry, Potter, Ostendorf (2014), pp. 358-359.

1394. A client has had a left mastectomy with axillary lymph node dissection. The nurse determines that the client understands postoperative restrictions and arm care if the client states to do which activity?
1. Use gloves when working in the garden.
2. Use a straight razor to shave under the arms.
3. Carry a handbag and heavy objects on the left arm.
4. Allow blood pressures to be taken only on the left arm.

Level of Cognitive Ability: Evaluating
Client Needs: Physiological Integrity
Integrated Process: Nursing Process/Evaluation
Content Area: Adult Health: Oncology
Priority Concepts: Client Education; Tissue Integrity

Answer: 1
Rationale: The client is at risk for edema and infection as a result of lymph node dissection. The client should use a variety of techniques to avoid trauma to the affected arm. Examples include using gloves when working in the garden, an electric razor to shave under the arm, and pot holders when cooking to prevent burns. The client should also avoid activities that increase edema, such as carrying heavy objects or having blood pressures taken on the affected arm.
Priority Nursing Tip: After mastectomy with axillary lymph node dissection, the client is at risk for lymphedema.
Test-Taking Strategy: Note the surgical procedure and focus on the subject, postoperative restrictions and arm care after left mastectomy with axillary lymph node dissection. Keeping this subject in mind, read each option, noting the potential risk related to edema or trauma. This will direct you to the correct option. Review: teaching points for the client after **mastectomy with axillary lymph node dissection.**
Reference(s): Ignatavicius, Workman (2013), p. 1608.

1395. The nurse is teaching a client about the modifiable risk factors that can reduce the risk for colorectal cancer. The nurse places **priority** on discussing which risk factor with this client?

1. Age older than 30 years
2. High-fat and low-fiber diet
3. Distant relative with colorectal cancer
4. Personal history of ulcerative colitis or gastrointestinal (GI) polyps

Level of Cognitive Ability: Applying
Client Needs: Health Promotion and Maintenance
Integrated Process: Teaching and Learning
Content Area: Adult Health: Gastrointestinal
Priority Concepts: Client Education; Health Promotion

Answer: 2
Rationale: Clients should be aware of modifiable risk factors as part of general health maintenance and primary disease prevention. Modifiable risk factors are those that can be reduced and include a high-fat and low-fiber diet. Common risk factors for colorectal cancer that cannot be changed include age older than 40, first-degree relative with colorectal cancer, and history of bowel problems such as ulcerative colitis or familial polyposis.
Priority Nursing Tip: Blood in stool is a common manifestation of colorectal cancer.
Test-Taking Strategy: Focus on the subject, modifiable risk factors related to colorectal cancer. Note the strategic word, *priority*. Recalling that modifiable risk factors are those that can be changed will direct you to option 2. Review: modifiable and nonmodifiable risk factors related to **colorectal cancer.**
Reference(s): Ignatavicius, Workman (2013), p. 1246.

1396. A client with gastroesophageal reflux disease (GERD) complains of chest discomfort that feels like heartburn, especially following each meal. After teaching the client to take antacids as prescribed, the nurse suggests that the client lie in which position during sleep?

1. Flat
2. Supine with the head of the bed flat
3. On the stomach with the head of the bed flat
4. With the head of the bed elevated 8 to 12 inches

Level of Cognitive Ability: Applying
Client Needs: Physiological Integrity
Integrated Process: Teaching and Learning
Content Area: Adult Health: Gastrointestinal
Priority Concepts: Client Education; Health Promotion

Answer: 4
Rationale: The discomfort of reflux is aggravated by positions that allow the reflux of gastrointestinal contents. The client is instructed to remain upright for 1 to 2 hours after a meal and sleep with the head of the bed elevated to approximately 30 degrees (usually on 8- to 12-inch blocks). Lying flat will increase the episodes of reflux, resulting in chest discomfort.
Priority Nursing Tip: Instruct the client with gastroesophageal reflux disease (GERD) to eat a low-fat, high-fiber diet and to avoid eating and drinking 2 hours before bedtime.
Test-Taking Strategy: Focus on the subject, sleeping position with GERD. Think about the physiology associated with this disorder. Eliminate options 1, 2, and 3 because they are comparable or alike and all indicate flat positions. Review: measures that will reduce discomfort in the client with **gastroesophageal reflux disease (GERD).**
Reference(s): Ignatavicius, Workman (2013), p. 1206.

1397. The nurse instructs a female client about collecting a midstream urine sample for culture and sensitivity. Which should the nurse include in client teaching?

1. Bathe before collecting the specimen.
2. Cleanse the perineum from front to back.
3. Label specimen with the provider's name.
4. Collect urine at the beginning of urination.

Level of Cognitive Ability: Applying
Client Needs: Physiological Integrity
Integrated Process: Teaching and Learning
Content Area: Fundamental Skills: Diagnostic Tests
Priority Concepts: Client Education; Elimination

Answer: 2
Rationale: To prepare properly for collection of a sterile urine specimen, the client cleanses the perineum from front to back using antiseptic swabs. Bathing before a midstream urine collection is unnecessary; however, proper specimen handling is critically important because improper specimen handling can yield inaccurate test results. The specimen should be labeled with the client's name, date, time, and medical record number in addition to the provider's name. The client should begin the flow of urine and collect the sample after starting the flow of urine, and then send the specimen to the laboratory as soon as possible.
Priority Nursing Tip: A sterile container needs to be used for the collection of urine for a midstream urine sample for culture and sensitivity.
Test-Taking Strategy: Focus on the subject, collecting a midstream urine sample. Recall the principles related to obtaining a midstream urine specimen. Noting the name of the type of sample, "midstream," will assist in eliminating option 4. From the remaining choices, use basic principles related to hygiene to assist in directing you to option 2. Review: **midstream urine sample.**
Reference(s): Ignatavicius, Workman (2013), p. 1479.

1398. The nurse is preparing to care for a client who has undergone esophagogastroduodenoscopy (EGD). After checking the vital signs, what should be the nurse's next priority?
1. Monitor for sharp epigastric pain.
2. Give warm gargles for sore throat.
3. Check for a return of the gag reflex.
4. Monitor for complaints of heartburn.

Level of Cognitive Ability: Applying
Client Needs: Physiological Integrity
Integrated Process: Nursing Process/Implementation
Content Area: Fundamental Skills: Diagnostic Tests
Priority Concepts: Gas Exchange; Safety

Answer: 3
Rationale: The nurse places highest priority on assessing for the return of the gag reflex, which is part of maintaining the client's airway. The nurse should also monitor the client for sharp pain (may indicate a potential complication) and heartburn. The client would receive warm gargles, but this cannot be done until the gag reflex has returned.
Priority Nursing Tip: Aspiration is a priority concern for a client who has had a procedure that involves the application of a local anesthetic to the throat.
Test-Taking Strategy: Note the strategic word, *priority*. Think about this procedure and what is done. Use the ABCs—airway, breathing, and circulation—to direct you to the correct option. Review: postprocedure care following an **esophagogastroduodenoscopy (EGD)**.
Reference(s): Pagana, Pagana (2013), p. 408.

1399. Methylphenidate (Ritalin) is prescribed for a child with a diagnosis of attention deficit hyperactivity disorder (ADHD). At which time should the nurse instruct the mother to administer the medication?
1. Before dinner and at bedtime
2. At the noontime and evening meals
3. In the morning after breakfast and at bedtime
4. Before breakfast and before the noontime meal

Level of Cognitive Ability: Applying
Client Needs: Physiological Integrity
Integrated Process: Teaching and Learning
Content Area: Pharmacology: Neurological Medications
Priority Concepts: Client Education; Safety

Answer: 4
Rationale: Methylphenidate is a central nervous stimulant and should be taken before breakfast and before the noontime meal. It should not be taken in the afternoon or evening because the stimulating effect causes insomnia. Options 1, 2, and 3 are incorrect.
Priority Nursing Tip: Inform the parents of a child taking a medication to treat attention deficit hyperactivity disorder (ADHD) that a drug-free period may be prescribed to allow growth of the child if the medication has caused growth retardation.
Test-Taking Strategy: Focus on the subject, the administration procedure for methylphenidate. Noting the name of the medication and the disorder and recalling that this medication is a central nervous system stimulant will direct you to the correct option. Review: the client teaching points related to the administration of **methylphenidate (Ritalin)**.
Reference(s): Hodgson, Kizior (2014), p. 759.

1400. A client has been scheduled for a barium swallow (esophagography) the next day. The nurse determines that the client understands preprocedure instructions if the client states to take which action before the test?
1. Take all oral medications as scheduled.
2. Eat a regular breakfast on the day of the test.
3. Monitor own bowel movement pattern for constipation.
4. Remove metal objects and jewelry, especially from the neck and chest area.

Level of Cognitive Ability: Evaluating
Client Needs: Physiological Integrity
Integrated Process: Nursing Process/Evaluation
Content Area: Fundamental Skills: Diagnostic Tests
Priority Concepts: Client Education; Safety

Answer: 4
Rationale: A barium swallow, or esophagography, is a radiograph that uses a substance called barium for contrast to highlight abnormalities in the gastrointestinal (GI) tract. The client is told to remove metal objects such as medals and jewelry before the test, so they will not interfere with radiographic visualization of the field. Some oral medications are withheld before the test, and the client should follow the health care provider's instructions regarding medication administration. The client should fast for a minimum of 8 hours before the test, depending on health care provider instructions. It is important after the procedure to monitor for constipation, which can occur as a result of the presence of barium in the GI tract.
Priority Nursing Tip: After a procedure that uses barium, inform the client of the importance of increasing oral fluid intake to help pass the barium.
Test-Taking Strategy: Focus on the subject, preprocedure instructions. Eliminate option 3 first because it is a part of aftercare. Knowing that the procedure is a type of radiographic study that involves barium and that the client needs to remain NPO will assist in eliminating options 1 and 2. Review: preprocedure care for a **barium swallow (esophagography)**.
Reference(s): Chernecky, Berger (2013), pp. 185-186, 328.

1401. A health care provider prescribes a chemotherapeutic medication dose that the nurse
believes is too high. The nurse calls the
health care provider, but the health care
provider has left the office for the weekend.
What action should the nurse take **next**?

1. Reschedule the client's chemotherapy until
the next week.
2. Telephone the answering service and confer with the on-call health care provider.
3. Withhold giving the medication until
the health care provider's partner makes
rounds the next day.
4. Check with the pharmacist, who agrees the
dose is too high, and then reduces the dose
accordingly.

Level of Cognitive Ability: Applying
Client Needs: Safe and Effective Care Environment
Integrated Process: Nursing Process/Implementation
Content Area: Leadership/Management: Ethical/
Legal
Priority Concepts: Collaboration; Health Care Law

Answer: 2
Rationale: If the nurse believes a health care provider's prescription to be in error, the nurse must clarify the dosage with the client's health care provider or the health care provider's substitute
before administering the medication. Rescheduling the client's chemotherapy is incorrect. Chemotherapy must be administered on a
specific schedule for maximum effect with minimum adverse effects.
Additionally, only a prescriber can withhold or reschedule chemotherapy. Withholding the medication until the next day is incorrect.
Chemotherapy agents must be administered in the proper combina-
tions or sequence in order to be effective. Checking with the pharmacist can assist the nurse in determining whether the dose prescribed is
incorrect, but the nurse or pharmacist cannot alter the dose without
a revised prescription from a licensed health care provider with pre-
scriptive authority.
Priority Nursing Tip: Regardless of the source or cause of a medication error, if the nurse gives an incorrect medication dose, the nurse is
legally responsible for the action.
Test-Taking Strategy: Focus on the subject, medication safety. Note
the strategic word, *next*. Use knowledge of the legal responsibilities
of the nurse in regard to a health care provider's prescriptions and
medication administration. Remember that the nurse cannot alter,
withhold, or reschedule a medication dose. Review: the legal implications regarding **medication administration**.
Reference(s): Potter et al (2013), pp. 578, 582-583.

1402. The nurse working in a long-term care
setting attended a workshop on creating a restraint-free environment for the
residents. Several coworkers firmly believe
that their current methods are satisfactory.
Which action should aid the nurse in being
effective in facilitating change?

1. Pointing out to coworkers the various mis-
takes that they are presently making in
adhering to outdated restraint procedures
2. Informing the nursing supervisor that current restraint policies must be changed
and requesting that all staff be required to
comply
3. Writing a new restraint policy over the
weekend and distributing it to coworkers for immediate implementation on
Monday morning
4. Asking coworkers to help gather data comparing the facility's restraint procedures
and outcomes with those of others using
revised procedures

Level of Cognitive Ability: Applying
Client Needs: Safe and Effective Care Environment
Integrated Process: Nursing Process/Implementation
Content Area: Leadership/Management: Ethical/
Legal
Priority Concepts: Collaboration; Professionalism

Answer: 4
Rationale: To be an effective change agent, the nurse must work collaboratively with others to solve common problems. The nurse who
works collaboratively with others to facilitate change has a much
greater chance of success than one who unilaterally demands or
implements change. By enlisting the assistance of others, there is a
greater chance that they will support proposed changes in procedures.
To focus on errors (perceived or real) serves only to alienate others
and is not effective in promoting change. A punitive atmosphere is
not effective in promoting change because it discourages people from
taking risks.
Priority Nursing Tip: Change is a dynamic process that leads to an
alteration in behavior. The nurse has the responsibility to identify situations in need of change that will improve the quality of care delivery to clients and the responsibility of initiating the change process.
Test-Taking Strategy: Note the strategic word, *effective*. Remembering
that to facilitate change, collaboration between the nurse and coworkers is important. Additionally options 1, 2, and 3 focus on unilateral
actions by the nurse. Review: the **change process**.
Reference(s): Huber (2014), pp. 45-47; Potter et al (2013), p. 36.

1403. A client being discharged from the hospital with a diagnosis of gastric ulcer has a prescription for sucralfate (Carafate) 1 gram by mouth 4 times daily. The nurse determines that the client understands proper use of the medication if the client states to take it at which time?
1. With meals and at bedtime
2. Every 6 hours around the clock
3. One hour after meals and at bedtime
4. One hour before meals and at bedtime

Level of Cognitive Ability: Evaluating
Client Needs: Physiological Integrity
Integrated Process: Teaching and Learning
Content Area: Pharmacology: Gastrointestinal Medications
Priority Concepts: Client Education; Safety

Answer: 4
Rationale: Sucralfate (Carafate) is an antiulcer medication. The medication should be scheduled for administration 1 hour before meals and at bedtime. This timing will allow the medication to form a protective coating over the ulcer before it becomes irritated by food intake, gastric acid production, and mechanical movement. The other options are incorrect.
Priority Nursing Tip: Sucralfate (Carafate) can cause constipation.
Test-Taking Strategy: Focus on the subject, medication administration times for sucralfate. Recalling the action of this medication, to form a protective coating, will direct you to the correct option. Review: client teaching points regarding sucralfate (Carafate).
Reference(s): Hodgson, Kizior (2014), pp. 1108-1109.

1404. The nurse is assisting a health care provider with abdominal paracentesis. What position should the nurse assist the client into for this procedure?
1. Prone
2. Supine
3. Semi-Fowler's on the back
4. Low Fowler's on the right side

Level of Cognitive Ability: Applying
Client Needs: Physiological Integrity
Integrated Process: Nursing Process/Implementation
Content Area: Fundamental Skills: Diagnostic Tests
Priority Concepts: Clinical Judgment; Safety

Answer: 3
Rationale: For abdominal paracentesis, the nurse should position the client in either a semi-Fowler's position or an upright position on the edge of the bed with the feet resting on a stool and the back well supported. This position allows the intestine to float posteriorly and helps prevent laceration during catheter insertion. Options 1, 2, and 4 are incorrect positions.
Priority Nursing Tip: The rapid removal of fluid from the abdominal cavity during paracentesis leads to a rapid decrease in abdominal pressure, which can cause vasodilation and resultant shock.
Test-Taking Strategy: Focus on the subject, abdominal paracentesis and the purpose of the procedure. Eliminate options 1 and 2 because they are comparable or alike and indicate a flat position. From the remaining choices, visualize this procedure and its associated complications to answer the question. Review: the procedure for abdominal paracentesis.
Reference(s): Chernecky, Berger (2013), pp. 849-850; Pagana, Pagana (2013), pp. 689, 692.

1405. A client was admitted to the hospital with a diagnosis of frequent symptomatic premature ventricular contractions (PVCs). After sitting up in a chair for a few minutes, the client complains of feeling lightheaded. Which finding should the nurse anticipate on auscultation of the heartbeat?
1. A regular apical pulse
2. An irregular apical pulse
3. A very slow regular apical pulse
4. A very rapid regular apical pulse

Level of Cognitive Ability: Analyzing
Client Needs: Physiological Integrity
Integrated Process: Nursing Process/Assessment
Content Area: Adult Health: Cardiovascular
Priority Concepts: Perfusion; Safety

Answer: 2
Rationale: The most accurate means of assessing pulse rhythm is by auscultation of the apical pulse. When a client has PVCs, the rate is irregular and if the radial pulse is taken, a true picture of what is occurring is not obtained. A very slow regular apical pulse indicates bradycardia. A very rapid regular apical pulse indicates tachycardia.
Priority Nursing Tip: If premature ventricular contractions (PVCs) occur, the health care provider is notified. The cause is determined and treatment is based on the cause.
Test-Taking Strategy: Focus on the subject, PVCs. Eliminate options 1, 3, and 4 because they are comparable or alike and indicate a regular pulse. Review: the manifestations associated with premature ventricular contractions (PVCs).
Reference(s): Ignatavicius, Workman (2013), p. 728.

1406. A client with a history of duodenal ulcer is taking calcium carbonate (Tums) chewable tablets. The nurse monitors the client for relief of which symptom?

1. Flatus
2. Heartburn
3. Rectal pain
4. Muscle twitching

Level of Cognitive Ability: Evaluating
Client Needs: Physiological Integrity
Integrated Process: Nursing Process/Evaluation
Content Area: Pharmacology: Gastrointestinal Medications
Priority Concepts: Pain; Safety

Answer: 2
Rationale: Calcium carbonate is used as an antacid for the relief of heartburn and indigestion. It can also be used as a calcium supplement or to bind phosphorus in the gastrointestinal tract in clients with renal failure. Options 1, 3, and 4 are unrelated to this medication.
Priority Nursing Tip: Calcium supplements can cause constipation. Instruct the client taking a supplement to increase fluid and fiber in the diet.
Test-Taking Strategy: Focus on the subject, calcium carbonate. Focusing on the client's diagnosis will direct you to the correct option. Review: the action of **calcium carbonate (Tums)**.
Reference(s): Hodgson, Kizior (2014), pp. 170-171.

1407. A child with Hirschsprung's disease is scheduled for surgery, and a temporary colostomy is performed on the child. Postoperatively, the nurse provides instructions to the parents about colostomy care at home. Which statement by the parents indicates their understanding of the instructions?

1. "We will give antidiarrheal medications."
2. "We will report signs of skin breakdown."
3. "We will give saline water enemas if my child doesn't pass stool."
4. "We will apply a heat lamp to any moist red tissue around the stoma."

Level of Cognitive Ability: Evaluating
Client Needs: Physiological Integrity
Integrated Process: Nursing Process/Evaluation
Content Area: Child Health: Gastrointestinal
Priority Concepts: Client Education; Tissue Integrity

Answer: 2
Rationale: The parents are instructed to report signs of skin breakdown or stomal complications, such as ribbonlike stools or failure to pass flatus or stools, to the health care provider or the nurse. Moist, red granulation tissue may grow around an ostomy site and does not require special treatment. Options 1 and 3 are incorrect actions and are contraindicated.
Priority Nursing Tip: Altered skin integrity is the primary concern for a client with a colostomy.
Test-Taking Strategy: Focus on the subject, colostomy care. Note the words *indicates their understanding of the instructions*. Careful reading of each option will direct you to the correct option. Review: **colostomy care.**
Reference(s): McKinney et al (2013), p. 1101.

1408. A client with Bell's palsy is distressed about the change in facial appearance. Which characteristic of Bell's palsy should the nurse tell the client about to help the client cope with the disorder?

1. It usually resolves when treated with vasodilator medications.
2. It is similar to stroke, but all symptoms will go away eventually.
3. It is not caused by stroke, and many clients recover in 3 to 5 weeks.
4. The symptoms will completely go away once the tumor is removed.

Level of Cognitive Ability: Applying
Client Needs: Psychosocial Integrity
Integrated Process: Teaching and Learning
Content Area: Adult Health: Neurological
Priority Concepts: Client Education; Intracranial Regulation

Answer: 3
Rationale: Clients with Bell's palsy should be reassured that they have not experienced a stroke and that symptoms often disappear spontaneously in approximately 3 to 5 weeks. The client is given supportive treatment for symptoms; the treatment does not involve administering vasodilators. Bell's palsy is not usually caused by a tumor.
Priority Nursing Tip: Bell's palsy results in paralysis of one side of the face.
Test-Taking Strategy: Focus on the subject, helping the client cope with Bell's palsy. Recalling that Bell's palsy is not a tumor and is not caused by a stroke or vasoconstriction will eliminate options 1, 2, and 4. Review: the characteristics associated with **Bell's palsy.**
Reference(s): Lewis et al (2014), p. 1467.

1409. A client has been given a prescription for propantheline as adjunctive treatment for peptic ulcer disease. How should the nurse tell the client to take this medication?
1. With meals
2. With antacids
3. Just after meals
4. 30 minutes before meals

Level of Cognitive Ability: Applying
Client Needs: Physiological Integrity
Integrated Process: Teaching and Learning
Content Area: Pharmacology: Gastrointestinal Medications
Priority Concepts: Client Education; Safety

Answer: 4
Rationale: Propantheline is an antimuscarinic anticholinergic medication that decreases gastrointestinal secretions. It should be administered 30 minutes before meals. The other options are incorrect.
Priority Nursing Tip: Medications with anticholinergic effects increase the potential for confusion in the surgical client.
Test-Taking Strategy: Focus on the subject, propantheline. Option 2 can be eliminated first using general medication guidelines because most medications cannot be administered with antacids because of interactive effects. Eliminate options 1 and 3 next because they are comparable or alike and indicate administering the medication with food. Review: **propantheline**
Reference(s): Kee, Hayes, McCuistion (2012), p. 718.

1410. The nurse obtains a finger-stick glucose of 400 mg/dL for a client who receives total parenteral nutrition (TPN). Which follow-up intervention should the nurse implement?
1. Discontinue the current TPN infusion.
2. Decrease the infusion rate of the TPN.
3. Replace TPN with 5% dextrose solution.
4. Confer with provider for glucose control.

Level of Cognitive Ability: Analyzing
Client Needs: Safe and Effective Care Environment
Integrated Process: Nursing Process/Implementation
Content Area: Critical Care: Parenteral Nutrition
Priority Concepts: Nutrition; Safety

Answer: 4
Rationale: Hyperglycemia is a complication associated with the administration of TPN because the base solution of TPN is 10% to 20% glucose in water. This client's capillary glucose is very high, and the hyperglycemia increases the risk of intravascular injury and hyperosmolar crisis. The nurse should not discontinue the infusion, decrease the rate, or replace the solution without a health care provider's prescription. Additionally these actions would not resolve the problem.
Priority Nursing Tip: Regular insulin may be prescribed for a client receiving total parenteral nutrition to maintain a normal blood glucose level.
Test-Taking Strategy: Focus on the subject, a complication of TPN. Eliminate options 1, 2, and 3 because they are counterproductive to the client's nutritional needs. Additionally, recalling the normal glucose level will direct you to the correct option. Review: care of the client receiving **total parenteral nutrition (TPN).**
Reference(s): Kee, Hayes, McCuistion (2012), pp. 251-252; Pagana, Pagana (2013), p. 478.

1411. Carbamazepine (Tegretol) is prescribed for a client in the management of generalized tonic-clonic seizures. The nurse is providing instructions to the client regarding the side and adverse effects of the medication and tells the client to inform the health care provider if which occurs?
1. Nausea
2. Dizziness
3. Sore throat
4. Drowsiness

Level of Cognitive Ability: Applying
Client Needs: Physiological Integrity
Integrated Process: Teaching and Learning
Content Area: Pharmacology: Neurological Medications
Priority Concepts: Client Education; Safety

Answer: 3
Rationale: Drowsiness, dizziness, nausea, and vomiting are frequent side effects associated with the medication. Adverse reactions include blood dyscrasias. If the client develops a fever, sore throat, mouth ulcerations, unusual bleeding or bruising, or joint pain, this may be indicative of a blood dyscrasia, and the health care provider should be notified.
Priority Nursing Tip: Serum liver and renal function tests and medication blood serum levels should be monitored when a client is taking an anticonvulsant.
Test-Taking Strategy: Focus on the subject, side and adverse effects of carbamazepine. Note the words *tells the client to inform the health care provider.* Recalling that blood dyscrasias can occur with the use of carbamazepine will direct you to the correct option. Remember that a sore throat is a sign of infection. Review: the side and adverse effects of **carbamazepine (Tegretol).**
Reference(s): Lehne (2013), p. 249.

1412. A medication nurse is supervising a newly hired nurse who is administering pyridostigmine (Mestinon) orally to a client with myasthenia gravis. Which observation by the medication nurse indicates safe practice by the newly hired nurse before administering this medication?
1. Asking the client to take sips of water
2. Asking the client to lie down on her right side
3. Asking the client to look up at the ceiling for 30 seconds
4. Instructing the client to void before taking the medication

Level of Cognitive Ability: Evaluating
Client Needs: Safe and Effective Care Environment
Integrated Process: Nursing Process/Evaluation
Content Area: Adult Health: Neurological
Priority Concepts: Mobility; Safety

Answer: 1
Rationale: Myasthenia gravis can affect the client's ability to swallow. The primary assessment is to determine the client's ability to swallow. Options 2 and 3 are not appropriate. In this situation, there is no reason for the client to lie down to swallow medication or look up at the ceiling. Additionally lying down could place the client at risk for aspiration. There is no specific reason for the client to void before taking the medication.
Priority Nursing Tip: For the client with a diagnosis of myasthenia gravis, determine the extent of neuromuscular dysfunction by assessing muscle strength, fatigue, ptosis, and ability to swallow.
Test-Taking Strategy: Focus on the subject, swallowing with myasthenia gravis. Note the diagnosis of the client and that the question addresses an oral medication. Recalling that myasthenia gravis can affect the client's ability to swallow will direct you to the correct option. Review: nursing care of the client with **myasthenia gravis**.
Reference(s): Hodgson, Kizior (2014), pp. 1004-1005; Ignatavicius, Workman (2013), p. 995.

1413. The home care nurse visits a client with chronic obstructive pulmonary disease (COPD) who is on home oxygen at 2 L per minute. The client's respiratory rate is 22 breaths per minute, and the client is complaining of increased dyspnea. What should the nurse do **initially**?
1. Determine the need to increase the oxygen.
2. Call emergency services to come to the home.
3. Reassure the client that there is no need to worry.
4. Collect more information about the client's respiratory status.

Level of Cognitive Ability: Analyzing
Client Needs: Physiological Integrity
Integrated Process: Nursing Process/Implementation
Content Area: Adult Health: Respiratory
Priority Concepts: Gas Exchange; Safety

Answer: 4
Rationale: Completing an assessment and collecting additional information regarding the client's respiratory status is the initial nursing action. The oxygen is not increased without validation of the need for further oxygen and the approval of the health care provider, especially because clients with COPD can retain carbon dioxide. Calling emergency services is a premature action. Reassuring the client is appropriate, but it is inappropriate to tell the client not to worry.
Priority Nursing Tip: Instruct the client with chronic obstructive pulmonary disease (COPD) that a Fowler's position and leaning forward aid in breathing.
Test-Taking Strategy: Note the strategic word, *initially*. Use the steps of the nursing process. Remember that assessment is the first step. Also, use the ABCs—airway, breathing, and circulation—to direct you to the correct option. Review: care of the client with **chronic obstructive pulmonary disease (COPD)**.
Reference(s): Ignatavicius, Workman (2013), pp. 621-622.

1414. A new breast-feeding mother is seen in the clinic with complaints of breast discomfort. The nurse determines that the mother is experiencing breast engorgement and provides the mother with instructions regarding care for the condition. Which statement by the mother indicates an understanding of the measures that will provide comfort for the engorgement?

1. "I will breast-feed using only one breast."
2. "I will apply cold compresses to my breasts."
3. "I will avoid the use of a bra while my breasts are engorged."
4. "I will massage my breasts before feeding to stimulate letdown."

Level of Cognitive Ability: Evaluating
Client Needs: Health Promotion and Maintenance
Integrated Process: Nursing Process/Evaluation
Content Area: Maternity: Postpartum
Priority Concepts: Health Promotion; Pain

Answer: 4
Rationale: Comfort measures for breast engorgement include massaging the breasts before feeding to stimulate letdown, alternating the breasts during feeding, taking a warm shower or applying warm compresses just before feeding, and wearing a supportive well-fitting bra at all times. Options 1, 2, and 3 are incorrect measures.
Priority Nursing Tip: The postpartum client who is breast-feeding should not use soap on the breasts because it tends to remove natural oils, which increases the chance of cracked nipples.
Test-Taking Strategy: Focus on the subject, breast engorgement. Visualize each of the descriptions in the options to assist in directing you to the correct option. Review: the measures to alleviate breast engorgement.
Reference(s): McKinney et al (2013), pp. 541, 543.

1415. The nurse fails to recognize that a client's vital signs have deteriorated over the past 4 hours after surgery. Later, the client requires emergency surgery. Which legal consequence does the nurse potentially face because of a failure to act?

1. Tort
2. Statutory law
3. Common law
4. Misdemeanor

Level of Cognitive Ability: Applying
Client Needs: Physiological Integrity
Integrated Process: Nursing Process/Implementation
Content Area: Leadership/Management: Ethical/Legal
Priority Concepts: Ethics; Heath Care Law

Answer: 1
Rationale: The nurse's inaction is consistent with a tort offense because a tort is a wrongful act intentionally or unintentionally committed against a person or the person's property. Option 2 describes laws that are enacted by state, federal, or local governments. Option 3 describes case law that has evolved over time via precedents. Option 4 is an offense under criminal law.
Priority Nursing Tip: The nurse must meet appropriate standards of care when delivering care to the client; otherwise the nurse would be held liable if the client is harmed.
Test-Taking Strategy: Focus on the subject, failure to act. Use knowledge regarding the definitions of the items identified in the options to answer this question. Review: tort offense.
Reference(s): Potter et al (2013), pp. 301-302.

1416. A postmastectomy client has been found to have an estrogen receptor–positive tumor. The nurse interprets after reading this information in the pathology report that the client will **most likely** have which common follow-up treatment prescribed?

1. Removal of the ovaries
2. Administration of estrogen
3. Administration of progesterone
4. Administration of tamoxifen (Soltamox)

Level of Cognitive Ability: Analyzing
Client Needs: Physiological Integrity
Integrated Process: Nursing Process/Planning
Content Area: Adult Health: Oncology
Priority Concepts: Cellular Regulation; Sexuality

Answer: 4
Rationale: A common treatment for women with estrogen receptor–positive breast tumors is follow-up treatment with tamoxifen. This medication is classified as an antineoplastic agent and competes with estrogen for binding sites in the breast and other tissues. The medication may be administered for years after surgery. Options 1, 2, and 3 are incorrect treatments.
Priority Nursing Tip: Estrogens are steroids that stimulate female reproductive tissue.
Test-Taking Strategy: Note the strategic words, *most likely*, this will assist in eliminating options 1 and 2. From the remaining choices, it is necessary to know the action of tamoxifen. Review: the action and use of tamoxifen (Soltamox) and an estrogen receptor–positive tumor.
Reference(s): Hodgson, Kizior (2014), pp. 1122-1123.

1417. The nurse reviews the client's health care record and notes that the client is taking donepezil hydrochloride (Aricept). Understanding the purpose of this medication, the nurse suspects this client has which medical problem?

1. Dementia
2. Seizure disorder
3. History of schizophrenia
4. Obsessive-compulsive disorder

Level of Cognitive Ability: Analyzing
Client Needs: Physiological Integrity
Integrated Process: Nursing Process/Analysis
Content Area: Pharmacology: Neurological Medications
Priority Concepts: Clinical Judgment; Cognition

Answer: 1
Rationale: Donepezil hydrochloride is a cholinergic agent that is used in the treatment of mild to moderate dementia of the Alzheimer's type. It enhances cholinergic functions by increasing the concentration of acetylcholine. It slows the progression of Alzheimer's disease. Options 2, 3, and 4 are not conditions that are treated with this medication.
Priority Nursing Tip: Donepezil hydrochloride, used to treat mild to moderate dementia of the Alzheimer's type, relieves some symptoms but does not cure or reverse the progression of the disease.
Test-Taking Strategy: Focus on the subject, donepezil hydrochloride. Specific knowledge regarding the use of donepezil hydrochloride is required to answer this question. Remember this medication is used in the treatment of mild to moderate dementia of the Alzheimer's type. Review: **donepezil hydrochloride (Aricept).**
Reference(s): Hodgson, Kizior (2014), pp. 376-377.

1418. A registered nurse (RN) is supervising a licensed practical nurse (LPN) providing care to a client with end-stage heart failure. The client is withdrawn, reluctant to talk, and shows little interest in participating in hygienic care or activities. Which statement by the LPN to the client indicates that the LPN **needs further teaching** in the use of therapeutic communication skills?

1. "You are very quiet today."
2. "What are your feelings right now?"
3. "Why don't you feel like getting up?"
4. "Tell me more about your difficulty with sleeping at night."

Level of Cognitive Ability: Evaluating
Client Needs: Psychosocial Integrity
Integrated Process: Teaching and Learning
Content Area: Mental Health
Priority Concepts: Communication; Leadership

Answer: 3
Rationale: When a "why" question is made to the client, an explanation for feelings and behaviors is requested, and the client may not know the reason. Requesting an explanation is a nontherapeutic communication technique. In option 1, the LPN is using the therapeutic communication technique of acknowledging the client's behavior. In option 2, the LPN is encouraging identification of emotions or feelings. In option 4, the LPN is using the therapeutic communication technique of exploring, which is asking the client to describe something in more detail or to discuss it more fully.
Priority Nursing Tip: Therapeutic communication techniques focus on encouraging the client to verbalize feelings.
Test-Taking Strategy: Note the strategic words, *needs further teaching.* These words indicate a negative event query and the need to select the incorrect statement by the LPN. Seek the option that is a block to communication. The word *why* in option 3 should guide you to this option. Review: **therapeutic communication techniques.**
Reference(s): Ignatavicius, Workman (2013), p. 749; Potter et al (2013), pp. 320-322.

1419. The nurse is administering a dose of ondansetron hydrochloride (Zofran) to a client for nausea and vomiting. Which frequent side effect of this medication should the nurse tell the client to report?

1. Dizziness
2. Blurred vision
3. A warm feeling
4. Urinary frequency

Level of Cognitive Ability: Applying
Client Needs: Physiological Integrity
Integrated Process: Teaching and Learning
Content Area: Pharmacology: Gastrointestinal Medications
Priority Concepts: Client Education; Safety

Answer: 1
Rationale: Ondansetron hydrochloride is a selective receptor antagonist used as an antinausea and antiemetic. Frequent side effects include anxiety, drowsiness, dizziness, headache, fatigue, constipation, diarrhea, urinary retention, and hypoxia. Occasional side effects include abdominal pain, diminished saliva secretion, fever, feeling cold, paresthesia, and weakness. Rare side effects include hypersensitivity reaction and blurred vision.
Priority Nursing Tip: Antiemetics can cause drowsiness; therefore, a priority intervention is to protect the client from injury.
Test-Taking Strategy: Focus on the subject, a frequent side effect. Noting that the medication is used to treat nausea and vomiting and that this medication is a selective receptor antagonist will direct you to the correct option. Review: **ondansetron hydrochloride (Zofran).**
Reference(s): Hodgson, Kizior (2014), p. 877.

1420. The nurse is reviewing a urinalysis report for a client with acute kidney injury and notes that the results are highly positive for proteinuria. The nurse determines that this client has which type of renal failure?
1. Prerenal failure
2. Postrenal failure
3. Intrinsic renal failure
4. Atypical renal failure

Level of Cognitive Ability: Analysis
Client Needs: Physiological Integrity
Integrated Process: Nursing Process/Assessment
Content Area: Adult Health: Renal and Urinary
Priority Concepts: Elimination; Fluid and Electrolyte Balance

Answer: 3
Rationale: With intrinsic (intrarenal) renal failure, there is a fixed specific gravity, and the urine tests positive for proteinuria. In prerenal failure, the specific gravity is high, and there is very little or no proteinuria. In postrenal failure, there is a fixed specific gravity and little or no proteinuria. There is no such classification as atypical renal failure.
Priority Nursing Tip: Monitor the urine output and urine color and characteristics closely for a client with renal insufficiency. Urine output should be at least 30 mL per hour.
Test-Taking Strategy: Focus on the subject, type of renal failure. Specific knowledge regarding the types of renal failure is required to answer this question. Remember with intrinsic renal failure, there is a fixed specific gravity, and the urine tests positive for proteinuria. Review: the manifestations associated with the classifications of renal failure.
Reference(s): Ignatavicius, Workman (2013), p. 1539.

❖ **1421.** A client has undergone a vaginal hysterectomy. Which appropriate interventions should the nurse write on the client's nursing care plan to decrease the risk of deep vein thrombosis or thrombophlebitis? **Select all that apply.**
❑ 1. Use pneumatic compression boots.
❑ 2. Maintain bed rest for 24 to 48 hours.
❑ 3. Assist with range of motion leg exercises.
❑ 4. Elevate the knees with the knee gatch on the bed.
❑ 5. Apply antiembolism stockings and removing them twice daily for assessment.

Level of Cognitive Ability: Analyzing
Client Needs: Physiological Integrity
Integrated Process: Nursing Process/Planning
Content Area: Adult Health: Cardiovascular
Priority Concepts: Clotting; Perfusion

Answer: 1, 3, 5
Rationale: The client is at risk for deep vein thrombosis or thrombophlebitis after this surgery, as for any other major surgery. For this reason, the nurse implements measures that will prevent this complication. Ambulation, pneumatic compression boots, range of motion exercises, and antiembolism stockings are all helpful. The nurse should avoid elevating the knees using the knee gatch in the bed, which inhibits venous return and places the client more at risk for deep vein thrombosis or thrombophlebitis.
Priority Nursing Tip: Monitor the amount of vaginal bleeding following hysterectomy. More than one saturated pad per hour may indicate excessive bleeding.
Test-Taking Strategy: Focus on the subject, the risk of deep vein thrombosis or thrombophlebitis. Thinking about the pathophysiology and the causes associated with this complication will direct you to the correct options. Review: care of the client after hysterectomy and deep vein thrombosis or thrombophlebitis.
Reference(s): Ignatavicius, Workman (2013), pp. 799-800; Lewis et al (2014), pp. 847-848, 1296.

1422. Sertraline (Zoloft) is prescribed for a client in the treatment of depression. Before administering the medication, the nurse reviews the client's record and consults with the health care provider if which finding was noted?
1. A history of diabetes mellitus
2. Use of phenelzine sulfate (Nardil)
3. A history of myocardial infarction
4. A history of irritable bowel syndrome

Level of Cognitive Ability: Analyzing
Client Needs: Safe and Effective Care Environment
Integrated Process: Nursing Process/Implementation
Content Area: Pharmacology: Psychiatric Medications
Priority Concepts: Mood and Affect; Safety

Answer: 2
Rationale: Sertraline is a serotonin reuptake inhibitor. Serious potentially fatal reactions may occur if sertraline is administered concurrently with a monoamine oxidase inhibitor (MAOI). Phenelzine sulfate is an MAOI. MAOIs should be stopped at least 14 days before sertraline therapy. Sertraline should also be stopped at least 14 days before MAOI therapy. Options 1, 3, and 4 are not concerns with the administration of this medication.
Priority Nursing Tip: Instruct the client and family that the therapeutic effect of an antidepressant medication may take 1 week or even longer.
Test-Taking Strategy: Focus on the subject, interactions and contraindications of sertraline. Knowledge regarding these interactions and contraindications is required to answer this question. Remember that serious potentially fatal reactions may occur if sertraline is administered concurrently with an MAOI. Review: sertraline (Zoloft).
Reference(s): Hodgson, Kizior (2014), pp. 1077-1078.

❖ **1423.** An adult client is admitted to the emergency department after a burn injury. The burn initially affected the upper half of the client's anterior torso, and there were circumferential burns to the lower half of both of the arms. The client's clothes caught on fire, and the client ran causing subsequent burn injuries to the entire face (anterior half of the head), and the upper half of the posterior torso. Using the rule of nines, the extent of the burn injury would be what percent? **Refer to the figure. Fill in the blank.**

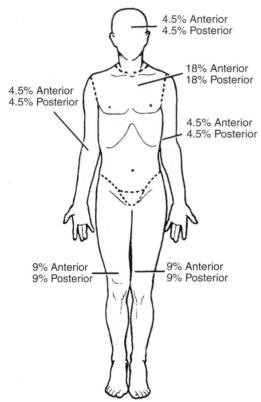

4.5% Anterior
4.5% Posterior

18% Anterior
18% Posterior

4.5% Anterior
4.5% Posterior

4.5% Anterior
4.5% Posterior

9% Anterior
9% Posterior

9% Anterior
9% Posterior

Figure from Ignatavicius D, Workman M: *Medical-surgical nursing: patient-centered collaborative care*, ed 7, Philadelphia, 2013, Saunders.

_____%

Level of Cognitive Ability: Applying
Client Needs: Physiological Integrity
Integrated Process: Nursing Process/Assessment
Content Area: Adult Health: Integumentary
Priority Concepts: Clinical Judgment; Tissue Integrity

Answer: 31.5%

Rationale: According to the rule of nines, with the initial burn, the upper half of the anterior torso equals 9% and the lower half of both arms equals 9%. The subsequent burn included the anterior half of the head equaling 4.5% and the upper half of posterior torso equaling 9%. This totals 31.5%.

Priority Nursing Tip: In addition to the rule of nines, the Lund-Browder chart is a method that can determine the extent of the burn injury. With this method, the client's age in proportion to relative body–area size is taken into account.

Test-Taking Strategy: Focus on the subject, the rule of nines to answer this question. Remember that the entire head equals 9%, each entire arm equals 9% (both arms 18%), anterior or posterior torso each equals 18% (36% for entire torso), each entire leg equals 18% (both legs equals 36%), and perineum equals 1%. Remember: 9% (head), 18% (arms), 36% (torso), 36% (legs), 1% (perineum) equaling 100%. Review: **rule of nines.**

Reference(s): Ignatavicius, Workman (2013), p. 523.

1424. The clinic nurse provides home care instructions to an adult client diagnosed with influenza. Which instructions should the nurse provide to the client? **Select all that apply.**
- ❑ 1. Practice frequent handwashing.
- ❑ 2. Remain at home until feeling better.
- ❑ 3. Sneeze or cough into the upper sleeve.
- ❑ 4. Return in 1 week for an influenza vaccine.
- ❑ 5. Take acetaminophen (Tylenol) for myalgia.
- ❑ 6. Completely isolate self in a room from other family members and use a separate bathroom until feeling better.

Level of Cognitive Ability: Analyzing
Client Needs: Safe and Effective Care Environment
Integrated Process: Teaching and Learning
Content Area: Fundamental Skills: Infection Control
Priority Concepts: Client Education; Infection

Answer: 1, 2, 3, 5
Rationale: Influenza (commonly known as the flu) refers to an acute viral infection of the respiratory tract. It is a communicable disease spread by droplet infection, and measures are instituted to prevent its spread. The client is instructed to practice frequent handwashing, remain at home, and cover the nose and mouth when sneezing and coughing. Supportive measures to relieve fever and myalgia such as the use of acetaminophen are also encouraged. It is unrealistic to completely isolate oneself in a room from other family members, and there is no useful reason to use a separate bathroom because the infection is spread through droplets. Influenza immunization is administered before the start of the "flu" season, not after developing the infection.
Priority Nursing Tip: For controlling the spread of influenza, the client is taught to sneeze or cough into the upper sleeve on the arm rather than into the hand. Respiratory droplets on the hands can contaminate surfaces and cause transmission to other people.
Test-Taking Strategy: Focus on the subject, the client's diagnosis, influenza. Recalling that this infection is spread by droplets will assist you in selecting the correct instructions. Also remember that the influenza immunization is administered before the start of the "flu" season, not after developing the infection. Review: home care measures for treating **influenza**.
Reference(s): Ignatavicius, Workman (2013), pp. 645-646.

1425. A client who has a positive sputum culture for *Mycobacterium tuberculosis* is receiving streptomycin as part of the treatment. The nurse determines that the client is experiencing a toxic effect of the medication if which result is abnormal?
1. Vision testing
2. Hepatic enzymes
3. Hemoglobin and hematocrit
4. Blood urea nitrogen (BUN) and creatinine

Level of Cognitive Ability: Analyzing
Client Needs: Physiological Integrity
Integrated Process: Nursing Process/Analysis
Content Area: Pharmacology: Respiratory Medications
Priority Concepts: Gas Exchange; Safety

Answer: 4
Rationale: BUN and creatinine are measured during therapy with streptomycin because the medication is nephrotoxic. Vision testing is done during treatment with ethambutol (Myambutol). The client taking isoniazid for tuberculosis is at risk for hepatotoxicity. Hemoglobin and hematocrit are not specifically related to tuberculosis.
Priority Nursing Tip: If the client with tuberculosis is taking streptomycin, instruct the client to notify the health care provider if hearing loss, changes in vision, or urinary problems occur.
Test-Taking Strategy: Focus on the subject, a toxic effect of streptomycin. To answer this question accurately you must be familiar with the various medications that are used to treat tuberculosis and their associated adverse or toxic effects. Remember that streptomycin is nephrotoxic. Review: the adverse effects of **streptomycin**.
Reference(s): Kee, Hayes, McCuistion (2012), p. 451.

❖ **1426.** The nurse is planning care for a client with a chest tube attached to a chest drainage system. Which actions should the nurse include as part of routine chest tube care? **Select all that apply.**
- ❑ 1. Encourage the client to cough and deep breathe.
- ❑ 2. Add water to the suction chamber as it evaporates.
- ❑ 3. Keep the collection chamber below the client's waist.
- ❑ 4. Clamp the chest tube when the client gets out of bed.
- ❑ 5. Tape the connection between the chest tube and the drainage system.

Level of Cognitive Ability: Analyzing
Client Needs: Physiological Integrity
Integrated Process: Nursing Process/Implementation
Content Area: Adult Health: Respiratory
Priority Concepts: Gas Exchange; Safety

Answer: 1, 2, 3, 5
Rationale: The client is encouraged to cough and deep breathe to assist in lung expansion. Water is added to the suction control chamber as needed to maintain the full suction level prescribed. The nurse keeps the drainage collection system below the level of the client's waist to prevent fluid or air from reentering the pleural space. Connections between the chest tube and system are taped to prevent accidental disconnection. To avoid causing tension pneumothorax, the nurse avoids clamping the chest tube for any reason unless specifically prescribed. In most instances, clamping of the chest tube is contraindicated by agency policy.
Priority Nursing Tip: Gentle, not vigorous, bubbling should be noted in the suction control chamber.
Test-Taking Strategy: Focus on the subject, chest drainage system. Think about the pathophysiology associated with a chest tube drainage system. Recalling that clamping chest tubes is contraindicated unless specifically prescribed will assist in answering correctly. Review: care of the client with a **chest tube.**
Reference(s): Ignatavicius, Workman (2013), pp. 636-637.

1427. Ibuprofen (Motrin IB) 400 mg orally four times daily has been prescribed for an older client with a diagnosis of rheumatoid arthritis. The client asks the nurse about the amount of medication prescribed. The nurse responds based on understanding what about this prescribed dosage?
1. It is the normal adult dose.
2. It is lower than the normal adult dose.
3. It is higher than the normal adult dose.
4. It is an unusual dose for this diagnosis.

Level of Cognitive Ability: Applying
Client Needs: Physiological Integrity
Integrated Process: Nursing Process/Implementation
Content Area: Pharmacology: Musculoskeletal Medications
Priority Concepts: Client Education; Safety

Answer: 1
Rationale: For acute or chronic rheumatoid arthritis or osteoarthritis, the normal oral adult dose for an older client is 200 to 800 mg 3 to 4 times a day. Therefore, options 2, 3, and 4 are incorrect.
Priority Nursing Tip: Hypoglycemia can result if ibuprofen (Motrin IB) is taken with insulin or an oral hypoglycemic medication.
Test-Taking Strategy: Focus on the subject, the normal dose for ibuprofen. Knowledge of the normal dosage for ibuprofen is required to answer this question. Remember that the normal oral adult dose for an older client is 200 to 800 mg 3 to 4 times a day. Review: the normal dosage for **ibuprofen (Motrin IB).**
Reference(s): Hodgson, Kizior (2014), p. 585.

1428. The nurse is monitoring a client with multiple sclerosis who is receiving baclofen (Lioresal). Which assessment finding would indicate a therapeutic response from the medication?
1. Decreased nausea
2. Decreased muscle spasms
3. Increased muscle tone and strength
4. Increased range of motion of all extremities

Level of Cognitive Ability: Evaluating
Client Needs: Physiological Integrity
Integrated Process: Nursing Process/Evaluation
Content Area: Pharmacology: Musculoskeletal Medications
Priority Concepts: Mobility; Safety

Answer: 2
Priority Nursing Tip: Baclofen (Lioresal) should be administered with caution in the client with renal or hepatic dysfunction or a seizure disorder.
Rationale: Baclofen is a skeletal muscle relaxant and acts at the spinal cord level to decrease the frequency and amplitude of muscle spasms in clients with spinal cord injuries or diseases, or multiple sclerosis. Options 1, 3, and 4 are unrelated to the effects of this medication.
Test-Taking Strategy: Focus on the subject, the client's diagnosis of multiple sclerosis and the therapeutic response of baclofen (Lioresal). Recalling that this medication is a skeletal muscle relaxant will direct you to the correct option. Review: the action of **baclofen (Lioresal).**
Reference(s): Hodgson, Kizior (2014), pp. 110-111.

1429. An intravenous dose of lorazepam (Ativan) is prescribed for a client. Which data from the client's history would indicate the need to consult with the health care provider before administering the medication?
1. History of glaucoma
2. History of hypothyroidism
3. History of diabetes mellitus
4. History of coronary artery disease

Level of Cognitive Ability: Analyzing
Client Needs: Physiological Integrity
Integrated Process: Nursing Process/Implementation
Content Area: Pharmacology: Psychiatric Medications
Priority Concepts: Collaboration; Safety

Answer: 1
Rationale: Lorazepam is a benzodiazepine and is contraindicated in clients who are comatose, with preexisting central nervous system (CNS) depression, with uncontrolled severe pain, and those with narrow-angle glaucoma. It is also contraindicated if hypersensitivity or cross-sensitivity with other benzodiazepines exists. It is also not prescribed for clients who are pregnant or breast-feeding.
Priority Nursing Tip: Flumazenil (Romazicon) reverses the effects of benzodiazepines.
Test-Taking Strategy: Focus on the subject, contraindications of lorazepam. Knowledge regarding the contraindications associated with the use of lorazepam is required to answer this question. Remember that this medication is contraindicated in the client with glaucoma. Review: **lorazepam (Ativan)**.
Reference(s): Lehne (2013), pp. 404-405.

1430. The nurse caring for a client immediately following transurethral resection of the prostate (TURP) notices that the client has suddenly become confused and disoriented. The nurse determines that this may be a result of which potential complication of this surgical procedure?
1. Hyponatremia
2. Hypernatremia
3. Hypochloremia
4. Hyperchloremia

Level of Cognitive Ability: Analyzing
Client Needs: Physiological Integrity
Integrated Process: Nursing Process/Analysis
Content Area: Adult Health: Renal and Urinary
Priority Concepts: Clinical Judgment; Fluid and Electrolyte Balance

Answer: 1
Rationale: The client who suddenly becomes disoriented and confused following TURP could be experiencing early signs of hyponatremia. This may occur because the flushing solution used during the operative procedure is hypotonic. If enough solution is absorbed through the prostate veins during surgery, the client experiences increased circulating volume and dilutional hyponatremia. The nurse needs to report these symptoms. The conditions noted in options 2, 3, and 4 are not complications of the procedure.
Priority Nursing Tip: If continuous bladder irrigation is prescribed for a client, use only sterile bladder irrigation solution or a prescribed solution to prevent water intoxication.
Test-Taking Strategy: Focus on the subject, that the client suddenly becomes confused and disoriented. Specific knowledge about the complications of this procedure is needed to answer correctly. Review: the complications related to **transurethral resection of the prostate (TURP)** and hyponatremia.
Reference(s): Ignatavicius, Workman (2013), pp. 181-182.

1431. A client hospitalized with a diagnosis of schizophrenia is prescribed risperidone (Risperdal) for the treatment of this disorder. Which laboratory study should the nurse anticipate to be prescribed before the initiation of this medication therapy?
1. Platelet count
2. Blood clotting tests
3. Liver function studies
4. Complete blood count

Level of Cognitive Ability: Analyzing
Client Needs: Physiological Integrity
Integrated Process: Nursing Process/Analysis
Content Area: Pharmacology: Psychiatric Medications
Priority Concepts: Psychosis; Safety

Answer: 3
Rationale: Risperidone is an antipsychotic medication that suppresses behavioral response in psychosis. Baseline assessment includes renal and liver function tests, and these studies should be done before the initiation of treatment. This medication is used with caution in clients with renal or hepatic impairment, clients with underlying cardiovascular disorders, and in older or debilitated clients. Options 1, 2, and 4 are unrelated to the administration of this medication.
Priority Nursing Tip: Instruct the client taking an antipsychotic medication to report signs of agranulocytosis, including sore throat, fever, and malaise.
Test-Taking Strategy: Focus on the subject, considerations with the administration of risperidone. Recalling that baseline liver and renal function studies should be done before therapy and that this medication is used cautiously in clients with renal or hepatic impairment will direct you to the correct option. Review: **risperidone (Risperdal)**.
Reference(s): Hodgson, Kizior (2014), pp. 1045-1046.

1432. The nurse has been working with an obese man and is evaluating a weight-reduction plan designed for the client. Which statement by the client indicates the **need for further teaching**?

1. "It is so difficult to find food exchanges that taste good and fill me up."
2. "This diet doesn't let me go out for lunch with my friends at work anymore."
3. "I wish my mother could have seen me lose the 60 pounds in the last 9 months."
4. "My wife was kidding me the other night about my being a whole new husband."

Level of Cognitive Ability: Evaluating
Client Needs: Health Promotion and Maintenance
Integrated Process: Teaching and Learning
Content Area: Fundamental Skills: Nutrition
Priority Concepts: Client Education; Health Promotion

Answer: 2
Rationale: Option 2 indicates that the client may be having difficulty in making appropriate dietary choices when going out for lunch or that he may perceive his coworkers are uncomfortable with his need to eat differently. A sense of not fitting in can leave the obese individual isolated and therefore make it more difficult for him to maintain his diet at work. In the absence of other data, option 1 is a normal response to the changes in eating habits. Both options 3 and 4 are responses indicating a positive perception of self, that another person has recognized these changes, and that the client wishes to have been able to share these changes with his mother.
Priority Nursing Tip: When developing a teaching plan, assess the client's motivation. If the client lacks motivation learning may not take place.
Test-Taking Strategy: Note the strategic words, *need for further teaching*. These words indicate a negative event query and the need to select the option that indicates client difficulty with the diet regimen and the need for teaching. Read each option carefully and determine whether it is a positive indicator or a negative one. This will assist in eliminating options 3 and 4 first. Option 1 is a common response by persons who have had to make dietary changes. Option 2 clearly states that the client perceives a definite barrier in pursuing his accustomed lifestyle. Review: dietary principles related to **weight reduction**.
Reference(s): Lewis et al (2014), pp. 914-915.

1433. A client is complaining of skin irritation from the edges of a cast that was applied the previous day, and the nurse notes that the skin is pink and irritated. Which corrective action should the nurse take?

1. Petal the edges of the cast with tape.
2. Massage the skin at the rim of the cast.
3. Shake a small amount of powder under the cast rim.
4. Use a hair dryer set on a cool high setting to soothe the irritation.

Level of Cognitive Ability: Applying
Client Needs: Physiological Integrity
Integrated Process: Nursing Process/Implementation
Content Area: Adult Health: Musculoskeletal
Priority Concepts: Mobility; Tissue Integrity

Answer: 1
Rationale: The nurse should petal the edges of the cast with tape to minimize skin irritation. Massaging the skin will not help the problem. Powder should not be shaken under the cast because it could clump, become moist, and cause skin breakdown. A hair dryer is used on a cool low setting if a nonplaster cast becomes wet or if the client's skin itches under a cast.
Priority Nursing Tip: Monitor the client with a cast for signs of infection such as increased temperature, hot spots on the cast, foul odor, or changes in pain.
Test-Taking Strategy: Focus on the subject of skin irritation from the edges of a cast. Because the question tells you that the cast edges are the cause of the irritation, you can eliminate options 2, 3, and 4. Review: the principles of **cast care**.
Reference(s): Ignatavicius, Workman (2013), pp. 1151, 1153.

1434. The nurse who has just begun the work shift is preparing to do tracheostomy care on a client. Which tracheostomy care items should the nurse obtain to perform this procedure?
1. Suction kit and tracheostomy dressing
2. Bottle of sterile saline and a tracheostomy care kit
3. Bottles of sterile saline and water and a tracheostomy dressing
4. Tracheostomy care kit, sterile saline and water, and a suction kit

Level of Cognitive Ability: Applying
Client Needs: Physiological Integrity
Integrated Process: Nursing Process/Implementation
Content Area: Adult Health: Respiratory
Priority Concepts: Clinical Judgment; Gas Exchange

Answer: 4
Rationale: Equipment needed to perform tracheostomy care includes a tracheostomy care kit, sterile water and saline solutions for cleansing and rinsing, and a suction kit for client suctioning. As part of tracheostomy care, the client's airway should be suctioned before cleansing the tracheostomy. New sterile solutions are obtained once per 24 hours, which is often done at the beginning of the workday. A tracheostomy care kit contains the needed supplies for cleaning the tracheostomy and for changing the dressing and holder (trach ties).
Priority Nursing Tip: A client with a respiratory problem should be placed in a semi-Fowler's to Fowler's position to assist in breathing easier.
Test-Taking Strategy: Focus on the subject, tracheostomy care. Visualize the procedure. Remember when an option contains more than one part, all parts of the option must be complete and correct. Recalling that the key items needed are the tracheostomy kit and suction kit will direct you to the correct option. Review: the procedure for **tracheostomy care.**
Reference(s): Perry, Potter, Ostendorf (2014), pp. 645, 1038.

1435. The nurse is observing an unlicensed assistive personnel (UAP) care for an older client who had a hip pinned following a fracture 4 days ago. To prevent client injury, the nurse should intervene in the care when which action is performed by the UAP?
1. Leaves both side rails down
2. Ensures that the nightlight is working
3. Answers the nurse call signal promptly
4. Places the nurse call signal within reach

Level of Cognitive Ability: Applying
Client Needs: Safe and Effective Care Environment
Integrated Process: Nursing Process/Implementation
Content Area: Fundamental Skills: Safety
Priority Concepts: Leadership; Safety

Answer: 1
Rationale: Safe nursing actions intended to prevent injury to the client include keeping one rail up (agency policy regarding side rails needs to be followed), bed in low position, and providing a call bell that is within the client's reach. Nightlights are usually built into the lighting systems of most facilities, and these bulbs should be routinely checked to see that they are functional. Responding promptly to the client's use of the call bell minimizes the chance that the client will try to get up alone, which could result in a fall.
Priority Nursing Tip: Always follow agency policies and procedures regarding the use of safety devices (restraints) and side rails.
Test-Taking Strategy: Note the words *nurse should intervene.* This creates a negative event query asking that the incorrect action by the UAP be selected. Focus on the subject, nurse intervening after an unsafe action by the UAP. Because options 3 and 4 are standard safety measures, they are eliminated first. Use of a nightlight would help prevent falls, which is also helpful, and can be eliminated next. Review: **basic safety measures.**
Reference(s): Potter et al (2013), pp. 384, 386.

1436. A client with chronic kidney disease (CKD) has received dietary counseling about potassium restriction in the diet. The nurse determines that the client has learned the information correctly if the client states he will do what when preparing vegetables?
1. Eat only fresh vegetables.
2. Boil them and discard the water.
3. Use salt substitute on them liberally.
4. Buy frozen vegetables whenever possible.

Level of Cognitive Ability: Evaluating
Client Needs: Physiological Integrity
Integrated Process: Nursing Process/Evaluation
Content Area: Adult Health: Renal and Urinary
Priority Concepts: Client Education; Nutrition

Answer: 2
Rationale: The potassium content of vegetables can be reduced by boiling them and discarding the cooking water. Options 1 and 4 are incorrect. Clients with CKD should avoid the use of salt substitutes altogether because they tend to be high in potassium content.
Priority Nursing Tip: Some foods high in potassium include avocado, bananas, cantaloupe, carrots, oranges, potatoes, raisins, spinach, strawberries, and tomatoes.
Test-Taking Strategy: Focus on the subject, potassium restriction in the diet. Recall which foods are high in potassium and how to reduce their potassium content. Options 3 and 4 can be eliminated first using basic principles of nutrition. Eliminate option 1 next, noting the close-ended word "only" in this option. Review: client teaching points related to **potassium restrictions** and **chronic kidney disease (CKD).**
Reference(s): Nix (2013), pp. 137-138.

1437. A client with chronic kidney disease has started receiving epoetin alfa (Epogen). The nurse reminds the client about the importance of taking which prescribed medication to enhance the effects of this therapy?
1. Aluminum carbonate
2. Ferrous gluconate (Ferate)
3. Calcium carbonate (Tums)
4. Aluminum hydroxide gel (AlternaGEL)

Level of Cognitive Ability: Applying
Client Needs: Physiological Integrity
Integrated Process: Nursing Process/Implementation
Content Area: Pharmacology: Renal and Urinary Medications
Priority Concepts: Client Education; Safety

Answer: 2
Rationale: In order to form healthy red blood cells, which is the purpose of epoetin alfa, the body needs adequate stores of iron, folic acid, and vitamin B_{12}. The client should take these ferrous gluconate (Ferate) supplements regularly to enhance the hematocrit-raising benefit of this medication. The other options are unnecessary medications.
Priority Nursing Tip: A major side effect of epoetin alfa (Epogen) is hypertension.
Test-Taking Strategy: Focus on the subject, epoetin alfa. Recall that this medication is used to stimulate red blood cell formation and that adequate body stores of vitamins and iron are needed to achieve this effect. Also, note that options 1, 3, and 4 are comparable or alike in that they are antacids. Review: client teaching points regarding epoetin alfa (Epogen) and ferrous gluconate (Ferate).
Reference(s): Hodgson, Kizior (2014), pp. 422-424, 476.

1438. A home care nurse is providing instructions to a client who is taking zolpidem (Ambien) for insomnia. To produce maximum **effectiveness** of the medication, how should the nurse tell the client to take the medication?
1. With milk or an antacid
2. At bedtime with a snack
3. Following the evening meal
4. With a full glass of water on an empty stomach

Level of Cognitive Ability: Applying
Client Needs: Physiological Integrity
Integrated Process: Teaching and Learning
Content Area: Pharmacology: Neurological Medications
Priority Concepts: Client Education; Safety

Answer: 4
Rationale: Zolpidem (Ambien) is a sedative. The client should be instructed to take the medication at bedtime and to swallow the medication whole with a full glass of water. For faster onset of sleep, the client should be instructed not to administer the medication with milk or food or immediately after a meal. Antacids should be avoided with the administration of the medication because of interactive effects.
Priority Nursing Tip: A lower than normal dose of zolpidem (Ambien) is usually prescribed for the older client.
Test-Taking Strategy: Focus on the subject, zolpidem. Note the word *maximum* and the strategic word *effectiveness* in the question. For maximal effectiveness of medications, medications should be taken on an empty stomach with water only. Also note that options 1, 2, and 3 are comparable or alike and indicate taking the medication with food or another substance. Review: the principles related to the administration of zolpidem (Ambien).
Reference(s): Skidmore-Roth (2014), pp. 1261-1262.

❖ **1439.** The nurse is performing an assessment on a client with a diagnosis of systemic lupus erythematosus (SLE). Which should the nurse expect to note? **Select all that apply.**
☐ 1. Fever
☐ 2. Bradycardia
☐ 3. Lymphadenopathy
☐ 4. Butterfly rash on the face
☐ 5. Muscular aches and pains

Level of Cognitive Ability: Analyzing
Client Needs: Physiological Integrity
Integrated Process: Nursing Process: Assessment
Content Area: Adult Health: Immune
Priority Concepts: Clinical Judgment; Immunity

Answer: 1, 3, 4, 5
Rationale: Manifestations of SLE may include fever, musculoskeletal aches and pains, butterfly rash on the face, pleural effusion, basilar pneumonia, generalized lymphadenopathy, pericarditis, tachycardia, hepatosplenomegaly, nephritis, delirium, seizures, psychosis, and coma.
Priority Nursing Tip: Lupus nephritis occurs early in the disease process of systemic lupus erythematosus (SLE).
Test-Taking Strategy: Focus on the subject, manifestations of SLE. Knowledge about the manifestations of SLE is needed to answer this question. Think about the pathophysiology associated with this disorder to assist in eliminating option 2. Review: the clinical manifestations of systemic lupus erythematosus (SLE).
Reference(s): Ignatavicius, Workman (2013), pp. 343-344.

1440. The nurse cares for a client who is pale and complains of fatigue, weakness, and dizziness. Which serum laboratory test result is the nurse's **priority** for planning care?

1. Hematocrit 43%
2. Sodium 130 mEq/L
3. Potassium 4.8 mEq/L
4. Hemoglobin of 7 g/dL

Level of Cognitive Ability: Analyzing
Client Needs: Physiological Integrity
Integrated Process: Nursing Process/Analysis
Content Area: Fundamental Skills: Laboratory Values
Priority Concepts: Clinical Judgment; Perfusion

Answer: 4
Rationale: The client's hemoglobin level and sodium level are low; however, the nurse uses the hemoglobin results to plan care because the client's clinical indicators are consistent with anemia. The client is pale because the serum hemoglobin is low; thus, the client's tissues are perfused with blood that has a low oxygen-carrying capacity. The client is weak and dizzy because the blood does not carry enough oxygen to meet tissue oxygen demands. The normal sodium level is 135 to 145 mEq/L. While a client who is hyponatremic can also feel weak and dizzy, a hyponatremic client is unlikely to be pale. The hematocrit and the potassium levels are within normal limits.
Priority Nursing Tip: The normal hemoglobin level for a woman is 12 to 15 g/dL. The normal level for a man is 14 to 16.5 g/dL.
Test-Taking Strategy: Note the strategic word, *priority*. Focus on the subject, signs and symptoms of anemia. Note that the client has several clinical indicators for anemia. Recalling the normal hemoglobin level will direct you to the correct option. Review: the **normal hemoglobin level** and the signs of **anemia**.
Reference(s): Ignatavicius, Workman (2013), p. 873.

1441. The nurse in the newborn nursery is performing vital signs on the newborn infant. Which finding indicates a normal respiratory rate?

1. 28 breaths per minute
2. 50 breaths per minute
3. 70 breaths per minute
4. 80 breaths per minute

Level of Cognitive Ability: Applying
Client Needs: Physiological Integrity
Integrated Process: Nursing Process/Assessment
Content Area: Maternity: Newborn
Priority Concepts: Development; Gas Exchange

Answer: 2
Rationale: The normal respiratory rate for a newborn infant is 30 to 60 breaths per minute. Therefore, options 1, 3, and 4 are incorrect.
Priority Nursing Tip: For a newborn, assess the heart rate and respiratory rate while the newborn is resting or sleeping.
Test-Taking Strategy: Focus on the subject, normal respiratory rate for a newborn. Knowledge of the normal respiratory rate for a newborn infant is required to answer this question. Remember that the normal respiratory rate is 30 to 60 breaths per minute. Review: newborn vital signs.
Reference(s): McKinney et al (2013), p. 479.

1442. The nurse is assessing a client with a diagnosis of polycythemia vera. Which clinical manifestation should the nurse expect to note in this client?

1. Pallor
2. Hypertension
3. A low hematocrit level
4. Pale mucous membranes

Level of Cognitive Ability: Analyzing
Client Needs: Physiological Integrity
Integrated Process: Nursing Process/Assessment
Content Area: Adult Health: Hematological
Priority Concepts: Clinical Judgment; Perfusion

Answer: 2
Rationale: Polycythemia vera is a myeloproliferative disease that causes increased blood viscosity and blood volume. Manifestations of polycythemia vera include a ruddy complexion, dusky red mucosa, hypertension, dizziness, headache, and a sense of fullness in the head. Signs of heart failure may also be present. The hematocrit level is usually greater than 54% in men and 49% in women.
Priority Nursing Tip: Conditions that cause increased blood viscosity and increased blood volume result in hypertension.
Test-Taking Strategy: Focus on the subject, polycythemia vera. Recalling that polycythemia vera is a myeloproliferative disease that causes increased blood viscosity and blood volume will direct you to the correct option. Review: **polycythemia vera**.
Reference(s): Ignatavicius, Workman (2013), p. 879.

1443. When reviewing the laboratory results of a client with leukemia who is receiving chemotherapy, the registered nurse (RN) notes that the neutrophil count is less than 500/mm³. The RN informs the new nurse caring for the client about the results. Which intervention identified by the new nurse indicates a **need for further teaching**?

1. Restricting visitors with colds or respiratory infections
2. Removing all live plants, flowers, and stuffed animals in the client's room
3. Placing the client on a low-bacteria diet that excludes raw foods and vegetables
4. Padding the side rails and removing all hazardous and sharp objects from the environment

Level of Cognitive Ability: Evaluating
Client Needs: Physiological Integrity
Integrated Process: Teaching and Learning
Content Area: Adult Health: Oncology
Priority Concepts: Cellular Regulation; Safety

Answer: 4
Rationale: Padding the side rails and removing all hazardous and sharp objects from the environment would be instituted if the client is at risk for bleeding. This client is at risk for infection. When the neutrophil count is less than 500/mm³, visitors should be screened for the presence of infection, and any visitors or staff with colds or respiratory infections should not be allowed in the client's room. All live plants, flowers, and stuffed animals are removed from the client's room. The client is placed on a low-bacteria diet that excludes raw fruits and vegetables.
Priority Nursing Tip: A client with a low platelet count should be placed on bleeding precautions.
Test-Taking Strategy: Note the strategic words, *need for further teaching*. These words indicate a negative event query and the need to select the incorrect intervention. Recalling that a low neutrophil count places the client at risk for infection will direct you to the correct option. Review: **neutrophil count** and **neutropenic precautions**.
Reference(s): Ignatavicius, Workman (2013), pp. 883, 891.

1444. The nurse is delivering care to a client who was diagnosed with toxic shock syndrome (TSS). Which complication of this syndrome should the nurse monitor the client for?

1. Pulmonary embolism
2. Vitamin K deficiency
3. Factor VIII deficiency
4. Disseminated intravascular coagulopathy (DIC)

Level of Cognitive Ability: Analyzing
Client Needs: Physiological Integrity
Integrated Process: Nursing Process/Assessment
Content Area: Adult Health: Cardiovascular
Priority Concepts: Clotting; Infection

Answer: 4
Rationale: Toxic shock syndrome (TSS) is caused by infection and is often associated with tampon use. DIC is a complication of TSS. The nurse monitors the client for signs of this complication, and notifies the health care provider promptly if signs and symptoms are noted. Options 1, 2, and 3 are not complications of TSS.
Priority Nursing Tip: The rapid and extensive formation of clots that occurs in disseminated intravascular coagulopathy (DIC) causes the platelets and clotting factors to be depleted. This results in bleeding and the potential vascular occlusion of organs from thromboembolus formation.
Test-Taking Strategy: Focus on the subject, TSS. Familiarity with TSS and knowledge that DIC is a complication is needed to answer this question. Remember DIC is a complication of TSS. Review: the complications of **toxic shock syndrome (TSS)** and **disseminated intravascular coagulopathy (DIC)**.
Reference(s): Ignatavicius, Workman (2013), pp. 1614-1615.

1445. The nurse is caring for a client with an acute head injury. Which neurological sign should the nurse carefully assess as the **primary** indicator of neurological status?

1. Vital signs
2. Motor function
3. Sensory function
4. Level of consciousness

Level of Cognitive Ability: Analyzing
Client Needs: Physiological Integrity
Integrated Process: Nursing Process/Assessment
Content Area: Adult Health: Neurological
Priority Concepts: Cognition; Intracranial Regulation

Answer: 4
Rationale: The level of consciousness is the primary indicator of neurological status. An alteration in the level of consciousness occurs before any other changes in neurologic signs or vital signs. Vital sign changes occur later.
Priority Nursing Tip: Assess the client's behavior to determine level of consciousness, such as confusion, delirium, unconsciousness, stupor, or coma.
Test-Taking Strategy: Noting the subject, neurological status, and the strategic word, *primary* will direct you to the correct option. Remember that the level of consciousness is the primary indicator of neurological status. Review: **neurological assessment**.
Reference(s): Ignatavicius, Workman (2013), p. 1021.

1446. A client is admitted to the hospital with Cushing's disease. The nurse should monitor the client's laboratory studies for which finding that occurs in this disorder?

1. Hypokalemia
2. Hyperglycemia
3. Decreased plasma cortisol levels
4. Low white blood cell (WBC) count

Level of Cognitive Ability: Analyzing
Client Needs: Physiological Integrity
Integrated Process: Nursing Process/Assessment
Content Area: Adult Health: Endocrine
Priority Concepts: Clinical Judgment; Glucose Regulation

Answer: 2

Rationale: The client with adrenocorticosteroid excess experiences hyperglycemia, hyperkalemia, elevated plasma cortisol and adrenocorticotropic hormone (ACTH) levels, and an elevated WBC count. These abnormalities are caused by the effects of excess glucocorticoids and mineralocorticoids on the body.

Priority Nursing Tip: Hypertension occurs in Cushing's disease.

Test-Taking Strategy: Focus on the subject, Cushing's disease. Recalling that an adrenocorticosteroid excess occurs in Cushing's disease will direct you to option 2. Also note that options 1, 3, and 4 identify decreased or low levels. Review: the manifestations associated with Cushing's disease.

Reference(s): Ignatavicius, Workman (2013), p. 1386.

1447. The nurse is going to suction an adult client with a tracheostomy who has copious amounts of secretions. Which action should the nurse take to accomplish this procedure safely and **effectively**?

1. Hyperoxygenate the client after the procedure only.
2. Apply continuous suction in the airway for up to 20 seconds.
3. Set the wall suction pressure range between 80 to 120 mm Hg.
4. Occlude the Y-port of the catheter while advancing it into the tracheostomy.

Level of Cognitive Ability: Applying
Client Needs: Physiological Integrity
Integrated Process: Nursing Process/Implementation
Content Area: Adult Health: Respiratory
Priority Concepts: Gas Exchange; Safety

Answer: 3

Rationale: The safe wall suction range for an adult is 80 to 120 mm Hg, making option 3 the action that is consistent with safe and effective practice. The nurse should hyperoxygenate the client both before and after suctioning. The nurse should use intermittent suction in the airway (not constant) for up to 10 to 15 seconds. The nurse should advance the catheter into the tracheostomy without occluding the Y-port to minimize mucosal trauma and aspiration of the client's oxygen.

Priority Nursing Tip: Hyperoxygenating the client both before and after suctioning is critical because suctioning not only removes respiratory secretions but also removes oxygen from the client's body.

Test-Taking Strategy: Note the strategic word, *effectively*. Focus on the subject, suctioning a client with a tracheostomy. Eliminate option 1 because of the closed-ended word "only." From the remaining choices, visualize the procedure to direct you to the correct option. Review: the procedure for suctioning and tracheostomy.

Reference(s): Ignatavicius, Workman (2013), p. 574.

1448. A client experiences postoperative blood loss. Which sign/symptom is an indication that the client is anemic?

1. Fatigue
2. Dyspnea
3. Bradycardia
4. Muscle cramps

Level of Cognitive Ability: Analyzing
Client Needs: Physiological Integrity
Integrated Process: Nursing Process/Assessment
Content Area: Adult Health: Hematological
Priority Concepts: Clinical Judgment; Gas Exchange

Answer: 1

Rationale: The client with anemia is likely to complain of fatigue caused by deficient hemoglobin leading to a decreased oxygen-carrying capacity of the blood and ability to meet tissue oxygen demands. The respiratory rate can increase to improve oxygenation; some shortness of breath can occur but dyspnea (option 2) related to anemia is uncommon. The client is more likely to have tachycardia than bradycardia (option 3), because the heart beats faster to deliver the same amount of oxygen to tissues in compensation for less oxygen in the blood. Muscle cramps (option 4) are an unrelated finding.

Priority Nursing Tip: Hemorrhage can cause a loss of circulatory fluid volume, which can result in shock.

Test-Taking Strategy: Focus on the subject, the signs/symptoms associated with anemia. Recalling that anemia causes a reduction in the oxygen-carrying capacity to the tissues will direct you to option 1. Review: the manifestations associated with anemia.

Reference(s): Ignatavicius, Workman (2013), p. 871.

1449. The nurse in a rehabilitation center is planning the client assignments for the day. Which client has needs that can be **most** safely met by the unlicensed assistive personnel (UAP)?
1. A client on strict bed rest for whom a 24-hour urine specimen is being collected
2. A client scheduled for transfer to the hospital for coronary artery bypass surgery
3. A client scheduled for transfer to the hospital for an invasive diagnostic procedure
4. A client who is going through rehabilitation after undergoing a below-the-knee amputation (BKA)

Level of Cognitive Ability: Creating
Client Needs: Safe and Effective Care Environment
Integrated Process: Nursing Process/Planning
Content Area: Leadership/Management: Delegating
Priority Concepts: Care Coordination; Leadership

Answer: 1
Rationale: The nurse must assign tasks based on the guidelines of nursing practice acts and the job description of the employing agency. Unlicensed assistive personnel are trained to care for the client on bed rest and to maintain 24-hour urine collections. The nurse should provide instructions to unlicensed assistive personnel regarding the tasks, but the tasks required for this client are within the role description of unlicensed assistive personnel. A client scheduled to be transferred to the hospital for coronary artery bypass surgery, a client scheduled for an invasive diagnostic procedure, and a client who had a BKA have both physiological and psychosocial needs.
Priority Nursing Tip: Maintain continuity of care as much as possible when assigning client care.
Test-Taking Strategy: Note the strategic word, *most.* Focus on the subject, activities that can be delegated to the unlicensed assistive personnel. When asked questions related to delegation, think about the role description of the employee and the client needs. This will direct you to option 1. Review: the responsibilities related to **delegation** and the job description of **unlicensed assistive personnel.**
Reference(s): Huber (2014), pp. 148-150; Potter et al (2013), pp. 282-283.

1450. The nurse is in the room with a client when a seizure begins. The client's entire body becomes rigid, and the muscles in all four extremities alternate between relaxation and contraction. Following the seizure, which type of seizure should the nurse document that the client had experienced?
1. Partial seizure
2. Absence seizure
3. Tonic-clonic seizure
4. Complex partial seizure

Level of Cognitive Ability: Applying
Client Needs: Physiological Integrity
Integrated Process: Communication and Documentation
Content Area: Adult Health: Neurological
Priority Concepts: Clinical Judgment; Intracranial Regulation

Answer: 3
Rationale: Tonic-clonic seizures are characterized by body rigidity (tonic phase) followed by rhythmic jerky contraction and relaxation of all body muscles, especially those of the extremities (clonic phase). Absence seizures are characterized by a sudden lapse of consciousness for approximately 2 to 10 seconds and a blank facial expression. There are two types of complex partial seizures: complex partial seizures with automatisms and partial seizures evolving into generalized seizures. Complex partial seizures with automatisms include purposeless repetitive activities such as lip smacking, chewing, or patting the body. Partial seizures evolving into a generalized seizure begin locally and then spread through the body.
Priority Nursing Tip: If a seizure occurs in a client, time the seizure and note the type, character, and progression of the movements during the seizure.
Test-Taking Strategy: Focus on the subject, the type of seizure. Eliminate options 1 and 4 first because they are comparable or alike. From the remaining choices, focus on the characteristics of the seizure in the question and recall that these characteristics do not occur in an absence seizure. This will direct you to the correct option. Review: tonic-clonic seizure.
Reference(s): Ignatavicius, Workman (2013), p. 932.

1451. The nurse is reviewing the nursing care plan of a client with a right-sided stroke who has left-sided deficits. The nurse notes documentation that the client has unilateral neglect. The nurse plans care with the understanding that which action would be least helpful?
1. Place bedside articles on the left side.
2. Approach the client from the right side.
3. Teach the client to scan the environment.
4. Move the commode and chair to the left side.

Level of Cognitive Ability: Applying
Client Needs: Safe and Effective Care Environment
Integrated Process: Nursing Process/Implementation
Content Area: Adult Health: Neurological
Priority Concepts: Intracranial Regulation; Safety

Answer: 2
Rationale: Unilateral neglect is an unawareness of the paralyzed side of the body, which increases the client's risk for injury. The nurse's role is to refocus the client's attention to the affected side. Personal care items, belongings, a bedside chair, and a commode are all placed on the affected side. The client is taught to scan the environment to become aware of that half of the body and is approached on that side by family and caregivers as well.
Priority Nursing Tip: Safety is a priority concern for a client experiencing unilateral neglect as a result of a stroke.
Test-Taking Strategy: Note the subject, unilateral neglect with left-sided deficits. Eliminate options 1 and 4 first because they are comparable or alike. For the remaining options, note the words *least helpful.* These words indicate the need to select the incorrect intervention. This will direct you to the correct option. Review: care of the client with **unilateral neglect.**
Reference(s): Ignatavicius, Workman (2013), pp. 1011, 1019.

1452. The nurse is evaluating the status of a client with myasthenia gravis. The nurse interprets that the client's medication regimen may not be optimal if the client continues to experience fatigue occurring at which time?
1. Early in the morning and before lunch
2. Before meals and at the end of the day
3. Early in the morning and late in the day
4. Following exertion and at the end of the day

Level of Cognitive Ability: Evaluating
Client Needs: Physiological Integrity
Integrated Process: Nursing Process/Evaluation
Content Area: Adult Health: Neurological
Priority Concepts: Clinical Judgment; Mobility

Answer: 4
Rationale: The client with myasthenia gravis has weakness after periods of exertion and near the end of the day. Medication therapy should assist in alleviating the weakness. The medication regimen may not be optimal if the client continues to experience fatigue. The nurse also works with the client to space out activities to conserve energy and regain muscle strength by resting between activities. The client is also instructed to take medication as prescribed.
Priority Nursing Tip: Myasthenia gravis is a neuromuscular disease characterized by considerable weakness and abnormal fatigue of the voluntary muscles.
Test-Taking Strategy: Note the subject, myasthenia gravis. Remember that when an option has two parts, both parts of the option must be correct for the option to be the correct answer. Remember that clients with any form of chronic condition characterized by fatigue experience the greatest amount of fatigue after exertion and at the end of the day. With this concept in mind, eliminate options 1, 2, and 3. Review: care of the client with **myasthenia gravis.**
Reference(s): Ignatavicius, Workman (2013), p. 996.

1453. What anatomical site and method should the nurse use to administer an injection of iron to a client?
1. Deltoid muscle using an air lock
2. Gluteal muscle using Z-track technique
3. Anterolateral thigh with ⅝ inch needle
4. Subcutaneous tissue of the abdomen with ⅝ inch needle

Level of Cognitive Ability: Applying
Client Needs: Physiological Integrity
Integrated Process: Nursing Process/Implementation
Content Area: Pharmacology: Hematological Medications
Priority Concepts: Clinical Judgment; Safety

Answer: 2
Rationale: The correct technique for administering parenteral iron is deep in the gluteal muscle using Z-track technique to minimize the possibility of staining or irritating the tissues. Administering iron subcutaneously or with a short needle (options 3 and 4) and using the deltoid muscle (option 1) is contraindicated because of iron's irritating nature.
Priority Nursing Tip: Because intramuscular iron solutions may stain the skin, separate needles should be used for withdrawing the solution and injecting the medication. The Z-track injection technique is used.
Test-Taking Strategy: Focus on the subject, medication administration of iron. Use principles of medication administration by the parenteral route and focus on the subject, an iron injection. Eliminate options 3 and 4 because they are comparable or alike and both indicate administering the medication subcutaneously. From the remaining choices, recall that iron irritates the tissues to direct you to option 2. Review: the procedure for **administering iron.**
Reference(s): Ignatavicius, Workman (2013), p. 877.

1454. A client is diagnosed with pernicious anemia. The nurse reviews the client's health history for disorders involving which organ responsible for vitamin B_{12} absorption?
1. Liver
2. Ileum
3. Kidney
4. Hepatobiliary

Level of Cognitive Ability: Applying
Client Needs: Physiological Integrity
Integrated Process: Nursing Process/Assessment
Content Area: Fundamental Skills: Nutrition
Priority Concepts: Clinical Judgment; Nutrition

Answer: 2
Rationale: Pernicious anemia can occur in a client who has a disease involving the ileum, where vitamin B_{12} is absorbed. The nurse checks the client's history for small bowel disorders to detect this risk factor. The liver and the kidney are not related to impaired B_{12} absorption. Hepatobiliary refers to the liver and gallbladder.
Priority Nursing Tip: The client should increase dietary intake of foods rich in vitamin B_{12}, such as meat and liver, if anemia is the result of a dietary deficiency of this vitamin.
Test-Taking Strategy: Focus on the subject, vitamin B_{12} absorption. Recalling that vitamin B_{12} is absorbed in the small intestine will direct you to the correct option. Review: **vitamin B_{12} absorption.**
Reference(s): Ignatavicius, Workman (2013), pp. 877-878.

1455. A client had a positive Papanicolaou smear and underwent cryosurgery with laser therapy. Which piece of information should the nurse provide the client before letting the client go home?
1. Pain can be relieved with opioid analgesics.
2. Sitz baths are soothing to the irritated tissues.
3. Vaginal discharge should be clear and watery.
4. There should be absolutely no odor or vaginal discharge.

Level of Cognitive Ability: Applying
Client Needs: Physiological Integrity
Integrated Process: Teaching and Learning
Content Area: Adult Health: Oncology
Priority Concepts: Client Education; Cellular Regulation

Answer: 3
Rationale: Cryosurgery is a procedure that involves freezing cervical tissues. Vaginal discharge should be clear and watery after the procedure. There is mild pain after the procedure, but opioid analgesics would not be required. Tub and sitz baths are avoided while the area is healing, which takes about 10 weeks. The client will begin to slough off dead cell debris, which may be odorous. This resolves within approximately 8 weeks.
Priority Nursing Tip: Instruct the client who underwent cryosurgery with laser therapy to avoid intercourse and the use of tampons while vaginal discharge is present.
Test-Taking Strategy: Focus on the subject, client information following cryosurgery. Specific knowledge about the purpose and effects of this procedure is needed to answer the question. Eliminate option 4 because of the closed-ended words "absolutely no." From the remaining choices, noting the word *clear* in option 3 will direct you to this option. Review: **cryosurgery with laser therapy** for a client with a positive **Papanicolaou smear.**
Reference(s): Ignatavicius, Workman (2013), pp. 1625-1626; Lewis et al (2014), pp. 442-443.

1456. The nurse is planning to do preoperative teaching with a client scheduled for a transurethral resection of the prostate (TURP). Which **most** frequent cause of postoperative pain should the nurse plan to include in the discussion?
1. Bladder spasms
2. Bleeding within the bladder
3. Tension on the Foley catheter
4. The lower abdominal incision

Level of Cognitive Ability: Applying
Client Needs: Physiological Integrity
Integrated Process: Teaching and Learning
Content Area: Fundamental Skills: Pain
Priority Concepts: Elimination; Pain

Answer: 1
Rationale: Bladder spasms can occur after this surgery because of postoperative bladder distention or irritation from the balloon on the indwelling urinary catheter. The nurse administers antispasmodic medications as prescribed to treat this type of pain. Options 2 and 3 are not frequent causes of pain. Some surgeons purposefully apply tension to the catheter for a few hours postoperatively to control bleeding. There is no incision with a TURP (option 4).
Priority Nursing Tip: Instruct the client who underwent transurethral resection of the prostate (TURP) to report dribbling or incontinence postoperatively.
Test-Taking Strategy: Focus on the subject, transurethral resection of the prostate. Note the strategic word, *most*, in the question. Eliminate option 4, knowing that there is no incision with this procedure. Eliminate options 2 and 3 because they are unrelated to the cause of pain. Review: the causes of pain after **transurethral resection of the prostate (TURP) surgery.**
Reference(s): Ignatavicius, Workman (2013), p. 1636.

1457. A client with gastroesophageal reflux disease (GERD) has just received a breakfast tray. The nurse setting up the tray for the client notices that which is the only food that will increase the lower esophageal sphincter (LES) pressure and thus lessen the client's symptoms?
  1. Coffee
  2. Nonfat milk
  3. Fresh scrambled eggs
  4. Whole wheat toast with butter

Level of Cognitive Ability: Applying
Client Needs: Physiological Integrity
Integrated Process: Nursing Process/Implementation
Content Area: Adult Health: Gastrointestinal
Priority Concepts: Health Promotion; Nutrition

Answer: 2
Rationale: Foods that increase the LES pressure will decrease reflux and lessen the symptoms of GERD. The food substance that will increase the LES pressure is nonfat milk. The other substances listed decrease the LES pressure, thus increasing reflux symptoms. Aggravating substances include chocolate, coffee, fatty foods, and alcohol and should be avoided in the diet of a client with GERD.
Priority Nursing Tip: The client with gastroesophageal reflux disease (GERD) should sleep with the head of the bed elevated on 6- to 8-inch blocks.
Test-Taking Strategy: Focus on the subject, foods that increase the LES pressure. Recall the effect of various food substances on LES pressure and GERD. Also noting the word *nonfat* in option 2 will assist in directing you to this option. Review: **lower esophageal sphincter (LES) pressure.**
Reference(s): Ignatavicius, Workman (2013), pp. 1204, 1206; Nix (2013), p. 356.

1458. The nurse is reviewing the serum laboratory test results for a client with sickle cell anemia. Which parameter should the nurse anticipate will be elevated?
  1. Sodium
  2. Hemoglobin-S
  3. Hemoglobin A1c
  4. Prothrombin time

Level of Cognitive Ability: Applying
Client Needs: Physiological Integrity
Integrated Process: Nursing Process/Assessment
Content Area: Adult Health: Hematological
Priority Concepts: Clinical Judgment, Gas Exchange

Answer: 2
Rationale: Sickle cell anemia is a severe anemia that affects African Americans predominantly and is characterized by sickled hemoglobin, or Hgb-S. The client must have two abnormal genes yielding hemoglobin-S to have sickle cell anemia. A client could have sickle cell trait by carrying one hemoglobin-A gene and one hemoglobin-S gene; then, the client has a less severe form of sickle cell anemia. Options 1, 3, and 4 are unrelated to sickle cell anemia.
Priority Nursing Tip: The primary symptom associated with sickling in sickle cell crisis is pain.
Test-Taking Strategy: Focus on the subject, sickle cell anemia. To answer this question you must know the pathophysiology of sickle cell anemia and how it is reflected in common laboratory studies. Remember that the client with sickle cell anemia must have two abnormal genes yielding hemoglobin-S to have sickle cell anemia. Review: the pathophysiology of **sickle cell anemia.**
Reference(s): Ignatavicius, Workman (2013), pp. 871-872.

1459. Which test result should the nurse examine to determine the compatibility of blood from two different donors?
  1. Rh factor
  2. ABO typing
  3. Direct Coombs'
  4. Indirect Coombs'

Level of Cognitive Ability: Applying
Client Needs: Physiological Integrity
Integrated Process: Nursing Process/Assessment
Content Area: Fundamental Skills: Laboratory Values
Priority Concepts: Clinical Judgment; Safety

Answer: 4
Rationale: The indirect Coombs' test detects circulating antibodies against red blood cells (RBCs) and is the screening component of a prescription to "type and screen" a client's blood. This test is used in addition to the ABO typing, which is normally done to determine blood type. The Rh factor is determined at the same time as the ABO type. The direct Coombs' test is used to detect idiopathic hemolytic anemia by detecting the presence of autoantibodies against the client's RBCs.
Priority Nursing Tip: The donor's blood and the recipient's blood must be tested for compatibility before administering a blood transfusion. If the blood is not compatible, a life-threatening transfusion reaction can occur.
Test-Taking Strategy: Focus on the subject, compatibility of blood. Eliminate options 1 and 2 because they are part of blood typing. From the remaining choices, it is necessary to know the difference between the two tests. Remember that the indirect Coombs' test is the screening component of a prescription to "type and screen" a client's blood. Review: the purpose of the direct and **indirect Coombs' test.**
Reference(s): Ignatavicius, Workman (2013), pp. 864-865.

1460. A client is being discharged to home after undergoing a transurethral resection of the prostate (TURP). The nurse teaches the client to expect which variation in normal urine color for several days after the procedure?
1. Dark red
2. Pink-tinged
3. Clear yellow
4. Cloudy amber

Level of Cognitive Ability: Applying
Client Needs: Physiological Integrity
Integrated Process: Teaching and Learning
Content Area: Adult Health: Renal and Urinary
Priority Concepts: Client Education; Elimination

Answer: 2
Rationale: The client should expect that the urine will be pink-tinged for several days after this procedure. Dark red urine may be present initially, especially with inadequate bladder irrigation, and if it occurs, it must be corrected. Clear urine it not expected after surgery; cloudy urine could indicate an infection.
Priority Nursing Tip: After transurethral resection of the prostate (TURP), the nurse should monitor the client closely for hemorrhage, bladder spasms, urinary incontinence, and infection.
Test-Taking Strategy: Note the subject, a client being discharged to home after a resection of the prostate. Nothing the words *several days after the procedure* will to direct you to the correct option. Review: transurethral resection of the prostate (TURP).
Reference(s): Ignatavicius, Workman (2013), p. 1636.

1461. A client is admitted to the hospital in sickle cell crisis. Which clinical indicator of the disorder should the nurse monitor the client?
1. Pain
2. Diarrhea
3. Bradycardia
4. Blurred vision

Level of Cognitive Ability: Analyzing
Client Needs: Physiological Integrity
Integrated Process: Nursing Process/Assessment
Content Area: Adult Health: Hematological
Priority Concepts: Gas Exchange; Pain

Answer: 1
Rationale: Sickle cell crisis usually causes severe pain in the bones and joints along with joint swelling. The pain develops as a result of microvascular occlusion from abnormal sickled hemoglobin that occurs with hypoxia. Therapy includes pain management with opioid analgesics, supplemental oxygen, and intravenous fluids. The remaining options are not associated with sickle cell crisis.
Priority Nursing Tip: Vaso-occlusive sickle cell crisis is caused by the stasis of blood with clumping of cells in the microcirculation, ischemia, and infarction.
Test-Taking Strategy: Note the subject, the client's diagnosis, sickle cell crisis. Recalling that the primary treatment of sickle cell crisis focuses on administering fluids and opioid analgesics will direct you to the correct option. Review: the manifestations associated with sickle cell crisis.
Reference(s): Ignatavicius, Workman (2013), pp. 873-874.

1462. Quinidine gluconate is prescribed for a client and the nurse reviews the client's medical record. Which is a contraindication in the use of this medication?
1. Asthma
2. Infection
3. Muscle weakness
4. Complete atrioventricular (AV) block

Level of Cognitive Ability: Analyzing
Client Needs: Physiological Integrity
Integrated Process: Nursing Process/Analysis
Content Area: Pharmacology: Cardiovascular Medications
Priority Concepts: Perfusion; Safety

Answer: 4
Rationale: Quinidine gluconate is an antidysrhythmic medication used as prophylactic therapy to maintain normal sinus rhythm after conversion of atrial fibrillation and/or atrial flutter. It is contraindicated in complete AV block, intraventricular conduction defects, abnormal impulses and rhythms caused by escape mechanisms, and myasthenia gravis. It is used with caution in clients with preexisting asthma, muscle weakness, infection with fever, and hepatic or renal insufficiency.
Priority Nursing Tip: Most antidysrhythmics should not be administered with food because food may affect absorption.
Test-Taking Strategy: Focus on the subject, a contraindication of quinidine gluconate. Recalling that this medication is an antidysrhythmic medication and has a direct cardiac effect will direct you to the correct option. Review: quinidine gluconate.
Reference(s): Lehne (2013), pp. 577, 586-587.

1463. A client with a ruptured intracranial aneurysm in which surgery is contraindicated is still maintained on bed rest with subarachnoid precautions in place. The nurse should question which medication if it is prescribed for this client?
1. Nicardipine (Cardene SR)
2. Heparin sodium (Heparin)
3. Docusate sodium (Colace)
4. Aminocaproic acid (Amicar)

Level of Cognitive Ability: Analyzing
Client Needs: Physiological Integrity
Integrated Process: Nursing Process/Implementation
Content Area: Critical Care: Emergency Situations
Priority Concepts: Collaboration; Intracranial Regulation

Answer: 2
Rationale: The nurse should question a prescription for heparin sodium, which is an anticoagulant. This medication could place the client at risk for rebleeding. Nicardipine is a calcium-channel blocking agent that is useful in the management of vasospasm associated with cerebral hemorrhage. Docusate sodium is a stool softener, which helps prevent straining. Straining would raise intracranial pressure. Aminocaproic acid is an antifibrinolytic agent that prevents clot breakdown or dissolution. It may be prescribed after ruptured intracranial aneurysm and subarachnoid hemorrhage if surgery is delayed or contraindicated.
Priority Nursing Tip: An intracranial aneurysm occurs because of dilation of the walls of a weakened cerebral artery.
Test-Taking Strategy: Focus on the subject, ruptured intracranial aneurysm. The question suggests that hemorrhage is occurring. It makes sense, knowing the action of heparin sodium, that this medication would be contraindicated. Review: care of the client with a ruptured intracranial aneurysm and heparin sodium (Heparin).
Reference(s): Ignatavicius, Workman (2013), pp. 794, 1014; Lehne (2013), pp. 658-659.

1464. A client who has a history of chronic ulcerative colitis is diagnosed with anemia. The nurse interprets that which factor is **most likely** responsible for the anemia?
1. Blood loss
2. Intestinal hookworm
3. Intestinal malabsorption
4. Decreased intake of dietary iron

Level of Cognitive Ability: Analyzing
Client Needs: Physiological Integrity
Integrated Process: Nursing Process/Analysis
Content Area: Adult Health: Gastrointestinal
Priority Concepts: Inflammation; Elimination

Answer: 1
Rationale: The client with chronic ulcerative colitis is most likely anemic as a result of chronic blood loss in small amounts that occurs with exacerbations of the disease. These clients often have bloody stools and are at increased risk for anemia. There is no information in the question to support options 2 or 4. In ulcerative colitis, the large intestine is involved, not the small intestine, where vitamin B_{12} and folic acid are absorbed (option 3).
Priority Nursing Tip: During an acute phase of ulcerative colitis, restrict the client's activity to reduce intestinal activity.
Test-Taking Strategy: Focus on the subject, the cause of the anemia in a client with a history of chronic ulcerative colitis. Note the strategic words, *most likely*, in the question. Focusing on the client's diagnosis and recalling the pathophysiology that occurs in this disorder will direct you to option 1. Review: the manifestations of ulcerative colitis.
Reference(s): Ignatavicius, Workman (2013), pp. 1273-1274.

❖ **1465.** A woman who thinks she is pregnant is being seen for her first prenatal visit. The nurse asks the woman how she has been feeling. Which signs of pregnancy should the nurse expect the woman to state? **Select all that apply.**
1. "I have been so nauseous."
2. "I am having so much trouble with diarrhea."
3. "I have not had a menstrual period in 2 months."
4. "It seems like I have to go to the restroom to urinate all the time."
5. "I have been going to the health club two times a day because I have so much energy."

Level of Cognitive Ability: Analyzing
Client Needs: Health Promotion and Maintenance
Integrated Process: Nursing Process/Assessment
Content Area: Maternity: Antepartum
Priority Concepts: Health Promotion; Reproduction

Answer: 1, 3, 4
Rationale: Because the nurse is asking the woman, she would expect presumptive signs of pregnancy to be vocalized. Specifically the presumptive signs of pregnancy are nausea, vomiting, breast changes, amenorrhea, urinary frequency, fatigue, and quickening.
Priority Nursing Tip: Presumptive signs of pregnancy are subjective signs and are body changes that are experienced by the woman.
Test-Taking Strategy: Focus on the subject, signs of pregnancy, and note the words *first prenatal visit*. Having knowledge of presumptive signs as subjective signs of pregnancy will lead you to the correct options. Other signs of pregnancy are probable signs of pregnancy, which are objective signs, and finally positive signs of pregnancy. Understanding the difference with presumptive, probable, and positive signs of pregnancy will lead you to the correct answers. Review: the signs of pregnancy.
Reference(s): McKinney et al (2013), pp. 242, 244.

1466. A client has been given a prescription to begin using nitroglycerin transdermal patches. The nurse instructs the client about this medication administration system and tells the client to expect which side effect?
1. Sweating
2. Headache
3. Dry mouth
4. Constipation

Level of Cognitive Ability: Applying
Client Needs: Physiological Integrity
Integrated Process: Teaching and Learning
Content Area: Pharmacology: Cardiovascular Medications
Priority Concepts: Client Education; Safety

Answer: 2
Rationale: Nitroglycerin is a coronary vasodilator used in the management of coronary artery disease. A common side effect of this medication is an intense headache. Clients should be instructed about this side effect and that acetaminophen (Tylenol) can be helpful in alleviating discomfort. Options 1, 3, and 4 are not associated with the use of this medication.
Priority Nursing Tip: Instruct the client using a nitroglycerin transdermal patch to apply the patch to a hairless area, using a new patch and different site each day.
Test-Taking Strategy: Focus on the subject, nitroglycerin and recall its action. Recalling that it is a vasodilator will direct you to the correct option. Review: the side effects of nitroglycerin.
Reference(s): Lehne (2013), p. 620.

1467. The nurse is visiting a client who has been started on therapy with topical clotrimazole (Lotrimin AF). The nurse should tell the client that this medication will alleviate which problem?
1. Pain
2. Rash
3. Fever
4. Sneezing

Level of Cognitive Ability: Applying
Client Needs: Physiological Integrity
Integrated Process: Teaching and Learning
Content Area: Pharmacology: Integumentary Medications
Priority Concepts: Client Education; Tissue Integrity

Answer: 2
Rationale: Clotrimazole is a topical antifungal used in the treatment of cutaneous fungal infections and will alleviate an associated rash. The nurse teaches the client that it is used for this purpose. It is not used for pain, sneezing, or fever.
Priority Nursing Tip: Topical medications should be applied to the affected area in a thin layer. They are not covered with occlusive dressings unless specifically prescribed.
Test-Taking Strategy: Focus on the subject, topical clotrimazole (Lotrimin AF). Recalling that this medication is an antifungal and noting the word *topical* in the question will direct you to the correct option. Review: the purpose of topical clotrimazole (Lotrimin AF).
Reference(s): Lehne (2013), pp. 1145-1146.

1468. The nurse is providing care to the client who has received medication therapy with tissue plasminogen activator (t-PA, Activase). Which item should the nurse have available for use as part of standard nursing care for this client?
1. Flashlight
2. Pulse oximeter
3. Suction equipment
4. Occult blood test strips

Level of Cognitive Ability: Applying
Client Needs: Physiological Integrity
Integrated Process: Nursing Process/Planning
Content Area: Pharmacology: Cardiovascular Medications
Priority Concepts: Clotting; Safety

Answer: 4
Rationale: Tissue plasminogen activator is a thrombolytic medication that is used to dissolve thrombi or emboli caused by thrombus. A frequent and potentially adverse effect of therapy is bleeding. The nurse monitors for signs of bleeding in clients receiving this therapy. Equipment needed by the nurse would include occult blood test strips to monitor for occult blood in the urine, stool, or nasogastric drainage. A flashlight may be used for pupil assessment as part of the neurological exam in the client who is neurologically impaired. Pulse oximeter and suction equipment would be needed if the client had evidence of respiratory problems.
Priority Nursing Tip: A client who has active internal bleeding should not receive tissue plasminogen activator (t-PA, Activase).
Test-Taking Strategy: Focus on the subject, tissue plasminogen activator (t-PA, Activase). Recalling that this medication is a thrombolytic and that bleeding is an adverse effect of this therapy will direct you to the correct option. Review: tissue plasminogen activator (t-PA, Activase).
Reference(s): Lehne (2013), pp. 654-655; Perry, Potter, Ostendorf (2014), pp. 1061, 1063.

1469. A client newly diagnosed with angina pectoris has taken two sublingual nitroglycerin tablets for chest pain. The chest pain is relieved, but the client complains of a headache. The nurse interprets that this **most likely** represents which response?
1. An early sign of medication tolerance
2. An allergic reaction to the nitroglycerin
3. An expected side effect of the medication
4. A warning that the medication should not be used again

Level of Cognitive Ability: Analyzing
Client Needs: Physiological Integrity
Integrated Process: Nursing Process/Analysis
Content Area: Pharmacology: Cardiovascular Medications
Priority Concepts: Clinical Judgment; Perfusion

Answer: 3
Rationale: Headache is a frequent side effect of nitroglycerin, because of the vasodilating action of the medication. It usually diminishes in frequency as the client becomes accustomed to the medication and is effectively treated with acetaminophen (Tylenol). The other options are incorrect.
Priority Nursing Tip: The nurse should offer a sip of water before giving a nitroglycerin tablet because mouth dryness may inhibit medication absorption.
Test-Taking Strategy: Focus on the subject, sublingual nitroglycerine tablets, and note the strategic words, *most likely*. Eliminate options 1 and 4 because they are comparable or alike and imply that the medication can no longer be used by the client. From the remaining choices, recalling that the medication vasodilates will direct you to option 3. Review: the effects of **nitroglycerin**.
Reference(s): Lehne (2013), p. 620.

1470. The nurse is evaluating a diabetic client's understanding of the signs of hyperglycemia. Which statement by the client reflects an understanding?
1. "I may become diaphoretic and faint."
2. "I may notice signs of fatigue, dry skin, and increased urination."
3. "I need to take an extra diabetic pill if my blood glucose is greater than 300."
4. "I should restrict my fluid intake if my blood glucose is greater than 250 mg."

Level of Cognitive Ability: Evaluating
Client Needs: Physiological Integrity
Integrated Process: Nursing Process/Evaluation
Content Area: Adult Health: Endocrine
Priority Concepts: Client Education; Glucose Regulation

Answer: 2
Rationale: Fatigue, dry skin, polyuria, and polydipsia are classic symptoms of hyperglycemia. Fatigue occurs because of lack of energy from the inability of the body to use glucose. Dry skin occurs secondary to dehydration related to polyuria. Polydipsia occurs secondary to fluid loss. Diaphoresis is associated with hypoglycemia. A client should not take extra hypoglycemic agents to reduce an elevated blood glucose level. A client with hyperglycemia becomes dehydrated secondary to the osmotic effect of the elevated glucose; therefore, the client must increase fluid intake.
Priority Nursing Tip: The normal blood glucose level is 70 to 110 mg/dL.
Test-Taking Strategy: Focus on the subject, signs of hyperglycemia. Eliminate options 3 and 4 first because they are incorrect client actions rather than signs of hyperglycemia. From the remaining options, discriminating between the signs of hypoglycemia and hyperglycemia will direct you to option 2. Remember that fatigue, dry skin, polyuria, and polydipsia are classic symptoms of hyperglycemia. Review: signs of **hypoglycemia** and **hyperglycemia**.
Reference(s): Ignatavicius, Workman (2013), p. 1452.

1471. A client is taking albuterol sulfate (Ventolin HFA) by inhalation but cannot cough up secretions. Which action should the nurse teach the client to do to **best** help clear the bronchial secretions?
1. Get more exercise each day.
2. Use a dehumidifier in the home.
3. Administer an extra dose before bedtime.
4. Increase the amount of fluids consumed every day.

Level of Cognitive Ability: Applying
Client Needs: Physiological Integrity
Integrated Process: Teaching and Learning
Content Area: Pharmacology: Respiratory Medications
Priority Concepts: Client Education; Gas Exchange

Answer: 4
Rationale: The client should take in increased fluids (2000 to 3000 mL/day unless contraindicated) to make secretions less viscous. This may help the client expectorate secretions. This is standard advice given to clients receiving any of the adrenergic bronchodilators, such as albuterol, unless the client has another health problem that could be worsened by increased fluid intake. Additional exercise will not effectively clear bronchial secretions. A dehumidifier will dry secretions. The client would not be advised to take additional medication.
Priority Nursing Tip: If the client needs to inhale two puffs of a bronchodilator, the client should wait at least 1 to 2 minutes before the second inhalation.
Test-Taking Strategy: Focus on the subject, clearing bronchial secretions, and note the strategic word, best. Use general guidelines related to administering medication to eliminate option 3. Next eliminate option 2, recalling that a dehumidifier will dry secretions. From the remaining choices, recalling basic respiratory principles will direct you to option 4. Review: **albuterol sulfate (Ventolin HFA)**.
Reference(s): Hodgson, Kizior (2014), p. 28.

1472. The nurse reviews the serum laboratory results for a client taking hydrochlorothiazide (HydroDIURIL). Which **most** frequent side effect of this medication should the nurse specifically monitor for?
1. Hypokalemia
2. Hypocalcemia
3. Hypernatremia
4. Hyperphosphatemia

Level of Cognitive Ability: Analyzing
Client Needs: Physiological Integrity
Integrated Process: Nursing Process/Assessment
Content Area: Pharmacology: Cardiovascular Medications
Priority Concepts: Fluid and Electrolyte Balance; Safety

Answer: 1
Rationale: The client taking a potassium-losing diuretic must be monitored for decreased potassium levels. Other fluid and electrolyte imbalances that occur with the use of this medication include hyponatremia, hypercalcemia, hypomagnesemia, and hypophosphatemia.
Priority Nursing Tip: Hyperglycemia is a side effect of thiazide diuretics. Instruct the client with diabetes mellitus to have the blood glucose level checked periodically.
Test-Taking Strategy: Focus on the subject, hydrochlorothiazide (HydroDIURIL) and note the strategic word, *most*. Recall that this medication is a potassium-losing diuretic. Remember that hypokalemia is a concern when a client is taking a potassium-losing diuretic. Review: **hydrochlorothiazide (HydroDIURIL).**
Reference(s): Lehne (2013), pp. 486-487.

1473. The nurse has administered a dose of diazepam (Valium) to the client. Which **most important** action should the nurse take before leaving the client's room?
1. Draw the shades closed.
2. Give the client a bedpan.
3. Turn the volume on the television set down.
4. Raise a side rail on the bed and instruct the client not to get out of bed without assistance.

Level of Cognitive Ability: Applying
Client Needs: Safe and Effective Care Environment
Integrated Process: Nursing Process/Implementation
Content Area: Fundamental Skills: Safety
Priority Concepts: Clinical Judgment; Safety

Answer: 4
Rationale: Diazepam is a sedative/hypnotic with anticonvulsant and skeletal muscle relaxant properties. The nurse should institute safety measures before leaving the client's room to ensure that the client does not injure self. The most frequent side effects of this medication are dizziness, drowsiness, and lethargy. For this reason, the nurse raises a side rail on the bed and instructs the client not to get out of bed without assistance. Note that agency policy regarding the use of side rails is always followed. Options 1, 2, and 3 may be helpful measures that provide a comfortable, restful environment. However, option 4 provides for the client's safety needs.
Priority Nursing Tip: Follow agency policies and procedures regarding the use of side rails. Some state laws indicate that only one side rail is to be raised on a client's bed.
Test-Taking Strategy: Note the strategic words, *most important*. Recalling that diazepam is a sedative/hypnotic and that safety is a major concern will direct you to the correct option. Review: **diazepam (Valium).**
Reference(s): Hodgson, Kizior (2014), pp. 344-345; Potter et al (2013), p. 386.

1474. The nurse provides home care instructions to a client who is taking lithium carbonate (Lithobid). Which statement by the client indicates a **need for further teaching**?
1. "I need to take the lithium with meals."
2. "My blood levels must be monitored very closely."
3. "I need to decrease my salt and fluid intake while taking the lithium."
4. "I need to withhold the medication if I have excessive diarrhea, vomiting, or diaphoresis."

Level of Cognitive Ability: Evaluating
Client Needs: Physiological Integrity
Integrated Process: Teaching and Learning
Content Area: Pharmacology: Psychiatric Medications
Priority Concepts: Client Education; Safety

Answer: 3
Rationale: A normal diet and normal salt and fluid intake (1500 to 3000 mL per day) should be maintained because lithium decreases sodium reabsorption by the renal tubules, which could cause sodium depletion. A low-sodium intake causes a relative increase in lithium retention and could lead to toxicity. Lithium is irritating to the gastric mucosa; therefore, lithium should be taken with meals. Because therapeutic and toxic dosage ranges are so close, lithium blood levels must be monitored very closely: more frequently at first, then once every several months after that. The client should be instructed to withhold the medication if excessive diarrhea, vomiting, or diaphoresis occurs, and inform the health care provider if any of these problems arise.
Priority Nursing Tip: If lithium toxicity is suspected, the medication is withheld and the health care provider is notified.
Test-Taking Strategy: Note the strategic words, *need for further teaching*. These words indicate a negative event query and the need to select the incorrect client statement. Remember that generally it is important that clients be taught to maintain an adequate fluid intake. This principle will direct you to the correct option. Review: **lithium carbonate (Lithobid).**
Reference(s): Skidmore-Roth (2014), pp. 748-750.

1475. A client is brought to the emergency department after a severe burn caused by a fire at home. The burns are extensive, covering greater than 25% of the total body surface area (TBSA). When the nurse reviews the laboratory results drawn on the client, which value should the nurse **most likely** expect to note?

1. Hematocrit 65%
2. Albumin 4.0 g/dL
3. Sodium 140 mEq/L
4. White blood cell (WBC) count 6000 cells/mm³

Level of Cognitive Ability: Analyzing
Client Needs: Physiological Integrity
Integrated Process: Nursing Process/Analysis
Content Area: Critical Care: Emergency Situations
Priority Concepts: Cellular Regulation; Fluid and Electrolyte Balance

Answer: 1
Rationale: Extensive burns covering greater than 25% of the TBSA result in generalized body edema in both burned and nonburned tissues and a decrease in circulating intravascular blood volume. Hematocrit levels elevate in the first 24 hours after injury (the emergent phase) as a result of hemoconcentration from the loss of intravascular fluid. The normal hematocrit is 42% to 52% in the male and 35% to 47% in the female. The normal albumin is 3.4 to 5 g/dL. The normal sodium level is 135 to 145 mEq/L. The normal WBC count is 4500 to 11,000 cells/mm³.
Priority Nursing Tip: Urinary output is the most reliable and sensitive noninvasive assessment parameter for cardiac output and tissue perfusion.
Test-Taking Strategy: Focus on the subject, laboratory values after burns and note the strategic words, *most likely*. Use the knowledge regarding physiological alterations and fluid and electrolyte balance during the first 24 hours after injury of a burn client. Note that the only abnormal laboratory value is option 1, the hematocrit. Review: **normal laboratory values** and the immediate postinjury period of **burns.**
Reference(s): Ignatavicius, Workman (2013), p. 524.

1476. The nurse is caring for a client with Parkinson's disease who is taking benztropine mesylate (Cogentin) daily. When assessing the client, what should the nurse specifically monitor that will assist in determining that the client is experiencing a side effect of this medication?

1. Pupil response
2. Prothrombin time
3. Skin temperature
4. Intake and output

Level of Cognitive Ability: Analyzing
Client Needs: Physiological Integrity
Integrated Process: Nursing Process/Assessment
Content Area: Pharmacology: Neurological Medications
Priority Concepts: Clinical Judgment; Safety

Answer: 4
Rationale: Urinary retention is a side effect of benztropine mesylate, an anticholinergic medication. The nurse needs to observe for dysuria, distended abdomen, voiding in small amounts, and overflow incontinence. Options 1, 2, and 3 do not relate to this medication.
Priority Nursing Tip: Anticholinergics can cause blurred vision; dryness of the nose, mouth, throat, and respiratory secretions; increased pulse rate; constipation; and urinary retention.
Test-Taking Strategy: Focus on the subject, benztropine mesylate (Cogentin). Remember that urinary retention is a concern with anticholinergics. This will direct you to the correct option. Review: **benztropine mesylate (Cogentin).**
Reference(s): Hodgson, Kizior (2014), pp. 123-125.

1477. A client has received electroconvulsive therapy (ECT). What intervention should the nurse perform **first** in the posttreatment area and upon the client's awakening?

1. Assist the client from the stretcher to a wheelchair.
2. Orient the client and monitor his or her vital signs.
3. Offer the client frequent reassurance and repeat orientation statements.
4. Check for a gag reflex and then encourage the client to eat breakfast and resume activity.

Level of Cognitive Ability: Applying
Client Needs: Physiological Integrity
Integrated Process: Nursing Process/Implementation
Content Area: Mental Health
Priority Concepts: Clinical Judgment; Safety

Answer: 2
Rationale: The nurse should first monitor vital signs, orient the client, and review with the client that he or she just received an ECT treatment. The posttreatment area should include accessibility to the anesthesia staff, oxygen, suction, pulse oximeter, vital sign monitoring, and emergency equipment. The nursing interventions outlined in options 1, 3, and 4 will follow accordingly.
Priority Nursing Tip: Following electroconvulsive therapy (ECT), the client may be confused. The nurse should provide frequent orientation that is brief, distinct, and simple and provide reassurance to the client.
Test-Taking Strategy: Note the strategic word, *first*. Use the ABCs—airway, breathing, and circulation—remembering that vital signs are a method of assessing the ABCs. Review: care of the client after **electroconvulsive therapy (ECT).**
Reference(s): Stuart (2013), p. 599.

1478. A client with acquired immunodeficiency syndrome who has cytomegalovirus retinitis is receiving ganciclovir (Cytovene). Which action should the nurse plan to take while the client is taking this medication?

1. Monitor blood glucose levels for elevation.
2. Administer the medication on an empty stomach only.
3. Apply pressure to venipuncture sites for at least 2 minutes.
4. Provide the client with a soft toothbrush and an electric razor.

Level of Cognitive Ability: Applying
Client Needs: Safe and Effective Care Environment
Integrated Process: Nursing Process/Planning
Content Area: Pharmacology: Immune Medications
Priority Concepts: Immunity; Safety

Answer: 4
Rationale: Ganciclovir causes neutropenia and thrombocytopenia as the most frequent side effects. For this reason, the nurse monitors the client for signs and symptoms of bleeding and implements the same precautions that are used for a client receiving anticoagulant therapy. These include providing a soft toothbrush and electric razor to minimize the risk of trauma that could result in bleeding. The medication may cause hypoglycemia, but not hyperglycemia. The medication does not have to be taken on an empty stomach. Venipuncture sites should be held for approximately 10 minutes.
Priority Nursing Tip: For the client taking ganciclovir (Cytovene), the nurse should monitor the client's white blood cell count (WBC) and platelet count. If the WBC or neutrophil count drops, neutropenic precautions should be instituted. If the platelet count drops, bleeding precautions should be instituted.
Test-Taking Strategy: Eliminate option 2 first because of the closed-ended word "only." Next, eliminate option 3 because of the words *2 minutes.* From the remaining choices, recalling that ganciclovir causes thrombocytopenia will direct you to the correct option. Review: **ganciclovir (Cytovene).**
Reference(s): Lehne (2013), p. 1169.

1479. A client is to be discharged from the hospital on quinidine to control ventricular ectopy, and the nurse provides medication instructions to the client. Which statement by the client would indicate the **need for further teaching**?

1. "The best time to schedule this medication is with my meals."
2. "I need to take this medication regularly, even if my heart feels strong."
3. "I should avoid alcohol, caffeine, and cigarettes while on this medication."
4. "If I get diarrhea, nausea, or vomiting, I need to stop the medication immediately."

Level of Cognitive Ability: Evaluating
Client Needs: Physiological Integrity
Integrated Process: Teaching and Learning
Content Area: Pharmacology: Cardiovascular Medications
Priority Concepts: Client Education; Safety

Answer: 4
Rationale: Diarrhea, nausea, vomiting, loss of appetite, and dizziness are all common side effects of quinidine. If these should occur, the health care provider or nurse should be notified, but the medication should never be stopped by the client. A rapid decrease in the medication level of an antidysrhythmic could precipitate dysrhythmia. Options 1, 2, and 3 are accurate client statements.
Priority Nursing Tip: Antidysrhythmic medications suppress dysrhythmias by inhibiting abnormal pathways of electrical conduction in the heart.
Test-Taking Strategy: Note the strategic words, *need for further teaching.* These words indicate a negative event query and the need to select the incorrect client statement. Noting that quinidine is used to control ventricular ectopy, and recalling that the client should not stop taking a medication without first consulting the health care provider will direct you to the correct option. Review: **quinidine.**
Reference(s): Lehne (2013), pp. 586-587.

1480. A client having a mild panic attack has the following arterial blood gas (ABG) results: pH 7.49, P_{CO_2} 31 mm Hg, Pa_{O_2} 97 mm Hg, HCO_3 22 mEq/L. The nurse reviews the results and determines that the client has which acid-base disturbance?

1. Metabolic acidosis
2. Metabolic alkalosis
3. Respiratory acidosis
4. Respiratory alkalosis

Level of Cognitive Ability: Analyzing
Client Needs: Physiological Integrity
Integrated Process: Nursing Process/Analysis
Content Area: Fundamental Skills: Acid-Base
Priority Concepts: Acid Base Balance; Gas Exchange

Answer: 4
Rationale: Acidosis is defined as a pH of less than 7.35, whereas alkalosis is defined as a pH of greater than 7.45. Respiratory alkalosis is present when the P_{CO_2} is less than 35, whereas respiratory acidosis is present when the P_{CO_2} is greater than 45. Metabolic acidosis is present when the HCO_3 is less than 22 mEq/L, whereas metabolic alkalosis is present when the HCO_3 is greater than 26 mEq/L. This client's ABGs are consistent with respiratory alkalosis.
Priority Nursing Tip: If the client has an acid-base imbalance, monitor electrolyte values, particularly the potassium level.
Test-Taking Strategy: Focus on the subject, ABG results, and note the words *panic attack*. This may help you anticipate that the client is having an increased respiratory rate, which makes the client prone to respiratory alkalosis. Otherwise, use the steps for interpreting blood gas results to answer the question. Review: steps in interpreting arterial blood gas (ABG) results.
Reference(s): Ignatavicius, Workman (2013), pp. 205, 207-208.

1481. Vasopressin (Pitressin) is prescribed for a client with diabetes insipidus, and the client asks the nurse about the purpose of the medication. The nurse responds, knowing that this medication promotes which action?

1. Vasodilation
2. Decrease in peristalsis
3. Decrease in urinary output
4. Inhibit smooth muscle contraction

Level of Cognitive Ability: Analyzing
Client Needs: Physiological Integrity
Integrated Process: Teaching and Learning
Content Area: Pharmacology: Endocrine Medications
Priority Concepts: Client Education; Fluid and Electrolyte Balance

Answer: 3
Rationale: Vasopressin is a vasopressor and an antidiuretic. It directly stimulates contraction of smooth muscle, causes vasoconstriction, stimulates peristalsis, and increases reabsorption of water by the renal tubules, resulting in decreased urinary output.
Priority Nursing Tip: Diabetes insipidus is characterized by polyuria of 4 to 24 liters per day. Therefore, monitor the client for signs of dehydration.
Test-Taking Strategy: Focus on the subject, vasopressin. Eliminate options 2 and 4 first because they are comparable or alike. From the remaining choices, recalling the pathophysiology associated with diabetes insipidus will direct you to option 3. Review: vasopressin (Pitressin).
Reference(s): Hodgson, Kizior (2014), pp. 1234-1235.

1482. The client has diabetes mellitus that has been well controlled with glyburide (DiaBeta), but recently, the client's fasting blood glucose has been reported to be 180 to 200 mg/dL. Which medication, if noted in the client's record, may be contributing to the elevated blood glucose level?

1. Prednisone
2. Ranitidine (Zantac)
3. Cimetidine (Tagamet)
4. Ciprofloxacin hydrochloride (Cipro)

Level of Cognitive Ability: Analyzing
Client Needs: Physiological integrity
Integrated Process: Nursing Process/Analysis
Content Area: Pharmacology: Endocrine Medications
Priority Concepts: Glucose Regulation; Safety

Answer: 1
Rationale: Corticosteroids, thiazide diuretics, and lithium may decrease the effect of glyburide, causing hyperglycemia. Options 2, 3, and 4 may increase the effect of glyburide, leading to hypoglycemia.
Priority Nursing Tip: Corticosteroids are used with extreme caution in clients with infections because they mask the signs and symptoms of an infection.
Test-Taking Strategy: Focus on the subject, glyburide, and the elevated blood glucose level. Knowledge regarding the medications that have an adverse effect if taken concurrently with glyburide is required to answer this question. Remember that corticosteroids can cause hyperglycemia. Review: glyburide (DiaBeta) and prednisone.
Reference(s): Lehne (2013), pp. 917-918.

1483. Buspirone hydrochloride (BuSpar) is prescribed for a client with an anxiety disorder. The nurse instructing the client should inform the client about which characteristic of this medication?
1. The medication is addicting.
2. Dizziness and nausea may occur.
3. Tolerance can occur with the medication.
4. The medication can produce a sedating effect.

Level of Cognitive Ability: Applying
Client Needs: Physiological Integrity
Integrated Process: Teaching and Learning
Content Area: Pharmacology: Psychiatric Medications
Priority Concepts: Anxiety; Client Education

Answer: 2
Rationale: Buspirone hydrochloride is used in the management of anxiety disorders. The medication has a more favorable side effect profile than do the benzodiazepines. Dizziness, nausea, headaches, lightheadedness, and paradoxical central nervous system excitement, which generally are not major problems, are side effects of the medication. The advantages of this medication are that it is not addicting, tolerance does not develop, and it is not sedating.
Priority Nursing Tip: Provide sugarless gum, hard candy, and frequent sips of water for the client who experiences dry mouth as a side effect of medications.
Test-Taking Strategy: Focus on the subject, buspirone hydrochloride. Knowledge regarding the side effects and advantages of buspirone hydrochloride is required to answer this question. Remember that dizziness and nausea may occur with this medication. Review: **buspirone hydrochloride (BuSpar).**
Reference(s): Hodgson, Kizior (2014), pp. 160-161.

1484. The nurse is teaching a client who is taking cyclosporine (Sandimmune) after renal transplant about medication information. The nurse should tell the client to be especially alert for which problem?
1. Hair loss
2. Weight loss
3. Hypotension
4. Signs of infection

Level of Cognitive Ability: Applying
Client Needs: Physiological Integrity
Integrated Process: Teaching and Learning
Content Area: Pharmacology: Immune Medications
Priority Concepts: Client Education; Immunity

Answer: 4
Rationale: Cyclosporine (Sandimmune) is an immunosuppressant medication used to prevent transplant rejection. The client should be especially alert for signs and symptoms of infection while taking this medication and report them to the health care provider if experienced. The client is also taught about other side/adverse effects of the medication, including hypertension, increased facial hair, tremors, gingival hyperplasia, and gastrointestinal complaints. Some weight loss may occur, but this is not as significant as the onset of an infection.
Priority Nursing Tip: Cyclosporine (Sandimmune) is usually administered via the oral route. Intravenous administration is reserved for clients who cannot take the medication orally.
Test-Taking Strategy: Focus on the subject, cyclosporine (Sandimmune). Recalling that this medication is an immunosuppressant will direct you to the correct option. Remember that the client is at risk for infection. Review: cyclosporine (Sandimmune).
Reference(s): Hodgson, Kizior (2014), p. 293; Ignatavicius, Workman (2013), p. 1570.

1485. Neuroleptic malignant syndrome is suspected in a client who is taking an antipsychotic medication. Which medication should the nurse prepare in anticipation of being prescribed to treat this adverse effect related to the use of an antipsychotic?
1. Protamine sulfate
2. Bromocriptine (Parlodel)
3. Phytonadione (Vitamin K)
4. Enalapril maleate (Vasotec)

Level of Cognitive Ability: Analyzing
Client Needs: Physiological Integrity
Integrated Process: Nursing Process/Planning
Content Area: Pharmacology: Psychiatric Medications
Priority Concepts: Psychosis; Safety

Answer: 2
Rationale: Bromocriptine is an antiparkinson prolactin inhibitor used in the treatment of neuroleptic malignant syndrome. Protamine sulfate is the antidote for heparin overdose. Vitamin K is the antidote for warfarin (Coumadin) overdose. Enalapril maleate is an angiotensin-converting enzyme inhibitor and an antihypertensive that is used in the treatment of hypertension.
Priority Nursing Tip: Monitor for extrapyramidal side effects in a client taking an antipsychotic medication.
Test-Taking Strategy: Focus on the subject, neuroleptic malignant syndrome. Recalling that option 3 is the antidote for warfarin overdose and option 1 is the antidote for heparin will assist in eliminating these options. From the remaining choices, focus on the medication classifications and eliminate option 4 because it is an antihypertensive. Review: **neuroleptic malignant syndrome.**
Reference(s): Hodgson, Kizior (2014), pp. 150-151; Lehne (2013), p. 195.

1486. A client with a fractured leg has learned how to use crutches to assist in ambulation. The nurse should determine that the client has a **need for further teaching** if the client makes which statement about using crutches?
1. "I will keep spare crutch tips available."
2. "I will keep crutch tips dry so they don't slip."
3. "I will inspect the crutch tips for wear from time to time."
4. "I will keep the set of crutches found in the basement of my home as a spare pair."

Level of Cognitive Ability: Evaluating
Client Needs: Safe and Effective Care Environment
Integrated Process: Teaching and Learning
Content Area: Adult Health: Musculoskeletal
Priority Concepts: Client Education; Safety

Answer: 4
Rationale: The client should use only crutches measured for the client. Crutches belonging to another person should not be used unless they have been adjusted to fit the client. Spare tips and crutches fitted to the client should be available if needed. Crutch tips should remain dry. Water could cause slipping by decreasing the surface friction of the rubber tip on the floor. If crutch tips get wet, the client should dry them with a cloth or paper towel. The tips should be regularly inspected for wear.
Priority Nursing Tip: When ambulating with a client with crutches, the nurse needs to stand on the client's affected side.
Test-Taking Strategy: Note the strategic words, *need for further teaching*. These words indicate a negative event query and the need to select the incorrect client statement. Option 2 relates to safety and is eliminated first. Eliminate options 1 and 3 next because they are comparable or alike and relate to the crutch tips. Review: client teaching points related to the use of **crutches**.
Reference(s): Perry, Potter, Ostendorf (2014), pp. 236-240.

1487. Disulfiram (Antabuse) is prescribed for a client who is seen in the psychiatric health care clinic. The nurse is collecting data from the client and is providing instructions regarding the use of this medication. Which datum is important for the nurse to obtain before beginning the administration of this medication?
1. When the last full meal was consumed
2. When the last alcoholic drink was consumed
3. If the client has a history of hyperthyroidism
4. If the client has a history of diabetes insipidus

Level of Cognitive Ability: Analyzing
Client Needs: Physiological integrity
Integrated Process: Nursing Process/Assessment
Content Area: Pharmacology: Psychiatric Medications
Priority Concepts: Addiction; Safety

Answer: 2
Rationale: Disulfiram may be used as an adjunct treatment for selected clients with chronic alcoholism who want to remain in a state of enforced sobriety. Clients must abstain from alcohol intake for at least 12 hours before the initial dose of the medication is administered. Therefore, it is important for the nurse to determine when the last alcoholic drink was consumed. The medication is used with caution in clients with diabetes mellitus, hypothyroidism, epilepsy, cerebral damage, nephritis, and hepatic disease. It is also contraindicated in severe heart disease, psychosis, or hypersensitivity related to the medication.
Priority Nursing Tip: If disulfiram (Antabuse) therapy is prescribed for the client, ensure that he or she agrees to abstain from alcohol and any alcohol-containing substances.
Test-Taking Strategy: Focus on the subject, disulfiram. Recalling that this medication is used as an adjunct treatment for chronic alcoholism will direct you to the correct option. Review: **disulfiram (Antabuse)**.
Reference(s): Lehne (2013), p. 449.

1488. A client with nephrotic syndrome states to the nurse, "Why should I even bother trying to control my diet and the swelling? It doesn't really matter what I do, if I can never get rid of this kidney problem anyway!" Which potential client problem should the nurse address based on the client's statement?
1. Anxiety
2. Difficulty coping
3. Feeling powerless
4. Negative body image

Level of Cognitive Ability: Analyzing
Client Needs: Psychosocial Integrity
Integrated Process: Nursing Process/Analysis
Content Area: Mental Health
Priority Concepts: Anxiety; Coping

Answer: 3
Rationale: Feeling powerless is a problem when the client believes that personal actions will not affect an outcome in any significant way. Anxiety occurs when the client has a feeling of unease with a vague or undefined source. Difficulty coping indicates that the client has impaired adaptive abilities or behaviors in meeting the demands or roles expected from the individual. Negative body image occurs when the way the client perceives body image is altered.
Priority Nursing Tip: Provide support for the client who is experiencing a negative body image. Embarrassment and shame may be associated with the altered appearance.
Test-Taking Strategy: Focus on the subject, potential client problem when client states, "It doesn't really matter what I do." This implies that the client has a sense of no control of the situation. This will direct you to the correct option. Review: the characteristics of feeling powerless.
Reference(s): Stuart (2013), pp. 204-205.

1489. Fluoxetine hydrochloride (Prozac) daily is prescribed for a client, and the nurse provides instructions to the client regarding the administration of the medication. Which statement by the client indicates an understanding regarding the administration of the medication?

1. "I should take the medication with food only."
2. "It is best to take the medication in the morning."
3. "I should take the medication at bedtime with a snack."
4. "I should take the medication at noontime with an antacid."

Level of Cognitive Ability: Evaluating
Client Needs: Physiological Integrity
Integrated Process: Nursing Process/Evaluation
Content Area: Pharmacology: Psychiatric Medications
Priority Concepts: Client Education; Safety

Answer: 2
Rationale: A daily dose of fluoxetine hydrochloride should be taken in the morning. If the medication is prescribed more than once daily, then the client is instructed to take the last dose of the day before 4:00 PM to avoid insomnia. It does not have to be taken with food. Antacids are avoided with its administration because the antacid will affect absorption.
Priority Nursing Tip: The client taking fluoxetine hydrochloride (Prozac) must avoid alcohol ingestion or other central nervous system depressants.
Test-Taking Strategy: Focus on the subject, fluoxetine hydrochloride. Eliminate option 1 because of the closed-ended word "only." Next, eliminate option 4, recalling that generally medications should not be administered with an antacid. From the remaining choices, recalling that the medication can cause insomnia will direct you to the correct option. Review: **fluoxetine hydrochloride (Prozac).**
Reference(s): Lehne (2013), p. 376.

1490. A new nurse is assigned to care for a client with a diagnosis of Tourette's syndrome who is receiving haloperidol decanoate (Haldol decanoate). The registered nurse asks the new nurse to describe the action of the medication. The new nurse responds correctly by stating that this medication has which action?

1. Is a serotonin reuptake blocker
2. Inhibits the breakdown of released acetylcholine
3. Blocks the uptake of norepinephrine and serotonin
4. Blocks the binding of dopamine to the postsynaptic dopamine receptors in the brain

Level of Cognitive Ability: Applying
Client Needs: Physiological Integrity
Integrated Process: Teaching and Learning
Content Area: Pharmacology: Psychiatric Medications
Priority Concepts: Psychosis; Safety

Answer: 4
Rationale: Haloperidol decanoate is a long-acting antipsychotic that acts by blocking the binding of dopamine to the postsynaptic dopamine receptors in the brain. Fluoxetine hydrochloride (Prozac) is a potent serotonin reuptake blocker. Donepezil hydrochloride (Aricept) inhibits the breakdown of released acetylcholine. Imipramine hydrochloride (Tofranil) blocks the reuptake of norepinephrine and serotonin.
Priority Nursing Tip: Some antipsychotic medications can cause a harmless change in urine color to pinkish to red-brown.
Test-Taking Strategy: Focus on the subject, haloperidol decanoate. Knowledge regarding the action of this medication is required to answer this question. Remember that this medication blocks the binding of dopamine. Review: **haloperidol decanoate (Haldol decanoate).**
Reference(s): Hodgson, Kizior (2014), pp. 557-558.

1491. The nurse is teaching a client how to mix regular insulin and NPH insulin in the same syringe. Which action should the nurse tell the client to take?

1. Draw up the NPH insulin into the syringe first.
2. Keep both bottles in the refrigerator at all times.
3. Rotate the NPH insulin bottle in the hands before mixing.
4. Take all of the air out of the insulin bottles before mixing.

Level of Cognitive Ability: Applying
Client Needs: Physiological Integrity
Integrated Process: Teaching and Learning
Content Area: Pharmacology: Endocrine Medications
Priority Concepts: Client Education; Glucose Regulation

Answer: **3**
Rationale: The NPH insulin bottle needs to be rotated for at least 1 minute between both hands. This resuspends the insulin. The nurse should not shake the bottles. Shaking causes foaming and bubbles to form, which may trap particles of insulin and alter the dosage. Regular insulin is drawn up before NPH insulin. Insulin may be maintained at room temperature. Additional bottles of insulin for future use should be stored in the refrigerator. Air does not need to be removed from the insulin bottles.
Priority Nursing Tip: Regular insulin is a type of insulin that can be administered intravenously.
Test-Taking Strategy: Focus on the subject, mixing regular insulin and NPH insulin in the same syringe. Eliminate options 2 and 4 first because of the closed-ended word "all." Visualize the procedure for mixing the insulins and remember *RN*, draw up the *R*egular before the *N*PH. This will direct you to option 3. Review: the steps in mixing **regular insulin** and **NPH insulin.**
Reference(s): Lehne (2013), pp. 733-734.

1492. A client has undergone mastectomy. The nurse determines that the client is having the **most** difficulty adjusting to the loss of the breast if which behavior is observed?

1. Performs arm exercises
2. Refuses to look at the dressing
3. Reads the postoperative care booklet
4. Requests pain medication when needed

Level of Cognitive Ability: Evaluating
Client Needs: Psychosocial Integrity
Integrated Process: Nursing Process/Evaluation
Content Area: Adult Health: Oncology
Priority Concepts: Coping; Sexuality

Answer: **2**
Rationale: The client demonstrates the most difficult adjustment to the loss if she refuses to look at the dressing. This indicates that the client is not ready or willing to begin to acknowledge and cope with the surgery. Performing arm exercises is an action-oriented behavior on the part of the client and is considered a positive sign of adjustment. Reading the postoperative care booklet indicates an interest in self-care and is a positive sign indicating beginning adjustment. Asking for pain medication is an action-oriented option that is helpful, although there is no direct connection to adjustment to the loss of the breast.
Priority Nursing Tip: If a breast reconstruction was performed after the mastectomy, the client will probably return from surgery with a surgical brassiere and prosthesis in place.
Test-Taking Strategy: Note the strategic word, *most*. Focus on the subject, the client is having difficulty adjusting to the loss of the breast. Note that options 1, 3, and 4 are comparable or alike and indicate a positive client action. Review: psychosocial responses related to **mastectomy.**
Reference(s): Ignatavicius, Workman (2013), pp. 1608-1609.

1493. A client has been taking lansoprazole (Prevacid) for 4 weeks. The nurse should monitor the client for relief from which problem?

1. Diarrhea
2. Heartburn
3. Flatulence
4. Constipation

Level of Cognitive Ability: Evaluating
Client Needs: Physiological Integrity
Integrated Process: Nursing Process/Evaluation
Content Area: Pharmacology: Gastrointestinal Medications
Priority Concepts: Pain; Safety

Answer: **2**
Rationale: Lansoprazole is a proton pump inhibitor and is classified as an antiulcer agent. The intended effect of the medication is relief of pain from gastric irritation, often referred to as heartburn by clients. The medication does not improve the other symptoms listed.
Priority Nursing Tip: Common side effects of proton pump inhibitors include headache, diarrhea, abdominal pain, and nausea.
Test-Taking Strategy: Focus on the subject, lansoprazole (Prevacid). Recalling that medication names that end with the letters "-zole" are gastric pump inhibitors will direct you to option 2. Review: **lansoprazole (Prevacid).**
Reference(s): Hodgson, Kizior (2014), p. 663.

1494. The nurse is preparing a client who had a total knee replacement with a metal prosthesis for discharge to home, and provides the client with discharge instructions. Which statement by the client indicates a **need for further teaching?**
1. "I can expect that changes in the shape of the knee will occur."
2. "I need to tell any future caregivers about the metal prosthesis."
3. "I need to report bleeding gums or tarry stools to the health care provider."
4. "I need to report fever, redness, or increased pain to the health care provider."

Level of Cognitive Ability: Evaluating
Client Needs: Physiological Integrity
Integrated Process: Teaching and Learning
Content Area: Adult Health: Musculoskeletal
Priority Concepts: Client Education; Mobility

Answer: 1
Rationale: After a total knee replacement, the client should be taught to report any changes in the shape of the knee. This is not an expected event during recuperation from surgery. The client must notify caregivers of the metal implant because the client will need antibiotic prophylaxis for invasive procedures, and will be ineligible for magnetic resonance imaging as a diagnostic procedure. With a metal prosthesis, the client must be on anticoagulant therapy and should report adverse effects of this therapy, such as evidence of bleeding from a variety of sources. Fever, redness, or increased pain may indicate infection.
Priority Nursing Tip: The client must avoid leg dangling after surgery for a total knee replacement.
Test-Taking Strategy: Note the strategic words, *need for further teaching.* These words indicate a negative event query and the need to select the incorrect client statement. Recalling that the client will be on prophylactic anticoagulant therapy will assist in eliminating option 3. Eliminate options 2 and 4 next because these are standard postoperative guidelines. Review: client teaching points after **total knee replacement.**
Reference(s): Lewis et al (2014), pp. 1534-1535.

1495. The nurse administers a dose of scopolamine to a preoperative client. The nurse should monitor the client for which common side effect of the medication?
1. Dry mouth
2. Diaphoresis
3. Excessive urination
4. Pupillary constriction

Level of Cognitive Ability: Analyzing
Client Needs: Physiological Integrity
Integrated Process: Nursing Process/Assessment
Content Area: Fundamental Skills: Perioperative Care
Priority Concepts: Clinical Judgment; Safety

Answer: 1
Rationale: Scopolamine is an anticholinergic medication that causes the frequent side effects of dry mouth, urinary retention, decreased sweating, and dilation of the pupils. Each of the incorrect options is the opposite of a side effect of this medication.
Priority Nursing Tip: If the client is taking an anticholinergic medication, monitor the client's bowel and urinary function and monitor for urinary retention, constipation, and paralytic ileus.
Test-Taking Strategy: Focus on the subject, scopolamine. Recalling that this medication is an anticholinergic will direct you to the correct option. Review: **scopolamine.**
Reference(s): Hodgson, Kizior (2014), pp. 1072-1073.

1496. The nurse is providing medication instructions to a client who is taking imipramine (Tofranil) daily. Which statement by the client indicates a **need for further teaching?**
1. "I need to avoid alcohol while taking the medication."
2. "I need to take the medication in the morning before breakfast."
3. "The effects of the medication may not be noticed for at least 2 weeks."
4. "If I miss a dose, I need to take it as soon as possible unless it is almost time for the next dose."

Level of Cognitive Ability: Evaluating
Client Needs: Physiological Integrity
Integrated Process: Teaching and Learning
Content Area: Pharmacology: Psychiatric Medications
Priority Concepts: Client Education; Safety

Answer: 2
Rationale: The client should be instructed to take the medication (a single dose) at bedtime and not in the morning because it causes fatigue and drowsiness. The client is told avoid alcohol or other central nervous system depressants during therapy and that medication effects may not be noticed for at least 2 weeks. The client is instructed to take the medication exactly as directed, and if a dose is missed, to take it as soon as possible unless it is almost time for the next dose.
Priority Nursing Tip: Cardiac toxicity can occur in a client taking a tricyclic antidepressant, and all clients should receive an electrocardiogram before treatment is started and periodically thereafter.
Test-Taking Strategy: Note the strategic words, *need for further teaching.* These words indicate a negative event query and the need to select the incorrect client statement. General principles related to medication administration will eliminate options 1 and 4. From the remaining choices, recalling that this medication is an antidepressant will eliminate option 3. Review: **imipramine (Tofranil).**
Reference(s): Lehne (2013), p. 377.

1497. The nurse is preparing to assess a client who was admitted to the hospital with a diagnosis of trigeminal neuralgia (tic douloureux). On review of the client's record, which symptom should the nurse expect to note that the client is experiencing?

1. Bilateral pain in the area of the sixth cranial nerve
2. Unilateral pain in the area of the sixth cranial nerve
3. Abrupt onset of pain in the area of the fifth cranial nerve
4. Chronic, intermittent pain in the area of the seventh cranial nerve

Level of Cognitive Ability: Analyzing
Client Needs: Physiological Integrity
Integrated Process: Nursing Process/Assessment
Content Area: Adult Health: Neurological
Priority Concepts: Client Education; Intracranial Regulation

Answer: 3
Rationale: Trigeminal neuralgia is a chronic syndrome characterized by an abrupt onset of pain. It involves one or more divisions of the trigeminal nerve (cranial nerve V). Options 1, 2, and 4 are incorrect.
Priority Nursing Tip: Instruct the client with trigeminal neuralgia to avoid placing hot or cold foods and fluids in the mouth because these can trigger episodes of acute pain.
Test-Taking Strategy: Focus on the subject, trigeminal neuralgia (tic douloureux). Recalling that trigeminal neuralgia affects the fifth cranial nerve will assist in eliminating options 1, 2, and 4. Review: the pathophysiology associated with trigeminal neuralgia (tic douloureux).
Reference(s): Ignatavicius, Workman (2013), pp. 912, 1000-1001.

1498. A client is taking docusate (Colace). The nurse should tell the client to monitor for which intended effect of the medication?

1. Abdominal pain
2. Decreased heartburn
3. Decrease in fatty stools
4. Regular bowel movements

Level of Cognitive Ability: Applying
Client Needs: Physiological Integrity
Integrated Process: Teaching and Learning
Content Area: Pharmacology: Gastrointestinal Medications
Priority Concepts: Client Education; Elimination

Answer: 4
Rationale: Docusate is a stool softener that promotes absorption of water into the stool, producing a softer consistency of stool. The intended effect is relief or prevention of constipation. The medication does not relieve abdominal pain, relieve heartburn, or decrease the amount of fat in the stools.
Priority Nursing Tip: The client who is receiving a laxative needs to increase fluid intake to prevent dehydration.
Test-Taking Strategy: Focus on the subject, docusate (Colace). Recalling that this medication is a stool softener will direct you to the correct option. Review: the action of docusate (Colace).
Reference(s): Hodgson, Kizior (2014), pp. 372-373.

1499. A client's laboratory test results reveal a decreased serum transferrin and total iron-binding capacity (TIBC). Which disorder is the **most likely** cause of the client's anemia?

1. Infection
2. Malnutrition
3. Iron deficiency
4. Sickle cell disease

Level of Cognitive Ability: Analyzing
Client Needs: Physiological Integrity
Integrated Process: Nursing Process/Analysis
Content Area: Fundamental Skills: Laboratory Values
Priority Concepts: Clinical Judgment; Nutrition

Answer: 2
Rationale: Malnutrition can cause reductions in the serum transferrin and the TIBC. Infection is an unrelated option. Iron-deficiency anemia is usually characterized by decreased iron-binding capacity but increased transferrin levels. Additionally, in clinical practice, the hemoglobin level is routinely used to detect iron-deficiency anemia. Sickle cell anemia is diagnosed by determining that the client has hemoglobin S.
Priority Nursing Tip: The normal serum iron level for a man is 65 to 175 mcg/dL. The normal level for a woman is 50 to 170 mcg/dL.
Test-Taking Strategy: Focus on the subject, serum transferrin and total iron-binding capacity (TIBC). Note the strategic words, *most likely*. Use these data and knowledge regarding the findings in malnutrition to direct you to the correct option. Review: the findings in malnutrition.
Reference(s): Ignatavicius, Workman (2013), pp. 1340, 1342.

1500. Which type of anemia is diagnosed with a Schilling test?
1. Aplastic
2. Pernicious
3. Megaloblastic
4. Iron deficiency

Level of Cognitive Ability: Applying
Client Needs: Physiological Integrity
Integrated Process: Nursing Process/Assessment
Content Area: Fundamental Skills: Laboratory Values
Priority Concepts: Clinical Judgment; Nutrition

Answer: 2
Rationale: The Schilling test is used to determine the cause of vitamin B_{12} deficiency, a potential precursor to pernicious anemia. This test involves the use of a small oral dose of radioactive B_{12} and a large nonradioactive intramuscular dose. A 24-hour urine specimen is then collected to measure the amount of radioactivity in the urine, and thus radioactive B_{12}. This test is not helpful in diagnosing aplastic, megaloblastic, or iron deficiency anemia.
Priority Nursing Tip: Vitamin B_{12} injections may be prescribed weekly initially and then monthly for maintenance (lifelong) if the anemia is the result of a deficiency of intrinsic factor or disease or surgery of the ileum.
Test-Taking Strategy: Focus on the subject, the Schilling test. Specific knowledge regarding the Schilling test and its purpose is needed to answer this question. Remember that the Schilling test is used to determine the cause of vitamin B_{12} deficiency. Review: **Schilling test** and the diagnostic tests associated with **pernicious anemia.**
Reference(s): Ignatavicius, Workman (2013), p. 1263.

1501. A health care provider has written a prescription for a client with diabetic gastroparesis to receive metoclopramide (Reglan) four times a day. The nurse schedules this medication to be given at which times?
1. With each meal and at bedtime
2. 30 minutes before meals and at bedtime
3. One hour after each meal and at bedtime
4. Every 6 hours spaced evenly around the clock

Level of Cognitive Ability: Applying
Client Needs: Physiological Integrity
Integrated Process: Nursing Process/Implementation
Content Area: Pharmacology: Gastrointestinal Medications
Priority Concepts: Clinical Judgment; Safety

Answer: 2
Rationale: Metoclopramide stimulates the motility of the upper gastrointestinal tract and is used to treat gastroparesis (nausea, vomiting, and persistent fullness after meals). The client should be taught to take this medication 30 minutes before meals and at bedtime. The before-meals administration allows the medication time to begin working before the client consumes food that requires digestion. The other options are incorrect.
Priority Nursing Tip: Metoclopramide (Reglan) can cause parkinsonian reactions. If this occurs, the medication will be discontinued by the health care provider.
Test-Taking Strategy: Focus on the subject, diabetic gastroparesis. Noting that the medication is used to treat gastroparesis will direct you to the correct option. Remember that it must be taken before meals to enhance digestion. Review: **metoclopramide (Reglan).**
Reference(s): Hodgson, Kizior (2014), pp. 763-764.

1502. The nurse is caring for a client who has just had a mastectomy. Which exercise should the nurse assist the client in doing during the **first** 24 hours after surgery?
1. Hand wall climbing
2. Pendulum arm swings
3. Elbow flexion and extension
4. Shoulder abduction and external rotation

Level of Cognitive Ability: Applying
Client Needs: Physiological Integrity
Integrated Process: Nursing Process/Implementation
Content Area: Adult Health: Oncology
Priority Concepts: Health Promotion; Mobility

Answer: 3
Rationale: During the first 24 hours after surgery, the client is assisted to move the fingers and hands, and to flex and extend the elbow. The client may also use the arm for self-care provided that she does not raise the arm above shoulder level or abduct the shoulder. The exercises identified in options 1, 2, and 4 are done once surgical drains are removed and wound healing is well established.
Priority Nursing Tip: In the postoperative period after mastectomy, initiate pain control measures before beginning prescribed exercises to promote participation in the exercise plan.
Test-Taking Strategy: Note the strategic word, *first.* Remember that options that are comparable or alike are not likely to be correct. In this situation, each of the incorrect options involves movement of the shoulder joint. Review: **mastectomy.**
Reference(s): Ignatavicius, Workman (2013), pp. 1603-1604.

1503. The nurse teaches a client about an upcoming endoscopic retrograde cholangiopancreatography (ERCP) procedure. The nurse determines that the client has a **need for further teaching** if the client makes which statement?

1. "An anesthetic throat spray will be used."
2. "A signed informed consent is necessary."
3. "Medication will be given orally for sedation."
4. "It is important to lie still during the procedure."

Level of Cognitive Ability: Evaluating
Client Needs: Physiological Integrity
Integrated Process: Teaching and Learning
Content Area: Fundamental Skills: Diagnostic Tests
Priority Concepts: Client Education; Safety

Answer: 3
Rationale: Intravenous sedation (not oral) is given to relax the client, and an anesthetic throat spray is used to help keep the client from gagging as the endoscope is passed. The client has to sign an informed consent form. The client also needs to lie still for ERCP, which takes about an hour to perform.
Priority Nursing Tip: After endoscopic retrograde cholangiopancreatography (ERCP), assess the client for the return of the gag reflex before offering the client anything to drink or eat.
Test-Taking Strategy: Note the strategic words, *need for further teaching* in the question. These words indicate a negative event query and the need to select the incorrect client statement. Recalling that this procedure is endoscopic and noting the word *orally* in option 3 will direct you to this choice. Review: preprocedure care for an **endoscopic retrograde cholangiopancreatography (ERCP).**
Reference(s): Pagana, Pagana (2013), pp. 388-390.

1504. A client has a prescription to take magnesium citrate (Citroma) to prevent constipation after upper and lower gastrointestinal (GI) barium studies. The nurse tells the client that which is the **best** way to take this medication?

1. With fruit juice only
2. At room temperature
3. With a tepid glass of water
4. Chilled with a full glass of water

Level of Cognitive Ability: Applying
Client Needs: Physiological Integrity
Integrated Process: Teaching and Learning
Content Area: Pharmacology: Gastrointestinal Medications
Priority Concepts: Client Education; Elimination

Answer: 4
Rationale: Magnesium citrate is available as an oral solution. It is commonly used as a laxative after certain studies of the GI tract. It should be served chilled and taken with a full glass of water. It should not be allowed to stand for prolonged periods. Allowing the medication to stand would reduce the carbonation and make the solution even less palatable. Options 1, 2, and 3 are incorrect.
Priority Nursing Tip: Magnesium citrate is an osmotic laxative that attracts water into the large intestine to produce bulk and stimulate peristalsis.
Test-Taking Strategy: Note the strategic word, *best*. Eliminate option 1 first because of the closed-ended word "only." Next, eliminate options 2 and 3 because they identify similar temperatures. Review: the procedure for administering **magnesium citrate (Citroma).**
Reference(s): Hodgson, Kizior (2014), pp. 723-725.

1505. A client has begun medication therapy with pancrelipase (Creon). The nurse should tell the client to expect which to occur from this medication?

1. Relieve heartburn
2. Eliminate abdominal pain
3. Help regulate blood glucose
4. Decrease the amount of fat in the stools

Level of Cognitive Ability: Applying
Client Needs: Physiological Integrity
Integrated Process: Teaching and Learning
Content Area: Pharmacology: Gastrointestinal Medications
Priority Concepts: Client Education; Safety

Answer: 4
Rationale: Pancrelipase is a pancreatic enzyme used in clients with pancreatitis as a digestive aid. The medication should reduce the amount of fatty stools (steatorrhea). Another intended effect could be improved nutritional status. It is not used to treat abdominal pain or heartburn. It does not regulate blood glucose; this is a function of insulin, a hormone produced in the beta cells of the pancreas.
Priority Nursing Tip: Pancreatic enzyme replacements should be taken with all meals and snacks.
Test-Taking Strategy: Focus on the subject, pancrelipase (Creon), which gives an indication of its possible uses. Also use knowledge of the physiology of the pancreas and recall that the suffix "-ase" in the medication name indicates an enzyme. This will assist in directing you to the correct option. Review: the action of **pancrelipase (Creon).**
Reference(s): Hodgson, Kizior (2014), pp. 903-904.

1506. The nurse is performing tracheostomy care and has replaced the tracheostomy tube holder (tracheostomy ties). Which is an **effective** measure for the nurse to use when checking that the holder is not too tight?
1. The client nods that he or she feels comfortable.
2. Two fingers can be slid comfortably under the holder.
3. Four fingers can be slid comfortably under the holder.
4. The tracheostomy does not move more than a half an inch when the client is coughing.

Level of Cognitive Ability: Evaluating
Client Needs: Physiological Integrity
Integrated Process: Nursing Process/Evaluation
Content Area: Adult Health: Respiratory
Priority Concepts: Gas Exchange; Safety

Answer: 2
Rationale: There should be enough room for two fingers to slide comfortably under the tracheostomy holder. This ensures that the holder is tight enough to prevent tracheostomy dislocation, while preventing excessive constriction around the neck. The other options are incorrect.
Priority Nursing Tip: Ensure that a tracheostomy tube of the same size and an obturator is at the bedside of a client with a tracheostomy.
Test-Taking Strategy: Note the strategic word, *effective*. Focus on the subject, that the tracheostomy holder is not too tight. Visualize each of the descriptions in the options to direct you to the correct option. Review: **tracheostomy care.**
Reference(s): Ignatavicius, Workman (2013), p. 576.

1507. The nurse has assisted the health care provider in placing a central (subclavian) catheter. Which **priority** action should the nurse take following the procedure?
1. Ensure that a chest radiograph is done.
2. Obtain a temperature reading to monitor for infection.
3. Label the dressing with the date and time of catheter insertion.
4. Monitor the blood pressure (BP) to check for fluid volume overload.

Level of Cognitive Ability: Applying
Client Needs: Physiological Integrity
Integrated Process: Nursing Process/Implementation
Content Area: Critical Care: Medications and IV Therapy
Priority Concepts: Clinical Judgment; Safety

Answer: 1
Rationale: A major risk associated with central catheter insertion is the possibility of a pneumothorax developing from an accidental puncture of the lung. Obtaining a chest radiograph and checking the results is the best method to determine if this complication has occurred and verify catheter tip placement before initiating intravenous (IV) therapy. While a client may develop an infection at the central catheter site, a temperature elevation would not likely occur immediately after placement. Labeling the dressing site is important, but it is not a priority action in this situation. Although BP assessment is always important in checking a client's status after an invasive procedure, fluid volume overload is not a concern until IV fluids are started.
Priority Nursing Tip: For central line insertion, tubing change, and line removal, place the client in the Trendelenburg position if not contraindicated or in the supine position.
Test-Taking Strategy: Noting the strategic word, *priority* and focusing on the subject, following the procedure, will assist in eliminating options 2 and 4. Option 3 will occur during the procedure. Review: central (subclavian) catheter insertion.
Reference(s): Ignatavicius, Workman (2013), p. 216.

1508. A client is complaining of gas pains after surgery and requests medication. The nurse reviews the medication prescription sheet to see if which medication is prescribed for the relief of gas pains?
1. Droperidol (Inapsine)
2. Simethicone (Mylicon)
3. Acetaminophen (Tylenol)
4. Magnesium hydroxide (MOM)

Level of Cognitive Ability: Analyzing
Client Needs: Physiological Integrity
Integrated Process: Nursing Process/Analysis
Content Area: Pharmacology: Gastrointestinal Medications
Priority Concepts: Elimination; Safety

Answer: 2
Rationale: Simethicone is an antiflatulent used in the relief of pain caused by excessive gas in the gastrointestinal tract. Droperidol is used to treat postoperative nausea and vomiting. Acetaminophen is a nonopioid analgesic. Magnesium hydroxide is an antacid and laxative.
Priority Nursing Tip: Instruct the client experiencing gas pains to avoid consuming carbonated beverages.
Test-Taking Strategy: Focus on the subject, postsurgery gas pains. Recalling the classifications of each of the medications listed in the options will direct you to the correct option. Review: the action and purpose of Simethicone (Mylicon).
Reference(s): Hodgson, Kizior (2014), pp. 1083-1084.

1509. A home care nurse notes that an older client is taking cimetidine (Tagamet). On assessment of the client, the nurse should check for which side effect of this medication?
1. Fatigue
2. Confusion
3. Constipation
4. Blurred vision

Level of Cognitive Ability: Analyzing
Client Needs: Physiological Integrity
Integrated Process: Nursing Process/Assessment
Content Area: Pharmacology: Gastrointestinal Medications
Priority Concepts: Cognition; Safety

Answer: 2
Rationale: Cimetidine is a gastric acid secretion inhibitor. Older clients are especially susceptible to the central nervous system side effects of cimetidine. The most frequent of these is confusion. Less common central nervous system side effects include headache, dizziness, drowsiness, agitation, and hallucinations. Options 1, 3, and 4 are not associated with the use of this medication.
Priority Nursing Tip: Cimetidine (Tagamet) and antacids should be administered at least 1 hour apart from each other.
Test-Taking Strategy: Focus on the subject, cimetidine (Tagamet). Recalling that cimetidine causes central nervous system side effects will direct you to the correct option. Review: the side effects of cimetidine (Tagamet).
Reference(s): Hodgson, Kizior (2014), pp. 242-243.

1510. A client is admitted to the hospital after sustaining a fall from a roof. The client has multiple lacerations and a right leg fracture, which has been treated with a plaster cast. How should the nurse position the client's leg to promote optimal circulation?
1. Flat or a level position
2. Flat for 3 hours and elevated for 1 hour
3. Elevated for 3 hours, and then flat for 1 hour
4. Elevated on pillows continuously for 24 to 48 hours

Level of Cognitive Ability: Applying
Client Needs: Physiological Integrity
Integrated Process: Nursing Process/Implementation
Content Area: Adult Health: Musculoskeletal
Priority Concepts: Mobility; Safety

Answer: 4
Rationale: A casted extremity is elevated continuously for the first 24 to 48 hours to minimize swelling and promote venous drainage. The other options are not part of standard positioning of the newly casted extremity.
Priority Nursing Tip: Monitor the casted extremity for signs of circulatory impairment. The health care provider is notified immediately if circulatory impairment is suspected.
Test-Taking Strategy: Focus on the subject, to promote optimal circulation of a casted fractured leg. Recalling that edema occurs after a fracture and can be increased by casting and using the principles of gravity will direct you to option 4. Review: casting of an extremity.
Reference(s): Ignatavicius, Workman (2013), pp. 1150-1151.

1511. A physical assessment is performed on a suicidal client upon admission to the inpatient unit. The nurse understands its importance because it provides information regarding which **priority** assessment data?
1. The presence of abnormalities
2. Evidence of physical self-harm
3. Both subjective and objective baseline data
4. Existing medical problems and complaints

Level of Cognitive Ability: Analyzing
Client Needs: Physiological Integrity
Integrated Process: Nursing Process/Assessment
Content Area: Mental Health
Priority Concepts: Mood and Affect; Safety

Answer: 2
Rationale: The physical assessment of a suicidal client should be thorough and should focus on the evidence of self-harm or the client's formulation of a plan for the suicide attempt. Although all of the choices are correct, option 2 is the priority in the context of the suicidal client. Clients with a history of self-harm are greater suicide risks.
Priority Nursing Tip: A client who is suicidal needs to be placed on suicide precautions. The nurse should ensure that visitors do not leave harmful objects in the client's room.
Test-Taking Strategy: Focus on the subject, a suicidal client. Note the strategic word, priority. Remember that assessing for physical evidence of harm is a priority component of the assessment process of a suicidal client. Review: the characteristics of the client at risk for suicide.
Reference(s): Stuart (2013), p. 335; Varcarolis (2013), p. 438.

1512. A client being mechanically ventilated after experiencing a fat embolus is visibly anxious. Which appropriate action should the nurse take?

1. Remain with the client and provide reassurance
2. Ask a family member to stay with the client at all times
3. Encourage the client to sleep until arterial blood gas results improve
4. Ask the health care provider to write a prescription for an antianxiety medication

Level of Cognitive Ability: Applying
Client Needs: Psychosocial Integrity
Integrated Process: Caring
Content Area: Adult Health: Respiratory
Priority Concepts: Anxiety; Coping

Answer: 1
Rationale: The nurse always speaks to the client calmly and provides reassurance to the anxious client. Family members are also stressed because of the severity of the situation; therefore, it is not beneficial to ask the family to take on the burden of remaining with the client at all times. Encouraging the client to sleep will not assist in relieving the client's anxiety. Antianxiety medications are used only if necessary and if other interventions fail to relieve the client's anxiety.
Priority Nursing Tip: It is important for the nurse to stay with a client who is anxious or fearful. Leaving the client alone will increase anxiety and fear.
Test-Taking Strategy: Focus on the subject, an anxious client. Remember that it is most important to address the client's feelings. Review: anxiety.
Reference(s): Ignatavicius, Workman (2013), p. 679.

1513. The nurse is caring for a client who is receiving colchicine (Colcrys). The nurse understands that the client is responding favorably to the medication if there is a decrease in which sign/symptom?

1. Headaches
2. Joint inflammation
3. Blood glucose level
4. Serum triglyceride level

Level of Cognitive Ability: Evaluating
Client Needs: Physiological Integrity
Integrated Process: Nursing Process/Evaluation
Content Area: Pharmacology: Musculoskeletal Medications
Priority Concepts: Inflammation; Safety

Answer: 2
Rationale: Colchicine is classified as an antigout agent. It interferes with the ability of the white blood cells to initiate and maintain an inflammatory response to monosodium urate crystals. The client should report a decrease in pain and inflammation in affected joints, as well as a decrease in the number of gout attacks. The other options are not related to the use of this medication.
Priority Nursing Tip: If gastrointestinal symptoms occur (nausea, vomiting, diarrhea, and abdominal pain) in a client taking colchicine, the medication is withheld and the health care provider is notified.
Test-Taking Strategy: Focus on the subject, colchicine (Colcrys). Recalling that this medication is used in the treatment of gout will direct you to the correct option. Review: the action of colchicine (Colcrys).
Reference(s): Hodgson, Kizior (2014), pp. 274-275.

1514. A client has a prescription to begin short-term therapy with enoxaparin (Lovenox). The nurse explains to the client that this medication is being prescribed for which action?

1. Dissolve urinary calculi
2. Relieve migraine headaches
3. Stop progression of multiple sclerosis
4. Reduce the risk of deep vein thrombosis

Level of Cognitive Ability: Applying
Client Needs: Physiological Integrity
Integrated Process: Teaching and Learning
Content Area: Pharmacology: Cardiovascular Medications
Priority Concepts: Client Education; Clotting

Answer: 4
Rationale: Enoxaparin is an anticoagulant that is administered to prevent deep vein thrombosis and thromboembolism in selected clients at risk. It is not used to treat urinary calculi, migraine headaches, or multiple sclerosis.
Priority Nursing Tip: The antidote to enoxaparin (Lovenox) is protamine sulfate.
Test-Taking Strategy: Focus on the subject, enoxaparin (Lovenox). Recalling that this medication is an anticoagulant will direct you to the correct option. Review: the action of enoxaparin (Lovenox).
Reference(s): Hodgson, Kizior (2014), pp. 409-410.

1515. A client takes aluminum hydroxide tablets as needed for heartburn. The nurse teaches the client that which is the **most** common side effect of this medication?
1. Dizziness
2. Excitability
3. Muscle pain
4. Constipation

Level of Cognitive Ability: Applying
Client Needs: Physiological Integrity
Integrated Process: Teaching and Learning
Content Area: Pharmacology: Gastrointestinal Medications
Priority Concepts: Client Education; Pain

Answer: 4
Rationale: Because of the antacid's aluminum base, aluminum hydroxide causes constipation as a side effect. The other side effect is hypophosphatemia, which is noted by monitoring serum laboratory studies. The other options are not side effects of this medication.
Priority Nursing Tip: Aluminum compounds contain significant amounts of sodium and should be used with caution in clients with hypertension or heart failure.
Test-Taking Strategy: Focus on the subject, aluminum hydroxide, and note the strategic word, *most*. Remember that this medication is an antacid. Recalling that aluminum-based antacids cause constipation will direct you to the correct option. Review: the side effects associated with **aluminum hydroxide**.
Reference(s): Lehne (2013), p. 996.

1516. The nurse is caring for a young adult client diagnosed with sarcoidosis. The client is angry and tells the nurse that there is no point in learning disease management because there is no possibility of ever being cured. Based on the client's statement, the nurse determines that the client is experiencing which potential problem?
1. Apprehension
2. Powerlessness
3. Intellectualization
4. Ineffective thought process

Level of Cognitive Ability: Analyzing
Client Needs: Psychosocial Integrity
Integrated Process: Nursing Process/Analysis
Content Area: Mental Health
Priority Concepts: Anxiety; Coping

Answer: 2
Rationale: The client with powerlessness expresses feelings of having no control over a situation or outcome. Apprehension is fearful or uneasy anticipation of something. Intellectualization is excessive reasoning to avoid feeling. Ineffective thought process involves interruption in normal thought.
Priority Nursing Tip: The cause of sarcoidosis is unknown, but a high titer of Epstein-Barr virus may be noted.
Test-Taking Strategy: Focus on the subject, anger about having sarcoidosis. Note the words *no point in learning disease management*. This will direct you to the correct option. Review: the characteristics of powerlessness.
Reference(s): Ignatavicius, Workman (2013), pp. 627-628, 632; Stuart, (2013), pp. 204-205.

1517. The nurse is providing instructions to the spouse of a client who is taking tacrine (Cognex) for the management of moderate dementia associated with Alzheimer's disease. Which instruction should the nurse give to the spouse?
1. Not to administer the medication with food.
2. If a dose is missed, double up on the next dose.
3. If a change in the color of the stools occurs, notify the health care provider.
4. If flulike symptoms occur, it is necessary to notify the health care provider immediately.

Level of Cognitive Ability: Applying
Client Needs: Physiological Integrity
Integrated Process: Teaching and Learning
Content Area: Pharmacology: Neurological Medications
Priority Concepts: Client Education; Safety

Answer: 3
Rationale: The client and caregiver are instructed to notify the health care provider if nausea, vomiting, diarrhea, rash, jaundice, or changes in the color of the stool occur. This may be indicative of the potential occurrence of hepatitis. Tacrine may be administered between meals on an empty stomach, and if gastrointestinal upset occurs, it may be administered with meals. Flulike symptoms without fever are frequent side effects that may occur with the use of the medication. The client or spouse should never be instructed to double the dose of any medication if it was missed.
Priority Nursing Tip: Tacrine (Cognex), a medication used to treat Alzheimer's disease, can cause ataxia, loss of appetite, nausea, vomiting, diarrhea, rash, jaundice, changes in the color of the stool, and hepatitis.
Test-Taking Strategy: Focus on the subject, the adverse effects of tacrine. Eliminate option 4 because of the word *immediately*. Flulike symptoms should not be a concern requiring immediate health care provider notification. Next, eliminate option 2 because of the words *double up on the next dose*. From the remaining choices, recalling that an adverse effect associated with the use of the medication is hepatitis will direct you to the correct option. Review: **tacrine (Cognex)**.
Reference(s): Kee, Hayes, McCuistion (2012), pp. 327-328.

1518. An older client has been using casanthranol (cascara sagrada) on a long-term basis to treat constipation. The nurse determines that which laboratory finding is a result of the side/adverse effects of this medication?
  1. Sodium 135 mEq/L
  2. Sodium 145 mEq/L
  3. Potassium 3.1 mEq/L
  4. Potassium 5.0 mEq/L

Level of Cognitive Ability: Analyzing
Client Needs: Physiological Integrity
Integrated Process: Nursing Process/Analysis
Content Area: Pharmacology: Gastrointestinal Medications
Priority Concepts: Clinical Judgment; Fluid and Electrolyte Balance

Answer: 3
Rationale: Hypokalemia can result from long-term use of casanthranol (cascara sagrada), which is a laxative. The medication stimulates peristalsis and alters fluid and electrolyte transport, thus helping fluid to accumulate in the colon. The normal range for potassium is 3.5 to 5.0 mEq/L. The normal range for sodium is 135 to 145 mEq/L. Options 1, 2, and 4 are normal values.
Priority Nursing Tip: A client with severe diarrhea is at risk for metabolic acidosis. Intestinal fluids are highly alkaline and excessive loss of these fluids places the client at risk for this acid-base disturbance.
Test-Taking Strategy: Focus on the subject, side/adverse effects of casanthranol. Recall knowledge regarding the normal laboratory values for sodium and potassium. The only abnormal value is option 3. Review: **casanthranol (cascara sagrada).**
Reference(s): Lilley, Rainforth Collins, Harrington, Snyder (2014), p. 841; Pagana, Pagana (2013), pp. 741-742.

1519. A client has been started on cyclobenzaprine (Flexeril) for the management of muscle spasms. The nurse should observe for which **most** frequent side effect?
  1. Fatigue
  2. Irritability
  3. Excitability
  4. Drowsiness

Level of Cognitive Ability: Applying
Client Needs: Physiological Integrity
Integrated Process: Nursing Process: Implementation
Content Area: Pharmacology: Musculoskeletal Medications
Priority Concepts: Mobility; Safety

Answer: 4
Rationale: The most frequent side effects of cyclobenzaprine are drowsiness, dizziness, and dry mouth. This medication is a centrally acting skeletal muscle relaxant used in the management of muscle spasms that accompany a variety of conditions. Fatigue, nervousness, and confusion are rare side effects of the medication.
Priority Nursing Tip: Safety is a priority for a client receiving a skeletal muscle relaxant because the medication can cause drowsiness.
Test-Taking Strategy: Note the strategic word, *most*. Eliminate options 2 and 3 first because they are comparable or alike. Recalling that this medication is a centrally acting skeletal muscle relaxant will direct you to option 4 from the remaining options. Review: **cyclobenzaprine (Flexeril),**
Reference(s): Hodgson, Kizior (2014), pp. 287-288.

1520. The nurse is caring for a client after shoulder arthroplasty for rheumatoid arthritis and is checking the client for brachial plexus compromise. To assess the status of the median nerve, which action would the nurse perform?
  1. Have the client spread all of the fingers wide and resist pressure.
  2. Monitor for flexion of the biceps by having the client raise the forearm.
  3. Have the client move the thumb toward the palm and back to the neutral position.
  4. Have the client grasp the nurse's hand while noting the client's strength of the first and second fingers.

Level of Cognitive Ability: Analyzing
Client Needs: Health Promotion and Maintenance
Integrated Process: Nursing Process/Assessment
Content Area: Adult Health: Musculoskeletal
Priority Concepts: Health Promotion; Mobility

Answer: 4
Rationale: To assess the median nerve status, the client should be instructed to grasp the nurse's hand. The nurse should note the strength of the client's first and second fingers. A weak grip may indicate compromise of the median nerve. Asking the client to spread all fingers wide and resist pressure assesses the ulnar nerve status. Monitoring for flexion of the biceps by raising the forearm assesses the cutaneous nerve status. Asking the client to move the thumb toward the palm and back to neutral position assesses the radial nerve status.
Priority Nursing Tip: Arthroplasty involves surgical replacement of a diseased joint with an artificial joint.
Test-Taking Strategy: Focus on the subject, assessment of the median nerve. Recalling the location and function of the median nerve will direct you to the correct option. Review: **median nerve.**
Reference(s): Ignatavicius, Workman (2013), p. 331.

1521. The nurse is preparing to administer heparin sodium 5000 units subcutaneously. Which indicates the accurate procedure for administering the medication?
1. Injecting the medication via an infusion device
2. Massaging the injection site after administration
3. Injecting the medication 1 inch from the umbilicus
4. Avoiding aspiration before administration of the medication

Level of Cognitive Ability: Applying
Client Needs: Physiological Integrity
Integrated Process: Nursing Process/Implementation
Content Area: Pharmacology: Hematological Medications
Priority Concepts: Health Promotion; Safety

Answer: 4
Rationale: Aspiration before administration of heparin sodium should be avoided. Heparin administered by the subcutaneous route does not require an infusion device. The injection site is above the iliac crest or in the abdominal fat layer. It is injected at least 2 inches from the umbilicus. After administration, the needle is withdrawn, pressure is applied to the injection site, and the site is not massaged. Injection sites are rotated.
Priority Nursing Tip: Instruct the client receiving heparin about the measures to prevent bleeding.
Test-Taking Strategy: Focus on the subject, accurate procedure to administer heparin sodium. Visualize the procedure as you read each option. Recalling the action and effects of heparin will direct you to the correct option. Review: **heparin sodium** subcutaneous administration.
Reference(s): Lilley, Rainforth Collins, Harrington, Snyder (2014), p. 437.

1522. What should the nurse assess for in a client who has pernicious anemia?
1. Constipation
2. Shortness of breath
3. Dusky lips and gums
4. Smooth, sore, red tongue

Level of Cognitive Ability: Analyzing
Client Needs: Physiological Integrity
Integrated Process: Nursing Process/Assessment
Content Area: Fundamental Skills: Nutrition
Priority Concepts: Clinical Judgment; Nutrition

Answer: 4
Rationale: Classic clinical indicators of pernicious anemia include weakness, mild diarrhea, and a smooth, sore red tongue. The client may also have neurological findings, such as paresthesias, confusion, and difficulty with balance. Constipation is not a common finding with pernicious anemia. Pernicious anemia does not affect tissue oxygenation, so the mucous membranes do not become dusky, and the client does not exhibit shortness of breath (options 2 and 3).
Priority Nursing Tip: Pernicious anemia results from a deficiency of intrinsic factor, necessary for intestinal absorption of vitamin B_{12}. Gastric disease or surgery can result in a lack of intrinsic factor.
Test-Taking Strategy: Focus on the subject, pernicious anemia. To answer this question you must be familiar with the clinical indicators of pernicious anemia. Remember that the classic clinical indicators of pernicious anemia include weakness; mild diarrhea; and a smooth, sore red tongue. Review: The assessment data related to **pernicious anemia.**
Reference(s): Ignatavicius, Workman (2013), p. 877.

1523. Benztropine mesylate (Cogentin) is prescribed for a client with a diagnosis of Parkinson's disease. Which instruction should the nurse provide to the client regarding the medication?
1. Sit in the sun for 30 minutes daily.
2. Avoid driving if drowsiness or dizziness occurs.
3. Expect difficulty swallowing while taking this medication.
4. Expect episodes of vomiting and constipation while taking this medication.

Level of Cognitive Ability: Applying
Client Needs: Safe and Effective Care Environment
Integrated Process: Teaching and Learning
Content Area: Pharmacology: Neurological Medications
Priority Concepts: Client Education; Safety

Answer: 2
Rationale: The client taking benztropine mesylate should be instructed to avoid driving or operating hazardous equipment if drowsy or dizzy. The client's tolerance to heat may be reduced because of the diminished ability to sweat, and the client should be instructed to plan rest periods in cool places during the day. The client should be instructed to contact the health care provider immediately if difficulty swallowing or speaking or vomiting occurs. The client should also inform the health care provider if central nervous system effects occur. The client is instructed to monitor urinary output and watch for signs of constipation.
Priority Nursing Tip: Benztropine mesylate (Cogentin) is an anticholinergic medication. Anticholinergic medications are contraindicated in clients with glaucoma.
Test-Taking Strategy: Focus on the subject, client instructions for benztropine mesylate. General principles related to safety and medications will direct you to the correct option. Review: client teaching points related to **benztropine mesylate (Cogentin).**
Reference(s): Hodgson, Kizior (2014), pp. 123-125.

1524. The nurse is preparing to do preoperative teaching with a client scheduled for radical neck dissection. Which should the nurse **initially** focus on?
1. The client's usual coping behaviors
2. The client's dependable support systems
3. Postoperative communication techniques
4. The information already supplied by the surgeon

Level of Cognitive Ability: Applying
Client Needs: Psychosocial Integrity
Integrated Process: Teaching and Learning
Content Area: Fundamental Skills: Perioperative Care
Priority Concepts: Client Education; Professionalism

Answer: 4
Rationale: The first step in client education is establishing what the client already knows. This allows the nurse to correct any misinformation or misunderstandings, determine the starting point for teaching, and plan and implement the education at the client's level. Although options 1, 2, and 3 can be a component of the plan, the first step in client education is establishing what the client already knows.
Priority Nursing Tip: The nurse must ensure that the client understands the surgical procedure or any other course of action prescribed. If the procedure has not been explained to the client, the nurse should contact the surgeon or other prescriber of the treatment.
Test-Taking Strategy: Note the strategic word, *initially*. It is likely that all of the options listed will be included in the teaching plan, but you need to determine what the nurse should focus on initially. Remember that in the teaching and learning process, client motivation and readiness to learn along with what the client already knows are initial assessment items. Review: the **teaching and learning process.**
Reference(s): Ignatavicius, Workman (2013), pp. 1199-1200.

1525. A client with refractory myasthenia gravis is told by the health care provider that plasmapheresis therapy is indicated. After the health care provider leaves the room, the client asks the nurse to repeat the health care provider's reason for prescribing this treatment. The nurse should tell the client that this therapy will **most likely** improve which problem?
1. Double vision
2. Difficulty breathing
3. Urinary incontinence
4. Pins and needles sensation in the legs

Level of Cognitive Ability: Applying
Client Needs: Physiological Integrity
Integrated Process: Teaching and Learning
Content Area: Adult Health: Neurological
Priority Concepts: Client Education; Gas Exchange

Answer: 2
Rationale: Plasmapheresis is a process that separates the plasma from the blood elements, so that plasma proteins that contain antibodies can be removed. It is used as an adjunct therapy in myasthenia gravis and may give temporary relief to clients with actual or impending respiratory failure. Usually three to five treatments are required. This therapy is not indicated for the reasons listed in options 1, 3, and 4.
Priority Nursing Tip: The nurse encourages the client with myasthenia gravis to sit up when eating or drinking fluids because of the difficulty with chewing and swallowing that occurs in this disorder.
Test-Taking Strategy: Note the strategic words, *most likely*. This tells you that the client with myasthenia gravis has severe disease, which is not adequately controlled with medication and other measures. Recalling the purpose of plasmapheresis and knowledge of the complications of this disease will direct you to option 2. Review: **plasmapheresis and myasthenia gravis.**
Reference(s): Ignatavicius, Workman (2013), pp. 988-989, 994.

1526. A client is admitted to the hospital in myasthenic crisis. The nurse should ask the client about which precipitating factor for this event?
1. Getting more sleep than usual
2. Not taking prescribed medication
3. A decrease in food intake recently
4. Taking excess prescribed medication

Level of Cognitive Ability: Analyzing
Client Needs: Physiological Integrity
Integrated Process: Nursing Process/Assessment
Content Area: Adult Health: Neurological
Priority Concepts: Mobility; Safety

Answer: 2
Rationale: Myasthenic crisis is often caused by undermedication and responds to the administration of cholinergic medications such as neostigmine (Prostigmin) and pyridostigmine (Mestinon). Increased sleep and change in diet are not precipitating factors. However, overexertion and overeating could possibly trigger myasthenic crisis. Cholinergic crisis is caused by excess medication and responds to withholding of medications.
Priority Nursing Tip: In myasthenic crisis, an increase in the cholinergic medication is usually prescribed.
Test-Taking Strategy: Focus on the subject, myasthenic crisis. Recalling that myasthenia gravis is treated with medication will direct you to the correct option. Not taking medication will lead to a crisis. Review: the causes of **myasthenia gravis.**
Reference(s): Ignatavicius, Workman (2013), p. 996.

1527. A client with trigeminal neuralgia asks the nurse what can be done to minimize the episodes of pain. The nurse's response is based on an understanding that what can trigger the pain?
1. Infection or stress
2. Hypoglycemia and fatigue
3. Facial pressure or extreme temperature
4. Excessive watering of the eyes or nasal stuffiness

Level of Cognitive Ability: Applying
Client Needs: Physiological Integrity
Integrated Process: Nursing Process/Implementation
Content Area: Adult Health: Neurological
Priority Concepts: Intracranial Regulation; Pain

Answer: 3
Rationale: The paroxysms of pain that accompany this neuralgia are triggered by stimulation of the terminal branches of the trigeminal nerve. Symptoms can be triggered by pressure from washing the face, brushing the teeth, shaving, eating and drinking, and yawning. Symptoms can also be triggered by thermal stimuli such as a draft of cold air. The items listed in the other options do not trigger the spasm.
Priority Nursing Tip: Provide small feedings of tepid liquids and soft tepid foods to the client with trigeminal neuralgia to prevent triggering the spasms and pain.
Test-Taking Strategy: Focus on the subject, trigeminal neuralgia. Recall the pathophysiology of this disorder and that precipitating factors such as pressure or thermal stimuli trigger the spasm. This will direct you to option 3. Review: **trigeminal neuralgia.**
Reference(s): Ignatavicius, Workman (2013), pp. 1000-1001.

1528. A client has been diagnosed with Bell's palsy. The nurse assesses the client to determine if which signs/symptoms are present?
1. Eye paralysis and ptosis of the eyelids
2. Chewing difficulties and one-sided facial droop
3. Fixed pupil and an elevated eyelid on one side
4. Twitching of one side of the face and ruddy cheeks

Level of Cognitive Ability: Applying
Client Needs: Physiological Integrity
Integrated Process: Nursing Process/Assessment
Content Area: Adult Health: Neurological
Priority Concepts: Intracranial Regulation; Mobility

Answer: 2
Rationale: Bell's palsy is a one-sided facial paralysis resulting from compression of the facial nerve (CN VII). There is facial droop from paralysis of the facial muscles; increased lacrimation; painful sensations in the eye, face, or behind the ear; and chewing difficulties. The other items listed are not associated with this disorder.
Priority Nursing Tip: Recovery from Bell's palsy usually occurs in a few weeks without residual effects.
Test-Taking Strategy: Focus on the subject, Bell's palsy. Remember that palsy is a type of paralysis. This will assist in eliminating option 4. Recalling that Bell's palsy results from dysfunction of the facial nerve (CN VII), not the nerves that govern eye movements (CN III, IV, VI), will help eliminate options 1 and 3. Review: the characteristics associated with **Bell's palsy.**
Reference(s): Ignatavicius, Workman (2013), pp. 1001-1002.

1529. A female client arrives at the emergency department and states she was just raped. In preparing a plan of care, which is the **priority** intervention?
1. Providing instructions for medical follow-up
2. Obtaining appropriate counseling for the victim
3. Providing anticipatory guidance for police investigations, medical questions, and court proceedings
4. Exploring safety concerns by obtaining permission to notify significant others who can provide shelter

Level of Cognitive Ability: Analyzing
Client Needs: Safe and Effective Care Environment
Integrated Process: Nursing Process/Planning
Content Area: Mental Health
Priority Concepts: Interpersonal Violence; Safety

Answer: 4
Rationale: After the provision of medical treatment, the nurse's next priority would be obtaining support and planning for safety. Option 1 is concerned with ensuring that the victim understands the importance of and commits to the need for medical follow-up. From the options provided, this is not a priority intervention. Options 2 and 3 seek to meet the emotional needs related to the rape and emotional readiness for the process of discovery and legal action.
Priority Nursing Tip: The rape victim is not required by law to report the assault or rape.
Test-Taking Strategy: Use Maslow's Hierarchy of Needs theory and note the strategic word, *priority*. Remember that physiological needs are the priority, followed by safety needs. Therefore, select option 4 because it addresses the safety needs. Review: **rape.**
Reference(s): Varcarolis (2013), pp. 427-428.

❖ **1530.** A client has health care provider instructions to take ibuprofen (Advil) 0.4 g for mild pain. The medication bottle contains ibuprofen (Advil) 200-mg tablets. How many tablets will the nurse instruct the client to take for each dose? **Fill in the blank.** _____ tablets

Level of Cognitive Ability: Applying
Client Needs: Physiological Integrity
Integrated Process: Nursing Process/Implementation
Content Area: Fundamental Skills: Medications/IV Calculations
Priority Concepts: Clinical Judgment; Safety

Answer: 2 tablets
Rationale: Convert 0.4 g to mg. In the metric system, to convert larger to smaller, multiply by 1000 or move the decimal three places to the right. Then follow the medication calculation formula.

Formula: 0.4 g = 400 mg

$$\frac{Desired}{Available} \times Quantity = Tablets\ per\ dose$$

$$\frac{400\ mg}{200\ mg} \times 1\ tablet = 2\ tablets$$

Priority Nursing Tip: Ibuprofen (Advil) is a nonsteroidal anti-inflammatory medication, and the client should be instructed to take the medication with food to prevent gastrointestinal irritation.
Test-Taking Strategy: Focus on the subject, ibuprofen tablets 0.4 g. Use the formula for the calculation of a medication dose. Remember to convert grams to milligrams. Make sure that the calculated dose makes sense, and recheck your answer using a calculator. Review: conversions and calculations.
Reference(s): Potter et al (2013), pp. 573-574.

1531. The nurse is admitting a client to the hospital who has a diagnosis of Guillain-Barré syndrome. During the history taking, the nurse should ask the family if the client has recently experienced which physical problem?
1. Meningitis
2. Seizures or head trauma
3. A back injury or spinal cord trauma
4. A respiratory or gastrointestinal (GI) infection

Level of Cognitive Ability: Analyzing
Client Needs: Physiological Integrity
Integrated Process: Nursing Process/Assessment
Content Area: Adult Health: Neurological
Priority Concepts: Gas Exchange; Intracranial Regulation

Answer: 4
Rationale: Guillain-Barré syndrome is a clinical condition of unknown origin that involves cranial and peripheral nerves. Many clients report a history of respiratory or GI infection in the 1 to 4 weeks before the onset of neurological deficits. Occasionally it has been triggered by vaccination or surgery. The other options are not associated with an incidence of this syndrome.
Priority Nursing Tip: The major concern with Guillain-Barré syndrome is difficulty breathing. The nurse must monitor the client's respiratory status closely.
Test-Taking Strategy: Focus on the subject, Guillain-Barré syndrome. Eliminate options 1, 2, and 3 because they are comparable or alike and relate to neurological problems. Review: the etiology associated with **Guillain-Barré syndrome.**
Reference(s): Ignatavicius, Workman (2013), p. 987.

1532. A client is using diphenhydramine (Benadryl) 1% as a topical agent for allergic dermatosis. The nurse evaluates that the medication is having the intended effect if the client reports relief of what complaint?
1. Pain
2. Urticaria
3. Headache
4. Skin redness

Level of Cognitive Ability: Evaluating
Client Needs: Physiological Integrity
Integrated Process: Nursing Process/Evaluation
Content Area: Pharmacology: Integumentary Medications
Priority Concepts: Clinical Judgment; Tissue Integrity

Answer: 2
Rationale: Diphenhydramine is an antihistamine medication that has many uses. When used as a topical agent on the skin, it reduces the symptoms of allergic reaction, such as itching or urticaria. It does not act to relieve pain, headache, or skin redness.
Priority Nursing Tip: Antihistamine medications can cause drowsiness. Instruct the client taking an antihistamine to avoid hazardous activities, alcohol, and other central nervous system depressants.
Test-Taking Strategy: Focus on the subject, diphenhydramine, and note the words, *intended effect.* Recalling that diphenhydramine is an antihistamine medication will assist in directing you to option 2. Review: the action of **diphenhydramine (Benadryl).**
Reference(s): Lehne (2013), pp. 887-888.

1533. A client is being treated in the emergency department for a fractured tibia. The skin is not broken, but the nurse can see on the x-ray viewer that the bone is completely fractured across the shaft and has small splintered pieces around it. What kind of fracture did the client sustain?
1. Simple fracture
2. Greenstick fracture
3. Compound fracture
4. Comminuted fracture

Level of Cognitive Ability: Analyzing
Client Needs: Physiological Integrity
Integrated Process: Nursing Process/Assessment
Content Area: Adult Health: Musculoskeletal
Priority Concepts: Clinical Judgment; Mobility

Answer: 4
Rationale: A comminuted fracture is a complete fracture across the shaft of a bone, with splintering of the bone into fragments. A simple fracture is a fracture of the bone across its entire shaft with some possible displacement but without breaking the skin. A greenstick fracture is an incomplete fracture, which occurs through part of the cross section of a bone. One side of the bone is fractured, and the other side is bent. A compound fracture, also called an open fracture, is one in which the skin or mucous membrane has been broken, and the wound extends to the depth of the fractured bone.
Priority Nursing Tip: If a fracture is suspected, the nurse should immobilize the affected extremity until further measures are implemented.
Test-Taking Strategy: Focus on the subject, fracture, and note the words *small splintered pieces*. Remember that a comminuted fracture is broken into minute (small) pieces. This will direct you to the correct option. Review: **comminuted fracture.**
Reference(s): Hammond, Zimmermann (2013), pp. 430-431.

1534. The nurse in the emergency department is providing care to a client with a leg fracture. The nurse ensures that which is done **first** before the fracture is reduced in the casting room?
1. Obtaining an anesthesia consent
2. Administering an opioid analgesic
3. Notifying the operating room staff
4. Obtaining an informed consent for treatment

Level of Cognitive Ability: Applying
Client Needs: Safe and Effective Care Environment
Integrated Process: Nursing Process/Implementation
Content Area: Adult Health: Musculoskeletal
Priority Concepts: Clinical Judgment; Health Care Law

Answer: 4
Rationale: Before a fracture is reduced, an informed consent for treatment is needed. The nurse should reinforce explanations according to the client's needs and ability to understand. Administration of anesthesia would only be done in the operating room for open reduction of fractures. Closed reductions may be done in the emergency department without anesthesia. An analgesic would be administered as prescribed because the procedure is painful, but the informed consent form must be obtained before administering the medication.
Priority Nursing Tip: Minors (clients younger than 18 years old) need a parent or legal guardian to sign an informed consent form.
Test-Taking Strategy: Focus on the strategic word, *first*. Note that the question specifically states that the procedure is going to be done in the cast room. This will assist in eliminating options 1 and 3. Recalling that an informed consent form must be obtained before administering sedating medication will direct you to option 4 from the remaining options. Review: **leg fracture.**
Reference(s): Ignatavicius, Workman (2013), p. 1150; Potter et al (2013), pp. 302-303.

1535. The nurse is monitoring a client with a fracture to the left arm. Which sign observed by the nurse is consistent with impaired venous return in the area?
1. Increasing edema
2. Weakened distal pulse
3. Pallor or blotchy cyanosis
4. Continued pain despite medication

Level of Cognitive Ability: Analyzing
Client Needs: Physiological Integrity
Integrated Process: Nursing Process/Assessment
Content Area: Adult Health: Musculoskeletal
Priority Concepts: Clinical Judgment; Perfusion

Answer: 1
Rationale: Impaired venous return is characterized by increasing edema. In the client with a fracture, this is most often prevented by elevating the limb. The other options identify signs of arterial damage, which can occur if the artery is contused, thrombosed, lacerated, or becomes spastic.
Priority Nursing Tip: The nurse needs to assess the neurovascular status of a casted extremity frequently for signs of impairment. If neurovascular impairment is suspected, the health care provider is notified immediately.
Test-Taking Strategy: Focus on the subject, impaired venous return. Use principles of blood flow to answer the question. Each of the incorrect options identifies difficulty with circulation to the extremity and is an arterial sign. The correct option identifies a sign that is consistent with impaired venous return. Review: the signs noted in **impaired venous return.**
Reference(s): Ignatavicius, Workman (2013), pp. 1148-1149.

1536. The nurse receives a client from the post-anesthesia care unit who has had skeletal traction applied in the operating room. The nurse should take **immediate** action to correct which problem noted with the traction setup?
1. Knots are secured tightly
2. Ropes are free of frays or shredding
3. Weights are resting against the foot of the bed
4. Ropes are centered in the wheel grooves of the pulleys

Level of Cognitive Ability: Applying
Client Needs: Physiological Integrity
Integrated Process: Nursing Process/Implementation
Content Area: Adult Health: Musculoskeletal
Priority Concepts: Mobility; Safety

Answer: 3
Rationale: The traction setup is checked to ensure that weights are hanging freely from the ropes, knots are tied securely, ropes are not frayed, and the ropes are in the grooves of the pulleys. Problems with any of these can interfere with maintenance of proper traction. If any problems are noted, they should be fixed immediately.
Priority Nursing Tip: Pin site care needs to be performed on the client with skeletal traction. Infection is a concern at the pin sites and the site should be monitored closely for signs of infection.
Test-Taking Strategy: Note the strategic word, *immediate*. Recalling that weights exert the pulling force needed in a traction setup will direct you to the correct option. Review: the principles of setting up traction.
Reference(s): Ignatavicius, Workman (2013), pp. 1153-1154.

1537. The nurse is monitoring for the presence of pitting edema in the prenatal client. The nurse presses the fingertips of the middle and index fingers against the shin and holds pressure for 2 to 3 seconds. The nurse notes that the indentation is approximately 1 inch deep. The nurse should document that the client has which level of pitting edema?
1. +1
2. +2
3. +3
4. +4

Level of Cognitive Ability: Applying
Client Needs: Physiological Integrity
Integrated Process: Nursing Process/Assessment
Content Area: Maternity: Antepartum
Priority Concepts: Clinical Judgment; Perfusion

Answer: 4
Rationale: When evaluating the presence of pitting edema, the nurse presses the fingertips of the index and middle fingers against the shin and holds pressure for 2 to 3 seconds. An indentation approximately 1-inch deep would be indicative of +4 edema. A slight indentation would indicate +1 edema. An indentation approximately ¼-inch deep indicates +2 edema. An indentation approximately ½-inch deep indicates +3 edema.
Priority Nursing Tip: Generalized edema in a pregnant client should be reported to the health care provider.
Test-Taking Strategy: Focus on the subject, pitting edema of an indentation approximately 1 inch deep. Knowledge regarding this technique and the interpretation of the findings will assist in directing you to option 4. Review: assessment for **pitting edema**.
Reference(s): McKinney et al (2013), pp. 248, 539, 596.

1538. A client has just been diagnosed with acute kidney injury. The laboratory calls the nurse to report a serum potassium level of 6.1 mEq/L on the client. Which **immediate** action should the nurse take?
1. Check the sodium level
2. Call the health care provider
3. Encourage an extra 500 mL of fluid intake
4. Teach the client about foods low in potassium

Level of Cognitive Ability: Applying
Client Needs: Physiological Integrity
Integrated Process: Nursing Process/Implementation
Content Area: Adult Health: Renal and Urinary
Priority Concepts: Clinical Judgment; Fluid and Electrolyte Balance

Answer: 2
Rationale: The client with hyperkalemia is at risk of developing cardiac dysrhythmias and resultant cardiac arrest. Because of this, the health care provider must be notified at once so that the client may receive definitive treatment. The nurse might also check the result of a serum sodium level, but this is not a priority action of the nurse. Fluid intake would not be increased because it would contribute to fluid overload and would not effectively lower the serum potassium level. Dietary teaching may be necessary at some point, but this action is not the priority.
Priority Nursing Tip: The normal potassium level is 3.5 to 5.0 mEq/L.
Test-Taking Strategy: Note the strategic word, *immediate*. Recalling the normal potassium level and noting that the level identified in the question is elevated will direct you to the correct option. Review: the normal **potassium level**.
Reference(s): Ignatavicius, Workman (2013), p. 1548.

1539. The nurse has received the client assignment for the day. Which client should the nurse care for **first**?
1. A client with a wound infection who has a temperature of 100.4° F
2. A client with a deep vein thrombosis who reports bleeding gums when brushing the teeth
3. A client who had a right arm casted 12 hours ago who is complaining of numbness in the fingers
4. A client with chronic obstructive pulmonary disease (COPD) who has a respiratory rate of 22 beats per minute

Level of Cognitive Ability: Analyzing
Client Needs: Safe and Effective Care Environment
Integrated Process: Nursing Process: Analysis
Content Area: Leadership/Management: Prioritizing
Priority Concepts: Clinical Judgment; Safety

Answer: **3**
Rationale: The client with a cast who experiences numbness in the fingers should be seen first because this could be a symptom of compartment syndrome. Compartment syndrome creates an emergency situation when it does occur. Within 4 to 6 hours after the onset of compartment syndrome, neurovascular and muscle damage are irreversible if treatment is not provided. The limb can become useless in 24 to 48 hours. It would be expected that the client with a wound infection will have an elevation in body temperature. A client on anticoagulant therapy for treatment of a deep vein thrombosis who experiences bleeding gums when brushing teeth should be evaluated but is not the priority. A respiratory rate of 22 breaths per minute in the client with COPD is considered normal.
Priority Nursing Tip: When considering priorities of care in regard to assessment, it is important to remember the letters A, B, and C for airway, breathing, and circulation. Note that CAB (circulation, airway, and breathing) is used to prioritize when cardiopulmonary resuscitation is necessary.
Test-Taking Strategy: Note the strategic word, *first* and focus on the subject, who to care for first. Look for the most critical client as the nurse's choice to care for first and use the ABCs—airway, breathing, and circulation. The client with a cast who is complaining of numbness in the fingers is experiencing a circulatory problem. Review: the principles related to **prioritizing care**.
Reference(s): Ignatavicius, Workman (2013), pp. 1145-1146; Potter et al (2013), pp. 238, 279.

1540. A client with glomerulonephritis is at risk of developing acute kidney injury. Which is a sign of this complication?
1. Bradycardia
2. Hypertension
3. Decreased cardiac output
4. Decreased central venous pressure

Level of Cognitive Ability: Analyzing
Client Needs: Physiological Integrity
Integrated Process: Nursing Process/Assessment
Content Area: Adult Health: Renal and Urinary
Priority Concepts: Fluid and Electrolyte Balance; Elimination

Answer: **2**
Rationale: Acute kidney injury caused by glomerulonephritis is classified as intrinsic or intrarenal failure. This form of acute kidney injury is commonly manifested by hypertension, tachycardia, oliguria, lethargy, edema, and other signs of fluid overload. Acute kidney injury from prerenal causes is characterized by decreased blood pressure or a recent history of the same, tachycardia, and decreased cardiac output and central venous pressure. Bradycardia is not part of the clinical picture for renal failure.
Priority Nursing Tip: In glomerulonephritis, destruction, inflammation, and sclerosis of the glomeruli of both kidneys occur.
Test-Taking Strategy: Focus on the subject, a client with glomerulonephritis who is at risk of developing acute kidney injury. Eliminate option 1 first because bradycardia will not occur. Remember that renal failure is accompanied by fluid overload. This will help you eliminate option 4 next. From the remaining choices, recall that hypertension accompanies acute kidney injury resulting from intrarenal causes, whereas decreased cardiac output accompanies acute kidney injury resulting from prerenal causes. Review: the manifestations associated with **acute kidney injury**.
Reference(s): Ignatavicius, Workman (2013), p. 1541.

1541. A client has been prescribed metoprolol (Lopressor) for hypertension. The nurse monitors client compliance carefully because of which common side effect of the medication?
1. Impotence
2. Mood swings
3. Increased appetite
4. Complete atrioventricular (AV) block

Level of Cognitive Ability: Analyzing
Client Needs: Physiological Integrity
Integrated Process: Nursing Process/Assessment
Content Area: Pharmacology: Cardiovascular Medications
Priority Concepts: Adherence; Sexuality

Answer: 1
Rationale: A common side effect of beta-adrenergic blocking agents, such as metoprolol, is impotence. Other common side effects include fatigue and weakness. Central nervous system side effects occur rarely and include mental status changes, nervousness, depression, and insomnia. Mood swings, increased appetite, and complete AV block are not reported side effects.
Priority Nursing Tip: Instruct the client taking a beta-adrenergic blocking agent to change positions slowly to prevent orthostatic hypotension.
Test-Taking Strategy: Focus on *subject*, metoprolol (Lopressor) and recall that medication names that end with the letters "-lol" are beta-adrenergic blocking agents. Note the nurse monitors client compliance, and the words, *common side effect.* Remember that a common side effect of beta-adrenergic blocking agents is impotence. This will direct you to option 1. Review: the expected side effects of **metoprolol (Lopressor).**
Reference(s): Hodgson, Kizior (2014), p. 768.

1542. The nurse is caring for a client with cancer of the lung who is receiving chemotherapy. The nurse reviews the laboratory results and notes that the platelet count is 18,000 cells/mm³. Based on this laboratory result, which should the nurse implement?
1. Contact precautions
2. Bleeding precautions
3. Respiratory precautions
4. Neutropenic precautions

Level of Cognitive Ability: Applying
Client Needs: Physiological Integrity
Integrated Process: Nursing Process/Implementation
Content Area: Adult Health: Oncology
Priority Concepts: Cellular Regulation; Safety

Answer: 2
Rationale: When the platelet count is less than 20,000 cells/mm³, the client is at risk for bleeding, and the nurse should institute bleeding precautions. Contact precautions are initiated in a client who has drainage from wounds that may be infectious. Respiratory precautions are instituted for a client with a respiratory infection that is transmitted by the airborne route. Neutropenic precautions would be instituted for a client with a low neutrophil count.
Priority Nursing Tip: Monitor the platelet count closely in clients receiving chemotherapy because of the risk for thrombocytopenia.
Test-Taking Strategy: Focus on the *subject,* a client with cancer and a low platelet count. Recalling that when the platelet count is low, the client is at risk for bleeding will direct you to option 2. Review: the **normal platelet count** and **bleeding precautions.**
Reference(s): Ignatavicius, Workman (2013), pp. 421-422, 864.

1543. A client with a leaking intracranial aneurysm has been placed on aneurysm precautions. A visiting family member wants to take the client to the unit lounge for "just a few minutes." Which concepts should the nurse use when explaining why the client must remain in the room?
1. A quiet environment promotes more rapid healing of the aneurysm.
2. Clients with aneurysms need isolation to cope with photosensitivity.
3. Reduced environmental stimuli are needed to prevent aneurysm rupture.
4. The client has disorganization of thoughts and feelings and needs reduced activity.

Level of Cognitive Ability: Applying
Client Needs: Physiological Integrity
Integrated Process: Nursing Process/Implementation
Content Area: Adult Health: Neurological
Priority Concepts: Intracranial Regulation; Safety

Answer: 3
Rationale: Subarachnoid precautions (or aneurysm precautions) are intended to minimize environmental stimuli, which could increase intracranial pressure and trigger bleeding or rupture of the aneurysm. The aneurysm will not heal more rapidly with reduced stimuli. The client does not need isolation to "cope" with photosensitivity (although photosensitivity may be a problem). No data indicate that the client has disorganization of thoughts and feelings.
Priority Nursing Tip: The client with a leaking intracranial aneurysm needs to be placed on aneurysm precautions. Visitors need to be limited and the client should be maintained in a private and darkened room (subdued lighting and avoid direct, bright, artificial lights) without stimulation.
Test-Taking Strategy: Focus on the *subject,* the purpose of aneurysm precautions. Recalling that the concern in this client is rupture will direct you to option 3. Review: **aneurysm precautions** and their purpose.
Reference(s): Ignatavicius, Workman (2013), p. 1014.

1544. A client has been taking metoclopramide (Reglan) on a long-term basis. A home care nurse calls the health care provider **immediately** if which side effect is noted in this client?

1. Excitability
2. Anxiety or irritability
3. Uncontrolled rhythmic movements of the face or limbs
4. Dry mouth not minimized by the use of sugar-free hard candy

Level of Cognitive Ability: Applying
Client Needs: Physiological Integrity
Integrated Process: Nursing Process/Implementation
Content Area: Pharmacology: Musculoskeletal Medications
Priority Concepts: Clinical Judgment; Safety

Answer: 3
Rationale: If the client experiences tardive dyskinesia (rhythmic movements of the face or limbs), the nurse should withhold the medication and call the health care provider. These side effects may be irreversible. Excitability is not a side effect of this medication. Anxiety, irritability, and dry mouth are milder side effects that are not harmful to the client.
Priority Nursing Tip: Metoclopramide (Reglan) stimulates upper gastrointestinal tract motility and is used to treat gastroesophageal reflux disease.
Test-Taking Strategy: Note the strategic word, *immediately*. Select the option that identifies the most serious effect. This will direct you to the correct option. Review: **metoclopramide (Reglan)** and the signs of **tardive dyskinesia**.
Reference(s): Hodgson, Kizior (2014), pp. 764-765.

1545. The nurse caring for a client taking clozapine (Clozaril) for the treatment of a schizophrenic disorder reviews the laboratory studies that have been prescribed for the client. Which laboratory study is the **priority** to monitor for an adverse effect associated with the use of this medication?

1. Platelet count
2. Cholesterol level
3. Blood urea nitrogen
4. White blood cell count

Level of Cognitive Ability: Analyzing
Client Needs: Physiological Integrity
Integrated Process: Nursing Process/Assessment
Content Area: Pharmacology: Psychiatric Medications
Priority Concepts: Psychosis; Safety

Answer: 4
Rationale: Hematological reactions can occur in the client taking clozapine and include agranulocytosis and mild leukopenia. The white blood cell count should be assessed before initiating treatment and should be monitored closely during the use of this medication. The client should also be monitored for signs indicating agranulocytosis, which may include sore throat, malaise, and fever. Options 1, 2, and 3 are unrelated to the use of this medication.
Priority Nursing Tip: Atypical antipsychotics are usually more effective for treating the negative symptoms of schizophrenia such as avolition, apathy, and alogia.
Test-Taking Strategy: Focus on the subject, clozapine, and note the strategic word, *priority*. Recalling that clozapine causes agranulocytosis will direct you to the correct option. Review: **clozapine (Clozaril)**.
Reference(s): Hodgson, Kizior (2014), pp. 272-273.

1546. A postoperative client has been placed on a clear liquid diet. Which items is the client allowed to consume? **Select all that apply.**
❏ 1. Tea
❏ 2. Broth
❏ 3. Gelatin
❏ 4. Pudding
❏ 5. Vegetable juice
❏ 6. Pureed vegetables

Level of Cognitive Ability: Applying
Client Needs: Physiological Integrity
Integrated Process: Nursing Process/Implementation
Content Area: Fundamental Skills: Nutrition
Priority Concepts: Clinical Judgment; Nutrition

Answer: 1, 2, 3
Rationale: A clear liquid diet consists of foods that are relatively transparent to light, and are clear and liquid at room and body temperature. These foods include such items as water, either regular or decaffeinated coffee or tea, bouillon, clear broth, gelatin, carbonated beverages, hard candy, lemonade, popsicles. The incorrect food items are items that are allowed on a full liquid diet.
Priority Nursing Tip: A clear liquid diet is easily digested and absorbed.
Test-Taking Strategy: Focus on the subject, a clear liquid diet. Recalling that a clear liquid diet consists of foods that are relatively transparent to light, and are clear and liquid at room and body temperature will assist in determining the correct food items. Review: foods that are on a **clear liquid diet**.
Reference(s): Perry, Potter, Ostendorf (2014), p. 765.

1547. A 30-week gestation client is admitted to the maternity unit in preterm labor. Betamethasone is prescribed to be administered and the client asks the nurse about the purpose of the medication. What should the nurse tell the client is the purpose for this medication?

1. Promote fetal lung maturity.
2. Delay delivery for at least 48 hours.
3. Stop the premature uterine contractions.
4. Prevent premature closure of the ductus arteriosus.

Level of Cognitive Ability: Applying
Client Needs: Physiological Integrity
Integrated Process: Teaching and Learning
Content Area: Maternity: Intrapartum
Priority Concepts: Development; Gas Exchange

Answer: 1
Rationale: Betamethasone, a corticosteroid, is administered to increase the surfactant level and increase fetal lung maturity, reducing the incidence of respiratory distress syndrome in the newborn infant. Surfactant production does not become stable until after 32 weeks' gestation. If adequate amounts of surfactant are not present in the lungs, respiratory distress and death are possible consequences. Delivery needs to be delayed for at least 48 hours after the administration of betamethasone in order to allow time for the lungs to mature. Options 2, 3, and 4 are incorrect.
Priority Nursing Tip: Betamethasone, administered to a preterm labor client, can decrease the mother's resistance to infection.
Test-Taking Strategy: Focus on the subject, betamethasone. Eliminate options 2 and 3 first because they are comparable or alike and both relate to stopping labor. Recalling that respiratory distress syndrome caused by immature lungs is a major concern of prematurity will direct you to option 1 from the remaining options. Review: betamethasone.
Reference(s): McKinney et al (2013), pp. 653-654.

1548. The nurse is performing a physical assessment on a client with rheumatoid arthritis. The nurse assesses the client's hands and notes which characteristic deformities? **Refer to the figure.**

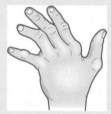

From Lewis S, Dirksen S, Heitkemper M, Bucher L: *Medical-surgical nursing: assessment and management of clinical problems*, ed 9, St. Louis, 2014, Elsevier.

1. Ulnar drift
2. Rheumatoid nodules
3. Swan neck deformity
4. Boutonniére deformity

Level of Cognitive Ability: Analyzing
Client Needs: Physiological Integrity
Integrated Process: Nursing Process/Assessment
Content Area: Adult Health: Musculoskeletal
Priority Concepts: Clinical Judgment; Mobility

Answer: 1
Rationale: Ulnar drift occurs when synovitis stretches and damages the tendons and eventually the tendons become shortened and fixed. This damage causes subluxation (drift) of the joints. All of the conditions that are identified in the options can occur in rheumatoid arthritis; however, the figure pictures ulnar drift.
Priority Nursing Tip: The nurse should provide range-of-motion exercises to the client with rheumatoid arthritis to maintain joint motion and promote muscle strengthening.
Test-Taking Strategy: Focus on the subject, characteristic deformities with rheumatoid arthritis. Note the relationship between the characteristics in the client's hands and option 1, ulnar drift. Review: rheumatoid arthritis and ulnar drift.
Reference(s): Jarvis (2012), p. 612.

1549. Which client could the nurse delegate to the unlicensed assistive personnel (UAP)?
  1. A client who needs teaching regarding the use of an incentive spirometer
  2. A client who needs to have a urine specimen collected for a clean catch urine
  3. A client who needs reinforcement of a dressing covering an abdominal incision
  4. A client who needs assessment of a newly identified area of pressure over the right hip

Level of Cognitive Ability: Analyzing
Client Needs: Safe and Effective Care Environment
Integrated Process: Nursing Process/Planning
Content Area: Leadership/Management: Delegating
Priority Concepts: Care Coordination; Leadership

Answer: 2
Rationale: The UAP can assist with specimen collection such as a clean catch urine because he or she is trained in this skill. Skills requiring nursing intervention such as dressing changes, teaching, and assessment cannot be delegated to unlicensed personnel.
Priority Nursing Tip: Understanding the training and limitations of unlicensed assistive personnel will assist the nurse in the delegation process. Licensed nurses must perform nursing interventions such as teaching, initial and ongoing assessment, and skills such as dressing changes.
Test-Taking Strategy: Focus on the subject, skills the UAP can perform. Understanding the scope of practice for the UAP should lead you to eliminate options 1, 3, and 4, as these require advanced nursing skills that are beyond the scope of practice of the UAP. Review: **unlicensed assistive personnel (UAP).**
Reference(s): Potter et al (2013), pp. 262, 282-283.

❖ **1550.** The nurse is preparing to perform a Mantoux tuberculin skin test. Which interventions apply in relation to this test? **Select all that apply.**
  ❑ 1. Explain the procedure to the client.
  ❑ 2. Obtain a 3-mL syringe with a ½-inch needle for the injection.
  ❑ 3. Mark the test area to locate it for reading 48 to 72 hours after injection.
  ❑ 4. Bunch up the skin and insert the needle with the needle bevel facing downward.
  ❑ 5. Cleanse the injection site on the lower dorsal surface of the forearm with alcohol and allow it to dry.
  ❑ 6. Ask the client about a previous history of receiving a positive purified protein derivative (PPD) reaction.

Level of Cognitive Ability: Analyzing
Client Needs: Physiological Integrity
Integrated Process: Nursing Process/Implementation
Content Area: Pharmacology: Respiratory Medications
Priority Concepts: Clinical Judgment; Safety

Answer: 1, 3, 5, 6
Rationale: The nurse should always explain the procedure to the client and then assess him or her for a previous history of a PPD reaction. The test should not be administered if the client has such a history. The nurse should use a tuberculin syringe (not a 3-mL syringe) with a ½-inch 26- or 27-gauge needle. The injection site on the lower dorsal surface of the forearm is cleansed with alcohol and allowed to dry. The skin is stretched taut and 0.1 mL of solution containing 0.5 tuberculin units of PPD is injected. The injection is made just under the surface of the skin with the needle bevel facing upward to provide a discrete elevation of the skin (a wheal) 6 to 10 mm in diameter. The test area is marked to locate it for reading and the test area is read 48 to 72 hours after injection.
Priority Nursing Tip: Once the Mantoux tuberculin skin test result for tuberculosis is positive, it will be positive in any future tests.
Test-Taking Strategy: Focus on the subject, administering a Mantoux tuberculin skin test. Visualize this procedure and remember that procedures are always explained to the client. Recalling that a Mantoux skin test is a tuberculin test will assist in determining that a tuberculin syringe, not a 3-mL syringe, is used for the injection. Also, recall that this injection is administered intradermally and that the needle bevel needs to face upward to provide a wheal. Review: the procedure for administering a Mantoux tuberculin skin test.
Reference(s): Pagana, Pagana (2013), pp. 933-934.

❖ **1551.** To maintain a safe milieu while addressing the needs of the cognitively impaired clients on the unit, which interventions should the psychiatric nurse do? **Select all that apply.**

❑ 1. Use distracting techniques when appropriate.
❑ 2. Be consistently visible and available to the clients.
❑ 3. Provide reality orientation to the clients as needed.
❑ 4. Anticipate the needs of the clients as much as possible.
❑ 5. Segregate potentially volatile clients from the other clients.

Level of Cognitive Ability: Analyzing
Client Needs: Safe and Effective Care Environment
Integrated Process: Nursing Process/Planning
Content Area: Mental Health
Priority Concepts: Cognition; Safety

Answer: 1, 2, 3, 4
Rationale: It is the nurse's responsibility to manage the safety of the milieu regardless of the client population, but it is particularly challenging when there are clients with poor impulse control resulting from cognitive impairment in the milieu. Because disorientation is often the trigger for agitation in the cognitively impaired client, frequent reality orientation is generally effective as is distraction for the client for whom re-orientation is ineffective. Maintaining a consistent presence on the unit and anticipating client needs also helps minimize agitation triggers for the cognitively impaired client. Keeping a potentially aggressive client away from the milieu is not necessary and should be done only when escalation of agitation actually occurs and cannot be managed with other techniques.
Priority Nursing Tip: Milieu safety is a primary nursing responsibility and is best achieved by consistently observing the clients, anticipating their needs, and effectively de-escalating any potentially aggressive clients.
Test-Taking Strategy: Focus on the subject, creating a safe milieu. Understanding the principles and techniques of therapeutic de-escalation of the cognitively impaired client will direct you to the correct options. It is not necessary to segregate clients with potential problems. Review: nursing care to the **cognitively impaired client.**
Reference(s): Stuart (2013), pp. 426, 429; Varcarolis (2013), pp. 32-33.

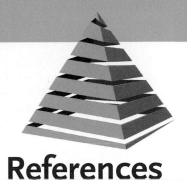

References

Baird, M., & Bethel, S. (2011). *Manual of critical care nursing, nursing interventions and collaborative management* (6th ed.). St. Louis: Mosby.

Bryant, R., & Nix, D. (2012). *Acute & chronic wounds: current management concepts* (4rd ed.). St. Louis: Mosby.

Centers for Disease Control and Prevention (CDC). (2011). *2011 Child & adolescent immunization schedules*. Retrieved February 6, 2011 from, http://www.cdc.gov/vaccines/recs/schedules/child-schedule.htm.

Chernecky, C., & Berger, B. (2013). *Laboratory tests and diagnostic procedures* (6th ed.). St. Louis: Saunders.

Dolan, B., & Holt, L. (2013). *Accident & emergency theory into practice* (3rd ed.). St. Louis: Elsevier.

Fortinash, K., & Holoday-Worret, P. (2012). *Psychiatric mental health nursing* (5th ed.). St. Louis: Mosby.

Gahart, B., & Nazareno, A. (2012). *2012 Intravenous medications* (28th ed.). St. Louis: Mosby.

Giger, J. (2013). *Transcultural nursing assessment & intervention* (6th ed.). St. Louis: Mosby.

Hammond, B., & Zimmermann, P. (2013). *Sheehy's manual of emergency care* (7th ed.). St. Louis: Elsevier.

Hockenberry, M., & Wilson, D. (2013). *Wong's essentials of pediatric nursing* (9th ed). St. Louis: Mosby.

Hockenberry, M., & Wilson, D. (2011). *Nursing care of infants and children* (9th ed.). St. Louis: Mosby.

Hodgson, B., & Kizior, R. (2014). *Saunders nursing drug handbook, 2014*. St. Louis: Saunders.

Huber, D. (2014). *Leadership and nursing care management* (5th ed.). St. Louis: Saunders.

Ignatavicius, D., & Workman, M. (2013). *Medical-surgical nursing: patient-centered collaborative care* (7th ed.). St. Louis: Saunders.

Jarvis, C. (2012). *Physical examination and health assessment* (6th ed.). St. Louis: Saunders.

Kee, J., Hayes, E., & McCuistion, L. (2012). *Pharmacology: A nursing process approach* (7th ed.). St. Louis: Saunders.

Lehne, R. (2013). *Pharmacology for nursing care* (8th ed.). St. Louis: Saunders.

Lewis, S., Dirksen, S., Heitkemper, M., Bucher, L., & Camera, I. (2011). *Medical-surgical nursing: Assessment and management of clinical problems* (8th ed.). St. Louis: Mosby.

Lewis, S., Dirksen, S., Heitkemper, M., & Bucher, L. (2014). *Medical-surgical nursing: Assessment and management of clinical problems* (9th ed.). St. Louis: Mosby.

Lilley, L., Rainforth Collins, S., Harrington, S., & Snyder, J. (2014a). *Pharmacology and the nursing process* (7th ed.). St. Louis: Mosby.

Lilley, L., Rainforth Collins, S., Harrington, S., & Snyder, J. (2014b). *Pharmacology and the nursing process* (7th ed.). St. Louis: Mosby.

Lowdermilk, D., Perry, S., Cashion, K., & Alden, K. (2012). *Maternity & women's health care* (10th ed.). St. Louis: Mosby.

McKinney, E., James, S., Murray, S., Nelson, K., & Ashwill, J. (2013). *Maternal-child nursing* (4th ed.). St. Louis: Elsevier.

Mosby's Dictionary of medicine nursing & health professions (2013). (9th ed.). St. Louis: Elsevier.

Nies, M., & McEwen, M. (2011). *Community/Public health nursing* (5th ed.). St. Louis: Elsevier.

Nix, S. (2013). *Williams' basic nutrition and diet therapy* (14th ed.). St. Louis: Mosby.

Pagana, K., & Pagana, T. (2013). *Mosby's diagnostic and laboratory tests reference* (11th ed.). St. Louis: Mosby.

Perry, A., Potter, P., & Elkin, M. (2012). *Nursing interventions & clinical skills* (5th ed.). St. Louis: Mosby.

Perry, A., Potter, P., & Ostendorf, W. (2014). *Clinical nursing skills & techniques* (8th ed.). St. Louis: Mosby.

Potter, P., Perry, A. G., Stockert, P. A., & Hall, A. M. (2013). *Fundamentals of nursing* (8th ed.). St. Louis: Mosby.

RxList, The internet drug index: Echinacea, retrieved July 22, 2013 from http://www.rxlist.com/echinacea/supplements.htm.

Skidmore-Roth, L. (2014). *Mosby's nursing drug reference* (27th ed.). St. Louis: Mosby.

Stuart, G. (2013). *Principles & practice of psychiatric nursing* (10th ed.). St. Louis: Mosby.

Swearingen, P. (2012). *All-in-one care planning resource: Medical-surgical, pediatric, maternity, & psychiatric nursing care plans* (3rd ed.). St. Louis: Mosby.

Varcarolis, E. (2013). *Essentials of psychiatric mental health nursing: a communication approach to evidence-based care* (2nd ed.). St. Louis: Saunders.

Yoder-Wise, P. (2011). *Leading and managing in nursing* (5th ed.). St. Louis: Mosby.

Zerwekh, J., & Zerwekh Garneau, A. (2015). *Nursing today: Transition and trends* (8th ed.). St. Louis: Elsevier.

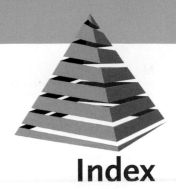

Index

A

ABCs (airway, breathing, and circulation), question prioritization based on, 24, 24*b*
Admission process, to testing center, 10
Analysis, in nursing process, 466, 467*b*
   question prioritization based on, 25–26, 26*b*
Answers, for test questions. *see* Options.
Anxiety, about NCLEX-RN exam, 15
   dealing with, 16–17
   graduate's perspective on, 17
Application, for NCLEX-RN exam. *see* Registration.
Appointment, for NCLEX-RN exam
   canceling of, 9
   foreign-educated nurse and, 14
   forfeiting of, 9
   rescheduling of, 9
   scheduling an, 9
Arrival time, at testing center, 9
Assessment, in nursing process, 466, 466*b*
   question prioritization based on, 24–25, 25*b*
Assignment of tasks guidelines, as test-taking strategy, 28–29, 29*b*
Audio questions, 7, 8*f*
Audio recordings, during testing, 10
Authorization to Test (ATT), for NCLEX-RN exam, 9, 19

B

Basic Care and Comfort, as Client Need, 32, 32*t*, 33*b*
Breaks, during test taking, 10, 19–20

C

Calculator, computer-based, use during testing, 21, 29
Candidate bulletin, NCLEX examination, 7–9, 11
Candidate identification number, on ATT, 9
Candidate performance report, for NCLEX-RN exam, 10–11
Candidate services, 9
Caring, as Integrated Process, 464, 464*b*
CAT (computer adaptive test), NCLEX-RN exam as, 3
Certification program, for foreign-educated nurses, 13–14
Chart questions, 6, 7*b*, 7*f*, 22
Client needs
   and NCLEX-RN® test plan, 4, 4*t*, 31–35
      categories of, 32, 32*t*. *see also* specific category, e.g., Physiological Integrity
      percentage of test questions on, 32*t*
      as test-taking strategy, 27–28
Closed-ended words, in options, 28, 28*b*
Cognitive ability, levels of, in NCLEX test plan, 4, 4*b*
Commission on Graduates of Foreign Nursing Schools (CGFNS), 13
Communication
   as Integrated Process, 464–465, 465*b*
   in nursing process, question prioritization based on, 27, 28*b*
Comparable or alike options, elimination of, 28, 28*b*
Computer adaptive test (CAT), NCLEX-RN exam as, 3
Confidence, and belief in yourself, 15*f*, 17
Contact information
   for candidate services, 9
   for Commission on Graduates of Foreign Nursing Schools, 13

Contact information *(Continued)*
   for National Council of State Boards of Nursing, 11, 12
   for NCLEX examination, 11
   for Pyramid to Success, 3
   for U.S. Citizenship and Immigration Services, 13
Content/concepts, nursing. *see* Nursing practice.
Control, developing, 15*f*, 16–17
   for anxiety, 16–17
   for physical readiness, 17, 17*b*
Credentialing agencies, for foreign-educated nurses, 12
Critical thinking, 467

D

Data analysis, in nursing process, question prioritization based on, 25–26, 26*b*
Delegation of tasks guidelines, as test-taking strategy, 28–29, 29*b*
Discipline, 16
Distractions
   during studying, 16
   during testing, 10
Documentation
   as Integrated Process, 464–465, 465*b*
   in nursing process, question prioritization based on, 26
   for test eligibility. *see* Legal documentation
Drag and drop questions, 2, 4–5, 22

E

Eating habits, healthy, 17*b*
Eligibility, for taking NCLEX examination, 9
   of foreign-educated nurses, 13
Elimination process, as test-taking strategy
   for closed-ended words, 28, 28*b*
   for comparable or alike options, 28
   for multiple-choice questions, 22
Emergency situation, in test questions, 25
English proficiency, of foreign-educated nurses, 12, 13
Environment, during test taking, 10
Evaluation, in nursing process, 467–468, 468*b*
   question prioritization based on, 27, 27*b*
Event, in test question, 21
Event query, in test question, 21
   negative, 23, 24*b*
   positive, 23, 23*b*
Exhibit questions, 6, 7*b*, 7*f*, 22

F

Fee(s)
   for NCLEX-RN exam, 9
   for Quick Results Service, 10
Figure questions, 5, 6*b*, 6*f*
Fill-in-the-blank questions, 5, 5*b*, 22
Fingerprint, digital, taken for NCLEX-RN exam, 9
Foreign-educated nurses, 12–14
   credentialing agencies for, 12
   licensure of
      general requirements for, 12–13, 13*b*
      general steps in process of, 13*b*
      state requirements for, 12
   National Council of State Boards of Nursing and, 12

Foreign-educated nurses *(Continued)*
   preparing to take the NCLEX exam, 14
   registering to take the NCLEX exam, 14
   VisaScreen for, 13–14
   work visa for, 13

G

Goals, identification of
   for exam preparation, 16
   in nurse planning, 26
Graduate's perspective, on NCLEX-RN® examination, 18–20
   answering question after question, 19
   anxiety and, 19
   application process, 19
   during the examination, 20
   final steps, 19–20
   passing the examination, 20
   planning a study routine that works, 18–19
      phase one, 18
      phase two, 18–19
   preparing for the examination, 18
Graphic options questions, 6, 7*b*, 7*f*

H

Health problems, client, categorization of, 466
Health Promotion and Maintenance
   as Client Need, 27–28, 32*t*, 33
   NCLEX-RN® content questions, 34*b*
HESI/Saunders Online Review for the NCLEX-RN® Examination, 2–3
Hot spot questions, 2

I

Identification (ID), for taking NCLEX-exam
   acceptable forms of, 9
   confirmation, 9
Immigration requirements, for foreign-educated nurses, 12
Implementation, in nursing process, 467, 467*b*
   question prioritization based on, 26–27, 26*b*
Infection control. *see* Safety and Infection Control.
Instructions, for registering to take the examination, 9
Integrated Processes, and the NCLEX-RN® test plan, 463–468, 4
   categories of, 464, 464*b*. *see also* specific category, e.g., Nursing process
Interstate endorsement, for NCLEX-RN exam, 11
Intravenous therapies. *see* Pharmacological and Parenteral Therapies.

L

Legal documentation
   for foreign-educated nurses, 12
      credentialing agencies review of, 12
      general licensure requirements and, 12–13, 13*b*
      state requirements for licensure and, 12
   for taking NCLEX-exam, 9
Licensed practical nurse, scope of practice of, 29
Licensing boards. *see* State Boards of Nursing.

683

Note: Page numbers followed by *b* indicate boxes, *f* indicate figures, and *t* indicate tables.